MW00395762

CLINICAL BIOMECHANICS
Musculoskeletal Actions and Reactions

Second Edition

CLINICAL BIOMECHANICS
Musculoskeletal Actions and Reactions

Second Edition

R. C. SCHAFER, DC, FICC

Developed in cooperation with the
ASSOCIATED CHIROPRACTIC ACADEMIC PRESS

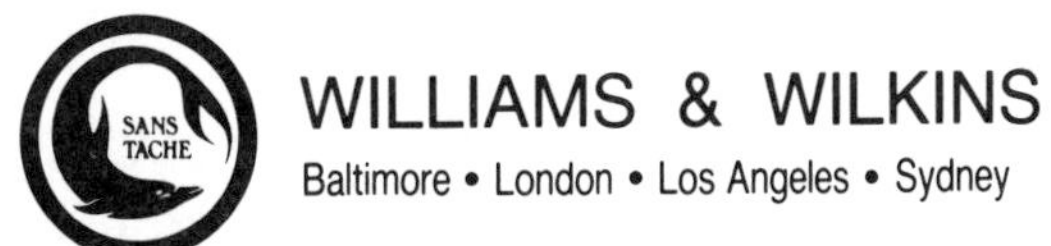

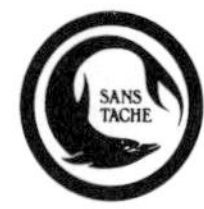

Senior Editor: Jonathan W. Pine, Jr.
Associate Editor: Victoria M. Vaughn
Copy Editor: Linda Hansford
Design: JoAnne Janowiak
Illustration Planning: Lorraine Wrzosek
Production: Anne G. Seitz

428 East Preston Street
Baltimore, MD 21202, U.S.A.

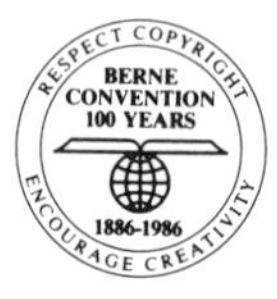

Printed in the United States of America

Second Edition

Library of Congress Cataloging-in-Publication Data

Schafer, R. C.
Clinical biomechanics.

"Developed in cooperation with the Associated Chiropractic Academic Press."
Bibliography: p.
Includes index.
1. Chiropractic. 2. Human mechanics. I. Title. [DNLM: 1. Biomechanics. 2. Chiropractic. 3. Neuromuscular Diseases—diagnosis. 4. Neuromuscular Diseases—therapy. WE 103 S296c]
RZ242.S33 1987 615.8′2 86-11134
ISBN 0-683-07584-5

Composed and printed at the
Waverly Press, Inc.

87 88 89 90 91
10 9 8 7 6 5 4 3 2 1

Foreword To First Edition

At last a book has been written for the general practitioner and advanced student that presents a basic understanding of the biomechanical approach to structure and function. Until now, our education has lacked any single composite source upon which to draw information with regard to our everyday commitment to musculoskeletal problems.

Unfortunately, much of our present knowledge is enmeshed in mathematical and engineering complexities that are irrelevant to the practitioner. *Clinical Biomechanics* allows us to apply biomechanical principles to common traumatic, pathologic, and postural disorders of the spine and extremities, and explains how these principles can be applied to speed patient recovery and rehabilitation. In essence, it offers a compendium of fundamental concepts that should be applied daily, as well as offering a basic understanding to comprehend more sophisticated literature.

This book presents information that allows doctors to review their personal approaches toward their treatment methods. It poses the questions: Does my method agree with current biomechanical principles? Are my results or failures occurring for the reasons I think they are?

We owe a great debt of gratitude to the author, Dr. Richard C. Schafer, who dedicated thousands of hours researching basic principles from over 500 books and technical papers. His ability to present this information in simple language and to unify rather than separate structure from function, as is routine in many orthopedic texts, should be welcomed throughout the health care field.

Warren I. Hammer, MS, DC, DABCO
Department of Biomechanics
New York Chiropractic College

Preface
To Second Edition

When this book was first introduced to the field in 1983, the subject of clinical biomechanics was not listed in the catalogs of any accredited chiropractic college within the United States. This is not true today. Within the last three years, many chiropractic colleges have incorporated specific courses on this subject. This reflects a tumid interest to apply more than a superficial knowledge of mechanical principles within the correction of applicable structural disorders.

This book has been widely described as the only comprehensive text on this subject that has been specially designed to meet the needs of the chiropractic physician. With this responsibility in mind, this second edition has been updated to include an abundance of new information that is felt to be especially helpful in chiropractic practice.

In Part 1, which describes the basic tenets of clinical biomechanics, new material regarding evaluation methodology, the effects of cyclic loading on the spine, postural and gait equilibrium and instability, muscle physiology, myalgia, managing muscle injuries, and differentiating confusing pathologic reflexes has been included. Recent data regarding the role of nociceptors have also been added.

In Part 2, which depicts the biomechanical principles of the spine and pelvis, new or expanded topics include factors affecting the stability of the vertebral motion unit, spinal coupling, the phases of spinal degeneration, upper and lower cervical biomechanics, and recent insights into the cause and correction of low-back pain. The subjects of vertebrobasilar insufficiency, whiplash syndromes, temporomandibular joint disorders, rib subluxations, lumbosacral and facet syndromes, spinal stenosis, and entrapment syndromes are also updated. Also new to this core material are expanded descriptions of vertebral fixation complexes, articular blocking, myofascial trigger points, and vertebrogenic pain. In addition, to enhance the practitioner's therapeutic skills, the management of soft-tissue injuries, pain control, transverse friction massage, the basis for mechanical traction and spinal supports, postural realignment, and new approaches in adjustive therapy are described.

The subject of scoliosis was covered throughout Parts 1 and 2 in the original book. In this edition, this material has been consolidated and expanded to form a new chapter on this important subject. Current diagnostic criteria, theories of causation, associated clinical syndromes, and some innovative clinical approaches are just a few of the new topics described.

In Part 3, which describes the clinical biomechanics of the extremities, new topics include recent data on extremity mechanics, diagnostic refinements, myofascial shoulder syndromes, research on articular and soft-tissue impingement syndromes, the iliotibial band syndrome, the meniscus-coronary ligament relationship in knee trauma, and the direction of current therapeutic approaches.

Many new figures have been added to support the topic descriptions, and several tables have been included to offer the reader quick, organized reference guides. In addition, the body of the text has been redesigned to improve the general format. To enhance the clinician's armamentarium during the differential diagnosis of spinal and extremity disorders, over 75 new clinical tests and signs have been added to the many previously portrayed. For those who have an appetency for sources of further information on specific topics, more than 4000 citations have been adduced within the text. Scores of uncited general references have also been listed as suggested readings.

In conclusion, I wish to extend special thanks to Dr. Tuan Tran of the Los Angeles College of Chiropractic, Dr. John Nash of Texas Chiropractic College, and Dr. Warren Hammer of New York Chiropractic College for their helpful suggestions during the development of this second edition. These dedicated educators, devoid of animadversion, set an example that is impossible for those of us with less sapient sentiments to follow.

Preface To First Edition

Clinical biomechanics has been a subject of interest within the chiropractic profession since its inception. In some instances within pioneer chiropractic, it was applied in a limited fashion as a logical approach to a mechanical problem. The historic writings of Carver, Reeves, Budden, Steinbach, Logan, Weiant, Grecco, Illi, and many others affirm this fact. During the last decade, this interest has been rapidly increasing on a much more sophisticated level, yet there has been little reliable literature available within the profession outside of specific papers on limited subjects.

For various reasons, much of the contemporary information pertinent to the biomechanical aspects of patient care has not been published in a readily available form. Most data have been brought forth in seminars or in technical bulletins and professional papers that were not widely distributed. In addition, considerable information important to general practice had to be sifted from literature aimed at the reconstruction surgeon or the prosthetic bioengineer. It is for these reasons that this book was initiated.

When biomechanical principles are incorporated into health care delivery, the physician has a clearer understanding of the muscular, skeletal, and articular components of the musculoskeletal system, its mechanisms, and how they determine gross human action and reaction. This requires analysis of both the internal specific and the external general aspects, an understanding of the mechanical principles involved, how they are influencing the person as a whole, and how the patient is adapting to these forces. Thus:

An understanding of clinical biomechanics is essential to the diagnosis and scientific application of adjusting fixed articular disrelationships and correcting those forces that tend to maintain abnormal musculoskeletal disorders and their neurologic, circulatory, and lymphatic ramifications.

This book for general practitioners and advanced students incorporates a practical state-of-the-art compilation of applied biostatics, biodynamics, kinesiology, kinematics, kinetics, and the related sciences to serve as a basis for clinical application and research. Emphasis is on the cause of articular disorders, the mechanisms involved, why they occur, how they interact, and how they can be corrected. This is not to say that physiatrists, osteopaths, physiotherapists, bioengineers, physical education students, and other members of the allied health sciences will not find many sections of extreme value in their respective disciplines.

The goal has been to offer a useful presentation for those who have a special health care interest in the neuromusculoskeletal system but do not have a broad background in physics, let alone biophysics, so that the "bottom line" conclusions of reliable research may be directly applied in patient care. Thus, advanced engineering language and the computation of mathematical equations of little usefulness to the clinician have been avoided. Great concern has been given to cause-and-effect principles rather than the solving of theoretical situations through geometric designs and trigonometric functions. For ease in comprehension, subjects are discussed from the general to the specific and from the simple to the more complicated whenever practical.

This is the first comprehensive text on this subject matter developed specifically for chiropractic physicians and the first such text to incorporate the findings of several chiropractic researchers in an orderly and sometimes comparative fashion. The research conclusions of scores of well-known figures and institutions within the profession are included with those of prominent orthopedic researchers in North America and Europe. It is also unique in that the book's Editorial Review Board incorporates representatives from the majority of recognized American chiropractic colleges to portray a wide scope of contemporary thought.

The text elucidates the role of biomechanics in the evaluation of numerous neuromusculoskeletal disorders and the anatomical basis of their conservative management. The discussions concentrate on essential clinical information primary to an understanding of biomechanical implications and applications. To make such an emphasis possible, pertinent mechanical laws and principles are included that are thought to be of value from a general education standpoint, without striving to weight the text with sometimes complicated physics that would be of interest only to the researcher.

The text is divided into three parts. Part 1 introduces the basic principles of clinical biomechanics and incorporates five chapters which offer a review of the pertinent basic sciences, mechanical terms, biodynamic principles, factors of clinical stability, static and dynamic postures, and the basic neuromuscular considerations involved in clinical application. These chapters have been designed to give the reader a fundamental and concise explanation of body structure, mechanical functions, kinematics, myokinetics, mechanical stress, tissue properties and responses, and their respective roles in clinical application. The emphasis is on systemic and multiregional considerations that do not easily fall into a regional category. The chapter on basic neuromuscular considerations is unusual in typical books on biomechanics, but it is vital in clinical practice to grasp the importance of the nervous system in holistic structural control. In health care, it would be folly to attempt to separate our understanding of function from structure in vivo.

Part 2, the core of the text, discusses in four chapters the biomechanical marvel of the human spine and pelvis. This part is introduced by a basic discussion of the general aspects of spinal biomechanics, which is followed by specific chapters on the cervical region, thoracic region, and the lumbar spine and pelvis. Herein, the practical application of biostatics, the science of the relationship of structure to function, is emphasized along with the biomechanical aspects of the resolution of common clinical problems.

Part 3 presents in two chapters the basic biomechanical factors of the upper and lower extremities. The emphasis here is on regional structure, kinesiology, biomechanical tests, and common clinical problems.

Rather than burden the book with numerous footnotes and reference numbers to multiple data sources, only the original author's name is mentioned in the text to guide the reader to the complete source in the bibliography. For rapid reference to specific points, a comprehensive index has been included.

Those of us who have been involved in the development of this book trust that this compilation will aid the reader in studying and treating the human body with greater insight.

—R.C.S

Acknowledgments

Deep appreciation is expressed to the members of the chiropractic educational community as well as scores of reputable practitioners and independent researchers. Because of their specialized ability and acknowledged expertise, the scope of this text has been enhanced by their suggestions to the basic manuscript and their constructive reviews.

While space does not allow mention of all contributors of information, special gratitude must be extended to the following, in alphabetical order:

Editors and Contributors of Information

J. G. Anderson, DC
Chairman, Clinical Sciences
Pasadena College of Chiropractic

Thomas F. Bergmann, DC
Chairman, Chiropractic Division
Northwestern College of Chiropractic

Arnold E. Cianciulli, DC, FICC
Member, Board of Governors
American Chiropractic Association

Richard L. Cohen, DC
Private Practice
Oklahoma City, Oklahoma

Frank Ferraro, DC
Assistant Professor, Clinical Sciences Division
Texas Chiropractic College

Robyn L. Finseth, DC
Chairperson, Clinical/Chiropractic Sciences
Western States Chiropractic College

Warren I. Hammer, MS, DC, DABCO
Instructor, Biomechanics
New York Chiropractic College

Andrew R. Jessen, DC
Private Practice
Salinas, California

Gary C. Johnson, DC
Professor of Body Mechanics
Logan College of Chiropractic

Wallace E. King, DC
Private Practice
Grand Forks, North Dakota

Edward I. Lynch, DC, DACBR
Private Practice
Oklahoma City, Oklahoma

John M. Nash, DC
Dean of Students
Texas Chiropractic College

Mary Jane Newcomb, DC, MA, PhD
Coordinator of Institutional Research
Cleveland Chiropractic College of Kansas City

C. A. Pinkenburg, DC, FICC
Private Practice
Hoisington, Kansas

Bruce D. Presnick, DC
Chairman, Clinical Sciences Division
Life Chiropractic College—West

T. L. Shrader, DC
Secretary, Council on Technic
American Chiropractic Association

Howard T. Silverstein, PhD, DC
Chairman, Department of Physiology and Chemistry
Palmer College of Chiropractic

Tuan A. Tran, PhD
Vice President of Research
Los Angeles College of Chiropractic

Cooperating Chiropractic Colleges

Cleveland Chiropractic College
Life Chiropractic College
Logan College of Chiropractic
Los Angeles College of Chiropractic
New York Chiropractic College
Northwestern College of Chiropractic
Palmer Chiropractic College
Pasadena College of Chiropractic
Texas Chiropractic College
Western States Chiropractic College

Cooperating Organizations

American Chiropractic Association
Associated Chiropractic Academic Press
Behavioral Research Foundation
The Chattanooga Corporation
Foot Levelers, Inc.
Motion Palpation Institute
Nu-Med Surgical/Dental Supply, Inc.
Posture Support Mfg., Inc.
Reedco Research
Therapeutic Products, Inc.

Illustration and Photography Credits

All drawings and photographs incorporated in this book unless credited to other sources have been reproduced with the permission of the Associated Chiropractic Academic Press (ACAP).

Contents

FOREWORD TO FIRST EDITION ... v
PREFACE TO SECOND EDITION ... vii
PREFACE TO FIRST EDITION ... ix
ACKNOWLEDGMENTS ... xi

PART 1: BASIC PRINCIPLES OF CLINICAL BIOMECHANICS

1: THE HUMAN MACHINE ... 3
- Introduction ... 3
- Osteologic Factors ... 6
- Connective Tissue ... 11
- Arthrologic Factors ... 13
- Myologic Factors ... 22
- Basic Anthropometry ... 30
- Evaluation Methodology: An Overview ... 36

2: MECHANICAL CONCEPTS AND TERMS ... 43
- Energy and Mass ... 43
- Newton's Laws of Mechanics ... 43
- Force ... 45
- Static Equilibrium ... 49
- Linear Forces ... 50
- Concurrent Forces ... 51
- Parallel Forces ... 52

3: BASIC PRINCIPLES OF BIODYNAMICS AND JOINT STABILITY ... 62
- Structural Motion ... 62
- Kinematics ... 64
- Kinetics ... 68
- Summary of Major Static and Kinetic Factors Influencing Mechanical Efficiency of Muscular Effort ... 72
- Biomechanical Stress ... 78
- Biomechanical Aspects of Articular Cartilage ... 84

4: BODY ALIGNMENT, POSTURE, AND GAIT ... 93
- Gravitational Effects ... 93
- Stance and Motion Postures ... 102
- Typical Effects of Balance Defects ... 129

5: BASIC NEUROMUSCULAR CONSIDERATIONS ... 143
- Background ... 143
- Skeletal Muscle Microstructure and Function ... 144
- Peripheral and Related Neural Considerations ... 150
- Central Neural Control Mechanisms ... 152
- Proprioception Mechanisms ... 154
- Training and Rehabilitative Considerations ... 159
- Selected Clinical Considerations ... 163

PART 2: CLINICAL BIOMECHANICS OF THE SPINE AND PELVIS

6: GENERAL SPINAL BIOMECHANICS 197
Background 197
The Vertebrae and Pertinent Osteology 201
The Spinal Joints and Pertinent Arthrology 211
The Vertebral Canal and Related Tissues 221
Spinal Circulation and Pertinent Angiology 225
The Spinal Muscles and Pertinent Myology 229
General Aspects of Vertebral Subluxations 233
Basic Biomechanical Considerations in Evaluating Spinal Pain 244

7: BASIC CLINICAL CONSIDERATIONS IN TREATING THE NECK AND BACK 257
General Aspects of Musculoskeletal Injury 257
Spinal Strains and Sprains 258
Myalgia (Fibrositis) 261
Myofascial Trigger Points in the Neck and Back 262
Bone Injuries 266
Arthrotic Pathology 266
Disc Degeneration, Protrusions, and Ruptures 268
Referred Pain and Reflexes 274
Spinal Fixations 277
Basic Neurobiomechanics in Conservative Spinal Therapeutics 280
Adjunctive Therapies 285

8: THE CERVICAL REGION 299
Background 299
Kinesiology of the Neck 299
Clinical Biomechanics of the Cervical Canal 303
General Aspects of Cervical Trauma 305
Clinical Biomechanics of the Upper Cervical Spine 312
Clinical Biomechanics of the Lower Cervical Spine 328

9: SELECTED CLINICAL PROBLEMS OF THE CERVICAL SPINE AND TEMPOROMANDIBULAR JOINT 347
Cervical Subluxation Syndromes 347
Neurovascular Deficit Syndromes 370
Traumatic Brachial Plexus Traction 374
Management of Cervical Strains, Sprains, and Whiplash 378
Cervical Disc and Related Disorders 380
Torticollis 386
Chronic Inflammatory Diseases of the Cervical Spine 389
Cervical Deformities and Anomalies 391
Temporomandibular Joint Disorders 394

10: THE THORACIC REGION AND RELATED CLINICAL PROBLEMS 410
Background 410
Functional Anatomy of the Thoracic Cage and Spine 410
Clinical Biomechanics of Thoracic Trauma 420
Gross Evaluation of the Thoracic Region 429

Structural Fixations and Motion Palpation . . . 431
Basic Therapeutic Considerations . . . 436
Pathology . . . 438
Selected Deformities and Anomalies . . . 440

11: THE LUMBAR SPINE AND PELVIS . . . 446
Prevertebral Function of the Abdominal Area . . . 446
The Lumbar Spine: Anatomical and Kinematic Considerations . . . 447
General Full Spine Postural Examination Considerations . . . 457
The Pelvis and Sacrum: Anatomical and Kinematic Considerations . . . 465

12: SELECTED DISORDERS OF THE LUMBAR SPINE AND PELVIS . . . 481
Clinical Problems of the Abdominal Muscles . . . 481
Postural Realignment of the Lumbar Spine . . . 482
Traumatic Disorders of the Lumbar Spine . . . 485
Lumbar Pain and Spasm . . . 490
Structural Fixation and Motion Palpation of the Lumbar Spine . . . 495
Lumbosacral Angle Syndromes . . . 496
Pathologic Displacements and Impingements . . . 503
Postural Realignment Problems of the Pelvis and Sacrum . . . 529
Traumatic Disorders of the Pelvis . . . 539
Structural Fixations and Motion Palpation of the Pelvis . . . 551
Entrapment Syndromes of the Pelvis . . . 556
Sacroiliac Pathology . . . 557

13: SCOLIOSIS . . . 570
General Considerations . . . 570
Selected Clinical Approaches: Some Old, Some New . . . 582
Cervical Scoliosis . . . 584
Considerations in Primary Thoracic Scoliosis . . . 586
Considerations in Primary Lumbar Scoliosis . . . 605
Lumbopelvic Considerations . . . 608
Effects of Chronic Pronation . . . 620

PART 3: CLINICAL BIOMECHANICS OF THE EXTREMITIES

14: THE UPPER EXTREMITY . . . 633
The Shoulder Girdle and Arm . . . 633
Selected Clinical Problems of the Shoulder Girdle . . . 640
Injuries of the Shoulder Joint . . . 647
The Elbow and Forearm . . . 662
Selected Clinical Problems of the Elbow and Forearm . . . 664
The Wrist . . . 670
Selected Clinical Problems of the Wrist Area . . . 672
The Hand and Thumb . . . 679
Selected Clinical Problems of the Hand and Thumb . . . 681
The Fingers . . . 681
Selected Clinical Problems of the Fingers . . . 685

15: THE LOWER EXTREMITY 696
The Hip and Thigh 696
Selected Clinical Problems of the Hip and Thigh 702
The Knee 711
Selected Clinical Problems of the Knee 717
The Leg and Ankle 732
Selected Clinical Problems of the Leg and Ankle 736
The Foot 748
Selected Clinical Problems of the Foot 750
Conclusion 757

INDEX 769

Part 1

BASIC PRINCIPLES OF CLINICAL BIOMECHANICS

CHAPTER 1
The Human Machine

CHAPTER 2
Mechanical Concepts and Terms

CHAPTER 3
Basic Principles of Biodynamics and Joint Stability

CHAPTER 4
Body Alignment, Posture, and Gait

CHAPTER 5
Basic Neuromuscular Considerations

CHAPTER 1

The Human Machine

In the study of clinical biomechanics, one should first be aware of the basic holistic, osteologic, arthrologic, and myologic factors involved, as well as the basic anthropometric systems frequently utilized. This chapter reviews these factors from their basic aspects so that it will be obvious that clinical biomechanics encompasses knowledge of a wide variety of related sciences.

Chiropractic's approach in health care is to establish and maintain optimal physiologic activity by correcting abnormal structural relationships. Its goal is to organize the body in such a manner as to enable it to utilize its own biologic resources for a return to normal function.[1,2] To this end, a thorough knowledge of clinical biomechanics is invaluable.

INTRODUCTION

Traditionally, although not limited to such, chiropractic health care is associated with the detection and correction of disrelated segments of the skeletal system, especially those of the spinal column and pelvis.[3] As the chiropractic profession has evolved during this century, it has become increasingly evident that disrelated structures, particularly certain spinal disorders, are a prime source of disturbance to the neurologic bed and constitute a threat to health that must not be ignored. Bronchial asthma, idiopathic dysmenorrhea, and essential hypertension are three of many visceral disorders frequently treated in a chiropractic office. Structural adjustments, nutritional therapy, and a variety of therapeutic modalities are commonly used.[4] Proper correction requires the careful blending of data gathered from a variety of specialized sciences so that practical applications can be made in a holistic manner.

Holistic Considerations

The musculoskeletal system can narrowly be looked at as a machine capable of performing mechanical work through its system of muscular forces, bony levers, centers of joint rotation, and body segments which provide weight and mass. In the study of biomechanics, there is a tendency to decompose a system and look at its part in isolation—the skeletal system alone can be thought of as a system of interconnected links. While this approach is helpful in specific biomechanical problem solving, such a purely mechanical concept is an oversimplification that is dangerous in health care. A far more holistic approach is necessary. The human body is not an object that accidentally gets disassembled and requires assembling.

Holism is the theory that the determining factors in nature as a whole are not reducible to the sum of their parts. A human being is still a mystery even after we add up all his or her tissues, organs, and systems in the laboratory. Chiropractic has recognized this in its approach to health care.[5] Unfortunately, there is an inherent danger in allopathic specialized health care of becoming "part" oriented. This danger must be avoided in chiropractic in any study or application of biomechanics. Our skeletal structure is more than an osseous cage to hold our vital organs or a bony hatrack on which nature has hung our muscles. Our muscles are more than pulleys, our nerves are more than wiring, and our vessels are more than fluid conduits. A person is more than an assortment of independent organs or a maze of sovereign systems. An individual is a carefully integrated biologic unit, not just the sum of its parts.[6]

From birth, the human as a biped enjoys an architectural opus magnum which allows for agility, strength, leverage, mobility, and balance against gravity's constant pull. When normal biomechanics are disturbed even slightly, distortion results because of the intricate interrelationship of our structural and functional systems.[7,8] Adaptation to stress depends upon the unifying, coordinating, and controlling forces within the body—the sum of *all* body systems, either directly or indirectly. Any dysfunction of one system may have a far-reaching effect upon the nervous system because of the inherent relationship between structure and function.[9] As structure cannot be separated from function, neither should health care fail to recognize the body's complex unification (Fig. 1.1). The term *biostatics* refers to the science of the relationship of structure and function.

There is another inherent danger in health care—to think of structure solely in its static sense, as shown on a textbook page. For example, and far too often, some think of the spine as a flexible rod that moves only on the command of will. Yet, humans are dynamic creatures, structurally as well as functionally. Body movement never ceases; motion is constant. With every breath, the skull, spine, pelvis, ribs, and attachments are in motion. Add this minimal motion to the gross movements of daily living, and we can appreciate the persistent motion, constant stress, and necessity for proper alignment. Mechanically, physiologically, and psychologically, the human body is compelled to struggle for a state of structural and functional equilibrium. The term *homeostasis* should not suggest a fixed state, but rather, a state of dynamic equilibrium—and the musculoskeletal system has a large role to play in maintaining systemic balance.[10]

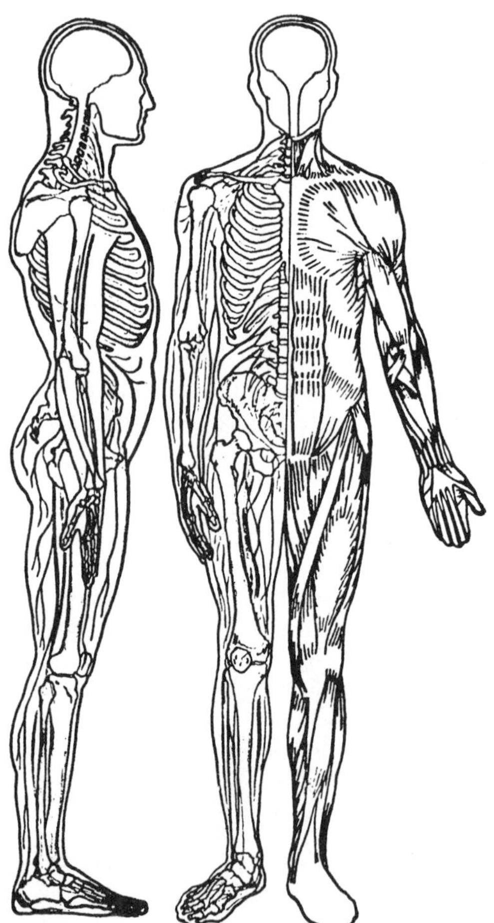

Figure 1.1. Artist's rendering of the overall relationship of the musculoskeletal system.

Related Sciences and Studies

Although the relationship of biomechanics to biodynamics has been emphasized by the chiropractic profession for almost a century, there is a continual need for more objective research to support clinical observations. Such research must incorporate the principles of several areas of related study.

Biomechanics and Associated Studies

A knowledge of either spinal or extravertebral joint action requires an understanding of such factors as power sources, segment speed and acceleration, axes and planes of motion, mass direction, leverage, muscle-length-tension relationships, and the neuromotor and sensory feedback integrative mechanisms.

Mechanics (the science of force and matter) is the study of forces and the effects of these forces. The terms biomechanics or bioengineering refer to these principles as applied to an organism at rest or during movement, incorporating the principles of engineering, anatomy, and physiology into health care goals. That is, *biomechanics* is the study of mechanical forces as they are applied to a living organism (bion), including those forces that arise internally or externally to the body. The general application of physical laws and theories to life force (bionergy), processes, and functions is called *biophysics*, while the science pertinent to life processes is referred to as *bionomy*. The general term of *biotics* is used to describe the science that deals with the functions and qualities of life.

In recent years, the term *bioengineering* has been restricted to the research and development of mechanical devices such as artificial parts, cardiac pacemakers, hearing aids, etc. Especially when such devices are computerized, the term *bionics* is used to describe the research, study, and application of such sophisticated apparatus. *Biometrics*, another related science, is the study of mathematics, statistics (biometry), and vital statistics (biostatistics) as applied to the analysis and solution of problems arising in the health sciences.

Kinesiology and Anthropometry

The broad term *kinesiology* (the study of muscles and muscular contraction) refers to the science of movement, particularly human movement and human movement problems.[11, 12] This encompasses all factors that influence or are influenced by movement. Such study is supported by such sciences as human anatomy and anthropometry.

Anthropometry, the science of measuring the human body, often utilizes such factors as height, gross size, weight, skin fold thickness, osteometry, craniometry, physique, body and part proportions, and segmental lengths and circumferences.

Biodynamics

Mechanics. The study of mechanics can be subdivided into two broad categories: statics and dynamics. The term *statics* refers to the study of bodies at rest or in equilibrium, whereas the study of *dynamics* is concerned with bodies in motion. The more restrictive term *biodynamics* refers to the scientific study of the nature and determinants of an organism's behavior during motion. Biodynamics can be subdivided into three categories: kinematics, kinetics, and kinesics.

Kinematics. Human kinematics (the science of body motion) is that part of biomechanics concerned with the possible motions of a body part. While not considering the forces involved in producing motion, kinematics deals with the various geometric relationships that exist among accelerations, velocities, and displacements during motion.[13–16] Kinematics, for example, describes body segment displacement (flexion, abduction, etc.), ranges of motion, and patterns of movement during motion such as of the ankle, hip, and spine. A kinematic study is performed when, for instance, such principles are applied to the analysis of scoliotic displacement.

Kinetics. The scientific study of the rate of change of a specific factor in the body is called *kinetics*. It is the study of the relationship between a force acting upon a body or body segment and the changes produced in body motion.[13, 14, 17, 18] In other words, kinetics is concerned with moving bodies and the forces that act to cause motion. It is commonly expressed as amount per unit of time. Kinetics, as contrasted to kinematics, analyzes forces such as those of muscles, gravity, and surface reactions that are involved in body propulsion, coordination, and segment displacement. For example, a kinetic study is performed when such principles are applied to analyze the forces necessary to change a scoliotic spine to a more normally aligned spine.

Kinesics. This field studies the body and its static and dynamic positions as a means of communication (body language). Body language is one's subconscious use of gestures, posture, and other forms of nonverbal expressions in communications. Its clinical application is found in diagnosis (gross inspection) and psychology. The form of kinesics most utilized in applied biomechanics is that of kinematography, in which the human form is analyzed during motion by such methods as photographic "stills."

Clinical Application

In traditional medical practice, the musculoskeletal system is the most overlooked system in the body, yet it contains over half the body mass. The relationship between structure and function, and the interrelationship between all body systems, cannot be denied. Muscles, bones, and connective tissues are involved in both local and systemic pathology and in a wide assortment of functional and referred disturbances. The scope of chiropractic practice is inexorably tied to the biologic concept that relates structure to function and how that concept relates to health and disease.[19]

An understanding of kinesiology and its related sciences helps the physician to better appreciate and analyze individual motor performance, differentiate performance in light of structure-function variables, understand the kinesiologic requirements of an individual's activities, and appreciate traumatic injuries. In addition, the physician is in a more advantageous position to manage kinetic injuries on a scientific basis, understand various handicapping disorders, apply musculoskeletal techniques, and prescribe therapeutic measures based on anatomic principles. As Osler, the great diagnostician, stated many times, the trained eye will learn more by observing the affected body in its dynamic patterns than by any other means.

OSTEOLOGIC FACTORS

As the total of all bones form the skeletal *system*, each bone can be considered as an *organ* and a highly complex tool. Biomechanically, the skeleton may be considered as an arrangement of levers which are moved by muscles or external forces. The type, range, and power of movement are governed by the nature of the joints between the moving parts, the lengths of the bony levers, the size and arrangement of the muscles acting on the levers, and the weight of the load to be moved. In review, the basic factors of bone function, structure, and classifications will be mentioned briefly.

Bone Function[20–22]

The skeletal system provides body framework, shape, and articulations (Fig. 1.2). It allows girder-like antigravity support for all vertebrates, it serves as points of attachment for muscles and tendons, and the long bones serve as levers to make movement and locomotion possible. It surrounds and provides protection for the internal organs, provides movement when acted upon by muscles, and manufactures blood cells. It serves as a storage source for mineral salts that would be toxic if free within the circulation. Bones also serve as clinical landmarks and reference points in measurements.

Bone Classifications[23–25]

A particular bone can be classified as long, short (polyhedral), flat, irregular,

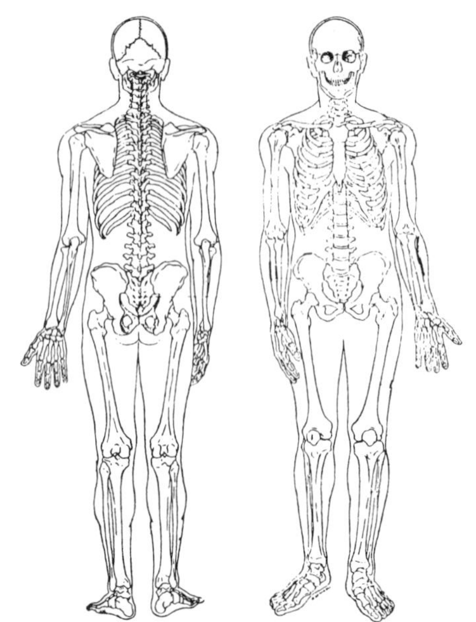

Figure 1.2. Posterior and anterior aspects of the human skeleton.

pneumatic (peculiar to the skull), or a special sesamoid. A long bone has a shaft that is coated with compact bone which contains a hollow tube lined with compact bone. These two layers surround an area of spongy bone. Long bones ossify intracartilaginously (especially) from at least the centers located in the diaphysis and each epiphysis. While the clavicles and ribs are usually considered long bones, they have no medullary cavity. Flat or plate-like bones consist of two plates of compact bone surrounding a layer of cancellous tissue. Flat bones ossify intramembranously. Short and irregular bones have a thin layer of compact bone encasing a core of spongy bone. They ossify intracartilaginously. A sesamoid is a small (usually) oval bone-like nodule embedded in a tendon over a bony surface or in a joint capsule. The patella is the largest sesamoid of the body. All bones except the clavicle and some bones of the skull develop from hyaline cartilage.

Physical Characteristics

Bone is about half water and half solid matter. Solid bone consists essentially of a cartilaginous model hardened by impregnated inorganic salts, chiefly carbonate and phosphate of lime crystals. The osteocytes which form bone have the ability to select calcium and other minerals from blood and tissue fluid and to deposit the salts in the connective tissue fibers between cells. Parathyroid tumors may cause the reduction of calcium from bone to such an extent that a slight sneeze or turn in bed will result in a fracture.

Bone is less resilient than cartilage. However, healthy adult bone has considerable resistance to being pulled apart, crumbled, or deformed.[26] Its compression strength (18,000–24,700 psi) and tensile strength (13,200–17,700 psi) exceed that of granite. It is the fibrous tissue that gives bone its resilience and toughness, while the mineral salts provide hardness and rigidity. If a long bone is demineralized by mineral acid, the remaining organic material displays the shape of untreated bone, yet it will be flexible enough to be tied in a knot.[27]

Using axial compression loads, the strength of the bone mineral content of L1–L4 vertebral bodies has been studied. Load resistance was found to increase linearly with increasing amounts of bone mineral content. While no difference appears to exist among L1–L4 vertebrae, a difference exists between male and female (weaker) specimens.[28]

Bones become harder and more brittle as age advances because there are higher proportions of minerals and fewer active osteocytes. This is probably not so much a factor of age itself but more a result of lack of exercise which affects bone's remodeling process. As age and/or inactivity increase, the proportion of lime imbedded in the matrix gradually increases and displaces water. This leads to bone brittleness and fracture from only moderate stress.

Bone Structure

From birth to the age of about 18 years, the average male body increases three times in height and 17 times in mass.

The combination of hard and dense compact bone and porous cancellous bone produces maximum strength with minimal weight. Keep in mind that a hollow shaft is lighter and stronger than a solid structure of equal length and mass. In addition, the shafts of long bones are not round; rather, they are triangular in cross section, like an angle iron, to resist bending.

Cancellous Bone[27,29–31]

The medullary canal of spongy bone is subdivided by thin bony trabeculae that join other plates at varying angles. The interstices between these plates contain relatively large spaces to form cancellous bone. Thus, while the degree of porosity varies considerably, the composition of compact and of cancellous bone is identical. The ratio of compact to cancellous bone normally varies according to the strength and function required of a particular bone. In a typical long bone of an adult limb (Fig. 1.3), the entire shaft between the exterior and the marrow cavity is cortical bone, except for the metaphyseal and epiphyseal areas.

Compact Bone[27,29,32,33]

Compact bone tissue is tunneled centrally by fine canals of the branching haversian system. Haversian canals (osteons) usually run parallel to the bone's long axis and consist of small blood and lymph vessels and nerve fibers. Bone-forming cells (oste-

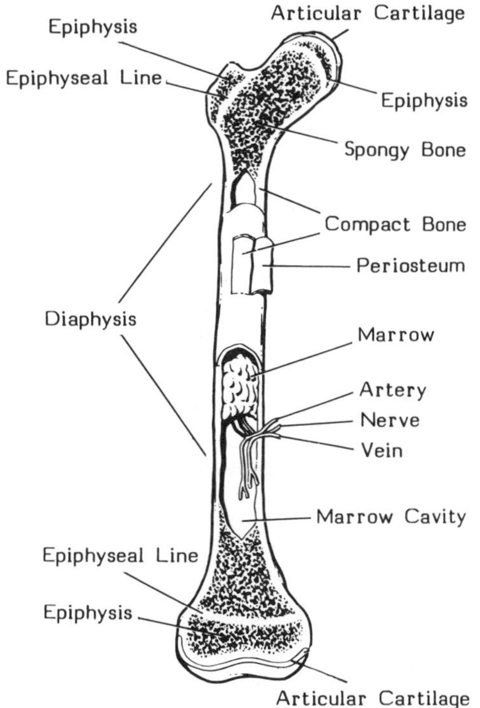

Figure 1.3. A typical long bone: the femur.

oblasts) around each haversian canal lay down bone in thin cylindrical layers (lamellae). These layers of bone correspond to lines of stress to offer greater strength. That is, a longitudinal section of a long bone reveals a fan-like arrangement with concentrations of lattice-like cancelli radiating in the directions of the major stresses to which the bone is subjected.

Wolff's Law. Bones in their external contour and internal architecture conform to the intensity and the stresses to which they are habitually subjected.[34, 35]

Between each layer of lamella are small cavities (lacunae) which contain a bone cell (osteocyte). Communication among lacunae and haversian canals is made by thread-like channels or passageways (canaliculi) which radiate from lacunae in all directions. These canaliculi, filled with blood and/or tissue fluid, also connect with Volkmann's canals which serve to join haversian canals with periosteal vessels.

Periosteum

Muscle tendons insert into periosteum, blend with it, and send many fibers fairly deep into bone tissue. This exterior, dense, fibrous connective tissue surface of bone (periosteum), which is firmly united to bony tissue by penetrating fibers, also contains a delicate, richly vasculated inner layer that extends the blood supply and provides cells adjacent to cortical bone that are bone forming. The osteocytes in periosteum are most active during growth and repair of injuries.

Influences of Stress

Throughout life, bone and muscle adapt to meet powerful stresses that occur during lifting, carrying, striking, throwing, kicking, catching, pulling, and other movements. The form of body structure alters continually during growth and is modified in accordance with the stresses placed upon it. During maturity, the body strongly reflects the sum of the demands that have been placed upon it since its conception.

The stresses and strains of activity and gravity influence the growth of all organs, but they especially influence joint and bone connective tissues and the nervous system. Even in adulthood, the strength of bone increases with the amount of strain stimulation to which it is subjected. The resistance of male bones is greater than female, because male bones are more dense and the skeleton is greater in mass. Likewise, the skeleton of the laborer is more dense than that of the sedentary worker. We often note that tall people become more affected by osseous age; they become more shrunken and bent because of the lifelong stress of the force of gravity and activity upon their relatively long bony levers.[36]

The relationship between bone development and the stresses it is subjected to is readily noted by examining trabeculae architecture. For example, a longitudinal section of the femur shows the trabeculae to closely resemble the supporting girders of a nonsuspension bridge. The bony design of the calcaneus closely resembles a wheel with crisscrossed spokes and a rim.

Bone Growth and Development[37–41]

The factors involving a bone's diameter growth and linear growth have clinical significance.

Diameter Growth

During cartilage growth, a blood vessel and its branches erode the cartilage and enter its central portion. The vessels also bring bone-forming cells that initiate the laying down of bone. Due to this erosion, solid cartilage is replaced by a hollow bone. So that diameter growth can be achieved, central erosion continues on the inside while bone is added to the exterior. Thus, such growth is not dependent upon cartilaginous plates; it is the result of successively deposited, solid-appearing, additional layers on bone already present.

Bone-forming cells, similar to those found within the inner periosteum, line the medullar cavity and haversian canals to form endosteum. Medullary endosteal cells can form bone, but their major function is to destroy bone to allow for diameter growth and to minimize bone weight without jeopardizing structural support.

Linear Growth

The end and middle parts of adult bones are firmly united. However, during infancy, portions of both ends of the larger long bones and a portion of one end of the small long bones of the hands and feet are chiefly cartilaginous. During childhood and adolescence, new bone is separated from the diaphysis by cartilaginous (epiphyseal) plates. While other cartilages may be involved, those near the ends of the long bones are the most responsible for growth in shaft length.

Growth subsides when the cartilage is being replaced by bone at a faster rate than new cartilage is being formed. In achondroplastic dwarfism, diameter growth continues while linear growth is inhibited. This results in child-like limbs attached to an adult trunk.

In spite of bone's strength, mechanical pressure may affect the development of epiphyseal cartilage. This is exhibited in disorders such as poliomyelitis, in which bone growth may be inhibited by the failure of paralyzed muscles to offer adequate support. However, growth abnormalities are usually attributed to thyroid, pituitary, and adrenal hormone disorders.

Some cranial bones are formed directly within a cellular membrane and are not related to a cartilaginous stage. Wrist, ankle, and rib bones, and many bones of the skull, do not contain epiphyses; thus, linear growth of these bones is similar to that of diameter growth.

Disorders of Growing Bone[42–44]

The so-called growing pains in children are usually the result of either joint overactivity, which disappears with rest, or of an epiphyseal disorder. Thus, it is important to diagnose joint and epiphyseal disorders early so that correction can be made before a young patient's future posture and well being are molded.

Types of Epiphyses

Normal postural balance depends to a great extent on the state of the epiphyses, because they form the future permanent skeleton. The epiphyses are functionally classed into three types: (1) the pressure epiphyses, found at the ends of long bones, which influence osseous growth and transmit body load from one structure to another; (2) the traction epiphyses, which serve as points of attachment for tendons and ligaments; and (3) the atavistic epiphyses, which serve to support and protect vital organs.

Epiphyseal lesions result from local ischemia that produces aseptic subchondral necrosis. They are most commonly found in the epiphyses of the femoral head, anterior tubercle of the tibia, head of the second metatarsal and tarsal navicular of the foot, and the lunate of the hand. Traumatic lesions of the epiphyses can range from a simple dislocation to a severe osteochondritis.

Classification of Growing Bone Disorders

Disorders of growing bone can be classified into three general groups: (1) disturbances in the general growth and development of bone such as premature ossification or delayed ossification, (2) acquired epiphyseal lesions, and (3) traumatic epiphyseal lesions.

Premature bone ossification is the result of an accelerated growth rate characterized by a large but otherwise normal skeleton such as that seen in giantism. Delayed cartilage growth or the conversion of cartilage into bone is seen in chondrodystrophy and cretinism.

Immobilization Effects

Immobilization not only weakens muscle tissue, it also contributes to osteoarthritis and abnormal bone formation. Studies with rabbits have shown that degenerative changes develop consistently with a severity proportional to the duration of immobilization. An increased turnover of osseous tissue in the immobilized limb compared to the nonimmobilized contralateral limb was also shown.[45]

Disorders of Bone Calcification

These conditions offer few physical signs until greatly advanced. They are usually diagnosed from roentgenography.

Local bone atrophy (osteoporosis) is seen most commonly as the result of disuse, posttraumatic bone atrophy, radiation atrophy, and peripheral vascular bone atrophy. Also in this class are gouty bone atrophy, arthritic atrophy, antibiotic bone atrophy, bone atrophy from celiac disease, and hemiatrophy. General bone atrophy is seen as the result of the physiologic changes occurring with senile osteoporosis and menopausal osteoporosis. Entities of generalized pathologic bone atrophy include osteomalacia, rickets, osteitis fibrosa cystica, osteoporosis melolytica, and osteogenesis imperfecta.[42]

A large number of disorders of calcified bone that are recognized on x-ray films are most difficult to detect by physical signs in the early stages. These conditions present a long list of disorders including osteosclerosis, ivory vertebra, calcified costal cartilages, soft tissue calcareous deposits, calcified lymph nodes, calcified hematoma, and calcification of blood vessels as in medial sclerosis of Mönckeberg, arteriosclerosis, and phleboliths. Calcification of muscle tissue is seen in traumatic myositis ossificans and myositis ossificans progressiva in children. Widespread calcific deposits are noted in Werner's syndrome, calcinosis, calcinosis circumscripta, and calcinosis interstitialis. Peritendonitis calcificans is often associated with various types of bursitis.

Bone Trauma

Musculoskeletal symptoms may be the first clues in the diagnosis of poor structural or stress adaptation. The most common musculoskeletal symptoms are joint stiffness, swelling, and pain.[46]

Joint structure represents the qualitative and quantitative ability of the chemical constituents of bone and associated tissues to cope with the action of external and internal forces. Bones, being essentially nonyielding structures, are damaged when excessive force is applied directly or indirectly (Fig. 1.4). The nature of the damage depends on the direction of the applied force and on the manner in which these bones are attached to other structures.[36] The most accurate diagnosis can be made immediately after injury, before swelling clouds the picture.

An applied stress that is greater than the structural resistance will fracture a bone or dislocate a joint. Stress is defined as the force exerted; ie, while it requires from about 1500–3000 lb to fracture the neck of the femur, a weight of only 20 lb dropped upon it will have the same result.

Normal bone has an excellent blood supply, with some exceptions in the metaphyseal area; but tendons, ligaments, discs and cartilage are poorly vascularized. Yet, both

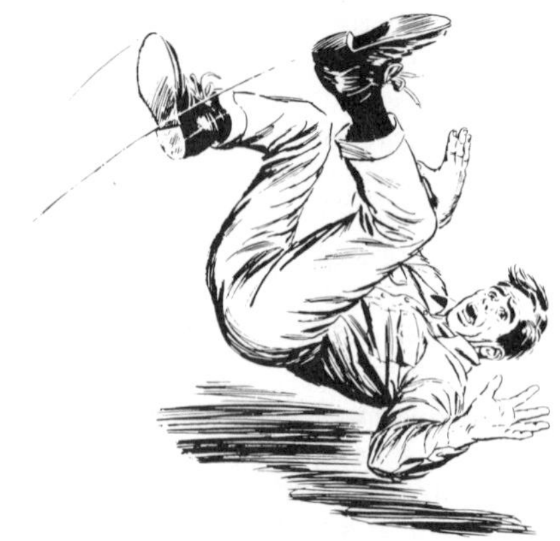

Figure 1.4. During a typical fall to the floor, a 200-lb person with a center of mass 40 inches above the ground would strike the bony prominence of a hip, for example, with an 867-lb force.

bone and joints challenge the host's reparative and defensive mechanisms. The pressure of pus under hard bone blocks circulation, and emboli and thrombosis can cause additional devascularization. When circulation is deficient, local phagocytic function and nutrition are deficient, and thus healing is inhibited.

When subjected to weight bearing or occupational and traumatic stress, bone demineralizes and undergoes degenerative changes, resulting in deformity of the articulating surfaces. Concurrently, the attending excoriation of the articular periosteal margins results in proliferative changes in the form of lipping and spur formations or eburnation.

Many fracture and dislocation complications such as nerve and vessel injury occur not from the trauma itself but from poor first aid which does not provide adequate splinting prior to movement. Traumatic bone injury rarely occurs without significant soft tissue damage.

The Repair Process in Fractures

A fracture is a rupture of living connective tissue. It repairs, as does all living tissue, by cellular growth, yet there are some unique characteristics due to bone's high mineral content. After fracture, a hematoma develops between the split ends. Within a few days, this space becomes invaded by granulation tissue, which in time becomes converted into fibrocartilage. This fibrocartilage is an osteoid tissue in which new bone is laid down for union. After this stage, resorption and remodeling to reduce the initial callus formation occur in an attempt to restore the bone to its original size and shape.[47–49]

While normal bone is highly vascular, readily repairs itself, and resists infection, avascular bone is defenseless in participating in the reparative process. Thus, after injury, treatment must be directed to prevent further devascularization and to encourage improved vascularity. Intra-articular and metaphyseal fractures have an abundant blood supply; thus early and active movement of the joint should be encouraged. However, proper stabilization of distal and proximal joints must be maintained in diaphyseal fractures because of the relatively poor blood supply. Thus, special care must be taken to increase circulation and prevent stiffness.

An abnormally slow healing fracture can almost always be attributed to a deficiency in minerals and vitamins, and rarely to endocrine or metabolic etiologies. However, too much site motion, joint distraction, infection, and other compound fracture complications can cause delayed union or nonunion.

Specific biomechanical implications may also be involved. As mentioned, layers of bone usually correspond to lines of normal stress to offer greater strength. If a fracture is poorly set, or when weight bearing or muscle-pull forces are drastically changed, the altered direction of stress upon trabeculae may necessitate drastic reorganization and rearrangement of the plates to withstand the new direction of forces. Another complication occurs during youth, when ossification is poorly advanced. The poorly mineralized fibrous bone tissue is tough but inadequately hard. Such bones tend to fracture irregularly and splinter as a green stick does when subjected to undue bending stress.

CONNECTIVE TISSUE

The functions of connective tissue, the largest tissue component of the body, are to connect, bind, serve as restraining straps and check bands, facilitate movement, support, sheathe, serve as pulleys, provide pathways and passageways, form sacs, defend, synthesize, nourish, and repair other tissues and parts. It is composed of a few widely dispersed cells in proportion to an abundance of intercellular material (Fig. 1.5). Bone and cartilage comprise the most dense connective tissues.[50]

Types

The various types of connective tissue include mucous, fibrous (white, yellow, and areolar), reticular, adipose, pigmented, and amorphous. Mucous tissue is the jelly-like substance from which connective tissue develops. White collagenous fibers, the most common type, are essentially inelastic. They are necessary at sites where some deformation is required and are often arranged in wavy bundles which allow them to slacken. Yellow fibers are elastic; they may be stretched and shorten upon relaxation of tension. Areolar tissue is a loose interlacing tissue consisting of collagenous and elastic fibers embedded in a semifluid network along with other cells and cellular elements. Reticular tissue consists of fine fibers which form a delicate interlacing network, while adipose tissue contains aggregations of closely packed fat cells.[51,52]

Muscle Fascia

Enveloping sheaths of fibrous connective tissue are well developed in the extremities. They surround a limb as a whole and cover

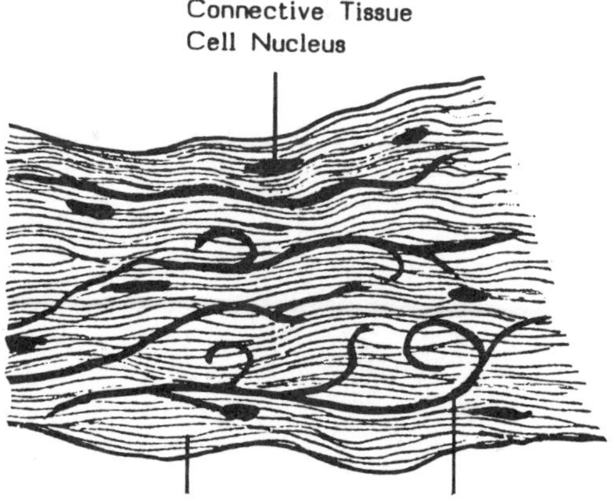

Figure 1.5. Schematic showing a longitudinal section of connective tissue consisting of many collagenous fibers and a few elastic fibers.

individual muscles (epimysium). Connective tissue septa pass from the epimysium into the muscle itself as perimysium to separate muscle tissue into bundles (fasciculi), and each muscle fiber is surrounded by delicate connective tissue (endomysium). The cellular units of skeletal muscle are the muscle fibers. The fluid between fascia and muscle acts as a lubricant. Fascias are joined by loose semifluid connective tissue, especially where lubrication is necessary, for instance, where muscles cross each other.

Bursae[53]

A bursa forms at various muscle-muscle, muscle-tendon, muscle-bone, tendon-bone, tendon-ligament sites and between the skin and bony prominences. A bursa, essentially, is a fascial pocket-like cavity of fluid where connective tissue spaces gather. This is usually in the vicinity of joints. Each bursa is lined with a synovia-secreting membrane to reduce friction.

Ligaments and Tendons[54-57]

Fascial fibers run in various directions to offer an interwoven architecture. However, in ligaments and tendons, the spiraling fibers run in one direction in closely packed cords to resist tension in that direction (Fig. 1.6). The heavy, dense collagenous bundles of tendons, which unite muscle to bone, blend with deep periosteum at one end and are firmly attached to muscle cells at the other end. These bundles contain a few elastic fibers.

Tendons are rarely ruptured, as they can sustain tension from 8,600–18,000 psi—far above that of muscle (about 77 psi). It is for this reason that a healthy tendon ruptured

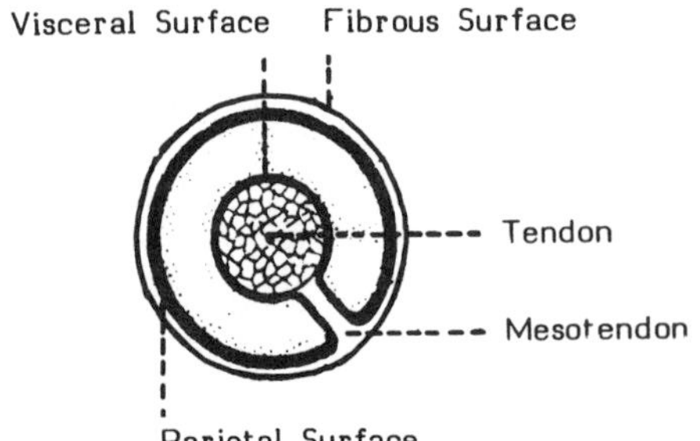

Figure 1.6. Schematic cross section of a tendon depicting a mesotendon and a synovial sheath.

by a sudden force fractures at its bony attachment, causing a bone fragment avulsion, or less frequently at its muscle insertion, rather than in the middle.

Tendons have great intrinsic strength and are capable of withstanding the action of strong muscle contraction, yet they are often incapable of withstanding an unexpected stretching force (eg, a misstep). For protection, the Golgi tendon stretch receptors have an inhibitory effect on muscle contraction. This tends to counterbalance the stretch receptors within muscle that excite contraction upon stretch.

Cartilage[56,58,59]

Cartilage (gristle) is a form of dense fibrous connective tissue in which the cells are embedded in a firm abundant matrix that adds greater toughness, hardness, and resistance to deformation than typical fibrous connective tissue. The three types are hyaline cartilage, elastic cartilage, and fibrocartilage. All types offer greater resilience and smoothness than bone. The fibers are especially heavy in areas where cartilage must withstand great crushing forces such as in the fibrocartilage of the intervertebral discs and the menisci of the knees. A thin layer of hard cartilage blankets the articular surfaces of bone to reduce friction and prevent excessive wear.

Symmetry and Asymmetry

Asymmetry of a part may be an important health clue, and it may have implications for physical performance when uncompensated. For example, atrophy of a muscle may be a clue that there is underlying joint abnormality. With slight variations, the normal human body is basically symmetrical and balanced around its center of gravity.

In general, if a limb is the same length as its partner, it is probable that bone is not involved and the condition occurred after bone maturity. If limb length is shortened, it is probable that the condition occurred prior to bone maturity.

Body asymmetry is greatly influenced by gender, and this has been attributed to the patterns and maturation of lateral asymmetries of the human brain differing between the sexes. A study has shown that asymmetries in the size of the feet were strongly related to sex and handedness. Right-handed males have larger right feet and right-handed females have larger left feet; and reverse is seen in non-right-handed individuals. Because these differences are apparent in early childhood, it has been suggested that fetal sex steroids may be critical in directing the maturation of both cerebral and pedal asymmetries.[60]

The Repair Process

Connective tissue bears the brunt of injury in moving parts and kinetic trauma. Any fibrous tissue of the body may be replaced by fibrocartilage if subjected to great pressures. When injured, cartilaginous and disc substances will progressively undergo degenerative change with possible dehydration and fragmentation.[61]

Connective tissue cells such as fibroblasts are responsible for the formation and repair of connective tissue fibers. They are located at intervals within the interstices between connective tissue fibers. During healing, new connective tissue fibers attempt to reunite separated parts. If destruction is severe or chronic, scar tissue tends to be produced in abundance. In time, the fibers tend to shorten and become densely packed to produce a hard mass that may interfere with motion of a part, produce a binding adhesion which often pulls tissue too closely to adjacent tissues, or create a stubborn contracture.

ARTHROLOGIC FACTORS

The evaluation of joint motion is often the starting point in the anatomic analysis of movement performance in acute or chronic joint malfunction resulting from either disease or injury. Most joints permit movement in the joint itself and/or fix a limb portion while another joint is in motion. They also function in transmitting stress when stabilized by musculature. This stabilization is necessary so that muscles can achieve their maximum leverage for joint motion (eg, angular, gliding, rotational).[62]

In essence, the joints, the bearings of the body machine, and their associated structures represent the functional units of the musculoskeletal system that allow motion.

Joint Classification[63–68]

A joint or articulation is a structure that holds together separate bones. Joints are classified according to the amount of movement they permit. Usually, the three types of human joints are grouped as the synarthroses (immovable), amphiarthroses (slightly movable), and diarthroses (freely movable) joints.

Nonaxial Joints

A nonaxial (plane) joint is an arthrodial or gliding joint in which the apposed bony surfaces are nearly flat, such as the carpal joints, small tarsal joints, or the vertebral articulations. Only slight motion is possible in each joint.

Uniaxial Joints

There are two types of uniaxial joints, *hinge* and *pivot,* in which movement is possible around only one axis (Fig. 1.7). In a uniaxial hinge (ginglymus) joint, there is a concave surface and a convex surface, and flexion and extension take place on a transverse axis. Such joints occur, for example, at the knee, ankle, elbow, and interphalangeal articulations. In a uniaxial pivot (trochoid) joint, a ring encircles a pivot set on a vertical axis so that only rotation may take

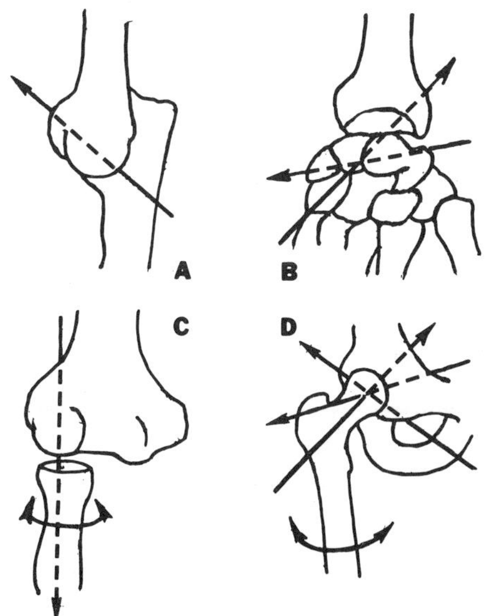

Figure 1.7. Some varieties of synovial joints. *A*, hinge joint; *B*, ellipsoid joint; *C*, pivot joint; *D*, ball-and-socket joint.

place on the longitudinal axis. Such a joint occurs between the atlas and odontoid process, and at the radioulnar articulation.

Biaxial Joints

There are two types of biaxial joints which allow movement around two axes and circumduction: *condyloid* and *ellipsoid*. In a condyloid joint, one bony surface serves as a ball and the other surface as a socket to allow a rolling or rocking action, but rotation is not a prominent feature. Such a joint occurs at the metacarpophalangeal junction. In a biaxial ellipsoid joint, one surface is oval and the other surface serves as a socket (like an egg resting in a spoon) such as at the radiocarpal articulation. Here, one axis is along the short diameter of the articular surface to permit abduction and adduction on one plane, and the other axis is along the long diameter of the articular surface to allow flexion and extension on the other plane.

Multiaxial Joints

There are two types of polyaxial joints which allow circumduction and axial rotation: *saddle* and *ball-and-socket*. In a multiaxial saddle (sellar) joint, the surfaces are reciprocally saddle-shaped such as in the carpometacarpal articulation of the thumb. The same movements are allowed as in an ellipsoid joint. In a multiaxial ball-and-socket joint, one surface is shaped like a ball which fits into the other surface shaped like a socket to provide a universal joint. A triaxial ball-and-socket (enarthrodial) joint occurs at the shoulder.

Joint Movements

Body joints are capable of various motions according to the structures involved. Selected joint movements and their innervation are listed in Table 1.1.

When the anatomic position is used as a reference point, joint movements occur in a definite plane and around a definite axis (Fig. 1.8). Flexion, extension, and hyperextension are movements in the sagittal plane about a frontal axis. Abduction and adduction are movements in the frontal plane about a sagittal axis. Rotation, pronation, and supination are movements in the transverse plane about a vertical axis. Circumduction is movement in both the sagittal and frontal planes.

Architecture of Synovial Joints[69–71]

During development, a synovial joint differs from a nonsynovial joint in that the interzonal mesenchyme liquifies between the articulating surfaces to form a joint cavity which maintains separate articulating surfaces. Such a freely movable joint is the most highly evolved articulation in human developmental history.[72–75]

All joints of the human appendicular skeleton are synovial with the exception of the pubic symphysis and tibiofibular syndesmosis. Synovial joints are found in the axial skeleton at the arches of consecutive vertebrae, at the occiput and C1 articulation, at the C1–C2 facets, and at the costovertebral and costosternal junctions. Although synovial joints are considered freely movable, the degree of motion possible varies according to the particular structural design, plane of articulation, primary function (motion vs stability), and age of the individual.

Because synovial joints are the most numerous in the body and are those most frequently affected by biomechanical disorders and disease, it is essential that the underlying anatomy be accurately visualized during examination and evaluation (Fig. 1.9).

The Articular Capsule

A typical synovial joint is completely enclosed by a sleeve-like fibrous joint capsule that is several millimeters thick. The capsule serves to protect the articulation, to hold the articulating bones in approximation while still affording motion freedom, and to provide a support for the synovial membrane. Except for the large joints, the capsule attaches to the circumference of bone near the margins of the articular surfaces, frequently making the epiphysis an intra-articular structure. Capsule attachment on the long bones is at or near the metaphysis.[56,76]

The capsule's outer fibrous layer (consisting chiefly of strong, interlaced, nonelastic collagen fibers) becomes continuous with periosteum. Associated reinforcing ligaments add to capsule strength. During flexion and extension, for instance, one side of the capsule is accordioned while the other

Table 1.1.
Selected Joint Movements and Their Innervation

Joint	Segments	Movement/Roots
Occiput	C1–C2	Extension (C1) Flexion (C1–C2) Rotation and abduction (C1–C2)
Neck	C2–C8	Flexion (C2–C7) Extension and rotation (C2–C8) Abduction (C3–C8)
Scapulae	C2–T1	Elevation and retraction (C2–C5) Depression and protraction (C5–T1)
Shoulder	C5–T1	Abduction (C5–C6) Extension (C5–C8) Abduction and flexion (C5–T1)
Elbows	C5–T1	Flexion (C5–C6) Extension (C6–T1)
Wrists	C6–T1	Supination, pronation, extension (C6–C7) Flexion (C7–T1)
Fingers	C6–T1	Extension (C6–8) Flexion (C7–T1)
Trunk (abdominals)	T5–L1	Flexion, lateral flexion, rotation (T5–L1)
Lumbosacral	T12–L3	Extension and lateral flexion (T12–L2) Flexion (L1–3)
Hips	L1–S2	Flexion (L1–S1) Extension and rotation (L4–S2) Adduction (L3–S1) Abduction (L4–S1)
Knees	L2–S2	Extension (L2–4) Flexion (L4–S2)
Ankles	L4–S2	Dorsiflexion (L4–S1) Plantar flexion (S1–2)

side is stretched taut to limit the range of movement. Rotation is allowed for by the oblique course of crisscrossing fiber bundles.[77]

Some capsules contain basic areas of weakness that become troublesome in biomechanical disorders. These deficits are most often seen where tendons penetrate or exit a joint, where the joint cavity communicates with a bursa, or where tendons fuse with and replace the capsule.

Capsular Tears. A capsule tear usually results from an unexpected joint force, often occurring in an abnormal plane of motion. The torn tissues produce hemorrhage and local tenderness. Damage to the synovial membrane is commonly associated, resulting in effusion and possible hemarthrosis. Unless joint stability is severely disrupted,

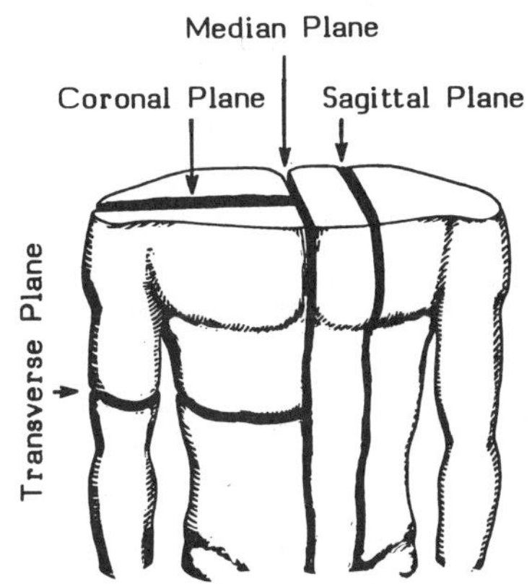

Figure 1.8. Cardinal planes of the body.

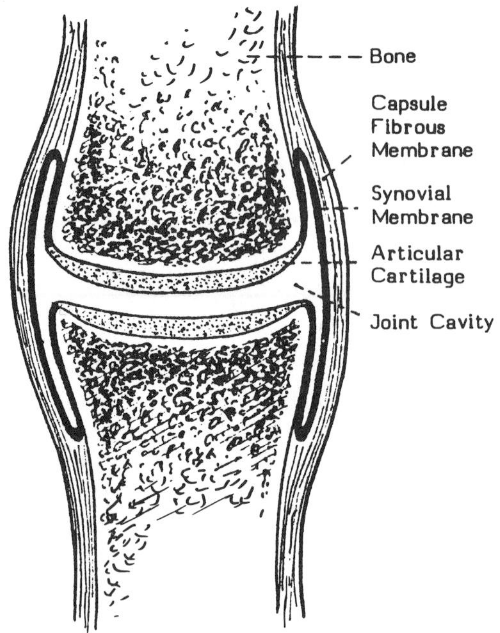

Figure 1.9. Main components of a typical synovial joint cut across the longitudinal midline of the joint. The synovial cavity has been exaggerated laterally to depict the potential space.

these disorders improve well with conservative care.[78]

Intracapsular Pinches. A sudden, usually rotational, joint stress may cause some soft tissue to be pinched within articular structures. This is most frequently seen in the knee where infrapatellar fat is nipped, resulting in effusion and possibly hemorrhage. Management is the same as that for sprain, but joint movement may be delayed because injured fat is slow to heal.

The Articular Surfaces[79,80]

The articulating surfaces are those hard bony portions in opposition that articulate during movement. These approximately reciprocally curved articular surfaces interlock at varying degrees depending upon the particular joint involved. For instance, reciprocity is slight in the knee and considerable in the hip. The surface of an articulating surface (articular lamella) is an especially hard form of compact bone, much denser than typical compact bone, which offers a tough support for the articular cartilage that covers its surface. Lamella contains neither periosteum nor haversian canals.

Articular Cartilage

Articular cartilage is a thin layer of cartilage on the articulating surface of bones that persists during maturation ossification; however, it tends to progressively reduce in thickness with age. When articular cartilage fails, flaking occurs, which may progress through the full thickness of the cartilage. If dislodged, flakes can live and grow in synovial fluid ("joint mice").[56,81–83]

Articular cartilage contains no nerves, blood vessels, or lymphatics and receives its nourishment essentially by matrix fluid ingress and egress during load demand and relief. It differs from other hyaline cartilage in that it does not ossify, contains no perichondrium, presents an extremely wear-resistant smooth surface, and its white fiber network is particularly adapted to bearing loads. Its function is to provide a smoother friction-reducing surface than does bone. The thickest aspect of articular cartilage is located at the site of normally greatest joint pressure. From a biomechanical standpoint, the collagen fibrils of articular cartilage are especially apt at binding proteoglycans into a fluid-filled resilient gel that is capable of resisting and distributing gravity-produced or muscle-action-initiated compression forces.[84–86]

The joint space viewed by roentgenography is occupied by articular cartilage. There are three zones of articular cartilage. In the adult, the deep zone is calcified. Its wavy surface becomes continuous with subchondral bone (Fig. 1.10). Collagen fibers originate from subchondral trabeculae, group at the calcified interface, and then radiate in a crisscross manner to "arcade" within the midzone of the cartilage. The smooth, more cellular, superficial armor layer contains a matrix of collagen bundles emitting from the deep layer.[87,88]

The Articular Disc

In addition to articular cartilage, several joints contain tough pad-like or shelf-like fibrocartilaginous discs with circumferences fused to their respective capsules. They are found in joints where the articular surfaces are never in complete contact and are interposed between articular surfaces. The typical disc, never loose within the joint, is

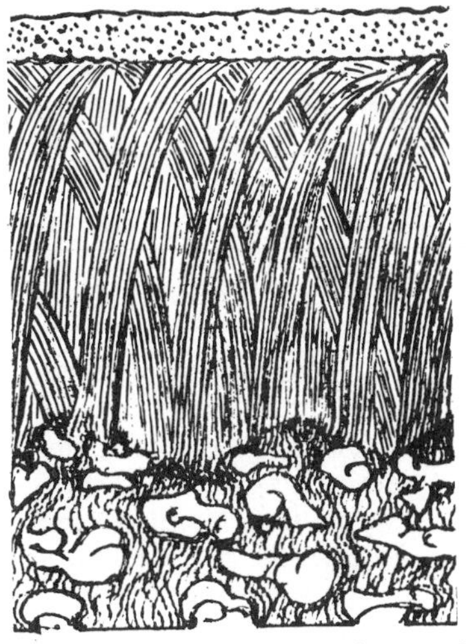

Figure 1.10. Diagram of a section of articular cartilage showing structure from armor layer to subchondral bone.

firmly anchored to one or both articulating bones. In some instances, the disc is penetrated by muscle fibers. Discs are devoid of nerves and vessels except at their peripheral attachments and are nourished by synovial fluid in the limbs.[56,85,89]

Variations. Examples of articular discs are found in the radioulnar, ulnocarpal, acromioclavicular, sternoclavicular, and temporomandibular joints. The discs of these joints are typical for sites where gliding, rotational, and angular displacements are necessary in combination. In some cases (eg, at the hip, shoulder), the sockets of the most freely movable joints are deepened by a pliable fibrocartilaginous ring (labrum) designed to improve the fit of the articulating surfaces. The disc is built up at the circumference to deepen the socket. In other cases (eg, sternoclavicular joint), the disc divides the joint into two sections. Somewhat different types of discs are found in the knee and the spine. The knee menisci are essentially incomplete crescent-shaped discs. Articular separation is often compensated for by a meniscus which tends to adapt the articulating surfaces. Intervertebral discs completely separate the articulating vertebral bodies.

Fibrocartilage Damage. Disc injuries are usually associated with the spine and knee but are occasionally related to the temporomandibular, sternoclavicular, and distal radioulnar joints. When injured, cartilaginous and disc substance progressively undergoes degenerative change with possible dehydration and fragmentation. Spinal disc damage results from repeated vertebral subluxations and the strain of mechanical and postural incompetence that tend to weaken the anulus, and, in the cervical and lumbar spine areas especially, weaken the posterolateral aspects with possible bulging into the intervertebral foramen.[90] According to Nelson, there may also be a visceral reflex associated that causes a slight vasospasm which leads to degeneration.[91]

Synovial Membrane[56,92–94]

The joint capsule and its synovium is usually collapsed; ie, a potential space. The pink, shiny synovium lines and is bounded by the capsule and adheres to the edges of the articulating surfaces. In contrast to a serous cavity, a synovial cavity lacks a basement membrane and the cells do not form a continuous epithelium. The synovial membrane within tendon sheaths and bursae is quite similar to that within synovial joints.

Synovial Zones. The synovium contains two zones: the *intima* and *subintima*. The intima, facing the joint cavity, consists of a matrix embedded with synovial cells. Some cells secrete viscous hyaluronic acids, some are involved in phagocytosis and pinocytosis, and some are intermediate transitory forms. The intima's surface has tissue folds exhibiting villous projections. The highly vascular subintima is composed of loose connective tissue with varying amounts of elastic fibers, microvessels, collagen, lymphatics, free lymphocytes, macrophages, mast cells, monocytes, and fat cells.[95]

Function. Synovial lining is slightly phagocytic, is regenerative if damaged, and secretes synovial fluid which is a nutritive lubricant that has bacteriostatic and anticoagulant characteristics. This anticoagulant effect may result in poor callus formation in an intra-articular fracture in which the fracture line is exposed to synovial fluid. Whenever synovial membrane becomes irritated, an excessive production of synovial fluid is produced.[96]

Synovial Folds. In some joints (eg, the knees), the synovial folds are quite pronounced and may project into the joint for a centimeter or more. The folds contain fat which serves as a space-occupying cushion against compression forces. If trauma detaches a large fold, joint locking may result. If injured, synovial membrane quickly regenerates from connective tissue. In fact, it may develop from any loose connective tissue in the body.[97,98]

Synovial Fluid[99–104]

The delicate, richly vascular, continuous, smooth synovium invests all intra-articular components except the articular cartilages; ie, nonarticulating bone, ligaments, tendons, and fat pads. However, only the labra, articular cartilage, and articular discs are directly bathed by this viscous, slimy, slippery joint fluid which resembles egg white. The function of synovial fluid, a dialysate of blood plasma plus a mucin, is to lubricate the articular cartilages and synovial folds. It also nourishes and clears metabolic wastes from articular discs and articular cartilages by molecular exchange between cartilage tissue and the synovial microvessels.

The Ligaments

Joint ligaments guide articular motion, assist tendons in restricting motion, and provide joint stability. Most ligaments lie in planes that require the greatest stability and serve to restrict excessive or undesirable motion. This function is obviously portrayed in the collateral ligaments of a hinge joint. As mentioned, the fibrous bands of joint ligaments tend to reinforce and thicken the capsule. However, accessory joint ligaments not directly related to the capsule are also found both within and without the capsule. Thin capsules such as those of hinge joints are invariably protected by adjacent tendons or muscles.[105]

The Fat Pads

Fat pads (haversian glands) are ensheathed by synovial membrane and located between the capsule and the synovial membrane as well as between the ligaments and tendons that cross the joint. Being quite pliant, they readily accommodate to changing positions.

The Blood and Nerve Supply

Circulation. All joints require a good blood supply. Fed by adjacent arteries, the branches of the periarticular anastomosis surround and penetrate the capsule to supply the capillary beds of the epiphyses and synovium.[106]

Innervation. Joints are richly innervated with vasomotor and afferent somatic sensory fibers for pain, temperature, pressure, vibration, and proprioception. A rule of thumb states that a joint is innervated by all major nerves that cross it. Nerve plexuses surround and penetrate the capsule to supply the capsule, ligaments, synovial membrane, and periosteum. Motor, sensory, and autonomic branches of adjacent muscles generally genetrate the joint. Almost all synovial membrane fibers provide a vasomotor function. *While articular cartilage is devoid of nerve fibers, the importance of joint nerve function to its structural integrity is readily shown in rapid degenerative changes following denervation.*[106,107]

Receptors. The joint capsule and its associated ligaments contain an abundance of pain and proprioceptive receptors and contain fibers that play an important role in reflex muscle contraction and inhibition. Capsular pain fibers become readily apparent when sprain, strain, infection, or arthritis cause swelling of the capsule and its related ligaments. For joint protection in most joints, that portion of the capsule that is stretched during function is supplied by a sensory branch of the nerve that supplies the antagonistic muscle(s).[108]

Joint Stability

Joint stability is essentially provided by (1) the shape of the articular surfaces, (2) the depth of the socket, (3) the muscle control and ligaments which restrict excessive movement, (4) the atmospheric pressure within the joint, and (5) the thick, sticky characteristics of synovial fluid that contribute to joint stability by way of adhesive surface tension. These factors have varying importance in particular joints. For example, in plane joints (eg, carpals) where the surfaces are fairly flat, gliding is allowed in all directions, but rotational and angular displacement is restricted; stability is provided essentially by the deep hip socket; the shallow shoulder joint is supported by strong muscles; the erect knee joint is stabilized by strong ligaments; and the small loosely packed joints are stabilized by the surface tension of synovial fluid.[96,109]

Joints may be injured from a direct blow leading to connective-tissue contusion and possible intra-articular fracture or a slipped growth plate in the young. The blow is often an unexpected one for which protective mechanisms have not been put in force, or it may be so excessive that protective mechanisms fail.

Joint Clicks

The importance of atmospheric pressure and surface tension of synovial fluid in joint stability is readily exhibited during the action of knuckle cracking or the audible click accompanying a chiropractic dynamic adjustment. A relaxed loosely packed joint may be moved several degrees to demonstrate that its collateral ligaments are relaxed. When the joint is distracted to the degree that a sound is heard, it is at this point that the articular surfaces suddenly separate, and a bubble of gas forms within the joint cavity which can often be demonstrated by roentgenography.

A distraction force applied transversely in the joint is resisted by both synovial surface tension and atmospheric pressure. The adhesiveness of synovial fluid attempts to maintain articular juxtaposition. But, once it is overcome, the intra-articular pressure is suddenly reduced to a level below atmospheric pressure so that gas is audibly released from the fluid. The larger the joint, the greater the force necessary for distraction. This is not only because of the proportionately greater contributions of surface tension and atmospheric pressure, but because of the stronger stabilizing muscles and ligaments.

Joint Stiffness

Joint stiffness is often the result of an overly stressed muscle in youth or a sign of degenerative changes in maturity and old age. It may be found in one joint or several, and it may last only a few moments or for several hours or days.

Joint stiffness is often caused by edema or structural changes. Edema around the joint capsule is found in inflammatory disorders such as rheumatism. Edema in the joint capsule secondary to inflammation is characterized by being more pronounced after rest; eg, in the morning or when standing after sitting for a long period. Stiffness that lasts for more than a half hour indicates the inflammatory arthritides, in which case it may last for several hours.[110,111]

Stiffness resulting from structural changes is usually traced to cartilage degeneration or capsule tears. Previous trauma or inflammation of a capsule or associated tendons and sheaths may have resulted in adhesion formation. Stiffness resulting from degenerative disease becomes pronounced when area muscle compensation fails to protect thinning cartilage. Here also the stiffness is more pronounced after rest; however, it is quickly relieved by mild exercise.

Joint Restrictions and Loose Bodies

Differentiation

Muscular spasm is distinguished from bony outgrowth as a cause of limited joint motion by several features. Bony outgrowths allow perfectly free motion up to a certain point, after which motion is arrested suddenly, completely, and without great pain. Muscular spasm, on the contrary, checks motion slightly from the onset. Resistance and pain gradually increase until the examiner's efforts are arrested at some point. This may be determined by the examiner's strength and heartlessness and by the patient's ability to bear the pain. Bony outgrowths within the joint are sometimes only recognized by the sudden arrest of an otherwise free joint motion at a certain point. In most cases, roentgenography is necessary. In true ankylosis, there is no mobility whatever.[112]

Motions limited by capsular thickening and adhesions are not, as a rule, as painful after limbering-up exercises. There is no sudden arrest after a range of free mobility, but motion is limited from the first and usually in all directions, although the muscles around the joint are not rigid. The possibility of more or less limbering-out after active exercise or passive motion distinguishes this type of limitation.

Free Bodies

Free bodies in the joint are not palpable externally and are recognized only by their symptoms, by roentgenography, and by operation. They are the result of trauma, degeneration, or an inflammatory process, and they may be singular or multiple, be free or attached, and be of bony, cartilaginous, or synovial origin. Loose-body formation is the outstanding symptom of osteochondritis dissecans and osteochondromatosis. These free bodies rarely present a problem; but if persistent joint "locking" occurs, surgery is usually advised.

There are certain other conditions in which loose bodies occur as a complication of a pathologic process: (1) breaking loose of new bone processes and cartilage in certain degenerative joint disorders (eg, osteoarthritis); (2) the organization of clots of fibrin forming rice bodies and melon-seed bodies; and (3) intra-articular fractures, especially compression fractures.

Motion Evaluation

Functional limitation may be the result of (1) pain associated with movement; (2) bone or joint instability (eg, muscle weakness, fracture, torn ligament); or (3) restricted joint movement by effusion, muscular spasm, ankylosis, thickening of or adhesions in the capsule and periarticular structures, obstruction by bony overgrowths, loose bodies, or gouty tophi.[113]

During examination, active and passive ranges of motion should be determined bilaterally and the joint simultaneously palpated to determine the presence of crepitation. Bone integrity is noted by its ability to resist a deforming pressure.

Goniometry

Measurement of joint motion offers an accurate record and extent of disability as part of a patient's permanent record. The most common method of measurement employs the goniometer, either the 180° system or the 360° system. Both systems depend on the fact that a long bone is like a lever rotating around a fulcrum; when it moves, it describes the arc of a circle. This arc is used in determining the amount of joint motion, and the goniometer is used to measure the angle produced between two bony segments when maximum motion in a particular plane has been made.[114]

Measurements are made of movements as it occurs around an axis perpendicular to one of the three body planes: sagittal, coronal, or transverse.

1. Motions in a sagittal plane around a coronal axis include shoulder flexion, extension, internal and external rotation; elbow flexion and extension; wrist flexion and extension; finger flexion and extension; hip flexion and extension; knee flexion and extension; ankle dorsiflexion and plantar flexion; and thumb abduction.
2. Motions in a coronal plane around a sagittal axis include shoulder abduction and adduction, wrist radial and ulnar deviation, thumb extension, hip abduction and adduction, and foot eversion and inversion.
3. Motions in a horizontal plane around a vertical axis include forearm supination and pronation, and hip internal and external rotation.

Differentiation should be made on the patient's record whether measurements are made on active or passive motion or both. When measurements are taken of a unilateral disabled joint, a comparison is made with the contralateral unaffected joint. Measurements can also be compared to established norms.

Joint Dysfunction

Joint dysfunction implies the loss of one or more movements within the normal range of motion with associated pain. It is but one possible problem that must be differentiated from other causes of joint pain. There may be many clues pointing to the diagnosis of joint disease and many strongly suggesting joint dysfunction. This may represent separate overlapping problems or one complex problem. Thus, joint and periarticular pain and discomfort must be fully understood to arrive at a correct diagnosis because they appear in such a large variety of dysfunctions and diseases which may underly an apparently acute disorder.[115]

Primary joint dysfunction is usually the result of intrinsic joint stress occurring at an unguarded moment when the joint is active within its normal range of motion. Another cause is that of extrinsic joint stress following a definite but minor trauma, often classified as sprain and/or strain. Secondary joint dysfunction is often overlooked in traditional medicine. Yet, joint dysfunction is the most common cause of residual symptoms after severe bone and joint injury and after almost every joint disease when the primary pathologic condition has been eradicated, has healed, or is quiescent. Immobilization after surgery, immobilization from a fracture cast even if the fracture is far from a joint, and immobilization from a taped sprain all cause residual symptoms of joint dysfunction.

Symptoms may follow joint inflammation or resolution of systemic joint disease with or without internal adhesions. When joint dysfunction causes residual symptoms after apparent recovery, the symptoms change from that of joint disease to joint dysfunction. That is, during the active process, rest increases joint pain and stiffness; during the residual dysfunction, rest relieves and action aggravates the pain. These points should be brought out during the case history.

The key history of points of primary joint dysfunction are: (1) the pain has a sudden onset and is sharp; (2) it usually follows stress at some unguarded joint motion, (3) pain is limited to one or adjacent joints, (4) pain is aggravated by movement and usually at some particular area of motion, (5) rest relieves the pain and does not produce stiffness, and (6) marked swelling or warmth is not associated.

Sprains

A sprain can be defined as a joint injury in which the ligaments, capsule, and surrounding tissues are partially torn or severely stretched without dislocation being present, but there may have been a partial dislocation that spontaneously reduced itself. The cause is primarily from forcing a range of motion beyond the power of a ligament to withstand the stress.[116–118] The extent of damage depends upon the amount and duration of the force and tissue strength.

Background

Ligaments play a much greater part in supporting loads than is generally thought. Electromyographic studies in situations involving fatigue from forces acting across a joint prove that muscles play only a secondary role. Such fatigue is basically a form of pain originating in the ligaments rather than the muscles. Thus, some researchers feel that if the muscles involved in a problem are weak to begin with, there is a more immediate ligamentous strain that produces the characteristic fatigue syndrome.

Acute Sprain. Ligaments are generally much stronger than necessary to resist normal forces. However, if overstress is chronic or occurs at an unguarded moment, the ligaments are stretched so as to allow the articulating bones to slide (subluxate) out of their normal positions.

Prolonged Sprain. In chronic conditions, the relatively rapid stretching of fibrous bands under continuous overtension is due partly to fiber elongation, but the majority of the stretching is a product of proliferative fibroblastic activity in which more collagenous tissue is produced to increase the length of the structure. This phenomenon is often seen in spinal subluxations of postural or occupational origin in which unilateral stress results in stretching and laxity of some supporting and check ligaments. It is for this reason, among others, that chronic subluxations are often difficult to hold in normal alignment. The site must be periodically adjusted and supported until ligament laxity is corrected. Just as unnecessary bone is resorbed, a ligament will not retain an unnecessary lengthened state. The same process is demonstrated in acquired flatfoot; weight is constantly applied on the medial aspect of the foot which leads to stretching of supporting ligaments and a flattening of the arch.

Effects of Acute Sprain Added to Chronic Sprain. When ligamentous or tendinous tissue is subjected to continuous pull, it becomes chronically inflamed and invaded by collagen substance and mineral salts. This results in sclerosing and varying degrees of calcification. In addition, when these tissues are subjected to acute traumatic stress, some of the comprising fasciculi rupture. This is attended by minute hemorrhages. Further attempts at repair result in collagen tissue deposition and mineral invasion which also produce sclerosing and calcification. If the involved ligament possessed elastic fibers, there will be a definite shortening.

Classification

Sprains are classified by severity, stage, or the area of involvement. In differentiating sprain and strain, keep in mind that sprain involves the ligaments of a joint and strain involves the muscular and tendinous structures. Sprain usually elicits pain on movement of the affected joint even without muscular effort; strain elicits pain on muscular effort even without movements as in resisted contraction.

Complications

The spine and extremity joints commonly suffer from sprains that may be uncomplicated or complicated. An uncomplicated sprain is a ligamentous injury unaccompanied by any pre-existing pathology of or injury to a synovial joint's contents, or the spinal column in case of vertebral sprain. A complicated sprain is accompanied by pre-existing pathology or injury to a synovial joint's contents.

Typically, complications result in sprains (or strains) when the tissues are abnormal or the general system is physiologically deficient at the time of injury, because the lowered vitality of the locally damaged cells and the accumulation of exudate may provide fertile soil for the invasion of inflammatory processes and delayed repair.

MYOLOGIC FACTORS

As the total of all muscles form the muscular system, each muscle can be considered an organ and a tool. No two muscles have exactly the same function. The quantity of muscle cells does not vary after birth, and, as with bone, muscle tissue develops according to need.

By examining the location of a muscle and noting the design of the structures to which the ends of the muscle are attached and by observing a muscle's color and studying its fiber arrangement, it is possible to describe the work of that muscle.[119] The deep-red highly vascular muscles are particular suitable for long-sustained, slow, static pulls (eg, soleus and other postural muscles).[120, 121] The pale muscles are especially adapted for fast movements but tire quickly under prolonged loads (eg, gastrocnemius).

A further examination of the size, fatty deposits, strength, and elasticity of a muscle allows one to accurately judge the amount of its use and the type of work to which it is subjected.[122, 123] Muscle which is worked frequently and rapidly is relatively free of fat. Because strenuous work demands a rich supply of capillaries, a microscopic count of the number of capillaries per unit reflects the work history of the muscle. Aging diminishes muscle elasticity, but stretching exercises can delay the stiffening process. Hard labor performed in a fixed position over a prolonged period (eg, shoveling) has a tendency to reduce elasticity of the muscles used; ie, a "muscle bound" state. Thus, the development of healthy muscle reflects its mechanical influences. Bones frequently warp if muscular pull is especially strong and prolonged.

Muscle Function

Muscles, the body's force generators, function because of five basic fiber properties. (1) *Excitability*: the ability to respond to stimulation (irritability). Muscle is second only to nerve tissue as the most highly excitable tissue of the body. (2) *Contractility*: the ability to shorten and thicken to produce tension (pull). (3) *Relaxation*: the ability to return to original form; the passive release of tension. Neither muscle contraction nor relaxation is instantaneous, both progress from zero to maximum within a time frame. (4) *Extensibility*: the ability to be distended. This is the ability to be lengthened or stretched by a force external to the muscle itself, such as another muscle, gravity, or some other external force (eg, weight, opponent). Distensibility is reversible as long as the fibers are not stretched beyond their physiologic limit. (5) *Elasticity*: the ability to be stretched and recoil from distended length to normal length at rest, unless the fibers have been stretched beyond their physiologic limit. Elasticity and distensibility are separate and opposite properties which coexist in muscular connective tissue.

These factors contribute to smooth performance and protect muscle tissue from injury during sudden changes in contraction or stretch.[124]

It is important to think of a skeletal muscle as one part of a three-part nerve-muscle-skeleton unit. For example, a motor nerve is needed to stimulate muscle contraction, the muscle itself must be able to contract and to relax, and the power of the contraction must be transmitted to a bone or other attachment to produce the desired movement. When any one part of this three-part unit cannot function normally, the other parts also lose their normal function.

Muscle Contraction

Skeletal muscle tissue constitutes almost half of the body's weight. Its primary property is that of contraction, and its main function is to generate force to either produce or prevent movement (Fig. 1.11).

Types of Movement. Movement of bone is produced by active isotonic contraction of muscles that cross a joint or by an external force (eg, gravity). Frequently, muscle contraction and external forces work together to accomplish a given motion. Movement may take place that reduces the joint angle (concentric contraction) or increases the joint angle (eccentric contraction).

Contraction Effects. When muscle fibers are stimulated by a nerve impulse to contract, the muscle shortens and pulls against its connective tissue attachment; ie, contraction approximates muscle sites of origin and insertion. One attachment (origin) is sometimes a fixed joint or anchor, and the direction of action is then toward it. If the fibers are in a spiral arrangement, contraction also brings the lines or origin toward the same place as the line of insertion. Thus, while a muscle's origin is fixed, its site of insertion arcs and possibly rotates during contraction. Many normal and abnormal mechanisms can be explained by the fact that a slightly stretched muscle contracts with a great amount of force, whereas a shortened muscle contracts with far less force.[125–128]

Mechanical Energy. Muscle contraction consumes nutrients and oxygen, produces acids, and is the major source of body heat. While machines convert thermal or chemical energy into mechanical energy, muscle tissue transforms nutrients directly into mechanical energy without a thermal intermediary. Thus, during contraction, muscular work reflects the consumption of mechanical energy. Some of this energy is unproductively used in internal friction, and some is stored for later use within elastic (contractile) tissues.

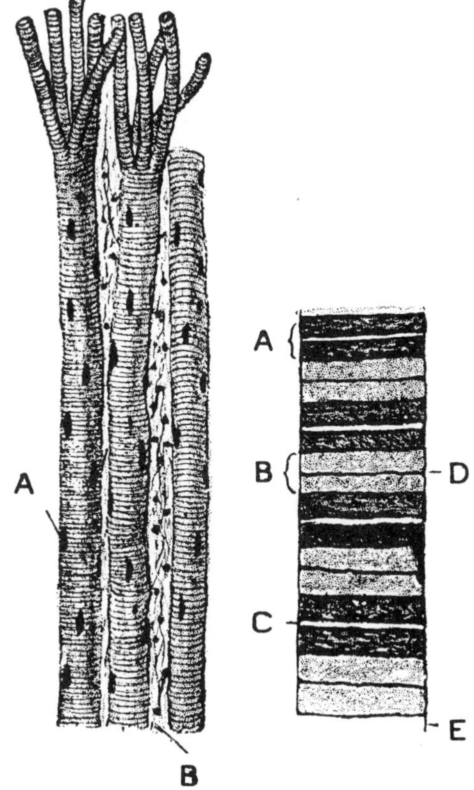

Figure 1.11. *Left*: three voluntary muscle fibers in long section. *A*, nuclei; *B*, fibrous tissue between fibers (endomysium). *Right*: structure of a muscle fiber. *A*, dark band; *B*, light band; *C*, median line of Hensen; *D*, membrane of Krause; *E*, sarcolemma.

Isometric and Isotonic Contractions[129–132]

Muscle contraction is classified into two general types: *isometric* and *isotonic*. These designations are made according to changes in muscle length as the result of either internal or external forces. Daily activity requires a continual shifting of and combination of these types of contraction to meet changing angles of pull and lever-arm length for both the load and muscle involved.

Isotonic Contraction. An isotonic contraction changes muscle length during action if the muscle force exceeds the external resistance force. In other words, an isotonic contraction is the result of greater energy utilization than is necessary to develop the tension necessary to equalize the load. The surplus energy is applied to shorten the muscle.

Types of Isotonic Action. Isotonic contraction can be subdivided into two forms: concentric and eccentric. *Concentric* (shortening) contraction shortens muscle while maintaining tension to effect movement of the bone to which it attaches. In *eccentric* (lengthening) contraction previously shortened fibers lengthen yet maintain tension when an external force is greater than the contraction. Eccentric contractions occur when muscles are used to oppose movement but not stop it. During human movement, eccentric contraction controls just about every movement in the direction of gravity; eg, bending, sitting, squatting, descending stairs, lowering a weight, etc. The active muscles during eccentric contraction are the antagonists of the identical movement when it is achieved against gravity. A muscle can maintain greater tension in eccentric contraction than it can during isometric contraction at any equivalent static length, and the force developed exceeds that of both concentric and isometric contraction at most muscle lengths. Electomyography shows that the electrical activity in these eccentrically contracted muscles is much lower than when the muscles are contracted concentrically with identical load, distance moved, and speed.

Isometric Contraction. A static contraction occurs when opposing muscles contract against each other, preventing movement. This fixating action of a muscle in a static contraction is called isometric action because the muscle develops tension without changing length. Thus, an isometric (static) contraction does not appreciably alter a muscle's *external* length because the internal contractile forces do not exceed the external forces of resistance. A state of equilibrium exists between the muscular energy expended and the tension produced as opposed to the resistance force. Actually, no body muscle contraction is isometric at the fibril level because there is a shortening of contractile components that is compensated for by the stretching of elastic components. Greater muscle tension develops from isometric than from isotonic contraction because no energy is lost in muscle shortening. Maximum tension against a load in isotonic contraction is only about 80% of that of maximum isometric tension.

Stabilization

Movement is produced when contraction shortens and broadens muscle. If contraction occurs without a change in muscle length, the joint becomes stabilized and movement by other forces is inhibited. However, the various body motions are not the sole result of muscular action alone; they are also the effect of the structure, balance, and position of the various bones forming the joints acted upon. This cooperative action of muscles and bones is the result of leverage, and levers operate according to mechanical laws. These laws will be described in Chapter 2.

Muscle Tone[133–135]

Healthy muscle is characterized by active contraction in response to the reaction of the nervous system to the environment. This readiness to act, resulting in firing of motor units as stimuli from the environment act upon the nervous system, is expressed as muscle tone. Muscles that have lost their tone through lack of activity, primary muscle disease, or nerve damage become flaccid. The tone of muscle is due to the constant, steady contraction and relaxation of different muscle fibers in individual muscles that help to maintain the "chemical engine" of the muscle cells. Even minor exercise helps to maintain tone by renewing blood supply to muscle cells.

Gross Body Movements

Muscular forces that result in body movements are classified as postural, ballistic, and tension movements.

Postural Movements. These are the motions of standing relatively still in a fixed position (eg, holding an erect military posture). While the body appears to be motionless, it is actually shifting form side to side and back and forth over its base of support. This slight but constant movement is the result of asynchronous muscle summations, controlled by countermovements, necessary to keep the body's center of gravity over its base of support. It is especially exhibited in any type of balance activity.[136]

Ballistic Movements. These are movements in which a strong muscle contraction begins motion, but the movement continues on its own momentum after the initial contraction (eg, kicking or throwing). Although strong muscle contraction is necessary to initiate the movement, constant contraction is not necessary throughout the full range of motion. A typical ballistic movement is demonstrated in skillfully pitching or kicking a ball.[137]

Tension Movements. These are movements that require constant muscle contraction throughout the range of motion (eg, handwriting, most gymnastics).

Jogging is an example of an activity that requires postural, ballistic, and tension movements. The trunk is fixed in an upright position by postural movements, and ballistic movements control the recovery leg resulting from the tension movement of the driving leg.

Voluntary Control[138, 139]

Skeletal muscle, under voluntary control, is activated by brain impulses that are transmitted to muscle tissue at specialized neuromuscular junctions. Intramuscular and intratendinous afferent impulses produce changes in muscle length, tension, and rapidity of movement, and the occurrence of these actions are fed back to the brain through a reflex arc. Such neural arcs monitor volitional motion and simultaneously inhibit undesirable contractions.

Typical volition controls whole movement, not that of single muscles. For example, if the forearm is voluntarily flexed, the biceps contracts to produce the movement. However, this will not occur when an attempt is made to contract the biceps voluntarily. Any movement requires a mental concentration on the desired movement and not on the specific muscle action involved. This is readily demonstrated by trying to walk while concentrating on how the muscles should be acting at a particular moment in stride.

In complex movements, all muscles of movement and stabilization must be coordinated. The complicated coordination of even a slow and simple motion makes voluntary control of each segment impossible. For example, the events that occur during a swing of a club or racket follow one another more rapidly than conscious directions can control. Integration of involuntary reflexes in complex movements occurs so rapidly that it is impossible for an individual to describe with accuracy the entire sequence of neuromuscular action which occurs during the action.

Neuromuscular Mechanisms[140–143]

Nerves containing both motor and sensory fibers pierce muscle fascia at the neurovascular hila. The terminal branches of an axon innervate each muscle fiber. The nerve cell body plus the long axon extending within the motor nerve (Fig. 1.12), plus all the terminal branches, and all the muscle fibers supplied by these branches comprise a nerve "motor unit." Each muscle is composed of a number of motor units (fasciculi) which in themselves are several muscle fibers linked to a motor nerve which, in turn, is joined to the central nervous system. Large motor units are required for powerful gross movements where the fasciculi are large and coarse, while precise fine movements require much smaller motor units where the fasciculi are relatively small.

The precision of muscle action in joint movement is limited by the quality of the neuromuscular system. Before movement of any joint can take place, there must be some relaxation of the muscles contralateral to the direction of movement. This process of relaxation is a combination of a decrease in nervous stimulation and a rearrangement of

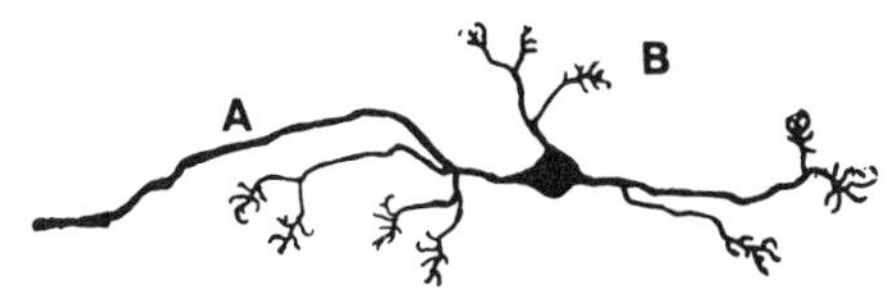

Figure 1.12. Nerve cell with dendrites ending in claw-like telodendria. *A*, neuraxis; *B*, telodendrion.

the molecules within the muscle fibers, and both of these phenomena are variable.

While one or more joints are being moved by muscles, other joints must be somewhat fixed or allowed to move to limit or extend the action. These muscles of stabilization may be brought into activity during any phase of movement, and more muscles are usually involved in stabilization than in movement.

Structural-Functional Relationships

Current evidence strongly suggests that sensory afferent impulses may play an important role in the maintenance of dynamic equilibrium of the human body with its environment. Overstress of muscles, tendons, and ligaments brings about a change in patterns of afferent nerve impulses that are fired from their nociceptors and mechanoreceptors and transmitted to the central nervous system. It can be hypothesized that, as a result of these changes, stress develops that not only affects the body's dynamic equilibrium with the forces of gravity but also can produce possible visceral dysfunction, and, in turn, visceral disorders influence the body's dynamic equilibrium.[144]

Movers, Synergism, and Antagonism[145–148]

Muscles almost always act in groups rather than singly, and the coordinated action of several muscles produces movement; ie, while one group contracts, the other group relaxes, and vice versa. The agonist muscle whose contraction contributes the most to a movement is the *prime mover.* Muscle offering an assistant or emergency role are *secondary muscles.* The muscle that relaxes during contraction of a prime mover or whose contraction results in a joint action that is the opposite to that of the prime mover is the *antagonist.* In flexion and extension of the forearm, for example, the biceps and triceps are alternately prime movers and antagonists.

Synergism. Muscles that act separately and in cooperation, and contract at the same time as the prime mover to produce a single movement are the synergists; for instance, shoulder adduction produced by contraction of the latissimus dorsi and pectoralis major. Such muscles often play a role in both limiting movement and enhancing power and coordination by acting isometrically to steady a bone against the contraction of another muscle. Synergism may exist in both simple and complex movements.

Types of Synergism. There are essentially three types of synergists: (1) *stabilizing synenergists,* which allow a greater amount of force to be exerted by the open end of a kinematic chain; (2) *neutralizing or counteracting synergists,* which cross multiple axial joints in a manner to allow more than one joint action; and (3) *cojoint synergists,* which are two muscles necessary to produce a movement that neither could accomplish alone.

Antagonism. The concept that there is a form of true antagonism between the muscles that move the joint in one direction as opposed to those that move the joint in another direction is not exact. The action is better termed a reciprocal inhibition because the "antagonistic" muscle relaxes completely. Most muscles that demonstrate a reciprocal pattern do not necessarily have an antagonistic role; it is closer to that of a synergistic partner. Nervous coordination is so precise there is no need for muscles to act on antagonism. Combined contraction is only seen in a hypertense individual, in a person using tremendous effort for which great stabilization is necessary, in a subject who is deliberately performing a movement having such an effect, or in pathologic states such as cerebral palsy and hemiplegia.

Control Grading. The central nervous system programs the work of synergist and antagonist muscles through contraction grading in four modes: (1) qualitatively, by muscle innervation; (2) intensively, by increasing intrinsic muscle tone; (3) spatially, by action within various optimal zones of contraction; and (4) temporally, by desynchronizing the action of various muscle bundles or muscles within a group.[149]

Adaptive Role Reversals

A muscle's fixed point of attachment during normal activity is considered the muscle's origin, and its mobile aspect is spoken of as the site of attachment. But this fact does not prevent role switching under special circumstances. Muscular attachments may reverse roles because of the effect of stabilization of a different set of muscles or of external forces.

For example, the usual role of the pectoralis major is to adduct the arm towards the thoracic cage. Here, the sternum and ribs are considered the muscle's origin and the humerus serves as the site of insertion. This typical function may be reversed in a situation of respiratory distress where we see a patient leaning on both elbows to stabilize the humeri. When this is done, the fixed humeri now serve as the origin of the pectoralis major as contraction lifts the ribs and expands the rib cage to assist in respiration. Thus, the muscle's origin and insertion have reversed roles. A similar situation is seen in "pull ups" on a horizontal bar where the hands are fixed and biceps contraction lifts the proximal aspect of the humerus. It is important that this principle be kept in mind during the analysis of unusual movements because any muscle that is primarily a prime mover may function as an antagonist or fixator, or synergically as a neutralizer, emergency assistant, or stabilizer.

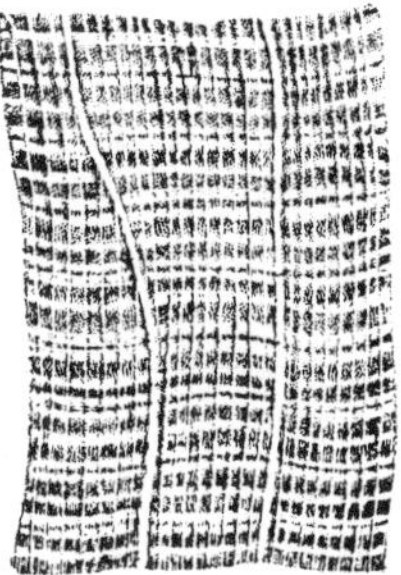

Figure 1.13. A section of striated muscle showing the intermediate discs bordering above and below the light isotropic discs.

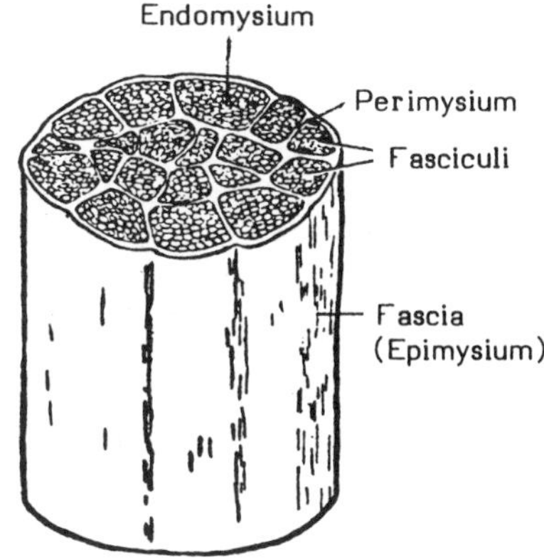

Figure 1.14. The connective tissue framework of a voluntary muscle.

Skeletal Muscle Classifications

Skeletal muscle can be classified by various criteria such as the magnitude of rotatory and stabilization components, position result, depth of fiber color, and primary function which is probably the most commonly utilized method.

Magnitude of rotatory and stabilization components: subclassed as the (1) largely rotatory "spurt" muscles, with their attachments close to the joint axis, and the (2) largely stabilizing "shunt" muscles, with their attachments far removed from the joint axis.

Position result: subclassed as the (1) expanders, which open and extend the body away from the fetal position such as the abductors, extensors, and external (lateral) rotators, and the (2) contractors, such as the adductors, flexors, and internal (medial) rotators, which pull the body into a fetal position.

Color: subclassed histologically as the (1) larger pale fibers which contract rapidly in comparison to the (2) small red fibers which contract slowly (Fig. 1.13).[150]

Function: subclassed as the (1) tonic, continuously low-level contracting, predominantly red and short penniform, deep, essentially stabilizing, antigravity (postural) muscles as opposed to the (2) rapidly contracting, predominantly pale, superficial, essentially mobilizing, phasic muscles utilized in motor skills.

Macroanatomy

Long slender muscle cells form fibers; these fibers are grouped together into bundles; and the bundles are united to form an individual skeletal muscle (Fig. 1.14). The biceps, for example, has some 600,000 fibers which are physiologically isolated and may act independently. Because muscle fibers act individually, it is thought that they probably never combine their action the same way twice in any intensity of muscular contraction.

Design[151–154]

The 640 muscles of the body can be placed in two general categories: longitudinal and penniform. The longitudinal group, with their lengthwise fibers, favors range of movement and speed rather than strength. Examples are the rhomboids, pectoralis major, biceps, and sartorius. The penniform group, with their feather-like shape, short fibers, and oblique angle favors strength rather than range of motion. Examples are the anterior tibialis, rectus femoris (bipenniform), and deltoid (multipenniform). Great power is achieved when multiple-headed muscles are placed at an angle on either side of a central tendon, as in the case of a bipenniform muscle (Fig. 1.15).

Fascia

The fascia and connective tissue stroma of skeletal muscle transmit muscle force to bone, serve as a spring element during contraction, determine the extent of muscle stretching and deformity, and provide pathways for nerves, blood vessels, and lymphatics. Extensions of muscle sheath become continuous with tough connective tissue attachments such as the cord-like tendons or sheet-like aponeuroses which bind muscles to bones or to adjacent muscles.[155]

Tendons

Tendinous tissue is always present at a muscle attachment even if it is not visible to the naked eye. In a few instances, the length of the tendon exceeds that of the muscle. Tendon cords are intertwined, and these in turn form intertwined bundles. In this manner, the effect of muscle pull is dispersed through many tough fibers. During muscle contraction, force begins at the muscle fibers, transfers to the endomysium, then to the tendon, and then progresses to the periosteum and into bone via Sharpey's fibers.

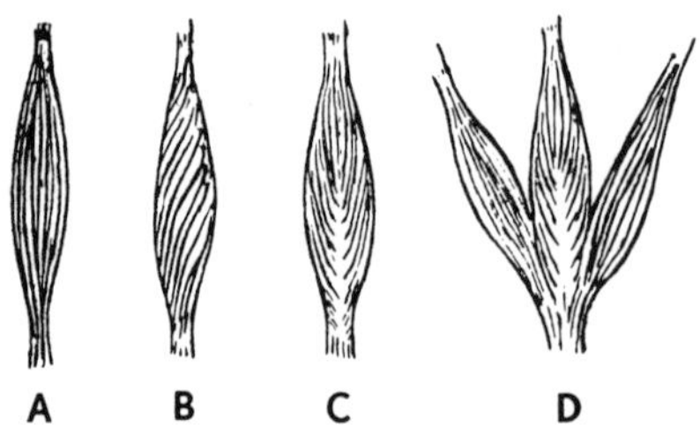

Figure 1.15. Typical skeletal muscle fiber arrangements. *A*, longitudinal; *B*, unipennate; *C*, bipennate; *D*, multipennate.

In a muscle with more than one tendon at its origin and/or insertion, the amount of pull against each tendon depends upon the number of fibers active in the part of the muscle pulling against the particular tendon. This often affects the angle of pull.[156]

Bony Prominences

The bony prominences that develop at tendon anchor points are due to the frequent tension created by muscle contraction which stimulates bone growth during development. Thus, the size and shape of tuberosities are directly related to the size of the musculature attached, and this bony architecture increases and decreases during a person's lifetime according to need.[157] Studies have shown that an increase in physical loading delays osseous aging, determines osseous hypertrophy, encourages linear growth of bone, and redistributes trabeculae design at the most loaded sites in an attempt to meet stress forces.

Vascularity

Blood vessels pierce muscle fascia at the neurovascular hila at one or two sites and then branch within the connective tissue septa. Endomysial capillaries surround each muscle fiber. The degree of vascularity of the capillary network between skeletal muscle fibers and in associated tissues depends greatly upon physical conditioning. Lymph vessels are not found within voluntary muscle.[158]

Muscle Injury and Dysfunction

All mechanical devices are subject to wear with use; this reflects their history of destructive forces. Unique to living tissue is its ability to heal and strengthen, providing a dialogue between destructive and constructive forces. Diseases and functional syndromes that affect the motor unit can be classified by their clinical symptoms and findings such as weakness or hypotonia, periodic paralysis, fatigue, cramping, stiffness, muscle contractions, and myotonia.

Soft tissue damage is usually more painful and can be more serious than bone injury. Bone heals with calcium, whereas soft tissue heals with fibrous or scar tissue. The latter is different from the original soft tissue and lacks the elasticity or viability of the original tissue. Soft tissue also takes longer to heal than bone tissue. Bone tissue may actually be stronger after the healing process has taken effect, whereas soft tissue is usually weaker after repair.

A muscle's strength is much less than its resistance to tearing. Some tissues can resist a tearing force of 175 psi, whereas the strength of the most powerful muscles seldom exceeds 85 psi. This factor of safety prevents a muscle from injuring itself during forceful contractions. Muscles are usually torn by a combination of the forces of antagonistic muscles, the force of momentum, and the force of external objects.

Muscle and Tendon Strains

A strain is defined as trauma to a muscle or tendon or to a portion of the musculotendinous unit from overuse or excessive stretching, direct trauma, and/or overcontraction against resistance. It can involve anything from a minor irritation of muscle fibers to an actual separation of the tendon from the bone structure. A strain cannot affect a muscle and not the tendon or vice versa: if it affects one part of the unit, it affects the other. Thus, the musculotendinous unit must be considered as a whole in cases of strain. The most common muscle injury is strain of a few muscle fibers and associated connective tissue. In strain, both intrinsic stress or extrinsic muscle load can produce torn muscle fibers, connective tissues, and vessels within a muscle belly or at its points of origin or insertion.

Chronic Strain. This is the result of prolonged overuse which produces an inflammation at the tendinous attachment, musculotendinous junction, or within the tendon itself. As activity continues, the inflammatory reaction progresses to calcification at the muscle origin or tendon insertion with possible spur development. Intramuscular hemorrhage is not uncommon in conditions of acute or chronic strain. Tendons with sheaths are more likely to become inflamed, with the inflammation spreading between the tendon proper and the sheath.

Incidence. The incidence of strain in the upper extremity is highest in the biceps and triceps (eg, glass arm), and in the elbow, wrist, and fingers in tennis players. Incidence is highest in the lower extremity in the quadriceps, hamstrings (eg, running), anterior tibial, adductors (eg, horseback riding), triceps surae (eg, tennis), and Achilles tendon (eg, older runners). Pulled spinal muscles are often seen in lifting, shoveling, and rowing activities. Pectineus and psoas strain is often seen in ballet dancers and athletes who do considerable kicking.

Complications. The spine and extremity joints commonly suffer strains that may be uncomplicated or complicated. For example, an uncomplicated spinal strain is a simple subluxation involving the muscular component primarily and does not contain a serious neurologic defect. A complicated strain is accompanied by mild autonomic disturbances and may be associated with pre-existing arthropathy or discopathy, congenital deformities, systemic diseases, myofascitis, or age. Tendons repair slowly and handle infection poorly because of their relative avascularity. Sheath trauma or infection can block nutrition, especially in those tendons that extend via long tunnels and are served with a long axis blood supply.

Classes of Strains

Strains are classified by either severity or by area. When classified by area, specific musculature are used such as gluteal, cervical paravertebral, intercostal, or abdominal. If the muscles involved are of a nonspecific multiple nature surrounding a joint, the general area may be used as a descriptor such as a right iliofemoral strain, left knee strain, or thoracocostal strain of T6–T11. When classified by severity, the terms first degree (mild), second degree (moderate), and third degree (severe) are generally applied.

Compartment Syndromes

Muscles enclosed and supported by strong fascial compartments may become involved in a compartment syndrome. This is any condition in which pressure within an anatomic space is increased resulting in circulatory embarrassment to the contents of the space. Any muscle crush or interference with circulation may result in muscle swelling restricted by the fascial sheath, leading to extreme pressure and cellular death.[159]

Compartment syndromes are seen in both

the upper and lower extremities, especially in the forearm and leg. Typical locations in the upper extremity include the volar and dorsal compartments of the forearm and the intrinsic compartments of the hand. Lower extremity locations are the anterior, lateral, and posterior superficial and deep compartments of the leg.

Increased pressure within a compartment may effect vascular closure, a reflex vasospasm and/or decreased perfusion pressure. The cause for the increased pressure may be traced to either an increase in compartment content or a decrease in compartment size by some factor(s). Hemorrhage, increased capillary permeability or capillary pressure, infusion, and hypertrophy are common causes of an increased compartment content. A decrease in compartment size is usually the effect of localized external pressure. Each syndrome has its individual clinical picture of pain, tenseness, weakened muscles, and sensory changes. The typical signs of lower extremity compartment syndromes are shown in Table 1.2.

A diminished peripheral pulse may point to either a compartment syndrome or arterial occlusion. Hot red skin overlying an affected compartment suggests a complication of thrombophlebitis or cellulitis. Kidney failure or myoglobinuria may add to and complicate the picture. A poorly responding case of shin splints with pain even on rest suggests a compartment syndrome.

BASIC ANTHROPOMETRY

Anthropometry—the science of measurement of weight, size, and proportions of the human body (general anthropometry) and its parts (regional anthropometry)—has many biomechanical implications.[160,161] The topics of physique, body composition, and body types are considered subdivisions of anthropometry.

Anthropometry helps in determining patterns of growth and development, helps in the investigation of variations in physique and body composition, helps in defining structural body type, and provides data for a physician's referential system.[162] These measurements essentially include measuring body dimensions such as lengths, weights, diameters, circumferences, and skin fold thickness. The instruments commonly used for conducting anthropometric measurements are weight and height scales, measuring tapes, bilateral (balance) scales, postural plumb line or grid, skin fold caliper, sliding caliper, and an anthropometer.

Body Size

A primary clinical consideration is an evaluation of an individual's size and proportion to (1) anticipate physial and functional performance capabilities, (2) anticipate potential weaknesses, and (3) isolate a potentially serious health disorder.

Body length (height), body width, and

Table 1.2.
Lower Extremity Compartment Syndromes

Sign	Compartment			
	Anterior	Lateral	Posterior	
			Superficial	Deep
Pain on passive movement	Toe flexion	Foot inversion	Foot dorsiflexion	Toe extension
Site of tissue tenderness	Between fibula and tibia, anteriorly	Lateral fibula area	Bulk of calf	Between tibia and Achilles in posterior-medial lower leg
Weakened muscles	Tibialis anterior, toe extensors	Peronei	Gastrocnemius, soleus	Tibialis anterior, toe flexors
Sensory change distribution	First web space (deep peroneal)	Dorsum of foot (deep and superficial peroneal)	No signs	Plantar surface (posterior tibial)

depth of parts are the concern of linear measurements.[163] These dimensions are usually obtained by calipers or grid photographs. Linear measurements offer us direct evidence of bony framework length. Ideal weight to height values are exhibited in Table 1.3.

Normal growth and development involve both an increase in size and a change in proportion. Proportionately, a child is not a minature adult. Growth and proportion effects are frequently indicators of genetic determinants, hormone balance, connective tissue health, and nutritional considerations.

Table 1.3.
Ideal Weight to Height Values

Height	Ecto-morphic (small) frame	Meso-morphic (medium) frame	Endo-morphic (large) frame
Males (Age 25 Years and Older)			
		pounds	
5′2″	116–125	124–133	131–142
5′3″	119–128	127–136	133–141
5′4″	122–132	130–140	137–149
5′5″	126–136	134–144	141–153
5′6″	129–139	137–147	145–157
5′7″	133–143	141–151	149–162
5′8″	136–147	145–156	153–166
5′9″	140–151	149–160	157–170
5′10″	144–155	153–164	161–175
5′11″	148–159	157–168	165–180
6′0″	152–164	161–173	169–185
6′1″	157–169	166–178	174–190
6′2″	163–175	171–184	179–196
6′3″	168–180	176–189	184–202
Females (Age 25 Years and Older)			
		pounds	
4′11″	104–111	110–118	117–127
5′0″	105–113	112–120	119–129
5′1″	107–115	114–122	121–131
5′2″	110–118	117–125	124–135
5′3″	113–121	120–128	127–138
5′4″	116–125	124–132	131–142
5′5″	119–128	127–135	133–145
5′6″	123–132	130–140	138–150
5′7″	126–136	134–144	142–154
5′8″	129–139	137–147	145–158
5′9″	133–143	141–151	149–162
5′10″	136–147	145–155	152–166
5′11″	139–150	148–158	155–169
6′0″	141–153	151–163	160–174

These ideal weight tables are based on maximum longevity data produced by the Metropolitan Life Insurance Company. Height is figured in men with 1-inch heels; women, with 2-inch heels. Weight in pounds is figured as ordinarily dressed in light clothing.

Biomechanical Factors

The rigid bones and mobile joints of the body along with the forces acting upon them represent a system of levers, and, as do all levers, transmit force and motion at a distance. In the body, muscle contraction normally constitutes the force, with resistance being supplied by a body part's center of gravity plus any extra weight that may be in contact with the part.

Greater height usually means longer limbs, which, during motor activities, means longer levers, longer stride, greater velocity, a wider arc of reach, a larger target, and height dominance over a shorter individual. Height presents a disadvantage in weight lifting because of the increased leverage and in any activity requiring quick changes in direction. Other disadvantages are in the lack of stability due to the higher center of gravity and in the lack of manipulative balance of the long limbs. Thus, long limbs are a disadvantage when equilibrium and strength are the priority and an advantage when range of motion and velocity are critical.

Body part depth and width affect motor activity as they affect body mass and relative size. For example, large feet offer a wide base of support.

Endocrine, Maturity, and Nutritional Factors

Several hormones influence body habitus. The growth hormone of the pituitary affects somatic growth. Thyroid hormone promotes linear growth and has a direct influence on cartilage ossification and epiphyseal maturation, and thus on skeletal proportions. In the young, overproduction of androgen stunts growth and underproduction removes the checks from linear growth. In the adolescent, however, androgens stimulate growth and muscular development and are responsible for the development of secondary sexual characteristics. The sex hormones influence epiphyseal maturation; if the growth plates in the long bones close too early, longitudinal growth is halted.

In addition to height and weight, it is

frequently helpful to determine the degree of a youth's progression through adolescence. This is simply done with males by rating pubic hair, axillary hair, facial hair, and genital development or with females by rating pubic hair and breast development. Skeletal maturity may be determined by x-ray evaluation of the bones of the wrist and hand and other joints, but exposure for this reason only is contraindicated.

Good or poor nutrition also has a distinct influence upon growth and development because of its influence upon hormone and connective tissue quality. Genetics, hormone balance, and nutrition manifest themselves in connective-tissue quality as seen in bone, cartilage, collagen, elastin, muscle, and fat.

Oxygen Intake Variants

Weight is the main determinant of oxygen consumption; the heavier the person, the higher the oxygen consumption. In contrast, the taller the person, the lower the oxygen consumption. In other words, if two people have the same weight, the shorter one will have the higher oxygen consumption. This is one reason why the tall, lean person appears to excel in events requiring endurance. Leg length has been shown to have an influence on energy costs in walking tests, but it is small in comparison to body weight. The obese show high oxygen consumption even at low effort levels.

Body Mass, Weight, and Height

Because of gravitational forces acting on the body, body weight in human movement is a significant structural and mechanical variable. Body mass is defined as body weight divided by the gravitational constant of 32 ft/sec.[2] Body weight is best measured in pounds or kilograms (2.2046 lb = 1 kg).

Body weight is a vital consideration in falls and contact sports because of the impact force. The greater the mass, the greater the amount of force required for movement. This may be an advantage or a disadvantage, depending upon motion objectives. For instance, greater mass is a distinct disadvantage in acceleration and an advantage in being difficult to move or stop once in motion.[164]

Dead Weight

Dead weight is the weight of the body not involved in locomotion (eg, fat, inactive muscles, viscera). It is for this reason that, when endurance and acceleration are the primary concerns, resistance exercises are used to develop strength without greatly increasing muscle bulk. Dead weight from inactive muscle mass is as useless in motor activity as fat. When weight is gained strictly through an increase in muscular weight, the undesirable effects of increasing body mass are offset by the increase in strength available for movement. On the other hand, an individual may employ his or her dead weight in gaining momentum (velocity × mass) and use the fat component to absorb the shock of impact.

Fat Content

In the well-developed adult, muscle tissue constitutes about 43% of body weight in the male and about 38% in the female. The relative proportions of the body's fat content and fat-free component (lean body mass) can roughly be determined by offering the below regression equation for estimating body density using fat calipers without applying more sophisticated measures:

$$D = 1.088468 - .007123A - .004834B - .005513C$$

where D is the estimated body density, A is the skin fold thickness of the chest at the midaxillary line at the level of the xiphoid, B is the skin fold measurement of the chest at a point near the nipple, and C is the skin fold measurement of the dorsum of the arm at a point midway between the tip of the acromion and the olecranon process.

Abnormal and Subnormal Body Weight

Overweight and obesity must be differentiated in physical assessment. Body weight is the total weight of four distinct body substances: protoplasm (50%), extracellular fluid (25%), adipose tissue (18%), and bone (7%). A loss or gain in weight therefore reflects a net loss or gain in one, several, or all of these substances.

Overweight. Obesity implies adipose tissue in excess of 20% above standard and comprises an unnecessary energy loss during motion. A state of overweight may be the result of excessive protoplasm, extracellular fluid, or bone mass as well. As obese people are less dense than the nonobese, body density is a good reference to estimate the contribution of fatty tissue to total body weight. Body density is ideally calculated by water displacement after removal of nonvital body air, but this is a cumbersome research method. The more common means is to caliper skin fold thickness such as back of the triceps (extremity fat) and below the scapula (truncal fat). More than an inch of tissue calipered in these areas is usually considered a sign of obesity. Other areas may also be recorded.

Underweight. Subnormal body weight is the result of protoplasm, extracellular fluid, or adipose tissue loss, all of which reduce skin fold thickness and weight/height indices. The most common cause is protoplasm loss associated with an abnormal nitrogen and potassium balance. Strength is approximately proportional to the quantity of body muscle, and lean muscle loss is calculated from urinary creatinine excretion and limb circumference measurements. Protein-caloric malnutrition affects physical performance early, long before results are seen in impaired cellular immunity and infection.

Body Height

Body height (length) is the distance from the highest body part to the lowest in the standing position and best measured in inches or centimeters (1 inch = 2.54 cm). Weight and height are related to the body's surface area, and surface area is related to heat dissipation and caloric needs. Proportional measurements aid in evaluation. A child's probable height at maturity can be estimated during development, as shown in Table 1.4.

Body Proportions and Physique

Assessment of physique and body composition should be based on anthropometric measurements, an analysis of body compartments, and an evaluation of maturation. The size and geometry of a person's body places individual constraints on one's capacity for physical activity. The effects naturally vary with the occupational and leisure activities involved.

Background

The major areas of concern are the individual's overall size and proportion, weight, height, degree of maturation, degree of symmetry, general body type, and demands of the anticipated activity. It is the physician's role to identify the extent of constraints present and their potential effect on physical fitness during rest and activity. Assessment begins with clues from the subject's history which may indicate genetic, congenital, nutritional, or connective tissue abnormalities.

Physique is defined as a person's physical structure, organization, and development; the characteristic appearance or physical power of an individual or a race. Body type greatly influences performance, and it is determined by weight, linear measurements, and girth dimensions.

Evaluation of body proportions is helpful in determining an individual's center of gravity. A person's common center of gravity affects one's motor equilibrium (kinetic and static). The center of gravity is defined as the point of application of the gravitational (vectorial) force acting on the body. In addition to the body as a whole, each part or segment has its individual center of gravity. Gravitational weight of the body as a whole or its segments differs from subject to subject depending upon body type, height, size, density, age, and sex. The position of a person's normal center of gravity may be slightly changed through the influence of training and conditioning, blood supply, and diet.

Basic Mensuration

For general screening, the examiner may measure (1) the lower body segment by recording the distance from the symphysis pubis to the floor; (2) the upper segment by recording the distance from the symphysis pubis to the highest point on the crown; and (3) the span by recording the distance from the laterally outstretched fingertip to the sternal notch. Normally, these three measurements should be equal after the age of 10 years. The measurements are made with the patient standing upright. A varia-

Table 1.4.
Height Estimation during Development

Age	Percent of mature height anticipated		Age	Percent of mature height anticipated	
	Males	Females		Males	Females
1.0 mo	30.2	32.4	7.0 yr	69.1	74.3
2.0 mo	32.4	34.5	7.5 yr	70.7	75.9
3.0 mo	33.9	36.0	8.0 yr	72.4	77.6
4.0 mo	35.2	37.5	8.5 yr	74.0	79.4
5.0 mo	36.5	38.8	9.0 yr	75.6	81.2
6.0 mo	37.7	39.8	9.5 yr	77.2	83.1
7.0 mo	38.4	40.7	10.0 yr	78.4	84.8
8.0 mo	39.2	41.8	10.5 yr	79.8	86.9
9.0 mo	40.1	42.2	11.0 yr	81.3	88.7
10.0 mo	40.8	43.1	11.5 yr	82.5	90.8
11.0 mo	41.5	44.1	12.0 yr	84.0	92.6
1.0 yr	42.2	44.7	12.5 yr	85.4	94.7
1.3 yr	44.0	46.9	13.0 yr	87.3	96.0
1.5 yr	45.6	48.8	13.5 yr	89.2	97.2
2.0 yr	48.6	52.2	14.0 yr	91.0	98.3
2.5 yr	51.1	54.8	14.5 yr	92.6	98.7
3.0 yr	53.5	57.2	15.0 yr	94.6	99.3
3.5 yr	55.6	59.5	15.5 yr	96.0	99.4
4.0 yr	57.7	61.8	16.0 yr	97.1	99.5
4.5 yr	59.8	64.0	16.5 yr	98.0	99.6
5.0 yr	61.6	66.2	17.0 yr	98.8	99.7
5.5 yr	63.4	68.2	17.5 yr	99.3	99.8
6.0 yr	65.3	70.3	18.0 yr	99.6	99.9
6.5 yr	67.1	72.0			

This list offers a means to estimate probable height during development. Multiply child's height in inches by 100 and divide by percentage figure listed at the right.

tion of this technique is to measure total span from fingertip to fingertip of the laterally outstretched upper extremities to arrive at the total span measurement. This should equal the distance from the top of the crown of the floor when the patient is standing upright.

These measurements offer significant maturation indices. For instance, during early youth, the trunk is normally longer than the limbs. However, as age increases, the extremities increase at a faster rate than the trunk until the limbs and trunk become the same length at about the age of 10 years and remain so throughout adulthood. It is an abnormal sign when the trunk is longer than the limbs after the age of 10 years and is usually an indication of hypothyroidism or certain chondrodystrophies. If the trunk is shorter than the limbs after the age of 10 years, gonadal hormone deficiency can be suspected to have failed to check longbone epiphyseal closing at the proper age. Abnormal ratios may be subtle, yet they are distinct diagnostic clues which should be noted by the examiner.

Minor degrees of atrophy are determined by comparing the circumference at corresponding levels of each arm, forearm, thigh, and calf. Care should be taken that the limbs are in a state of relaxation. It is also helpful to measure and record the circumference of the head, thorax, abdomen, and obviously asymmetrical parts. If thoracic inflexibility is suspected, it is well to record chest circumference at full inspiration and full expiration. If flexibility is the sole question, one need only record the difference in inches between inspiration and expiration measurements, and compare findings periodically to record degree of improvement.

Body Types

In anthropometry, two general physique classifications are made: biotypes and phenotypes. For many years, these terms were used interchangeably. In recent years, however, they have been differentiated. The term *biotype* is now used to refer solely to the basic *genetic* constitution of an individual or those possessing such a *genotype* (basic combination of genes); ie, a group of individuals who resemble each other in hereditary makeup. The term *phenotype*, when used restrictively, refers solely to *external* physical appearance; ie, a group of individuals who resemble each other in outward appearance. The term *body type* is used in this text as a collective for both genetic biotype and its manifested phenotype.

Background

An analysis of body type is helpful in determining adequacy for certain occupations and activities, as well as predispositions to certain types of injury.[165] By general definition, body type (constitution) is the morphologic, physiologic, and psychologic result of the properties of all cellular and humoral influences of the body which are determined by genetic and environmental influences.

Anatomically, physiologically, mentally, and emotionally, no two people are exactly alike. However, three major general body types are recognized: (1) the mesomorphic or intermediate type, (2) the ectomorphic type, and (3) the endomorphic type.[166]

The size and location of the various abdominal organs vary considerably from one person to another, depending upon the particular body build and posture. The visceral organs are usually placed high in the endomorph and low in the ectomorph as compared to the intermediate mesomorphic build.[162–169]

Regardless of body type, the viscera are dynamic and not completely fixed structures as seen on the printed page. They move with the movements of the diaphragm and anterior abdominal wall. They move when posture changes, being highest when the patient is recumbent, lower when he stands, and lower yet when he sits. They rise when the anterior wall is voluntarily retracted. These points must be remembered during health examination and performance evaluation. The structures that appear to vary the most are the pyloric stomach (the cardiac orifice is nearly stationary), duodenum, head of the pancreas, liver, spleen, and kidneys.

Any close observation of people shows a wide variation in human form. Few will truly fit textbook descriptions. Of the variations from the intermediate body form, the two most easily distinguishable types are the ectomorphic (lean) and endomorphic (heavy) types (Fig. 1.16). While most people are of mixed types, it is useful to describe the basic characteristics of the mesomorphic, ectomorphic, and endomorphic body types.[170]

The Mesomorph

The intermediate type is characterized by good muscle, fat, and connective tissue development. The trunk is the same length as the limbs after the age of 10 years, and total span is equal to height. Other general proportions are that the arms are three times the length of the outstretched hands, the length of the leg is three times the length of the foot, and the torso is three times the height of the head. In the female, the limbs are slightly shorter, the carrying angle of the forearm is greater, and the thighs are more obliquely placed as the result of the wider pelvis than in the male. The thorax is full and rounded in the intermediate type, and the upper abdomen is rounded. All abdominal viscera, except a small portion of the large and small intestine, are above the umbilicus. The lower abdomen is flat. The stomach is pear shaped and placed well up under the ribs.

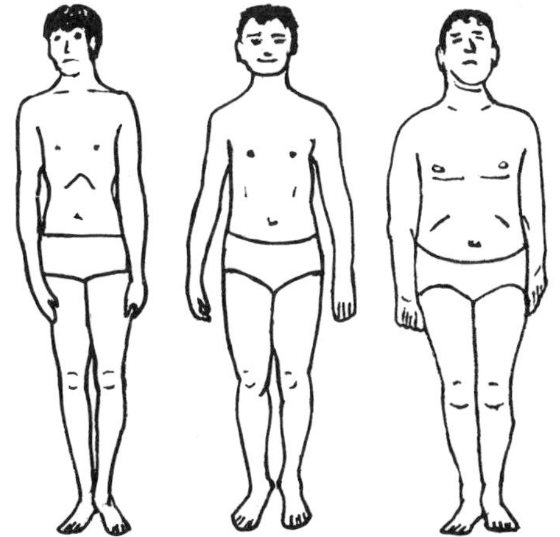

Figure 1.16. Body types. *Left*, ectomorph; *middle*, mesomorph; *right*, endomorph.

The Ectomorph

This is the tall-thin, lean-lanky build. The body design is slender, and the physical frame is frail. Musculature, subcutaneous fat, and tissues are often deficient. The neck is long, thin, and the larynx protrudes. The clavicles, ribs, and spinous processes protrude because of the deficiency of subcutaneous fat. The extremity bones are long and thin, and the thighs are placed widely apart. This asthenic build presents a frail slender physique, light body weight, and delicate body structure. The thorax is long and narrow, and the abdomen is short. There is disproportion between the pelvic cavity and that of the upper abdomen. The false pelvis is often as wide and capacious as that of an endomorph twice as tall, but chest expansion is limited. The ectomorph's gastrointestinal tract is low. The stomach is long, tubular, atonic, and largely pelvic when the subject is standing. The tone of the gastrointestinal tract is poor, and its motility is slow. There is a tendency toward visceroptosis. Ectomorphic females are prone to pelvic organ prolapse.

The Endomorph

This is the stocky-sturdy, chubby-heavy type. The neck is short and thick. The shoulders and chest are broad, and there is good thoracic expansion. The extremities are large and sturdy. The vertebrae are large and strong, and the lumbar spine is short. Spinal motion is more restricted than that seen in the ectomorph or mesomorph. The musculature is well developed and powerful, and connective tissue and fat are abundant. This hypersthenic build presents a powerful and massive physique, great body weight, and heavy bony framework. The thorax is short, deep, and wide. The abdomen is long and of great capacity in its upper zone. The endomorph's gastrointestinal tract is high. Gastric and colonic motility is fast, and the whole tract presents marked tone. Strong, short mesenteric attachments hinder the development of visceroptosis.

EVALUATION METHODOLOGY: AN OVERVIEW

Several analyses of data from Worker's Compensation Board cases have indicated that a significant reduction in costs and time loss from work has been achieved under chiropractic care compared to medical services for the same condition.[171,172] A recent Wisconsin population survey indicated that the major differences between users and nonusers of chiropractic services are that users are older, report more chronic health problems, and have used medical physicians frequently.[173] For the elderly, chiropractic services do not appear to substitute for medical services. In fact, some elderly chiropractic users consume more physician services than do other elderly persons of equal health status, in addition to visiting chiropractors.[174] While great gains have been made within chiropractic, it would be a gross error to rest on past achievements.

Because it has been estimated that from 50% to 85% of adults seek medical attention for low-back pain at one time or another, attention has been brought to increasing effective treatment and rehabilitation programs. Toward this goal, the "back school" concept has been initiated in recent years in both North America and Europe, and it appears to be playing an increasing role in the nonsurgical management of patients with low-back pain in its emphasis on physical therapy, exercise, and patient education.[175,176] Although early studies of results do not indicate a statistical difference between back-school patients and those treated in the traditional medical fashion, a challenge has been presented to the chiropractic profession to maintain ever increasing standards in diagnosis and therapy. Clinical routines cannot be allowed to become "routine."

History Data. The initial patient history is the cornerstone of the ensuing relationship between the clinician and the patient,[177] yet it can be severely compromised by the pressures of time in a busy practice. In the majority of cases, however, the following physical and laboratory examinations will (1) confirm an accurate case history or (2) indicate case history inadequacies. Without question, the ability to develop a case history data base relevant to the total care of a patient is a requisite skill for clinical problem solving.[178,179]

Physical Data. It is obvious that any physical examination should be structured to detect those health problems and disorders that can be corrected or modified to improve the patient's health status.[180] Emphasis should be on seeking objective signs of those symptoms brought forth in the patient interview and case history so that a comprehensive patient profile can be formulated.

Laboratory Data. The yield of a laboratory test for a chronically ill patient is best interpreted by analyzing the prognostic information it furnishes.[181] Facts determined by the case history, physical examination, roentgenography, and other clinical procedures should be used in assessing the yield of any new test.

Adjustive and Adjunctive Therapy. Armed with the facts revealed by the history, physical examination, and laboratory data, and supported by the principles of the basic and clinical sciences and of applied biomechanics, the physician can arrive at a working diagnosis and determine (1) the best method(s) to initially use with the patient, (2) how activating forces are to be applied, (3) the direction and amount of force to be used, and (4) the anticipated frequency of applications.[182,183]

Jamison defines *optimal health care* to include the supposition that the health care consumer should be provided with the best proven diagnostic and therapeutic intervention currently available.[184] Toward this goal, the information gathered from static and dynamic biomechanical analyses of physical activities has been invaluable in expanding our knowledge about the mechanical bases for function and dysfunction.[185–187] Thus, the goal of this text is to present the core material of this vast area of interest in a manner that allows it to be incorporated into clinical practice and to spur further research so that continually increasing levels of competence can be achieved.

REFERENCES

1. Schafer RC: Chiropractic: A challenge for health education. *Journal of School Health* January 1975, pp 52–53.
2. Evans GD: The role of the chiropractor at the primary care level. *Journal of the California Chiropractic Association* December 1975.
3. American Chiropractic Association: *Chiropractic State of the Art.* Arlington, Va, American Chiropractic Association, 1983, pp 4–5.
4. Wiles MR, Diakow P: Chiropractic and visceral disease: A brief survey. *Journal of the Canadian Chiropractic Association* 26:65–68, 1982.
5. Schafer RC: *Chiropractic Health Care,* ed 3. Des Moines, The Foundation for Chiropractic Education and Research, 1979, p 51.
6. Northup GW: *Osteopathic Medicine: An American Reformation.* Chicago, American Osteopathic Association, 1972, pp 22–23, 32.
7. Janse J: *Principles and Practice of Chiropractic.* Lombard, Ill, National College of Chiropractic, 1976, pp 45–46.
8. Jaquet P: The upright position of man: Its phylogenetic and psychological aspects and some therapeutic considerations of interest. *Annals of the Swiss Chiropractic Association* 4:185–195, 1969.
9. Branton P: Behavior, body mechanics, and discomfort. *Ergonomics* 12:316–327, 1969.
10. Hoag JM: The musculoskeletal system: A major factor in maintaining homeostasis. *Journal of the American Osteopathic Association* 78:562, 1979.
11. Craig AS: Elements of kinesiology for the clinician. *Physical Therapy* 44:470–473, 1964.
12. Barham JN, Wooten EP: *Structural Kinesiology.* New York, Macmillan, 1973, p 4.
13. LeVeau B: *Williams and Lissner: Biomechanics of Human Motion,* ed 2. Philadelphia, W.B. Saunders, 1977, p 4.
14. Gowitzke BA, Milner M: *Understanding the Scientific Basis of Human Movement,* ed 2. Baltimore, Williams & Wilkins, 1980, p 150.
15. Barham JN, Wooten EP: *Structural Kinesiology.* New York, Macmillan, 1973, p 95.
16. Cochran GVB: *A Primer of Orthopaedic Biomechanics.* New York, Churchill Livingstone, 1982, pp 6–7.
17. White AA, Panjabi MM: *Clinical Biomechanics of the Spine.* Philadelphia, J.B. Lippincott, 1978, p 482.
18. Cochran GVB: *A Primer of Orthopaedic Biomechanics.* New York, Churchill Livingstone, 1982, p 6.
19. Vear HC: An assessment of chiropractic scope of practice. In Coyle BA, Martinez DP: *Proceedings of the Second Conference on Current Topics in Chiropractic: Reviews of the Literature,* May 4–5, 1985. Sunnyvale, Cal, Palmer College of Chiropractic—West, 1985, pp C1–C2.
20. Moore KL: *Clinically Oriented Anatomy.* Baltimore, Williams & Wilkins, 1980, pp li–lii.
21. Brashear HR, VanderWiel CJ: Histology and growth of bone. In Wilson FC (ed): *The Musculoskeletal System: Basic Processes and Disorders,* ed 2. Philadelphia, J.B. Lippincott, 1983, p 90.
22. Barham JN, Wooten EP: *Structural Kinesiology.* New York, Macmillan, 1973, pp 15–16.
23. Basmajian JV (ed): *Grant's Method of Anatomy,* ed 9. Baltimore, Williams & Wilkins, 1975, pp 4–6.
24. Moore KL: *Clinically Oriented Anatomy.* Baltimore, Williams & Wilkins, 1980, pp xlv–xlvii.
25. Barham JN, Wooten EP: *Structural Kinesiology.* New York, Macmillan, 1973, pp 18–19.
26. Burstein AH et al: The ultimate properties of

bone tissue: The effects of yielding. *Journal of Biomechanics* 5:35, 1972.
27. Basmajian JV (ed): *Grant's Method of Anatomy*, ed 9. Baltimore, Williams & Wilkins, 1975, p 4.
28. Hansson T, Roos B, Nachemson A: The bone mineral content and ultimate compressive strength of lumbar vertebrae. *Spine* 5:46–55, 1980.
29. Rosse C, Ross R: Tissues of the musculoskeletal system. In Rosse C, Clawson DK: *The Musculoskeletal System in Health and Disease*. Hagerstown, Md, Harper & Row, 1980, p 21.
30. Williams JGP, Sperryn PN (eds): *Sports Medicine*, ed 2. Baltimore, Williams & Wilkins, 1976, p 252.
31. Hollingshead WH, Jenkins DB: *Functional Anatomy of the Limbs and Back*. Philadelphia, W.B. Saunders, 1981, pp 12–14.
32. Barham JN, Wooten EP: *Structural Kinesiology*. New York, Macmillan, 1973, pp 20–21.
33. Albright JA: Bone: Physical properties. In Albright JA, Brand RA (eds): *The Scientific Basis of Orthopaedics*. New York, Appleton-Century-Crofts, 1979, pp 142–149.
34. Ogden JA: The development and growth of the musculoskeletal system. In Albright JA, Brand RA (eds): *The Scientific Basis of Orthopaedics*. New York, Appleton-Century-Crofts, 1979, p 69.
35. Brashear HR, VanderWiel CJ: Histology and growth of bone. In Wilson FC (ed): *The Musculoskeletal System: Basic Processes and Disorders*, ed 2. Philadelphia, J.B. Lippincott, 1983, p 96.
36. McElhaney JH: Dynamic response of bone and muscle tissue. *Journal of Applied Physiology* 21:231–236, 1966.
37. Albright JA: Bone: Physical properties. In Albright JA, Brand RA (eds): *The Scientific Basis of Orthopaedics*. New York, Appleton-Century-Crofts, 1979, p 174.
38. Rosse C, Ross R: Tissues of the musculoskeletal system. In Rosse C, Clawson DK: *The Musculoskeletal System in Health and Disease*. Hagerstown, Md, Harper & Row, 1980, pp 19–26.
39. Barham JN, Wooten EP: *Structural Kinesiology*. New York, Macmillan, 1973, pp 23–24.
40. Hooker CW, Greene WB: Normal development of the musculoskeletal system. In Wilson FC (ed): *The Musculoskeletal System: Basic Processes and Disorders*, ed 2. Philadelphia, J.B. Lippincott, 1983, pp 6–8.
41. Salter RB: *Textbook of Disorders and Injuries of the Musculoskeletal System*. Baltimore, Williams & Wilkins, 1981, pp 3–6.
42. Schafer RC: *Chiropractic Physical and Spinal Diagnosis*. Oklahoma City, Associated Chiropractic Academic Press, 1980, p IV-20.
43. Hooker CW, Greene WB: Congenital malformations. In Wilson FC (ed): *The Musculoskeletal System: Basic Processes and Disorders*, ed 2. Philadelphia, J.B. Lippincott, 1983, pp 20–30.
44. Ogden JA: The development and growth of the musculoskeletal system. In Albright JA, Brand RA (eds): *The Scientific Basis of Orthopaedics*. New York, Appleton-Century-Crofts, 1979, p 89.
45. Michelsson JE, Videman T, Langenskiold A: Changes in bone formation during immobilization and development of experimental osteoarthritis. *Acta Orthopaedica Scandinavica* 48:444–449, 1977.
46. Mennell JMcM: *Joint Pain*. Boston, Little, Brown, 1964, pp 13–16.
47. Williams JGP, Sperryn PN (eds): *Sports Medicine*, ed 2. Baltimore, Williams & Wilkins, 1976, p 253–256.
48. Schafer RC: *Chiropractic Management of Sports and Recreational Injuries*. Baltimore, Williams & Wilkins, 1982, p 225.
49. Iverson LD, Clawson DK: *Manual of Acute Orthopaedic Therapeutics*. Boston, Little, Brown, 1977, pp 8, 10–11.
50. Hollingshead WH, Jenkins DB: *Functional Anatomy of the Limbs and Back*. Philadelphia, W.B. Saunders, 1981, pp 9–12.
51. Rosse C, Ross R: Tissues of the musculoskeletal system. In Rosse C, Clawson DK: *The Musculoskeletal System in Health and Disease*. Hagerstown, Md, Harper & Row, 1980, pp 3–6.
52. Cailliet R: *Soft Tissue Pain and Disability*. Philadelphia, F.A. Davis, 1980, pp 4–8.
53. Basmajian JV (ed): *Grant's Method of Anatomy*, ed 9. Baltimore, Williams & Wilkins, 1975, p 24.
54. Rosse C, Ross R: Tissues of the musculoskeletal system. In Rosse C, Clawson DK: *The Musculoskeletal System in Health and Disease*. Hagerstown, Md, Harper & Row, 1980, pp 13, 17.
55. Basmajian JV (ed): *Grant's Method of Anatomy*, ed 9. Baltimore, Williams & Wilkins, 1975, p 23.
56. Barham JN, Wooten EP: *Structural Kinesiology*. New York, Macmillan, 1973, p 32.
57. Williams JGP, Sperryn PN (eds): *Sports Medicine*, ed 2. Baltimore, Williams & Wilkins, 1976, pp 282–283.
58. Rosse C, Ross R: Tissues of the musculoskeletal system. In Rosse C, Clawson DK: *The Musculoskeletal System in Health and Disease*. Hagerstown, Md, Harper & Row, 1980, pp 17, 19.
59. Basmajian JV (ed): *Grant's Method of Anatomy*, ed 9. Baltimore, Williams & Wilkins, 1975, p 11.
60. Levy J, Levy JM: Human lateralization from head to foot: Sex-related factors. *Science* 200:1291–1292, 1978.
61. Rosse C, Ross R: Tissues of the musculoskeletal system. In Rosse C, Clawson DK: *The Musculoskeletal System in Health and Disease*. Hagerstown, Md, Harper & Row, 1980, pp 29–32.
62. Barham JN, Wooten EP: *Structural Kinesiology*. New York, Macmillan, 1973, pp 38–39.
63. Cailliet R: *Soft Tissue Pain and Disability*. Philadelphia, F.A. Davis, 1980, pp 10–12.
64. Basmajian JV (ed): *Grant's Method of Anatomy*, ed 9. Baltimore, Williams & Wilkins, 1975, p 17.
65. Gowitzke BA, Milner M: *Understanding the Scientific Basis of Human Movement*, ed 2. Baltimore, Williams & Wilkins, 1980, p 4.
66. Salter RB: *Textbook of Disorders and Injuries of the Musculoskeletal System*. Baltimore, Williams & Wilkins, 1981, p 9.
67. Rosse C, Simkin PA: Joints. In Rosse C, Clawson DK: *The Musculoskeletal System in Health & Dis-*

ease. Hagerstown, Md, Harper & Row, 1980, pp 77, 84–87.
68. Barham JN, Wooten EP: *Structural Kinesiology*. New York, Macmillan, 1973, pp 29–32.
69. Esch D, Lepley M: *Musculoskeletal Function: An Anatomy and Kinesiology Laboratory Manual*. Minneapolis, University of Minnesota Press, 1974, pp 40–41.
70. Kendall HO, Kendall FP, Wadsworth GE: *Muscles: Testing and Function*, ed 2. Baltimore, Williams & Wilkins, 1971, pp 20–21.
71. Barham JN, Wooten EP: *Structural Kinesiology*. New York, Macmillan, 1973, pp 27–29, 38–40.
72. Rosse C, Simkin PA: Joints. In Rosse C, Clawson DK: *The Musculoskeletal System in Health and Disease*. Hagerstown, Md, Harper & Row, 1980, pp 77–79.
73. Hooker CW: Histology of cartilage and synovium. In Wilson FC (ed): *The Musculoskeletal System: Basic Processes and Disorders*, ed 2. Philadelphia, J.B. Lippincott, 1983, pp 209–210.
74. Salter RB: *Textbook of Disorders and Injuries of the Musculoskeletal System*. Baltimore, Williams & Wilkins, 1981, pp 10–11.
75. Hollingshead WH, Jenkins DB: *Functional Anatomy of the Limbs and Back*. Philadelphia, W.B. Saunders, 1981, pp 28–29.
76. Rosse C, Simkin PA: Joints. In Rosse C, Clawson DK: *The Musculoskeletal System in Health and Disease*. Hagerstown, Md, Harper & Row, 1980, p 79.
77. Rosse C, Simkin PA: Joints. In Rosse C, Clawson DK: *The Musculoskeletal System in Health and Disease*. Hagerstown, Md, Harper & Row, 1980, p 81.
78. Schafer RC: *Chiropractic Management of Sports and Recreational Injuries*. Baltimore, Williams & Wilkins, 1982, p 239.
79. Rosse C, Simkin PA: Joints. In Rosse C, Clawson DK: *The Musculoskeletal System in Health and Disease*. Hagerstown, Md, Harper & Row, 1980, pp 79–80.
80. Barham JN, Wooten EP: *Structural Kinesiology*. New York, Macmillan, 1973, p 31.
81. Edwards CC, Chrisman OD: Articular cartilage. In Albright JA, Brand RA (eds): *The Scientific Basis of Orthopaedics*. New York, Appleton-Century-Crofts, 1979, pp 313–314.
82. Grieve GP: *Common Vertebral Joint Problems*. New York, Churchill Livingstone, 1981, p 36.
83. Rosse C, Simkin PA: Joints. In Rosse C, Clawson DK: *The Musculoskeletal System in Health and Disease*. Hagerstown, Md, Harper & Row, 1980, pp 80–81.
84. Turek SL: *Orthopaedics: Principles and Their Application*, ed 3. Philadelphia, J.B. Lippincott, 1977, pp 14–19.
85. Basmajian JV (ed): *Grant's Method of Anatomy*, ed 9. Baltimore, Williams & Wilkins, 1975, p 20.
86. Salter RB: *Textbook of Disorders and Injuries of the Musculoskeletal System*. Baltimore, Williams & Wilkins, 1981, pp 11, 22–23.
87. Edwards CC, Chrisman OD: Articular cartilage. In Albright JA, Brand RA (eds): *The Scientific Basis of Orthopaedics*. New York, Appleton-Century-Crofts, 1979, pp 315–319.
88. Hooker CW: Histology of cartilage and synovium. In Wilson FC (ed): *The Musculoskeletal System: Basic Processes and Disorders*, ed 2. Philadelphia, J.B. Lippincott, 1983, pp 210–213.
89. Hooker CW: Histology of cartilage and synovium. In Wilson FC (ed): *The Musculoskeletal System: Basic Processes and Disorders*, ed 2. Philadelphia, J.B. Lippincott, 1983, pp 213–215.
90. Schafer RC: *Chiropractic Management of Sports and Recreational Injuries*. Baltimore, Williams & Wilkins, 1982, p 238–239.
91. Nelson WA, personal communication, 1980. Based on Bennett TJ: *A New Clinical Basis for the Correction of Abnormal Physiology*. Burlingame, Cal, TJ Bennet, 1960.
92. Rosse C, Simkin PA: Joints. In Rosse C, Clawson DK: *The Musculoskeletal System in Health and Disease*. Hagerstown, Md, Harper & Row, 1980, p 80.
93. Hooker CW: Histology of cartilage and synovium. In Wilson FC (ed): *The Musculoskeletal System: Basic Processes and Disorders*, ed 2. Philadelphia, J.B. Lippincott, 1983, pp 214–215.
94. Taft TN, Hooker CW: The lower limb. In Wilson FC (ed): *The Musculoskeletal System: Basic Processes and Disorders*, ed 2. Philadelphia, J.B. Lippincott, 1983, pp 61–62.
95. Rosse C, Simkin PA: Joints. In Rosse C, Clawson DK: *The Musculoskeletal System in Health and Disease*. Hagerstown, Md, Harper & Row, 1980, p 82.
96. Schafer RC: *Chiropractic Management of Sports and Recreational Injuries*. Baltimore, Williams & Wilkins, 1982, p 229.
97. Barham JN, Wooten EP: *Structural Kinesiology*. New York, Macmillan, 1973, p 33.
98. Salter RB: *Textbook of Disorders and Injuries of the Musculoskeletal System*. Baltimore, Williams & Wilkins, 1981, p 24.
99. Turek SL: *Orthopaedics: Principles and Their Application*, ed 3. Philadelphia, J.B. Lippincott, 1977, pp 161–164.
100. Rosse C, Simkin PA: Joints. In Rosse C, Clawson DK: *The Musculoskeletal System in Health and Disease*. Hagerstown, Md, Harper & Row, 1980, pp 83, 87–88.
101. Brand RA: Joint lubrication. In Albright JA, Brand RA (eds): *The Scientific Basis of Orthopaedics*. New York, Appleton-Century-Crofts, 1979, pp 355–363.
102. Cochran GVB: *A Primer of Orthopaedic Biomechanics*. New York, Churchill Livingstone, 1982, pp 135–138.
103. VanderWiel CJ: Chemistry and biochemistry of cartilage and synovial fluid. In Wilson FC (ed): *The Musculoskeletal System: Basic Processes and Disorders*, ed 2. Philadelphia, J.B. Lippincott, 1983, pp 222, 224.
104. Grieve GP: *Common Vertebral Joint Problems*. New York, Churchill Livingstone, 1981, pp 36–38.
105. Hollingshead WH, Jenkins DB: *Functional Anatomy of the Limbs and Back*. Philadelphia, W.B. Saunders, 1981, pp 29–30.
106. Rosse C, Simkin PA: Joints. In Rosse C, Clawson DK: *The Musculoskeletal System in Health and*

Disease. Hagerstown, Md, Harper & Row, 1980, p 83.
107. Hooker CW: Histology of cartilage and synovium. In Wilson FC (ed): *The Musculoskeletal System: Basic Processes and Disorders*, ed 2. Philadelphia, J.B. Lippincott, 1983, p 215.
108. Grieve GP: *Common Vertebral Joint Problems*. New York, Churchill Livingstone, 1981, pp 10–11.
109. Rosse C, Simkin PA: Joints. In Rosse C, Clawson DK: *The Musculoskeletal System in Health and Disease*. Hagerstown, Md, Harper & Row, 1980, p 88.
110. Cochran GVB: *A Primer of Orthopaedic Biomechanics*. New York, Churchill Livingstone, 1982, p 136.
111. Schafer RC: *Chiropractic Physical and Spinal Diagnosis*. Oklahoma City, Associated Chiropractic Academic Press, 1980, p II-15.
112. Schafer RC: *Chiropractic Management of Sports and Recreational Injuries*. Baltimore, Williams & Wilkins, 1982, p 235.
113. D'Ambrosia RD: Evaluation of the patient. In D'Ambrosia RD (ed): *Musculoskeletal Disorders: Regional Examination and Differential Diagnosis*. Philadelphia, J.B. Lippincott, 1977, pp 6–7.
114. Schafer RC (ed): *Basic Chiropractic Procedural Manual*, ed 4. Arlington, Va, American Chiropractic Association, 1984, pp 286–287.
115. Mennell JMcM: *Joint Pain*. Boston, Little, Brown, 1964, pp 5, 9–10, 20–21.
116. Iverson LD, Clawson DK: *Manual of Acute Orthopaedic Therapeutics*. Boston, Little, Brown, 1977, pp 15–16.
117. Schafer RC: *Chiropractic Management of Sports and Recreational Injuries*. Baltimore, Williams & Wilkins, 1982, pp 236–237.
118. Cailliet R: *Soft Tissue Pain and Disability*. Philadelphia, F.A. Davis, 1980, p 36.
119. Morehouse LE, Cooper JM: *Kinesiology*. St. Louis, C.V. Mosby, 1950, p 26.
120. Jokl P: Muscle. In Albright JA, Brand RA (eds): *The Scientific Basis of Orthopaedics*. New York, Appleton-Century-Crofts, 1979, pp 372–374.
121. Gowitzke BA, Milner M: *Understanding Scientific Basis of Human Movement*, ed 2. Baltimore, Williams & Wilkins, 1980, pp 102–103.
122. Bennett RL: Muscle testing: A discussion of the importance of accurate muscle testing. *Physiotherapy Review* 27:242–243, 1947.
123. Brunnstrom S: Muscle group testing. *Physiotherapy Review* 21:3–21, 1941.
124. Barham JN, Wooten EP: *Structural Kinesiology*. New York, Macmillan, 1973, p 52.
125. Huxley HE: The mechanism of muscular contraction. *Scientific American* 213:18, 1965.
126. Morehouse LE, Cooper JM: *Kinesiology*. St. Louis, C.V. Mosby, 1950, pp 19–22, 28.
127. Williams JGP, Sperryn PN (eds): *Sports Medicine*, ed 2. Baltimore, Williams & Wilkins, 1976, p 292.
128. Hollingshead WH, Jenkins DB: *Functional Anatomy of the Limbs and Back*. Philadelphia, W.B. Saunders, 1981, pp 16–17.
129. Elftman H: Biomechanics of muscle. *Journal of Bone and Joint Surgery* 48A:363–377, 1966.
130. Granger CV: The clinical discernment of muscle weakness. *Archives of Physical Medicine* 44:430–438, 1963.
131. Gordon AM, Rosse C: Skeletal muscle. In Rosse C, Clawson DK: *The Musculoskeletal System in Health and Disease*. Hagerstown, Md, Harper & Row, 1980, p 48.
132. Gowitzke BA, Milner M: *Understanding the Scientific Basis of Human Movement*, ed 2. Baltimore, Williams & Wilkins, 1980, p 94.
133. Hunt CC (ed): *Handbook of Sensory Physiology*. New York, Springer-Verlag, 1974, vol III.
134. Morehouse LE, Miller AT Jr: *Physiology of Exercise*. St. Louis, C.V. Mosby, 1948, p 30.
135. Karvinen E, Koma PV: Neuromuscular performance. In Larson LA (ed): *Fitness, Health, and Work Capacity*. New York, Macmillan, 1974, pp 85–86.
136. Daniels L, Worthingham C: *Therapeutic Exercise*, ed 2. Philadelphia, W.B. Saunders, 1977, p 6.
137. Barham JN, Wooten EP: *Structural Kinesiology*. New York, Macmillan, 1973, pp 66–67.
138. Basmajian JV, Baeza N, Fabrigar C: Conscious control and training of individual spinal motor neurons in normal human subjects. *Journal of New Drugs* 5:78–85, 1965.
139. Elftman H: The action of muscles in the body. *Biological Symposium* 3:191–209, 1941.
140. Hoyle G: How is muscle turned on and off? *Scientific American* 222:84, 1970.
141. Ogden JA: The development and growth of the musculoskeletal system. In Albright JA, Brand RA (eds): *The Scientific Basis of Orthopaedics*. New York, Appleton-Century-Crofts, 1979, pp 50–51.
142. Taylor RG, Fowler WM Jr: Electrodiagnosis of musculoskeletal disorders. In D'Ambrosia RD: *Musculoskeletal Disorders: Regional Examination and Differential Diagnosis*. Philadelphia, J.B. Lippincott, 1977, pp 84–86.
143. Hollingshead WH, Jenkins DB: *Functional Anatomy of the Limbs and Back*. Philadelphia, W.B. Saunders, 1981, pp 44–45.
144. Pinkenburg C: A basis for the theory of manipulative medicine. *Journal of Manipulative and Physiological Therapeutics* 3(2):81–85, June 1980.
145. Barham JN, Wooten EP: *Structural Kinesiology*. New York, Macmillan, 1973, pp 65–66.
146. Rosse C: Muscle action and its control. In Rosse C, Clawson DK: *The Musculoskeletal System in Health and Disease*. Hagerstown, Md, Harper & Row, 1980, pp 57–58.
147. Gowitzke BA, Milner M: *Understanding the Scientific Basis of Human Movement*, ed 2. Baltimore, Williams & Wilkins, 1980, pp 106–109.
148. Hollingshead WH, Jenkins DB: *Functional Anatomy of the Limbs and Back*. Philadelphia, W.B. Saunders, 1981, pp 36–38, 42–43.
149. Williams JGP, Sperryn PN (eds): *Sports Medicine*, ed 2. Baltimore, Williams & Wilkins, 1976.
150. Brown MD: Role of activity in the differentiation of slow and fast muscles. *Nature* 244:178, 1973.
151. Morehouse LE, Cooper JM: *Kinesiology*. St. Louis, C.V. Mosby, 1950, pp 28–30.
152. Barham JN, Wooten EP: *Structural Kinesiology*. New York, Macmillan, 1973, p 62.

153. Fowler WM Jr, Taylor RG: Differential diagnosis of muscle diseases. In D'Ambrosia RD: *Musculoskeletal Disorders: Regional Examination and Differential Diagnosis*. Philadelphia, J.B. Lippincott, 1977, pp 93–94.
154. Cochran GVB: *A Primer of Orthopaedic Biomechanics*. New York, Churchill Livingstone, 1982, pp 230–231.
155. Barham JN, Wooten EP: *Structural Kinesiology*. New York, Macmillan, 1973, p 64.
156. Hollingshead WH, Jenkins DB: *Functional Anatomy of the Limbs and Back*. Philadelphia, W.B. Saunders, 1981, pp 31–32.
157. Gowitzke BA, Milner M: *Understanding the Scientific Basis of Human Movement*, ed 2. Baltimore, Williams & Wilkins, 1980, p 110.
158. Morehouse LE, Cooper JM: *Kinesiology*. St. Louis, C.V. Mosby, 1950, p 30.
159. Turek SL: *Orthopaedics: Principles and Their Application*, ed 3. Philadelphia, J.B. Lippincott, 1977, pp 609–618.
160. Sills FD: Anthropometry in relation to physical performance. In Johnson WR: *Science and Medicine of Exercise and Sports*. New York, Harper & Brothers, 1960.
161. Keith A: Man's posture: Its evolution and disorders. Hunterian Lectures. *Clinical Orthopaedics* 62:5–14, 1969.
162. Walters GC, Hoth M: Aid for recording gross evaluation. *Physical Therapy* 44:179, 1964.
163. Barham JN, Wooten EP: *Structural Kinesiology*. New York, Macmillan, 1973, pp 132–134.
164. Barham JN, Wooten EP: *Structural Kinesiology*. New York, Macmillan, 1973, pp 130–132.
165. Dempster WT: The anthropometry of body action. *Annals of the New York Academy of Science* 63:559–585, 1955.
166. Basmajian JV (ed): *Grant's Method of Anatomy*, ed 9. Baltimore, Williams & Wilkins, 1975, pp 201–204.
167. Breitmann MJ: Endocrine anthropometry. In Piersol GM, Bortz EL (eds): *The Cyclopedia of Medicine, Surgery and Specialties*, Philadelphia, F.A. Davis, 1949, vol 5, pp 563–573.
168. Pende N: Biotypology. In Piersol GM, Bortz EL (eds): *The Cyclopedia of Medicine, Surgery and Specialties*, Philadelphia, F.A. Davis, 1949, vol 5, pp 592–600.
169. Sheldon WH: *Atlas of Man*. New York, Harper & Brothers, 1954.
170. Sheldon WH et al: *The Varieties of Human Physique*, ed 4. New York, Harper & Brothers, 1940.
171. American Chiropractic Association: *Chiropractic State of the Art*. Arlington, Va, American Chiropractic Association, 1983, pp 29–32.
172. Bergemann B, Cichote A: Cost-effectiveness of medical vs chiropractic treatment of low-back injuries. *Journal of Manipulative and Physiological Therapeutics* 3:143–147, 1980.
173. Cleary PD: Chiropractic use: A test of several hypotheses. *American Journal of Public Health* 72:727–729, 1982.
174. Sharpiro E: The physician visit pattern of chiropractic users: Health-seeking behavior of the elderly in Manitoba, Canada. *American Journal of Public Health* 73:553–557, 1983.
175. Fisk JR, DiMonte P, McKay CS: Back schools: Past, present, and future. *Clinical Orthopaedics and Related Research* 179:18–23, 1983.
176. Lankhorst GJ et al: The effect of the Swedish back school in chronic idiopathic low back pain. *Scandinavian Journal of Rehabilitation Medicine* 15:141–145, 1983.
177. Walker HK: Introduction to the history. In Walker HK, Hall WD, Hurst JW (eds): *Clinical Methods*, Woburn, Mass, Butterworth, 1976, vol 1, p 19.
178. Wolliscroft JO et al: Evaluating the medical history: Observation versus write up review. *Journal of Medical Education* 59:19–23, 1984.
179. Rozeiu AM: Clinical decisions: A normative approach. *Journal of the Canadian Chiropractic Association* 26:102–106, 1982.
180. Heck RS, Brueschke EE: The yearly physical examination. *Female Patient* 4:75–80, 1979.
181. Harrell FE et al: Evaluating the yield of medical tests. *Journal of the American Medical Association* 247:2543–2546, 1982.
182. Schafer RC: *Chiropractic Health Care*, ed 3. Des Moines, The Foundation for Chiropractic Education and Research, 1979, pp 41–44, 46–47.
183. Kimberly PE: Formulating a prescription for osteopathic manipulative treatment. *Journal of the American Osteopathic Association* 79:506–513, 1980.
184. Jamison JR: Optimal health care: An Australian version. *Journal of the Australian Chiropractors' Association* 13:11–14, 1983.
185. Deausinger RH: Biomechanics in clinical practice. *Physical Therapy* 64:1860–1868, 1984.
186. Miller GF: Clinical evaluation and treatment of common musculoskeletal disorders. *ACA Journal of Chiropractic* April 1963.
187. Grieve GP: *Common Vertebral Joint Problems*. New York, Churchill Livingstone, 1981, p 39.

SUGGESTED READINGS

Barham JN, Thomas WL: *Anatomical Kinesiology*. New York, Macmillan, 1969.

Barnett CH et al: *Synovial Joints: Their Structure and Mechanics*. Springfield, Ill, Charles C Thomas, 1961.

Basmajian JV: *Muscles Alive: Their Function Revealed by Electromyography*, ed 2. Baltimore, Williams & Wilkins, 1967.

Bolis L et al (eds): *Comparative Physiology*. New York, American Elsevier, 1973.

Bourne GH (ed): *The Structure and Function of Muscle*. New York, Academic Press, 1973.

Cheraskin E: The musculoskeletal disease proneness profile. *ACA Journal of Chiropractic* May 1977.

Cooper JM, Glassow RB: *Kinesiology*, ed 3. St. Louis, C.V. Mosby 1972.

Ishiko T: The organism and muscular work. In Larson LA (ed): *Fitness, Health, and Work Capacity*. New York, Macmillan, 1974, chapter 3.

Jensen CR, Schultz GW: *Applied Kinesiology*. New York, McGraw-Hill, 1970.

Kelsey JL et al: The impact of musculoskeletal disorders on the population of the United States. *Journal of Bone and Joint Surgery* 61A:959–964, 1979.

Lindahl O: Methods for evaluating the therapeutic

effect of nonmedical treatment. *Scandinavian Journal of Rehabilitation Medicine* 11:151–155, 1979.

Lockhart RD et al: *Anatomy of the Human Body*. Philadelphia, J.B. Lippincott, 1965.

Logan AL, McKinney WC: *Kinesiology*. Dubuque, W.C. Brown, 1970.

Rash PJ, Burke RK: *Kinesiology and Applied Anatomy*. Philadelphia, Lea & Febiger, 1967.

Romanes GJ: *Cunningham's Textbook of Anatomy*, ed 10. New York, Oxford University Press, 1964.

Steingisser AR: Chiropractic orthopedics in general practice. *New England Journal of Chiropractic* Winter 1979.

Thompson CW: *Manual of Structural Kinesiology*, ed 6. St. Louis, C.V. Mosby, 1969.

Wells KF: *Kinesiology*, ed 5. Philadelphia, W.B. Saunders, 1971.

CHAPTER 2

Mechanical Concepts and Terms

All motor activities such as walking, running, jumping, pushing, pulling, lifting, and throwing are examples of dynamic musculoskeletal mechanics. To better appreciate the sometimes simple and often complex factors involved, this chapter reviews the basic concepts and terms involved in maintaining static equilibrium. Static equilibrium is the starting point for all dynamic activities.

ENERGY AND MASS[1-3]

Biomechanics is constantly concerned with a quantity of matter (whatever occupies space, a mass) to which a force has been applied. Such a mass is often the body as a whole, a part of the body such as a limb or segment, or an object such as a load to be lifted or an exercise weight. By the same token, the word "body" refers to any mass, ie, the human body, a body part, or any object.

Energy[4,5]

Energy is the power to work or to act. Body energy is that force which enables it to overcome resistance to motion, to produce a physical effect, and to accomplish work. The body's kinetic energy, the energy level of the body due to its motion, is reflected solely in its velocity, and its potential energy is reflected solely in its position. Mathematically, kinetic energy is half the mass times the square of the velocity, $m/2 \times V^2$. In a closed system where there are no external forces being applied, the law of conservation of mechanical energy states that the sum of kinetic energy and potential energy is equal to a constant for that system.

Potential energy (PE), measured in newton meters or joules, is also stored in the body as a result of tissue displacement or deformation, like a wound spring or a stretched bowstring or tendon. It is expressed mathematically in the equation PE = mass × gravitational acceleration × height of the mass relative to a chosen reference level (eg, the earth's surface). Thus, a 100-lb upper body balanced on L5 of a 6-ft person has a potential energy of about 300 ft-lb relative to the ground.

The Center of Mass[6,7]

The exact center of an object's mass is sometimes referred to as the object's center of gravity. When an object's mass is evenly distributed throughout, the center of mass is located at the object's geometric center. In the human body, however, this is infrequently true, and the center of mass is located toward the heavier, often larger, aspect. When considering the body as a whole, the center of mass in the anatomic position, for instance, is constantly shifted during activity when weight is shifted from one area to another during locomotion or when weight is added to or subtracted from the body.[8-10]

The term *weight* is not synonymous with the word *mass*. Body weight refers to the pull of gravity on body mass. Mass is the quotient obtained by dividing the weight of a body by the acceleration due to gravity (32 ft/sec^2). Each of these terms has a different unit of measurement. Weight is measured in pounds or kilograms, while mass is measured by a body's weight divided by the gravitational constant. The potential energy of gravity can be simply visualized as an invisible spring attached between the body's center of mass and the center of the earth. The pull is always straight downward so that more work is required to move the body upward than horizontally (Fig. 2.1).[11,12]

NEWTON'S LAWS OF MECHANICS[13-16]

Sir Isaac Newton's three laws of mechanics apply in any movement or injury and serve as the basis for the science of mechanical engineering. They are applied through-

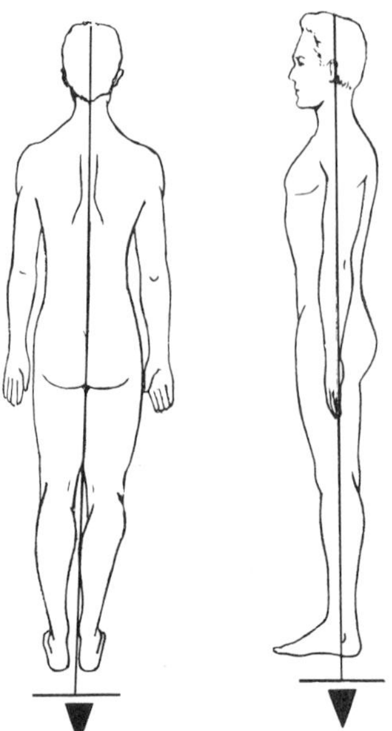

Figure 2.1. The median (*left*) and frontal (*right*) planes of the body.

out the study of biomechanics and deserve definition and explanation.

The Law of Inertia[17,18]

Newton's First Law

A body remains at rest or in a state of uniform motion in a straight line until acted upon by an unbalanced or outside force. When a body is at rest, the forces acting upon it are completely balanced. When the body or a part is in motion, it will continue to move until some force causes it to stop. All objects express inertia in that they resist change whether at rest or in motion. The force necessary to overcome the inertia of a body depends upon the weight of the body and the rate at which it is moving. It is for this reason that more effort is required to put a shot than throw a baseball the same distance.[19]

An object does not move unless a force has been applied that is greater than the object's inertia. A body at rest may have many forces acting upon it; and if their magnitudes and directions completely cancel one another, there is zero *net* force and a state of static equilibrium. If these forces are unbalanced and result in a net force other than zero, movement (dynamics) occurs.

The Law of Acceleration

Newton's Second Law (Proportionality)

The acceleration of an object is proportional to the unbalanced forces acting upon it and inversely proportional to the object's mass.[18] In other words, the net force acting on a body gives it an acceleration that is proportional to the force in both direction and magnitude and inversely proportional to the mass of the body.

Acceleration Measurement

A forceful push moves a small object rapidly; a light push on a large object moves it slowly. Acceleration is a quantity that refers to the rate of change of linear velocity, which may be a change in direction or magnitude. It is measured by its magnitude in feet or meters per second per second. Mathematically, acceleration = force/mass, or final velocity minus original velocity divided by time.[20]

The Law of Reaction

Newton's Third Law (Interaction)

For every action there is an equal and opposite reciprocal reaction. Inertia is manifest as a reaction equal and opposite to the action that created the acceleration. Thus, forces are always in pairs that are equal in magnitude but opposite in direction. It is arbitrary which force is called the *action* and which the *reaction*, but usually in biomechanics we refer to internal body forces as actions and external forces applied to the body as reactions (eg, weights, floor reactions).

Examples of Reaction

Regardless of what degree of force is induced upon a part, there is always a counteracting stress because for every action there must be a reaction. For instance, a downward pressure equals an opposing upward thrust (eg, as that of a rocket). When an individual pushes against or lifts up any object, the object pushes against the person or pulls down with equal force in a line directly opposite to that of the individual's force. A force pulling right is equal to a pull toward the left, expressed in terms of centripetal and centrifugal force. A spiraling force in one direction must be accompanied by an equal twisting force in the opposite direction. A force permitting a part to slide downward must be resisted by an adequate upward force. And a force tending to bend a structure along its axis must be resisted by a force equal to prevent such bending.

FORCE[21-26]

Force, simply, is any push or pull produced by one object acting upon another. It is anything that tends to cause or change the yield movement acceleration of an object. For example, when an object at rest is pushed (or pulled), it moves in the direction of the push at a speed relative to the strength and time of the pushing force. Linear movement without turning is called *translation*, and it is the result of the force passing through the center of mass. Some degree of *rotation* will accompany translation if the line of push or pull does not pass through the center of mass. The further the line of force is from the center of mass, the greater is the rotational component.

Force is measured in gravitational units, pounds or kilograms. It has two components: strength (magnitude of force) and direction.

Moments[27-29]

The term *moment* in mechanics refers to the tendency, or measure of tendency, to produce motion, especially about a point or axis. The *moment of inertia* is greatest in all axes of the body that go through the center of gravity of the body, and it is less through axes that pass outside this center of gravity. Thus, it is easier to topple an upright object by striking it high or low than in the midsection.

It is easier to spin a person around by striking his outstretched arm than by striking his shoulder. When a force produces rotation, the measure of this rotational effect is called a moment of force or torque. The *rotation moment* of such a force can be computed by the force applied times the perpendicular distance from the center of rotation.

Types of Force[30,31]

Load and Stress

Forces and moment (torque) external to a particular structure such as gravity, another muscle contraction, inertia, wind, water resistance, and surface reaction are referred to as *loads*. The applied weight used in traction or an adjustment and the resistance offered to an exercise are external mechanical loads. Interior resistance forces such as tendon tensile strength and muscle stretch which react to a load are referred to as biomechanical *stress*.

Newtons

Loads are often measured by *newtons*, the universal measure of force based on Newton's second law of motion. A newton is the quantity of force necessary to give a 1-kg mass an acceleration of 1 meter per second per second: 1 newton = 0.2248 pound force; 1 pound force = 4.48 newtons. Note that, unlike pounds and kilograms, a newton's definition does not depend on the earth's gravitational field.

Substance Mechanical Properties

The mechanical properties of a substance determine how it will react to load and stress. If a substance's mechanical properties are identical in all directions, such as a metal, it is *isotropic*. A sample portion of an isotropic material shows the same characteristics of strength and elasticity as any other sample portion. As every human tissue is specialized to resist customary loads, the human body contains no isotropic structures.[32]

All body tissue is *anisotropic*; ie, its mechanical properties differ with varying area orientations. As an example, a bone will vary in its strength and elasticity to a load depending upon whether the load is applied transversely, axially, at an angle, or with a twist.[33]

External Loads

The resistance offered to the forces of musculoskeletal structures and joints is commonly derived from gravitational pull, the resistance of a fixed structure, manual resistance, environmental factors (eg, swimming in water, running against wind), elasticity, and friction factors. Gravity is the most common external force to which the body is subjected, and it always offers a force directed in a straight line downward. In determining the effect of gravity, the weight and position of resistance must be considered (Fig. 2.2).[34,35]

Sample Clinical Applications

Such factors have common applications in therapeutics. When the resistance of gravity is not desired (eg, in weakness), the resistance of the body can be reduced by immersion in water where the body is buoyed up by a force equal to the weight of the water displaced to balance the gravitational force on the body. Canes and crutches also help to reduce gravitational forces on a weak or tender body part.

When resistance is desired, stationary or resistant structures and manual loads are utilized in developing isometric muscle contraction. In therapeutic exercise, for instance, friction devices to offer load resistance against muscle contraction are popular. A variety of elastic materials are used, such as springs and tubes, in which the line of resistance lies along the length of the elastic material.[36]

Stress on Weight-Bearing Joints

The pull of supporting muscles frequently increases joint pressure in weight-bearing joints.[37] For example, if a 200-lb person leans so that his weight is supported on one limb, the hip joint is subjected to all the person's weight above the hip, plus the weight of the other limb, and it also withstands the pull of the muscles necessary to maintain equilibrium. As one lower limb is typically 15% of total body weight, this would mean the support of 170 lb of body weight plus 425 lb of balance force for a total force on the hip of almost 600 lb. This happens during quiet standing; running or holding a weight would greatly add to the stress.[38,39]

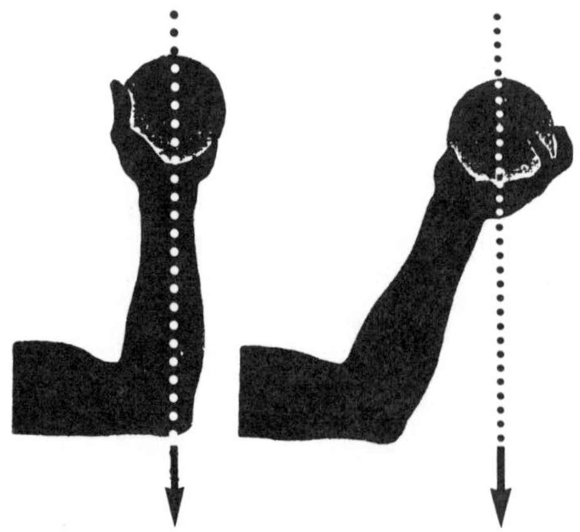

Figure 2.2. Balancing a weight with the forearm in a vertical position takes little effort. When the arm is not vertical, the same weight exerts a downward pull, causing strain on muscles and tendons throughout the upper extremity, shoulder girdle, and spine.

Spinal Load Considerations

Typical spinal loads offer another example of the effects of external forces on the musculoskeletal system. When the spine is loaded in lifting a weight, the lumbosacral area is subjected to weight forces from both the upper body plus the weight being lifted. It is also being subjected to the bending torque caused by these forces because they are some distance from L5's center of mass. The load on the lumbosacral disc is the sum of the weight of the upper body, the weight held, the spinal muscle forces, and their lever arms respective to the disc.[40]

The importance of spinal cord loads is underscored in such activities as lifting, bowling, rowing, and even in lordotic joggers. It has been estimated that when an object is held 14 inches away from the spine, the load on the lumbosacral disc is 15 times the weight lifted. Thus, a mother lifting a 20-lb child at arm's length theoretically places a 300-lb load on her lumbosacral disc.

Another example is a dead lift of 200 lb by a 170-lb person, for which it has been shown that a 2000-lb force is exerted on the lumbosacral disc (Fig. 2.3). This load, of course, must be dissipated, otherwise the L5 vertebra would be crushed. The load is dissipated through the paraspinal muscles and, importantly, by the abdominal cavity, which acts as a hydraulic chamber to absorb and thus diminish the load applied.

These observations on spine loading emphasize the vulnerability of the spine to the mechanical stresses placed upon it, especially in people with poor muscle tone. Bony compression of the emerging nerve roots arises as a result of subarticular entrapment,

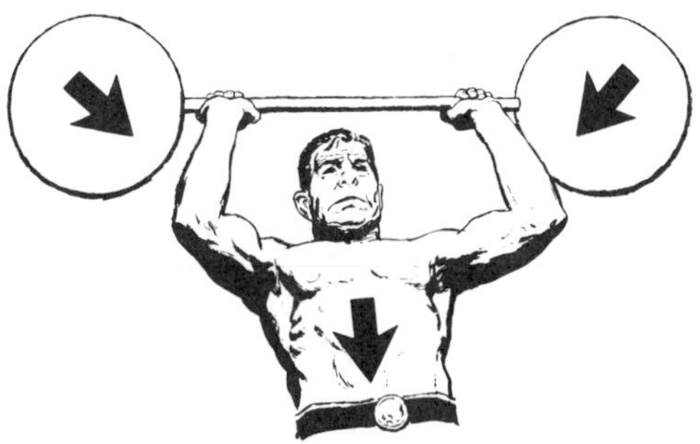

Figure 2.3. During lifting, the load vector at L5, for example, is equivalent to all the forces acting upon it, including upper body weight, the lifted load, and the bending moment caused by those forces that are distal to the center of L5.

pedicular kinking, or foraminal impingement due to posterior vertebral subluxation.

Stress on Non-Weight-Bearing Joints

Even joints that do not bear weight can be subjected to tremendous pressure. For example, when the extended forearm is flexed, the flexors exert a line of pull that is almost parallel to the ulnar and radius. Thus, much of the muscular force is exerted at the elbow joint which compresses the articular surfaces. Because of the lack of complete articular reciprocity, this pressure is concentrated onto an area far less than that of the whole apposed articular faces. If the hand holds a weight during this flexion, the contraction must be of greater force, which in turn causes greater pressure.

Other Factors

The total stress on the body during lifting is not completely determined by mechanical factors, however. It has been found that the combined effect of biomechanical and physiologic stresses leads to an overall measure of lifting-task acceptability as expressed by the psychophysical stress involved. One study has found that there are conditions for which the acceptability measures of the combined biomechanical and physiologic stresses and the psychophysical stress involved are close to one another.[41]

The Characteristics of Force[42]

The four features of a force are its magnitude, action line, direction, and point of application. A force cannot be described unless these factors are known because any variation of one or more of these factors changes the result.

Magnitude and Action Line

Magnitude is a scalar quantity such as time, speed, temperature, volume, and length that has no direction. More factors must be known besides magnitude if a force involving a stress is to be accurately described. For example, a 5-lb weight held in a hand when the arm is held vertically produces a far different effect in the shoulder joint than the same weight held in the hand when the arm is held horizontally. Thus, the action line (line of force application) must be known.

Direction and Point of Application

Since a pulling force has a different effect than a pushing force, it is important to know the direction of force along the action line. In addition, the site where the force is applied must be known to complete the picture.

Biomechanical Descriptions

Many basic considerations in biomechanics involve time, mass, center of mass, movement, force, and gravity—all of which operate in accordance with the laws of physics. However, while numerous parameters of movement are interrelated, no one factor is capable of completely describing movement by itself. For example, acceleration and velocity involve displacement and time, but they are insufficient unless force and movement are considered.

Vectors[43–45]

Although force is usually applied over an area, it is usually described in biomechanical drawings as a summarized point force by an arrow. Any quantity that gives both magnitude and direction is a *vector* (eg, a force) that can be described by a straight line. Quantities that involve only magnitude are referred to as *scalars*. When illustrating a force, the vector's length should be proportional to the magnitude of the force. For example, if 1 inch is used to represent a 10-lb force, a 2-inch line would represent a 20-lb force.

A vector can be used to define a force in a simple line drawing if the vector drawn to scale represents magnitude by the line's *length*, if the vector's *tail* indicates the point where the force is applied on the object, and if the direction of force is indicated by the vector's *arrowhead*. If the magnitude of a vector is known, it should be indicated (eg, 1 inch = 20 lb). If the magnitude is not known, it is indicated by the capital letter *F* (force) or *P* (pressure) to designate the unknown magnitude. Distances are usually represented by lower case letters.

The force of gravity is always directed toward the center of the earth. Thus, gravity's line of action and direction are constants. In the upright "rigid" body, the gravitational force on the entire mass can be thought of as a single vector through the center of mass which represents the sum of many parallel positive and negative coordinates (Fig. 2.4).[46] If a weight is held in the outstretched hand, the quantity of gravitational force is governed by the weight of the extremity plus the weight held.

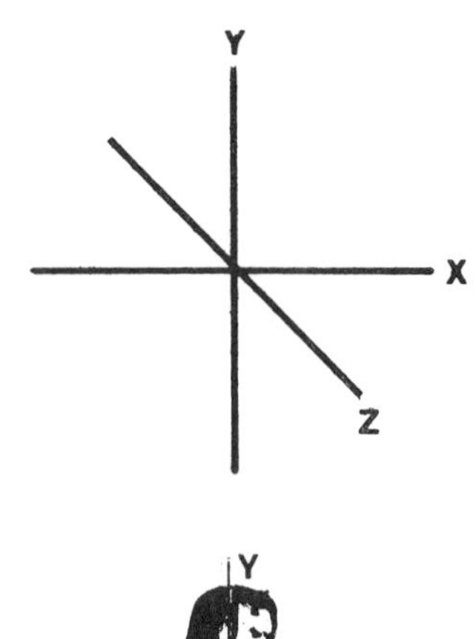

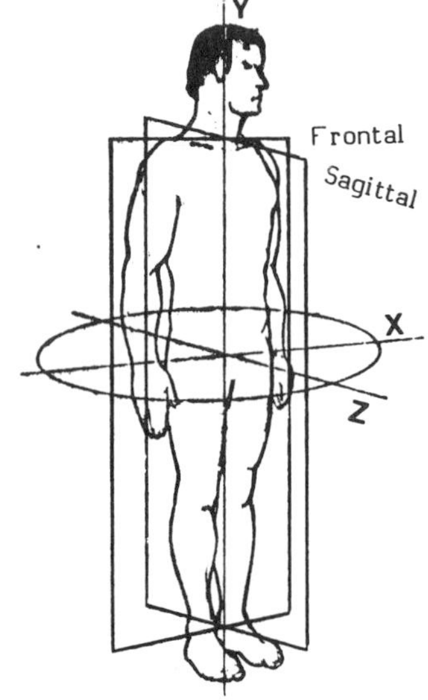

Figure 2.4. The *X*, *Y*, and *Z* planes of the body.

Space

As a force may act along a single line in a single plane or in any direction in space, this must be considered to provide an illustrative reference system. In a two-dimensional system, the plane is simply divided into four quadrants by means of a perpendicular vertical ordinate line (*Y* axis) and a horizontal abscissa line (*X* axis). The point of axial intersection is referred to as the system's origin (Fig. 2.5). Abscissa (X) measurements to the right of the origin are considered positive, while those to the left are negative.[47] Ordinate (*Y*) measurements above the origin are considered positive, while those below the origin are negative. By this method, any point on the plane can be given an *X* and *Y* value.

The term *coordinate* refers to a specific point location from the origin which has been given a value. For example, a point located 5 units to the right of the origin and 3 units down from the origin would be defined as $X = 5$, $Y = -3$.

A third axis (usually titled Z) can be introduced to locate points in three dimensions. Such an axis crosses the origin and is perpendicular to the other two planes (X and *Y*). All Z points in front of the *X-Y* plane are positive, while those behind are negative (Fig. 2.6). By utilizing *X*, *Y*, and Z coordinates, any point in space can be located and depicted. However, a minimum of six coordinates is necessary to specify the position of a rigid body. Force and moment are three-dimensional vectors having three components each; thus load may be considered a six-component vector.

In biomechanics, the body's origin is located at the body's center of mass which is usually anterior to the S2 segment. When this point is known, gross body space can be visualized as being in the sagittal (right-left) *Y-Z* plane, frontal and coronal (anterior-posterior) *X-Y* plane, or horizontal or transverse (superior-inferior) *X-Y* plane. With such a reference system, any movement of any body segment in these planes

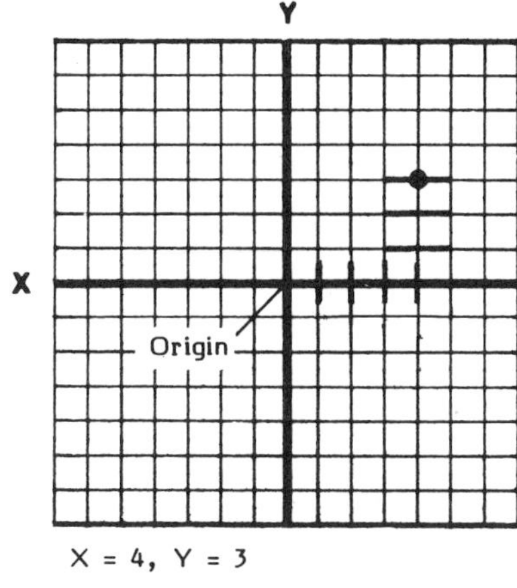

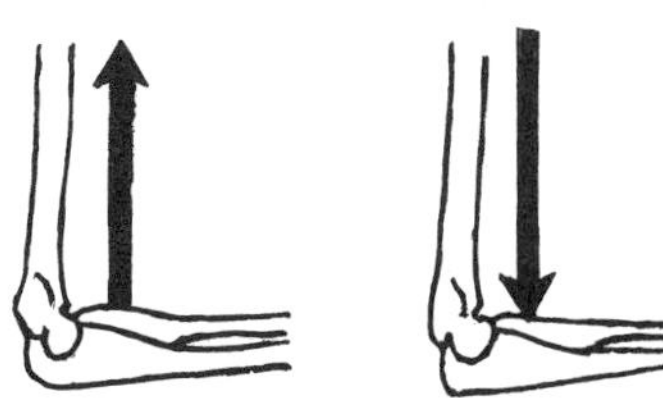

Figure 2.5. *Top*, plotting points relative to *X* and *Y* axes. *Bottom*, vectors should be identified by a label indicating force magnitude.

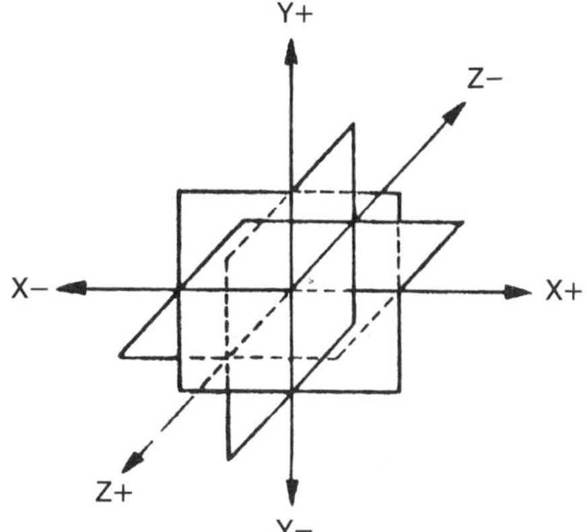

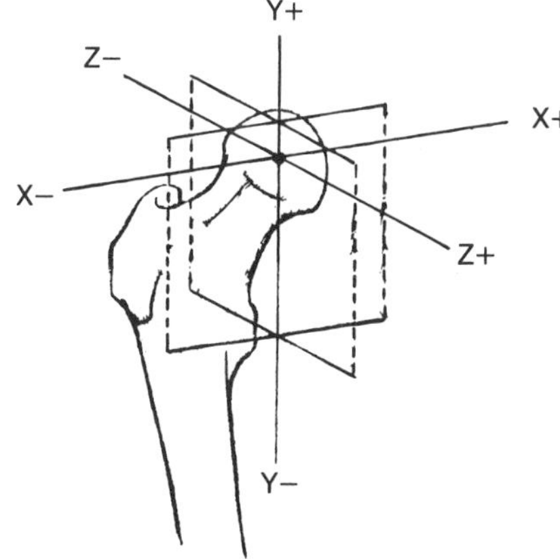

Figure 2.6. *Top*, positive and negative *X*, *Y*, and *Z* axes. *Bottom*, system of coordinates pertinent to the hip joint's mechanical axis.

can be approximately described by placing a coordinate system at the axis of a joint and projecting the action lines of the muscles involved.

STATIC EQUILIBRIUM[48-52]

Statics

According to Newton's first law, a body remains at rest in static equilibrium when its velocity is zero or remains in a state of motion (dynamic equilibrum) when its velocity is other than zero. The study of bodies at rest, as the result of forces acting upon them simultaneously balancing each other so that the resultant velocity is zero, is referred to as *statics*. This balanced state is one of translational equilibrium. That is, during motion, if a body moves in a direction in which a straight line in the body always remains parallel to itself, the motion is called *translation*. It is a vector quantity measured in feet or meters.

Major Principles of Statics

Two conditions of equilibrium summarize the principles of statics: (1) For an object to be in linear equilibrium, the total of all *X* components must equal zero and the sum of all *Y* components must equal zero. (2) For an object to be in rotatory equilibrium, the total of all torque forces that tend to produce a rotation in one direction (eg, clockwise) must be counterbalanced by the total of torque forces that tend to produce a rotation in the opposite direction (eg, counterclockwise).

Free-Body Analysis

Clinically, free-body analysis of statics is used whenever traction force is applied; eg, during a manual adjustment of the spine or extremities, or in the use of therapeutic equipment. Other applications are found, for instance, in determining stresses at particular points during activity positions (Fig. 2.7). Free-body analysis is a mathematical

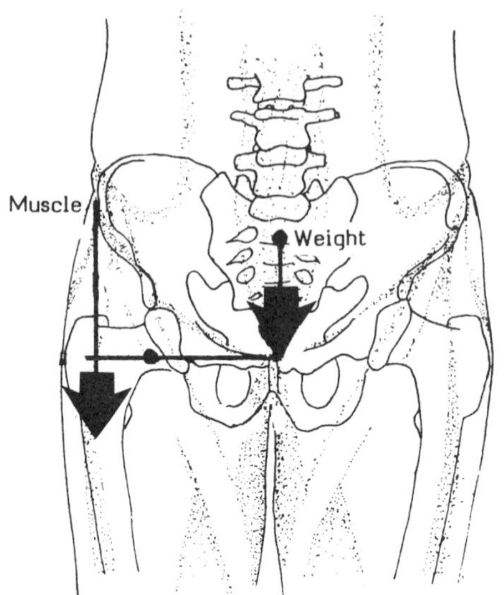

Figure 2.7. Diagram of the static forces acting about the axis of the femoral head during unilateral stance or the weight-bearing phase of locomotion.

technique of utilizing equilibrium equations to determine the internal stresses at a structural point that is being subjected to external load. Such equations can be used to calculate the magnitude of force and moments acting on a vertebral area, for example, at a known position and load.[53–55]

Equilibrium

While forces of all types may cause subluxations, dislocations, fractures, strains and sprains, etc, the biomechanical mechanisms involved determine the type and extent of the injury produced, depending upon the applications of force and its resistance.[56] For example, different applications of force may cause bending, stress, or compression fractures. When the examiner understands how an injury was caused, the tissues involved are more readily located and the extent of injury is more quickly ascertained.

LINEAR FORCES[46, 57–59]

Linear forces are those acting in the same straight line (Fig. 2.8). If two forces are to be in equilibrium in a linear system, the forces must be equal in magnitude and exactly opposite in direction.

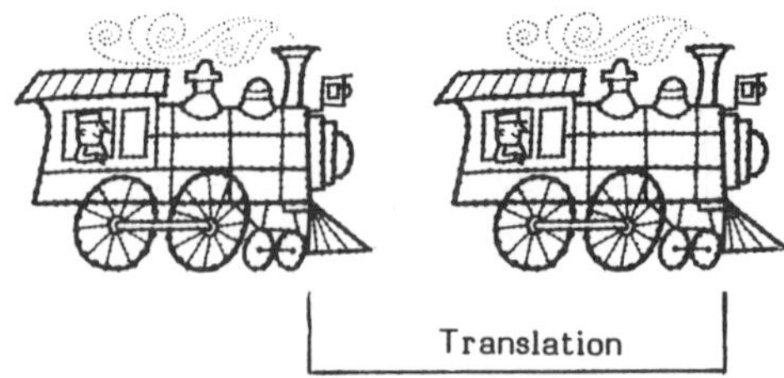

Figure 2.8. Linear force, translation.

Pressure

Pressure refers to how a force is distributed over a surface. Pressure (P) can be defined as the action of a force (F) against some opposing force distributed over an area (A) as in the equation $P = F/A$, which gives the units of force per unit area such as in pounds per square inch (psi).[60]

Pressure during Manipulation

This principle of force is used throughout therapy. In manual adjustment procedures, for example, a patient can withstand a broad palm contact with considerable force without discomfort, yet the same force exerted by a thumbtip or pisiform contact becomes quite painful because the pressure per unit of surface area is now much greater. Thus, whenever pain or skin damage is the priority consideration, the contact forces should be applied over as large an area as possible.

Pressure of Supports

The same principle must be applied in taping procedures to avoid circulatory and neural impairment, in applying traction slings to distribute force, and in fitting supports if pressure sores are to be avoided. The noxious effects of continuous pressure can be reduced by using somewhat elastic materials such as felt or foam rubber padding as an underlay beneath supports to spread force from prominent bony areas. In large-area supports such as for scoliosis, an underlying water-inflated football bladder has shown to offer automatic pressure distribution and good reciprocity to surface shape. The modern use of air splints during transportation of extremity fractures is another example of this principle applied in health care.

Compression

A pressure always results in a compression stress. Tensile and compression stresses (axial stresses) operate along the axis of a part without altering it. Both of these stresses are measured in newtons.[61] A compression force within the body tends to push substances closer together. When a muscle crossing a joint contracts, it produces a compression force into the joint, and the bones must produce a reactive force to withstand the compression force. Within the spine, the vertebrae and the intervertebral discs are the major compression-carrying components which must support the weight of the body above a particular disc, the initial tension in other ligaments, the additional tension in the muscles and ligaments that are necessary to balance eccentric trunk weight, plus any added external load.

Tension

A pull causes a tensile stress that is an action directly opposed to compresson. When tension is applied to connective tissue fibers, the fibers elongate to their physiologic limit, somewhat like a stretched rubber band, unless a cut or weakness produces a fracture. During torsion (shear) stress, fibers at 45° to the long axis are placed in tension. When a long structure is subjected to bending stress, tension is exhibited in the fibers on the convex side of the curvature.[62]

Motion Tension[63–65]

Examples of tension are exhibited during all spinal movements. Anulus fibers of the intervertebral discs are placed in tension during disc torsion when the spine is rotated axially, and ligaments posterior to the instantaneous axis of rotation are tensed during spinal flexion. A spinal curvature in any direction involves a constant state of abnormal tension and compression of bones, cartilages, and muscles.

During work, muscles do not maintain a constant tension or length, or move with a constant rate of shortening. The strength of muscle action is affected markedly by the amount of tension in the muscle at the start of movement, the degree of muscle stretch at the beginning of contraction, and the rate at which shortening takes place.

Poisson's Ratio

Similar to a piece of rubber, elastic connective tissue fibers thin during stretch and thicken during compression. In both cases, however, the volume remains constant. The ratio between axial strain in length from compression to transverse strain in diameter from tension is Poisson's ratio.[66]

CONCURRENT FORCES[67,68]

In a concurrent force system, as contrasted to a linear system, the forces acting on the body meet at a certain point rather than lie along the same line of action. These forces may be applied to the body from different angles so that their action lines cross either interior or exterior to the body (Fig. 2.9). For example, if two coplanar nonparallel muscles are acting on a bone, a third concurrent force, passing through the point of intersection of the two original muscle forces, must act to maintain equilibrium and avoid rotation.

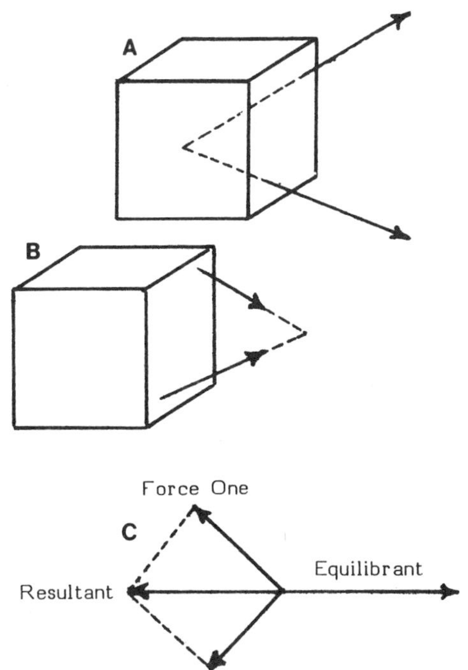

Figure 2.9. Concurrent forces intersecting *A*, within a body or *B*, outside a body. *C*, the resultant and equilibrant of two concurrent forces.

PARALLEL FORCES[69–72]

When parallel forces some distance from each other act upon a body, these forces must be completely nullified by each other if the body is to maintain equilibrium. If forces do not coincide at the same point, such as in a concurrent system, the result is rotation around a stationary axis. A simple form of this action is a force system in which the forces lying in the same plane are parallel. Any force acting on an object at a distance from a fixed point tends to rotate the object. Forces producing clockwise rotation are arbitrarily referred to as positive, while counterclockwise forces are termed negative.

The distance from the point of force application (pivot point) to the point of rotation is called the *moment arm* or lever arm. When a force acts at a distance from a pivot point, its effectiveness is determined by both its magnitude and its location.[73]

The tendency of a force to cause rotation about an axis that is equal to the magnitude of the force times the perpendicular distance from the action line of the force to that point is referred to as a *moment* (torque) of force. Mathematically, it is expressed as moment = force × distance, and its unit of measure is foot-pounds (ft-lb), kilogram-centimeters (kg-cm), or an equivalent measure.

Lever Actions[74–76]

A lever system is a good example of moments developed by coplanar forces. Simply, a lever is a rigid bar turning about an axis. The three components of a lever are the *fulcrum* upon which the lever turns, the *resistance* or weight load that is to be moved, and the *effort* that moves the lever.

The articulating surfaces of joints are usually used as fulcrums, the rigid bone shafts extending from axis to axis serve as lever arms, and the source of effort to move the lever arms is the muscles. That is, in the body, we have an effort force and a resisting force acting around a pivot axis (fulcrum) which serves as a supporting force (Fig. 2.10). When a muscle contracts, the bony lever arm to which it is fixed is pivoted about the fulcrum. Work is done when resistance is overcome by a lever system. Here again is an example that the resistance to be overcome by the body is generally the sum of the load of the lever segment plus the load of the object to be moved.[77,78]

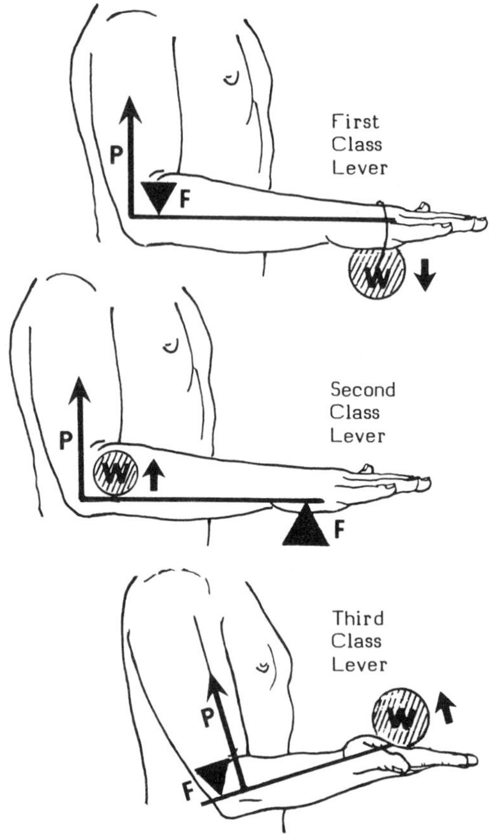

Figure 2.10. Mechanical arrangement of bones as levers and muscles as sources of power; *P*, power; *W*, weight; *F*, fulcrum; *arrow*, direction of movement. *Top*, the arm is used as a first-class lever in pressing weight downward, with the triceps serving as the power source. *Center*, the arm is used as a second-class lever in elevating the body as in doing push-ups, with the triceps serving as the source of negative power. *Bottom*, the arm is used as a third-class lever in lifting a weight vertically, with the biceps serving as the source of power.

Mechanical Advantage

The force developed when a muscle contracts is determined by the *mechanical advantage* of the levers employed. The position of the attachment of the muscle in relation to the position of the center of the resistance and the position of the fulcrum are important in deciding the mechanical advantage of any lever. Mechanical advantage is the ratio of output force delivered to the input force applied by a mover. If the resistance is placed near the fulcrum, the mechanical advantage is good. If the same resistance is placed further from the fulcrum, the mechanical advantage lessens and a greater effort is required to overcome the resistance.

Mechanical advantage is computed by dividing force into resistance: R/F. If a 150-lb individual wishes to lift a 1200-lb weight by means of a lever, the mechanical advantage required of the lever would be $R/F = 1200/150 = 8$. Thus, the force arm must be eight times as long as the resistance arm of the lever.

Types of Levers[79]

At one time or another, every bone in the body, acting alone or in combination, acts as a lever, and the human machine offers many examples of first- and third-class levers. Most of the joints of the body can be used as levers of more than one class.

First-Class Levers. An example of a first-class lever in which the fulcrum is located between the applied load and the resisting weight is seen in tapping the toes on the floor and in the action of the triceps on the ulnar when the arm is held over the head. Other examples are found (1) when the spleni act to extend the skull across the atlanto-occipital joints (Fig. 2.11) and (2) when the soleus tendon force behind and the gravity force in front of the ankle fulcrum are utilized in standing erect. In a first-class lever system, the longer the lever arm, the less is the force required to move or resist the applied load.

Second-Class Levers. A second-class lever has the resistance weight located between the applied force and the fulcrum. Since most of the muscles moving each joint are inserted near the joint and the resistance is usually at the long end of the body levers, levers of the first and third classes are the most commonly used in the body. There are no positive second-class levers in the body because the length of the resistance arm of the movement is always greater than that of the effort arm when movement is produced by muscle shortening. Some kinesiologists refer only superficially to the action of the brachioradialis on the forearm during elbow flexion and the action of the calf plantar flexors when one stands on the toes as second-class lever actions. A true second-class lever system can be demonstrated, however, when muscle tension becomes a resistance to a reversal of joint action caused by an outside force so that a third-class lever system is reversed and becomes a second-class lever system. In such cases, the eccentric muscular contraction is performing negative rather than positive work. An example of this is seen when one stands on tiptoes with the fulcrum located on the ball of the foot, and force is applied through the gastrocnemius at the ankle to lift body weight.

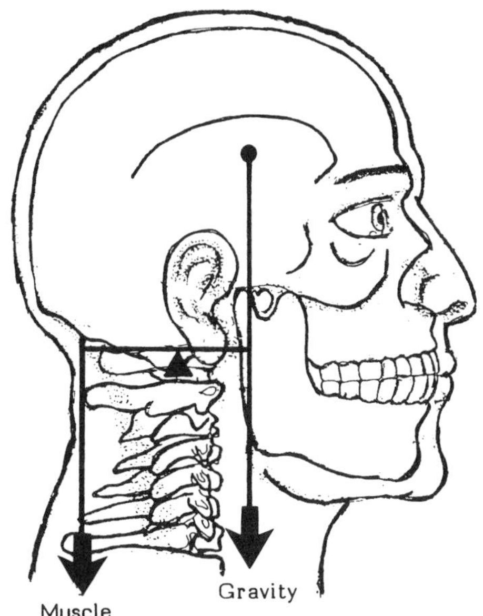

Figure 2.11. An example of a first-class lever in the atlas region.

Third-Class Levers. A third-class lever, in which the applied force is always located between the fulcrum and the supported weight (resistance), is seen in the action of the biceps in flexing the forearm. The biceps inserts between the elbow and hand; thus, when the biceps contracts, the elbow joint serves as a fulcrum. The same mechanism is seen in lifting a weight with the foot.

The resolution of the force of gravity or muscle contraction into components must include a rotary component. Also, the distance from the point of application of the rotary component to the axis of motion in the joint must be considered. The joints that serve as fulcrums also limit the range of movement of the body lever.

The Levers Principle

The mechanical advantage derived by the three different lever classes depends on the relative distances between the components, and the *levers principle* has been established upon this relationship. The resistance is to the effort inversely as the relative distances of the resistance and the effort from the fulcrum. The equation representing the levers principle is: effort × effort arm = resistance × resistance arm. The distance from the resisting force to the fulcrum is called the *resistance arm*, and the distance from the effort force to the fulcrum is the *force arm*.[80]

Calculating Effort. The levers principle is used to calculate the effort required to overcome a resistance within a lever system of any class. It is also used to calculate the advantages gained by shifting the position of the resistance, the point of application of effort, and the position of the fulcrum. In the body, the points of application of effort and the position of the fulcrums are somewhat fixed by the anatomic location of the origin or insertion of the muscles in relation to the joints. In some instances, however, changes of posture make effective improvements in mechanical advantage due to shifts in position of the point of application of force and the position of the fulcrum.

Muscle Force. In the musculoskeletal system, all muscle moment arms are short in proportion to the bony levers they move. The moment arm of the muscle is the perpendicular distance from the muscle's action line of force to the axis of the joint involved. This distance must be used to calculate muscle force rather than the length of the lever arm (distance from the muscle's point of attachment from the joint axis).

Human Potential vs Stability. While our lever-like extremities transmit forces and motion at a distance, they also favor musculoskeletal injuries by amplifying forces (usually external, occasionally internal) acting on the body's biomechanical system. Statistics indicate that excessive stress appears greatest on the short arm of first-class levers (eg, elbow, knee).

Linear and Angular Velocity Relationships

The linear velocity of an object at the end of a lever is the product of the lever's length and angular velocity. Thus, an increase in angular velocity and lever length increases the linear velocity because the end of the lever travels further per unit of time. In addition to a longer lever's increased velocity, it takes greater force to move it because the torque exerted by an object at the end of the lever is the product of the length of the lever and its weight.[81]

Wheel-and-Axle Mechanisms

The wheel-and-axle machine, consisting of a wheel attached to a central axle about which it revolves, works on the lever principle (Fig. 2.12).[82] Rotational force may be applied to either the rim (eg, a steering wheel) or axle (eg, a drive shaft).

Numerous examples of such mechanisms are found within the human machine. For instance, all joint rotation movements in the body involve such a mechanism. On cross section, one readily sees that a long bone of an extremity serves as an axle and its surrounding muscles as a wheel. In the thorax, the rib cage serves as a wheel and the spine as the axle. Here, force is applied to the ribs by the oblique abdominal muscles and to the vertebrae by the deep spinal muscles.

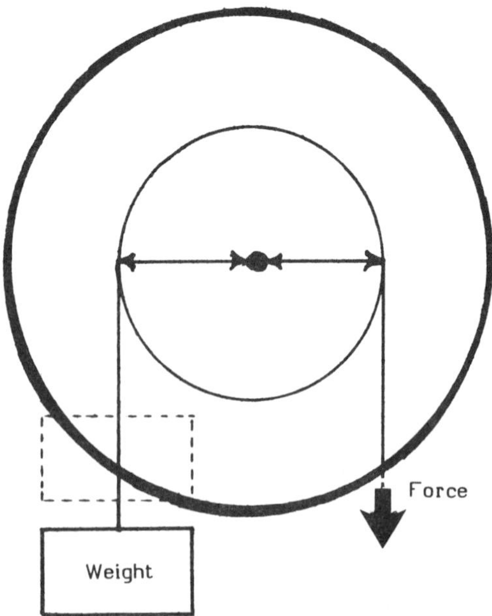

Figure 2.12. A wheel-and-axle mechanism.

Pulley Systems

A pulley system may be constructed as either a linear or concurrent force system. A pulley functions as that of a first-class lever with equal arms. Within the body, various fixed pulley systems that may act in any direction are utilized to alter the angle of action on the body by providing resistance and stabilization, and/or to assist movement (Fig. 2.13).[83]

An example of a fixed single pulley in the body is the patella. The position of the patella changes the direction of quadriceps pull on the tibial tuberosity so as to increase the mechanical advantage. Another example can be found in how the external malleolus of the ankle serves to change the pull of the peroneus longus muscle.

Force Couples

A mechanical couple represents a special case of a pair of parallel forces of equal magnitude that act in opposite directions some distance apart and tend to produce rotation (Fig. 2.14). Two noncolinear parallel forces that are equal in magnitude and opposite in direction have a net force of zero. While no linear motion would occur in the body, these forces, representing a couple, produce a rotation effect on the body. The torque (T) of a couple is expressed mathematically as T = force in newtons × perpendicular distance in meters. Pure rotation cannot take place unless there is a couple.[84]

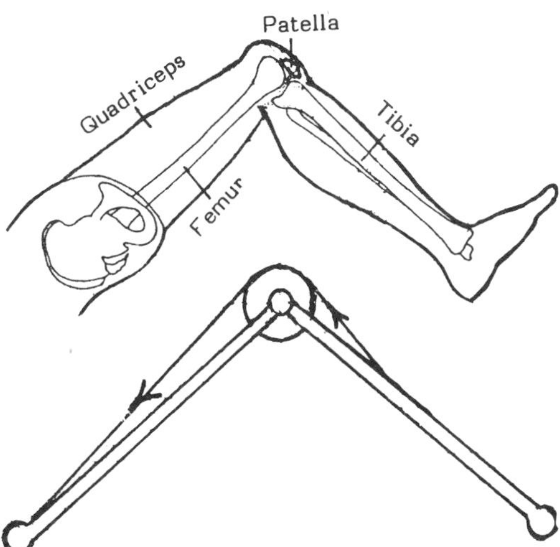

Figure 2.13. A typical biomechanical pulley mechanism within the body (*top*) compared to a mechanical pulley.

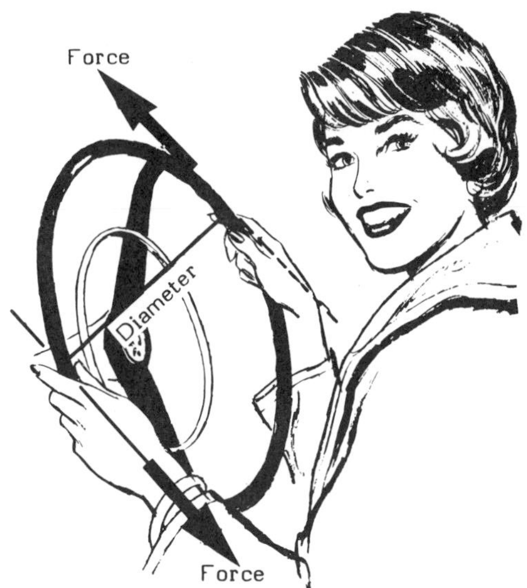

Figure 2.14. A steering wheel offers an example of a couple in which two parallel forces are separated by a distance to produce torque. Torque equals two parallel forces times distance.

Typical Applications

Examples of muscle actions that have a couple-like action are exhibited in anterior pelvic tilting by contraction of the lumbar extensors and hip flexors, thoracic rotation on the pelvis by contraction of the latissimus dorsi and contralateral external oblique muscles, and rotation of the head about the axis between C1 and C2 by contraction of the splenius capitis and contralateral sternocleidomastoideus muscles. Scapulohumeral rhythm and the depression action of the rotator cuff muscles on the humerus are two other examples of couple mechanisms. An interruption in either of these two couples compromises shoulder girdle motion. Typical side-position lumbar and pelvic adjustments and cervical rotatory adjustments incorporate twisting forces to the spine in opposite directions by action of the adjustor's stabilizing and contact points.

A couple consisting of small forces with a large distance between them is just as effective in producing rotation as one in which the forces are great and the distance between them is small. For example, in rotatory adjustment, a lesser force is necessary to produce the same effect when contact is taken well on a transverse process than when one is taken closer to the spinous process.

Coupling

A coupling is a device that serves to connect the ends of adjacent parts of objects to produce a phenomenon of consistent association of one motion about an axis with another simultaneous motion about a second axis. In the spine, for example, axial rotation is coupled with lateral bending, vertebral anterior translation is coupled with flexion rotation, lateral scoliotic deformity is coupled with axial rotation to rotate the posterior vertebral elements toward the concavity of the curvature, and vertebral movements toward and from the sagittal plane are coupled with associated rotatory and translatory movements.[85]

Bending[86]

If a load is applied to a relatively long structure that is not directly supported at the point where the load is applied, the resulting deformity is called bending. During bending, the fibers on the concave side of a connective-tissue structure are compressed, while those on the convex side are stretched.

Two effects are seen when a force acts on an object. First, the object tends to move in the direction that the force is applied (translation). Second, the force will cause the object to rotate (bending moment).

Bending Moment

A bending moment (torque) is a quantity, usually measured in newton-meters, at a point in a structure that is equal to the product of the applied force and the shortest distance from the point to the force direction (Fig. 2.15). For example, think of the trunk of a person sitting as a tree trunk and a laterally abducted arm as a branch of the tree. If a heavy book is placed on an outstretched hand, the bending moment increases in magnitude from zero at the hand to a maximum at the junction of the tree trunk and branch (shoulder). In the same manner, relatively small weights placed on horizontal limbs apply substantial bending

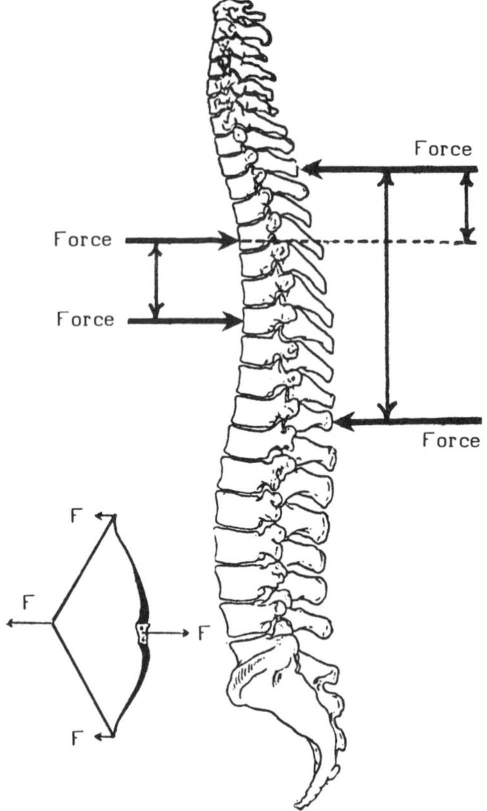

Figure 2.15. *Lower left*, a bow loaded in three-point bending. *Right*, the spine loaded in four-point bending.

moment at the thoracic and lumbar discs because of the long lever arm. If equilibrium is to be maintained, this stress must be compensated by the bending moment produced by large magnitudes of muscle and ligament force because of the much shorter lever arms of these tissues.

Body weight acting through the center of gravity and the first-class lever system of the hip tends to rotate the trunk toward the midline.[87] To maintain equilibrium, this turning effect abut the hip from the force of body weight must be resisted by an equal and opposite turning effect produced by the abductors pulling the pelvis downward. The bending moment is the product of force times the perpendicular distance from the force to the center of rotation.

Spinal bending involves the multiple actions of tension, compression, and torsion. The amount of this fiber stress (S) equals the bending moment (B) divided by the sectional moment (I) of inertia times the fiber distance from the neutral axis (Y): $S = B/I \times Y$. If the radius (R) of the curvature is desired, it may be computed by $R = E/B \times I$, where E is the modulus of elasticity of the material.

The moment of inertia of an elliptical object is greatest for bending loads in the direction that is parallel to its major axis. For this reason, the elliptical cross section of a vertebra's pedicle is seen to be most suitable for taking up bending loads in the sagittal plane where such loads are common.

Multipoint Bending

Both three-point and four-point bending occur within the body. *Three-point bending* is a form of bending in which one force is applied to one side of a structure and two forces are applied on the other side. Examples are seen with a seesaw or a drawn bowstring. In *four-point bending,* two transverse forces are applied on one side of a structure and two are applied on the other. If the forces are equal and symmetrical, the structure between the inner two forces is constantly subjected to bending moment.

The Neutral Axis

When a long fibrous structure is subjected to bending, the longitudinal line along which normal axial stress is zero is referred to as the neutral axis (Fig. 2.16). The plane of the neutral axis is that area situated between the fibers under tension on the convex side of the curvature and the compressed fibers on the concave side. However, there is usually shear stress along the neutral axis resulting from transverse forces, even though the tension-compression stress is zero. In cases of torsion stress applied about the neutral axis, the fibers at the neutral axis will have zero shear stress.

Torsion[88-91]

The mechanical internal moment or couple of restitution that arises in a cord or rod when twisted is referred to as torsion (Fig. 2.17). That is, torsion or torque is the load that is applied by force couples about the long axis of a structure. The *moment of torque* is the product of a force and its perpendicular distance from the fulcrum. Thus torque (T) is synonymous with force (F) times the length of the lever arm (a): $T = Fa$.

If the torques on either side of the fulcrum are equal, the lever is in equilibrium. As mentioned previously, when a lever is in equilibrium, the sum of the moments of force or torques tending to turn it in one direction (eg, clockwise) about a given point must equal the sum of the moments of the torques tending to turn it in the opposite direction (counterclockwise) about the same point.[92]

Application Principles

Practically all muscles pull obliquely and some pull with a slight twist. The oblique insertion of the pectoralis major into the humerus, for example, causes the humerus to be rotated as well as adducted during contraction of the muscle. In addition, all angles of pull against the bones change with each fraction of a degree of movement. For instance, the angle of pull of the biceps upon the radius changes with each degree of flexion of the elbow.

If torque is applied to the ends of a curved structure, each cross section of the structure is subjected to both torsion and bending forces. Many researchers feel that this principle is responsible for the low-back pain

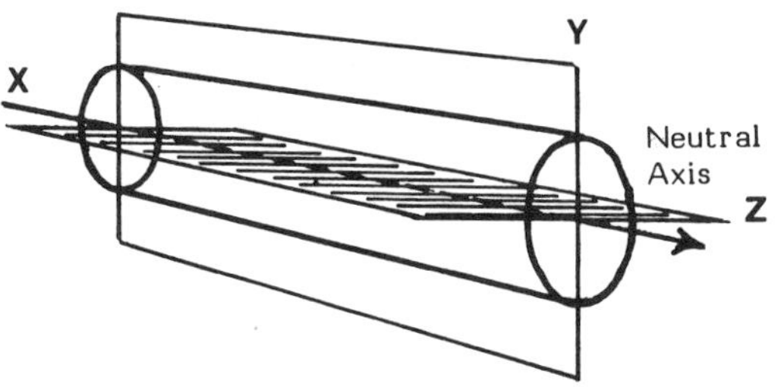

Figure 2.16. Torsion represents the force applied by couples about a long axis of a structure.

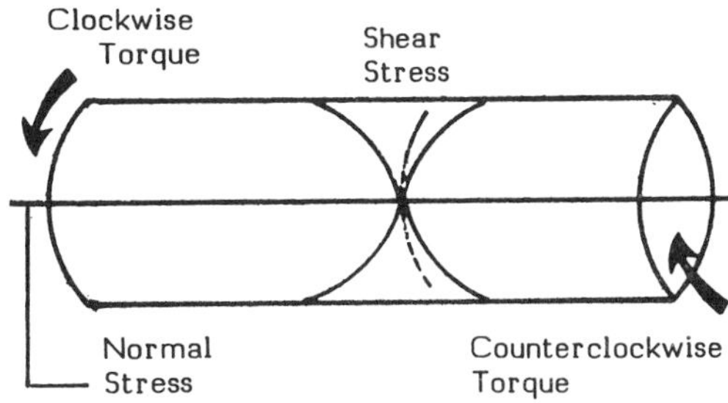

Figure 2.17. The stress effects of torsion.

from disc failure because simple axial rotation of the trunk (load) produces severe torsion and bending stress on the lumbosacral disc.

When considering rotational movement, torque fills the same role that force does for motion in a straight line. That is, the magnitude of the moment increases or decreases the angular velocity of an object to produce acceleration or deceleration of the rotation involved.

Torsion Terms[93]

Torsional Rigidity. Rotatory stiffness is called torsional rigidity in mechanics and represents the torque per unit, measured in newton-meters per radian, of angular deformation. This rotatory stiffness is a characteristic of all body joints.

Area Moment of Inertia. According to Newton's first law, the terms mass and inertia can be used interchangeably. The term "moment of inertia" describes the degree to which a material's shape influences its strength. There are two types: area and polar. The area moment of inertia refers to a measure, in feet or meters to the fourth power, of the distribution of material about its center which determines its bending and torsion strength (ie, its bending resistance). It is for this factor that a hollow tube such as a long bone is many times stronger in bending and torsion than a solid tube of identical mass (Fig. 2.18).

Polar Moment of Inertia. This is that characteristic of the transverse section of a long object that gives a measure of the distribution of the substance about its axis to increase its torsional strength (resistance). It is also measured in feet or meters to the fourth power. The greater distance a mass is from its axis of torsion, the greater its polar moment of inertia. The reason that the tibia spiral fractures most frequently at the junction of its middle and distal third is because this site has a low polar moment of inertia, even though the cortex is especially thick at this point.

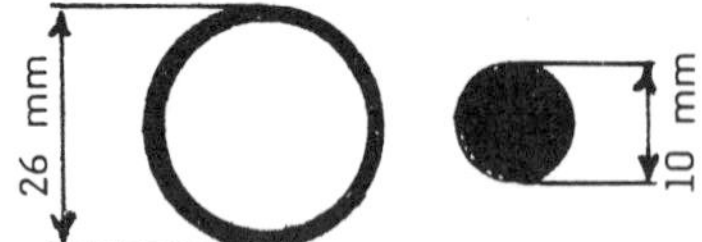

Figure 2.18. Although both tubes contain the same amount of material, the hollow tube (eg, a long bone) is more than twice as strong in bending and over five times stronger in torsion than the solid tube because of its area moment of inertia.

Shear Stress. A force directed against a structure at an angle to its axis that permits one part to slide over the other is called a shearing stress. Typical examples are that of the cervical and thoracic vertebral articular facets and that occurring at the intervertebral disc and vertebral body junction. In shear stress, both articulating parts may be movable with the parts sliding in opposite directions or one part may be fixed. Shear stress represents the intensity of force parallel to the surface upon which it acts and is measured in newtons per square meter or pascals. Because bone is weaker in tension than in shear, torsional overstress produces spiral fractures in long bones.

Shear Modulus. Shear modulus is a material property that represents the ratio of a substance's shear stress to its shear strain. As is shear stress, it is measured in newtons per square meter. Materials such as rubber and ligamentous tissue with their low modulus of elasticity also have a lower, about 38% lower, modulus of shear.

With these concepts and terms in mind, we shall be able to proceed to those of dynamics and stability.

REFERENCES

1. Williams JGP, Sperryn PN (eds): *Sports Medicine*, ed 2. Baltimore, Williams & Wilkins, 1976, pp 119–123.
2. Alley PW, Sells RL: *Introduction to Physics*. Boston, Allyn & Bacon, 1971.
3. Madley R, Winter R: *Modern Physics: A Student Study Guide*. New York, John Wiley & Sons, 1971.
4. Wilkie DR: Man as a source of mechanical power. *Ergonomics* 3(1), 1960.
5. Barham JN, Wooten EP: *Structural Kinesiology*. New York, Macmillan, 1973, pp 85–86.
6. Clauser CE, McConville JT, Young JW: *Weight, Volume, and Center of Mass of Segments of the Human Body*, Wright-Patterson Air Force Base, Ohio, AMRL-TR-69-70, 1969.
7. Dumbleton JH, Black J: Principles of mechanics. In Black J, Dumbleton JH (eds): *Clinical Biomechanics: Case History Approach*. New York, Churchill Livingstone, 1981, pp 367–368.
8. Schenck JM, Cordova FD: *Introductory Biomechanics*, ed 2. Philadelphia. F.A. Davis, 1980, pp 1–7.
9. Kendall HO, Kendall FP, Wadsworth GE: *Muscles:*

Testing and Function, ed 2. Baltimore, Williams & Wilkins, 1971, p. 18.

10. Squire PJ: Centre of gravity height and its relation to anthropometric measurements in female physical education students. *Journal of Human Movements Studies* 3:214–220, 1977.
11. Cochran GVB: *A Primer of Orthopaedic Biomechanics*. New York, Churchill Livingstone, 1982, pp 14–15.
12. Barham JN, Wooten EP: *Structural Kinesiology*. New York, Macmillan, 1973, pp 87, 129–130, 134–135.
13. Gowitzke BA, Milner M: *Understanding the Scientific Basis of Human Movement*, ed 2. Baltimore, Williams & Wilkins, 1980, p 55.
14. Williams JGP, Sperryn PN (eds): *Sports Medicine*, ed 2. Baltimore, Williams & Wilkins, 1976, pp 108–110.
15. LeVeau B: *Williams and Lissner: Biomechanics of Human Motion*, ed 2. Philadelphia, W.B. Saunders, 1977, p 10.
16. Barham JN, Wooten EP: *Structural Kinesiology*. New York, Macmillan, 1973, pp 99–100.
17. Edwards S: *Physics: A Discovery Approach*. New York, John Wiley & Sons, 1971.
18. Straley JW: *Basic Physics*. Englewood Cliffs, NJ, Prentice-Hall, 1974.
19. Cochran GVB: *A Primer of Orthopaedic Biomechanics*. New York, Churchill Livingstone, 1982, pp 1, 13, 16, 152–153.
20. Barham JN, Wooten EP: *Structural Kinesiology*. New York, Macmillan, 1973, p 131.
21. Schenck JM, Cordova FD: *Introductory Biomechanics*, ed 2. Philadelphia. F.A. Davis, 1980, pp 22–24.
22. LeVeau B: *Williams and Lissner: Biomechanics of Human Motion*, ed 2. Philadelphia, W.B. Saunders, 1977, pp 4–6.
23. Dumbleton JH, Black J: Principles of mechanics. In Black J, Dumbleton JH (eds): *Clinical Biomechanics: Case History Approach*. New York, Churchill Livingstone, 1981, pp 360–364.
24. White HE: *Modern College Physics*, ed 5. New York, Van Nostrand Reinhold, 1966.
25. Fowler RG, Myer DI: *Physics for Engineers and Scientists*. Boston, Allyn & Bacon, 1958.
26. Fuchs WR: *Physics for the Modern Mind*. New York, Macmillan, 1967.
27. Schenck JM, Cordova FD: *Introductory Biomechanics*, ed 2. Philadelphia. F.A. Davis, 1980, pp 7–9, 25–26.
28. Gowitzke BA, Milner M: *Understanding the Scientific Basis of Human Movement*, ed 2. Baltimore, Williams & Wilkins, 1980, p 78.
29. Black J, Dumbleton JH (eds): *Clinical Biomechanics: Case History Approach*. New York, Churchill Livingstone, 1981, pp 364–365.
30. Cochran GVB: *A Primer of Orthopaedic Biomechanics*. New York, Churchill Livingstone, 1982, pp 5, 12–17.
31. Williams JGP, Sperryn PN (eds): *Sports Medicine*, ed 2. Baltimore, Williams & Wilkins, 1976, pp 107–108.
32. White AA, Panjabi MM: *Clinical Biomechanics of the Spine*. Philadelphia, J.B. Lippincott, 1978, pp 480–481, 457.
33. Gonzna ER, Harrington IJ: *Biomechanics of Musculoskeletal Injury*. Baltimore, Williams & Wilkins, 1982, p 12.
34. Daniels L, Worthingham C: *Therapeutic Exercise for Body Alignment and Function*, ed 2. Philadelphia, W.B. Saunders, 1977, pp 101–102.
35. LeVeau B: *Williams and Lissner: Biomechanics of Human Motion*, ed 2. Philadelphia, W.B. Saunders, 1977, pp 1–2.
36. Dumbleton JH, Black J: Principles of mechanics. In Black J, Dumbleton JH (eds): *Clinical Biomechanics: Case History Approach*. New York, Churchill Livingstone, 1981, pp 360–361.
37. Hollingshead WH, Jenkins DB: *Functional Anatomy of the Limbs and Back*. Philadelphia, W.B. Saunders, 1981, pp 28–29.
38. Strait LA, Inman VT, Ralston HJ: Sample illustrations of physical principles selected from physiology and medicine. *American Journal of Physics* 15:375–382, 1947.
39. White AA, Panjabi MM: *Clinical Biomechanics of the Spine*. Philadelphia, J.B. Lippincott, 1978, pp 330–332.
40. Cailliet R: *Low Back Pain Syndrome*, ed 3. Philadelphia, F.A. Davis, 1981, pp 132–137.
41. Karwowski W: Fuzzy modelling of stresses in manual lifting tasks. *Ergonomics* 27:641–649, 1984.
42. LeVeau B: *Williams and Lissner: Biomechanics of Human Motion*, ed 2. Philadelphia, W.B. Saunders, 1977, pp 23–32.
43. Cochran GVB: *A Primer of Orthopaedic Biomechanics*. New York, Churchill Livingstone, 1982, pp 5–6, 54–58.
44. Gowitzke BA, Milner M: *Understanding the Scientific Basis of Human Movement*, ed 2. Baltimore, Williams & Wilkins, 1980, pp 42–43.
45. Barham JN, Wooten EP: *Structural Kinesiology*. New York, Macmillan, 1973, pp 91–93.
46. White AA III, Panjabi MM: Spinal kinematics. In Goldstein M (ed): *The Research Status of Spinal Manipulative Therapy*, NINCDS Monograph No. 15, DHEW Publication No. (NIH) 76-998, Stock No. 017-049-0 0060-7. Washington, DC, U.S. Government Printing Office, 1975, p 93.
47. LeVeau B: *Williams and Lissner: Biomechanics of Human Motion*, ed 2. Philadelphia, W.B. Saunders, 1977, pp 6–7.
48. Dumbleton JH, Black J: Principles of mechanics. In Black J, Dumbleton JH (eds): *Clinical Biomechanics: Case History Approach*. New York, Churchill Livingstone, 1981, pp 359–360.
49. Barham JN, Wooten EP: *Structural Kinesiology*. New York, Macmillan, 1973, pp 100–101.
50. Gowitzke BA, Milner M: *Understanding the Scientific Basis of Human Movement*, ed 2. Baltimore, Williams & Wilkins, 1980, p 75.
51. McCormick WW: *Fundamentals of College Physics*. New York, Macmillan, 1965.
52. Shames IH: *Engineering Mechanics—Statics and Dynamics*, ed 2. Englewood Cliffs, NJ, Prentice-Hall, 1967.
53. Dempster WT: Free-body diagrams as an approach to the mechanics of human posture and locomotion. In Evans FG (ed): *Biomechanical Stud-*

ies of the MusculoskeletaL System. Springfield, Ill, Charles C Thomas, 1961.
54. Dumbleton JH, Black J: Principles of mechanics. In Black J, Dumbleton JH (eds): *Clinical Biomechanics: Case History Approach.* New York, Churchill Livingstone, 1981, pp 368–369.
55. White AA, Panjabi MM: *Clinical Biomechanics of the Spine.* Philadelphia, J.B. Lippincott, 1978, pp 476–477.
56. Dumbleton JH, Black J: Principles of mechanics. In Black J, Dumbleton JH (eds): *Clinical Biomechanics: Case History Approach.* New York, Churchill Livingstone, 1981, pp 365–367.
57. Schenck JM, Cordova FD: *Introductory Biomechanics,* ed 2. Philadelphia. F.A. Davis, 1980, pp 76–81, 85.
58. Sears FW, Zemansky MW: *University Physics,* ed 4. Reading, MA, Addison-Wesley, 1960.
59. Halliday D, Resnick R: *Fundamentals of Physics.* New York, John Wiley & Sons, 1974.
60. LeVeau B: *Williams and Lissner: Biomechanics of Human Motion,* ed 2. Philadelphia, W.B. Saunders, 1977, p 9.
61. White AA, Panjabi MM: *Clinical Biomechanics of the Spine.* Philadelphia, J.B. Lippincott, 1978, p 462.
62. White AA, Panjabi MM: *Clinical Biomechanics of the Spine.* Philadelphia, J.B. Lippincott, 1978, p 504.
63. Jokl P: Muscle. In Albright JA, Brand RA (eds): *The Scientific Basis of Orthopaedics.* New York, Appleton-Century-Crofts, 1979, pp 380–381.
64. Karvinen E, Komi PV: Neuromuscular performance. In Larson LA (ed): *Fitness, Health, and Work Capacity.* New York, Macmillan, 1974, pp 85–86.
65. Morehouse LE, Miller AT Jr: *Physiology of Exercise.* St. Louis, C.V. Mosby, 1948, pp 21–22.
66. Dumbleton JH, Black J: Principles of mechanics. In Black J, Dumbleton JH (eds): *Clinical Biomechanics: Case History Approach.* New York, Churchill Livingstone, 1981, p 387.
67. Lehman RL, Swartz C: *Foundations of Physics.* New York, Holt, Rinehart & Winston, 1965.
68. LeVeau B: *Williams and Lissner: Biomechanics of Human Motion,* ed 2. Philadelphia, W.B. Saunders, 1977, pp 15–16.
69. Schenck JM, Cordova FD: *Introductory Biomechanics,* ed 2. Philadelphia. F.A. Davis, 1980, pp 76–81, 83.
70. Benedek GB, Villars FMH: *Physics.* Reading, Penn, Addison-Wesley, 1973.
71. Kenedi RM (ed): *Biomechanics and Related Bioengineering Topics.* Oxford, Pergamon Press, 1965.
72. Sayers BMcA et al: *Engineering in Medicine.* London, Oxford University Press, 1974.
73. Morehouse LE, Miller AT Jr: *Physiology of Exercise.* St. Louis, C.V. Mosby, 1948, pp 224–225.
74. Hollingshead WH, Jenkins DB: *Functional Anatomy of the Limbs and Back.* Philadelphia, W.B. Saunders, 1981, pp 34–36.
75. Williams JGP, Sperryn PN (eds): *Sports Medicine,* ed 2. Baltimore, Williams & Wilkins, 1976, pp 114–118.
76. Gonzna ER, Harrington IJ: *Biomechanics of Musculoskeletal Injury.* Baltimore, Williams & Wilkins, 1982, pp 34–35.
77. Morehouse LE, Cooper JM: *Kinesiology.* St. Louis, C.V. Mosby, 1950, pp 101–102
78. Morehouse LE, Miller AT Jr: *Physiology of Exercise.* St. Louis, C.V. Mosby, 1948, pp 223–224.
79. Cochran GVB: *A Primer of Orthopaedic Biomechanics.* New York, Churchill Livingstone, 1982, pp 18, 225–227.
80. Morehouse LE, Cooper JM: *Kinesiology.* St. Louis, C.V. Mosby, 1950, pp 103–106.
81. Gowitzke BA: Milner M: *Understanding the Scientific Basis of Human Movement,* ed 2. Baltimore, Williams & Wilkins, 1980, pp 44–47.
82. Barham JN, Wooten EP: *Structural Kinesiology.* New York, Macmillan, 1973, pp 82–83.
83. LeVeau B: *Williams and Lissner: Biomechanics of Human Motion,* ed 2. Philadelphia, W.B. Saunders, 1977, pp 41–42.
84. Cochran GVB: *A Primer of Orthopaedic Biomechanics.* New York, Churchill Livingstone, 1982, pp 19–20.
85. White AA III, Panjabi MM: Spinal kinematics. In Goldstein M (ed): *The Research Status of Spinal Manipulative Therapy,* NINCDS Monograph No. 15, DHEW Publication No. (NIH) 76-998, Stock No. 017-049-0 0060-7. Washington, DC, U.S. Government Printing Office, 1975, p 98.
86. White AA, Panjabi MM: *Clinical Biomechanics of the Spine.* Philadelphia, J.B. Lippincott, 1978, pp 457–458, 476.
87. Gonzna ER, Harrington IJ: *Biomechanics of Musculoskeletal Injury.* Baltimore, Williams & Wilkins, 1982, pp 37–38.
88. Dumbleton JH, Black J: Principles of mechanics. In Black J, Dumbleton JH (eds): *Clinical Biomechanics: Case History Approach.* New York, Churchill Livingstone, 1981, pp 374–376, 394, 398.
89. Williams JGP, Sperryn PN (eds): *Sports Medicine,* ed 2. Baltimore, Williams & Wilkins, 1976, pp 125–126
90. Gowitzke BA, Milner M: *Understanding the Scientific Basis of Human Movement,* ed 2. Baltimore, Williams & Wilkins, 1980, pp 73, 77.
91. White AA, Panjabi MM: *Clinical Biomechanics of the Spine.* Philadelphia, J.B. Lippincott, 1978, p 506.
92. Morehouse LE, Cooper JM: *Kinesiology.* St. Louis, C.V. Mosby, 1950, pp 109–110.
93. White AA, Panjabi MM: *Clinical Biomechanics of the Spine.* Philadelphia, J.B. Lippincott, 1978, pp 485, 491–492, 496–487, 507.

Suggested Readings

Alt F (ed): *Advances in Bioengineering and Instrumentation.* New York, Plenum Press, 1966.

Bernstein N: *The Coordination and Regulation of Movements.* New York, Pergamon Press, 1967.

Bick EM: *Source Book of Orthopaedics.* New York, Hafner, 1968.

Bootzin D, Muffley HC: *Biomechanics.* New York, Plenum Press, 1969.

Bowen WP, Stone HA: *Applied Anatomy and Kinesiology,* ed 6. Philadelphia, Lea & Febiger, 1949.

Casper JM (ed): *Biomechanics*. Chicago, Athletic Institute, 1970.

Clarke HH: *Development and Adaptive Physical Education*. New York, Prentice-Hall, 1963.

Crenshaw AH (ed): *Campbell's Operative Orthopaedics*, ed 5. St. Louis, C.V. Mosby, 1971.

Dyson G: *The Mechanics of Athletics*, ed 2. London, University of London Press, 1970.

Frankel VH, Nordin M: *Basic Biomechanics of the Skeletal System*. Philadelphia, Lea & Febiger, 1980.

Fung YC et al (eds): *Biomechanics: Its Foundation and Objectives*. Englewood Cliffs, NJ, Prentice-Hall, 1972.

Nelson RC, Morehouse CA (eds): *Biomechanics IV*. Baltimore, University Park Press, 1974.

CHAPTER 3

Basic Principles of Biodynamics and Joint Stability

The techniques used for analyzing static positions of the body are only approximate, inasmuch as forces accompanying movement incorporate such *dynamic* factors as acceleration, momentum, friction, the changing positions of rotational axes, and the resistance and support offered by tissues other than muscles. This chapter discusses the basic concepts and terms of biodynamics, biomechanical stress, and the biomechanical aspects of articular cartilage pertinent to the clinical setting.

STRUCTURAL MOTION

The study of dynamics is concerned with loads and the motions of bodies (kinematics) and the action of forces in producing or changing their motion (kinetics). *Kinematics* lets us describe the *characteristics* of motion position, acceleration, and velocity such as in gait or scoliotic displacements. Here we are concerned with the position of the center of mass of the body and its segments, the segmental range of motion, and the velocity and direction of their movements. In *kinetics,* we become concerned with the *forces* that cause or restrict motion such as muscle contraction, gravity, and friction. A complete biomechanical analysis of human motion or motion of a part would include both kinematic and kinetic data.[1]

While linear motion is readily demonstrated in the body as a whole as it moves in a straight line, most joint motions are combinations of translatory and angular movements that are more often than not diagonal rather than parallel to the cardinal planes. In addition to muscle force, joint motion is governed by factors of movement freedom, axes of movement, and range of motion.

Degrees of Freedom[2–5]

That motion in which an object may translate to and fro along a straight course or rotate one way or another about a particular axis equals one degree of freedom. From a purely biomechanical viewpoint, joint motion can be reduced to just two types: (1) ovoid, which permits motion in one plane, *X*; and (2) sellar, which permits motion in two planes, *Y* and *Z* (Fig. 3.1).[6]

Joint Freedom[7,8]

To know the actual degrees of freedom available to a part of the body, one must sum the available degrees of adjacent joints to appreciate the amount of free motion of one part relative to another part. The degrees of freedom of a fingertip relative to the trunk, for example, are the sum of the degrees of freedom of all the joints from the distal phalanges to the shoulder girdle. While the distal phalanges have only one degree of freedom, the entire extremity has 17 degrees in total. This summation process is an example of a living, *open kinematic chain.*

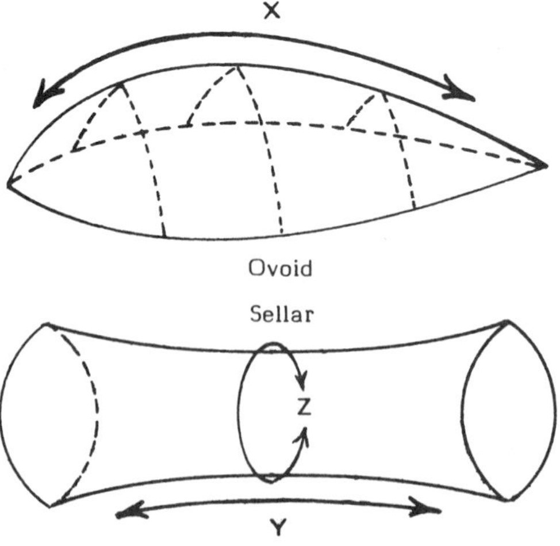

Figure 3.1. Ovoid and sellar joint motion.

Combined Movements

Simple translatory motions of a body part involve movements of more than one joint. This requires reciprocating actions of three or more segments at two or more joints if parallel lines are to be followed. For example, a fingertip cannot be made to follow the straight edge of a ruler placed in front if the wrist and elbow joints are locked. If the wrist and elbow are fixed, the fingertip must follow an arc and not a straight line. Thus, human motion can be described as translatory motion that has major contributions from linear, angular, and curvilinear motions. The term general or three-dimensional motion implies that an object may move in any direction by combining multidirectional translation and multiaxial rotation.[9]

Plane and Out-of-Plane Motion[10–12]

Plane Motion

Any motion in which all coordinates of a rigid body move parallel to a fixed point is referred to as *plane motion.* Such motion has three degrees of freedom; eg, sliding anterior or posterior, sliding lateral, and spinning. In other words, plane motion has two translatory degrees of motion along two mutually perpendicular axes and one rotatory degree of motion around an axis perpendicular to the translatory axes. For instance, if a person curves his trunk forward, the thoracic vertebrae flex and rotate in a single plane about an axis that is perpendicular to the sagittal plane (Fig. 3.2). In such plane motion, various points on a particular vertebra move in parallel planes.

The Instantaneous Axis of Rotation

Plane motion is described by the position of its *instantaneous axis of rotation* and the motion's rotatory magnitude about this axis.

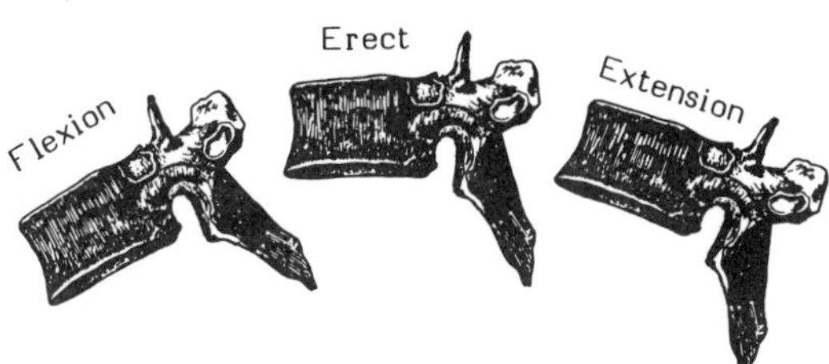

Figure 3.2. Vertebral plane motion.

In the above example of cervical flexion, for instance, as a vertebra moves in a plane, there is a point at every instant of motion somewhere within or without the body that does not move. If a line is drawn from that point so that it perpendicularly meets the line of motion, the point of intersection is called the instantaneous axis of rotation for that motion at that particular point in time (Fig. 3.3). Most joint movement is to a great degree rotatory motion, but the axis of motion may change its location and/or its orientation during a complete range of motion.

Out-of-Plane Motion

In contrast to plane motion, *out-of-plane motion* is a version of general body motion with three degrees of freedom consisting of two rotations about mutually perpendicular axes and a translation perpendicular to the plane formed by the axes. Thus, in out-of-plane motion, the body moves more than in a single plane. For example, if a person bends laterally, a midthoracic vertebral body translates from the sagittal plane toward the horizontal plane (Fig. 3.4). This is not plane motion because various points on the vertebra do not move in parallel planes.

Range of Motion

A freely moving body such as a vertebra has six degrees of freedom as it moves in three-dimensional space: eg, translations along and rotations about each of the three cardinal axes. The range of motion (ROM)

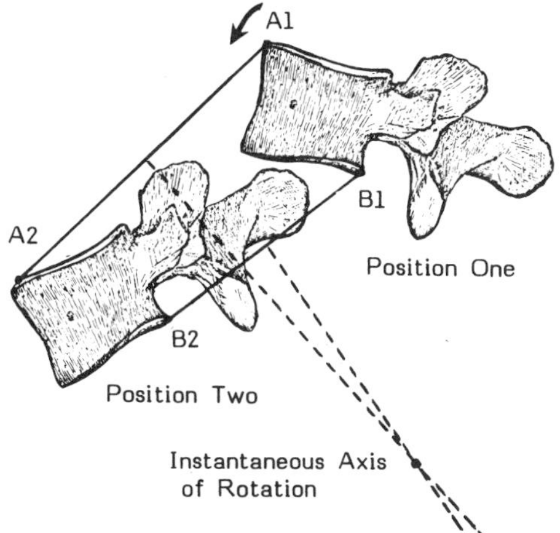

Figure 3.3. Determining the instantaneous axis of rotation of a vertebra from one position to another.

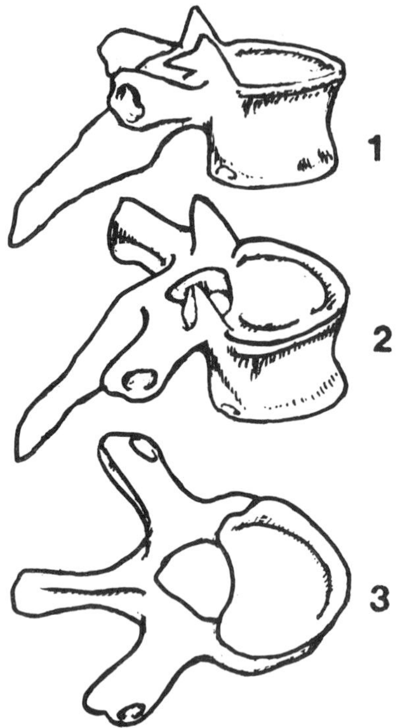

Figure 3.4. Vertebral out-of-plane motion.

of a joint is the quantities that indicate two points at the extreme range of physiologic rotation and translation for each of the joint's six degrees of freedom. Thus, the range of motion is the difference between the extremes of physiologic motion. It is measured in linear units for translation and in degrees for rotation.[13]

An articulation may have several degrees of freedom and a most limited range of motion, and a joint with one degree of freedom may have a large range of motion. Keep in mind that degrees of freedom refer to the ability to move in planes (ie, the number of axes), while range of movement is dependent upon soft tissue restraints, the number of joint axes, the joint architecture, and the size and position of adjacent tissue which may affect motion of a part (eg, biceps hypertrophy restricting forearm flexion). The knee joint has one degree of freedom and a relatively large range of motion; L5 has six degrees of freedom and a most restricted range of motion. In a joint having one or more degrees of motion, a range of motion can be expressed for each degree.

KINEMATICS[12, 14, 15]

Kinematics, without considering the forces involved, is the study of the motion of objects with emphasis on displacement, acceleration, and velocity.[16] Many of the concepts previously discussed such as coordinate systems, translation, rotation, coupling, degrees of freedom, range of motion, and axes of motion are major concerns within kinematics. The importance of this sometimes complex study is underscored in the analysis and management of structural problems of the body, in understanding trauma and clinical stability, in coping with spinal imbalance and other postural problems, and in evaluating orthopedic x-ray films.

It might be helpful here to review some major terms of kinematics. *Motion* implies a continuous change (displacement) of position. *Translation* refers to movement in which various points in an object at a specific interval of time have the same direction of displacement relative to some fixed point. *Rotation* (spinning or angular motion) refers to movement in which various points in a straight line in an object (or a hypothetical extension of such a line) at a specific interval of time have a velocity of zero relative to some fixed point. Rotation involves angular displacement of an object about some axis that is located within or exterior to the revolving object, and in which the points of the object describe concentric circles around an axis. *Coupling* is motion in which translation or rotation of an object along or about an axis is constantly related to simultaneous translation along or rotation about another axis.[17]

Acceleration

The application of Newton's second law is an important facet of kinematic studies. That is, a net force acting on the body gives it an acceleration that is proportional to the force in both direction and magnitude and inversely proportional to the body's mass.[18]

Linear Acceleration[19–22]

During human movement, the importance of body weight as a variable is explained in Newton's second law. Acceleration is the rate of change in velocity of an object. The greater a person's mass, the greater his or her equilibrium as measured by the quantity of force necessary to accelerate it positively or negatively. Thus, a heavy body has the advantage in maintaining a state of equilibrium, but it has a disadvantage in producing acceleration. This is exhibited in the weight need of a wrestler vs that of a sprinter. Also, the analysis and treatment of gait disorders and the application of braces and supports, for example, depend on the mechanical parameters of acceleration, displacement, and velocity.

Angular Acceleration[23–26]

Angular acceleration is produced by a force when its line of action does not pass through the center of rotation. The further the distance between the line of action and the center of rotation, the more effective is the force in producing angular motion (moment, torque). The same factors involved in kinematic and kinetic translational relationships apply to rotational motion if we substitute moment of inertia for mass, moment of force for force, angular change for displacement, and moment for force.

Angular acceleration is the rate of change of angular velocity. Neither a body in linear motion nor a rotating body needs to have a uniform angular velocity. If a body's angular velocity changes to a new value in a time frame, the angular velocity is changed (Fig. 3.5). The unit of measurement of angular acceleration's magnitude is degrees or radians per second per second. Mathematically, angular acceleration equals the new angular

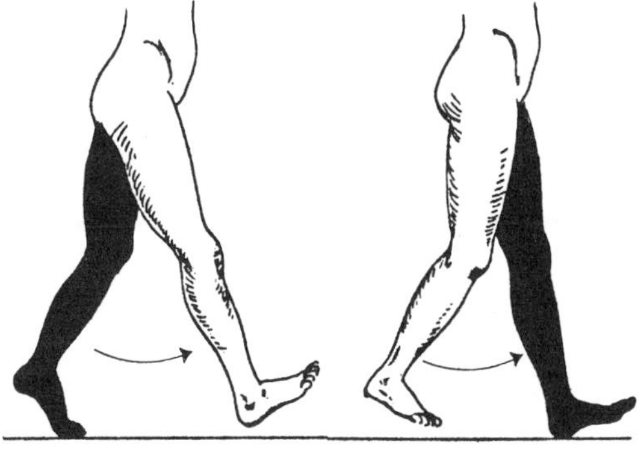

Figure 3.5. During locomotion, angular acceleration changes from positive to negative in a cyclic manner during gait.

velocity minus the original angular velocity times the time involved.

In rotational movements, moment = mass moment of inertia × angular velocity. This physical property reflects how mass is distributed about an axis, and it is concerned with differences in motion by various rotating body segments. The moment of inertia of a body will differ about its various axes because the motion of any one segment for a specific angular rotation is determined by the distance of that part from the center of rotation. For example, when an automobile is struck from the rear, the trunk of a person in the car is accelerated forward in relation to the head. The head responds more slowly than the trunk because of its inertia, and it is angularly accelerated backward. Thus, the mechanism of cervical whiplash injury is determined by the angular acceleration of the head and its inertia.

Velocity

Kinematic analyses invariably incorporate the concepts of linear velocity, angular velocity, and instantaneous velocity. When velocity increases, acceleration is said to be positive; when velocity decreases, acceleration is negative.

Linear Velocity[27]

Linear velocity is an object's rate of linear position change. The term *speed* refers to velocity's magnitude. If acceleration is constant and an object starts moving from rest, the final velocity that will be required will be directly proportional to the duration of the event. As a position change is measured by changes in distance or length, linear velocity = distance/time. If a muscle shortens 3 inches in half a second during contraction, the contraction's linear velocity is 6 inches/sec.

Angular Velocity[28,29]

Angular velocity occurs when the motion is rotation. A thrown ball always has a linear velocity, and it may have an angular velocity if it spins. A spinning top always has an angular velocity, and it may have a linear velocity if it simultaneously moves across a surface.

When a bony lever is moved by a muscle, the length of the lever can be considered the radius of a circle. The difference between a starting position and a stopping position can be measured by the angle formed. Thus, angular velocity equals the angle turned through per unit of time. A radian is a unit of angular measurement commonly used to describe angular velocity and is defined as the ratio of arc length to the length of the radius.

All but a few body movements are rotations of bones about their joints, and these rotations are seldom confined to one simple arc. Rather, they tend to vary irregularly to compensate for the restrictions of other joints and for the transfer of power from one set of muscles to another. During such irregular rotations, the bones also twist about their own axes. For example, during walking, the legs not only move forward and backward, they also rotate laterally during the forward swing, during contact of the foot with the ground, and again during the recovery phase of the stride.

In addition, all human movement is governed by the positive and negative acceleration of joint actions. During locomotion, for instance, the thigh changes its linear and angular positions and its velocities during gait. Linear acceleration during straight-line locomotion is partially produced by the increased angular velocity (angular acceleration) of the lower extremities. In all joint movements, the principle applies that linear acceleration equals the product of the radius and the angular acceleration.

Instantaneous Velocity[30,31]

Both linear and angular velocity are vector quantities because they have magnitude and direction. The term *instantaneous velocity* is the average velocity when the time interval approaches zero. It is measured in linear units per second. An object moving toward a goal may not have consistent speed and direction, eg, an automobile driving up a winding and dipping road to reach the summit of a hill. At any instant in time, both acceleration and direction may be above or below the average for the journey. Thus, an accurate description of velocity may necessitate the full plotting of its instantaneous velocity vectors.

Kinematic Analyses of Human Motion

Frame-by-frame motion pictures of a body or cineroentgenography of a region in motion can be analyzed to gain a great appreciation of human movement.[32–35] The problem is often to determine the levers involved in each joint action and compute the types of external load and internal stress involved. This analysis should incorporate at least the following data:[36]

1. The name of the movement under study, the time frame (frame number) at which the movement is initiated and concludes, and the joint or joints at which movement occurs.

2. A description of the segment or segments (lever) making up the kinematic chain being moved that are the effect of joint action.

3. A description of the force or forces causing the movement and the point of force application. These forces would include such factors as gravity, isotonic or concentric muscle shortening, or some other force contributing to the production of movement.

4. A description of the force or forces offering resistance to the movement and the point of force application. These forces would include such factors as gravity, eccentric muscle lengthening while exerting tension, or some other force contributing to movement resistance.

5. A description of the stabilized and/or relaxed joints *in* the lever and the forces that stabilize these articulations.

6. A description of the adjacent stabilized and/or relaxed joints *outside* the lever and the forces that stabilize these articulations.

When more sophisticated data are desired, body markers (often illuminated), specialized photographic equipment, timing devices, and electromyographic and electrogoniometric appliances can be used to:

1. Plot the trajectory (X vs Y axes) for each body marker, and Y coordinate for each marker in relation to time.

2. Plot velocity and/or acceleration of each marker relative to time.

3. Plot joint angles, angular velocity, and/or angular acceleration relative to time or instant of movement cycle.

4. Plot average velocity in terms of direc-

tion, movement length, and range of movement.

5. Plot the angle of one joint against angle of another at various intervals of time.

Body Links[37–40]

During human motion, several moving segments are involved in each study—one segment moves on an adjacent segment, which moves on another. This is similar to engineering links that involve overlapping segments held together by pins (joints) that serve as axes of rotation. Such overlapping does not occur in the human body except in a few places such as at the ankle and the C1-odontoid articulation.

A link is a straight line (eg, a rod) of constant length that extends from axis to axis (Fig. 3.6). Such a system of links can serve as a geometric model to analyze motion. If power is to be transmitted, the links of a machine must form a closed system in which each link has a particular relation to every other link in the system. The closed system guarantees that forces are transmitted in a positive and predictable manner.

Open Body Systems

The body can be thought of as a system of body links that form one or more kinematic chains. Most skeletal links are open chains rather than closed systems. This is because the distal ends of the extremities are free (unconnected to another link).

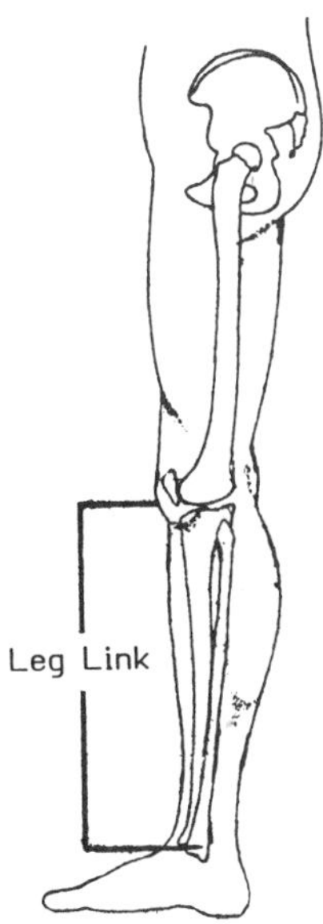

Figure 3.6. Leg link.

The dimensions of human links are determined by the length of bone from joint axis to joint axis. The joint axes are used because few articulations have overlapping bones. In kinematic analysis of human motion, the rotational axes are *not* located at the bony junctures. For example, the axis of the shoulder is within the humeral head; that of the hip, within the femoral head. In the knee and elbow, the axes are proximal to the articulating surfaces.

As mentioned earlier in the discussion of degrees of freedom, a proximal link in a segmental chain cannot be moved without causing displacement in one or more adjacent links. Thus, the "lever" in gross body movements is the kinematic chain involved, which is made up of a number of linked levers. Hip flexion and extension, for example, are not determined solely by the skeletal lever of the femur. When a person takes a step, the pelvis, hip, thigh, knee, leg, ankle, foot, and toes are involved.

In addition to the segmental levers involved in body movement and the forces producing the movement, consideration must be given to muscular and other soft tissue forces that stabilize a segment involved in the kinematic chain. It is for this reason that a kinematic analysis must include a description of the stabilized joint both within and without the lever and the forces that stabilize the involved articulations.[41]

Closed Body Systems

While kinematic chains in the body are open systems, there are two excellent examples of closed systems which are of special interest in chiropractic. One is found in the thoracic cage where the dorsal spine, upper 10 ribs, and sternum are united by the costovertebral and costosternal joints to form a closed kinematic chain. No movement of one segment can be made that does not affect the other in a predictable manner. The other example is found in the pelvic girdle where the ilia and sacrum are united by the sacroiliac and pubic joints to form a closed kinematic chain. Again, no movement of one segment can be made that does not affect the others.

Of course, the body as a whole or a part could be considered a closed system if the ends of the system are fixed. For instance, when a person tries to dislodge the overlapping bumpers of two cars, the person's feet are fixed to the ground by body weight and lifting compression and the hands are fixed by the weight of the car being lifted. The same principle applies when trying to displace any firmly fixed object (Fig. 3.7). One can appreciate that this concept has several implications in the analysis of fixated and ankylosed vertebrae during spinal movement.

Segmental Parameters

It is frequently important in kinematic and kinetic studies to know the center of mass for a particular body part as well as for the body as a whole, for which the center of mass is located slightly anterior to S2. Many researchers utilize the segmental centers of mass loci determined by Dempster, with slight adaptations.[42,43] (See Table 3.1.) The average weight percentages for body segments are shown in Table 3.2.[44,45]

KINETICS[46–49]

Muscles are the primary source of force within the body and gravity the primary source of force without that produce motion of the body. As with kinematics, kinetic analyses are essentially based on Newton's laws of motion.

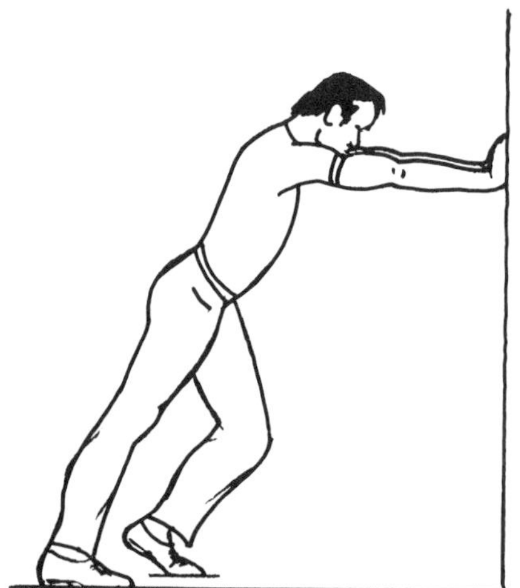

Figure 3.7. An example of the body as a closed system when an immovable object and the floor offer strong resistance at the distal extremites.

Several methods are used by the research scientist in analyzing kinetic problems. Briefly, these include the application of acceleration, impulse-momentum, and work-energy factors.[50] An acceleration approach is used in kinetics to analyze either linear or rotational forces and instantaneous acceleration problems. An impulse-momentum approach is used to analyze force acting over a specific time, and it is essential in problems of falls or when two or more objects collide. A work-energy approach is used in kinetics to analyze forces known as a function of body position and which are acting over a distance.

Momentum[51–53]

The quantity of a body's motion is its momentum. *Linear momentum* (L) is the product of an object's mass (M) and velocity (v): $L = Mv$. Its units of measure are pound-feet (lb-ft) per second or kilogram-meters per second (kg-mps). When a body is acted upon by a force, the momentum of that body is changed in the *direction* of the force. Also, the momentum is proportionate to the *amount* of the force applied and to the *duration* of the force acting upon the body (Fig. 3.8).[54] Momentum is directly associated with inertia. The greater the inertia of the body, the greater the force that must be applied to change the momentum.

Momentum and Power[55]

Momentum affects the amount of power that must be applied in moving, stopping, or changing the direction of a load. A greater amount of power must be applied to overcome the stationary object's inertia than to maintain the spped of the moving object. Likewise, a greater amount of power is necessary to stop a moving object quickly than to stop it by gradually reducing the speed. A greater momentum can be imparted to a movable object if the weight arm is lengthened. Less power is necessary to change the direction of a moving object if the object is kept moving than if the object is brought to a stop before it is moved in the new direction. Thus, the turn in swimming is a continuous motion through a short circle, not an abrupt reversal of the direction of movement.

Table 3.1.
Locations of Segmental Centers of Mass

Segment(s)	Center of mass
Head, neck, and trunk	Slightly anterior to the vertebral body of T11.
Head and neck	On the bottom surface of the basioccipital bone or within ¾–1⅛ inches from the crest of the dorsum sellae.
Head	Within the sphenoid sinus, about 3⁄16 inch past the anterioinferior edge of the sella turcica.
Upper limb	Slightly above the elbow joint.
Arm	Within the medial head of the triceps adjacent to the radial groove, about 3⁄16 inch proximal to the far end of the deltoid insertion.
Forearm	About ½ inch proximal to the distal aspect of the insertion of the pronator teres and ⅜ inch anterior to the interosseous membrane.
Hand	On the axis of the 3rd metacarpal, nearly centered between the volar and palmar skin at the angle formed between the radial longitudinal and proximal transverse crease of the palm.
Lower limb	Slightly above the knee joint.
Thigh	Within the adductor muscles, ½ inch medial to the linea aspera, below the adductor canal, 13⁄16 inches beneath the apex of the femoral triangle, and ¾ inch proximal to the farthest fibers of the adductor brevis.
Leg	About 1½ inches under the popliteus at the posterior aspect of the posterior tibialis, ⅝ inch superior to the proximal aspect of the Achilles tendon, and ⅜ inch posterior to the interosseous membrane.
Foot	On a line between the center of the ankle joint and the ball of the foot in the plane of the 2nd metatarsal; either within the plantar ligaments or just superficial to the adjacent deep foot muscles, below the proximal halves of the 2nd and 3rd cuneiform bones.

Table 3.2.
Average Weight of Body Segments

Segment	Percentage of total body weight
Head	7.3
Trunk	50.7
Arm	2.6
Forearm	1.6
Hand	0.7
Thigh	10.3
Leg	4.3
Foot	1.5

Note: The above computations are based on a 150-lb male mesomorph. Figures do not add up to 100% because limbs are not computed bilaterally in the above tabulation.

Momentum Transference[56]

When an object receives a force, the momentum lost by one object is gained by another. Thus, the momentum of a jumper's landing is transferred to the landing pad and then to the earth. The momentum of a fly ball is transferred to the outfielder's glove and body and then to the earth. The momentum of a dynamic adjustment is transferred to the patient's body, to the ad-

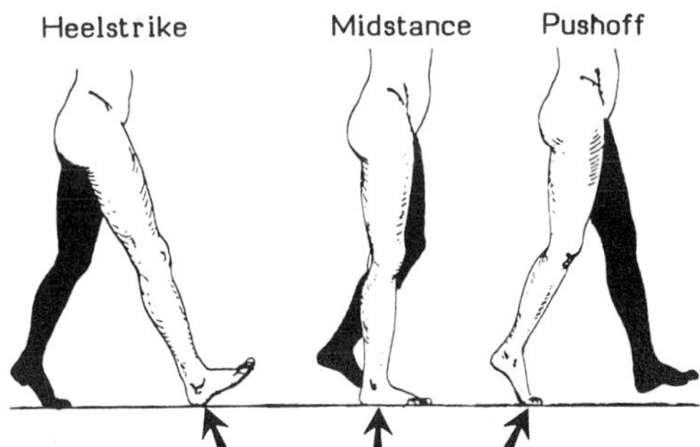

Figure 3.8. During locomotion, the reaction force of the floor is equal in action line and magnitude but counter in direction. Heelstrike force is greater than that of midstance force because of the momentum of the body. Pushoff force is greater than midstance force because of the force produced by calf contraction to plantar flex the foot and propel the body forward.

justing table, to the floor, and then to the ground.

The Moment of Inertia[57–59]

As previously discussed, the *moment of inertia* is the measure of resistance of an object at rest to rotation or of a rotating object to change in state of rotation. This is the quantitative measure of inertia for change in angular velocity, measured in lb-ft^2 or kg-m^2, and this inertia is equal to the mass of the object (lb) times the square of its radius of gyration (ft). Torque (T) exerts a turning force that is equal to the product of the moment of inertia (I) and the angular acceleration (a): $T = Ia$.

Angular Momentum[60–62]

An object's *angular momentum* (A) is the product of its mass moment of inertia (I) and its angular velocity (w): $A = Iw$. Its unit of measure is lb-ft^2/sec or kg-m^2/sec. If there is no external torque acting on a closed system, the total of angular momentum remains unchanged even when the moment of inertia is changed.

This principle is often expressed in athletics. An acrobat, tumbler, high diver, or free-fall parachutist can regulate his or her speed as the body rotates about its center of gravity by the postures assumed. If the limbs are tucked in, the radius of gyration is shorter than when the limbs are abducted, the moment of inertia will be relatively small, and the body will spin rapidly about a transverse axis in the coronal plane. It is for this reason that the spinning figure skater can increase rotational speed by bringing the arms toward the center of the body. Conversely, the speed of rotation can be slowed by opening the extremities to increase the radius of gyration and increase the moment of inertia.

The sum total of momentum also has many clinical implications. For example, the physician often sees signs showing evidence that a small force applied for a sustained period of time can cause momentum changes that are comparable to a much larger force applied for a shorter interval.

Friction[63–66]

In the action of one object pressing against another, *friction* is the resistance to relative lateral motion between the two objects in contact (Fig. 3.9). The resistance to the force that develops at the contact surfaces has a magnitude called *frictional force*, and the quantity of force necessary to produce motion of one surface relative to the other is governed by the physical properties of the materials in contact (eg, roughness), how tightly the surfaces are compressed, lubrication, and the type of movement between the surfaces. When mechanical work is done by moving against frictional forces, one effect is heat production between the articulating surfaces.

The Coefficient of Friction

The *coefficient of friction* is the ratio of tangential force to interbody pressure necessary to start a sliding motion between two objects.[67] One can skate more easily on a

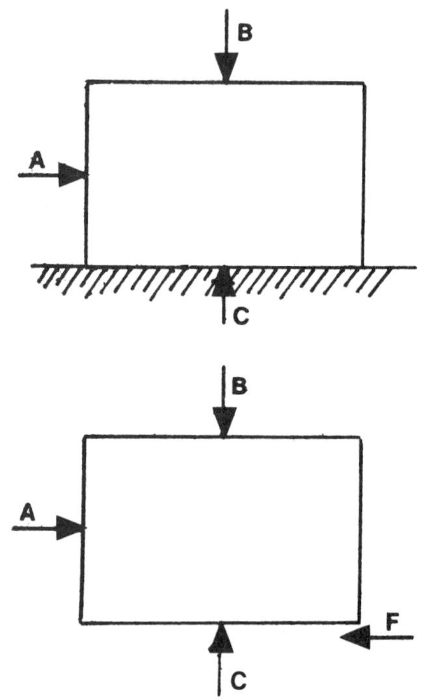

Figure 3.9. In this example of friction forces, force *A* pushes laterally against weight *B* which is pushing downward. The object's weight is vertically opposed by the normal force *C* which is perpendicular to the surface. In the *bottom diagram*, the friction force (*F*) counters the horizontal force (*A*). Actually, force *C* does not lie in the same line as *B* as drawn because the couple created by *A-F* forces must be balanced by the *B-C* couple.

hard, smooth surface than a soft, rough surface because the ratio of effort to body weight is smaller on the firm, flat surface. This action between the skater and the flat surface demonstrates a low coefficient of friction, whereas the action between the skater and the rough surface demonstrates a high coefficient of friction (Fig. 3.10).

Principles of Friction

It is well to keep in mind two points about friction. The first point is that once an object is set in motion (eg, an adjusted vertebrae), it takes less force to keep it moving. The friction effect of contacting surfaces at rest is constant, but this friction effect is greatly reduced once motion takes place. Just as it takes more force to get a heavy box sliding than to keep it sliding, it takes more force to free a fixated-subluxated articulation in its initial position than to adjust it to its "normal" site. This concept is demonstrated in the quick "dynamic" chiropractic adjustments as opposed to the relatively slow "leveraged" adjustment of osteopathy.

The second point is that contacting surfaces (eg, articular surfaces) produce a frictional effect that has no relation to the size of the contact area. Thus, a certain contacting force produces a given frictional effect whether the contact surfaces are large or small.

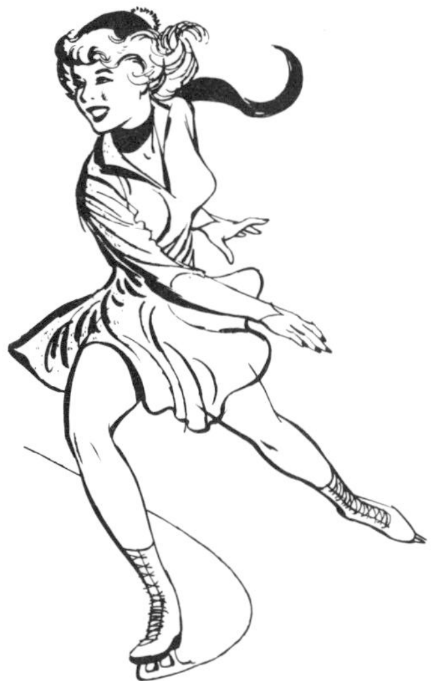

Figure 3.10. An ice skater can glide easily on ice because of the low coefficient of friction. Also, the skater's radius of gyration in turning is shortened if the limbs are abducted, allowing the body to spin more rapidly about a transverse axis in the coronal plane because of the decreased inertia.

Intrinsic Friction[68–70]

Friction is also a factor between flexible and rigid objects such as between a tendon and a bony prominence or between the soft tissues within the intervertebral foramen and its bony borders. Forces of friction in the body are especially important between articulating surfaces and layers of tissue, and around structures that glide upon each other. At common sites of friction wear, bursae are genetically located to decrease the effects of friction. At uncommon sites, a bursa will form by physiologic demand. In acute situations, traumatic effects of friction are seen both macroscopically and microscopically.

Clinical Applications

There are many instances in practice in which the effects of friction are desirable and undesirable. Lubricants are used in deep tissue goading to reduce skin friction. A felt or foam rubber pad is used under an elastic bandage to enhance firm gripping of the area and to more evenly distribute the compressive forces of the bandage.[71] The frictional forces within joints help greatly in stabilizing the body at rest. However, these forces must be assisted, especially by the stabilizing forces of muscles and ligaments and the deformation of articular cartilage under load.

Damping

Damping is the property of material that offers resistance to speed. For example, it takes more force to move a bicycle pump's plunger quickly than to move the plunger slowly. This principle is also exhibited in an automobile's shock absorbers, in the body's ligaments and joints, and dramatically in the viscoelastic intervertebral discs. The blood within the vertebral capillaries also offers a damping effect in rapid spinal loading because the blood has difficulty in rapidly escaping through the foramina.[72]

The *damping coefficient* (measure of damping) is the ratio of force exerted to the deformation speed when the damping resistance is proportional to the speed. For translatory motion, it is measured in pound force seconds per foot or newton seconds per meter. For rotatory motion, it is measured in pound force seconds per degree or newton seconds per radian. The term viscous damping refers to a situation in which damping resistance is proportional to the speed.

Work and Power[73–76]

Work is accomplished when the velocity of the body is increased as the result of an applied force. It can be measured in various ways, but the most common is to consider it the product of the force applied and the distance moved in the direction of force. For example, when a force (F) is applied to the body so that it moves a distance (d), the energy expended by the body or the work (W) done is expressed by the equation $W = Fd$. If a muscle lifts a 20-lb weight through a distance of 3 ft, the mechanical work accomplished is 60 ft-lb.[77]

Note that *work* should not be confused with the *effort* expended; great force may be used against an immovable object that would result in zero work. Work, in the specific mechanical sense, is the result of a force overcoming a resistance and moving an object through a distance: work = force × distance.[78]

Work Capacity

The work capacity of muscle has been variously estimated to be from 80–85 psi of cross-sectional area. Work capacity varies from muscle to muscle and in various conditions of fatigue, training, temperature, and state of nutrition. The computation of the force exerted by a muscle is a function of the work capacity, size, and shortening of the muscle. For example, if a sartorius with a work capacity of 80 psi of cross-sectional area has a cross-sectional area of 2 inches and fibers 18 inches long, and contracts one-third of its length during a movement against maximal resistance, the work accomplished will be: cross section in inches × strength psi × distance muscle contracts in inches divided by 12 = force exerted in foot-pounds.[79]

Although torque is measured in similar units and also equals force × distance, it should not be confused with work. Work concerns displacement and lies in the same plane as the distance the object is displaced, while torque is perpendicular to a lever arm distance. However, torque can produce work; ie, torque × angular displacement = work.

Types of Work

The term *energy* means the capacity to do work. *Positive work* is accomplished when a muscle contracts and shortens (eg, in lifting a load). *Negative work* is achieved when an external force overcomes internal muscle contraction force to the extent that the muscle lengthens during contraction (eg, in lowering a load). That is, negative work occurs when a force acts parallel to the movement but in a direction that is opposite to the movement.[80]

There is a close association in the same unit of time between the work accomplished by a weight lifter and by a sprinter.

Power

Muscle contraction force is synonymous with strength; ie, that energy which tends to produce motion or work. The term *power*, as used in biomechanics, should not be confused with *strength*. Power relates to the time element of the work; ie, the rate at which energy is expended, the rate at which work is done.[81] Power = force × distance/time, and it is expressed in foot-pound horsepower (1 hp = 55 ft-lb/sec), or joules per second.[82] When force is measured in newtons and distance in meters, the unit of work is a *joule* (J): 1 J = 1 newton continuously applied during 1 m of displacement.

SUMMARY OF MAJOR STATIC AND KINETIC FACTORS INFLUENCING MECHANICAL EFFICIENCY OF MUSCULAR EFFORT

The different size, quantity, and length of muscle fiber structures govern the force that a muscle can produce and the distance that a muscle can contract. Most of these characteristics are genetically determined by usual body needs such as the strength and range of motion required.

When muscles act upon a bone segment,

the result depends on (1) the length of the lever arms, (2) the range and force developed by each muscle, (3) the stretched condition of the contracting muscle, (4) the individual angles of muscle pull, (5) the site of the muscle relative to the joint axis, and (6) the action of synergic and antagonistic muscles.

Lever Arm Length and Mechanical Advantage[83–87]

To a great extent, the human body has been designed for speed rather than for overcoming great loads.[88] In most of the levers of the body, the distance between the fulcrum and the point where force is applied (the power arm of the lever) is relatively shorter than the distance between the fulcrum and the center of the weight (load arm). In man-made mechanical levers, the power arm is relatively long and the load arm is short so that great loads can be overcome by the application of minimum force. Thus, the source of body power is placed at a mechanical disadvantage, and strong forces must be applied through short power arms that act through short distances. The muscles that are the source of power must be strong and efficient to work effectively at such a mechanical disadvantage.

A long power arm in comparison with the length of the load arm gives the lever a mechanical advantage that enables heavy loads to be lifted. A short power arm results in a mechanical disadvantage in lifting loads, but it imparts speed to the movement if the muscular force is sufficient. For example, the calcaneus presents a long power arm that enables a person to rise on the toes while carrying a heavy weight, and the olecranon is a short power arm that allows great speed in throwing.

A long load arm is a disadvantage in lifting heavy loads, but it is an advantage in movements of speed and in imparting momentum to light objects. A short load arm in relation to the power arm gives the lever a mechanical advantage in lifting loads. The farther a light object is held from the fulcrum, the greater is the advantage for speed. Thus, a light weight is thrown with the arm extended, while a heavy weight (eg, shot put) is put near the shoulder.

Muscle Range of Movement and the Force Developed[89–94]

A primary attribute of muscle tissue is its ability to develop tension against resistance. When a muscle contracts, it does so in the direction of the muscle fibers; ie, fiber arrangement determines the line of pull of an individual muscle.

Range of Movement

Muscles with long parallel fibers produce the greatest range of movement. Some muscle fibers extend the entire length of a muscle, while others terminate intramuscularly in connective tissue stroma. While fiber length helps govern the overall range of effective movement, other factors are important, such as the shape of the articular surfaces, leverage, and the degree of stabilizing, antagonistic, and synergistic action. Because contraction may shorten a muscle's length by half, the long muscles in which the fasciculi are fairly parallel produce the greatest range of movement.[95]

Contraction Force and Anatomic Fiber Length[96–99]

Pennate fibers, which attach at an angle to the line of pull, have shorter fibers (Fig. 3.11). Thus, the distance that a muscle can shorten is not related to the length of the muscle as a whole but to the length of its fibers. However, the strength of contraction is determined by the size and number of contraction fibers (cross-sectional mass) and

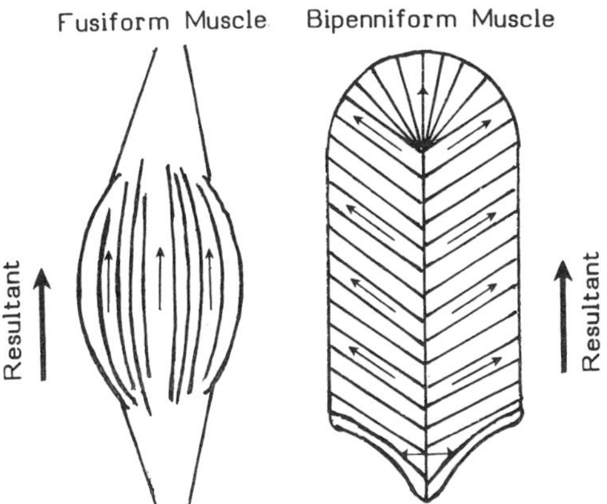

Figure 3.11. A schematic comparison of fusiform and bipenniform muscle fiber architecture and action lines.

not by the distance over which a muscle contracts. Thus, in most instances, there are more fibers in a cross section of pennate muscle than in nonpennate muscle. The range of muscle motion is dependent on fiber length, strength on size and quantity. The loss of range of movement efficiency in oblique fibers is usually compensated for by an increased quantity of fibers. This allows for powerful short-range movements. The inverse relationship between movement strength and range of movement follows the mechanics of levers; a bone serves as a rigid bar, the joint as a fulcrum, the muscle furnishes the force, and the load or resistance serves as the force that must be overcome to move the lever.

Contraction Force and Physiologic Fiber Length[100,101]

As discussed previously, *tension*, a scalar quantity, and *force*, a vector quantity, are not synonymous. Tension has magnitude but not direction. Under load, the tension developed in the body is produced to the physiologic maximum in proportion to the number of links in the kinematic chain. Internal muscle force (stress) implies a tension magnitude acting in the direction of a muscle's action line under various conditions to resist a load. The elastic components within muscle shorten during contraction, but whether or not the muscle shortens in toto depends on the relation of the internal force developed to the force of the external load.

In addition to a muscle's length at rest, its length at the instant of activation greatly affects its ability to develop tension. The maximum quantity of this tension can be judged as the greatest load that can be overcome. Many normal and abnormal mechanisms can be explained by the fact that a slightly stretched muscle at the time of stimulation contracts with a great amount of force, whereas a shortened muscle contracts with much less force. This is true regardless of the type of contraction. It is for this reason of greater force under stretch that isotonic contraction, which increases tension during stretch, can produce more work with a lower energy cost than the other types of contraction. When fibers are parallel, maximum tension is produced at lengths that are only slightly longer than those at rest. Nonparallel fibers develop their maximum tension at a somewhat greater stretch.

Two-Joint Muscles[102,103]

Muscles of the thigh and upper arm that cross two joints are called two-joint muscles by Morehouse and Cooper. There are several mechanical advantages offered by this arrangement, for the two-joint muscle can act as a towline. During motion in one joint, two-joint muscles exert a contrary action on the second joint so that the origin and insertion move in the same direction and energy can be transferred from one part to another (Fig. 3.12).

The duplication of effort saved when two-joint muscles act instead of two separate muscles has been calculated to be the algebraic sum of the rates of work of the one-joint muscles they replace. This relationship exists whether the work is done by the tissue during shortening or during stretching. With a two-joint muscle, the change in length is less rapid. This slower rate of shortening puts the muscle in a more favorable state for the production of muscle tension.

The length at rest of a two-joint muscle is inadequate to allow full motion in the opposite direction at the same time in both joints over which it passes. Extension cannot take place naturally at any one of the articulations without also occurring at the other. Because of two-joint muscle tension, the articulations are moved to about the same extent. For example, the trunk and lower leg are usually parallel in movement. It is

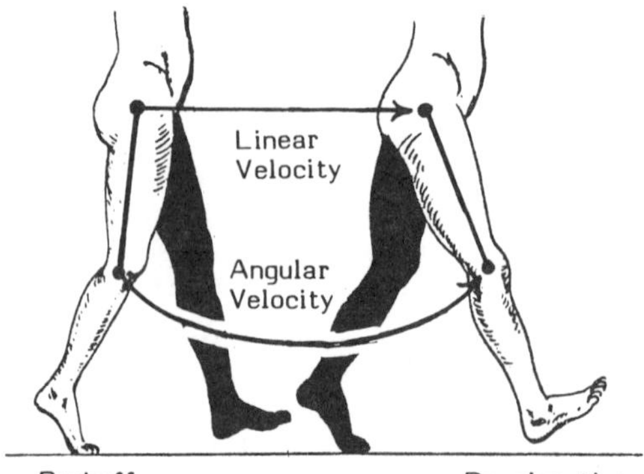

Figure 3.12. Linear and angular velocity of the femur during gait.

difficult to bend the knees and keep the trunk erect.

During action, the distance between the origin and insertion of these pluriarticular muscles may be changed. This change in length of the muscle involves a change by either shortening or lengthening to maintain constant tension. For instance, when the distance between origin and insertion of the biceps is shortened by raising the arm above the shoulder, the stretch of the biceps is reduced and the strength of its maximum contraction is diminished.

Muscle Speed and Velocity[104–107]

Most muscles at rest shorten to about half their resting length when loaded to the maximum. The distance to which a particular muscle can shorten is essentially determined by the length and arrangements of its fibers, the resistance of antagonists, the joint architecture, and the amount of resisting load.

In addition to the biochemical reactions involved, the speed of muscle contraction varies inversely with the load; ie, the speed approaches maximum when the load decreases. Thus, the magnitude of the load determines the speed at which the lever can be moved. The heavier the load, the slower the movement. If a fast movement is required, the weight must be relatively light. A heavy weight can be moved faster if it is held closer to the fulcrum of the lever system. In the case of heavy loads, the quantity of load determines the distance through which it can be lifted.

The importance of the most effective application of muscular power and mechanical efficiency becomes greater as the load increases. A load that is difficult to lift by the use of inefficient movements becomes less difficult if efficient mechanical principles are applied. Some investigators have shown that even the chemical reactions associated with contraction are governed by the degree of load and force capabilities of the tissue involved.

The velocity at which a muscle shortens (ie, the rate of shortening in a direction) is governed biomechanically by the force necessary to overcome a load, thus contraction velocity is maximum with zero load. Whenever more fibers are put into action than are necessary to overcome a load, the excess force is expressed as an increase in velocity and the distance of movement. This is exhibited when one lifts a light object that was perceived to be much heavier.

Angle of Pull[55, 108]

Mechanical efficiency is more important than muscular efficiency in determining strength of body force. A pull at right angles to the lever gives maximum mechanical efficiency. The greater the deviation from the right angle, the less efficient is the *angle* of the pull. Thus, the effect of the angle of pull of a muscle upon the force imparted to the lever is generally a decrease in the efficiency of the pull because the angle made by the bones on either side of a joint is either decreased or increased from a right angle. The reason that efficiency of pull is greatest when the joint is at a right angle is that in this position the muscle is pulling directly against bone. In this position of direct pull, none of the force of the muscle is wasted in pulling the bone of its insertion either toward or away from the joint.

A muscle that is pulling at an angle less than 90° has a stabilizing effect upon the joint. The smaller the angle of pull, the greater will be the portion of the total force that will be devoted to the stabilizing effect. This stabilizing effect relieves the stress and strain on the body, but it represents only a loss of effort in the accomplishment of external work.

Consider the strongest pull in flexion of the forearm. The strongest pull by the forearm can be made when placed in 90° flexion, even if the flexor muscles are not stretched enough to give their most powerful contraction, for it is in its position of maximum mechanical efficiency. If the forearm is extended to 180°, the muscle is in a position for a powerful pull, but the pull in this position is at such a mechanical disadvantage that only a small force can be applied to a load. In the flexion of the fully extended arm, considerable force is wasted by pulling the radius and ulna against the humerus.

This principle is commonly demonstrated in professional sports when we observe the position of the body joints during different physical activities that require strong movements. (See Figure 3.13.)

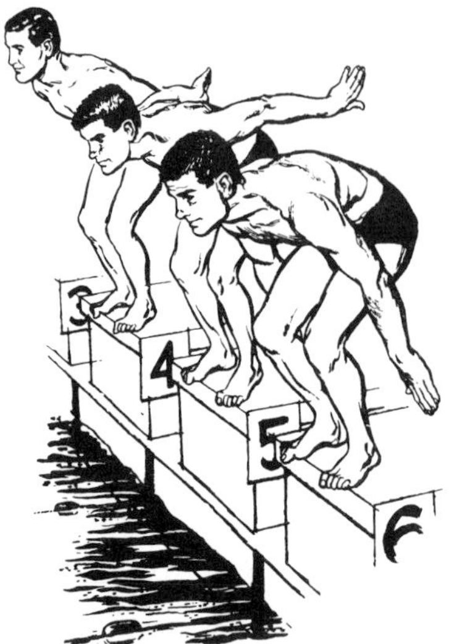

Figure 3.13. At the instant of greatest stress, the lever should be at a right angle to its working muscle. Note the knee and hip in the swimming start.

Composition of Forces[109–111]

As previously discussed, the effect produced when a force is applied to a lever is that of moving the lever in the direction of the force. If several forces act upon a single lever, the movement that results depends upon (1) the magnitude of the forces, and (2) the direction of the forces.

Obviously, the design of the musculoskeletal system is such that the majority of muscles pull at an angle against the bones they move. The resultant of two forces acting at an angle to each other can be computed rather simply by constructing a *parallelogram of forces*. This method is demonstrated in Figure 3.14, which shows the anterior and posterior fibers of the deltoid acting through a common tendon inserted into the humerus to abduct the humerus. The diagonal of the parallelogram represents the resultant of the two forces. If the resultant force of 100 lb in Figure 3.14 is in the direction of the pull of the middle deltoid, and if it is exerting an additional force of 60 lb, then the total force of all three deltoid parts acting on the common tendon is 160 lb.

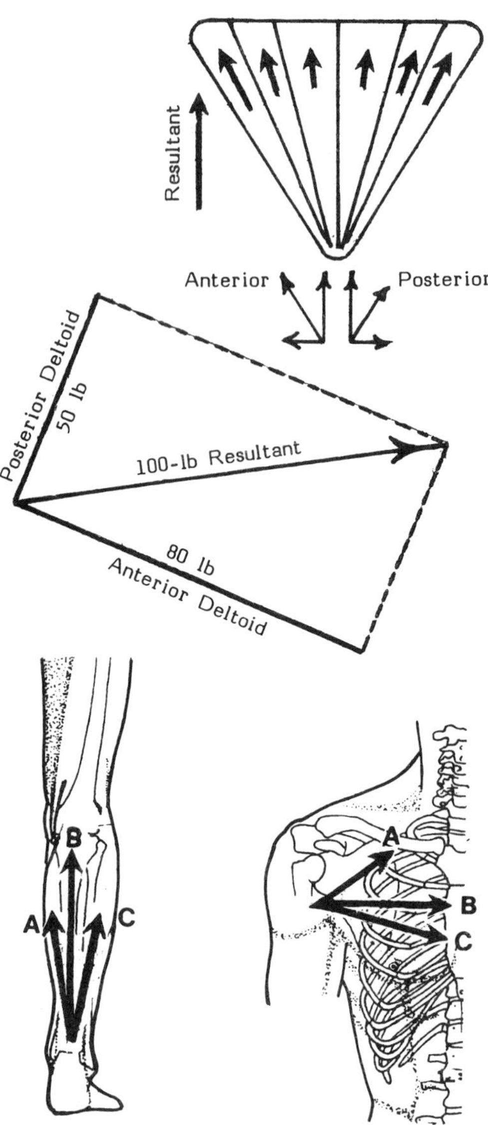

Figure 3.14. *Top*, resultant of deltoid (a triangular muscle) forces. *Center*, parallelogram of deltoid forces. *Bottom left*, graphic demonstration of the forces exerted by the two heads of the gastrocnemius. *Bottom right*, composition of forces by the sternal and clavicular heads of the pectoralis major.

Attachment Site[112–114]

The amount of a muscle's in toto maximum stretch and shortening is determined by the maximum degree of angular displacement of the body part at a particular joint. In joints where rotation is customary, the muscle fibers are coiled. During contraction, they unwind to produce bone rotation. All muscles crossing a single joint, but not those crossing two or more joints, are affected by the degree of angular displacement to the extent that they are normally capable of contracting sufficiently enough to move the attached segment through its maximum angular displacement and extensible enough to allow the full range of opposite-directed motion. If a muscle crosses two or more joints, tension creates force movements at each joint crossed to an extent that depends on the amount of muscle force exerted and the instantaneous length of the moment arm at each joint.

How a muscle is attached to a bone influences the effect of muscle contraction because the rotational and stabilizing components of force are determined by the angle at which a muscle pulls the bony lever (Fig. 3.15). Quite frequently, this factor is determined by the passage of the muscle tendon over one or more bony prominences that moves the muscle's action line distal to the joint axis and increases the muscle's moment arm.

A muscle's anatomic position determines the action line of a muscle producing motion about a joint. The perpendicular distance from the action line of the musculotendinous unit to the axis of rotation of the joint constitutes the lever arm. Also, the torque may be determined by the muscle force that is perpendicular to the length of the bony rod times the distance from its site of attachment to the axis of the joint. Thus, the moment of force it is possible to produce is determined by the distance of the muscle attachmernt from the axis of the particular lever system. A muscle attached close to a joint sacrifices range of movement for strength. The farther a tendon lies from the joint's axis, the better will be its turning effect on the segment about the joint.

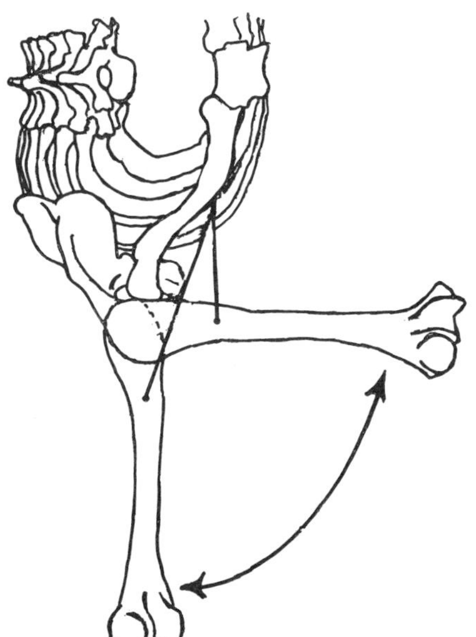

Figure 3.15. Although the clavicular head of the right pectoralis major has shortened only less than 1 inch, the humerus is moved through almost a 90° arc in this view from above. Thus, a small amount of contraction can effect a wide range of movement if the muscle attaches near the joint.

The Action of Synergic and Antagonistic Muscles[110, 115–117]

If the pull of a muscle is not directly away from its point of insertion, additional muscles must be called into action to hold the lever in the desired position during the movement. Most arm movements in swimming, for example, are angular and require the contraction of synergic muscles.

The reciprocal action of synergic and antagonistic muscles increases the steadiness and accuracy of a movement. The greater the quantity of muscles engaged in a movement, the more accurate and graceful is the movement. The more complete the relaxation of the antagonistic muscles, the more rapid and powerful is the movement. The more angular the direction of pull, the greater is the importance of the action of the synergic muscles in controlling the direction of the movement.

Opposing Forces on Joints[118]

Newton's third principle, that for every action there must be an equal and opposite reaction, is the basis upon which muscle moment is based. If the muscles acting on a joint produce movement, there must be forces acting to oppose this movement. These opposing forces essentially consist of gravity, exterior reaction forces, and inertia:

1. *Gravity.* Although the gravitational force acting at the center of mass of any body segment is a constant, the moment produced is governed by the segmental centers of rotation and the locations of the centers of the segmental masses. As the body in motion is constantly changing the

position of its segments, the gravitational moments are constantly changing.

2. *Reaction force*. In simple walking, this is expressd as the reaction force exerted by the ground surface against the foot.

3. *Inertia*. The inertial force of a body segment is proportional to segmental acceleration, but it acts in the opposite direction of the segmental acceleration.

Opposing muscle mechanisms are readily seen during the walking cycle. Just prior to heelstrike, for example, gravity, surface reaction forces, and inertia are producing an extension (counterclockwise) moment about the knee. However, the knee flexors, principally the hamstring group and gastrocnemius, are essentially two-joint muscles so that when knee flexion is produced they also produce hip extension (hamstrings) and plantar flexion (gastrocnemius).

Genetic Influences[119–121]

It is not unusual to find an individual endowed with bony levers that have exceptional mechanical arrangements. Their muscles are inserted further than normal from the joints about which the levers move (Fig. 3.16). When this occurs, it seems to be characteristic of all joints in that particular person. The result is that the mechanical advantage of the various levers is greater than normal, and the individual appears to have superior muscular power.[122] In this instance, the superior power is not due to the integrity of the muscle fibers, but rather to an improved application of force.

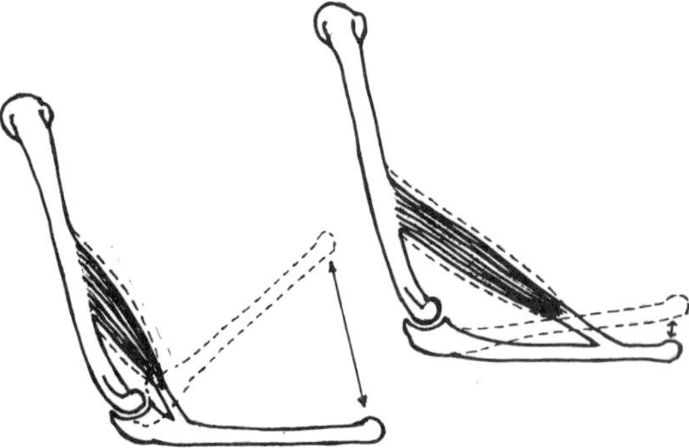

Figure 3.16. These diagrams show how muscles shortening the same amount but attached at different sites of a long bone have far different effects on range of movement. The muscle on the left moves the lever further because it is attached much closer to the jont, but the muscle on the right has a mechanical advantage.

An example of this principle is seen with a 12-inch forearm used to raise a 20-lb weight. If the insertion of the biceps is 2 inches from the center of the elbow rather than only 1½ inches, the mechanical advantage of the lever is increased from 0.125 to 0.166. This small increase in mechanical advantage would reduce the effort required by the biceps to lift a 20-lb load from 160 lb to 120 lb, an advantage of 40 lb. The total effective strength of a muscle is thus enhanced when the inherent mechanical advantage is greater.

Mechanical advantage and disadvantage have a distinct relationship with performance.[123] For example, pace varies with limb length, thus long limbs are an advantage in running, especially in long-distance events. But tall individuals possessing long body levers can use these levers to an advantage only against light loads unless the muscles moving them are extremely strong. The strength of the muscles moving these long levers becomes the limiting factor in their use. Weak muscles place the long levers at a disadvantage. A higher center of gravity is a disadvantage in that it takes extra postural effort to maintain balance such as in gymnastics or skating, but it has its advantages in sports such as basketball in which increased height places one closer to the goal.

BIOMECHANICAL STRESS

Clinical stability refers to the body's ability under load to limit various patterns of potential displacement in order to prevent damage or irritation to its components. In the spine, for instance, this is the ability of the vertebral column and its associated tissues to avoid cord, nerve, vascular, lymphatic, ligament, disc, or muscle irritation, stretch, pressure, deformation, or pain as the result of structural changes from loads (Fig. 3.17). Thus, any disruption of a musculoskeletal unit decreases the unit's stability in proportion to the degree of structural and physiologic impairment.

The body functions in accordance with its basic design—a relatively unstable-jointed frame, precariously balanced about a small

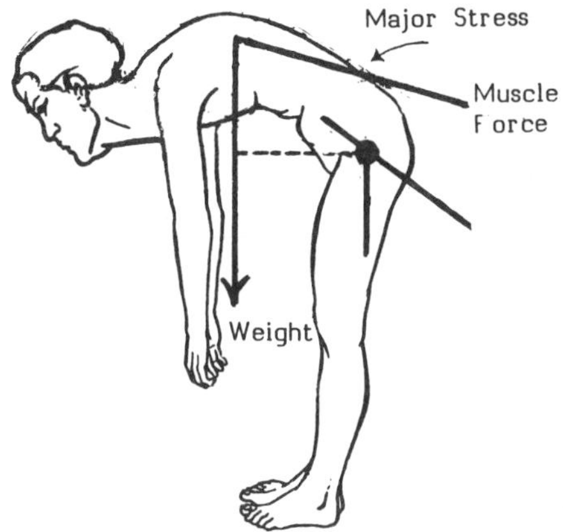

Figure 3.17. Forces acting on the lower back when the trunk is inclined 45° from the vertical.

base of support from the purely biomechanical viewpoint. Even slight movement requires tension adjustments of the muscles surrounding a joint. However, this inherent instability affords considerable mobility and a means for rapid change of direction. Work is fairly restricted to anterior tasks due to the ventral placement of most sense organs and the design of the extremity joints and their associated muscles, tendons, and ligaments.

Joint Stability vs Mobility[124–126]

Joint stability depends primarily upon its resistance to displacement. Biomechanically, it is the opposite of joint mobility. Joint flexibility is determined by osseous structures, soft tissue bulk, restraining ligaments, synovial fluid viscosity, muscle tone, nonelastic connective tissue of muscle, and the restraint action of the skin. Joint stability, on the other hand, is determined by mechanical and anatomic factors.

Mechanical Factors

Joint stability is provided mechanically by the biomechanical principles (eg, Newton's laws of motion) that govern the degree of stability of a particular joint by interacting with structural factors such as mass, the lateral distance of the common line of gravity to the joint's center, height of the joint's partial centers of gravity, the line of action, acceleration, size and position of the base of support, etc. Regarding the base of support, it is well to keep in mind that each segment of an articulated system has as its base of support the structure immediately underneath it, which in turn often has another base of support beneath it.

Anatomic Factors[127]

Joint stability is provided anatomically by the design of the articular surfaces, the joint capsule, the associated ligaments and fascia, joint fibrocartilage, atmospheric pressure, synovial fluid viscosity, and the site and function of muscles. Joints with poorly mated articular surfaces usually have strong collateral ligaments to resist forces transmitted across the joint (eg, the knee). Besides providing movement, muscles absorb energy during load transmission, provide smooth load transmission from one joint to another (reduce jar), and help to stabilize the joint.

Biomechanical Stress and Strain[128–130]

The terms stress and strain have specific meanings in mechanics which differ from their popular interpretations.

Stress[131–133]

Stress equals load divided by the original cross-sectional area. In mechanics, measurement is recorded by pounds per square inch (psi), newtons per square meter, or pascals. The two types of stress are *normal stress* and *shear stress*. Any stress normal to a cardinal plane is referred to as a *principal stress*.

Normal and Shear Stress. Normal stress is that which is perpendicular to a cross-sectional plane (eg, compression, tension), while shear stress is parallel to a cross-sectional plane. Thus, the intensity of any normal or shear stress on any site of the body at any particular time is relative to the stress direction through the cross-sectional plane. For example, the axial fibers of a bone are subjectd to normal stress during compression (negative stress), tension (positive stress), or bending (concave negative and convex positive stress). (See Figure 3.18.)

The Angle and Area of Application. The change in angle of the application of force has a distinct effect on stress. When the sacral angle changes, for instance, there must be changes in the shear and compression components of the force upon

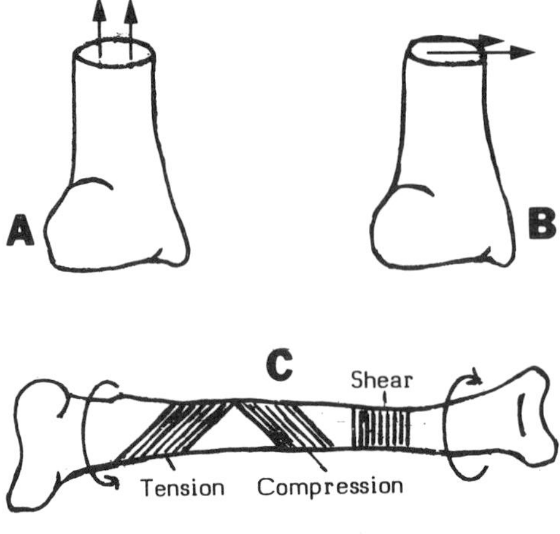

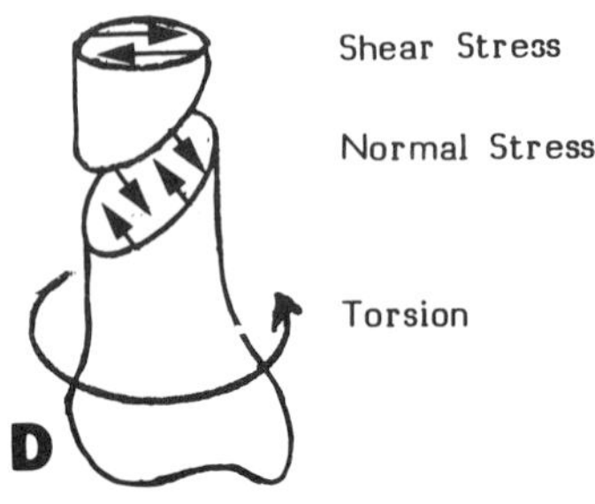

Figure 3.18. Examples of bone stress. *A*, normal stress; *B*, shear stress; *C*, the tension, compression, and shear stresses involved in torsion; *D*, mechanisms involved in typical torsion fracture of the tibia.

the sacrum (Fig. 3.19). In addition, the area over which stress is applied governs the magnitude of stress (force concentration). For example, a pisiform contact has a higher stress concentration than a broad contact. Joint stress concentration is determined by shape (articular congruity) and the articular tissue's plasticity. The better the articular mating and the tissue plasticity, the lower the stress concentration because these factors increase the bearing surface under load.

Stress and bending moments are related. For instance, when a load is applied to the head of the femur, the bending effect causes the bone's inner cortex to be under compression and its lateral cortex to be under tension. This places considerable compression and tensile stress in the subtrochanteric area.

Strain and Deformation

Normal and Shear Strain. Strain equals a change in shape or length divided by the original length of the structure; thus it represents a change in angle (Fig. 3.20). This alteration of shape or length is called *deformation*. There is no unit of measurement for strain as there is with stress. As with stress, the two types of strain are *normal strain* and *shear strain*. Stress is usually plotted on the *Y* axis, while strain is plotted on the *X* axis.

Ultimate Loads and Stresses. When a load is increased upon a structure to the point of fracture, that point of maximum load is called the *ultimate load* of the structure. The *ultimate stress* of a structure is computed by dividing the ultimate load by the original cross-sectional area.

Yield Factors[136, 137]

Such factors as flexibility, viscosity, elasticity, stiffness, plasticity, viscoelasticity,

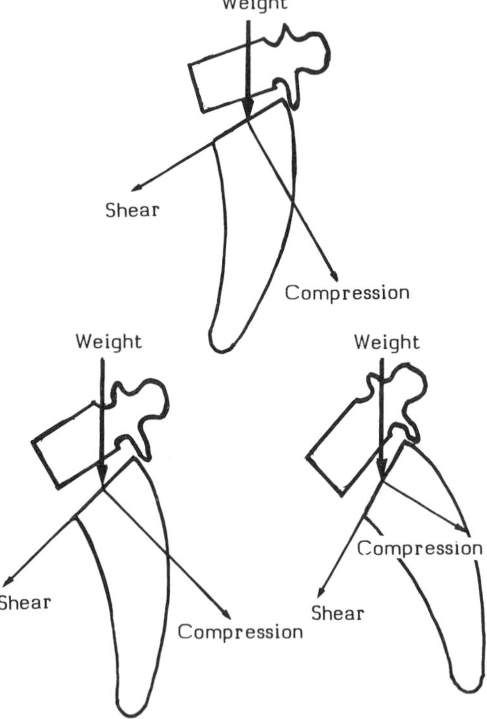

Figure 3.19. When the sacral angle is changed, there are changes in the compression and shearing force components. *Top*, Ferguson's angle is 30°; *bottom left*, 45°; *bottom right*, 60°. As the angle increases, greater weight is carried on the articular processes and associated tissues to resist shearing, and less weight is carried by the sacrum itself.

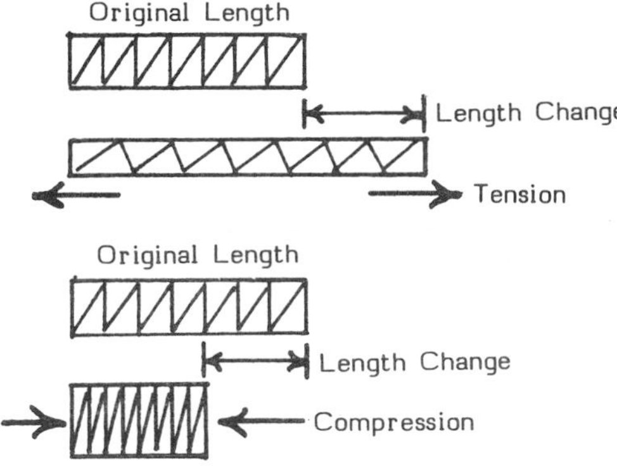

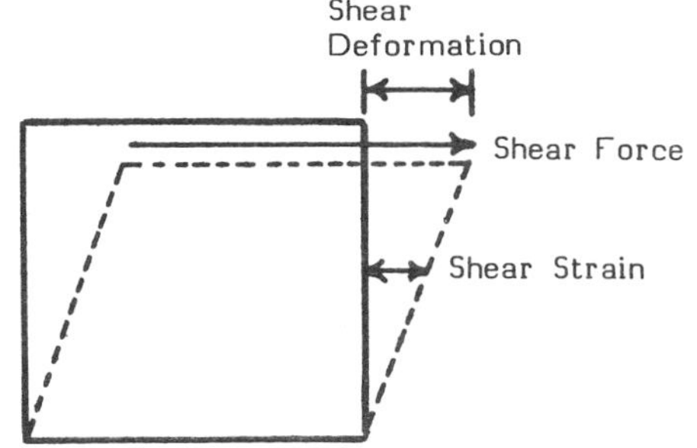

Figure 3.20. Diagrams of normal strain (*top*) and shear strain (*bottom*).

and structural fatigue are important considerations when dealing with mechanical reactions to structural load.

Flexibility

Flexibility refers to a substance's ability to be flexed and yield without fracture; thus, its pliability and nonrigidity. The ratio of the quantity of displacement produced to the load applied is the *flexibility coefficient* (responsiveness) of the structure.[138] A relatively high flexibility coefficient is seen in a readily yielding physiologic scoliosis in which only small forces result in large deformities.

Viscosity

Viscosity refers to that property of a substance whereby, when flow occurs within it, forces arise in such a direction as to oppose the flow. For example, when the viscosity of synovial fluid becomes higher than normal, friction increases and movement is inhibited. Mathematically, viscosity is expressed as the ratio of the shearing stress to the shearing strain rate for viscous solids or the shearing stress to the velocity gradient for fluids.[139,140]

Elasticity

In the mechanical sense, elasticity is that springiness or resilience property of a substance that causes it to resist deformation by storing energy and thereby recovering its original shape and size without permanent deformation by releasing energy when the deforming forces are removed.[141]

The Range of Elasticity. All substances are elastic to some degree, but the elastic range under load to the point of permanent deformation and fracture varies widely. For most practical purposes, the vertebrae are considered rigid bodies compared to the easily deformed intervertebral discs even though both bone and fibrocartilage have elastic characteristics under load.

The Modulus of Elasticity. The degree of stiffness is the ratio of the normal stress to the normal strain of a substance. The lower the value, the less stiff is the substance.

Stiffness

Stiffness is that property of a substance that resists deformation when the substance is under load. Although similar, stiffness and elasticity are not opposites. Elasticity is a *property* of the substance, while stiffness represents the *mechanical behavior, size,* and *shape* of a substance under load. The brittleness of bone is due to its high mineral content.[142,143]

Coefficient of Stiffness. The *coefficient of stiffness* varies with the magnitude of the load; ie, a stiff (eg, ankylosed) adult spine has a higher stiffness coefficient than that of an infant. The stiffness coefficient equals the applied load divided by the displacement produced (Fig. 3.21).

Torsional Rigidity. The term *torsional rigidity* refers to a substance's rotational stiffness; ie, the torque per unit of angular deformation. All joints present this characteristic.

Plasticity

Plasticity refers to the ability of a substance to retain a permanent shape attained by pressure deformation beyond its elastic

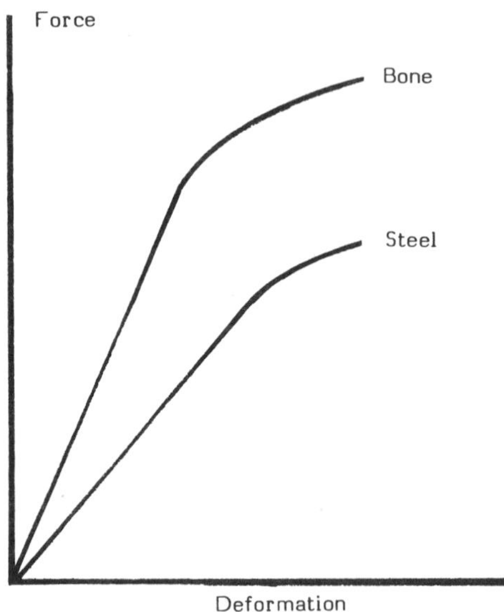

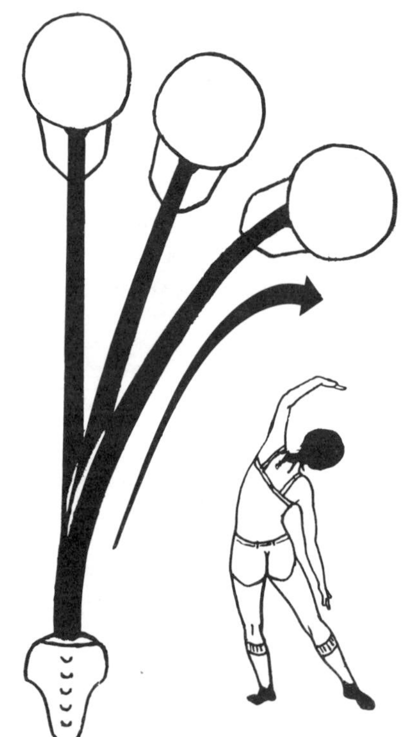

Figure 3.21. Stiffness. *Top*, curves show that although steel is stiffer than cortical bone, it has a higher modulus of elasticity. *Bottom*, the stiffness coefficient is much higher in an ankylosed spine than in a healthy, supple spine.

range in any direction without fracture.[144–146]

The Range of Plasticity. Any range beyond the elastic range to the point of rupture is referred to as the *plastic range of deformation.*

Yield Stress. A substance's *yield stress* is that point at which appreciable deformation occurs without an appreciable load increase; ie, that point at which plastic deformation begins. After the load is removed, the deformation that occurs after the point of yield stress is relatively permanent (Fig. 3.22).

Allowable Stress. The term *allowable stress* refers to a value of stress that is above that of normal loads but lower than that of the yield stress; ie, that margin of safety necessary to withstand accidental overloads during exceptional activities. For example, an athlete's body is commonly subjected to stresses far above that necessary for average activity but which are within the range of allowable stress for that particular individual.

Ductility. That ability of a substance to absorb relatively large amounts of plastic deformity energy prior to fracture, either in elongated length or decreased cross section, is called ductility. Substances with low ductility (less than 5%) are referred to as brittle (eg, cortical bone). Substances with high ductility have a high energy absorption capacity.

Viscoelasticity

All biologic materials have a loading rate for which, for example, a slow gradual pull will produce considerable deformation be-

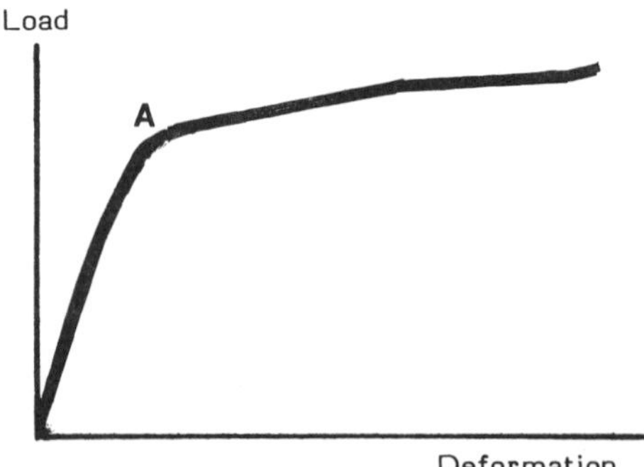

Figure 3.22. Diagram of yield stress. At point *A* the load has been removed, yet the yield stress is relatively permanent.

fore fracture in contrast to a fast pull that produces fracture with little deformation. This loading rate characteristic concerns the viscoelastic nature of the substance in question such as bone, fibrocartilage, ligaments, muscles, and tendons. Thus, any material whose mechanical properties vary depending upon the rate at which load is applied is a viscoelastic material.[147,148]

Relaxation. The combined components of viscosity and elasticity allow for relaxation and creep. To measure *relaxation,* a load is applied to produce a deformation which is then fixed. Relaxation, sometimes popularly called "give," is a steady deformation that occurs with less force over a period of time (Fig. 3.23). This is demonstrated in a tissue being stressed at a constant magnitude when the force necessary to maintain the deformation decreases with time.

Creep. To measure *creep,* a load is applied suddenly and sustained at a constant magnitude. Creep is a steady deformation that occurs over a period of time. This is exhibited in the loss in an individual's height from many hours in the upright position due to creep phenomena occurring in the intervertebral discs where a constant weight has been borne over a period of time.

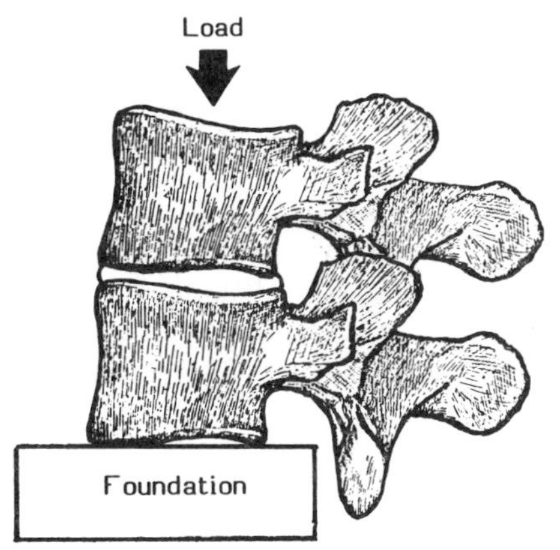

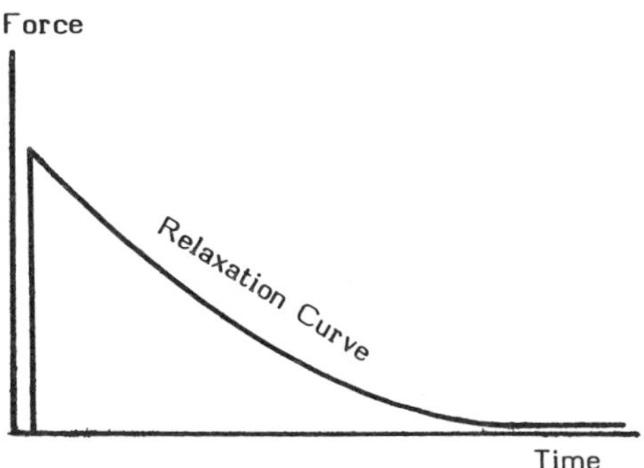

Figure 3.23. *Top*, vertebrae subjected to load. *Bottom*, if a constant deformation force is applied, the force in the vertebrae and disc decreases with time.

The implications of creep and hysteresis within the lumbar spine have been brought out in a number of studies. In 1982, for example, Twomey and Taylor applied a standard test with fresh lumbar spines from nine male subjects (aged 6–71 years). The columns were loaded with 3.5 kg for 1 hour using a weight-pulley apparatus.[149] Other tests were conducted using 1 kg and 5.5 kg for varying durations. The four oldest columns exhibited a pronounced decrease in flexion movement but a consistent increase in flexion creep deformation. After the load was removed, hysteresis recovery time was greater in the older lumbar columns than in the young.

Viscoelastic Stability. As mentioned, the critical factor in elastic stability is the magnitude of the load. However, the critical factor in *viscoelastic stability* involves both load and a time element. That is, a viscoelastic material may withstand a certain load for a certain period of time and then fail without the load being altered. Thus, all musculoskeletal structures have a time-dependent stability factor, but this is often structurally adapted to in living tissue if the time element is prolonged (eg, redesign of trabeculae).

Hysteresis. During cyclic loading and unloading, a viscoelastic substance shows a loss of energy in the form of heat. This phenomenon is called *hysteresis* (Fig. 3.24). For example, when an intervertebral disc is subjected to repetitive cycles of load and unload (eg, hopping), the shock waves directed from the feet to the head are substantially dissipated by disc hysteresis. Hysteresis decreases when the load-unload cycle is prolonged (eg, constant bumping) and during old age when viscoelasticity diminishes.

Biomechanical Fatigue and Endurance[150,151]

The process of developing structure cracks when subjected to cyclic loading is

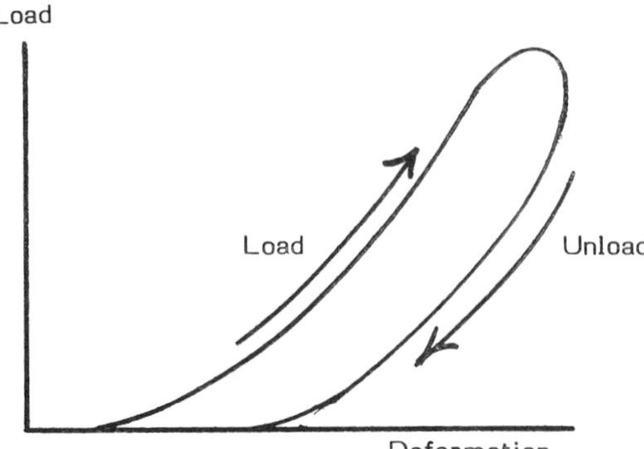

Figure 3.24. A diagram of hysteresis. The area between the two curves represents the energy loss during a single cycle of load/unload.

called *fatigue*. The magnitude of the load is usually far below that of the ultimate load of the particular structure, and thus well within the elastic range. The result is a summation effect, in which a fatigue crack reaches a size that causes the remainder of the structure to become so stressed that the entire structure fails. This factor is popularly called the *time* or *aging factor* of a body structure, and the time of failure decreases as the magnitude of the load increases. The term *endurance limit* refers to the least load that produces a failure from structural fatigue.

If healing processes are inhibited or do not have adequate time to repair structural cracks in bone, for example, a *fatigue fracture* occurs. From a biomechanical standpoint, the term *stress fracture* is a misnomer, because all fractures are the result of excessive stress.

BIOMECHANICAL ASPECTS OF ARTICULAR CARTILAGE[8, 152–155]

The principal mechanical functions of articular cartilage are exhibited in its ability to control joint motion by its shape, sustain a load (absorb energy), reduce friction during movement, transmit load from adjacent limb segments, and maintain joint stability by the specific shape of the bearing surfaces.

Load Carriage[156, 157]

All articulating bony surfaces possess a variety of incongruities and small projections where dynamic stress would be concentrated if not for the smoothing effect of articular cartilage. These small projections are the minute bony asperities that produce surface roughness. This characteristic of articular cartilage allows deformation during loading to increase the contact area and significant recovery during the unloaded stage. Load carriage is particularly enhanced by the ability of cartilage's hydrophilic proteoglycans to retain matrix water as a result of Donnan osmotic pressure and by the ability of cartilage collagen to resist matrix tensile forces.

Joint Reactive Force[158]

When any joint in the body is subjected to loading, certain internal reactive forces act at the surfaces in contact. Clinically, we see this exhibited in most low-back strains from lifting (Fig. 3.25).

Normal and Shear Forces. At a finger, for example, one major reaction (normal) is perpendicular and compressive to the contact surfaces, and the other much smaller secondary tensile reaction (tangential) is parallel to the contact surfaces (Fig. 3.26). This tangential force is opposite to the sliding movement, and the low coefficient of friction at the contact surfaces is the ratio between normal and tangential components.

Direction of Force. Articular cartilage is predominantly loaded perpendicular to the articulating surfaces. Tensile forces in all

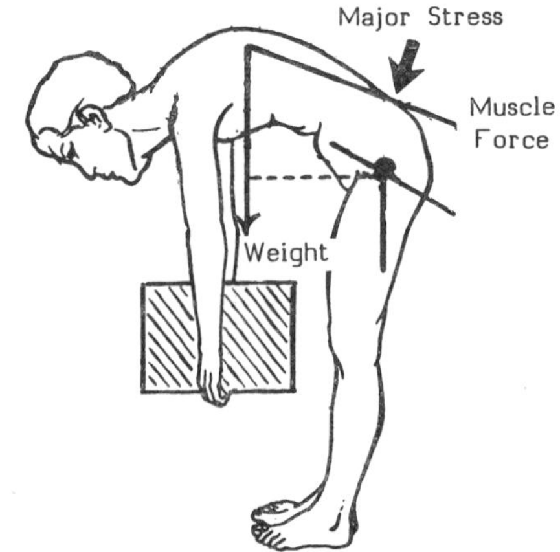

Figure 3.25. Forces acting on the lower back when the trunk is inclined anteriorly 45° while lifting a load. The added external load creates a much greater force on the lumbosacral articular processes.

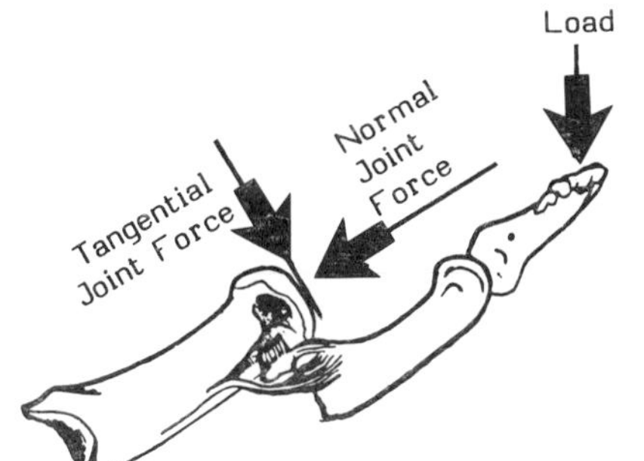

Figure 3.26. An example of joint reaction forces in a dislocated joint.

directions within the matrix are secondary to the perpendicular compressive forces. The magnitude and direction of these forces are governed by varieties of load application and the area of application, which are dependent on the joint's point in its range of movement.

Fiber Arrangement. When articular cartilage is tensile, loaded in planes parallel to the articulate surface, the stiffness of the tissue (far below that of bone) is closely related to the quantity and arrangement of collagen fibers lying parallel to the direction of the tensile force. Fibers in the midzone are randomly oriented to accommodate the tensile stresses occurring in different directions. In the deepest zones, the collagen fibers have a distinct tendency to be perpendicular to the direction of tensile force and help tether the matrix to subchondral bone.

Deformation from Loading[159–161]

When articular cartilage is subjected to loading, deformation develops instantaneously according to the tissue's stiffness. This initial rapid deformation stage has a negligible matrix fluid flow, and tissue contour changes but not its volume. This stage is followed by a slower time-dependent creep that is related to the flow of water through the matrix according to the magnitude of the load, the fiber elasticity, the quantity of surface area loaded, the uniformity of force distribution, the matrix permeability which is low even when unloaded, the osmotic pressure of the matrix colloid, and the length of the flow path.

When the load is removed during rest, the stressed cartilage begins to return to its original thickness, quickly at first (90%) because of the elastic recoil of the collagen fibers and then slowly from the absorption of water that is governed by the Donnan osmotic pressure of the proteoglycans in the matrix gel. This recovery by absorption is enhanced by oscillation of the unloaded joint and limited by the collagen fiber's stiffness and strength that are subjected to increasing tensile forces as the swelling develops.

Responses to Cyclic Loading[162–164]

A *dynamic load,* in contrast to a static load, is any load that varies with time. If a dynamic load has a repetitive pattern of variation, it is referred to as a *cyclic load.* For example, all weight-bearing structures are subjected to dynamic load as body weight is shifted from one limb to the other during locomotion. Because this weight has a repetitive pattern, it is also a cyclic load.

Cyclic Loading Magnitude and Duration. Almost all weight-bearing joints are continually subjected to high loads of short duration that are rapidly applied. During a normal walking cycle, for instance, the weight-bearing surfaces of the sacrum are subjected to loads up to five times body weight at an approximate rate of one time per second. The typical cycle time between heelstrike and toeoff is about half a second. These and greater load forces are sustained by mechanical forces and liquid pressures within the matrix and bone. Although shock-absorbing articular cartilage is quite thin, peak forces, often twice the compressible strength of bone, would undoubtedly produce bone failure if not for the damping and attenuating viscoelastic properties of articular cartilage.

Recovery during Cyclic Loading. Because fluid flow within the matrix is time-dependent, cartilage response to compression depends upon the magnitude of the load, the length of time the load is applied, and if the load is applied statically or cyclically. A small amount of water is expressed through the matrix even during a briefly applied load, and its absorption is time-dependent. If a second load is applied before the matrix is fully reimbibed, as during cyclic loading, the result is incomplete recovery which summates as the cyclic loading continues. In addition, all cartilage can be considered fatigue-prone.

Effects of Cyclic Loading on the Spine

There appears to be strong, yet not definitive, evidence that spines exposed to dynamic loads may have an increased risk of low-back disorders. Current evidence suggests that chronic low-back pain relates to disc degeneration and that this, in turn, may be accelerated by mechanical failure in the region of the end-plate and subchondral bone.

Two hypotheses are proposed by Sandover that relate fatigue-induced failure of vertebral tissues to disc degeneration.[165] After an investigation of the extent of dynamic stresses on the vertebral column motion segment arising from transport, the results indicated that fatigue-induced failure is a distinct possibility.

Liu and associates conducted a study of low-cycle fatigue on 11 lumbar intervertebral joints placed under axial compression in the range of 37%–80% of failure load.[166] The maximum deformation, measured in terms of the number of cycles applied, showed two distinct results: one group showed a gradual-stable increase, and the other group showed an abrupt-unstable increase in deformation. Before-and-after radiographs showed a 1:1 correspondence between unstable specimens and generalized bony failure. Subsequent roentgenography of end-plate slices showed crack propagation from the periphery of the subchondral bone centrally. When the organic matrix from the cracked specimens was removed, it disintegrated into small particles. The normal controls and stable specimens in the experiment, however, retained their normal size and shape.

Adams and Hutton flexed and fatigue loaded 41 cadaveric intervertebral joints from 18 spines to simulate a vigorous day's activity.[167] Post-test examination showed that 23 out of the 41 discs exhibited distortions in the lamellae of the anulus fibrosus and, in a few of these, complete radial fissures in the posterior anulus were found.

Joint Lubrication[63, 168–171]

During articulation, movement is restricted by frictional forces at the contact surfaces, and its coefficient is the ratio of frictional force to load weight. The coefficient of friction is governed by the extent of the area in contact and the shear strength of the contacting surfaces. According to Newton's first law, a greater force is necessary to start a joint's movement (static frictional force) than is necessary to keep it moving (sliding frictional force) at a constant velocity.

Surface Irregularities[172]

As the load is increased and the area of contact increases, friction increases. Any apposing surface irregularities of articular cartilage, or bone in its absence, have the highest points sheared off as the articulating surfaces slide on one another.

The more congruous (well mated) the articulating surfaces, the more stress force per unit of surface area can be distributed uniformly. It is for this reason that incongruous (trauma, disease) weight-bearing joints (hip, knee, ankle) are more apt to exhibit degenerative changes.

Body Bearings[173]

Every machine with moving parts, including the body, requires lubrication to prevent wear of articulating parts, reduce friction, and minimize heat production. If the synovial membrane is injured, hemarthrosis and a thick, boggy, blood-stained synovium result. Later, adhesions may develop to produce stiffness and restrict movement, but these effects can be reduced or eliminated by early mobilization.

The complex lubrication system of human joints far exceeds that of similarly designed man-made bearings. Much of this is due to (1) the renewable coating of glycoprotein molecules that blanket the surface of articular cartilage, (2) the ingress and egress of fluid from the cartilage's matrix, (3) the porosity and elasticity of cartilage which also affords fluid imbibement and expulsion during load compression and relief, and (4) the unique folding and sliding action of synovial folds during movement.

Factors of Self-Lubrication[174]

An important factor in joint lubrication is the fact that the curves of the articulating surfaces are not exactly congruous (ie, do not fit reciprocally). This is necessary to afford better lubrication of the joint. Self-lubrication depends on a thin wedge-shaped space (provided by the slight incongruity), a viscous fluid, and a degree of rapid movement. During loading, the hydrostatic pressure developed in the matrix counteracts the pressure of the lubricant trapped within the area of surface deformation.

Joint lubrication is greatly diminished in prolonged immobilization such as in post-traumatic support or paralysis. The effect is atrophy of muscle, cartilage, and subcutaneous fat, along with chronic circulation disturbances, capsular contraction, and bone decalcification.

The Viscosity Factor in Joint Lubrication

There are several possible lubrication mechanisms for living joints. One such mechanism, the squeeze film compliant bearing, has been indirectly studied by the use of a computational model.[175] It was found that changes in viscosity of the lubricant had a greater influence than changes in the cartilage stiffness, and the lubrication qualities of the compliant system were superior to those of the system with rigid surfaces. It was also found, however, that a compliant system with a low viscosity has poorer lubrication properties than a rigid system with a higher viscosity.

Factors Disturbing Normal Function[176-178]

Aging

Aging decreases articular cartilage permeability up to the age of about 40 years, after which, an increase in permeability begins to develop. However, aging has little or no influence on the elastic properties of articular cartilage. The effect of aging on tensile strength is unknown.

Trauma and Inflammation

Both trauma and inflammation increase permeability of synovial vessels, which allows large molecules of plasmin to enter the joint and act on articular cartilage to adversely alter its mechanical properties. Sustained joint blood, such as that associated with prolonged trauma, also tends to alter the physical and chemical properties of articular cartilage. Any joint malalignment (eg, subluxation, genu distortions) produces abnormal unilateral loads which tend to break down articular cartilage.

Tension

Normal cartilage may fail mechanically when the collagen network is overly tensed. This usually requires a single impact of great magnitude sufficient to burst the aqueous gel. High loads of continual pressure produce cartilage degeneration and chondrocyte necrosis which contribute to cartilage failure. In cyclic loading, tension failure results from fatigue.

Tissue Nutrition

The nutrition of articular cartilage is provided by the ingress and egress of matrix fluid during cycles of loading and relief. Thus, either sustained compression or sustained relief invites degeneration from lack of nutrition.

Even in a well-lubricated joint, continuous cartilage-against-cartilage pressure results in a irreparable pressure necrosis in a few days due to the prevention of synovial nutritive elements from entering surface pores of the cartilage. When this occurs, such as in immobilization in a forced position, chondrocytes die and degenerative arthritis is encouraged and its extent, from superficial to deep involvement, is proportional to the duration of the compression. In addition, the protein-polysaccharide complexes become depleted. The cartilage becomes unable to withstand stress as movement occurs, and degenerative changes develop. In osteoarthritis, articular cartilage loses its stiffness, especially at the surface.

The role of exercise on the nutrition of intervertebral discs was studied by Holm and Nachemson.[179] Experiments on dogs under a supervised exercise program utilizing moderate, violent, or specific regimens showed a distinct increase in aerobic metabolism in the outer part of the IVD anulus and the central portion of the nucleus pulposus, which resulted in a reduction of lactate concentration. The conclusion of their findings was that prolonged spinal movements effect positive nutritional variations and that these changes might be significant for human disc problems inasmuch as several studies have demonstrated nutritional similarities between the discs of humans and canines.

Drug Effects

Certain drugs and biologic deficiencies have been shown to have a harmful effect on articular cartilage. Injections of corticosteroids especially tend to soften and fibrillate articular cartilage. Midzone areas of cell degeneration, failure of chondrocyte proliferation, abnormal patterns of subchondral ossification, suppression of intracytoplasmic metabolic processes, and matrix weakening have been described by some researchers. Proteoglycan-deficient cartilage is more deformable, and the matrix is more permeable than usual under loading. It also fatigues earlier than normal under cyclic loading.

REFERENCES

1. Hakim NS, King AI: A three dimensional finite element dynamic response analysis of a vertebra with experimental verification. *Journal of Biomechanics* 12:277–292, 1979.
2. Steindler A: *Kinesiology of the Human Body*. Springfield, Ill, Charles C Thomas, 1973.
3. White AA, Panjabi MM: Spinal kinematics. In Goldstein M (ed): *The Research Status of Spinal Manipulative Therapy*. NINCDS Monograph No. 15, DHEW Publication No. (NIH) 76-998, Stock No. 017-049-00060-7, Washington, DC, U.S. Government Printing Office, 1975, pp 93–94.
4. Williams JGP, Sperryn PN: *Sports Medicine*, ed 2. Baltimore, Williams & Wilkins, 1976, pp 113–114.
5. Cochran GVB: *A Primer of Biomechanics*. New York, Churchill Livingstone, 1982, pp 9–10.
6. Cailliet R: *Soft Tissue Pain and Disability*. Philadelphia, F.A. Davis, p 10.
7. Gowitzke BA, Milner M: *Understanding the Scientific Basis of Human Movement*, ed 2. Baltimore, Williams & Wilkins, 1980, p 4.
8. Gonzna ER, Harrington IJ: *Biomechanics of Musculoskeletal Injury*. Baltimore, Williams & Wilkins, 1982, pp 31–32.
9. LeVeau B: *Williams and Lissner: Biomechanics of Human Motion*, ed 2. Philadelphia, W.B. Saunders, 1977, pp 159, 160, 223.
10. Dumbleton JH, Black J: Principles of mechanics. In Black J, Dumbleton JH (eds): *Clinical Biomechanics: Case History Approach*. New York, Churchill Livingstone, 1981, pp 374–376.
11. White AA, Panjabi MM: *Clinical Biomechanics of the Spine*. Philadelphia, J.B. Lippincott, 1978, pp 479, 489.
12. White AA, Panjabi MM: Spinal kinematics. In Goldstein M (ed): *The Research Status of Spinal Manipulative Therapy*. NINCDS Monograph No. 15, DHEW Publication No. (NIH) 76-998, Stock No. 017-049-00060-7, Washington, DC, U.S. Government Printing Office, 1975, pp 93–101.
13. White AA, Panjabi MM: *Clinical Biomechanics of the Spine*. Philadelphia, J.B. Lippincott, 1978, p 63.
14. Tyson HN: *Kinematics*. New York, John Wiley & Sons, 1966.
15. Frankel VH, Nordin M: *Basic Biomechanics of the Skeletal System*. Philadelphia, Lea & Febiger, 1980.
16. LeVeau B: *Williams and Lissner: Biomechanics of Human Motion*, ed 2. Philadelphia, W.B. Saunders, 1977, pp 4, 159, 223.
17. LeVeau B: *Williams and Lissner: Biomechanics of Human Motion*, ed 2. Philadelphia, W.B. Saunders, 1977, pp 159–160.
18. LeVeau B: *Williams and Lissner: Biomechanics of Human Motion*, ed 2. Philadelphia, W.B. Saunders, 1977, pp 10, 162.
19. Morehouse LE, Cooper JM: *Kinesiology*. St. Louis, C.V. Mosby, 1950, pp 122–123.
20. Barham JN, Wooten EP: *Structural Kinesiology*. New York, Macmillan, 1973, pp 98, 131.
21. Gowitzke BA, Milner M: *Understanding the Scientific Basis of Human Movement*, ed 2. Baltimore, Williams & Wilkins, 1980, p 46.
22. White AA, Panjabi MM: *Clinical Biomechanics of the Spine*. Philadelphia, J.B. Lippincott, 1978, pp 455–456.
23. Grieve DW: The assessment of gait. *Physiotherapy* 55:452–460, 1975.
24. Barham JN, Wooten EP: *Structural Kinesiology*. New York, Macmillan, 1973, p 99.
25. LeVeau B: *Williams and Lissner: Biomechanics of Human Motion*, ed 2. Philadelphia, W.B. Saunders, 1977, pp 165, 167.
26. White AA, Panjabi MM: *Clinical Biomechanics of the Spine*. Philadelphia, J.B. Lippincott, 1978, pp 456–457.
27. Barham JN, Wooten EP: *Structural Kinesiology*. New York, Macmillan, 1973, p 96.
28. LeVeau B: *Williams and Lissner: Biomechanics of Human Motion*, ed 2. Philadelphia, W.B. Saunders, 1977, pp 164, 165.
29. Barham JN, Wooten EP: *Structural Kinesiology*. New York, Macmillan, 1973, pp 95, 96–97.
30. Gowitzke BA, Milner M: *Understanding the Scientific Basis of Human Movement*, ed 2. Baltimore, Williams & Wilkins, 1980, p 45.
31. White AA, Panjabi MM: *Clinical Biomechanics of the Spine*. Philadelphia, J.B. Lippincott, 1978, pp 479–480.
32. Plagenhoef SC: Computer programs for obtaining kinetic data on human movement. *Journal of Biomechanics* 1:221–234, 1968.
33. Plagenhoef SC: *Patterns of Human Motion: A Cinematographical Analaysis*. Englewood Cliffs, NJ, Prentice-Hall, 1971.
34. Dilman CJ: A kinetic analysis of the recovery leg during sprint running. In Cooper JM (ed): *Selected Topics on Biomechanics*. Chicago, The Athletic Institute, 1971.
35. Carlsoo S: *How Man Moves*. London, William Heinemann, 1972.
36. Gowitzke BA, Milner M: *Understanding the Scientific Basis of Human Movement*, ed 2. Baltimore, Williams & Wilkins, 1980, p 152.
37. LeVeau B: *Williams and Lissner: Biomechanics of*

Human Motion, ed 2. Philadelphia, W.B. Saunders, 1977, p 206.
38. Gowitzke BA, Milner M: *Understanding the Scientific Basis of Human Movement*, ed 2. Baltimore, Williams & Wilkins, 1980, p 3.
39. Cochran GVB: *A Primer of Biomechanics*. New York, Churchill Livingstone, 1982, p 6.
40. Dumbleton JH, Black J: Principles of mechanics. In Black J, Dumbleton JH (eds): *Clinical Biomechanics: Case History Approach*. New York, Churchill Livingstone, 1981, pp 369–372.
41. Hatze H: A complete set of control equations for the human musculoskeletal system. *Journal of Biomechanics* 10:799–805, 1977.
42. Dempster WT: The anthropometry of body action. *Annals of the New York Academy of Science* 63:559–585, 1955.
43. Dempster WT: Free-body diagrams as an approach to the mechanics of human posture and locomotion. In Evans FG (ed): *Biomechanical Studies of the Musculoskeletal System*. Springfield, Ill, Charles C Thomas, 1961.
44. Clauser CE, McConville JT, Young JW: Weight, volume, and center of mass of segments of the human body. AMRL-TR-69-70, Wright-Patterson Air Force Base, Ohio, 1969.
45. Drillis R, Contini R: Body segment parameters. Technical Report 1166.03. New York, New York University, 1966.
46. Stish EE: Anthropokinetics. *Journal of Health, Physical Education, and Recreation* 35:33, November/December 1964.
47. Barham JN, Wooten EP: *Structural Kinesiology*. New York, Macmillan, 1973, pp 101–102.
48. Eberhart HD, Inman VT, Bresler B: The principal elements in human locomotion. In Klopsteg PE, Wilson PD (eds): *Human Limbs and Their Substitutes*. New York, McGraw-Hill, 1954.
49. Wartenweiler J, Wettstein A: Basic kinetic rules for simple human movements. In *Biomechanics II*. Medicine and Sports Series. Baltimore, University Park Press, 1971, pp 134–145.
50. LeVeau B: *Williams and Lissner: Biomechanics of Human Motion*, ed 2. Philadelphia, W.B. Saunders, 1977, p 172.
51. Morehouse LE, Cooper JM: *Kinesiology*. St. Louis, C.V. Mosby, 1950, p 120.
52. Gowitzke BA, Milner M: *Understanding the Scientific Basis of Human Movement*, ed 2. Baltimore, Williams & Wilkins, 1980, pp 65–66.
53. White AA, Panjabi MM: *Clinical Biomechanics of the Spine*. Philadelphia, J.B. Lippincott, 1978, pp 483–486.
54. Elftman H: The force exerted by the ground in walking. *American Journal of Physiology* 10:485–491, 1939.
55. Morehouse LE, Miller AT Jr: *Physiology of Exercise*. St. Louis, C.V. Mosby, 1948, p 225.
56. Paul JP: Bio-engineering studies of the forces transmitted by joints. In Kenedi RM (ed): *Biomechanics and Related Bio-engineering Topics*. Oxford, Pergamon, 1965, pp 351–357.
57. Gonzna ER, Harrington IJ: *Biomechanics of Musculoskeletal Injury*. Baltimore, Williams & Wilkins, 1982, pp 13, 120.
58. LeVeau B: *Williams and Lissner: Biomechanics of Human Motion*, ed 2. Philadelphia, W.B. Saunders, 1977, p 176.
59. Gowitzke BA, Milner M: *Understanding the Scientific Basis of Human Movement*, ed 2. Baltimore, Williams & Wilkins, 1980, p 78.
60. Dapena J: A method to determine the angular momentum of a human body about three orthogonal axes passing through its center of gravity. *Journal of Biomechanics* 11:251–256, 1978.
61. Gowitzke BA, Milner M: *Understanding the Scientific Basis of Human Movement*, ed 2. Baltimore, Williams & Wilkins, 1980, pp 78–80.
62. LeVeau B: *Williams and Lissner: Biomechanics of Human Motion*, ed 2. Philadelphia, W.B. Saunders, 1977, p 182.
63. Dumbleton JH, Black J: Principles of mechanics. In Black J, Dumbleton JH (eds): *Clinical Biomechanics: Case History Approach*. New York, Churchill Livingstone, 1981, pp 396–399.
64. LeVeau B: *Williams and Lissner: Biomechanics of Human Motion*, ed 2. Philadelphia, W.B. Saunders, 1977, pp 143–144.
65. Cochran GVB: *A Primer of Biomechanics*. New York, Churchill Livingstone, 1982, pp 128–131.
66. Gowitzke BA, Milner M: *Understanding the Scientific Basis of Human Movement*, ed 2. Baltimore, Williams & Wilkins, 1980, pp 80–81.
67. White AA, Panjabi MM: *Clinical Biomechanics of the Spine*. Philadelphia, J.B. Lippincott, 1978, p 462.
68. Barnett CH, Cobbold AF: Lubrication within living joints. *Journal of Bone and Joint Surgery* 44B:662–784, 1962.
69. Linn FC: Lubrication of animal joints. *Journal of Biomechanics* 1:193–205, 1968.
70. Jackson R: *The Cervical Syndrome*, ed 2. Springfield, Ill, Charles C Thomas, 1958.
71. Knocke FJ, Knocke LS: *Orthopaedic Nursing*. Philadelphia, F.A. Davis, 1945.
72. Markolf KL: Stiffness and damping characteristics of the thoracic-lumbar spine. *Proceedings: Workshop on Bioengineering Approaches to the Problems of the Spine*. National Institutes of Health, September 1970.
73. Travers PR, Campbell WR: The organism and speed and power. In Larson LA (ed): *Fitness, Health, and Work Capacity*. New York, Macmillan, 1974, pp 100–110.
74. Barham JN, Wooten EP: *Structural Kinesiology*. New York, Macmillan, 1973, pp 107–108.
75. Morehouse LE, Cooper JM: *Kinesiology*. St. Louis, C.V. Mosby, 1950, pp 196–204.
76. Richards JG, Cooper J: Implementation of an online isokinetic analysis system. *Journal of Orthopedics and Sports* 4:36–38, 1982.
77. Barham JN, Wooten EP: *Structural Kinesiology*. New York, Macmillan, 1973, pp 82, 85.
78. LeVeau B: *Williams and Lissner: Biomechanics of Human Motion*, ed 2. Philadelphia, W.B. Saunders, 1977, pp 184–185.
79. Morehouse LE, Cooper JM: *Kinesiology*. St. Louis, C.V. Mosby, 1950, p 115.
80. Barham JN, Wooten EP: *Structural Kinesiology*. New York, Macmillan, 1973, p 86.
81. LeVeau B: *Williams and Lissner: Biomechanics of*

Human Motion, ed 2. Philadelphia, W.B. Saunders, 1977, p 193.

82. Gowitzke BA, Milner M: *Understanding the Scientific Basis of Human Movement*, ed 2. Baltimore, Williams & Wilkins, 1980, pp 69–70.
83. Morehouse LE, Cooper JM: *Kinesiology*. St. Louis, C.V. Mosby, 1950, pp 101, 103.
84. Barham JN, Wooten EP: *Structural Kinesiology*. New York, Macmillan, 1973, pp 78–81.
85. LeVeau B: *Williams and Lissner: Biomechanics of Human Motion*, ed 2. Philadelphia, W.B. Saunders, 1977, pp 48, 50, 64.
86. Gowitzke BA, Milner M: *Understanding the Scientific Basis of Human Movement*, ed 2. Baltimore, Williams & Wilkins, 1980, pp 123–130.
87. Morehouse LE, Miller AT Jr: *Physiology of Exercise*. St. Louis, C.V. Mosby, 1948, pp 223–224.
88. Lipovetz FJ: *Medical Physical Education*, rev ed. Minneapolis, Burgess, 1946.
89. McCloy CH: Some notes of differential actions of partite muscles. *Research Quarterly, American Association of Health, Physical Education, and Recreation* 17:254, 1946.
90. Travers PR, Campbell WR: The organism and speed and power. In Larson LA (ed): *Fitness, Health, and Work Capacity*. New York, Macmillan, 1974, pp 99–100.
91. Elftman H: Biomechanics of muscle. *Journal of Bone and Joint Surgery* 48A:363–377, 1966.
92. Morehouse LE, Miller AT Jr: *Physiology of Exercise*. St. Louis, C.V. Mosby, 1948, pp 217–218.
93. Morehouse LE, Cooper JM: *Kinesiology*. St. Louis, C.V. Mosby, 1950, pp 189–191.
94. Barham JN, Wooten EP: *Structural Kinesiology*. New York, Macmillan, 1973, pp 108–111.
95. Gowitzke BA, Milner M: *Understanding the Scientific Basis of Human Movement*, ed 2. Baltimore, Williams & Wilkins, 1980, p 95.
96. Huxley AF, Niedergerke R: Structural changes in muscle during contraction; interference microscopy of living muscle fibers. *Nature* 173:971, 1954.
97. LeVeau B: *Williams and Lissner: Biomechanics of Human Motion*, ed 2. Philadelphia, W.B. Saunders, 1977, pp 23–24.
98. Hollingshead WH, Jenkins DB: *Functional Anatomy of the Limbs and Back*. Philadelphia, W.B. Saunders, 1981, pp 32–34.
99. Rosse C, Clawson DK: *The Musculoskeletal System in Health and Disease*. Hagerstown, Md, Harper & Row, 1980, pp 39–47, 51–52.
100. Henneman E, Olson CB: Relations between structure and function in the design of skeletal muscle. *Journal of Neurophysiology* 28:581, 1965.
101. Huxley HE: The mechanism of muscular contraction. *Science* 164:1356, 1969.
102. Morehouse LE, Cooper JM: *Kinesiology*. St. Louis, C.V. Mosby, 1950, pp 111–113, 188–189.
103. Gowitzke BA, Milner M: *Understanding the Scientific Basis of Human Movement*, ed 2. Baltimore, Williams & Wilkins, 1980, p 115.
104. Walker SM, Schrodt GR: Contraction of skeletal muscle. *American Journal of Physical Medicine* 46:151, 1967.
105. Jordan HE: The structural changes in striped muscle during contraction. *Physiology Review* 13:301, 1933.
106. Lupton H: An analysis of the effects of speed on the mechanical efficiency of human muscular movement. *Journal of Physiology* 57:337, 1923.
107. Gowitzke BA, Milner M: *Understanding the Scientific Basis of Human Movement*, ed 2. Baltimore, Williams & Wilkins, 1980, pp 97–102.
108. Barham JN, Wooten EP: *Structural Kinesiology*. New York, Macmillan, 1973, pp 90–91.
109. Gowitzke BA, Milner M: *Understanding the Scientific Basis of Human Movement*, ed 2. Baltimore, Williams & Wilkins, 1980, pp 61–65, 117–118.
110. LeVeau B: *Williams and Lissner: Biomechanics of Human Motion*, ed 2. Philadelphia, W.B. Saunders, 1977, pp 22, 23.
111. Morehouse LE, Cooper JM: *Kinesiology*. St. Louis, C.V. Mosby, 1950, pp 113–114.
112. Rosse C, Clawson DK: *The Musculoskeletal System in Health and Disease*. Hagerstown, Md, Harper & Row, 1980, p 57.
113. Gowitzke BA, Milner M: *Understanding the Scientific Basis of Human Movement*, ed 2. Baltimore, Williams & Wilkins, 1980, pp 109–112.
114. Morehouse LE, Cooper JM: *Kinesiology*. St. Louis, C.V. Mosby, 1950, pp 114–115.
115. Rosse C, Clawson DK: *The Musculoskeletal System in Health and Disease*. Hagerstown, Md, Harper & Row, 1980, pp 57–58.
116. Morehouse LE, Miller AT Jr: *Physiology of Exercise*. St. Louis, C.V. Mosby, 1948, pp 225–226.
117. Morehouse LE, Cooper JM: *Kinesiology*. St. Louis, C.V. Mosby, 1950, p 193.
118. Williams JGP, Sperryn PN: *Sports Medicine*, ed 2. Baltimore, Williams & Wilkins, 1976, pp 109–110.
119. Tanner JM: *The Physique of the Olympic Athlete*. London, George Allen and Unwin, 1964.
120. Williams JGP, Sperryn PN: *Sports Medicine*, ed 2. Baltimore, Williams & Wilkins, 1976, pp 9, 23, 145.
121. De Garay A, Carter L: *Genetic and Anthropological Studies of Olympic Athletes*. New York, Academic Press, 1974.
122. Hollinshead WH, Jenkins DB: *Functional Anatomy of the Limbs and Back*. Philadelphia, W.B. Saunders, 1981, p 35.
123. Schafer RC: *Chiropractic Management of Sports and Recreational Injuries*. Baltimore, Williams & Wilkins, 1982, p 101.
124. Salter RB: *Textbook of Disorders and Injuries of the Musculoskeletal System*. Baltimore, Williams & Wilkins, 1981, p 396.
125. Rosse C, Clawson DK: *The Musculoskeletal System in Health and Disease*. Hagerstown, Md, Harper & Row, 1980, p 88.
126. Barham JN, Wooten EP: *Structural Kinesiology*. New York, Macmillan, 1973, pp 119–121.
127. Gonzna ER, Harrington IJ: *Biomechanics of Musculoskeletal Injury*. Baltimore, Williams & Wilkins, 1982, p 32.
128. Dumbleton JH, Black J: Principles of mechanics. In Black J, Dumbleton JH (eds): *Clinical Biomechanics: Case History Approach*. New York, Churchill Livingstone, 1981, pp 382–385.

129. Evans FG: *Stress and Strain in Bones*. Springfield, Ill, Charles C Thomas, 1957.
130. White AA, Panjabi MM: *Clinical Biomechanics of the Spine*. Philadelphia, J.B. Lippincott, 1978, pp 496–497, 500–501.
131. Gonzna ER, Harrington IJ: *Biomechanics of Musculoskeletal Injury*. Baltimore, Williams & Wilkins, 1982, pp 41, 120, 171.
132. LeVeau B: *Williams and Lissner: Biomechanics of Human Motion*, ed 2. Philadelphia, W.B. Saunders, 1977, pp 4, 223.
133. Cochran GVB: *A Primer of Biomechanics*. New York, Churchill Livingstone, 1982, pp 30–38.
134. Gonzna ER, Harrington IJ: *Biomechanics of Musculoskeletal Injury*. Baltimore, Williams & Wilkins, 1982, p 120.
135. Cochran GVB: *A Primer of Biomechanics*. New York, Churchill Livingstone, 1982, pp 27–30.
136. Frankel VH, Nordin M: *Basic Biomechanics of the Skeletal System*. Philadelphia, Lea & Febiger, 1980.
137. White AA, Panjabi MM: *Clinical Biomechanics of the Spine*. Philadelphia, J.B. Lippincott, 1978, pp 470–472, 475, 484, 498–499, 507, 513.
138. Panjabi MM, Krag MH, Goel VK: A technique for measurement and description of three-dimensional six degree-of-freedom motion of a body joint with an application to the human spine. *Journal of Biomechanics* 14:447–460, 1981.
139. Cochran GVB: *A Primer of Biomechanics*. New York, Churchill Livingstone, 1982, pp 76–78, 131–132.
140. Black J, Dumbleton JH (eds): *Clinical Biomechanics: Case History Approach*. New York, Churchill Livingstone, 1981, pp 18–19, 21, 387, 388.
141. Cochran GVB: *A Primer of Biomechanics*. New York, Churchill Livingstone, 1982, pp 73–75, 84–85.
142. Dumbleton JH, Black J: Principles of mechanics. In Black J, Dumbleton JH (eds): *Clinical Biomechanics: Case History Approach*. New York, Churchill Livingstone, 1981, p 393.
143. Cochran GVB: *A Primer of Biomechanics*. New York, Churchill Livingstone, 1982, pp 84, 147.
144. White AA, Panjabi MM: *Clinical Biomechanics of the Spine*. Philadelphia, J.B. Lippincott, 1978, pp 212, 456, 469–470, 490, 514, 515.
145. Cochran GVB: *A Primer of Biomechanics*. New York, Churchill Livingstone, 1982, pp 75–76, 158–159, 192.
146. Burstein AH et al: The ultimate properties of bone tissue: The effects of yielding. *Journal of Biomechanics* 5:35, 1972.
147. Cochran GVB: *A Primer of Biomechanics*. New York, Churchill Livingstone, 1982, pp 87, 91–96.
148. White AA, Panjabi MM: *Clinical Biomechanics of the Spine*. Philadelphia, J.B. Lippincott, 1978, pp 347–348, 352, 478, 511–513.
149. Twomey L, Taylor J: Flexion creep deformation and hysteresis in the lumbar vertebral column. *Spine* 7:116–122, 1982.
150. Cochran GVB: *A Primer of Biomechanics*. New York, Churchill Livingtone, 1982, pp 89–90, 170–172.
151. White AA, Panjabi MM: *Clinical Biomechanics of the Spine*. Philadelphia, J.B. Lippincott, 1978, pp 474–475.
152. Rosse C, Clawson DK: *The Musculoskeletal System in Health and Disease*. Hagerstown, Md, Harper & Row, 1980, pp 80–81, 82.
153. Salter RB: *Textbook of Disorders and Injuries of the Musculoskeletal System*. Baltimore, Williams & Wilkins, 1981, pp 22–23, 194.
154. Goldie IF, Dumbleton JH: Intertrochanteric osteotomy of the femur. In Black J, Dumbleton JH (eds): *Clinical Biomechanics: Case History Approach*. New York, Churchill Livingstone, 1981, pp 83, 84, 87.
155. Goldie IF, Dumbleton JH: Intertrochanteric osteotomy of the femur. In Black J, Dumbleton JH (eds): *Clinical Biomechanics: Case History Approach*. New York, Churchill Livingstone, 1981, p 83.
156. Edwards CC, Chrisman OD: Articular cartilage. In Albright JA, Brand RA (eds): *The Scientific Basis of Orthopaedics*. New York, Appleton-Century-Crofts, 1979, pp 329–330.
157. King AI, Vulcan P: Elastic deformation characteristics of the spine. *Proceedings: Workshop on Bioengineering Approaches to Problems of the Spine*. National Institutes of Health, September 1970, p 15.
158. Cochran GVB: *A Primer of Biomechanics*. New York, Churchill Livingstone, 1982, p 231.
159. Dumbleton JH, Black J: Principles of mechanics. In Black J, Dumbleton JH (eds): *Clinical Biomechanics: Case History Approach*. New York, Churchill Livingstone, 1981, pp 377–382, 388–389.
160. White AA, Panjabi MM: *Clinical Biomechanics of the Spine*. Philadelphia, J.B. Lippincott, 1978, p 468.
161. Cochran GVB: *A Primer of Biomechanics*. New York, Churchill Livingstone, 1982, pp 23, 26–27, 82, 190–193.
162. McElhaney JH: Dynamic response of bone and muscle tissue. *Journal of Applied Physiology* 21:231–236, 1966.
163. Gonzna ER, Harrington IJ: *Biomechanics of Musculoskeletal Injury*. Baltimore, Williams & Wilkins, 1982, pp 10, 32.
164. White AA, Panjabi MM: *Clinical Biomechanics of the Spine*. Philadelphia, J.B. Lippincott, 1978, p 470.
165. Sandover J: Dynamic loading as a possible source of low-back disorders. *Spine* 8:652–658, 1983.
166. Liu YK et al: Fatigue response of lumbar intervertebral joints under axial cyclic loading. *Spine* 8:857–865, 1983.
167. Adams MA, Hutton WC: The effect of fatigue on the lumbar intervertebral disc. *Journal of Bone and Joint Surgery* 65B:199–203, 1983.
168. Brand RA: Joint lubrication. In Albright JA, Brand RA (eds): *The Scientific Basis of Orthopaedics*. New York, Appleton-Century-Crofts, 1979, pp 349–363.
169. Cochran GVB: *A Primer of Biomechanics*. New York, Churchill Livingstone, 1982, pp 125, 133–138.
170. Rosse C, Clawson DK: *The Musculoskeletal Sys-*

tem in Health & Disease. Hagerstown, Md, Harper & Row, 1980, pp 87–88.

171. Wright V: *Lubrication and Wear in Joints*. Philadelphia, J.B. Lippincott, 1969.
172. Edwards CC, Chrisman OD: Articular cartilage. In Albright JA, Brand RA (eds): *The Scientific Basis of Orthopaedics*. New York, Appleton-Century-Crofts, 1979, pp 330–331.
173. Jones ED: Joint lubrication. *Lancet* 1:1426, 1934.
174. Gonzna ER, Harrington IJ: *Biomechanics of Musculoskeletal Injury*. Baltimore, Williams & Wilkins, 1982, pp 32–33.
175. Rybicki EF et al: Effects of cartilage stiffness and viscosity on a nonporous compliant bearing lubrication model for living joints. *Journal of Biomechanics* 12:403–409, 1979.
176. Edwards CC, Chrisman OD: Articular cartilage. In Albright JA, Brand RA (eds): *The Scientific Basis of Orthopaedics*. New York, Appleton-Century-Crofts, 1979, pp 319, 331, 334.
177. Turek SL: *Orthopaedics: Principles and Their Application*, ed 3. Philadelphia, J.B. Lippincott, 1977, pp17–19, 331–332, 347.
178. Cochran GVB: *A Primer of Biomechanics*. New York, Churchill Livingstone, 1982, pp 124–125.
179. Holm S, Nachemson A: Variations in the nutrition of the canine intervertebral disc induced. *Spine* 8:866–874, 1983.

Suggested Readings

Benedek GB, Villars FMH: *Physics*. Reading, Mass, Addison-Wesley, 1973, vol 1, Mechanics.

Halliday, D, Resnick R: *Fundamentals of Physics*. New York, John Wiley & Sons, 1974.

Kramer DJ: *Kinematics for the Handicapped*. New York, Exposition Press, 1973.

Metheny E: *Body Dynamics*. New York, McGraw-Hill, 1952.

Miller DI, Nelson RC; *Biomechanics of Sport*. Philadelphia, Lea & Febiger, 1973.

Miller F Jr: *College Physics*, ed 3. New York, Harcourt, Brace, Jovanovich, 1974.

Ralston HJ, Lukin L: Energy levels of human body segments. *Ergonomics* 12:39, 1969.

Ripley JA: *The Elements and Structure of the Physical Sciences*. New York, John Wiley & Sons, 1964.

Ruch TC, Patton HD: *Physiology and Biophysics*. Philadelphia, W.B. Saunders, 1974.

Schenck JM, Cordova FD: *Introductory Biomechanics*, ed 2. Philadelphia. F.A. Davis, 1980.

Straley JW: *Basic Physics*. Englewood Cliffs, NJ, Prentice-Hall, 1974.

Wells KF: *Kinesiology*, ed 5. Philadelphia, W.B. Saunders, 1971.

CHAPTER 4

Body Alignment, Posture, and Gait

With the background material offered in the basic principles of the musculoskeletal system, statics, dynamics, and joint stability, this chapter discusses how these factors are exhibited in body alignment and posture during static and dynamic positions.

GRAVITATIONAL EFFECTS[1–4]

Improper body alignment limits function, and thus it is a concern of everyone, regardless of occupation, activities, environment, body type, sex, or age. To effectively overcome postural problems, therapy must be based upon mechanical principles. In the absence of gross pathology, postural alignment is a homeostatic mechanism that can be voluntarily controlled to a significant extent by osseous adjustments, direct and reflex muscle techniques, support when advisable, therapeutic exercise, and kinesthetic training.

Gross Posture Analysis[5–12]

It has long been felt in chiropractic that spinal subluxations will be reflected in the erect posture and that spinal distortions result in the development of subluxation syndromes. Consequently, an array of different methods and instrumentations has been developed for this type of analytical approach, such as plumb lines with foot positioning plates to allow for visual evaluation relative to gravitational norms, transparent grids, bubble levels, silhouettographs, posturometer devices to measure specific degrees in attitude, multiple scale units to measure the weight of each vertical half or quadrant of the body, electromyography, and moire contourography.[13–15]

Objectives

Such procedures yield useful information; however, there is a great deal of possible subjective error in the interpretation of findings. Nevertheless, recorded analyses of body alignment serve as a guide to a patient's holistic attitude, structural balance or imbalance, hypertonicity, need for therapeutic exercises, habitual stance, postural fatigue, and basic nutritional status, and they offer a comparative progress record.[16]

Eye Dominance

One source of analytical error that can be easily corrected is that of eye dominance. It is important to realize that the examiner's peripheral vision is used for judging the body bilaterally. This is true in posture analysis as well as in the physical examination when, for instance, bilateral motion of the rib cage is assessed. If the examiner has a dominant eye, the reclining patient should be observed with the dominant eye over the midline of the patient's body.[17]

Test. An examiner may determine eye dominance by the following procedure: (1) Hold the index finger of the right hand at arm's length directly in front of the nose at the level of the eyes. (2) Place the tips of the left index finger and thumb to form a circle. (3) Place this circle directly in front of the nose about elbow distance away. (4) Sight the tip of the right index finger in the center of the circle using both eyes. (5) Close the left eye to see if the right index finger stays in the center of the circle. If it does, the right eye is dominant. (6) Close the right eye to see if the right index finger stays in the center of the circle. If it does, the left eye is dominant.

Inspection[18–23]

Have the patient stand with his heels together, with his hands hanging normally at his sides. Encourage the patient to stand normally and not to try to assume "good posture" or the "military stance." Note body type and then the following checkpoints relative to a lateral plumb line falling just anterior to the external malleolus (Fig. 4.1) and an anterior or posterior vertical line bisecting the heels.[24]

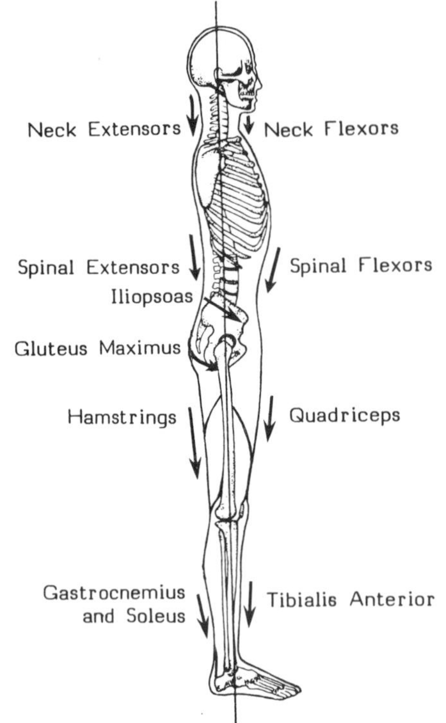

Figure 4.1. The major antigravity muscles that maintain the erect position.

Head and Neck. From the side, forward or backward shifting of body weight (not normal sway) can be judged by the position of the line from the ear. From the rear, note the position of the patient's head by comparative ear level. If the head is tilted to the right, the chin will tilt to the left. Note the bilateral development of the sternocleidomastoideus and suboccipital muscles. Asymmetrical fullness of the suboccipital musculature indicates upper cervical rotation.

Shoulder Girdle. From the side, note the prominence, rotation, or tilting of the inferior angles of the scapulae. From the rear, observe the comparative height of the scapulae, comparing one to the other. The cervicobrachial spine is always scoliotic toward the side of the high shoulder. Check for winged scapulae or for scapulae failing to lie smoothly on the chest wall. Note the distance of the scapulae vertebral borders from the spine. The midthoracic spine is always scoliotic toward the side on which the vertebral margin of the scapula is more prominent and flaring. If the shoulder is high on the right and the scapula flares on the right, the entire cervicobrachial and thoracic spine is scoliotic toward the right. If the shoulder is high on the right yet the left scapula flares, the cervicobrachial spine is scoliotic to the right and the midthoracic spine is scoliotic to the left.[25,26]

Thorax. From the front, observe any signs of hollow chest, sternal or rib depression, or pathologic signs such as Harrison's groove, funnel chest, barrel chest, or pigeon chest. From the rear, note the contours of the trapezius muscles for normal development or for abnormal tightness or tenderness. Note the angles of the ribs. A difference in the height of the scapulae and the iliac crests usually indicates a scoliosis. Lateral positions of the spinous processes and anterior or posterior positions of the transverse processes together with an elevation of the angles of the ribs indicate a rotation of vertebrae.

Abdomen. From the side, check the degree of abdominal muscle relaxation. Keep in mind that children normally have a prominent abdomen and adult women have a deposit of superficial fat lying transversely below the umbilicus.

Spine. From the side, check the curvatures of the spine. Evaluate as normal or abnormal, lordotic or kyphotic. Note the degree of sacral tilt and lumbosacral angle. From the rear, compare the line of the spinous processes. Bear in mind the possibility of a spinous process being asymmetrical, deviated to the right or left, without the body of the vertebra being involved. Evaluate any degree of scoliosis.[27,28]

Pelvis. In pelvic mechanical pathologies on the side of involvement, there is a reduction in the height and depth of the body angle as observed from the posterior. A low and less prominent iliac crest will be best observed from the front. Note the comparative height of the iliac crests and greater trochanters. Check the comparative height and depth of the sacral dimples, the position of the gluteal cleft, and the bilateral buttock height. If chronic sciatic neuralgia is on the high iliac crest side, degenerative disc weakening with posterolateral protrusion should be suspected. If it occurs on the side of the low iliac crest, one must consider the possibility of a sacroiliac slip and lumbosacral torsion as the causative factor.

Legs. From the side, note the degree of knee hyperextension. From the front, check for any degree of genu valgum or genu varum by the space between the knees. Seek possible tibial torsion or lateral rotation of the tibia (usually unilateral) by noting the position of the patellae.[29]

Feet. From the rear, note the degree of foot pronation by the line of the Achilles tendon. From the front, check for flattening of the longitudinal arch by noting the position of the navicular tubercles. Seek evidence of hallux valgus or hammer toes.

Postural Changes during Growth[30–34]

Spinal contour changes drastically during the various stages of maturation. As space becomes limited during the second half of prenatal life, the uterine walls act as restricting barriers to fetal extension To adapt, the fetus adopts a position of flexion for maximum comfort. This results in a gently kyphotic spinal curve which extends from the atlas to the sacrum (Fig. 4.2).

From Birth to 1 Year of Age

In the newborn, the spine remains "C" curved; throughout the first year of life, flexor tone is predominant in the extremities in the horizontal position. The first attempt to defy gravity occurs when the baby tries to raise his head in the prone position.[35] This usually becomes successful at about 3 months of age. The first anteroposterior (A-P) curve develops in the neck as the head is held erect and strength for cervical extension develops (Table 4.1). The ability to roll from prone to supine is usually established by 5 months, and from supine to prone at 6 months. The typical child is able to sit unsupported for the first time between 6 and 8 months. Straightening of the thoracic spine occurs when sitting can be maintained, and the normal lumbar lordosis begins to develop parallel with the ability to walk without assistance at about 13 months.[36]

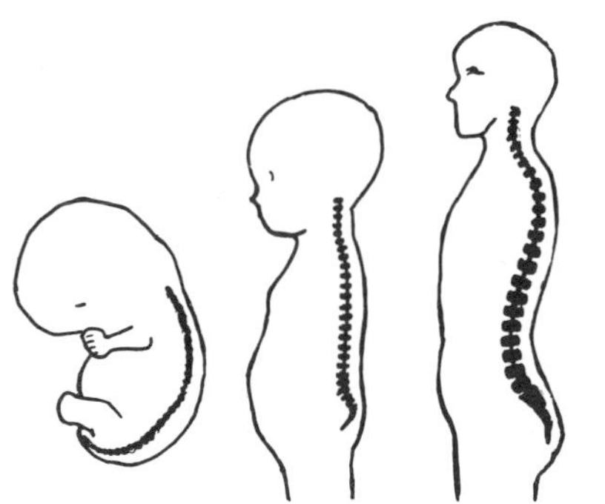

Figure 4.2. Variations of the spinal curve at different age levels from embryo, to infant, to adult.

Between 1 and 2 Years of Age

During the second year of life, the child learns to stand upright and to balance both A-P and laterally. For stability, he stands and walks with a wide stance to widen the base of support. This is enhanced by diapers, which increase the distance between the upper thighs. During early totter when walking is insteady, the child leans forward to help forward progression, the legs are partly flexed, and the arms are abducted and slightly flexed at the elbows similar to unfolded wings. By the end of the second year, postural reflexes are well established, allowing for greater skill in propulsion and

Table 4.1.
Developmental Progress

Skill	Average age
Head up, prone	3.2 mo
Puts hands together	3.7 mo
Grasps small objects	4.1 mo
Sits, head steady	4.2 mo
Arm support	4.3 mo
Rolls over	4.7 mo
Reaches for objects	5.0 mo
Bears some weight on legs	6.3 mo
Accepts objects in hands	7.5 mo
Pulls to sitting position	7.7 mo
Sits without support	7.8 mo
Resists toy pull	10.0 mo
Pulls to standing position	10.1 mo
Thumb-finger grasp	10.6 mo
Stands briefly, no support	13.0 mo
Walks forward	13.3 mo
Walks backward	21.5 mo
Kicks ball	2.0 yr
Throws ball	2.6 yr
Rides tricycle	3.0 yr
Hops on one foot	4.9 yr
Catches ball	5.5 yr

This list shows selected normal motor skills at average ages from 3–65 months.

balancing in the erect position. At this age, the legs will be held closer together, but there will still be a degree of flatfootedness, a prominent abdomen, and an exaggerated lordosis.

Between 2 and 6 Years of Age

Between the ages of 2 and 6 years, the necessity for lateral balance is maintained by torsion of the tibia. This is exhibited by a degree of knock-knees which should correct itself by the age of 6 years. The abdomen becomes less prominent and the foot develops a longitudinal arch. Height increases steadily, but at a constant rate. During the early years of school, the child's posture is one of extreme mobility. The knees may show distinct hyperextension in standing, the pelvis is tilted downward and forward 30–40°, the abdomen protrudes, the lumbar area is usually lordotic, but may lean back sharply from the lumbosacral area, the scapulae are braced back by the trapezius muscles, often winged, the dorsal area is mildly kyphotic, and the buttocks protrude. A mild "sway-back" condition during this developmental stage should not be confused with a developmental defect.

Early Locomotion

Bipedal locomotion appears to be a learned skill rather than an inherited reflex. According to Inman and co-workers a child that is blind at birth never attempts to stand or walk unless carefully trained to do so.[37] Without assistance, such a child will travel as a quadriped, coordinating his or her four limbs so that three limbs are on the floor at the same time to offer the stability of a tripod. Thus, walking upright can be considered a trial-and-error translational learning process. This translation is the product of measurable angular displacements of body segments about joint axes.

The characteristic walking pattern of the adult is not acquired until the child is about 7–9 years of age. Prior to this, the child conducts progressively more difficult neuromusculoskeletal experiments that tend to improve neural control of motor skills that help to modify segmental displacements.

Puberty

Prior to puberty, the limbs grow faster than the trunk. The rate of trunk and extremity growth is about the same at puberty. The trunk continues to grow after the extremities slow their rate of growth in the postpuberty period.[38] This changes the ratio of sitting to standing height. Sitting height is about 70% of total height at birth and about 52% for 16-year-old girls and 14-year-old boys. Thus, postural adjustments must be made during the growth period to adapt to gravitational forces (Figs. 4.3 and 4.4).

Adolescence

During the adolescent spurt of growth, changes in body proportions occur to adjust to gravity. The pelvic tilt decreases to 20–30°. The knees are slightly bent, but the earlier hyperextension is not necessary to balance a prominent abdomen. Posture becomes less mobile, and the postural patterns become stabilized. If proper adaptive mechanisms fail, an adolescent "round shoulders" condition may be present with a neck projected forward and a head that is extended.

Gravitational Forces[39–44]

The success that a person has in meeting the constant stress of gravity may have a

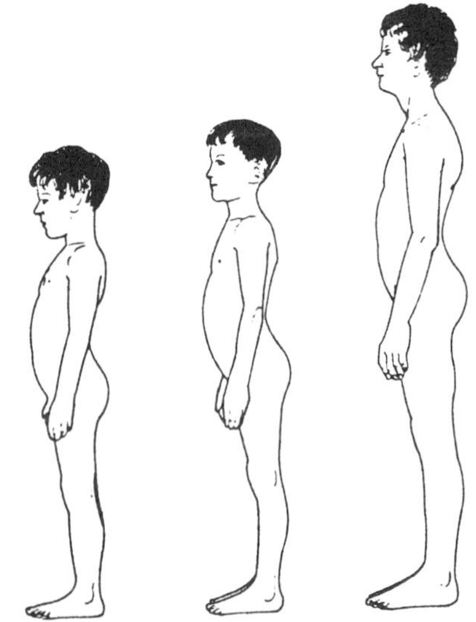

Figure 4.3. Typical postures of boys during the primary school period. *Left*, age 7, pelvic tilt 34°; *center*, age 8, pelvic tilt 35°; *right*, age 12, pelvic tilt 39°.

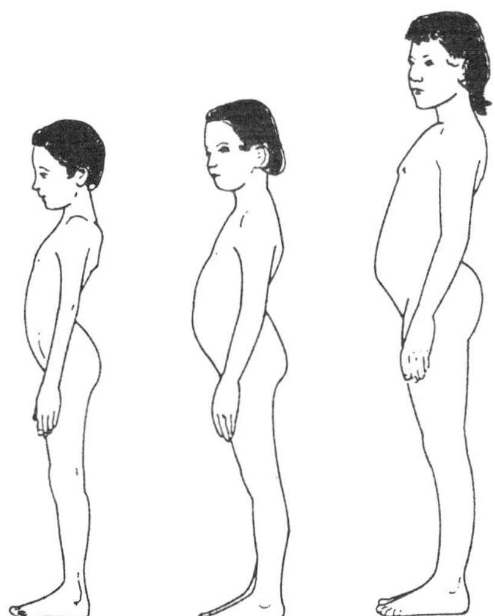

Figure 4.4. Typical postures of girls during the primary school period. *Left*, age 7, pelvic tilt 40°; *center*, age 8, pelvic tilt 35°; *right*, age 12, pelvic tilt 36°.

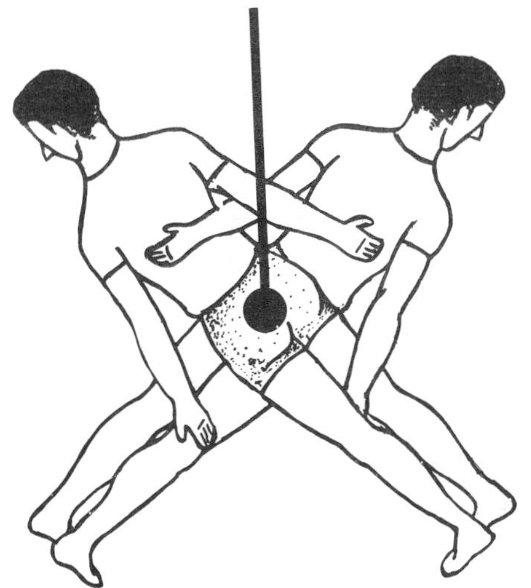

Figure 4.5. If the body could be suspended from its exact center of gravity, it could be oriented in any direction.

subtle yet profound influence on his or her quality of health and performance. While gravity stabilizes the lower extremities in standing and provides friction for locomotion, it also places considerable stress on those body parts responsible for maintaining the upright position. Without appropriate neuromusculoskeletal compensation and accommodation, such actions result in imbalance and often falling. Thus, postural deviations resulting in balance problems lead to frequent strain and injury to antigravity structures.

Center of Gravity[45–49]

As gravity acts on all parts of the body, one's entire weight can be considered as concentrated at a point where the gravitational pull on one side of the body is equal to the pull on the other side. This point is the body's *center of gravity*, and it constitutes the exact center of body mass[50] (Fig. 4.5). When the center of gravity is above the base of support and the pull of gravity is successfully resisted by the supporting members, an equilibrium of forces or a state of balance is reached and no motion occurs.

In a model subject, the center of gravity is located in the region just anterior (about 1½″) to the top of the second sacral segment; ie, about 55% of the distance for women, and 57% for men, from the plantar surfaces to the apex of the head in the erect position.[51] Its location will vary somewhat according to body type, age, and sex, and move upward, downward, or sideward in accordance with normal position movements and abnormal neuromusculoskeletal disorders.

The accumulation of fat and the loss of soft tissue tone are common factors in altering one's center of gravity. Thus, the center of gravity shifts with each change in body alignment, and the amount of weight borne by the joints and the pull of the muscles varies within reasonable limits with each body movement. Adequate compensation is provided for in the healthy, structurally balanced person.

Line of Gravity[52–57]

Reference Points. The vertical *A-P line of gravity* of the body, as viewed laterally in the erect model subject, falls from above downward through the earlobe, slightly posterior to the mastoid process, through the odontoid process, through the middle of the shoulder joint, touches the midpoint of the anterior borders of T2 and T12, then falls just slightly anterior to S2, slightly behind the axis of the hip joint, slightly anterior to the transverse axis of rotation of the knee (slightly posterior to the patella), crosses anterior to the lateral malleolus and through the cuboid-calcaneal junction to fall between the heel and metatarsal heads. When viewed from the back, the *lateral line of gravity* passes through the occipital protuberance, the C7 and L5 spinous processes, the coccyx and pubic cartilage, and bisects the knees and ankles. Thus, the A-P and lateral lines of gravity divide the body into four quarters (Fig. 4.6).

Plumb Line Analysis. The plumb line, as used in postural analysis, serves as a visual comparison to the line of gravity. For example, when the plumb line is centered over S1, it should fall in line with the occipital protuberance. In uncompensated scoliosis, however, it will be seen to fall lateral to the occipital protuberance.[44,58]

Weight Bearing. The most economical use of energy in the standing position is when the vertical line of gravity falls through a column of supporting bones. If the weight-bearing bony segments are aligned so that the gravity line passes directly through the center of each joint, the least stress is placed upon the adjacent ligaments and muscles. This is the ideal situation, but it is impossible in the human body because the centers of segmental links and the movement centers between them cannot be brought to accurately meet with a common line of gravity.[59]

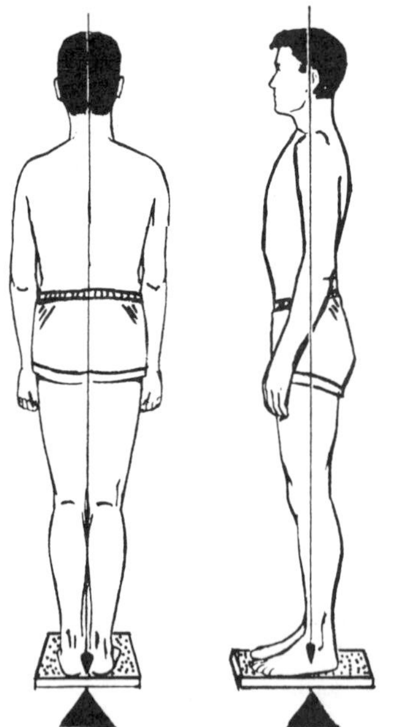

Figure 4.6. *Left*, lateral gravity line; *right*, anterior-posterior gravity line.

Stability. Because the body is a segmented system, the stability of the body depends upon the stability of its individual segments. The force of gravity acting upon each segment must be individually neutralized if the body as a whole is to be in complete gravitational balance. That part of balance contributed by an individual segment is called the segment's *partial equilibrium*, in contrast to the total equilibrium of the whole body. Thus, each segment has its own partial center of gravity and partial gravity line.

Position Changes. Any change in position of a partial center of gravity produces a corresponding change in the common center of gravity. When the arms are raised overhead and lowered, the center of gravity is respectively raised and lowered within the body. When the arms are stretched forward or backward, the center of gravity is respectively moved anteriorly or posteriorly within the body. When the trunk is flexed severely forward or laterally, the center of gravity shifts outside the body.

Body Balance and Equilibrium[60–63]

Active and Passive States. Positions of the body that require muscular forces to maintain balance are said to be in *active equilibrium*, while those that do not require muscular effort are in *passive equilibrium*. In passive equilibrium, all segmental centers of gravity and the centers of all joints fall within the gravity line of the body which must fall within the base of support. This requires complete neutralization of all linear and rotary components of gravitational force by joint surfaces and the base of support. Thus, such a state is impossible in the erect position but possible in the horizontal position.

Balance. When the forces of gravity on a body are in a balanced position, the pull is equal on all sides about the center of gravity; ie, its center of gravity is directly above its base of support and the body is quite stable (Fig. 4.7). The amount of body mass outside this base does not affect the equilibrium unless the center of gravity of the mass is altered. If a part is laterally shifted to one side without a compensatory

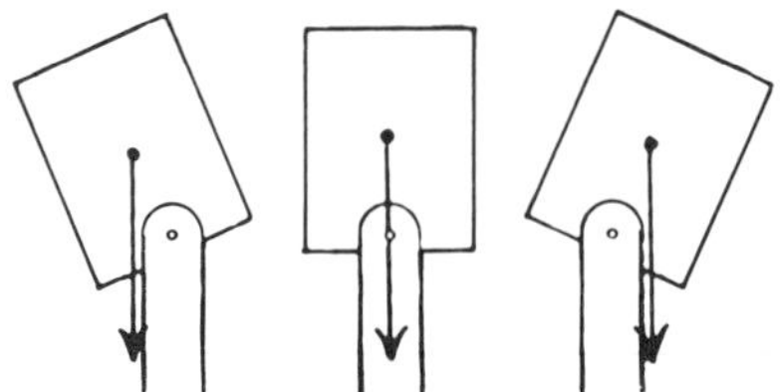

Figure 4.7. Optimal body balance is achieved as in the mechanical object in the *center*, with its center of gravity directly over its base of support.

shift of another part of equal weight, the center of gravity is displaced sideward. The body will topple if the center of gravity is displaced outside its base of support because gravity pulls greater on the side of weight displacement.[64] Because males generally have a larger thorax, broader shoulders, and heavier arms than females, they are toppled with less force than are females of the same size.

Common Torques. In the body, all partial centers of gravity or their axes of motion do not coincide with the common line of gravity. In fact, many partial centers are quite distant from the common line, and this causes active rotary torques in many joints because of gravitational pull which must be neutralized by antigravity muscles. A weight-bearing joint is considered to be in equilibrium if the gravity line of the supported structure is equal to the joint's axis of rotation. If the gravity line is posterior to the joint's axis of rotation, the superior segment tends to rotate posteriorly in compensation. If it is anterior to the axis, the superior segment tends to rotate anteriorly.[65, 66]

Toppling Rate. The rate of movement of an unbalanced body that is toppling depends on the amount of lateral displacement of the center of gravity from its base of support. For this reason, a toppled tree falls slowly at first because of trunk resistance and then rapidly as its center of gravity is further displaced from the tree trunk. A tall person falls harder than a short person. For the same reason, the further the body's center of gravity is displaced from the midline of its base of support, the more force is necessary to return it to the balanced position.

Action Lines

Segmental weight offers resistance to movement because gravity is acting on the part only in a downward direction with the part's mass acting as if it were at its center of mass (Fig. 4.8). The effectiveness of this weight for rotating a part can be changed by shifting its position in relation to the fulcrum, because the farther the gravity line falling through the center of mass is from the axis of motion, the longer will be the moment arm and the greater will be the moment.

During motion, the gravitational action line of a part can be moved near to or away from the axis of a joint simply by changing the part's position. For example, it is easier to raise a flexed leg in the horizontal position than a straight leg. This flexion does not change the limb's weight. The straight knee increases the moment of the gravita-

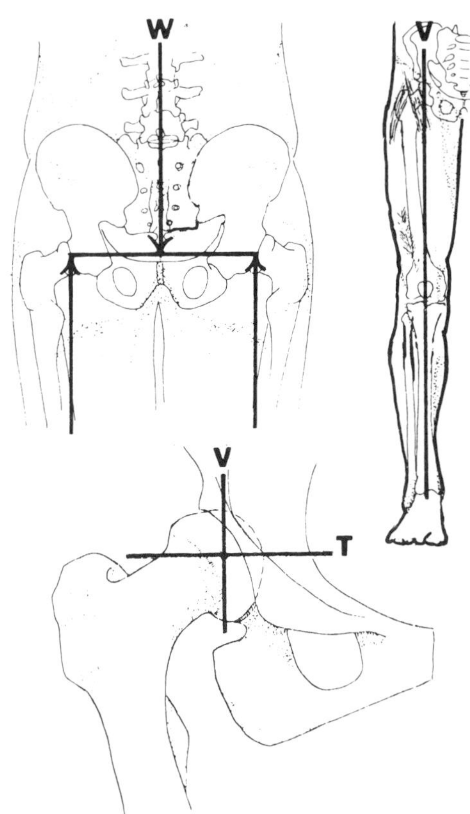

Figure 4.8. *Top left*, schematic of the static weight forces (*W*) that act on the femoral heads during bilateral stance. *Top right*, vertical axis (*V*) for movement, from the hip through the lower tibia. *Bottom*, transverse (*T*) axis at the hip for thigh flexion and extension, and vertical (*V*) axis at the hip for abduction and adduction.

tional force because the distance from the action line of the gravitational force on the hip has been shortened. For the same reason, it is much easier to do situps with the hands at the sides than when the hands are extended overhead.

Clinical Applications. These principles are commonly applied in therapeutic exercises. They are also applied in muscle testing and muscle stretching procedures. In muscle testing, resistance applied at the most distal aspect of the segment gives the resistance force a better lever arm and greater advantage than one applied more proximally. In muscle stretching, a much more proximal grip should be taken. This reduces the chance of joint or soft-tissue injury and affords better control of the movement.

Stabilization Mechanisms[67–70]

Electromyograph studies have shown that very little muscle activity is required in the normal relaxed standing position. Most action involves those muscles that act around the ankle. The minimal activity necessary is attributed to the elastic properties of muscle, joint locking, and the tension from the passive stretch of muscles, ligaments, and fascia which act prior to muscle contraction of joint stabilizers.[71–74]

The body's stability is greatest when its center of gravity is low and its base of support is wide. Knee and hip joints are fully extended during weight bearing, and the knee joint "screws home" by slightly rotating on the fully extended joint to provide firm joint locking.

Position of the Center of Gravity

The closer the body's center of gravity to its base of support the more stable it is: resisting moment = weight × distance. That is, the stability of an object is indirectly proportional to the height of its center of mass above its base. For example, a book laid flat upon a table is difficult to upset compared to one standing on a narrow end.

Size of the Base of Support[75, 76]

Both the size and position of the base of support are important in maintaining equilibrium. Regardless of toe position in the standing position, stability is provided if the gravity line falls approximately midway along the base of support. That is, the body is stable until the center of gravity falls perpendicularly outside the base of support. The larger the base of support, the greater the displacement of the center of gravity from a midpoint before balance is lost. The use of a cane or crutches increases stability because they provide an increased base of support.

Stance and Stability. The erect body is a poorly engineered model from a strict biomechanical viewpoint because the heavier portions are placed upon a narrow base of support, similar to an inverted cone. Obviously, this position is far less stable than that of the four-legged vertebrates. When the feet are parallel and close together, the upright body is least stable. When a chiropractor delivers an adjustment, a wide stance enhances his stability to the resistance force. Likewise, balance is maintained during reaching and stooping when one foot is advanced to the other. When standing on a ship deck or moving bus, stability is improved by widening the stance. Thus, during stance and locomotion, stability varies greatly as the feet are placed close together, further apart, or at an angle to each other to increase or decrease the size of the base of support.

Segmental Bases. Each segment in an articulated system rests upon the one beneath it. The interposed joint surfaces serve as the support base of the separate segments. From this viewpoint, one can see that joint stability is partially dependent on (1) the size of the joint surfaces, (2) the height of the segmental centers of gravity above the joint surface, and (3) the horizontal distance of the common gravity line to the joint's center.[77]

Head Weight. The head has a small base of support, ie, the atlas. In the erect position, the relatively small atlas must provide an upward push equal to the weight of the head plus added weight such as that of a hat, helmet, glasses, etc. In a 200-lb person, the atlas offers about a 14-lb resistance force to the skull[78] (Fig. 4.9). When the occiput is tilted so that its center of mass is not in line with both atlantal articulations, cervical muscles opposite to the direction of tilt must contract to maintain equilibrium. The muscles and ligaments at the base of

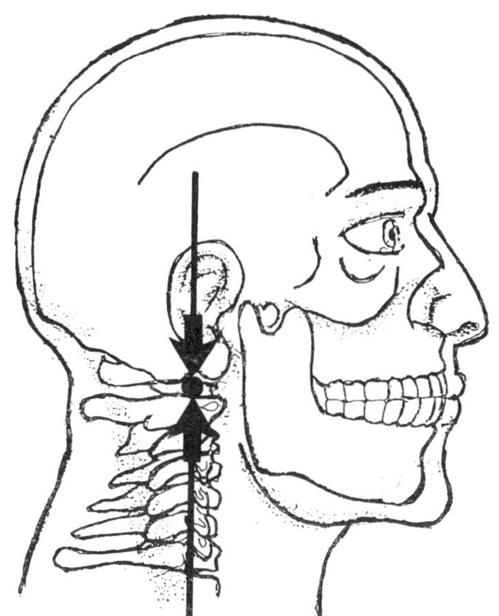

Figure 4.9. Schematic of forces established by the weight of the head upon the atlas.

the skull serve to check the compression and shear forces. When these mechanisms fail, a degree of subluxation must result. A similar situation occurs in the lower back where a great deal of weight is borne by the L5 vertebra.

Balance Sway[79, 80]

In most joints, the line of gravity is not identical to the center line of the joint; ie, most joint centers are some distance from the weight line. This requires constant muscle forces to combat rotational forces to maintain equilibrium by equalizing all translational and torque forces. Even when there is no movement, the antigravity muscles cannot be at rest. To maintain balance, the body is slightly but constantly swaying involuntarily anteroposteriorly, laterally, diagonally, and in rotation.

The body is always in motion. Minute oscillatory movements occur in all body parts, whether awake or asleep, and gross movements are not started until they are in phase with normal oscillations.[81, 82]

Control. The normal A-P sway of the body is controlled essentially by slight intermittent soleus and tibialis anterior action. The neuromechanisms are not completely understood, but one theory holds that body sway is under intermittent autonomic control: a geotropic reflex said by some to be initiated by position shifts that stretch antigravity muscles and stimulate tonic contractions to bring the joint toward balance.

Direction and Rates. Most sway occurs near the A-P plane. During A-P sway, weight is invariably anterior to the axis of hip, knee, and ankle. It is composed generally of slower and larger movements than other oscillations. In the average mature adult, it has about a 1⅝-inch range. Lateral sway has about a 1⅛-inch range. Body sway is generally to that degree sufficient to produce stimuli to evoke a righting reflex.

Shifting. During prolonged stance, normal body sway is altered. Weight is distributed symmetrically only 25% of the time, with a mean time factor of half a minute. This periodic shifting allows intermittent rest periods for the antigravity tissues. However, certain occupations and other physical attitudes may by necessity interfere with this shifting, and this may contribute to postural distortions.

Functional Effects. The frequent contraction and relaxation of the postural muscles during sway and minute weight shifting has a beneficial influence in milking blood and lymph through the muscles. In this manner, circulation is assisted. The working fibers are supplied with nutrients and are prevented from becoming choked by their own metabolic wastes.

The Alexander Technique[83–86]

F. M. Alexander, an Australian actor, made an important discovery about posture which was published in 1924. His findings were confirmed in 1926 by Professor Coighill of the Wistar Institute in London and in 1937 by Dr. Mungo Douglass in his text on anatomy. Sir Charles S. Sherrington, the Nobel prize–winning physiologist, praised Alexander for his discovery, as did educator John Dewey and Dr. Frank P. Jones, Research Associate at the Tuffs Institute for Psychological Research. Raymond A. Dart, Professor Emeritus of Anatomy and Dean Emeritus of a South African medical school, wrote a paper entitled "Anatomist's Tribute to F. Matthias Alexander." *The British Medical Journal* once published a letter endorsing the technique that was signed by 19 prominent physicians. In 1973, Professor

Nikolas Tinbergen of Oxford, upon receiving the Nobel prize for medicine, devoted half his acceptance speech to the technique.

Claims have been made that utilization of this technique keeps one feeling one's best, streamlines physical appearance, changes mental attitudes, cures neurotic tendencies, reduces periods of depression, reduces high blood pressure, helps symptoms of rheumatism and arthritis, aids the asthmatic, improves circulation and heart function, corrects fallen arches, reduces migraine attacks, improves digestion, corrects insominia, reduces stress, keeps one young, and much more.

It was Alexander's belief that the mind and body are inextricably bound together to form an inseparable whole: "A physical act is an affair not of this or that limb solely, but of the total neuromuscular activity of the moment." He showed that in every day physical acts, from the most trivial to the most strenuous, every motion begins with a slight motion at the base of the skull.

And what were Alexander's findings that have such a wide influence on health? It can be concisely stated: *As you begin any movement or act, move your head as a whole upward and away from your whole body, and let your whole body lengthen effortlessly by following that upward direction.* If this is done, ideal posture will be assumed in any position (Fig. 4.10). Alexander looked to the body segments as a train with the head as its engine. He felt the key postural reflex or major site of the kinesthetic sense was located at the atlanto-occipital area, the "crown of the senses." Undoubtedly, Alexander's findings had an influence on B. J. Palmer's emphasis on the upper cervical area.[87]

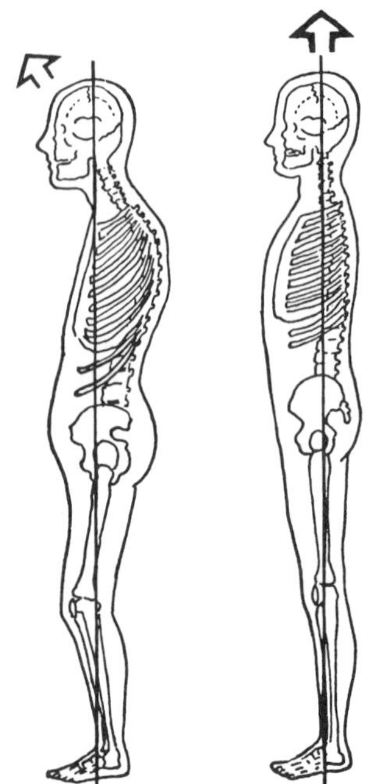

Figure 4.10. *Left*, poor posture from excessive sagging, producing joint centers out of alignment and resulting in increased muscle activity. *Right*, good postural alignment of body centers as the result of utilizing the Alexander technique.

The Perry Technique

Several variations of the Alexander technique have been developed that have the same or similar objective. For example, Perry, a chiropractor who has gained a wide reputation in treating Olympic and professional athletes, feels that poor running technique can be attributed to poor habits in posture and walking. One method that he uses to improve the technique of such athletes is through "imagery to improve posture." He instructs patients to close their eyes and imagine five helium-filled balloons attached to their body. A balloon is attached to the vertex of the head, to each pectoral muscle, and to the top of each side of the pelvis. As a reinforcement trigger, he asks patients to select their favorite color and every time they see that color, or any derivative of that color, to imagine the balloons inflating with gas.

> As a result, your pelvis starts to rise, your chest starts to lift, your neck elongates, you feel taller. As your pelvis lifts, your back will become less tense; as your chest rises, your shoulders and upper back relax; as your head lifts, the back of your neck relaxes.[88]

STANCE AND MOTION POSTURES[89–92]

Static Stance and Sitting Postures

The term static posture is used in its relative sense, referring to a position of rest rather than one of gross movement. As discussed previously, the body is always dynamic because of such factors as body sway, respiration, and restless shifting.[93]

Individual Differences in Stance Posture[94–97]

Racial Differences. Certain races tend to have characteristic rigid or relaxed static postures accompanied by various degrees of kyphosis and/or lordosis. These postures appear to be related to differences in nutrition, climate, training, and social customs.

Weight. Body weight has a distinct influence on the erect posture. The obese have the most erect posture as a result of supporting the load over the relatively small base of support. This posture features twisting while walking with short, stiff steps. A large abdomen requires a compensatory posterior torso leaning and acute lumbosacral angle to balance the anterior weight. More weight is borne by the heels. Conversely, the slim person may assume an overly relaxed stance.

Height. A short person tends to have an erect posture in an attempt to appear taller. This is especially true in the short stocky person because the erect posture tends to make the physique both taller and slimmer. Conversely, the especially tall individual often slouches to appear shorter by developing a habitual kyphosis and knee flexion.

Military Postures. The military position of attention is an unnatural, immobile position in which the chin is drawn in, the neck and chest are elevated, the scapulae are rotated towards the spine, the spine is held vertical, the abdomen is sucked in, the pelvis is tilted posteriorly, and the feet are placed close together with body weight distributed bilaterally. In this position, considerable stress is placed on the erectors of the back and the extensors of the hip and calf. The knee extensors are more relaxed because the center of gravity falls more anterior to the axis of the knee joint. This posture is difficult to maintain for long periods because of the constant muscular tension and the functionally impaired circulation, which can result in pooling within the lower extremities that leads to cerebral anemia.

Pelvic Tilt. In the typical relaxed stance, pelvic weight falls anterior to the gravity line and trunk weight falls posterior to the gravity line. The degree increases in proportion to the degree of "sway back" present. In contrast, during a tensed stance (eg, military posture), trunk weight is placed further posteriorly and balanced over the hips in the sagittal plane. This state is also seen in a patient with a flattened lumbar region with the pelvis rotated posteriorly.

Effects of Pregnancy. During the advanced stages of pregnancy, the center of gravity is displaced considerably forward from the normal because of the increased anterior weight from the fetus, amniotic fluid, and enlarged uterus. Postural compensation is made similar to that seen in the obese with a large abdomen, but there is a more exaggerated compensatory backward lean which is adapted to by a customary upper torso slouch.

Effects of High Heels. As heel height is increased, the center of gravity is moved posteriorly. When the calcaneus is elevated about a half inch above the level of the base of the ball of the foot, its shaft is brought to a tangent with the Achilles tendon. Thus, the gastrocnemius and soleus are able to exert a greater force in plantar flexion. High heels, habitually worn, tend to shorten these muscles and stretch the anterior ankle muscles.

Occupational Effects. Habitual strenuous work results in postural adaptations due to the over-development of asymmetrical musculature or to asymmetries between one part of the body and another.

Shoes. As mentioned, prolonged standing with little movement results in lower extremity pooling. The local effect is that the feet may increase up to about two sizes. A common adaptation is the wearing of loose fitting shoes, but this encourages pronation. A well-fitted shoe should be constructed so that most of the weight is borne on the outside of the foot, which is supported by strong ligaments. The inside of the foot is supported by long thin muscles which easily fatigue and allow the arch to drop and the foot to pronate.

Standing Surfaces. An elastic floor surface, as opposed to a hard surface, becomes slightly compressed by body weight to exert a continual force against the foot in an attempt to recover its original shape. Thus, change of position is assisted by an elastic floor surface.

Postures of Readiness[98]

The anticipation of a forthcoming event affects one's static posture, and the position assumed is in accord with the immediate goal at hand to be achieved (Fig. 4.11). When one is about to perform a rapid or strong movement, the posture of readiness is an alert one, reaching its peak between 1 and 2 seconds after thought is concentrated on the situation. After this peak, posture either becomes relaxed or becomes unstable because of an exaggerated tremor resulting from fatigue of the coordinating centers of the nervous system. If no action is anticipated or if the environment is nonexciting, the result is a relaxed posture. This posture is so well recognized that the relaxed posture is often used in sports as a ploy to deceive an opponent.

Applications. During a posture of alert readiness, the center of gravity is shifted toward the anticipated direction of movement. There is a slight head and plantar flexion that causes equilibrium instability to facilitate this shift. Then arm and leg positions are adjusted to the action that is to follow. The baseball infielder leans forward and rises on his toes as the ball is pitched. The base runner taking a lead off a base will also lean toward the next base and rise on his toes as the ball is pitched. The football quarterback crouches with arms forward and heels and hands together in a position of readiness to catch the ball. Somersaults are started forward and backward by a throw of the head. In each instance, the mechanical equilibrium of the body is disturbed and movement is started.

Proprioceptive Mechanisms. Postures of alert readiness should not be held motionless for a long period because proprioceptive sensations, which govern position sense and the relationship of body parts, will be diminished and must be re-established before accurate movement can be achieved. It is for this reason that the golfer and batter waggle their club while adjusting position.

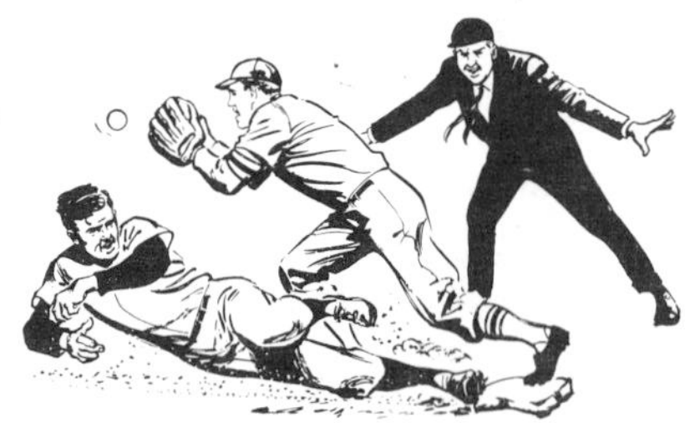

Figure 4.11. Note the postures of readiness of the baseman and referee, with their wide stance and forward lean toward the point of action.

Stability vs Balance. Postures of alert readiness are often superimposed on postures adapting to mechanical forces. Most movements involve lateral shifts of weight which disturb balance and require the application of opposing forces to regain balance. Postural shifts of the body's center of gravity in the vertical direction alter stability but not balance. An ice skater racing forward in the straightway leans forward to maintain equilibrium between gravitational force and the driving action of the legs. If the torso is held erect, the driving action of the legs would soon topple the skater backward. When skating around a curve at high speed, the skater must lean forward to compensate for the driving action of the legs and lean toward the inside of the curve to counteract centrifugal forces.

Sitting Postures[99–102]

In the relaxed sitting position, the head is held erect, balanced over the neck, with the head's center of gravity situated slightly anterior to the atlanto-occipital joint. Body weight should be supported upon the ischial tuberosities and the adjacent soft tissues. The degree of the lumbar curve during the sitting posture depends upon sacral angulation which is governed by pelvic posture and the degree of mobility/fixation of the involved segments.

Center of Gravity. In the erect sitting position, the center of gravity is forward of the ischia, the lumbar lordosis is but slightly flattened, and about 25% of body weight is transmitted to the floor through the lower extremities. However, in the slouched sitting position, the center of gravity is posterior to the ischia, the lumbar lordosis is reversed, and far less body weight is transferred to the floor through the lower extremities[103] (Fig. 4.12).

Disc Pressure. Lumbar intervertebral disc pressure is increased during sitting as compared to the erect posture. The reason for this is that disc pressure increases with

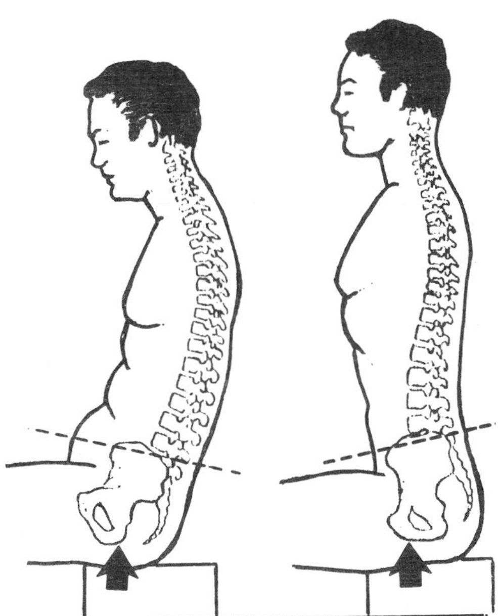

Figure 4.12. Two positions of the pelvis during sitting. Sitting posture essentially depends on the relationship of the body's center of gravity to the ischia. *Left*, it is far posterior; *right*, it is well balanced over the ischial prominences.

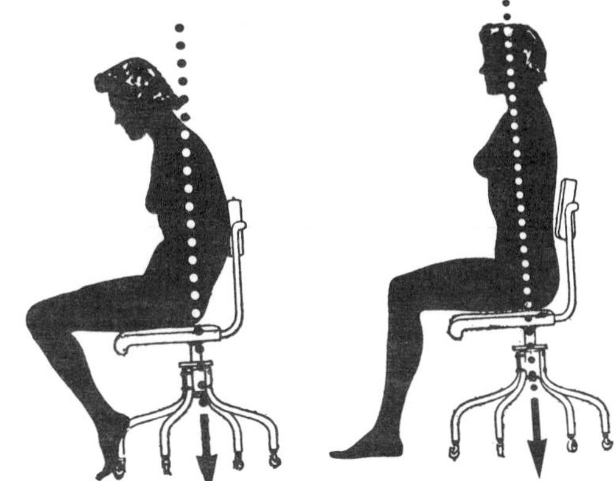

Figure 4.13. *Left*, a slumped sitting attitude that is typical of balance-disturbing posture. Note distortion of the spine compared with the properly balanced figure on the *right*.

the tendency toward lumbar kyphosis.[104] This increased pressure while sitting can be diminished by arm rests on the chair, back support to maintain the lumbar lordosis, and reclining the back of the chair from 90–120°.

Fatigue. Prolonged sitting (eg, typing, driving) can be quite fatiguing if strains from imbalance are not avoided. If the head is allowed to protrude forward, the posterior muscles of the neck soon become tired because continuous tension on the erectors interferes with their circulation (Fig. 4.13). This is sometimes a cause of residual neuromuscular hypertension.

Pressure Points in the Sitting Posture. Drummon and associates developed an instrument that measures the pressure distribution during normal and unbalanced sitting. The data collected showed that during sitting approximately 18% of body weight is distributed over each ischial tuberosity, 21% over each thigh, and 5% over the sacrum.[105]

Chairs and Desks

Chair Design. Chair height should allow the hips, knees, and ankle joints to form an approximate right angle. The seat should deepen slightly to conform to the increasing thickness of the thigh as it meets the buttocks. The seat of the chair should be wide enough so that body weight can be distributed over a wide area and long enough to support the buttocks and lengths of the femurs. Bucket-type seats have a tendency to closely confine the body and restrict restless movements necessary to improve circulation.

Optimal Support. A reading chair is most comfortable if it is inclined slightly backward and has arm rests at elbow height. The backrest of the chair should provide support at the hips, lumbar curve, and shoulders. The upper aspect of the lumbar curve should be supported by a slight convex curve in the back of the chair. These factors contribute to relaxation of trunk muscles. However, the hollows and curves that make a desk chair comfortable are not desired in an adjustable chair because the hollows and curves no longer fit the body when the chair is tilted backward. If a head rest is provided, it should incline slightly forward so that the head and neck are supported in an upright position. If a leg rest is provided, it should be placed at nearly the height of the seat with a slight tilt forward to enhance venous blood and lymph drainage of the lower extremities.

Seat and Table Height and Inclination. A number of studies have been undertaken in recent years to determine the ideal seat height and inclination for school children and office workers. Studies by Bendix indicate that the lumbar spine tends to decrease the thoracic kyphosis when a tiltable seat is inclined upward 5°, especially if this is combined with a slightly increased seat height.[106] Although inclinations of the pelvis and trunk as well as the posture of the cervical spine did not change systematically with variable chair-table heights, it was determined in an earlier study that the cervical and lumbar regions of the spine extended and the head and trunk changed toward a more upright posture when the desk slope was increased during reading. This reaction occurred even though electromyography (EMG) analyses of the trapezius showed a low muscular load that did not change with varying desk slopes during reading and writing. The conclusion of the study indicated that a steep slope of the desk is most favorable for reading and a horizontal surface is most favorable for writing.[107]

Desks. Both desks and chairs must be adapted to meet individual biomechanical requirements. If a person is seated at a desk that is too low, there is a tendency to lean forward and suspend the head by force of the posterior neck and upper back muscles. If the desk is too high, there is a tendency to spread the elbows and bring the work too close to the eyes.

Reclining Postures[108, 109]

The reclining posture requires little energy expenditure because most gravitational pull is counteracted by the mattress. Circulatory stress is minimal because energy demands are low and the horizontal position assists venous return and lymph drainage.

Pillows. Elevation of the head, neck, and upper back helps to relieve respiratory congestion. A soft pillow aids in preventing chill of the neck and shoulders during cold weather. When a person is lying in the side position, a pillow helps to maintain vertical alignment of the neck if it is depressed to the same thickness as the distance from the neck to the tip of the shoulder. However, a pillow of this thickness used by a person in the supine position would stretch the posterior neck muscles, and this tension allows little rest for these muscles. Thus, a soft pillow that can be flattened or bunched to accommodate changes in position is better than a firm pillow. Reading in bed requires a near-sitting position supported by at least two pillows—the back should be supported by a horizontal pillow with the neck supported by a vertical pillow.

Developmental Defects and Posture[110]

During health evaluation, overall posture should be inspected for early signs of spinal curvature, subluxations, leg-length discrepancies, foot pronation (Fig. 4.14), and other subtle or gross deformities. Both structural and functional deformities result in postural compensations. This is readily apparent in a patient with either a physiologic or structural short leg resulting in a scoliosis that is improved by a shoe lift. Pronated feet result in a tilted pelvis and lordosis which are corrected when the pronation is corrected.

Few if any adult spines are free of defects that involve several vertebrae. In many instances, the entire spinal column labors under the strain of improper balance. In this sense, however, the defects of balance referred to are something less than the classical conditions of clinical kyphosis, lordosis, and scoliosis.

Nature, through genetic factors and its difficulty with phylogenetic increments, commonly leaves the skeleton in defect and instability, and the gross and subtle implications of anteroposterior balance, lateral balance, and rotational balance are manifold (Fig. 4.15).[111] The incidence of neck and low-back involvements of a protracted and recurring nature is much higher in those patients (especially younger people) whose spines show evidence of developmental defects and anomalies.

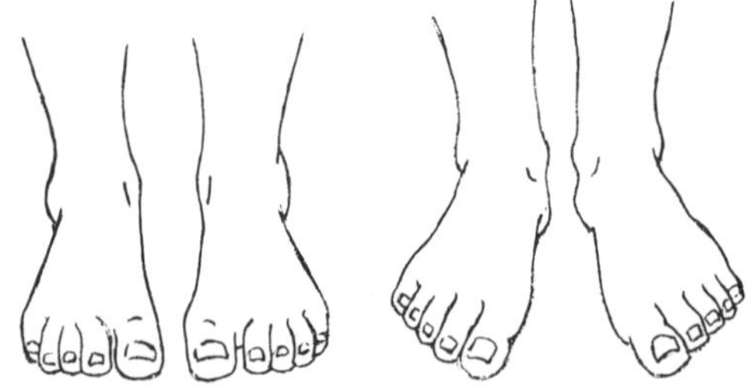

Figure 4.14. Excessive toe-out shown in the right diagram may be either the cause or the effect of a chronic pronation disorder.

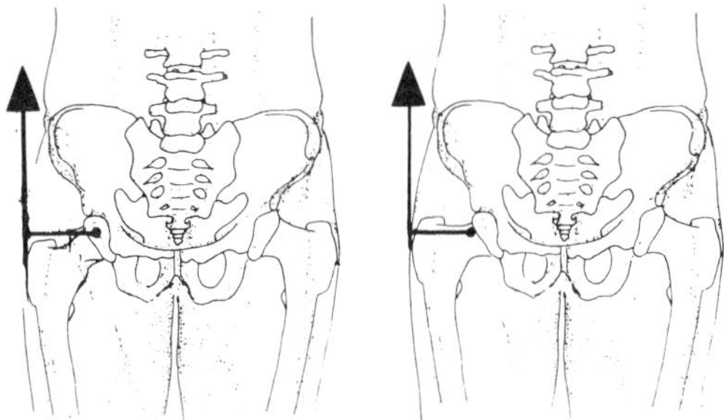

Figure 4.15. A shortening and change in angulation of the femoral neck greatly modifies the lever length of the abductor muscles acting on the lateral hip.

Bipedism greatly augments the mechanical and neurologic complications of the lumbosacral complex. As the low back and sciatic syndromes are evaluated, no clinician should disregard this fact. Lumbosacral defects and complications such as asymmetrical facet facing, imbrication, sacralization (especially the pseudo type), lumbarization, pars defect, discopathy, iliotransverse ligament sclerosing, retrolisthesis, and L5–S1 reverse rotation are priorities of clinical importance.

Dynamic Postures[112–117]

The appreciation of the basic biomechanics involved in dynamic posture is the first step in the analysis of movement. During gross movements, postural changes affect mechanical equilibrium. Thus it can be said that instability is a basic characteristic of body movement. As a result of body instability, rotary forces are developed. These may be beneficial or a hindrance, depending on how they are applied and controlled. Efficient analysis assumes an understanding of biomechanical applications and of neuromuscular control of the forces of motion in successive postures of movement.

Morehouse and Cooper classify all body movements into (1) preliminary movements, (2) a main action, and (3) a follow-through.[118] However, the degree of each component varies considerably from action to action. These factors are clearly demonstrated in athletics because they are often exaggerated for advantage, but they are utilized in all body movements. Thus, the sports-oriented examples that follow should also be identified with nonathletic activities.

Preliminary Movements[119–122]

All main muscle actions are preceded by some degree of preliminary preparatory movement. Generally, the purposes of preliminary movement are to overcome inertia, control the range of motion, set the direction of force, achieve mechanical advantage, and initiate speed to gain the momentum desired.

Head Motion and Footwork. Preliminary action serves to overcome inertia, initiate motion, and to place body position advantageously for the main action to come. Frequent shifts in body position, both in and out of sports, are started essentially by head motion (Fig. 4.16). Footwork takes over in importance once the body becomes balanced and is moving in the direction of the force to be applied. Good footwork reduces uneconomical vertical and horizontal motions that are not directly related to the task. Thus, footwork can be used to gain optimal momentum by traveling smoothly with minimal dipping and waddling. Movements that do not contribute to the main action are wasted efforts that decrease movement efficiency.

Range of Motion. The importance of range of motion is readily demonstrated in the golfer's or batter's preliminary movements. In both instances, the player extends his backswing according to the force with which he wants to hit the ball. When a long hit is desired, the player will shift the hips, rotate the trunk, turn the shoulders, lift his arms, and abduct his wrist to allow the club

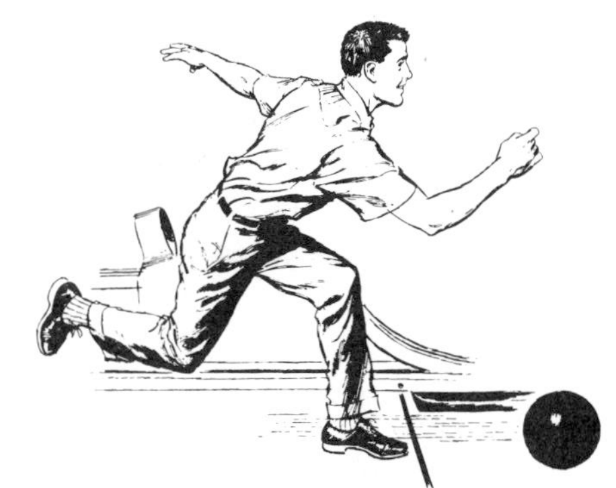

Figure 4.16. All shifts in body position are initiated by head motion, whereafter footwork becomes vital once the direction of force has been established.

to arc behind his head before the forward (main action) power movement takes place. All these preliminary actions determine the range of circumferential movement of the club or bat. Likewise, a baseball pitcher or javelin thrower increases his range of motion by extending his active arm, turning his shoulder, twisting his trunk, lifting his contralateral foot, and leaning backward so that a large forward step can be made during the main forward action. In some actions, time is not sufficient to allow for wide preliminary movements, for example, in a catcher's throw to second base, net play in tennis doubles, or other rapid defensive actions for which the backswing is shortest.

Positioning the Center of Gravity. The closer the body's center of gravity is to its base of support, the more stable it is. For this reason, a tightrope walker holds the pole low and the pole is weighted at both ends. During a somersault, an acrobat lands in a deeply crouching position with the hands held low to keep his center of gravity low. Likewise, a shot putter helps to maintain his balance after a throw by lowering himself to a squat. Flexed knees, a forward crouch, and hands held low help the surfboard rider maintain balance by maintaining a low center of gravity. During a slow run, there is little body lean; but when speed is to be increased, a greater forward lean must be started before powerful leg action is initiated if balance is to be maintained. Conversely, a backward lean must be initiated before a fast run is reduced or stopped. The greater the lean during a fast run, the more difficulty there is in changing direction without a loss in balance. If direction is to be changed, the center of gravity must be shifted toward the new direction and shorter strides must be taken. In most cases, these changes in direction are initiated by a head movement, eg, forward in increasing speed and backward in decreasing speed.

Leverage. Preliminary movements can employ body parts for optimal mechanical advantage. Several examples of this are demonstrated in sports techniques. It is much easier to push or pull when the body is slightly leaning anteriorly than when it is erect.[123] This forward lean contributes weight and leverage to the arms and lowers the body's center of gravity. A gymnast grips rings with the proximal aspect of the palms rather than the fingers to shorten the resistance lever arm about 3 inches. During a swimming start or a basketball center jump, the athlete crouches, flexing his hips, knees, and ankles at a right angle so that the joint extensors are placed at their best mechanical advantage. In throwing, the elbow placed at a preliminary right angle offers optimal mechanical advantage to the triceps and anconeus muscles for elbow extension. In baseball, the batter's forward elbow is carried high so that the triceps can pull forcibly on the bat.

Stabilization. If the trunk is held loosely during arm and leg actions, some extremity forces will be diverted to stabilize the torso. It is for this reason that efforts in jumping, lifting, pushing, pulling, and throwing are enhanced if the breath is held and the abdominal muscles fixed during the main action.

Utilizing Large Muscles. Preliminary movements bring the most advantageous muscle grups quickly into action. When the larger muscles are used for a main action, the result is a powerful action. A chinup, for instance, is more easily performed when the palms are supinated to allow the powerful biceps to be the major force. If the hands are pronated, the weaker brachialis and brachioradialis must overcome the load. During hand wrestling, a far greater force can be exerted if the large muscles of the shoulder, back, thigh, and legs are utilized than if only the muscles of the arm and forearm are used.

Coordination. Coordination may be defined as the ability to integrate separate abilities in a complex task. Limb motion or the addition of a load shifts an individual's center of gravity and changes body balance; how one copes with gravitational influences may be witnessed in one's degree of coordination. Well-coordinated movement, usually involving the large muscles in sports, requires perfect timing between the nervous and muscular systems, for example, as seen in the biologic teamwork expressed in bowling, gymnastics, badminton, throwing, jumping hurdles, handball, tennis, ice hockey, hitting a baseball or golf ball, or kicking a soccer ball. In fast movement of light loads, the antagonists must relax before the prime movers contract. In slow movement of heavy loads, the antagonists stabilize the levers involved in the movement. During fatigue, muscles become tensed and are unable to exhibit efficient teamwork; thus optimal skill, force, speed, steadiness, accuracy, and endurance are lost.

Momentum. A left-handed batter in baseball can effectively utilize the momentum of the bat to overcome inertia and start his run to first. Likewise, if a fielder can catch a fly ball on the forward run, this momentum will add to the force of his throw. In the basketball jump, the player should extend his tipping arm before the main action or the movement during the main action will produce an equal downward force toward the torso and reduce the force of pushoff. During throwing, the arm is first driven sharply backward to initiate the forward movement (Fig. 4.17). The swimming start requires that both arms be thrown backward.

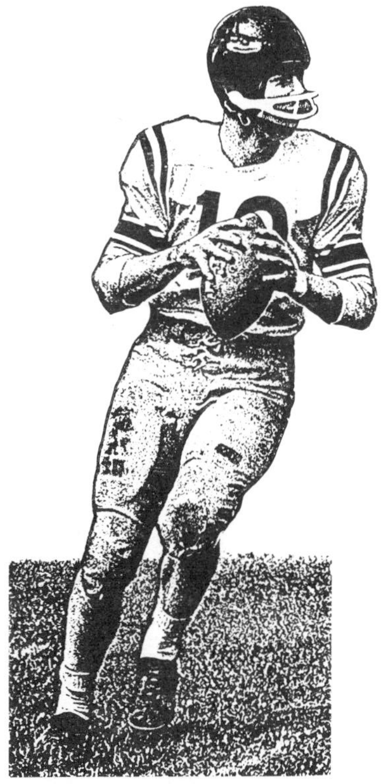

Figure 4.17. To add body momentum to the power of a throw, body weight is shifted toward the goal.

Main Actions[124–126]

Body Bulk. Body bulk has both advantages and disadvantages. Muscle bulk, especially in contact sports, provides both force inertia and protection for bones and joints. Body weight is less a consideration in rowing and swimming sports because the weight is supported, but it offers some buoyancy advantages, or it provides necessary insulation from subcutaneous fat (eg, open-water swimming). Due to gravitational pull, a heavy bulk is a disadvantage in running sports because it must be raised at each pace. There are also disadvantages in bulky hypertrophy because it increases viscous resistance to movement, produces problems from physical apposition, and increases the body mass to be moved. Thus, to avoid mass accumulation in an irrelevant part of the body, muscle training should be specific for the use desired. Indiscriminate muscle hypertrophy is likely to impair performance in endurance events.

The Critical Moment. In any movement there is a critical moment. This is seen at the instant when a hockey stick contacts a puck, when a bat contacts a baseball, when the throwing hand is about to release a bowling ball, or when the foot of a soccer player is in contact with a ball. In each case, the critical moment is very brief and the forces are usually great. There is little time for correction at the moment of contact or release. At this critical moment, the forces are resolved so that they act in a straight line; thus, the force must be in line with that desired, for a fraction of error during impact or release will be magnified by the distance the object travels.

Agility. Agility involves speed with the addition of a sudden change in direction or height such as in a defensive maneuver or a change in attack—the ability to change positions in space. The number of positional changes available is obviously almost endless, and thus agility is most difficult to evaluate. Good agility is demanded in the sports of hockey, gymnastics, diving, boxing, and karate, and in the positions of running back and infielder.

Base of Support. The larger the base of support (eg, large feet or wide stance), the greater the impact that can be received without toppling. Thus, a boxer who stands with his feet spread in the direction of a blow is more difficult to knock down. This is because the center of gravity can prescribe a wide arc about the center base before it falls perpendicularly outside the base of support. When the legs are outspread, the angle of maximum lean is enlarged.[127]

Balance. Balance is a necessary attribute whenever one's base of support is reduced yet body position must be maintained. Standing, walking, running, bending, throwing, and contact sports all require constant voluntary loss and regain of body balance. The human body tries to maintain its upright position with the head positioned so that the field of vision is parallel to the horizon and straight ahead. During linear motion, balance is maintained only if forces acting in other directions are in equilibrium. If balance in the direction of action is not maintained during motion, the accuracy of striking or throwing will be reduced. Once balance is lost, force economy and direction are interfered with, neuromuscular coordination and speed are inhibited by tension, and agility is reduced. Rarely can an imbalanced preliminary movement be corrected during the main action unless the person is highly trained in achieving instantaneous alterations in timing or form. Even then, the muscular attempts to re-establish equilibrium dilute the muscle force necessary for the main action. Precise ballet-like balance is required in such sports as tight-rope walking, hand standing, surfing, karate, hockey, skiing, and to a varying degree in most ball-handling, hitting, kicking, etc, sports in which movement is required in an "off-balance" position.

Delivering Impact. Whether impact is delivered or received, its force will be in accord with the relative velocities and mass of the colliding bodies. Thus, greater impact force can be made with a hip than an elbow because the trunk has greater mass. When impact is made by elbow or knee extension, such as in throwing or kicking, a greater velocity must be developed. The summation of forces can be used (eg, in boxing) to increase impact force by adding a second blow at the instant of the peak of the force from the first blow, which will be much greater than blows delivered simultaneously or separately.

Receiving Impact. Postural adjustments just prior to receiving an impact (eg, utilizing one's center of gravity, going with the direction of force, and prolonging the duration of impact) can diminish its force. For example, a toppling force can be minimized by receiving the impact as close to one's center of gravity as possible. An impact force can be reduced by moving in the same direction as the force; ie, rolling with the punch. The peak force of impact can be lessened by prolonging the duration of impact, such as allowing the hand to be carried backward when catching a ball or changing direction toward the line of a body block. Rolling on impact or hitting an elastic surface can reduce the peak force of a fall (Fig. 4.18).

Follow-Through

Follow-through has no effect on an object after impact, but it has an important function in preventing injury. It is for this reason that the baseball pitcher's arm must be allowed to continue its horizontal arc and the softball pitcher's arm to follow its vertical arc to dissipate the forces initiated within the arm. In all powerful movements, the

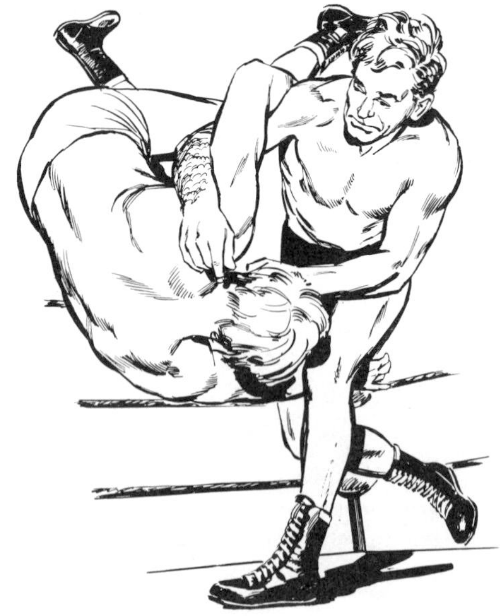

Figure 4.18. The force of a fall can be reduced by prolonging the duration of impact and rolling upon impact.

main action should be allowed to continue and gradually decelerate within the range of motion to save injury or fatigue to check ligaments and muscles.

The Walking Function[128–134]

Biomechanically, walking can be considered as a series of continuous losses and recoveries of balance in which the rhythmic play of muscles narrowly averts toppling. Steindler refers to the basic sequence of movements in walking as a "series of catastrophies narrowly averted."[135] This is a constantly changing process that includes starting, speed and directional changes, adaptive changes to slope or surface conditions, modifications to neuromusculoskeletal disorders and energy requirements, physical proportions, adaptations to heel height and footwear, and stopping movements. However, all these motions are transitory movements that are superimposed on individual basic patterns of rhythmic displacement whose objective is progression toward a goal.

On level ground, walking can be considered biomechanically as forward translation of the body's center of mass. This requires an external force, provided essentially by the extensors of the hip and knee and the ankle plantar flexors, whose efficiency is governed by the friction produced between the foot and the floor during pushoff.

Background[136]

It is typical during the chiropractic examination to study the patient in the static standing position and during gross movements with the feet relatively fixed in the standing or Adams positions and the pelvis relatively fixed in the sitting position. While these procedures offer vital information, they fail to detect many subtle adaptive mechanisms brought out by carefully viewing the patient during progression. This latter technique requires training and experience because the alternating movements occur rapidly even during slow walking. Attention must be directed to many aspects simultaneously. Photographic stills are helpful but impractical in the typical clinical situation.

A walking cycle equals one stride: two steps, one with each lower limb. During a walking cycle, stride length determines the body's segmental displacements and the frequency of duration of the stride governs the time involved. Stride length is essentially determined by an individual's leg length. These two factors, time and distance, are the major factors contributing to a person's particular gait.

Newton's second law should be kept in mind when analyzing gait. The floor pushes up against the plantar surface in locomotion with an equal force and along the same line of action as that of the force of the foot. However, this counterforce of the floor or ground may fail (eg, loose rug, gravel, sand, soft mud). In addition, an equal and opposite horizontal force, usually supplied by friction, must accompany pushoff if progression is to take place. This is greatly reduced or fails to happen on a slippery surface. When walking on a slippery surface, a long stride is more apt to lead to a fall because of the angle at which the heel hits the surface. A short stride allows the foot to descend in a more vertical direction.

Walking is the result of muscle action developing tension and producing joint rotations (angular changes). Body weight is balanced over the hip joint by the abductor muscles acting through the greater trochanter—a first-class lever system. In walking, body weight acts medial to the knee in such a manner that the center of rotation or fulcrum is centered over the medial condyle. Equilibrium is controlled by forces acting in the lateral ligaments, biceps femoris.

Individual Differences in Walking Patterns

Ectomorphic, mesomorphic, and endomorphic body types have differnt types of gait, and there is great variation within these general categories. It is not unusual to recognize a person at a distance strictly by his or her gait. Each of us has a characteristic walking pattern that is altered by both mood and environment. In addition, injury frequently alters normal axes of movement, restricting some and exaggerating others. Thus, any description of gait is a generalization that points out gross similarities of segmental motion.

The Gait Cycle[137–139]

The normal gait presents smoothness of function without any sign of impairment or affliction of parts of the body. The normal walking cycle is considered to have two phases: (1) a *stance phase*, when the foot is in contact with the ground; and (2) a *swing phase*, when the foot is moving forward in the air (Fig. 4.19). During normal walking, one leg is in the stance phase while the other is in the swing phase. Muscles must contract to counterbalance the forces of gravity, to offer acceleration or deceleration to momentum forces, and to overcome the resistance of the walking surface.

The Stance Phase. About 60% of the walking cycle is spent in the stance phase. Because the stance phase is the weight-bearing phase requiring the greatest stress, most problems will become apparent in its analysis. The stance phase is subdivided into (1) heelstrike, (2) footflat, and (3) toe pushoff. Midstance is that weight-bearing period between footflat to toeoff. The duration of gait is usually measured from heelstrike to heelstrike, but any two identical points can be taken.

The Swing Phase. This is subdivided into (1) initial acceleration, (2) midswing, and (3) final deceleration—depending upon the intent. The swing phase, about 40% of the gait cycle, begins with toeoff and ends with heelstrike. Midswing represents the transition period between acceleration and deceleration.

Body Oscillation[140]

A wheel is efficient in forward translation because its center of mass is kept parallel to the ground. In the human, however, there is considerable up and down, side-to-side, and rotational oscillation as well as linear translation (Fig. 4.20). Thus, force is required for vertical, lateral, and rotational displacement that must be added to the force necessary for forward movement. Any disorder that increases oscillation is energy-consuming and linear speed-reducing.

High Points. As previously explained, the center of mass of the body is the point at which the mass movements on one side of any plane are equal to the mass movements on the other side. During gait, the high point of vertical oscillation (about 2 inches) and lateral displacement are reached when unilateral weight is greatest and the lower extremity is in full extension. This occurs near midstance of the single-supporting limb and midswing of the non-weight-bearing limb. Also, the highest point in elevation of the center of mass occurs when body velocity is lowest, and vice versa. This upward movement begins just after the center of mass has passed anterior to the weight-bearing foot as the body's momentum carries the body up and over the leg in stance. Immediate fall of the center of mass after it has passed over and in front of the weight-bearing foot is delayed by the relative lengthening of the weight-bearing leg by knee extension, ankle plantar flexion, and foot supination. These mechanisms tend to produce a smoother translational pathway.

Low Points. The low point is reached when the distance between the two feet is greatest, ie, during the middle of double-support bilateral weight bearing. The greater the stride length, the greater the vertical excursion. This low point, at which both feet are in contact with the ground, one foot at toeoff and the other at heelstrike, normally accounts for 15% of the gait cycle.

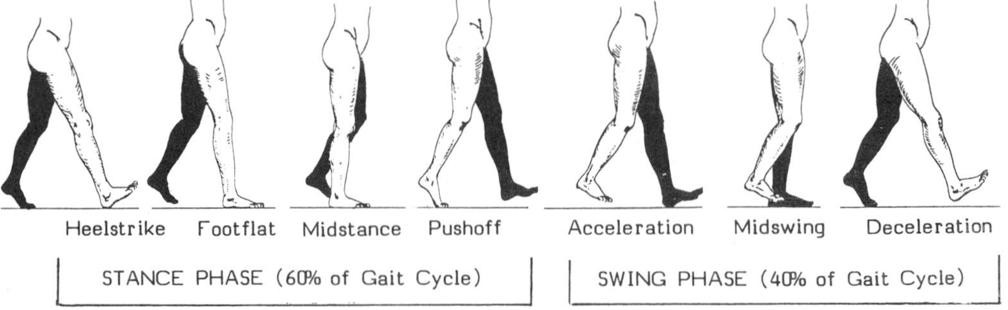

Figure 4.19. The complete gait cycle: stance and swing. Walking is a purposeful disturbance in body equilibrium during which alternating leg displacement sustains body weight.

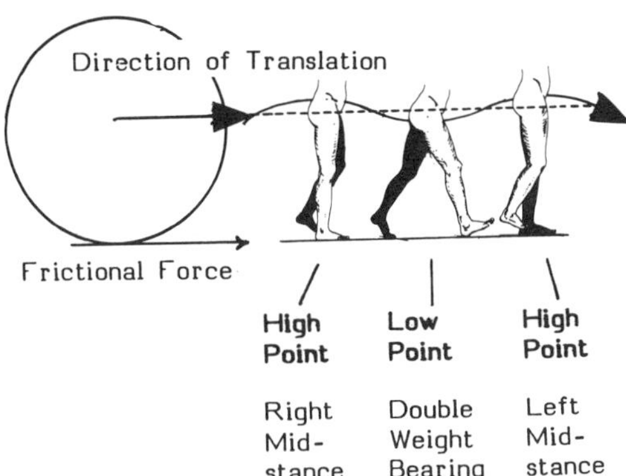

Figure 4.20. A wheel has no oscillation in its direction of translation, except for that caused by a rough surface. During gait, the high point is reached during midstance and the low point between toeoff and heelstrike.

This is the period of double support, and its duration shortens as walking speed increases. In running, the period of double support is zero.

Stress Points. The depth of the low point depends on the degree of pelvic rotation and lateral shifting during the period of double support, while the height of the high point depends on the degree of pelvic tilt and knee flexion during footflat. The high point places stress on both the weight-bearing hip and knee; the low point places stress only on the hip as the knee is relatively locked in extension. Flattening the arc of the body's center of mass during translation is maintained by three basic elements (1) *pelvic tilt,* which depresses the high point; (2) *pelvic rotation,* which elevates the ends of the arc; and (3) *knee flexion,* which also reduces the high point.[141]

Pelvic Tilt. During normal gait, the pelvis lists coronally downward a few degrees (4–6°) away from the leg in stance and toward the leg in swing from the force of gravity (positive Trendelenburg). This alternating angular displacement at the hip joint is maximum at midswing on the side of the swinging leg. Pelvic tilt is essentially controlled by contraction of the hip adductors of the stance side. By dipping the center of gravity, it has an effect of minimizing (flattening) the summit of the vertical oscillation arc during gait. The knee of the leg in swing must flex so that the foot will clear the floor. Tilting appears exaggerated in the female because of the wider pelvis and greater superficial fat.

Pelvic Rotation. Relative to the line of progression, the pelvis alternately rotates toward the right and left about a vertical axis during typical gait. This somewhat stabilizes the center of mass by reducing abrupt changes in oscillation arcs, which tends to reduce the severity of impact at surface contact. During hip extension and flexion, angular displacement is reduced and the force necessary to change direction of the body's center of mass in the following arc of translation is reduced. Pelvic rotation occurs anteriorly on the side of the advancing limb during the swing phase and posteriorly during midstance. These alternating rotations occur essentially at the hip joints due to the relative rigidity of the pelvis. The movement is maximum just before heelstrike, moving 3–5° on either side of the central axis. As speed is increased, this value increases because there is a corresponding increase in stride length.

Pelvic rotation in the transverse plane when walking on a fairly level surface has long been known as an instinctive energy-saving mechanism—it increases stride length with minimal effort during gait. This mechanism of pelvic rotation has been considered by some to be lost during the metabolically expensive exercise of walking or running uphill or downhill. Wall and associates, however, have shown that this belief is not true.[142] Data recorded from subjects walking on a treadmill that was sloped plus or minus 20% showed that pelvic rotation on a 20% incline was substantially the same as that on a level surface.

Lateral Sway. Besides pelvic tilt and rotation, a degree of alternating horizontal displacement occurs to replace the gravity line nearer the hip of stance (Fig. 4.21) during the period of single support. Its rhythm is one-half the frequency of vertical displacement. It reaches its greatest degree following midstance on the weight-bearing leg and constitutes about a 2-inch lateral movement of the center of mass with each complete stride. This is seen as an adduction movement of the stance side, as is pelvic tilt. Once its peak of lateral displacement is reached, the pelvis begins to reverse direction. This horizontal sway increases the base

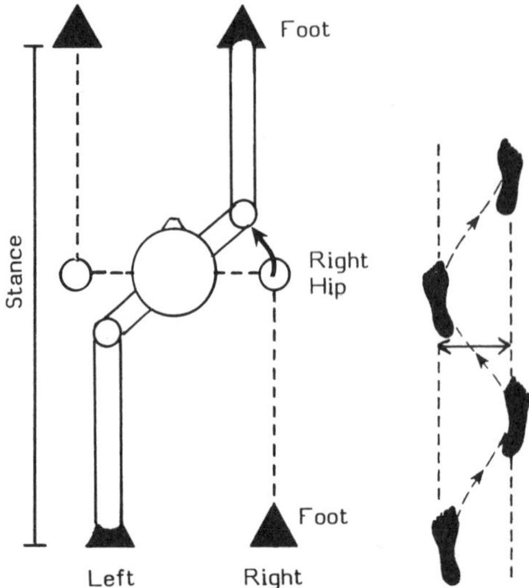

Figure 4.21. *Left*, schematic of stride length. *Right*, the extent of sway depends upon the width of the base of support.

of support about 4–8 inches as the feet pass each other. There is normally a slight degree of genu valgum that allows the leg to remain essentially vertical and the feet close together during gait hip movements. When the lateral distance between the feet is increased or decreased, the degree of lateral sway is increased or decreased.

Hip and Knee Flexion and Extension. The high point of vertical oscillation is also minimized by slight flexion of the hip and knee during midstance. This flexion moves the gravity line anterior to the hip and posterior to the knee. The greater the degree of this flexion, the greater is the effort required by the hip and knee extensors to maintain equilibrium. During a walking cycle, extension and flexion occur alternately. Knee extension (nonlocking) occurs at heelstrike. Following heelstrike, slight flexion occurs and continues through midstance. Midstance is followed by extension and then flexion occurs again during pushoff and swing. The knee joint is almost fully extended at heelstrike and then begins to flex to about a maximum of 15° until footflat. Just prior to full weight bearing, the knee again passes into extension. Note that the center of mass is in a state of dropping at the point of heelstrike. This drop is decelerated by slight knee flexion against quadriceps resistance.

Ankle and Foot Flexion and Extension. At the ankle, dorsiflexion, plantar flexion, and rotation occur alternately during a gait cycle. The ankles display maximum dorsiflexion at the end of stance and maximum plantar flexion at the end of pushoff. The ankles rotate forward in an arc around the radius formed by the heel at heelstrike and about a center point in the forefoot at pushoff. That is, the foot is plantar flexed against tibialis anterior resistance after heelstrike around a point where heelstrike occurs. Rotation about this point tends to shorten the leg relatively and causes the ankle to be carried slightly forward until footflat is achieved. Deceleration of these movements is the result of quadriceps contraction acting on the knee and tibialis anterior contraction acting on the foot. Added to these mechanisms is the fact that the ankle pronates slightly during full weight-bearing midstance. During a typical walking cycle, heel elevation changes are about twice those of the ankle and toes, while ankle and toe changes are 2–3 times those of the knee and hip.

Thigh and Leg Rotation. There is a slight medial (clockwise) rotation of the femur at the hip and knee during swing and from heelstrike to near midstance. This is followed by a change to lateral (counterclockwise) rotation which continues through stance to pushoff. That is, the thigh and leg reach their maximum clockwise rotation at heelstrike of the opposite limb and their maximum counterclockwise rotation during stance. There is a close relation between stride length and the degree of thigh/leg rotation. As opposed to arm swing, these transverse rotations of the thigh and leg are in phase with pelvic rotations and increase progressively in degree of displacement from below upward. As with the pelvis, the thigh and leg begin to rotate internally toward the leg in stance as the swing phase begins, and this rotation continues during double weight bearing. However, at midstance the leg abruptly begins to rotate externally, and this external rotation continues until the next swing phase is initiated.

Arm Swing and Spinal Rotation. Although swinging the arms has no effect upon shifting the center of mass during body oscillation, it provides a means of neutralizing total angular momentum (Fig. 4.22). That is, the leg advance and pelvic rotation that produce an angular momentum to the lower body are balanced by a reverse angular momentum of the upper body, which is aided by arm swing resulting from shoulder rotation. During normal gait, these rotations are about 180° out of phase with rotation of the pelvis. That is, maximal forward arm swing occurs contralateral to swing, and backward arm swing occurs contralateral to stance. This helps to control weight over the stance hip, maintain forward momentum, and smooth forward progression of the body as a whole.[143] The inertia of the arms is overcome essentially by the alternating lumbar rotation toward the side of the low pelvis which is compensated by a reverse rotation of the thoracic spine.

Vertebral Motion. Because of out-of-phase shoulder and pelvic rotations during gait, there must be points of minimum and maximum transverse rotation. Keep in mind that the pelvis rotates anteriorly and the shoulder rotates posteriorly on the side of the swinging leg, and vice versa. Studies have shown that the upper thoracic vertebrae rotate to a degree about equal to that of the shoulder girdle and the lower lumbar vertebrae rotate to a degree about equal to that of the pelvis. The point of rotational transition, and the site of greatest rotation between vertebrae, is typically between T6 and T7. When weights are carried in the hands, however, this point of transition tends to move upward.

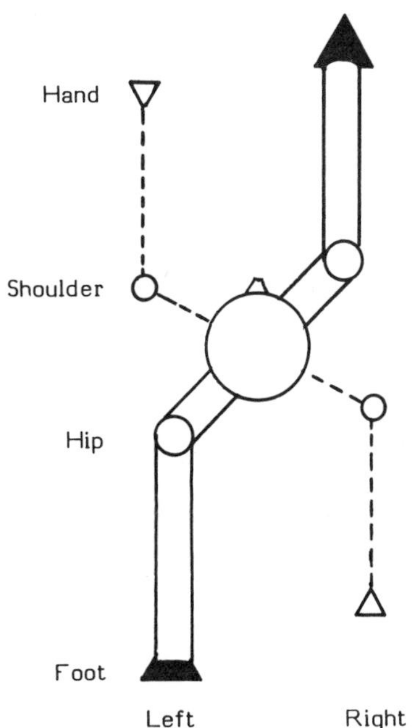

Figure 4.22. During normal gait, arm position is alternately coordinated with contralateral leg position.

Ankle Rotation. When the foot is free during the swing phase, the toes point inward on plantar flexion and outward on dorsiflexion. When the foot is fixed on the surface during stance, relative plantar flexion produces external rotation of the leg and dorsiflexion causes internal rotation. The primary mechanism here is the subtalar joint, a single-axis hinge joint whose axis is inclined about 45°, which allows transverse rotation of the tibia. Without this, the foot would have to slip upon the walking surface. It is interesting to note that the foot must change from a flexible structure at the beginning of stance to a rigid lever at pushoff.

Foot Rotation. The foot tends to rotate medially after heel strike and prior to flatfoot. Pronation occurs as the foot is increasingly loaded. When body weight is transferred from the heel to the forefoot during stance and the person rises on his metatarsal heads prior to pushoff, the heel inverts, the foot supinates, and the leg rotates externally. This raises the longitudinal arch medially and depresses it laterally, tending to shift body weight laterally during maximum weight bearing. At pushoff, the foot deviates laterally to distribute weight between all the metatarsal heads. Evidence of this is shown by the oblique crease in the shoe where the vamp and the cap join. This crease is over the metatarsophalangeal joints and will vary with individual differences in the long axis of the foot and the angle of the metatarsal heads.

Added Loads. Vertical displacement and length of stride are decreased when the walking individual is carrying a load. Body weight shifts laterally to relieve the load over the oscillating leg[144] (Fig. 4.23). The knees and hips are flexed to decrease vertical oscillation and to reduce the jar at footstrike. It is also because of these factors that obese people tend to walk with a waddle.

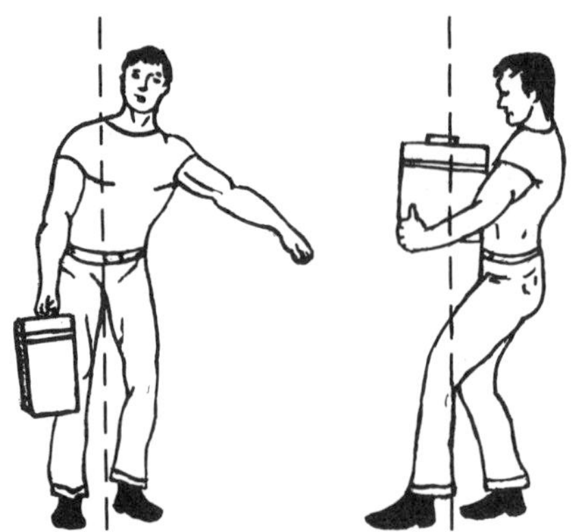

Figure 4.23. When external loads are added to the body in gait, automatic postural mechanisms center the total mass of the base of support as efficiently as possible.

A mother often carries a young child between her hip and ribs (or on the lower back or top of the head in some cultures) because this is the most economical position for the added load.

Effect of Manipulation on Gait

A surface electromyographic study conducted by Hibbard showed that significant amplitude changes occurred in the electrical activity of gait muscles following manipulation of the lower extremity articulations to reduce malposition, while the electrical activity of gait muscles in control subjects decreased only slightly.[145] Hibbard also cites the work of Rebechini-Zasadny and associates who had previously found a significant difference in the electrical activity of peripheral muscle following manipulation of just the cervical spine.

Examination of Gait[146–153]

Every person has a gait, or manner of progressive locomotion, that is peculiar to that individual. However, there are also various modes of walking peculiar to certain diseases which provide important diagnostic clues. The range of movements in the lower extremities assists in recognizing specific diseases and helps the doctor of chiropractic determine postural changes resulting from an unnatural gait. For instance, a shortened leg gives a characteristic limp. A stiff knee causes the affected limb to swing outward while walking. Intermittent claudication or limping is observed in chronic peripheral vascular diseases such as endarteritis because muscular activity requires more blood than muscular inactivity.

As the walking gait is the most fundamental form of dynamic posture, it should form the basis of holistic biomechanical analysis. In health, most locomotive adjustments are conducted at an unconscious level. This is not true with the patient suffering a neuromusculoskeletal disability affecting gait. Every motion may require a frustrating conscious effort such as that taken by a healthy person stepping into a canoe where the support is unfamiliar.

Although children emulate adult gait in many respects, there are differences that must be considered in analyzing a pathologic or functionally impaired gait during childhood. Foley and associates, utilizing a television-computer system of data gathering and analysis, found that joint-angle ranges were the same in children as in adults.[154] However, accelerations, velocities, and linear displacements were consistently larger in children aged from 6 to 13 years (mean 10.2 years) than in adults.

Sitting and Ascent

During examination, have the subject sit in a chair, arise, and then walk across the room if you have not had an opportunity to witness this previously.[155] The chair should be one that gives firm sitting support and provides for 90° flexion of the knees and hips.

While the patient is sitting, note from the front the patient's sitting balance, levelness of ears, shoulders, and pelvis. From the side, note head, shoulder, and pelvic carriage. Observe how the patient rises from the chair to the standing position. Note the needed base of support: how far the knees are apart and how far the forward foot is from the back foot. If the chair has arms, note the degree to which the hands are used in the change from sitting to standing to assist weak knees or weak hip extensors, or to maintain stability, balance, and coordination.

Normal Stance and Swing Phases[156]

Noting a gait deformity and in what phase it occurs is most helpful to diagnosis.

Many subtle but significant points are frequently missed in the fully clothed patient, thus the patient should be minimally clothed and examined in a private environment. Immediately after analysis, make a graphic or mental record of your impressions of the subject's gait. Osler, the great diagnostician, warned that more can be learned by observing the body in dynamic action than can be learned upon the autopsy table when it is too late to help.

During normal ambulation, the normal range of motion at the ankle is from 20° plantar flexion to 15° dorsiflexion. The knee moves 65° from flexion to extension. At the hip, about 6° of adduction occurs and a 45° range is necessary from flexion to extension.

After the walking sequence has been initiated, the movements are normally continued in a rhythmic manner solely by reflex actions. The stretch reflex of the antagonistic extensor muscles is reflexly inhibited as the flexors of the hip, knee, and ankle are stretched. Walking actions are maintained by the reflexive interplay of muscles acting around the joints in motion (Fig. 4.24).

During the stance phase, the heelstrike to footflat, footflat to midstance, midstance to heeloff, heeloff to toeoff, toeoff to midswing, and midswing to heelstrike actions should be analyzed. During the swing phase, which is only about a third of the cycle, the acceleration to midswing and midswing to deceleration actions should be analyzed.

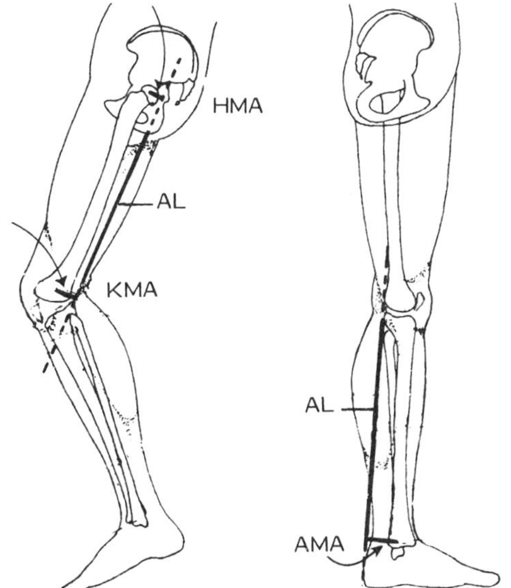

Figure 4.24. Muscle moment arms, *left*, of the biceps femoris at the hip and knee; *right*, of the soleus at the ankle. *AL*, action line; *HMA*, hip moment arm; *KMA*, knee moment arm; *AMA*, ankle moment arm.

Heelstrike[157]

Inspection. At heelstrike, the ankle is between dorsiflexion and plantar flexion, the knee is fully extended, the hip flexes to about 25°, and the head and trunk are vertical. The right arm is posterior to the midline of the body with the elbow extended, and the left arm is anterior to the midline with the elbow partially flexed. The pelvis is slightly rotated anteriorly, the knee is extended, and the leg is vertically aligned with the pelvis. The foot is near a right angle to the leg on the side of heelstrike, and the plantar surface of the forefoot is visible from the front (Fig. 4.25).

Mechanisms. The reactive force of the ground tends to plantar flex the foot so that a large surface contacts the ground, to flex the knee, and to drive the hip into greater flexion. This reactive force is checked by extensor action of the joints involved; ie, contraction of the ankle dorsiflexors, eccentric quadricep contraction at the knee, and contraction of the gluteus maximus and hamstrings at the hip. These mechanisms prevent flexion collapse under body weight and absorb the impact jar at heelstrike.

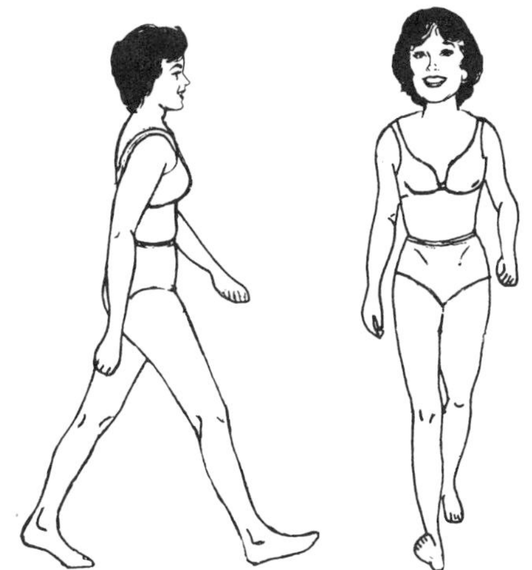

Figure 4.25. *Left*, lateral view of heelstrike; *right*, frontal view of heelstrike.

There is also some contraction of the posterior hamstrings at heelstrike, but this is considered only to prevent hyperextension of the knee.

Joint Reaction. At heelstrike, it has been calculated that the magnitude of the joint reaction at the foot is 5.8 times body weight for a heavy, energetically walking male. It is 2.3 times body weight for an average female walking slowly. For both male and female, the maximum joint reaction at the knee during walking is about four times body weight. The posterior cruciate ligaments carry more than twice the shearing forces carried by the anterior cruciates.

Footflat

Inspection. In weight bearing, the pelvis rotates on its vertical axis, the femur rotates on the pelvis, and the tibia rotates laterally on the femur.

Mechanisms. During footflat, maximum stabilization of the foot occurs during stance when body weight is directly above the foot. Forward momentum eliminates the need for active hip and ankle flexion or extensor stabilization, but there is some knee flexion by quadriceps contraction. When body weight is placed on the stance side, the plantar flexors of the foot contract to counterbalance the reactive force of the walking surface, which forces the foot into dorsiflexion up to 15° at heeloff, and the adductors of the hip contract to counterbalance the pelvic adduction resulting from pelvic tilt.

Midstance

Inspection. At midstance, the head and trunk are vertical with the arms near the midline of the body and at an equal distance from the body. The elbows are partially flexed. On the weight-bearing side, the pelvis is rotated slightly anteriorly, the knee is in slight flexion, the leg is in slight lateral rotation at the hip, and the ankle is in slight dorsiflexion. There is a downward pelvic tilt on the contralateral side (Fig. 4.26).

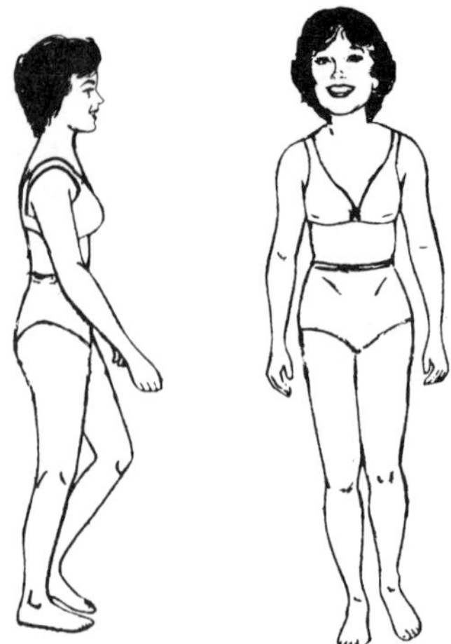

Figure 4.26. *Left*, lateral view of midstance; *right*, frontal view of midstance.

Mechanisms. Following full vertical weight bearing, the line of gravity moves forward on the stabilized plantar surface to produce a reactive force that contributes to ankle, knee, and hip extension. Hip extension reaches about 15° at the time of heeloff. This takes place without any active extensor muscle action, but some stabilization effect occurs by the iliopsoas. During this process, the gravity line falls anterior to the knee so that quadriceps action is no longer necessary. The ground reaction moves from the midfoot to the forefoot as toeoff approaches, which increases the moment of dorsiflexion. In reaction, plantar flexion contraction peaks at heeloff to drive the body forward. While this tends to extend the knee, full extension is restricted by the gastrocnemius–an ankle and knee flexor.

Energy Absorption. During gait, peak activity of the joints of the lower extremity is reached during the period of double support. At this period, the knee muscles are absorbing energy while the other joints are producing energy. As the hamstring group and gastrocnemius are two-joint muscles, much of this energy can be transferred to produce energy at other joints.

Compensation. When the power output of one segment exceeds the power required, the surplus energy must be absorbed by other segments. Likewise, when the power requirement of one segment exceeds muscle output, the energy necessary must come from other segments.

Effect of Shoe Lift. Although unsymmetrical lower extremity length has long been known to have adverse effects in the spine, only recently has its effects on contributing to depletion of the body's energy stores been measured. Delacerda and Wikoff have shown that the equalization of leg length by a shoe lift equalized the time durations for the four phases of gait and decreased the kinetic energy of the lower extremity segments for both legs in spite of the bilateral difference in segmental masses of the legs.[158]

Pushoff

Inspection. On the side of pushoff, the arm is anterior to the midline of the body and the elbow is partially flexed. On the contralateral side, the arm is posterior and the elbow is slightly extended. Both arms are equally distant from the body. On the side of pushoff, the femur is slightly rotated laterally at the hip, the knee is slightly flexed, the ankle is plantar flexed, and the toes are hyperextended at the metatarsophalangeal joint. The plantar surface of the heel and midfoot should become visible from the posterior during pushoff (Fig. 4.27).

Mechanisms. The later part of stance occurs between heeloff and toeoff and provides the major portion of forward and vertical propulsion force. The hip adductors and iliopsoas begin to contract in anticipation of the swing phase, but most action occurs at the ankle and knee. The ankle changes from about 15° dorsiflexion at heeloff to about 35° plantar flexion at toeoff, and the extended knee flexes to about 40° as the quadriceps contract. At toeoff, the segments begin to reverse the lateral rotation attained during footflat, and this medial rotation of the pelvis, thigh, and leg continues to 20–35°, depending on walking speed, until the next footflat is reached. Once the toes leave the ground, hip and calf muscles relax.

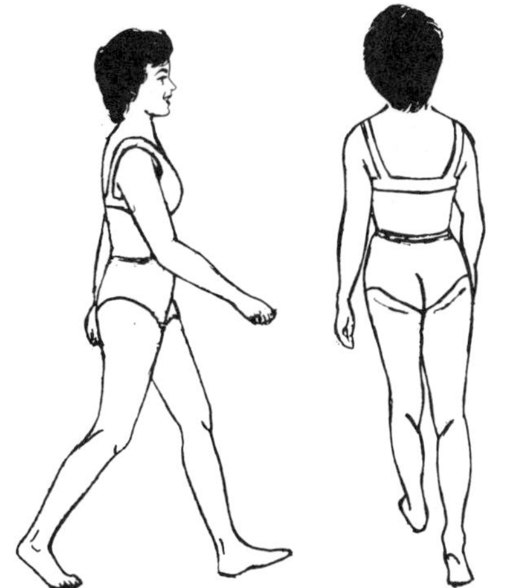

Figure 4.27. *Left*, lateral view of pushoff; *right*, posterior view of pushoff.

Acceleration

Inspection. The period of acceleration of the advancing leg occurs during the first part of the swing phase when the limb is between toeoff and midswing. The swing phase involves almost simultaneous hip flexion, knee flexion, ankle dorsiflexion, and usually a concomitant forward swing of the hip that rotates the pelvis contralaterally to some degree.

Mechanisms. The primary forces are generated by the hip flexors and ankle dorsiflexors. Hip flexion is governed by the tensor fasciae latae, the pectineus, and the sartorius. The most powerful hip flexor, the iliopsoas, and the adductor magnus are not active during swing, according to electromyographic evaluations. Knee flexion is aided by sartorius contraction, gravity, and passive pull of the posterior hamstrings. The flexion of the knee after toeoff is passive while the thigh accelerates forward from action by the hip flexors. As the hip and knee continue to flex and the ankle dorsiflexes, the leg "shortens" so that it can clear the ground.

Midswing and Deceleration

Inspection. The head and trunk are vertical, and both arms are near the midline of the body and held at an equal distance from the body. On the weight-bearing side, the pelvis is rotated slightly anteriorly and tilted downward, the hip and knee are flexed, the femur is rotated slightly medially at the hip, the leg is vertically aligned with the pelvis, and the foot is at a right angle to the leg and slightly everted (Fig. 4.28).

Mechanisms. At heelstrike, the ankle is held in its neutral position by its dorsiflexors, especially the anterior crural muscles, the knee rapidly moves from flexion to full extension by hamstring contraction, and this hamstring contraction also slows hip flexion. During the swing phase, there is a ballistic movement of hip flexion in which the thigh is first accelerated by the hip flex-

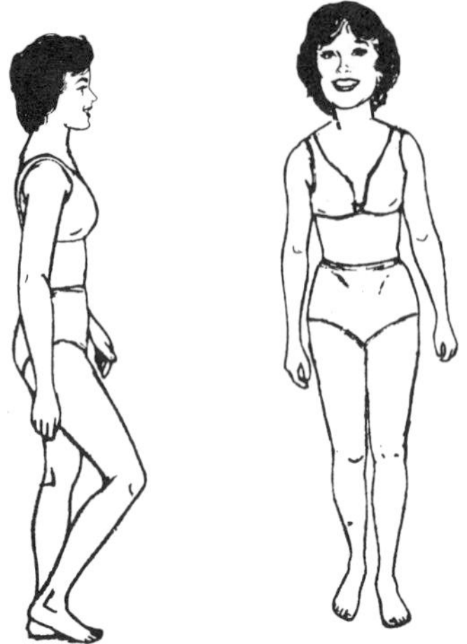

Figure 4.28. *Left*, lateral view of midswing; *right*, frontal view of midswing.

ors at the beginning of swing and then decelerated by the hip extensors.

Lateral Observation[159–161]

From the side note rhythm, symmetry, speed, and stride lengths of cadence. Vertical excursion is best viewed from the side. Check if the duration of the stance phase is the same bilaterally. As the patient walks, note all deviations from normal gait. Normally, the head and trunk are vertical, stride length is even, and the arms swing freely and alternate with the leg swing.

Note the foot at heelstrike and pushoff. The foot is about at a right angle to the leg and the knee is extended but not locked at heelstrike. At pushoff, the foot is firmly flexed and the toes are hyperextended. The foot easily clears the floor during the swing phase of the gait.

Displacement. The trunk should be vertical at stance. Observe the degree of lurch during flexion and extension, and during the swing phase. Note the degree of hip, knee, and ankle flexion. If the head is carried far forward, seek further evidence of atlanto-occipital fixation, subluxation, costoclavicular or neurovascular syndrome, upper dorsal lesion, or shoulder disorder. These malfunctions would also be suspect if the head were tilted to one side, but lateral carriage is found more commonly in torticollis, in visual defects, and in primary or secondary scoliosis.

Pathologic Postures. If pain is present, determine where and when it is greatest. Check for trunk fixation in flexion or extension. Fixed lordotic and kyphotic spines will be evident during both stance and swing, but posterior pelvic tilts are difficult to observe. Shoulders drooping forward may be an indication of cardiac dysfunction, lung or pleural pathology, depression, or a dorsal lesion. Diabetics and those suffering from cardiorenal disorders often have pot bellies. Due to the lack of tone in the abdominal musculature, the viscera sag downward which results in organ malposition and disturbed function contributing to the problem.

Anterior-Posterior Observation

From the front and rear note rhythm, symmetry, and speed of cadence. Lateral motions are best viewed from the front or rear. As the body advances, note smoothness of the body's vertical oscillation. Pathology may express itself in increased vertical oscillation and disrupt the normally smooth pattern. Normally, the pelvis is centrally positioned over the line of progression at toeoff and begins its movement toward the side of the weight-bearing limb.

Pelvic Displacement. Note the degree of pelvic tilt and drop on each side. This is more easily noted by watching the top horizontal line of the underwear. A lateral shift of the pelvis and hip of about one inch to the weight-bearing side is normal to center the weight over the hip. Maximum pelvic tilt is usually reached just after midstance. Its degree is normally determined by *stride width,* which corresponds to the lateral shear forces acting on the pelvis, and *walking speed,* which determines how long these shear forces are acting on the body. Lateral shifting is accentuated in gluteus medius weakness and should be noted. A gait exhibiting bending to one side may be the result of a pericardial or pleural friction rub, a sacroiliac lesion, shoulder condition, affection of the brachial plexus, or lesion in the upper dorsal section of the spine. On the other hand, a ram-rod gait is a sign of a thoracic lesion, sacralization, or spasm of the lumbar paravertebral musculature—all of which may or may not be associated with an abnormal lumbar curve. A fixed pelvic tilt or elevation will not change from stance to swing. The pelvis is normally level at heel contact, drops to its maximum on the side approaching toeoff during double support, then returns to a level position shortly after toeoff and remains there until heelstrike. As speed increases, the degree of drop increases on the side in the swing phase.

Base Width. Check the walking base width for broadness, stability, and consistency (Fig. 4.21, *right*). From heel to heel, base width is normally not more than 2–4 inches. If wider, dizziness, unsteadiness from a cerebellar problem, or numbness of a foot's plantar surface may be a cause for the wider base. An abnormally decreased base usually produces a crossover "scissor" action after midswing.

Limp. Any articular malfunction from the spine to the foot may result in a limp. Muscular weakness or spasm, fascial contraction, fracture, a torn ligament or tendon, bone disease, or a neurologic affection may be cause for a limp. Generally, an uncomplicated limp can be traced to a knee, ankle, or foot dysfunction or deformity, a hip disorder, or a sacroiliac or lumbar lesion. A female gait exhibiting rigid buttocks is a sign of a uterus retroflexed or prolapsed, or of a lumbosacral lesion.

Diagnostic Stance and Swing Clues[162]

Heelstrike. Inability of a foot to heelstrike is an indication of a heel spur and associated bursitis or a blister. Failure of the knee to fully extend during heelstrike is a sign of weak quadriceps or a flexion fusion of the knee. A harsh heelstrike, usually associated with knee hyperextension, is a frequent sign of weak hamstrings.

Footflat. When the foot slaps down sharply after heelstrike, weak dorsiflexors should be suspect.

Midstance. Fused ankles will prevent a midstance flat foot. Weak quadriceps display themselves in excessive flexion and poor knee stability during midstance. A midstance forward lurch of the hip is a typical indication of a weak gluteus medius, while a midstance backward lurch is a sign of a weak gluteus maximus.

Pushoff and Swing. If the patient must rotate the pelvis severely anteriorly to provide a thrust for the leg, the cause is most likely weak quadriceps. If the hip is flexed excessively to bend the knee and thus prevent the toe from scraping the floor as in a steppage gait, weak ankle dorsiflexors are the usual cause. Failure to hyperextend the foot during pushoff is a sign of arthrosis. Pushing off with the lateral side of the front of the foot is usually seen in disorders involving the great toe. A flat-footed calcaneal gait during pushoff is symptomatic of weak gastrocnemius, soleus, and flexor hallucis longus muscles.[163] The foot will have trouble clearing the floor if the ankle dorsiflexors are weak or the knee is unable to flex properly.

Antalgic Gaits[164, 165]

Guarded Limps. A limp may be a sign of disease, malfunction, or both. It may also be in compensation for another condition such as a sprained ankle, injured knee, old fracture malunion or hip surgery. However, the majority of limps seen are those described as "guarded" limps. Guarded limps frequently point to specific musculoskeletal disorders. These limps are the result of the patient walking in a manner that protects or relieves stress upon an area that would otherwise be uncomfortable or painful. The term "antalgic position" describes that static posture assumed by the patient to produce the same pain-diminishing effect as does a guarded gait.

Midspinal and Bilateral Spinal Pain. When pain is in the midline of the spine, the gait pattern is guarded, symmetrical, and slow, with a short stride and restricted trunk rotation and pelvic tilt. If paraspinal muscle spasm is present, the patient will tend to lean backward throughout the gait in compensation. However, if the irritation is located at the posterior aspect of the spinal column (eg, articular facets), the patient will tend to lean forward throughout gait in an attempt to gain relief by reducing weight on the sensitive area. Walking on the toes, as if walking on eggs, is often seen in cases of lumbosacral or cervical lesions to reduce jar. To avoid jarring any sensitive joint, the heel strike is usually eliminated and the length of stride is shortened by reducing the swing phase.

Unilateral Spinal Pain. Walking in a stooped position with one hand supporting the back is a frequent sign seen in a lumbar lesion. During both stance and swing in mild or moderate irritations, the trunk usually leans toward the affected side in compensation for muscle splinting. However, in pronounced intervertebral disc or sacroiliac lesions, the lean is usually away from the site of irritation to reduce pressure.

Hip Pain. While the hip joint of one extremity is in the stance phase and acts as the fulcrum for rotation, the other hip in the swing phase rotates about 40° forward. This normal hip rotation is not seen in patients suffering a stiff or painful hip. When a hip is painful, the gait is asymmetrical, the base is widened during swing, the stance phase is reduced on the affected side and made longer on the unaffected side, the trunk is thrown forward during stance to shift the center of mass, and the affected hip is lifted so the limb will clear the floor. The affected hip is quite fixed in flexion and abduction, and is rotated laterally to reduce joint tension. As a consequence of the hip flexion, the knee and ankle flex. Keep in mind the cyclic load on the hip during gait (Fig. 4.29).[166]

Knee Pain. If a knee joint is effused, with or without pain, 25° flexion offers the largest capsule volume, and thus the least tension. This flexion is compensated by ankle plantar flexion and an absent heelstrike, so that the patient will walk on the toes of the affected side. This guarded gait minimizes quadriceps function and thus reduces knee compression.

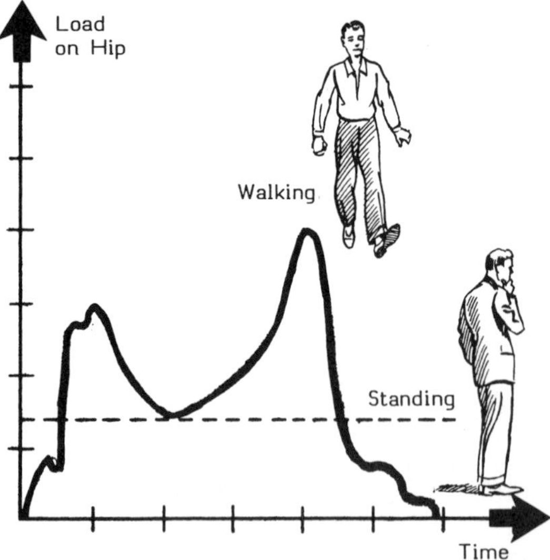

Figure 4.29. The dynamic load on the femoral head, for example, varies considerably during gait compared to the static standing position.

Ankle Pain. In any painful disorder of the ankle, ankle motion will be guarded and the most comfortable position will be assumed. There is little, if any, plantar flexion during footflat or heelstrike, or dorsiflexion during heeloff. This will be compensated for by an exaggerated knee flexion after heeloff and a restricted heel rise before toeoff. The patient will reduce his base and shift his trunk so that more weight falls directly over the joint during weight bearing.

Common Stance Phase Problems. Most stance phase problems are the result of pain and characterized by an antalgic gait wherein the patient spends as little time on the affected extremity as possible. Gait patterns vary according to the type and location of the disorder present. A shoe problem should not be overlooked, being one of the more common causes. Pain in a foot during midstance may be caused by corns, calluses from a fallen transverse arch, rigid pes planus, a plantar wart, bunion, subtalar arthritis, or poor-fitting shoes. Heelstrike will be eliminated and toe walking will be seen if a lesion is present in the heel or posterior aspect of the foot. Lesions of the forefoot such as metatarsal or phalangeal disorders are characterized by heel walking, reduced pushoff, and an exaggerated forward hip thrust and knee flexion in compensation. Sharp pain on pushoff is often caused by corns between the toes or metatarsal callosities. In longitudinal arch disorders, weight will be borne on the lateral plantar surface during weight bearing. If chronic, excessive wear on the lateral sole of the shoe will be noted.

Neurologic Gaits[167–171]

Neurologic gaits are usually the result of unilateral flexor or extensor spasticity. The clinical picture is the result of exaggerated stretch reflexes, reflex impairment of the antagonists, and poor flexor-extensor coordination. Almost all spastic gaits present a slow cadence and a repetitive pattern during each cycle.

Unilateral Flexor Spasticity. This gait is characterized by a distinct forward lurch of the trunk, a narrow base of support, a decreased stride length, and an absent heelstrike. Usually, adductor tone is normal.

Unilateral Extensor Spasticity. A spastic gait is common in upper motor neuron diseases that have a spastic paralysis of the extensor muscles. It is a feature of spinal paralysis, lateral sclerosis, and some other forms of myelitis and anterior tract or brain damage. The upper body is flexed while the lower extremity is extended. The locomotion pattern is characterized by a short stride length, a narrow base of support, and pelvic elevation during swing so that the foot will clear the floor. The legs are firmly extended, the foot is dragged along in a shuffling manner with the toes scraping upon the ground to permit one foot to pass the other, and the pelvis is tilted slightly. There is little knee flexion during the swing phase if the quadriceps are spastic. Heelstrike is absent and the knee is hyperextended in midstance if the plantar flexors are spastic or if the ankle dorsiflexors are weak. Usually, adductor tone is normal. In some cases, the adductors contract to cause the legs to cross (scissors gait), and the knees often rub each other, as seen in Little's disease.

Mowing Gait. In spastic hemiplegia, there is a unilateral spastic gait in which the pelvis is tilted and the leg is swung around in front of the other with the toes often scraping the ground. It is sometimes referred to as the mowing gait. The most common cause is hemiplegia due to cerebrovascular disease, but any condition that would result in an upper motion neuron lesion can produce the gait.[172]

Proprioception Impairment. In this gait, named an "ataxic gait" because it occurs in locomotor ataxia, the patient walks in a stooped posture with the eyes looking at the feet. The foot is raised unusually high, thrown forward with force, and brought to the ground flat-footedly with a stamp to increase sensory awareness. While in the air and before being lowered, the foot wavers as if there is a degree of uncertainty in bringing it down. The patient walks with his feet wide apart and is constantly looking at them. This is done for the purpose of supplementing the loss of proprioception. To maintain a large area of foot contact throughout weight bearing, heelstrike is usually eliminated. It is sometimes called the "tabetic gait," and characteristic of a lesion in the dorsal ganglia, dorsal roots, or posterior column of the cord—rarely in higher levels. The ataxis is increased when the eyes are closed or when the patient must walk in a darkened room. The gait is seen in tabes dorsalis, pernicious anemia, and other disorders involving proprioceptive pathways.[173,174]

Basal Ganglia Dysfunction. This gait is characteristic of paralysis agitans or Parkinson's disease. It is sometimes called a "propulsive gait" or festination (increasing speed). The hurried "sissy" toddle of parkinsonism is due to the forward tilt of the trunk in the attitude of a stoop and the attempt of the patient to maintain balance.[175,176] As the center of mass is anterior to the base of support, the patient appears to be chasing his center of gravity. Almost all joint motion is restricted, as is arm swing, pelvic tilt, pelvic rotation, and knee flexion. The body and head lean far forward. The trunk, hips, knees, and ankles are flexed to some degree, and the subject walks with short, hurried, shuffling steps, which makes it appear as if he is being pushed from the rear and is about to fall. Heelstrike is absent, and the toe is dragged during the swing phase. It is difficult for such a patient with this gait to stop suddenly or to turn a corner. Thus, falls are frequent. Progression is slow at first, and then increases rapidly.[177]

Cerebellar Dysfunction. This gait, a sign of cerebellar ataxia, resembles the actions of an intoxicated person. The patient walks with the feet wide apart, takes short steps, and sways to and fro to such an extent that progression in a straight line is almost impossible. The gait resembles that of a person trying to walk on a rolling ship, constantly trying to maintain equilibrium with little success. The gait is found in tumor of the cerebellum and disease of the semicircular canals. Cerebellar lesions are invariably associated with vertigo. It may be indicative of long-term use of alcohol or other drugs ("Jake legs") or neurosyphilis. If the causative factor is unilateral, deviation is to the involved side because of the hypotonia.[178–180]

Paralytic Gaits[167,181–183]

Paralytic or paretic gaits with varying patterns are the result of spinal root lesions, brain lesions, nerve compression syndromes, peripheral mononeuritis, abnormal reflexes, and trauma. Table 4.2 shows the common gait deviations associated with specific muscle weakness.

If the quadriceps are extremely weak, locomotion is usually impossible because the knee is too unstable during stance. If knee flexion and plantar flexion are weak during swing, compensation is made by hip elevation. The two typical patterns are referred to as the "steppage gait" and the "waddling gait."

Steppage Gait. This gait—also called the prancing, highstepping, or footdrop gait—is commonly found in infantile paralysis, multiple neuritis, peroneal nerve injury, and arsenic poisoning paralysis. The gait resembles that of a person walking in tall grass; hence its name.[184] The flexor muscles of the foot are subject to a flaccid paralysis so that the toes hang downward when the foot is raised from the floor. To prevent the toes

Table 4.2.
Common Gait Deviations Associated with Specific Muscle Weakness

Major muscle weakness	Gait sign (deviation from normal)
Spinal extensors, hip flexors	Posterior pelvic rotation at heelstrike.
Hip flexors	Toes drag on floor during midswing. Trunk shifts to swing side, pelvis lifts on weight-bearing side, and leg is circumducted during swing phase.
Hip extensors	Posterior shifting of head and trunk at midstance with pelvis rotated posteriorly. Arms are at an uneven distance from the midline and both elbows are flexed at pushoff. Femur in exaggerated lateral rotation at hip during pushoff. Forefoot not in contact with floor when heel is lifted in pushoff.
Abdominals and hip extensors	Exaggerated anterior pelvic rotation at midstance and pushoff.
Hip adductors	Femur abducted at hip at heelstrike. Head and trunk tip to weight-bearing side and pelvis tips downward on the contralateral side at midstance. Exaggerated outward rotation of femur during midstance.
Medial rotators of hip, knee extensors, foot evertors	Short step, trunk displaced to right, femur rotated laterally at hip at heelstrike and midstance. The femur is laterally rotated at the hip at midswing.
Knee extensors	Anterior shift of head and trunk at heelstrike, and at midstance with exaggerated anterior rotation of pelvis. Arms are at an uneven distance from the midline and both elbows are flexed at pushoff. Femur in exaggerated lateral rotation at hip during pushoff. The forefoot does not keep contact with the floor when heel is lifted during pushoff.
Knee flexors	Toes drag on floor during midswing. Trunk shifts to swing side, pelvis lifts on weight-bearing side, and leg is circumducted during swing phase.
Knee extensors and flexors, and ankle dorsiflexors	Knee locked or hyperextended at heelstrike and/or at midstance.
Ankle dorsiflexors	No heelstrike, slapping forefoot, and plantar surface of forefoot is not visible at heelstrike. At midswing, hip and knee flexion are exaggerated and forefoot drops (ie, steppage gait). Toes may drag on floor during midswing. Trunk shifts to swing side, pelvis lifts on weight-bearing side and leg is circumducted during swing phase.
Ankle plantar flexors	Knee is in exaggerated flexion and ankle is in calcaneal position at midstance. Knee partially flexed at pushoff. Arms are not at an equal distance from midline and both elbows are flexed at pushoff. Plantar flexion limited with ankle in possible dorsiflexion, and metatarsophalangeal joints are straight at pushoff. Femur is in exaggerated lateral rotation at hip during pushoff. Forefoot not in contact with floor when heel is lifted during pushoff.
Foot invertors	Foot is in valgus position at midstance.
Foot evertors	Foot is in varus position at midstance. Forefoot drops during midswing.

from dragging on the floor or catching upon objects, the foot is raised high and brought to the floor forcibly before the toes can drop. Thus the foot strikes the floor heel first or flat-footed.[185] The gait is especially suspect in tertiary syphilis.

Waddling Gait. This occurs when there is extreme muscular weakness in the thigh and hip muscles as commonly found in pseudohypertrophic muscular paralysis and muscular atrophy or dystrophy. In this gait, the shoulders are thrown back, the lower section of the spine is lordotic, the pelvis is tilted greatly, and, while in this state, the leg is brought around and placed on the floor. When walking, the subject swings from side to side in a very noticeable manner; thus it is often referred to as the goose gait. This gait is also seen in bilateral hip dislocation. In gaits involving muscle weakness, the compensatory pattern is largely the result of the patient's attempt to alter the center of gravity relative to the base of support.[185–187]

Hip Disorders. Extension weakness, flexion weakness, or abductor weakness of the hip offer characteristic gait patterns:

1. *Extension weakness.* During extension paralysis, the gait is grossly altered in weight bearing after heelstrike when the extensors normally contract. Due to the weakness, the trunk is thrown backward to maintain balance by keeping the center of gravity behind the axis of the hip.

2. *Flexion weakness.* Weak hip flexors affect acceleration during swing, the pelvis is usually elevated, the trunk is thrown backward toward the unaffected side in compensation, but stance is rarely affected. The stride is usually short on the involved side.

3. *Abductor weakness.* In upper motor neuron weakness of the hip abductors, the trunk is thrown toward the affected side during weight bearing. If uncompensated, the pelvis distinctly lunges laterally toward the affected side and dips on the side of swing. At midswing, hip and knee flexion is exaggerated on the unaffected side. In less severe cases, there is little sideward lunging because of trunk compensation. Use of a cane on the contralateral side of involvement also eliminates this lateral lurch.

Knee Disorders. As with the hip, extension weakness or flexion weakness offer characteristic gait patterns:

1. *Extensor weakness.* This pattern is often difficult to see. In stance, the knee is normally fully extended. The features of the weakness are most prominent after heelstrike when the quadriceps normally contract and the knee flexes. Signs of excessive heel lift during gait and excessive knee flexion during the swing phase should be sought. Knee extension is maintained at heelstrike and throughout stance by hip extension (eg, gluteus maximus via the iliotibial tract) and plantar flexion. This is assisted by throwing the trunk forward at heelstrike to move the center of gravity anterior to the axis of the knee. In pronounced cases, the patient will push the affected thigh backward with his hand to assist extension.

2. *Flexor weakness.* Weak hamstrings allow full knee extension and inhibit deceleration as heelstrike approaches. This produces a quite hard heelstrike, often called an "overshot." Near the end of the stance phase, the knee fails to flex until pushoff. In prolonged conditions, the result is often the development of distinct knee hyperextension (genu recurvatum) that is most difficult to correct without the use of a check brace until the ligaments tighten.

Ankle Disorders. Ankle plantar flexion weakness and dorsiflexion weakness exhibit characteristic patterns:

1. *Plantar flexion weakness.* If these muscles are weak, propulsion is inhibited because heeloff is impaired. The foot leaves the floor as a unit, the knee is fully extended, and the hip flexes at pushoff to begin the swing phase. As pushoff is controlled essentially by foot plantar flexion, triceps surae paralysis or Achilles tendon trauma will force some compensation by the gluteus maximus and posterior hamstrings.

2. *Dorsiflexion weakness.* When the ankle dorsiflexors are mildly weak, it is possible to lift the foot from the floor, but during the swing phase, relaxation occurs, which causes the foot to be slapped down during flatfoot. In severe weakness, toestrike replaces heelstrike. This requires a compensatory increase in hip and knee flexion during the swing phase so that the foot clears the floor (steppage gait).

Restricted Motion Gaits

Movement restricted within either the passive or active range of motion of the hip, knee, or ankle exhibits changes in locomotive patterns. The picture is usually attributable to soft tissue contractures and/or bony deformities (Fig. 4.30). In pure anklyosis, from either bone fusion or excessive fibrosis, there is no joint motion whatever. The terminology in describing these conditions is often confusing, because abduction contracture refers to adduction limitation, flexion deformity refers to extension limitation, etc.

Restricted Hip Flexion. At heelstrike, the lumbar area is flexed to compensate for the pelvis being rotated and elevated, and a distinct backward trunk lunge is seen if the spine is not flexible. Stride length is shortened on the involved side. Pelvic elevation, hip flexion, and knee flexion become exaggerated during swing to help the involved limb to clear the floor.

Restricted Hip Extension. The stride length is shortened on the uninvolved side, and midstance of the involved limb shows exaggerated knee flexion. When the disorder is severe, toe walking is seen, early heeloff occurs, a compensatory lumbar lordosis is produced after midstance, and the trunk is often thrown forward, especially if the spine is not flexible.

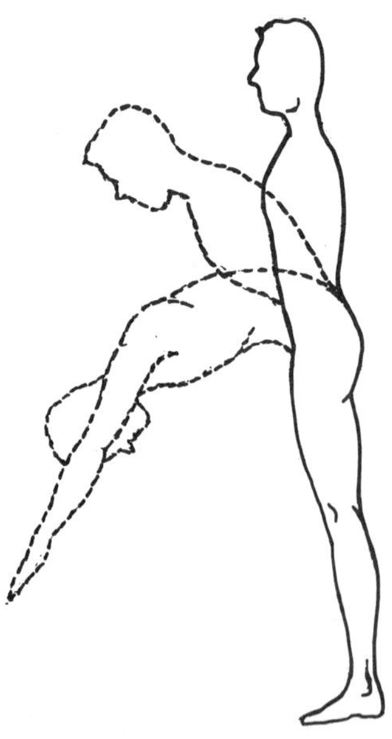

Figure 4.30. The Adams maneuver: the round forward trunk bend in evaluation of hip and spinal flexibility.

Restricted Hip Rotation. Once this occurs, stride length is greatly diminished. The foot pivots laterally on the involved side during weight bearing, especially between flatfoot and toeoff.

Restricted Hip Abduction. On the uninvolved side, the pelvis is elevated during swing and stance. A compensatory functional sciolosis that curves *toward the involved side* is common. A broad base is constantly attempted.

Restricted Hip Adduction. During stance, the trunk is thrown toward the affected side. In contrast to restricted abduction, the base is kept small, and a scissor motion is usually made when the involved limb is in the swing phase. A compensatory functional sciolosis that curves *toward the uninvolved side* is common. This is necessary to maintain the center of gravity over the limb during weight bearing. Contracture is exhibited by a functional short-leg that is compensated for by exaggerated hip and knee flexion on the uninvolved side and toe walking during stance on the involved side.

Restricted Knee Flexion. When knee flexion is limited, the pelvis must be elevated and the extremity circumducted so that the foot can avoid the ground during the swing phase. To assist this, there is usually a distinct toe stance during weight bearing on the uninvolved side.

Restricted Knee Extension. If the knee is unable to fully extend, the stride length shortens on the involved side, and heelstrike is usually eliminated. The heel remains raised during flatfoot, propulsion is weak at pushoff, and hip and knee flexion is exaggerated on the uninvolved side during swing.

Restricted Ankle Dorsiflexion. Heelstrike is absent, toe contact is seen throughout the stance phase, and the knee is forced into hyperextension. The propulsive force at pushoff is lessened. During swing, hip and knee flexion is exaggerated on the involved side and the affected limb is swung outward to help clear the ground.

Senile Gait. This gait is caused by shortening and loss of elasticity of ligaments and tendons, and a stiffening of cartilage, muscle, and fascia as a result of the degenerative aging process. Steps are short, shuffling, and assumed in a stooped position if osteoporosis is present to cause a marked dorsal kyphosis. Whenever the passive range of joint motion is limited by structural changes, the compensatory pattern usually reflects an exaggerated motion at noninvolved joints.

Short-Leg Syndrome. A difference in leg lengths increases the vertical oscillatory amplitude of the body's center of gravity. In compensation on the involved side, the pelvis drops on heelstrike and remains tipped throughout stance, heelstrike reduces in proportion to the leg deficiency, stride length is shortened, and toe walking is seen throughout the stance phase. On the side of the long limb, increased hip and knee flexion occurs during both the swing and stance phases.

Functionally Inhibited Gaits[188]

In addition to those gaits discussed, locomotion may be restricted by various types of psychomotor disorders. The two major types are those due to hysteria or higher center apraxia.

Hysteria. These gaits rarely have a repetitive pattern, and many movements are highly exaggerated. It is difficult to match gait signs with neurologic and musculoskeletal findings. Tremor usually appears during observed active exercise, and strength rapidly fades when passive movements are resisted by the patient. Although the motions are gross and unpredictable, falling is rare. If falling occurs, it is well protected. In some cases, the pattern is repetitive. This is the result of a "gait habit" that persists long after the cause of malfunction has been eliminated. The clinical picture is often confusing because persistent atrophy, edema, and vasomotor instability may be solely the result of disuse.[189]

Gait Apraxia. In this condition, motor power is present but the *memory* of how to use the power is lacking or diminished. Steps are small, slow, and uncertain, and the patient must be urged or assisted to initiate progress. This gait is characteristic of frontal lobe lesions or bilateral lesions of the corticospinal tract in the internal capsule, cerebral peduncles, or high brainstem. It is often seen immediately following prolonged bed confinement, but in this situation it is quickly overcome.

Laboratory Mensuration of Gait

The analysis of gait impairments in the office of a general practitioner is conducted almost exclusively through gross observation, inspection, muscle testing, range of motion analyses, electrodiagnosis, and, sometimes, electromyography. The research laboratory, however, offers many advantages in objectively quantifying gait patterns, functional deficits, and patient response to therapy. The data obtained from frame-by-frame motion picture of a body or cineroentgenography of a region in motion, for example, were described in Chapter 3. Other means are being developed each year.

To measure relative joint rotation of the ankle, knee, and hip, instrumentation at the Mayo Gait Laboratory includes three-dimensional electrogoniometers. Instrumented mats are used to measure step length and width, footswitches are used to record foot-floor contact sequences, piezoelectric force plates are used to measure floor-reaction forces, and two walkways are used to simulate variable ground conditions. The data obtained are then analyzed with the aid of a computer to assess patient progress under prescribed exercise and gait training regimens.[190]

Running and Jumping[191]

The mechanics of running are similar to those of walking in several respects. Both walking and running require (1) weight to be projected forward and the legs carried alternately under the body for brief periods of support, and (2) the weight-bearing limb to provide the propulsive action after the center of body weight has passed over it. Walking becomes a running gait at that point in acceleration when a period of nonsupport appears. During the phase of nonsupport in which there is no surface friction, the body can be considered a missile.

Jumping is essentially the act of propelling the body into the air by rapid leg extension. It is usually considered in three phases: takeoff, flight, and landing. Jumping is governed by the same principles that govern missiles. Thus, the motions made during flight have little influence on direction, height, or distance. Their main purpose is to prepare the body for landing.

Biodynamics

During running, angular knee flexion displacement increases to reduce the effective radius of the limb as the hip of the recovery thigh begins to flex (Fig. 4.31). This decreases the limb's moment of inertia to allow a faster recovery on the swing-through with less effort. The flexing hip transfers angular momentum to the leg and foot as the limb continues to swing forward. The knee continues to extend until the foot reaches its most anterior position. At footstrike, the body's center of mass is carried over the weight-bearing foot by combined hip extension and the forward momentum of the body. Arm swing, trunk rotation, and position and forces of the contralateral limb help to counteract the undesirable moments established during footstrike.

Running speed is essentially limited by (1) the forces necessary to accelerate and then decelerate the recovery limb, and (2) the inertia of the lower limbs during recovery. Other contributing factors include poor strength or endurance, excessive arm or lower-extremity antagonistic muscle tension, excessive leg weight, short leg length, decreased flexibility, poor timing and coordination, slow reaction speed, and inhibited pace or motivation.

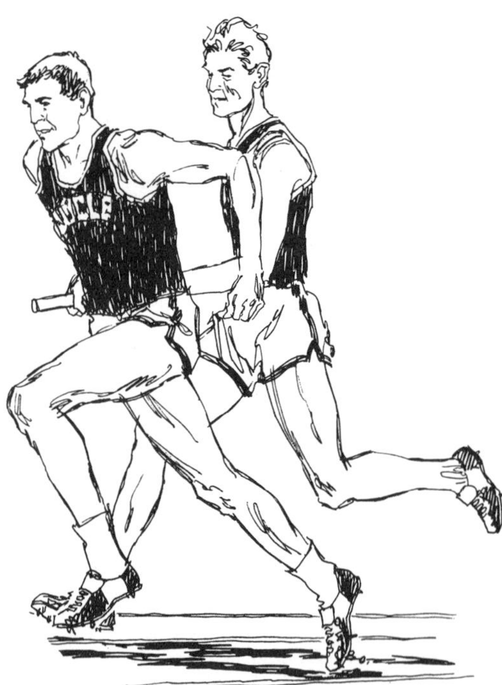

Figure 4.31. Portrayal of the biodynamics of running at pushoff by the front figure and the period of nonsupport by the back figure.

The muscle contractions occurring near the extreme of movement initiate a mechanical impulse to the limb segments that causes the limb to decelerate and reverse direction. This, in turn, gives the limb sufficient momentum to swing through its range of motion without the assistance of muscular action. It should be noted that hamstring injury usually occurs when this muscle group is attempting to reduce the speed of the extending knee.

The foot changes velocity in short periods as it accelerates and decelerates. Powerful hip and knee extension occur during the running cycle, and the gastrocnemius and soleus contract strongly before the foot strikes the ground. This prevents heelstrike by transferring body weight to the ball of the foot which subjects the arch to enormous forces when the impact force of footstrike is added to body weight. The same is true during pushoff. These forces must be absorbed by the body through the joints.

Arm Swing

While it was once thought that the arms simply act as pendulums during gait, it has recently been established that they play an active integrated part in locomotion. The angular momentum of the arms helps to counteract the rapid changes in the angular momentum of the trunk. When walking increases to running, the elbows remain flexed and the amplitude of arm swing is increased to compensate for the necessary angular momentum of the arm.

Practical Fluid Mechanics and Buoyancy

The human body commonly moves through the fluid media of air and water. Air resistance has little effect in normal activities at slow speeds. However, in such activities as distance runs at maximum speed, skiing, kite gliding, and sky diving, air resistance and force interactions are factors to be considered.

While man is essentially a land animal,

many human characteristics are useful in aquatic activity. Mechanical forces increase as the density of the fluid medium increases. For example, the force of fluid friction is readily exhibited in the energy consumed when one tries to walk or run within waist-deep water.[192]

Buoyancy

A person's specific gravity is usually slightly less than water when the lungs are inflated. The buoyancy force on a body submerged wholly or partially in water is equal to the weight of the volume of water displaced (Archimedes' principle).[193]

The Center of Buoyancy. The center of buoyancy is the center of gravity of the volume of fluid displaced *prior* to displacement. This volume of displaced fluid is the same shape as the submerged body. In biomechanical problems, buoyancy force is considered to act at the body's center of buoyancy just as gravitational force is considered to act at the body's center of gravity. However, these lines will not coincide because the body is not of uniform density. Once emerged partially or wholly in water, the body's center of buoyancy is in the center of the region that displaces the most water. Thus, for a swimmer, it is in the center of the torso (lower thorax).

Equilibrium[194]

Static Equilibrium in Water. When the relaxed body attempts to float within water, the swimmer's body rotates until his center of buoyancy and center of gravity are in the same plane, whether it be horizontal, diagonal, or vertical (Fig. 4.32).

Dynamic Equilibrium in Water. Dynamic equilibrium is not difficult to maintain as long as the swimmer stays in a relatively horizontal position. The higher the body position in the water, the lesser is the resistance. The lower the body position, the greater is the energy economy.

Drag. The other biomechanical forces that affect performance are *form drag* and *surface drag.* Form drag depends on the cross-sectional area of the body that is perpendicular to the direction of water flow and the smoothness (waviness) of the water surface. Surface drag is the resistance generated between the surface of the body and the water adjacent to it, and its end result depends upon the surface area of the body, the body's velocity, and the properties of the fluid medium.

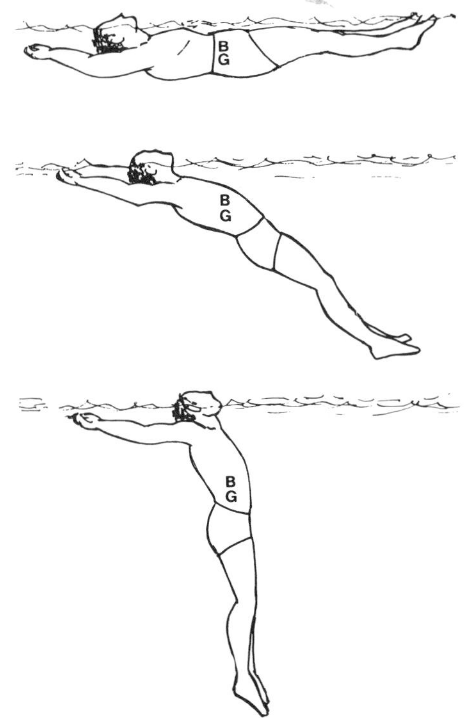

Figure 4.32. Various floating positions depend on the relationship between the individual's centers of gravity and buoyancy. In the drawings, *B* is the approximate center of buoyancy, *G* is the approximate center of gravity.

TYPICAL EFFECTS OF BALANCE DEFECTS[195, 196]

Normal posture is that posture which best suits an individual according to his or her internal and external environmental conditions. An erect posture reflects self-confidence, a readiness to act, and shows the physique to a better advantage. Clothes are designed for such a posture.

A relaxed or slouched posture usually connotes laziness, incompetence, and an inferior self-image. However, this is not always the case. That is, superior energy potential and intellectual capacity is often housed in a body that is habitually slouched. Some individuals assume habitual postures of great relaxation during periods of nonactivity. This is because one will assume an energy-conserving posture during a state of fatigue.

There is no clear symptomatic picture of balance defects, because individuals vary so much in response to mechanical insult. Some people present immediate symptoms upon slight deviation, while others offer no symptoms until pathologic changes are in progress. Much of this is determined by how the body is used; eg, occupational and athletic considerations.[197]

Effects of Bipedism[198-201]

Bipedism requires certain anatomic considerations to appreciate the fact that the spine and pelvis are of commanding clinical importance because of their intimate involvement with the nervous system. In the human biped, there is a unique relationship between the musculoskeletal mechanism and the neurologic bed.[202] The neurologic factors that relate to bipedism represent the rationale of clinical chiropractic that is often readily portrayed during dynamic postures.

Derangements in the musculoskeletal system in the human are much more common than in the quadriped. Consequently, the human biped is heir to those elements that are the consequence of disturbed body mechanics. For example, the sacroiliac articulations at the time of birth are amphiarthrodial. But as standing and locomotion are acquired, the joints are induced to assume diarthrodial movements and come to possess encompassing ligaments, articulating cartilages, and a bed of proprioceptors.[203]

Effects of Bipedal Stress[204-206]

The human torso is much like a "skyscraper" wherein strain and stress are greater at certain points than at others[207] (Fig. 4.33). Within the zone of these points of primary function and stress, there is a relatively heavy deposition of sensory nerve endings and motor end plates. When these areas, heavily populated with neuronal and vascular ramifications, are subject to trauma, occupational stress, the strains of postural fatigue, and abnormal viscerospinal reflexes, the process of transudation, fibrin precipitation, and adhesion formation ensues to establish an intramuscular and myofascial plane trigger point.[208] To this must be added the principle of neurologic facilitation and spread. Not uncommonly, there is a musculoskeletal syndrome complex that challenges the clinical capacity of the most healthy.

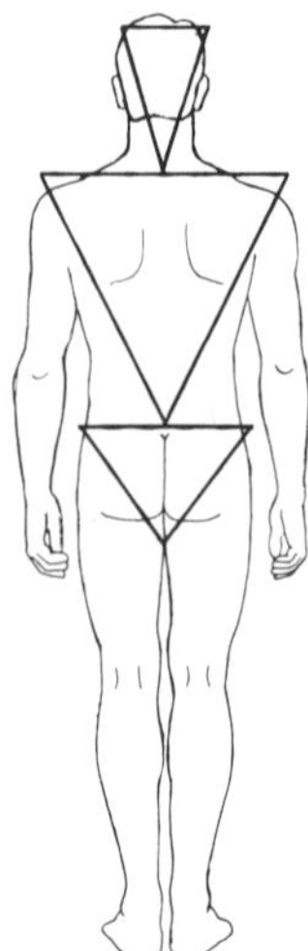

Figure 4.33. The inverted pyramid design of the body predisposes it to instability and chronic stress to maintain balance.

Bipedism augments the concern of gravity and weight bearing, postural faults, strains and stresses of occupation and play, and trauma.[209] Because of such stress, the articular, syndesmotic, and myologic proprioceptive complex is often disturbed, which results in the development of many common spinosomatic and spinovisceral syndromes. The intervertebral disc, especially in certain areas of the spine, becomes a most vulnerable unit of disturbance, discogenic extension, and resultant disc syndromes. A deranged spinal or pelvic segment within its motor bed will always result in disturbance of the proprioceptive bed with facilitation of the discomfort and pain phenomenon.

Functional tension (whether it be of emotional, infectious, traumatic, or immobilization origin) leads to irritation and pain. Pain leads to muscle tension, edema, inflammation, a fibrotic reaction, and ultimately to functional disability (Fig. 4.34). When a muscle is under constant tension, the retained metabolites from stasis and internal tissue ischemia create a vicious circle enhancing tension and inflammation.[210]

Body Type and Balance Defects[211-221]

Balance defects tend to differ somewhat in the classic body types. They are especially

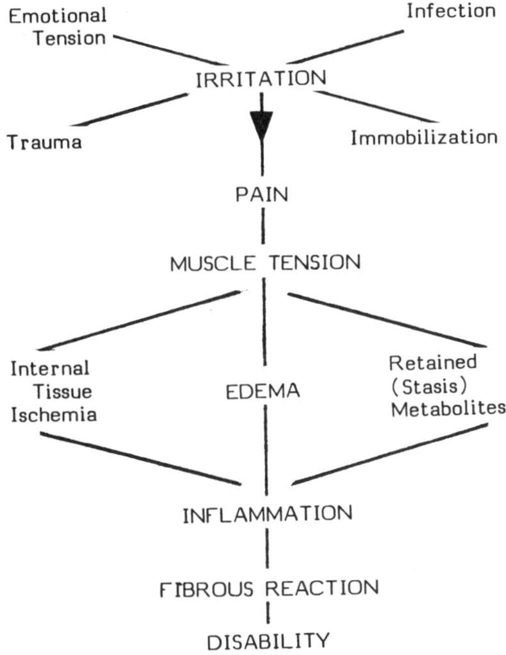

Figure 4.34. Basic mechanisms by which irritation can lead to functional disability, as adapted from Cailliet.

difficult to differentiate during youth (Fig. 4.35).

The Ectomorph

In the lean ectomorph, the anatomic design has a tendency to encourage poor body mechanics. Postural relaxation is the rule unless the person has had specialized training or makes a conscious effort. Habitual relaxation leads to a forward head carriage, flat chest, and narrow subcostal angle. The ribs and diaphragm are low, and the vital capacity is decreased. The abdomen is small above and protrudes just above the symphysis pubis, while retroperitoneal fat is slight. Visceroptosis is usually evident. The spine presents sharp bends in the midcervical and upper dorsal areas. There is a sharp lumbosacral curve with some accompanying lordosis. The pelvis inclines more than 60°, and the knees are often hyperextended.

The Endomorph

Such extremes of relaxation do not usually occur in the stocky endomorph because the anatomic construction is not so favorable to strain. However, the endomorph's shorter ligaments and restricted range of joint motion allow symptoms to appear with only moderate deviations from the ideal. It is common to see sagging of the large, heavy viscera in the poorly conditioned individual, compensated for by a backward inclination of the trunk. Because of the limited range

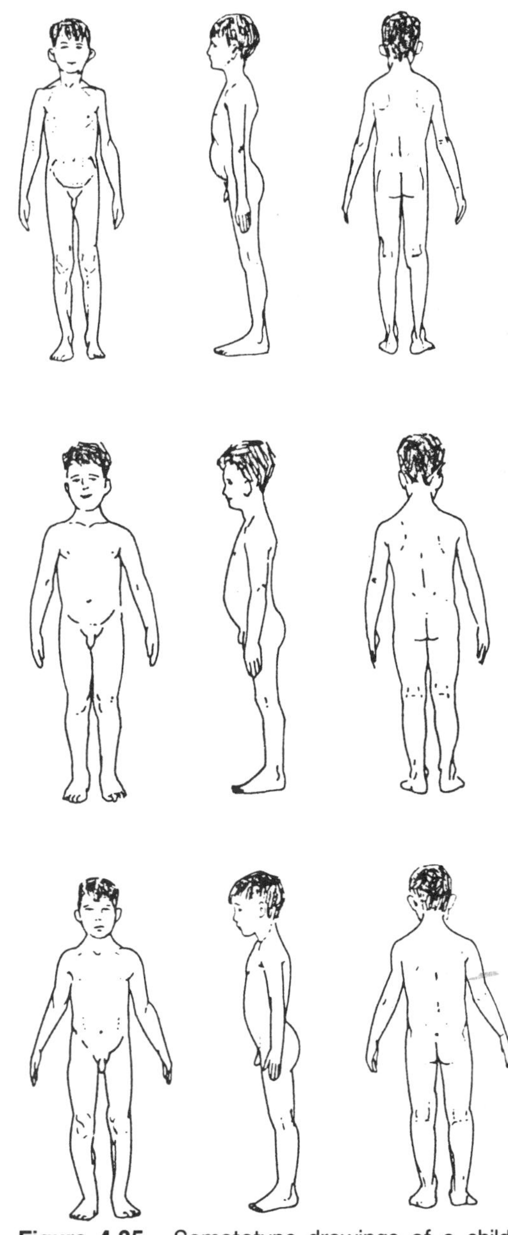

Figure 4.35. Somatotype drawings of a child exhibiting *top*, a high degree of ectomorphism; *center*, a high degree of endomorphism; *bottom*, a high degree of mesomorphism.

of spinal motion, bending to maintain the center of gravity over the feet usually comes either at the hips or dorsolumbar junction. Thus, both areas are common points of stress and fatigue.

The Mesomorph

Faulty body mechanics also occur in the intermediate body type, resembling either an overly relaxed ectomorph or endomorph, and thus are difficult to profile.

Biomechanical Properties of Different Body Types

By using a mathematical model to estimate the size and inertial properties of the segments and the whole body of three boys, Jensen has shown that varying biomechanical properties have important implications for the development of motor skills and efficiency in children of different body types.[222] Comparisons were made between an endomorph and an ectomorph who had similar link dimensions, and between the endomorph and a mesomorph who had a similar body mass. For the endomorph, some of the segment masses were substantially greater than would be expected by comparing the total body masses of the endomorph and ectomorph, suggesting significant constraints on the development of upper- and lower-extremity linear momentum. These differences were even more pronounced when the segmental and whole body principal moments of inertia were compared; the greatest differences were for the longitudinal axes. When comparing the inertial properties of the endomorph and mesomorph, it was found that they were similar. The mesomorph in this study, however, was older and more physically developed than the endomorph, and was thus more able to accommodate to the constraints.

Etiology of Postural Faults[223-227]

From a physiologic standpoint, "normal" posture is that condition in which the body functions the most efficiently. From a structural standpoint, a population's normal posture is more difficult to judge. That shown in most illustrations is an "ideal" posture, not normal posture. Posture is constantly shifting to rest active muscles and to adapt to various conditions such as ground surface, heat and cold, sickness and health, sadness and joy, clothing, and social customs.

A few influences on human posture are (1) gravity; (2) environment, eg, occupation, weather; (3) architecture of the vertebral column, upper and lower appendages, and organs and tissues that attach to or are suspended from the spinal column; (4) physiology, normal and abnormal; (5) pathology; (6) emotional states; and (7) pain.

Subluxations are often the forerunners of balance defects brought about through the effort of the spinal column to compensate for the stress and thus to reduce the more serious effects. Balance defects may also originate from habitual faulty postures in standing, sitting, and lying, as well as from activities that constantly employ the forces of the large muscles in asymmetrical action.[228] When created, such defects serve to lessen the power of the body to withstand shock and are, in turn, the precursors to subluxations.

Other causes of defects in balance are found in the frequent occurrence of unequal lower extremities, in faulty development of vertebrae and the sacrum, and from the effects of abnormal reflexes. The least common causes of balance defects can be attributed to inheritance. Constitutional stress, visceral malfunction, nutritional status, fatigue and debility, neuromuscular tension, a large variety of psychologic factors, height, weight and body type all combine to express themselves in one's posture, body balance, and motor ability.

Basic Physiologic Reactions to Postural Faults[225, 229-233]

No two individuals react in an identical manner to actual or potential loss of body balance. All vary somewhat in the accomodation process, depending upon gross structure and functional capabilities, the momentary potential for redistributing body mass, and the visual efficiency necessary to guide correct accommodations.

Most balance faults witnessed in practice will be within "physiologic" limits without obvious structural deformity, yet it should be appreciated that abnormal function leads to reduced performance capabilities early and to pathology later if left uncorrected. Isolated muscle weakness should be suspected especially in situations of head or pelvic tilt, trunk imbalance, scoliosis, and uneven gait or limp.

Basic Factors

Tolerance. Poor posture from habit, disease, or abnormal reflexes results in constant structural malalignment which allows a disproportionate amount of weight and muscle pull to fall upon some parts. This alters the normal locomotion apparatus and functions of the internal organs as well. While these changes may develop insidiously, the resulting static abnormalities produce pathologic changes in the body during standing, sitting, lying, and motion. Such abnormalities are tolerated for a short time, but sooner or later, serious, and often subtle, maladjustments result when the body's compensation resources become exhausted. These factors, in total, may predispose an individual to injury or hinder performance.

Endurance. An important factor in health care is that, with good postural body mechanics, balance is maintained with the least amount of muscular effort, thus encouraging longer endurance, with less strain on any one part. Locomotion can be made without wasted time or energy. Muscle pull in maintaining an erect carriage is more direct, thus avoiding strain. A natural balance is maintained between the iliopsoas group and the hip extensors, and a similar condition exists at the knee and ankle joints.

Effort. Energy requirements vary considerably with different postures. The rigid "military" posture requires about 20% more energy than the relaxed standing posture. In this rigid posture, blood pressure rises because of the muscular effort required. A completely relaxed standing position requires little more energy than that required for the sitting position.[234]

Regional Effects. Postural faults can lead to a number of regional disorders. For example, a round-shouldered posture alters the glenohumeral articulating mechanism by depressing the overhanging acromion in front and rotating the dependent arm internally. Both of these conditions encourage cuff entrapment and attrition. An exaggerated cervical or lumbar lordosis decreases the size of the intervetebral foramina, frequently resulting in chronic radiculitis and degenerative changes. Exaggerated thoracic kyphosis decreases rib excursion and alters the functional motion of the shoulder girdle. These and many other postural disorders will be discussed further in later chapters.

Functional Stress and Fatigue[235]

In chronic balance defects, physiologic stress and fatigue cannot be discussed in unrelated terms. Stress arises when the body is forced to be used in a position that is not favorable to muscle balance or when the joints are at their physiologic limit of articulation. Thus, pull comes from ligaments rather than muscles. The result is tissue insult leading to edema, pain, and physical deformity that is referred to (1) the structures upon which the strain is imposed, or (2) the cutaneous branches of the spinal nerve root supplying the strained tissues. Long-term muscle strain results in adaptive changes occurring in the joints and ligaments to meet the needs of the malalignment. Thus, low-key chronic sprain is a part of the picture. Abnormal fatigue is the result of wasted energy.

In the spine, for example, the more pronounced an abnormal curvature, the greater becomes the mechanical disadvantage to which the supporting structures are subjected. Thus, the process is a vicious circle. Along with chronic stress and fatigue, constant pull causes small tears in ligamentous attachments. This results in a series of subperiosteal hemorrhages which later may calcify into exostoses, becoming extremely painful upon further stress. Such a situation may occur in any joint that is subjected to prolonged strain, but it is especially common in the spine and other weight-bearing joints.

Neuralgia

In spinal imbalance, there always appears to be some degree of intervertebral foramina (IVF) insult present. Neuralgic pains in the thorax and legs are common.[227] Less common, because it mimics visceral disease, is intercostal neuralgia. If originating in the cervical region and associated with hypertrophic changes, pain is often referred about the shoulders and down the arms, frequently being mistaken for angina pectoris. Similar neuralgic pains in the chest walls can be mistaken for pleurisy, pleural adhesions, or pulmonary lesions. Auscultation will serve in the differentiation.

Intrafascicular Adhesions

A muscle in spasm or under strain from any cause (or a stressed tendon or ligament) will become congested. This congestion always results in some degree of transudation and the conversion of fibrinogen into fibrin, which acts as a cobweb-like adhesion or interfascicular gluing that impedes fascicular glide. As a result in muscles, tendons, and ligaments under strain, painful interfascicular constrictions occur, leading to the common algias of these structures.[236] If permitted to continue, collagenic infiltration and even calcific deposition may take place. When a tendon is likewise involved or when a ligament is subject to strain, similar changes take place, with an invasion process resulting in possible fibrosis and calcific tendonitis or syndesmitis.

Trigger Points

Concurrently, similar events occur in the myofascial planes at a point of major tensile stress leading to the development of "trigger points" and the resulting delta or spread effect. All muscles have their fascial encasements (epimesium, perimesium, endomesium); and, as muscles lie and move one upon the other, the myofascial planes are described. The number of fasciculi involved in the all-or-none contraction effort determines the tone or strength of muscle contraction. Furthermore, a muscle usually does more work at one point of its composite than at another.

Circulatory Implications[227,237]

Circulatory disturbances are rarely absent in gross postural faults. The low diaphragm results in venous congestion by its failure to assist blood returning to the heart. Sagging viscera stretch mesenteric vessels and narrow their lumina. Thus, circulatory symptoms may manifest throughout the body. For instance, medical researchers have recorded the relief of eyestrain and mild myopia in children by postural correction alone. They explain this as a relief of venous congestion in the head.

In extreme cases, impaired circulatory inefficiency may be sufficient to produce a marked fall in blood pressure and loss of consciousness. This is said to be the result of general muscle relaxation with pooling of blood in the venous reservoirs, especially in the abdomen, thus reducing the practical blood volume. More often it causes only dyspnea and weakness, sometimes accompanied by palpitation. Precordial pain resembling angina pectoris is not rare.

Drainage Impairments

Faulty posture mechanics may cause the liver to rotate anteriorly and to the right. Traction is thereby exerted on the common duct and in some cases seriously interferes with biliary drainage. Ptosis of the kidneys, especially the left kidney, results in traction on the renal veins which may obstruct venous outflow to cause passive congestion and albuminuria.[238]

Visceral Implications

It is unwise to consider the various parts of the body as separate entities. All parts share responsibility in the orthograde posture. Any disturbance in one part causes an immediate and definite functional change in other parts.[239]

Extreme curvature and malalignment produce physiologic changes and are considered to be pathologic, but how much deviation is possible without causing severe impairment of health? The opinion on the effect on function varies in the research literature. Most research workers agree, however, that poor body mechanics predisposes to certain visceral disorders; ie, the viscera are held in their optimum position for function in good body mechanics. If mechanics are good, the abdominal cavity is shaped like an inverted pear with adequate space above L4 for the abdominal viscera of an intermediate body type.

Nature provides good support for the abdominal organs when the body is normally erect. In the ideal attitude, tissue ledges and shelves exist to partially support the abdominal organs. However, if the lumbar and dorsal curves increase and the abdominal wall relaxes, these vital supports are lost.

The Stomach. With the stomach lying mainly to the left of the spine and supported by a diaphragmatic attachment behind the transverse sagittal plane, there is little tendency for downward displacement if there is no rib cage deformity or abdominal muscle weakness.

The Liver. The liver is generally posterior to the transverse sagittal plane. It is partly supported by the surrounding organs and its attachments to the diaphragm, but most of its weight is borne by the concave space at the side of the spine and by the curves of the lower ribs.

The Spleen and Pancreas. The spleen is well back and held in place by peritoneal folds, and the pancreas depends chiefly on the surrounding organs for support.

The Kidneys. The kidneys normally rest in definite depressions that begin around the level of L4 and are supported by the psoas muscle, quadratus lumborum, and retroperitoneal fat.

The Colon. The attachments of the hepatic and splenic flexures of the colon are external to the kidney and attached to the posterior surface of the abdominal cavity. About 87% of the weight of the abdominal organs is borne by the psoas shelf and the muscles of the abdominal wall.

Digestive Disturbances. Mild digestive symptoms may be present in the apparently healthy person. This is sometimes traced to a degree of visceroptosis which results in dysfunction of the displaced organs. Abdominal dilatation and motility disturbances are not infrequent occurrences. This is most likely the outcome of stretching of the sympathetic nerves. Pottenger points out that stretched nerves within involuntary or voluntary muscles usually produce a temporary paralysis.[240] In addition, when the abdominal cavity becomes shortened longitudinally, the viscera become crowded as do the glands of internal secretion and the nerve ganglia.[241] Thus, orthostatic albuminuria, dysmenorrhea, and constipation may sometimes be associated.

Effects of Prolapse. As a result of visceroptosis, a compensating lumbar lordosis, and the insult at the intervertebral foramina, symptoms can be diffuse and subtle.[242] Duodenal stasis may be attributed to increased tension on the superior mesenteric vessels. One study has shown that postural correction relieved 65% of cases exhibiting a picture of duodenal obstruction, and 75% of cases presenting gastric distress, nausea, and abdominal pain associated with visceroptosis. Narrowing of the IVF may cause severe pain that has a segmental distribution and is evidenced in the skin, muscle, or parietal peritoneum. This condition is usually misleading as to origin because it suggests the presence of some intra-abdominal disorder.

Respiratory Considerations

Most physical activities require good lung capacity, and respiratory balance and the maintenance of proper intra-abdominal pressure are dependent upon good body mechanics.[243,244]

The Diaphragm. In the ideal physical attitude, the position of the head well poised and the chest held high is important because the anterior mediastinal ligaments attached to the diaphragm originate in the deep cervical fascia and are attached to the lower cervical vertebrae. When mechanics are poor, a lowered diaphragm is the rule, and proper coordination of the muscles of respiration is lost. This abnormal position may decrease vital capacity by more than half. Venous and lymphatic return is greatly assisted by the rhythmic contractions of the diaphragm. When the diaphragm has been lowered, it has a much shorter range of excursion and is thus much less effective as a circulatory aid.

Respiratory Efficiency. Because only a small part of available lung tissue is ample for the minimal requirement of gaseous exchange in the relaxed state, respiratory efficiency is difficult to measure during the nonactive state. The small gain in maximal diaphragmatic excursion and vital capacity resulting from postural changes can be considered inconsequential. Thus, the physiologic efficiency in the erect posture, relaxed or rigid, should not be considered "normal" because the efficiency of the metabolic and circulatory systems is reduced.

Postural Instability: Precursor to Low-Back Pain

Porterfield considers most low-back strains and sprains to originate in tissues that have been chronically stressed by poor posture. He states that many patients have decreased overall fitness, asymmetrical skeletal forces, and an unstable lumbopelvic region that is highly vulnerable to injury, and thus are "accidents waiting to happen." If normal function and postural biomechanics are not restored, frequent reinjury and chronic symptoms often occur.[245]

It is Micheli's opinion that much of the postural instability that leads to low-back pain in adolescents represents a transient overgrowth syndrome in which, during the second growth spurt, the bony elements develop faster than the ligaments, tendons, and strong dorsal fascia. The result is a combination of taut weak abdominal muscles anteriorly and lumbosacral fascia and hamstrings posteriorly, which produces a posterior decompensation of the trunk over the pelvis. The typical compensation mechanism for this structural imbalance is to develop a mild round back, which helps to rebalance the trunk more anteriorly over the pelvis, and this can lead to wedged vertebral bodies at the apex of the compensatory thoracic kyphosis.[246]

REFERENCES

1. Stish EE: Anthropokinetics. *Journal of Health, Physical Education, and Recreation* 35:33, November/December 1964.
2. Scott MG: *Analysis of Human Motion: A Textbook in Kinesiology*, ed 2. New York, Appleton-Century-Crofts, 1963.
3. Dempster WT: Free-body diagrams as an approach to the mechanics of human posture and locomotion. In Evans, FG (ed): *Biomechanical Studies of the Musculoskeletal System*. Springfield, Ill, Charles C Thomas, 1961.
4. Sills FD: Anthropometry in relation to physical performance. In Johnson WR: *Science and Medicine of Exercise and Sports*. New York, Harper & Brothers, 1960.
5. Clawson DK, Rosse C, Stolov WC: Screening examination of the musculoskeletal system. In Rosse C, Clawson DK: *The Musculoskeletal System in Health and Disease*. Hagerstown, Md, Harper & Row, 1980, pp 431–434.
6. Grieve GP: *Common Vertebral Joint Problems*. New York, Churchill Livingstone, 1981, pp 307–308.
7. Appleton AB: Posture. *Practitioner* 156:48, 1946.
8. Fisk JW: *The Painful Neck and Back*. Springfield, Ill, Charles C Thomas, 1977, pp 54–62.
9. Trubenbach HL: The distortion graphometer. In Johnson AC: *Postural Correction*. Los Angeles, Chiropractic Educational Extension Bureau, pp 15–16 (undated).
10. Turek SL: *Orthopaedics: Principles and Their Application*, ed 3. Philadelphia, J.B. Lippincott, 1977, pp 1413–1414.
11. Masters, RO Sr: Spinalzing: Reading body language. *The Digest of Chiropractic Economics* November/December 1983, pp 66, 68–69.
12. West HG Jr: Physical and spinal examination procedures utilized in the practice of chiropractic. In Haldeman S (ed): *Modern Developments in the Principles and Practice of Chiropractic*. New York, Appleton-Century-Crofts, 1980, pp 277–279.
13. Hellebrandt FA, Kelso LEA, Fries C: Devices useful to the physiological study of posture. *Physiotherapy Review* 22:10–16, 1942.
14. Schafer RC (ed): *Basic Chiropractic Procedural Manual*, ed 4. Arlington, Va, American Chiropractic Association, 1984, p 176.
15. Grice AS, Fligg DB: Class notes: Spinal dynamics. Department of Biomechanics/Kinesiology, BK202. Toronto, Canadian Memorial Chiropractic College, p 88 (undated).
16. Daniels L, Worthingham C: *Therapeutic Exercise for Body Alignment and Function*, ed 2. Philadelphia, W.B. Saunders, 1977, pp 8–9.
17. Schafer RC: *Chiropractic Physical and Spinal Diagnosis*. Oklahoma City, Associated Chiropractic Academic Press, 1980, p IV-54.
18. Hoppenfeld S: *Physical Examination of the Spine and Extremities*. New York, Appleton-Century-Crofts, 1976, p 238.
19. De Jarnette MB: *Subluxation Patterns*. Sacro Occipital Technic Seminar notes, published by the author, 1975.
20. Verner JR: *The Science and Logic of Chiropractic*. Englewood, NJ, published by the author, 1941, pp 281–283.
21. Burnside JW: *Adams' Physical Diagnosis*, ed 15. Baltimore, Williams & Wilkins, 1974, pp 187–189.
22. Cailliet R: *Scoliosis: Diagnosis and Management*. Philadelphia, F.A. Davis, 1975, p 5.
23. LACC Technic Department: Multiposition spinal examination. *The Chirogram* April 1976.
24. Barham JN, Wooten EP: *Structural Kinesiology*. New York, Macmillan, 1973, pp 123–124.
25. Fowler WM, Taylor RG: Differential diagnosis of muscle diseases. In D'Ambrosia RD (ed): *Musculoskeletal Disorders: Regional Examination and Differential Diagnosis*. Philadelphia, J.B. Lippincott, 1977, p 108.
26. Riggins RS: The shoulder. In D'Ambrosia RD (ed): *Musculoskeletal Disorders: Regional Examination and Differential Diagnosis*. Philadelphia, J.B. Lippincott, 1977, pp 331–332.
27. Finneson BE: *Low Back Pain*. Philadelphia, J.B. Lippincott, 1973, pp 41–42.
28. During J et al: Toward standards for postural characteristics of the lower back system in normal and pathologic conditions. *Spine* 10:83–87, 1985.
29. Daniels L, Worthingham C: *Therapeutic Exercise for Body Alignment and Function*, ed 2. Philadelphia, W.B. Saunders, 1977, p 14.
30. Asher C: *Postural Variations in Childhood*. London, Butterworths, 1975, pp 40–47.

31. Roper N: *Man's Anatomy, Physiology, Health and Environment*, ed 5. New York, Churchill Livingstone, 1976, pp 54, 57–58.
32. Kenel F: The body posture of children and adolescents. *Annals of the Swiss Chiropractic Association* vol II, 1961.
33. Vear H: A survey of postural indices in adolescents. *Journal of the Canadian Chiropractic Association* April 1970.
34. Vilholm F: Statistical evaluation of posture in 1000 school children. *Annals of the Swiss Chiropractic Association* vol 5, 1971.
35. Daniels L, Worthingham C: *Therapeutic Exercise for Body Alignment and Function*, ed 2. Philadelphia, W.B. Saunders, 1977, pp 3–4.
36. Hughes JG: *Synopsis of Pediatrics*, ed 3. St. Louis, C.V. Mosby, 1971, pp 23–24.
37. Inman VT, Ralston HJ, Todd F: *Human Walking*. Baltimore, Williams & Wilkins, 1981, p 1.
38. Asmussen E, Heeboll-Nielsen K: Posture, mobility, and strength of the back in boys 7–16 years old. *Acta Orthopaedica Scandinavica* 2:174–189, 1959.
39. Grieve DW, Gear RJ: The relationships between length of stride, step frequency, time of swing, and speed of walking for children and adults. *Ergonomics* 5:379, 1966.
40. Van Dusen LG: *Chiropractic Relationship to Gravitational Force*. Sodus, NY, published by the author, 1968, pp 5–9.
41. Morehouse LE, Cooper JM: *Kinesiology*. St. Louis, C.V. Mosby, 1950, pp 130–138.
42. Triano JJ: The use of instrumentation and laboratory examination procedures in chiropractic. In Haldeman S (ed): *Modern Developments in the Principles and Practice of Chiropractic*. New York, Appleton-Century-Crofts, 1980, pp 232–234.
43. Levine M: *The Structural Approach to Chiropractic*. New York, published by the author, 1964, pp 51–53.
44. Grice AS, Fligg DB: Class notes: Spinal dynamics. Department of Biomechanics/Kinesiology, BK202. Toronto, Canadian Memorial Chiropractic College, p 87 (undated).
45. Palmer CE: Studies of the center of gravity in the human body. *Child Development* 15:99–180, 1944.
46. Daniels L, Worthingham C: *Therapeutic Exercise for Body Alignment and Function*, ed 2. Philadelphia, W.B. Saunders, 1977, pp 1–2.
47. Murray MP, Seireg A, Scholtz RC: Center of gravity, center of pressure, and supportive forces during human activities. *Journal of Applied Physiology* 23:831–838, 1967.
48. Williams JGP, Sperryn PN (eds): *Sports Medicine*, ed 2. Baltimore, Williams & Wilkins, 1976, pp 119–125.
49. Cailliet R: *Low Back Pain Syndrome*, ed 3. Philadelphia, F.A. Davis, p 72.
50. White AA, Panjabi MM: *Clinical Biomechanics of the Spine*. Philadelphia, J.B. Lippincott, 1978, p 461.
51. Gowitzke BA, Milner M: *Understanding the Scientific Basis of Human Movement*, ed 2. Baltimore, Williams & Wilkins, 1980, p 124.
52. Kendall HO, Kendall FP, Wadsworth GE: *Muscles: Testing and Function*, ed 2. Baltimore, Williams & Wilkins, 1971, pp 18–19, 30–31.
53. Fox MG, Young OG: Placement of the gravital line in anteroposterior standing posture. *Research Quarterly*, 25:277–285, 1954.
54. Daniels L, Worthingham C: *Therapeutic Exercise for Body Alignment and Function*, ed 2. Philadelphia, W.B. Saunders, 1977, pp 10, 12.
55. Barham JN, Wooten EP: *Structural Kinesiology*. New York, Macmillan, 1973, pp 134–135.
56. Johnson AC: *Postural Correction*. Los Angeles, Chiropractic Educational Extension Bureau, pp 15–16 (undated).
57. Basmajian JV (ed): *Grant's Method of Anatomy*, ed 9. Baltimore, Williams & Wilkins, 1975, p 15.
58. Kendall HO, Kendall FP, Boynton DA: *Posture and Pain*. Huntington, NY, Robert E. Krieger, 1977, pp 5–14.
59. Yoels J: *Re-Shape Your Body, Re-Vitalize Your Life*. Englewood Cliffs, NJ, Prentice-Hall, 1972, pp 63–70.
60. Walters GC, Hoth M: Aid for recording gross evaluation. *Physical Therapy* 44:179, 1964.
61. Gowitzke BA, Milner M: *Understanding the Scientific Basis of Human Movement*, ed 2. Baltimore, Williams & Wilkins, 1980, pp 75, 77.
62. Ward LE: *The Dynamics of Spinal Stress*. Long Beach, Cal, SSS Press, 1980, pp 9–17.
63. Carver W: *Carver's Chiropractic Analysis*, ed 4. Oklahoma City, Paul O. Parr, 1921, vol 1, pp 143–148.
64. LeVeau B: *Williams and Lissner: Biomechanics of Human Motion*, ed 2. Philadelphia, W.B. Saunders, 1977, p 73.
65. Cochran GVB: *A Primer of Orthopaedic Biomechanics*. New York, Churchill Livingstone, 1982, pp 18, 19.
66. Barham JN, Wooten EP: *Structural Kinesiology*. New York, Macmillan, 1973, p 80.
67. Basmajian JV: Man's posture. *Archives of Physical Medicine* 46:26–36, 1965.
68. Daniels L, Worthingham C: *Therapeutic Exercise for Body Alignment and Function*, ed 2. Philadelphia, W.B. Saunders, 1977, pp 4–7.
69. Hollingshead WH, Jenkins DB: *Functional Anatomy of the Limbs and Back*. Philadelphia, W.B. Saunders, 1981, pp 207–209.
70. D'Ambrosia RD: The hip. In D'Ambrosia RD: *Musculoskeletal Disorders: Regional Examination and Differential Diagnosis*. Philadelphia, J.B. Lippincott, 1977, pp 409, 411.
71. Hooker CW: The back. In Wilson FC (ed): *The Musculoskeletal System: Basic Processes and Disorders*, ed 2. Philadelphia, J.B. Lippincott, 1983, p 85.
72. Fisk JW: *The Painful Neck and Back*. Springfield, Ill, Charles C Thomas, 1977, p 40.
73. Joseph J: *Man's Posture: Electro-myographic Studies*. Oxford, England, Blackwell, 1960.
74. Basmajian JV: *Muscles Alive: Their Functions Revealed by Electromyography*. Baltimore, Williams & Wilkins, 1962.
75. Wooten EP: The structural base of human movement. *Journal of Health, Physical Education, and Recreation* 36:59, October 1965.
76. Cochran GVB: *A Primer of Orthopaedic Biome-*

chanics. New York, Churchill Livingstone, 1982, p 62.
77. Barham JN, Wooten EP: *Structural Kinesiology*. New York, Macmillan, 1973, pp 119–123.
78. LeVeau B: *Williams and Lissner: Biomechanics of Human Motion*, ed 2. Philadelphia, W.B. Saunders, 1977, p 90.
79. Stevens DL, Tomlinson GE: Measurement of human postural sway. *Proceedings of the Royal Society of Medicine* 64:653–665, 1971.
80. Hellebrandt FA, Riddle S, Fries C: Influence of postural sway on stance photography. *Physiotherapy Review* 22:88–97, 1952.
81. Coplans CW: The Conservative treatment of low back pain. In Helfet AJ, Gruebel Lee DM (eds): *Disorders of the Lumbar Spine*. Philadelphia, J.B. Lippincott, 1978, pp 178–179.
82. Lay EM: The osteopathic management of temporomandibular joint dysfunction. In Gelb H (ed): *Clinical Management of Head, Neck and TMJ Pain and Dysfunction*. Philadelphia, W.B. Saunders, 1977, pp 514–519.
83. Maisel E (ed): *The Alexander Technique: The Resurrection of the Body*. New York, Dell Publishing, 1969.
84. Barlow W: *The Alexander Principle*. London, Victor Gollancz, 1973.
85. Barker S: *The Alexander Technique: The Revolutionary Way to Use Your Body for Total Energy*. New York, Bantam, 1978.
86. Walther DS: *Applied Kinesiology*. Pueblo, Col, Systems DC, 1981, vol 1, pp 196–197.
87. Goodheart GJ: *Collected Published Articles and Reprints*. Montpelier, Ohio, Williams County Publishing, 1969, pp 75–77.
88. Perry L Jr: Learn to walk before you run: A matter of body mechanics, posture and technique. *Today's Chiropractic* pp 9–10, November/December 1984.
89. Keith A: Man's posture: Its evolution and disorders (Hunterian Lectures). *Clinical Orthopaedics* 62:5–14, 1969.
90. Grice AS: Mechanics of walking, development and clinical significance. *Journal of the Canadian Chiropractic Association* 16(3), 1972.
91. Tricker RAR, Tricker BJK: *The Science of Movement*. New York, American Elsevier, 1967.
92. Grice AS: Posture and postural mechanics. *Journal of the Canadian Chiropractic Association* July 1970.
93. Coplans CW: The Conservative treatment of low back pain. In Helfet AJ, Gruebel Lee DM: *Disorders of the Lumbar Spine*. Philadelphia, J.B. Lippincott, 1978, pp 178–180.
94. Morehouse LE, Cooper JM: *Kinesiology*. St. Louis, C.V. Mosby, 1950, pp 139–147.
95. Morehouse LE, Miller AT Jr: *Physiology of Exercise*. St. Louis, C.V. Mosby, 1948, pp 308–314.
96. Hviid H: Erect working posture. *Annals of the Swiss Chiropractors' Association* 6:71–90, 1976.
97. Jaquet P: The upright position of man: Its phylogenetic and psychological aspects and some therapeutic considerations of interest. *Annals of the Swiss Chiropractic Association* 4:185–195, 1969.
98. Morehouse LE, Cooper JM: *Kinesiology*. St. Louis, C.V. Mosby, 1950, pp 147–149.
99. Kroemer KH: Seating in plant and office. *American Industrial Hygiene Association Journal* 32:633–652, 1971.
100. Hooton EA: *A Survey in Seating*. Gardner, Mass, Heywood-Wakefield, 1945.
101. Morehouse LE, Cooper JM: *Kinesiology*. St. Louis, C.V. Mosby, 1950, pp 149, 154.
102. Yoels J: *Re-Shape Your Body, Re-Vitalize Your Life*. Englewood Cliffs, NJ, Prentice-Hall, 1972, pp 55–62, 99–102.
103. Cailliet R: *Low Back Pain Syndrome*, ed 3. Philadelphia, F.A. Davis, 1981, pp 131–132.
104. White AA, Panjabi MM: *Clinical Biomechanics of the Spine*. Philadelphia, J.B. Lippincott, 1978, pp 329–330.
105. Drummond DS et al: A study of pressure distributions measured during balanced and unbalanced sitting. *Journal of Bone and Joint Surgery* 64A:1034–1039, 1982.
106. Bendix T: Seated trunk posture at various seat inclinations, seat heights, and table heights. *The Human Factor* 26:695–703, 1984.
107. Bendix T, Hagberg M: Trunk posture and load on the trapezius muscle whilst sitting at sloping desks. *Ergonomics* 8:873–882, 1984.
108. Fisk JW: *The Painful Neck and Back*. Springfield, Ill, Charles C Thomas, 1977, p 196.
109. Morehouse LE, Cooper JM: *Kinesiology*. St. Louis, C.V. Mosby, 1950, pp 154, 156.
110. Ogden JA: The development and growth of the musculoskeletal system. In Albright JA, Brand RA (eds): *The Scientific Basis of Orthopaedics*. New York, Appleton-Century-Crofts, 1979, pp 75–86, 93–99.
111. LeVeau B: *Williams and Lissner: Biomechanics of Human Motion*, ed 2. Philadelphia, W.B. Saunders, 1977, pp 70–71.
112. Yamada K: The dynamics of experimental posture. *Clinical Orthopaedics* 25:20–31, 1962.
113. Brooks V: Motor control: how posture and movements are governed. *Physical Therapy* 63:664–673, 1983.
114. Johnson AC: *Postural Correction*. Los Angeles, Chiropractic Educational Extension Bureau, p 7 (undated).
115. Carlsoo S: *How Man Moves*. London, William Heinemann, 1972.
116. Bernstein N: *The Coordination and Regulation of Movements*. New York, Pergamon, 1967.
117. Broer M: *Efficiency of Human Movement*, ed 3. Philadelphia, W.B. Saunders, 1973.
118. Morehouse LE, Cooper JM: *Kinesiology*. St. Louis, C.V. Mosby, 1950, p 158.
119. Thomas DP, Whitney L: Postural movements during normal standing in man. *Journal of Anatomy* 93:524–539, 1959.
120. Rogers MH: Basic body mechanics: An interpretation. *Journal of Health, Physical Education, and Recreation* 32:12–20, 1961.
121. Morehouse LE, Cooper JM: *Kinesiology*. St. Louis, C.V. Mosby, 1950, pp 158–181.
122. Tucker WE: *Active Alerted Posture*. London, Livingstone, 1960.
123. White AA, Panjabi MM: *Clinical Biomechanics of*

the Spine. Philadelphia, J.B. Lippincott, 1978, pp 332–333.
124. Gowitzke BA, Milner M: *Understanding the Scientific Basis of Human Movement*, ed 2. Baltimore, Williams & Wilkins, 1980, pp 65–66.
125. Morehouse LE, Miller AT Jr: *Physiology of Exercise*. St. Louis, C.V. Mosby, 1948, p 225.
126. Kelley DL: *Kinesiology: Fundamentals of Motion Descriptions*. Englewood Cliffs, NJ, Prentice-Hall, 1971.
127. Wooten EP: The structural base of human movement. *Journal of Health, Physical Education, and Recreation* 36:59, October 1965.
128. Yack HJ: Techniques for clinical assessment of human movement. *Physical Therapy* 64:1821–1829, 1984.
129. Haller JS, Gurewitsch AO: An approach to dynamic posture based on primitive motion patterns. *Archives of Physical Medicine* 31:632–640, 1950.
130. Perry J: The mechanics of walking. *Physical Therapy* 47:778, 1967.
131. Morehouse LE, Cooper JM: *Kinesiology*. St. Louis, C.V. Mosby, 1950, pp 221–223, 226–230.
132. Medeiros J: Automated measurement systems for clinical motion analysis. *Physical Therapy* 64:1846–1850, 1984.
133. Walther DS: *Applied Kinesiology*. Pueblo, Col, Systems DC, 1981, vol 1, pp 157–159.
134. Hooper BJ: *The Mechanics of Human Movement*. New York, American Elsevier, 1973.
135. Steindler A: *Kinesiology of the Human Body Under Normal and Pathological Conditions*. Springfield, Ill, Charles C Thomas, 1955.
136. Inman VT, Ralston HJ, Todd F: *Human Walking*. Baltimore, Williams & Wilkins, 1981, pp 2–21.
137. Hollingshead WH, Jenkins DB: *Functional Anatomy of the Limbs and Back*. Philadelphia, W.B. Saunders, 1981, pp 335–337.
138. Daniels L, Worthingham C: *Muscle Testing: Techniques of Manual Examination*, ed 4. Philadelphia, W.B. Saunders, 1980, pp 167–177.
139. Grice AS, Fligg DB: Class notes: Introductory Concepts to Clinical Analysis of Joint Movement and Muscle Testing. Department of Biomechanics/Kinesiology, BK101. Toronto, Canadian Memorial Chiropractic College, pp 92–93 (undated).
140. Stolov WC: Normal and pathologic ambulation. In Rosse C, Clawson DK (eds): *The Musculoskeletal System in Health and Disease*. Hagerstown, Md, Harper & Row, 1980, pp 318–328.
141. Grice AS, Fligg DB: Class notes: Introductory Concepts to Clinical Analysis of Joint Movement and Muscle Testing. Department of Biomechanics/Kinesiology, BK101. Toronto, Canadian Memorial Chiropractic College, pp 103–104 (undated).
142. Wall JC, Nottrodt, Charteris J: The effects of uphill and downhill walking on pelvic oscillations in the transverse plane. *Ergonomics* 24:807–816, 1981.
143. LeVeau B: *Williams and Lissner: Biomechanics of Human Motion*, ed 2. Philadelphia, W.B. Saunders, 1977, p 198.
144. LeVeau B: *Williams and Lissner: Biomechanics of Human Motion*, ed 2. Philadelphia, W.B. Saunders, 1977, p 78.
145. Hibbard D: Effects of manipulation on gait muscle activity: preliminary electromyographic research. *ACA Journal of Chiropractic* 17(10):104–106.
146. Grieve DW: The assessment of gait. *Physiotherapy* 55:452–460, 1975.
147. Cochran GVB: *A Primer of Orthopaedic Biomechanics*. New York, Churchill Livingstone, 1982, pp 269–290.
148. Hoppenfeld S: *Physical Examination of the Spine and Extremities*. New York, Appleton-Century-Crofts, 1976, pp 134–141.
149. Inman VT, Ralston HJ, Todd F: *Human Walking*. Baltimore, Williams & Wilkins, 1981, pp 103–117.
150. Schafer RC: *Chiropractic Physical and Spinal Diagnosis*. Oklahoma City, Associated Chiropractic Academic Press, 1980, pp I-30–I-32.
151. Turek SL: *Orthopaedics: Principles and Their Application*, ed 3. Philadelphia, J.B. Lippincott, 1977, pp 1521–1522.
152. Drillis R: Objective recording and biomechanics of pathological gait. *Annuals of the New York Academy of Science* 17:86, 1958.
153. Beardall AG: Additional gait tests. *Digest of Chiropractic Economics* 19(5), March/April 1977.
154. Foley CD, Quanbury AO, Steinke T: Kinematics of normal child locomotion: A statistical study based on TV data. *Journal of Biomechanics* 12:1–6, 1979.
155. Finneson BE: *Low Back Pain*. Philadelphia, J.B. Lippincott, 1973, pp 42–43.
156. Taft TN, Hooker CW: The lower limb. In Wilson FC (ed): *The Musculoskeletal System: Basic Processes and Disorders*, ed 2. Philadelphia, J.B. Lippincott, 1983, pp 71–72.
157. Perry JA: Clinical interpretation of the mechanics of walking. *Physical Therapy* 47:778–801, 1967.
158. Delacerda FG, Wikoff OD: Effect of lower extremity asymmetry on the kinematics of gait. *Journal of Orthopaedics and Sports* 3:105–107, 1982.
159. Cerny K: Pathomechanics of stance: Clinical concepts for analysis. *Physical Therapy* 64:1851–1859, 1984.
160. Rosse C: The vertebral column. In Rosse C, Clawson DK (eds): *The Musculoskeletal System in Health and Disease*. Hagerstown, Md, Harper & Row, 1980, pp 138, 140.
161. Wiles P: Postural deformities of the antero-posterior curves of the spine. *Lancet* April 17, 1937.
162. Schafer RC: *Chiropractic Management of Sports and Recreational Injuries*. Baltimore, Williams & Wilkins, 1982, pp 471, 516, 527.
163. Sutherland DH, Baumann JU: Correction of paralytic foot drop by external orthoses. In Black J, Dumbleton JH (eds): *Clinical Biomechanics: Case History Approach*. New York, Churchill Livingstone, 1981, p 308.
164. Plastridge AL: Gaits. *Physiotherapy Review* 21:24–29, 1941.
165. Kirby JD; *Essentials of Physical Diagnosis*. North Hollywood, Cal, Chiropractic Business Services, 1978, p 17.

166. White AA, Panjabi MM: *Clinical Biomechanics of the Spine*. Philadelphia, J.B. Lippincott, 1978, p 471.
167. Saunders JB, Inman VT, Eberhart HD: The major determinants in normal and pathological gait. *Journal of Bone and Joint Surgery* 35A:543–558, 1953.
168. Walker HK: The motor system. In Walker HK, Hall WD, Hurst JW (Eds): *Clinical Methods*. Boston, Butterworths, 1976, vol 2, pp 815–816.
169. Bogardh E, Richards CL: Gait analysis and relearning of gait control in hemiplegic patients. *Canadian Physiotherapy* 33:223–230, 1981.
170. D'Ambrosia RD: Evaluation of the patient. In D'Ambrosia RD (ed): *Musculoskeletal Disorders: Regional Examination and Differential Diagnosis*. Philadelphia, J.B. Lippincott, 1977, pp 8–9.
171. Cabot RC: *Physical Diagnosis*, ed 7. New York, William Wood, 1919, pp 481–484.
172. Firth JN: *A Text-Book on Chiropractic Diagnosis*, ed 5. Indianapolis, published by the author, 1948, pp 13–14.
173. Landau WM, O'Leary JL: Disturbances of movement. In MacBryde CM, Blacklow RS (eds): *Signs and Symptoms*, ed 5. Philadelphia, J.B. Lippincott, 1970, pp 703–704.
174. Heilman KM, Watson RT, Greer M: *Handbook for Differential Diagnosis of Neurologic Signs and Symptoms*. New York, Appleton-Century-Crofts, 1977, p 106.
175. Kirby JD; *Essentials of Physical Diagnosis*. North Hollywood, Cal, Chiropractic Business Services, 1978, p 18.
176. Firth JN: *A Text-Book on Chiropractic Diagnosis*, ed 5. Indianapolis, published by the author, 1948, pp 14, 419.
177. Schafer RC (ed): *Basic Chiropractic Procedural Manual*, ed 4. Arlington, Va, American Chiropractic Association, 1984, p 39.
178. Holmes G: The cerebellum of man. *Brain* 62:1–30, 1939.
179. Brown JR: Diseases of the cerebellum. In Baker AB, Baker LH (eds): *Clinical Neurology*. New York, Harper & Row, 1975, vol 2, chap 29.
180. Carver W: *Carver's Chiropractic Analysis*, ed 4. Oklahoma City, published by the author, 1922, vol 2, pp 302–306.
181. Schafer RC: *Chiropractic Physical and Spinal Diagnosis*. Oklahoma City, Associated Chiropractic Academic Press, 1980, pp I-32–I-33.
182. Heilman KM, Watson RT, Greer M: *Handbook for Differential Diagnosis of Neurologic Signs and Symptoms*. New York, Appleton-Century-Crofts, 1977, pp 105–106.
183. Ducroquet R, Ducroquet J, Ducroquet P: *Walking and Limping: A Study of Normal and Pathological Walking*. Philadelphia, J.B. Lippincott, 1968.
184. Firth JN: *A Text-Book on Chiropractic Diagnosis*, ed 5. Indianapolis, published by the author, 1948, p 13.
185. Teranel JA: *Chiropractic Orthopedics and Roentgenology*. Newark, NJ, Medusa Press, 1953, p 35.
186. D'Ambrosia RD: The hip. In D'Ambrosia RD (ed): *Musculoskeletal Disorders: Regional Examination and Differential Diagnosis*. Philadelphia, J.B. Lippincott, 1977, pp 422–423.
187. Turek SL: *Orthopaedics: Principles and Their Application*, ed 3. Philadelphia, J.B. Lippincott, 1977, p 1083.
188. Kendall HO, Kendall FP: Normal flexibility according to age groups. *Journal of Bone and Joint Surgery* 33A:690–694, July 1948.
189. Engel GL: Conversion symptoms. In MacBryde CM, Blacklow RS (eds): *Signs and Symptoms*, ed 5. Philadelphia, J.B. Lippincott, 1970, p 663.
190. Laughman RK et al: Objective clinical evaluation of function. *Physical Therapy* 64:1839–1845, 1984.
191. Morehouse LE, Cooper JM: *Kinesiology*. St. Louis, C.V. Mosby, 1950, pp 226–227, 229–230, 235, 238–250.
192. Morehouse LE, Cooper JM: *Kinesiology*. St. Louis, C.V. Mosby, 1950, p 375.
193. Gowitzke BA, Milner M: *Understanding the Scientific Basis of Human Movement*, ed 2. Baltimore, Williams & Wilkins, 1980, pp 81–82.
194. Gowitzke BA, Milner M: *Understanding the Scientific Basis of Human Movement*, ed 2. Baltimore, Williams & Wilkins, 1980, pp 82, 84.
195. Lorez E: Some fundamentals of human locomotion. *Annals of the Swiss Chiropractors' Association* 6:7–36, 1976.
196. Dempster WT: The anthropometry of body action. *Annals of the New York Academy of Science* 63:559–585, 1955.
197. Mac Ewan CC, Howe EC: An objective method of grading posture. *Research Quarterly, American Association of Health, Physical Education, and Recreation* 3:144–157, 1932.
198. Hamerton JL: Bipedalism. *Cytogenetics* 15:99, 1962.
199. Mennell JMcM: *Joint Pain*. Boston, Little, Brown, 1964, pp 160–163.
200. Brennan MJ: Adaptations to bipedalism. *ACA Journal of Chiropractic* 14:24–31, November 1980.
201. Krogman WM: The scars of human evolution. *Scientific American* 185(6):54–57, 1951.
202. Illi FW: *The Vertebral Column: Life-line of the Body*. Chicago, National College of Chiropractic, 1951, p 11.
203. Janse J: The concepts and research of Dr. Fred W. Illi. *Notes on Correlative Techniques*. An informal compilation of various notes and articles Chicago, National College of Chiropractic (undated).
204. Keith A: Man's Posture: Its evolution and disorders (Hunterian Lectures). *Clinical Orthopaedics* 62:5–14, 1969.
205. Olsen GA, Hamilton A: The lateral stability of the spine. *Clinical Orthopaedics* 65:143, 1969.
206. Goodheart GJ: *Collected Published Articles and Reprints*. Montpelier, Ohio, Williams County Publishing, 1969, p 28.
207. De Jarnette MB: *Sacro-Occipital Technic*. Seminar notes, published by the author, 1977.
208. Riggins RS: The shoulder. In D'Ambrosia RD (ed): *Musculoskeletal Disorders: Regional Examination and Differential Diagnosis*. Philadelphia, J.B. Lippincott, 1977, p 332.

209. Schafer RC: *Chiropractic Health Care*, ed 3. Des Moines, The Foundation for Chiropractic Education and Research, 1979, p 55.
210. Cailliet R: *Soft Tissue Pain and Disability*. Philadelphia, F.A. Davis, 1980, pp 23–24.
211. Davenport CB: *Body, Build, and Its Inheritance*. Washington, DC, Carnegie Institute Publication No. 329, 1924.
212. Teranel JA: *Chiropractic Orthopedics and Roentgenology*. Newark, NJ, Medusa Press, 1953, pp 45–50.
213. Asher C: *Postural Variations in Childhood*. London, Butterworths, 1975, pp 8–12.
214. Daniels L, Worthingham C: *Therapeutic Exercise for Body Alignment and Function*, ed 2. Philadelphia, W.B. Saunders, 1977, p 8.
215. Williams JGP, Sperryn PN (eds): *Sports Medicine*, ed 2. Baltimore, Williams & Wilkins, 1976, pp 142–149.
216. Barham JN, Wooten EP: *Structural Kinesiology*. New York, Macmillan, 1973, pp 135–136.
217. Schafer RC: *Chiropractic Physical and Spinal Diagnosis*. Oklahoma City, Associated Chiropractic Academic Press, 1980, p I-28.
218. Basmajian JV (ed): *Grant's Method of Anatomy*, ed 9. Baltimore, Williams & Wilkins, 1975, pp 201–204.
219. Sheldon WH, Dupertuis, McDermott E: *Atlas of Men*. New York, Harper & Brothers, 1954.
220. Sheldon WH: *The Varieties of Human Physique*. New York, Harper & Row, 1940.
221. Peterson G: *Atlas for Somatotyping Children*. Netherlands, Van Gorcum, 1967.
222. Jensen RK: Estimation of the biomechanical properties of three body types using a photogrammetric method. *Journal of Biomechanics* 11:349–358, 1978.
223. D'Amico JC: The postural complex. *Journal of the American Podiatry Association* August 1976.
224. Freyberg RH: Back pain. In MacBryde CM, Blacklow RS (eds): *Signs and Symptoms*, ed 5. Philadelphia, J.B. Lippincott, 1970, pp 213–214.
225. Burt HA: Effects of faulty posture. *Proceedings of the Royal Society of Medicine* 43:187, 1950.
226. Daniels L, Worthingham C: *Therapeutic Exercise for Body Alignment and Function*, ed 2. Philadelphia, W.B. Saunders, 1977, pp 1, 7.
227. Johnson AC: *Postural Correction*. Los Angeles, Chiropractic Educational Extension Bureau, p 11 (undated).
228. Freyberg RH: Back pain. In MacBryde CM, Blacklow RS (eds): *Signs and Symptoms*, ed 5. Philadelphia, J.B. Lippincott, 1970, p 205.
229. Schafer RC: *Chiropractic Physical and Spinal Diagnosis*. Oklahoma City, Associated Chiropractic Academic Press, 1980, pp I-28–I-30.
230. Cyriax E: Some common postural deformities and their treatment by exercise and manipulation. *British Journal of Physical Medicine* June 1938.
231. Verner JR: *The Science and Logic of Chiropractic*. Englewood, NJ, published by the author, 1941, pp 137–138.
232. Teranel JA: *Chiropractic Orthopedics and Roentgenology*. Newark, NJ, Medusa Press, 1953, pp 46–50.
233. Lowman CL, Young CH: *Posture and Fitness: Significance and Variances*. Philadelphia, Lea & Febiger, 1960.
234. Morehouse LE, Miller AT Jr: *Physiology of Exercise*. St. Louis, C.V. Mosby, 1948, pp 247–248.
235. Kendall HO, Kendall FP: Developing and maintaining good posture. *Journal of the American Physical Therapy Association* 48:319–336, 1968.
236. Schafer RC: *Chiropractic Physical and Spinal Diagnosis*. Oklahoma City, Associated Chiropractic Academic Press, 1980, pp IV-29–IV-30.
237. Schafer RC: *Chiropractic Management of Sports and Recreational Injuries*. Baltimore, Williams & Wilkins, 1982, p 69.
238. Janse J: *Principles and Practice of Chiropractic*. Lombard, Ill, National College of Chiropractic, 1976, pp 160–161.
239. Schafer RC: *Chiropractic Management of Sports and Recreational Injuries*. Baltimore, Williams & Wilkins, 1982, pp 64–65.
240. Pottenger FM: *Symptoms of Visceral Disease*. St. Louis, C.V. Mosby, 1944.
241. Verner JR: *The Science and Logic of Chiropractic*. Englewood, NJ, published by the author, 1941, pp 235–236.
242. Goldthwait JE et al: *Essentials of Body Mechanics in Health and Disease*, ed 5. Philadelphia, J.B. Lippincott, 1952.
243. Lewit K: Relation of faulty respiration to posture, with clinical implications. *Journal of the American Osteopathic Association* 79:525–529, 1980.
244. Schafer RC: *Chiropractic Management of Sports and Recreational Injuries*. Baltimore, Williams & Wilkins, 1982, pp 65–66.
245. Porterfield JA: Dynamic stabilization of the trunk. *Journal of Orthopaedics and Sports Physical Therapy* 6:271–276, 1985.
246. Micheli LJ: Low back pain in the adolescent: Differential diagnosis. *American Journal of Sports Medicine* 7:362, 1979.

SUGGESTED READINGS

Anderson RT: New instrumentation for anthropometry. *ACA Journal of Chiropractic* 15:43–47, June 1981.

Bendix T et al: Lumbar curve, trunk muscles, and line of gravity with different heel heights. *Spine* March 1984. pp 223–227.

Gajdosik R et al: Pelvic tilt: Intratester reliability of measuring the standing position and range. *Physical Therapy* 65:169–174, 1984.

Goodheart GJ: Observation of sonagraphic computerized analysis. *Journal of the Council on Sports Injuries* 1(1):13–16, January 1982.

Greenawalt MH: Who are you? You are the posture specialist. *Digest of Chiropractic Economics* September/October 1985, pp 40, 42–43.

Hadler NM: *Medical Management of the Regional Musculoskeletal Diseases*. Orlando, Fla, Grune & Stratton, 1984.

Holden JM et al: Clinical gait assessment in the neurologically impaired: Reliability and meaningfulness. *Physical Therapy* 64:35–40, 1984.

Hosek RS: Computerized leg check: A computer-aided gravity weight line analyzer. *Today's Chiropractic* January/February 1985, pp 9–13.

Jones L: *The Postural Complex: Observations as to Cause, Diagnosis, and Treatment*. Springfield, Ill, Charles C Thomas, 1955.

Moore KL: *Clinically Oriented Anatomy*. Baltimore, Williams & Wilkins, 1980.

Nottrodt JW, Charteris J, Wall JC: The effects of speed on pelvic oscillations in the horizontal plane during level walking. *Journal of Human Movement Studies* 8:27–40, 1982.

O'Connell AL, Gardner EB: *Understanding the Scientific Basis of Human Movement*. Baltimore, Williams & Wilkins, 1972.

Perry L Jr: Advice for runners, parts 1, 2, and 3. *Today's Chiropractic* January/February 1985, pp 17–18; May/June 1985, pp 14–15; September/October 1985, pp 45–46.

Reid JG, Costigan PA: Geometry of adult rectus abdominis and erector spinae muscles. *Journal of Orthopaedics and Sports Physical Therapy* 6:278–280, 1985.

Schafer RC: *Symptomatology and Differential Diagnosis*. Arlington, Va, American Chiropractic Association, to be published 1986.

Schmorl G, Junghanns H: *The Human Spine in Health and Disease*, ed 2. New York, Grune & Stratton, 1971.

Simonelli C, Eaton RP: Cardiovascular and metabolic effects of exercise—the strong case for conditioning. *Postgraduate Medicine* 63:71–77, 1978.

Squire PJ: Centre of gravity height and its relation to anthropometric measurements in female physical education students. *Journal of Human Movement Studies* 3:214–220, 1978.

Stiga J: Postural chiropractic. *Today's Chiropractic* July/August 1984, pp 9–11; September/October 1984, pp 11–12.

Wells KF: *Kinesiology: The Scientific Base of Human Motion*. Philadelphia, W.B. Saunders, 1971.

Wright R: The concept of posture. *Digest of Chiropractic Economics* September/October 1985, p 124.

CHAPTER 5

Basic Neuromuscular Considerations

The principal aspects of the osseous and muscular systems have been discussed in previous chapters, as have the fundamental mechanical principles underlying their function. In this chapter, we shall review those neuromuscular principles that govern the dynamic human "machine" to better appreciate muscle action, control, and coordination. Certain pathologic disorders will also be discussed that may be underlying or superimposed on biomechanical difficulties.

BACKGROUND[1]

A discussion of neuromuscular function is not usually included in a text about biomechanics. However, this subject cannot be ignored when biomechanics is approached from a clinical basis. The motor system and its sensory feedback mechanisms are expressed holistically in three integrated systems: (1) the osseous system, which supplies the bony levers that generate motion; (2) the muscular system, which provides the power to move these levers; and (3) the nervous system, which directs and regulates muscle power.

In myology, muscles are usually studied as separate entities with specific actions. However, when the body is studied holistically, we note that it is much more than a machine composed of many parts. It is a complex organism with many variables, and this requires many concessions before applying mechanical laws. Obviously, there are individual variations of age, sex, body type, race, and physiologic and psychologic function. Some more subtle variations are listed below.[2,3]

1. A single muscle usually acts in conjunction with one or more others as a group. It rarely works alone. The manner in which muscle groups are stimulated by a variable number of neurons generating variable asynchronous firing rates produces group reactions not seen in isolated laboratory reactions. Individual fibers probably never combine the same way twice in any intensity of muscular contraction. This means that in a repetitive action, the muscle power behind the movement will always vary to some extent.

2. In muscles that span more than one joint, the action distance between origin and insertion is a variable that depends on the position of the part when action is initiated. That is, joint angles vary considerably when contractions are initiated, and the angles of muscle pull against bone change with each fraction of a degree of movement.

3. Certain muscles have multiple tendons at origin or insertion, and the amount of pull against each tendon depends on a variable number of fibers acting to affect the angle of pull. Also, some muscles have a broad origin or insertion, and muscular segments are functionally independent and can act individually, in groups, or as a whole.

4. Most joints are moved by more than one muscle and their combined interaction determines a movement's strength and direction. The quality of individual neuromuscular mechanisms governs the precision of such movements and is expressed in a wide variance of motor skills.

5. The length of muscle fibers at the time of stimualtion and the effect of their prior elongation offer many performance variables. After a muscle has been stretched, it is in its optimum state to offer maximum contraction force with a minimum energy cost. It is not uncommon for a muscle to be stretched by forces exterior to it during the process of contraction (ie, lengthening contraction). Even during moderate activity such as casual locomotion, myographic studies indicate that prolonged submaximal contractions as the result of low-rate excitations are common in the body.

6. Prior to joint movement, there must be antagonist relaxation. The process of this relaxation is a variable combination of decreased or inhibited stimulation and molecular rearrangement within muscle fibers.

7. Most body movements are rotations about joint axes and are rarely confined to a simple neural arc. Motions vary to compensate for muscle-joint restrictions, bones twisting about their axes, and the transfer of power from one set of muscles to another during the range of movement.

8. During joint motion, other joints are usually fixed to control the action. Usually, more muscles are involved in fixation than movement, and these muscles may be brought into action at any phase of movement. This requires intricate coordination of involuntary reflexes subject to variable functional, training, and conditioning effects.

9. Specific features of striated muscle limit its ability to develop tension, such as the state of fatigue, nutritional status, and whether the muscle is warm or cool. Maximum effort can be either enhanced or diminished by these conditions.

10. The body is constantly in motion. Whether asleep or awake, minute oscillatory movements occur in all body parts. Gross movements are not initiated until they are in phase with an individual's normal oscillation.[4]

SKELETAL MUSCLE MICROSTRUCTURE AND FUNCTION

To give an appreciation of the underlying factors involved in gross movement, this section will review muscular microanatomy, muscle contraction, and neurosynaptic function as it pertains to movement.

It is well to think of a skeletal muscle as one part of a three-part nerve-muscle-skeleton unit. That is, a motor nerve is necessary to stimulate muscle contraction, the muscle itself must be able to contract and to relax, and the power of the contraction must be transmitted to a skeletal attachment to produce the desired movement. When any one part of this three-part unit cannot function normally total function suffers.

Pertinent Anatomy[5–8]

The approximately 640 muscles of the huamn body have many shapes, sizes, joint relations, and action lines that determine their gross function. Muscle mass consists of 75% water, 20% protein, and 5% miscellaneous materials, and striated muscle mass constitutes the far greater part of body mass. Microscopic and electronmicroscopic features offer us insight into the mechanisms involved.

Structure[9–12]

Basic muscle tissue consists of both (1) active contractive elements within the muscle fibers and (2) inactive spring-like yielding connective tissue that allows muscle tension to be transmitted smoothly and allows elongated fibers to recover. The quantity of noncontractile connective tissue decreases and the length of muscle fibers increases as muscles are located more proximally in a limb.

In a cross section of a muscle belly, the active and inactive elements are readily discernible. Muscle strength is considered proportional to the diameter of its cross section.[13,14] Near the myotendinous junction, muscle bundles and collagen bundles of the tendon blend to form a strong continuous union, which offers a harness between fiber contraction and the body lever and offers a buffer against muscle fiber rupture from rapid contraction forces.

Much of the connective tissue element of muscle tissue is quite elastic. During work, there is no load on or shortening of the active contractile fibers until the load first stretches the inactive elastic connective tissue components.

Blood Supply[15–18]

Muscle tissue is rich in blood vessels. Arteries and veins course through the epimysium, arterioles and venules travel along the perimysia, and capillaries run longitudinally between muscle fibers in the endomysia. There are many collateral links and tiny reservoirs between many of these vessels to form a rich pool-like network that supplies necessary oxygen and other nutrients during prolonged effort when severe contraction may restrict capillary flow. During rest, many of these pools are closed, but they open when contraction makes it necessary. In this manner, the blood supply to a muscle is normally in accord with the degree of physical activity.

Nerve Supply[15,19–22]

For the skeletal and muscular systems to function properly and in harmony, the nervous system gives the body awareness of its environment, enables it to react to stimuli from the environment, and allows the body to work as a unit by coordinating its activities. Nerves containing both motor and sensory fibers pierce muscle fascia at the site of the primary arterial branch (the neurovascular hila).[23] These nerves then fan out to supply both motor and sensory nerve fibers to each muscle spindle. Figure 5.1 illustrates cross-sectional nerve structure.

Types. There are two categories of motor fibers: (1) large α-fibers, whose cell bodies are located in the spinal cord's ventral horn, which bifurcate several times to richly supply numerous muscle fibers; and (2) small γ-fibers that supply the muscle spindles and provide indirect central control via a neural loop.[24] A longitudinal section through a nerve fiber is depicted in Figure 5.2.

There are also two types of sensory neurons: (1) large neurons whose fibers supply sensory terminals in the muscle spindles and tendon receptor organs, and (2) smaller neurons that transmit muscle pain. These nerve endings are stimulated by muscle tension and send messages centrally to monitor muscle tone, part position, and movement rate and extent.

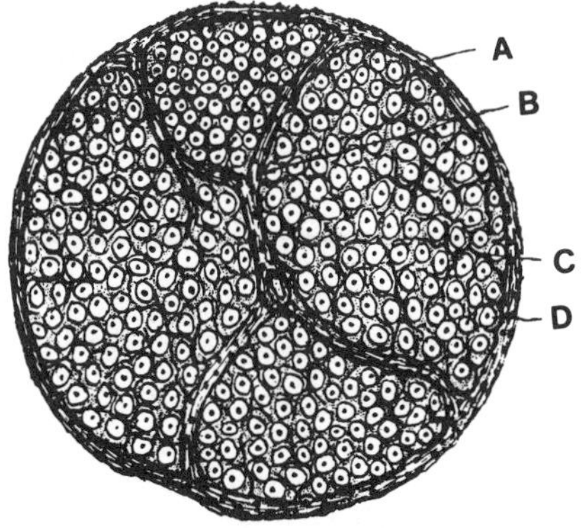

Figure 5.1. Transverse section of a nerve. *A*, epineurium; *B*, perineurium; *C*, endoneurium; *D*, section of a single fiber.

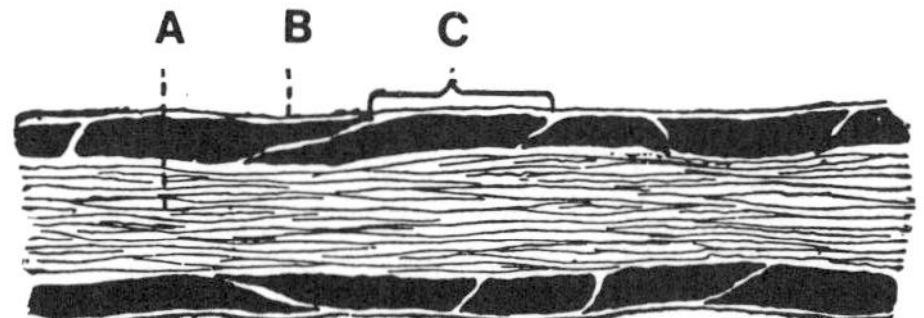

Figure 5.2. Longitudinal section through a nerve fiber. *A*, fibrils of axis cylinder; *B*, neurolemma; *C*, segment of Lantermann.

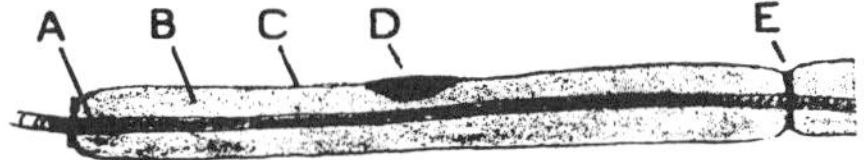

Figure 5.3. Longitudinal section of a nerve fiber depicting *A*, axis cylinder; *B*, medullary sheath; *C*, neurolemma; *D*, nucleus; *E*, node of Ranvier.

Myelination. Many peripheral nerves have an inseparable insulating myelin sheath and a neurolemma (Fig. 5.3), both of which are products of Schwann cells. The fibers located within the white matter of the brain and spinal cord have a myelin sheath but no neurolemma. In contrast, postganglionic autonomic fibers have a neurolemma but no myelin sheath.

Motor Units[25]

The nerve cell body, the long axon, all the terminal branches, and all the muscle fibers supplied to these branches comprise a nerve *motor unit*.[26] Each muscle is composed of a number of motor units that in themselves are several muscle fibers linked to a motor nerve which, in turn, is joined to the central nervous system. Different motor units respond differently to identical stimulus intensities and present different frequency peaks and discharge rhythms.[27]

The motor unit is the functional unit of striated muscle, since an impulse descending from its axon causes all muscle fibers of a particular motor unit to contract simultaneously. With the arrival of nerve impulses, usually below 50 per second, all fibers of a motor unit contract synchronously and contract to their maximum (all-or-none law).

When several motor units are stimulated by asynchronous firings, the attached fibers contract and voluntary body movement occurs. However, because motor units fatigue after several stimulations, other units must be called into play to allow for smooth movement. While it appears during normal muscle contraction that all muscle fibers are in a smooth continuous muscle contraction, they are not. This appearance results from the sum of a series of small groups of fibers contracting at the same moment.

All muscle fibers of a motor unit do not lie in an adjacent position. They are spread throughout the muscle belly so that excitation will produce a weak contraction in a broad area of the muscle, rather than a strong contraction at a relatively isolated area. This allows delicate manipulations.

Large motor units are required for powerful gross movements and the fasciculi are large and coarse. Fine precise movements require much smaller motor units with fasciculi that are relatively small in proprotion to the connective tissue.

Muscular Contraction[28–32]

Histology

Each cylindrical muscle fiber is covered with a specialized layer of sarcolemma which covers a peripheral longitudinal layer of nuclei and cylindrical myofibrils. Sarcolemma insulates each fiber from adjacent fibers so that excitation of one fiber does not affect its neighbors.[33,34]

Within each muscle fiber, there are a thousand or more longitudinal myofibrils arranged in bundles that constitute about 80% of fiber volume. Each myofibril contains many white *I bands* and many dark, short, thick *A bands,* and each of these isotropic and anisotropic bands contains specialized zones. It is the stacking of myofibrils in register that gives voluntary muscle its microscopic transverse striations[35–37] (Fig. 5.4).

The thin white bands of myofibrils contain smaller myofilaments composed of actin, tropomyosin, and troponin protein (Fig. 5.5); the thick dark bands consist essentially of myosin protein. An A band contains a central *H zone* composed solely of myosin filaments that interdigitate with the thin active filaments on either side.[38] The midpoints of the myosin filaments are secured to one another transversely by connections whose line of cross links is termed the *M line* at the middle of the H zone.

Gross muscle shortening should not be confused with filament shortening. During excitation, the contractile elements do shorten.

The Contraction Process[18,39–41]

When a nerve impulse reaches the neuromuscular junction, a chemical transmitter is released which diffuses through the barrier to excite the muscle fiber. The energy potential enters the muscle fiber through minute T tubules, then travels to the A and I band junctions where it triggers the release of calcium, which initiates the process of fiber activity. Myofibril contractile elements tense as the action potential travels across the sarcolemma. The rate is 1–3 m/sec.

During rest, the thick myosin myofilaments only slightly overlap the thin actin myofilaments. During excitation, the A and I bands increasingly slide into an overlapping position to a degree proportional to the chemical interactions beween filaments. The light bands appear to shorten and finally disappear as the thin filaments slide toward each other between the dark myofilaments. When the action potential ceases, calcium returns to storage, the elastic elements recoil, and the thin I bands draw back to their relaxed state (Fig. 5.6).

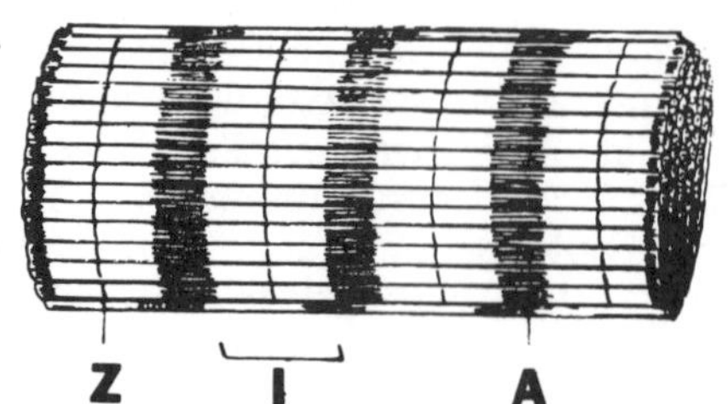

Figure 5.4. Muscle fiber schematic showing arrangement of dark A bands and light I bands.

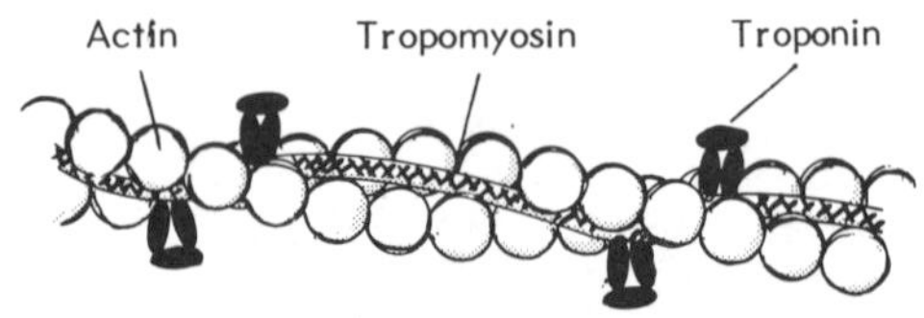

Figure 5.5. Diagram of the probable double helix arrangement of actin molecules along the minute strings of tropomyosin (*cross-hatched*) and occasional troponin (*black*) within the thin I bands of a muscle fiber.

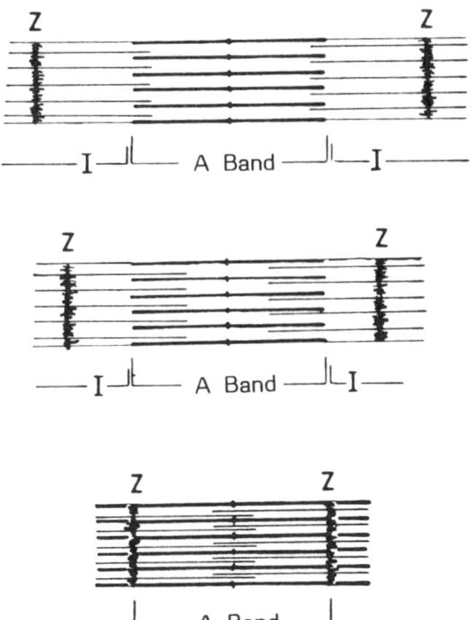

Figure 5.6. The probable arrangement of muscle filaments during stretch (*top*), relaxation (*center*), and strong contraction (*bottom*).

Contraction Strength[42–44]

Muscle power is equal to the load moved times the speed at which the load is moved. The amount of shortening (strength) of a muscle fiber following a stimulus depends on a combination of such complex variables as: (1) the number of nerve fibers employed in carrying stimuli to the muscle fibers, (2) the specific characteristics of the stimulus, (3) the speed at which the muscle is required to act, (4) the rate of flow of nerve impulses arriving from each active nerve fiber, (5) the degree of stretched fiber elongation at the beginning of contraction, (6) whether the muscle tissue is warm or cool, and (7) the state of local fatigue and nutrition. Although maximum effort may be applied to a task, biomechanical performance will be either enhanced or diminished by these conditions.

In addition to the above seven factors, the mechanism of the generation of motor nerve impulses in the brain is so susceptible to environmental and psychologic influences that the absolute stength of stimuli (number of nerve fibers and rate of nerve impulses) in two similar situations is unpredictable; eg, motivation affects work output. Different people respond differently to an identical stimulus.

Factors Affecting Muscle Contraction

MacDonald and Stanish point out that the mechanical factors governing muscle contraction are (1) the angle of pull, (2) the length of the muscle, and (3) the velocity of muscle shortening.[45] The optimum angle of pull is at a 45° joint angle, and a muscle fiber's contractile force is greatest during extension. Obviously, a long muscle fiber can shorten more than a short fiber. Parallel to this is the fact that a suddenly prestretched muscle has an increased contractile capacity. The studies of A. V. Hill showed that the optimum speed at which a muscle can produce its greatest power and efficiency is approximately one-third of its maximum speed.[46]

Besides these mechanical factors, temperature and flexibility should be considered. Hill's studies also showed that a muscle's speed of contraction can be increased 20% by raising body temperature 5°F, thus the benefit of adequate warmup before athletic participation is underscored. Reducing muscle temperature appears to increase the threshold of irritability, which causes weakened and more sluggish contractions. Improved flexibility through static stretching exercises, which do not activate the stretch reflex, appears to reduce soft-tissue restrictions and enhance the relaxation of antagonists.

Mechanical Efficiency[47,48]

As in any mechanical process, the mechanical efficiency of muscle fibers is measured by the ratio of the work accomplished relative to the energy expended. The energy that is not used during muscle activity in performing work is expressed ultimately as heat. The total amount of body energy expended is usually calculated clinically from the respiratory exchange, from which the energy value of the chemical reactions occurring in musculature may be estimated.

The metabolic cost of negative work is 3–9 times less than that of positive work. This is because muscle motor-unit activity for a given load is much lower when contraction occurs during elongation.

Contraction Speed. A muscle's speed of contraction is one of the factors that determines its mechanical efficiency. Shortening speed is determined by muscle length, fiber arrangement, and load. For a rapid contraction, there is an especially large fraction of energy used to overcome tissue viscosity. An opposing consideration is the fact that a slowly contracting muscle requires considerable energy to maintain a prolonged state of tension, and this diminishes mechanical efficiency. Thus, there is an optimum rate at which most effort can be made with the greatest efficiency.[49,50]

Heat. In addition to the energy loss in overcoming tissue viscosity and in maintaining tension, it is the nature of the chemical reactions governing muscle contraction to produce a degree of heat that cannot be converted into mechanical work.[51–53]

Neuron Structure[54–59]

Rather than think of neuron fibers as an electric extension cord, Inman and associates feel it would be better to think of them as living, squirming, moving streams through which a peristaltic flow of chemical supplies is driven from the cell body.

Each neuron consists of four specialized functional parts: the receiving area, the nerve cell body, the axon, and its transmitting area.

The Reception Area. The receiving pole of the nerve cell body has multiple, short, branches (dendrites), usually situated close to the cell body. Once the tree-like dendrites are stimulated, excitation develops by graded depolarization that travels over the dendrites and nerve cell body.

The Cell Body. The rounded nerve cell body proper (perikaryon) serves as the metabolic center of activity. Nerve cell bodies outside the brain and spinal cord are usually located in groups (ganglia), in the cortex of the brain as extensive laminated sheets, and elsewhere in the brain and spinal cord as groups of various shapes and sizes known as nuclei, which comprise the gray matter. Impulses are initiated by an ionic change in the cell's cytoplasm following an influx of sodium, which produces a polarity reversal so that the inner cell is briefly positive relative to the negative cell exterior. This afferent process continues along the axon. The speed of the impulse varies in proportion to the fiber's diameter: faster in large fibers, slower in small axons. During action, materials are transported from the cell body into and along the neuronal processes via the endoplasmic reticulum, microtubules, and neurofilaments.

The Axon. The thread-like conducting axon segment is usually long, singular, and covered by an insulating myelin sheath whose thickness is generally proportional to axon length and diameter. Action potentials are produced and conducted along the axon if its initial segment is sufficiently depolarized. Efferent nerve impulses are produced in the axon near the nerve cell body at an unmyelinated low-threshold area, and they are transmitted in an all-or-none manner in both velocity and magnitude. Figure 5.7 illustrates the major components of a multipolar neuron.

The Transmitters. The transmitting pole of the axon ends in branching terminal telodendria with unmeylinated tips. When the energy impulse reaches the terminals, a chemical transmitter substance (excitatory or inhibitory) is secreted into the synapse in proportion to the magnitude of the impulse, diffuses across the synaptic space, and chemically affects the receptor sites at the postsynaptic neuron membranes. It is likely that neural impulses accelerate on-going transmitter secretory processes, rather than

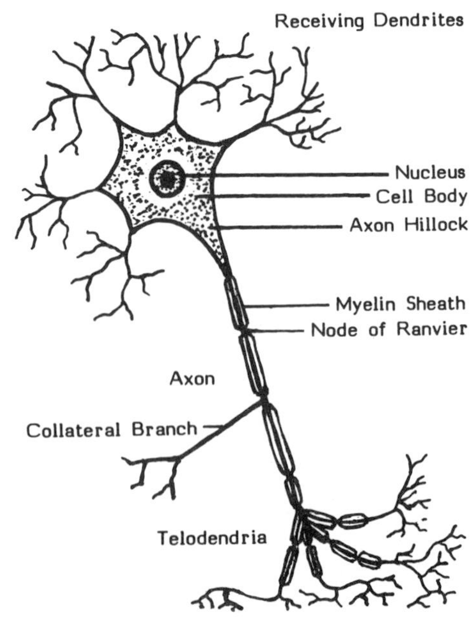

Figure 5.7. Schematic of a multipolar neuron.

initiate them from a completely inactive state.[60]

Impulse Variables. Essentially, muscle reacts in proportion to the quantity of fibers activated and the frequency of impulse bombardment. A neural impulse, to be adequate for muscle contraction, must consist of several appropriate variables. These include sufficient stimulus intensity, frequency of impulse bombardment, rate of wave rise, and duration to activate the contractile elements within the muscle fibers.[61]

Synaptic Processes[62–67]

An illustration of three synapses is shown in Figure 5.8. At the synapse, action potential transmission is not in the all-or-none fashion. It may be inhibited or amplified here according to the specific type of transmitter substance produced. Inhibitory factors can also be produced presynaptically in the axon or produced by fatigue (hypoxia) and drugs.

It is generally accepted, with a few exceptions, that each neuron releases the same type of transmitter substance at all of its terminals (Dale-Feldberg law) and that the substance will have either an excitatory or inhibitory influence on all associated postsynaptic receptors, depending on their properties and on local hormonal influences. As synaptic function is based upon a carefully controlled integration of chemical influences, a slight chemical imbalance (eg, unwise medication, nutrition imbalance) may produce a distinct effect upon synaptic transmission in terms of noxious systemic and behavioral effects.

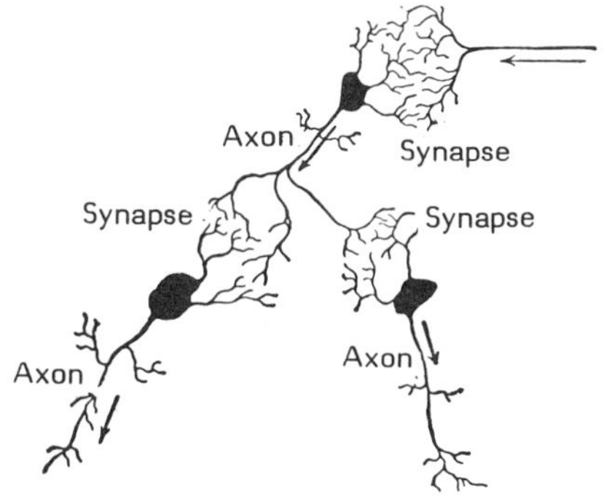

Figure 5.8. A diagram of three synapses. Nerve impulse is indicated by *arrows*.

The Neuromuscular Junction[65, 68–72]

The neuromuscular junction can be considered a specialized type of neuroeffector synapse. The myelin sheath of the terminal axon narrows and then ceases just prior to the motor end-plate. At the site of the end-plates, capillary anastomoses are especially well developed to maintain good nutrition.

Nerve fibers enter the endomysium but do not penetrate the sarcolemma; their terminal branches appose the surface of the muscle fiber (Fig. 5.9). This site is a specialized area of axolemma and sarcolemma where the subneural apparatus is folded into clefts and the sarcolemma is abundant with mitochondria. It is a specialized area that serves as a minute structural barrier where the nerve impulse must be transmitted chemically.

Axon terminals contain mitochondria and numerous vesicles that store the chemical bridge acetylcholine that allows the nerve impulse to be transmitted across the synapse (Fig. 5.10). It is thought that the transmitter substance changes sarcolemma permeability to allow an influx of sodium ions, which generates the electric potential to release the calcium, which is necessary for the acetylcholine release that allows the interaction of myosin and actin filaments to produce muscle contraction.

The enzyme cholinesterase has a dual function. It can activate nerve sheath acetylcholine into its active form or degrade it into acetic acid and choline. Thus, a lack of

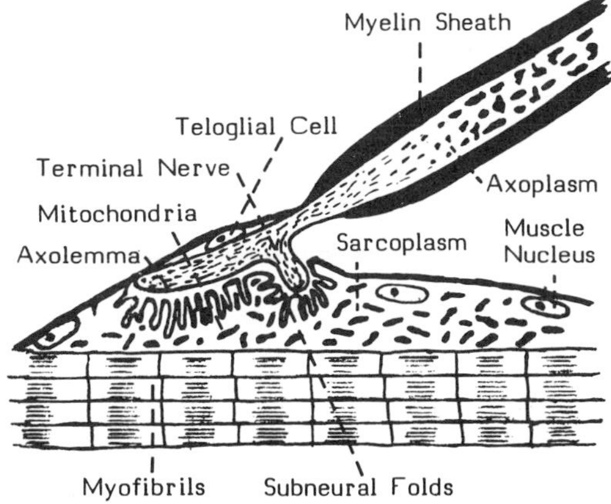

Figure 5.9. Diagram of a neuromuscular junction, its major components, and its relationship with myofibrils.

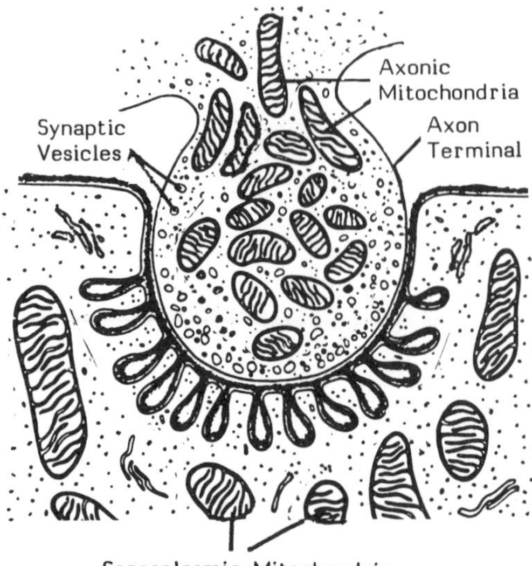

Figure 5.10. Illustration of the bulbous axon terminal, its vesicles and mitochondria, and its relationship to the subneural trough, clefts, and sarcoplasmic mitochondria.

cholinesterase can either produce abnormal or subnormal function. This is often expressed as a sudden jerking of various skeletal muscles many times just prior to or during sleep. This symptom is thought to be due to a lack of cholinesterase which prevents residual acetylcholine from being properly inactivated. A complaint of frequently dropping objects involuntarily may also represent a shortage of cholinesterase failing to inactive acetylcholine. Such symptoms may be a clue to otherwise subclinical riboflavin and/or niacin deficiency that may be expressed in neuromuscular biomechanical mechanisms.[73]

PERIPHERAL AND RELATED NEURAL CONSIDERATIONS

The human nervous system is a marvel in organizing adaptation to internal and external environmental changes: (1) The receptors and afferent neurons of the sensory input system are necessary to detect internal and external environmental changes. (2) The efferent neurons and the muscles of the motor output system must be stimulated if action is to be taken. (3) The integrative system serves as intermediary stations via a complex arrangmenet of interneurons whose synapses control impulse strength and signal direction from the sensory system to the motor system.[74]

Sensory-Motor Segmental Mechanisms[75]

Sensory impulses initiated from receptors in muscles, joints, skin, or viscera travel to the dorsal root ganglia by way of unipolar neurons and then to the spinal cord. Some of these impulses are transmitted to higher control centers where they may or may not reach conscious awareness. The majority of these sensory impulses are instantly relayed via cord interneurons (flexor, extensor, excitatory, inhibitory) to motor neurons located at the same segmental level (ipsilaterally or contralaterally) as the entering dorsal root to determine whether muscles will act as prime movers, accessories, antagonists, or synergists. A minority of sensory impulses synapse directly with motor neurons without assistance from interneurons; these allow the *stretch reflex*.[76]

Because most afferent impulses travel a multisynaptic course, each motor neuron at the segmental level is subject to numerous contralateral and ipsilateral influences, communications from superior and inferior adjacent segments, and influences from higher centers transmitted through the descending pathways. The integrating net effect of these influences determines motor neuronal membrane potential and the resulting state of excitability.

Each muscle spindle contains a few muscle fibers whose purpose is *not* to help in contracting the whole muscle but to control the sensitivity of the muscle spindle to stretch. Spindle fibers are controlled by gamma motor neurons, while other muscle fibers are activated separately by alpha motor neurons. The more contracted muscle spindles become, the more sensitive they are to stretch stimuli.[77]

Muscle Tone[78–81]

Normal muscle firmness is the result of a slight sustained flow of low-frequency asynchronous impulses from the spinal cord generating slight contractions of a small fraction of skeletal muscle fibers plus any degree of active tension. If the function of the ventral roots is impaired, a muscle loses its basic tone immediately; and the same is true if the dorsal roots containing sensory fibers from the muscle are damaged. Thus, tone must be considered not a property of muscle itself but of reflex activity.

In evaluating physical performance, the basic nervous mechanisms that operate during stance and locomotion to provide distribution of postural tension throughout the musculoskeletal system should be understood. There are two fundamental types of neuromuscular activity. One type is the reflex *postural contractions* which are the basis of posture and physical attitudes and maintain muscle tone. The other type is the *phasic contractions* which produce movement and may be either reflex or volitional in origin. While reflex actions are always purposeful, predictable, and involuntary, cortical activity is not.[82]

Phasic and Tonic Motor Neuron Characteristics[83, 84]

Phasic motor neurons are large in size, have a rapid conduction velocity, have a relatively high threshold of physiologic excitability, present large impulses of short duration, and are electrically silent during rest. In contrast, tonic motor neurons are smaller in size, have a slower conduction velocity, have a lower threshold of physiologic excitability, present smaller impulses of longer duration, and are electrically active during rest.

Postural Tone and Balance[85]

Postural tonus refers to the sustained contraction of muscles supporting the upright position. The stimuli producing the volley of nerve impulses that continually excite the postural muscles can arise from every sense organ of the body. For example, postural tone is increased by loud noises, bright lights, strong odors, and jarring shocks. When such stimuli are absent, postural tone diminishes.[86]

Muscle tone is essentially sustained by the stretch reflex.[87] Gravity pulls on all antigravity muscles, and this stretch elicits muscular tone which reflexively helps maintain the body erect. It is on the foundation of postural muscle tone that voluntary movements are superimposed.

As mentioned, the stretch reflex is a major component of maintaining muscle tone and is well developed in the antigravity muscles to control body posture. However, although basic muscle tone and postural patterns involve local cord reflexes, they are definitely under brain control (eg, cerebral cortex, cerebellum, inner-ear proprioceptors). This is readily apparent in states of unconsciousness when the body quickly gives in to the force of gravity.

Reciprocal Inhibition

Every movement starts from a certain posture and ends with a certain posture. While postural tone is necessary in opposing gravity to maintain a static posture, this control must temporarily give way to allow movement. That is, a volley of impulses capable of exciting or inhibiting certain motor neurons must also direct a simultaneous opposite effect on those motor neurons that supply the antagonists (Fig. 5.11). Thus, phasic contractions are accompanied by a reciprocal decrease in antagonist tone. This temporary abolition of postural tone is called *reciprocal inhibition,* and it calls for

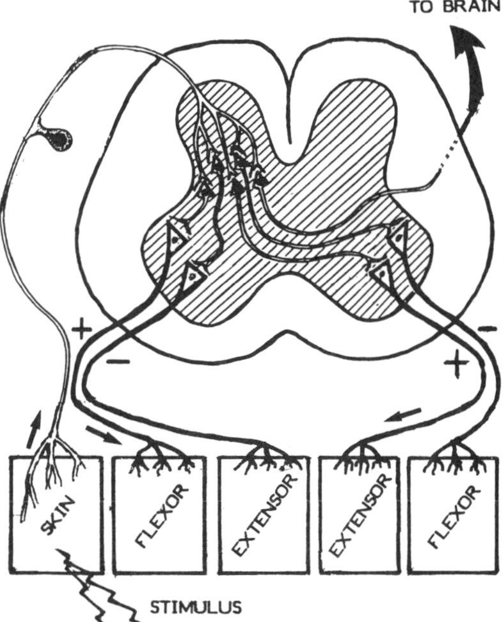

Figure 5.11. Reciprocal innervation mechanism, showing a single interneuron between the afferent and efferent fibers where there normally are many. In this example, a painful stimulus on the skin produces unilateral flexor excitation and extensor inhibition, and contralateral extensor excitation and flexor inhibition, as seen in a typical nocifensive response.

intricate neuromuscular coordination to adjust to the speed and range of contraction of the desired movement.[88,89]

In bilateral activities such as gait, we see that this reciprocal process extends to motor neurons in the contralateral aspect of the segment. For example, when impulses produce flexor action and extensor inhibition on the right side of the body, interneurons relay this message to the left side of the segment to produce reciprocal extensor action and flexor inhibition. When fixation of a joint is required through dual action by both flexors and extensors, higher motor centers take control to balance the synaptic input of the involved circuits.

Without reciprocal inhibition, there would be constant conflict between prime movers and antagonists. This neuromuscular coordination process is enhanced by a period of physical "warmup." Without this, the antagonist muscles may fail to completely relax promptly, resulting in undesired consequences.

The Nocifensive Reflexes

A skin receptor that is stimulated by injury (nociceptor) or the anticipation of traumatic stimuli will induce a protective reflex response. For example, a limb will automatically withdraw from a stimulus that is irritating or perceived to be irritating. This usually unilateral, and usually contractile response will also involve an opposite reaction in the ipsilateral antagonist and contralateral limb's flexors and extensors.[90]

CENTRAL NEURAL CONTROL MECHANISMS[91–94]

Whether a person is awake or asleep, the brain is constantly bombarded by input from all skin and internal receptors. This barrage of incoming messages is examined, valued, and translated relative to a framework composed of instincts, experiences, and psychic conditioning. In some yet to be discovered manner, an appropriate decision is arrived at that is transmitted to all pertinent muscles necessary for the response desired. By means of varying synaptic facilitation and restraints within the appropriate circuits, an almost limitless variety of neural integration and signal transmission is possible. A diagram of a typical motor and sensory circuit is shown in Figure 5.12.

In terms of motor function, the cerebral cortex can be discussed as three distinct regions that control specific muscle groups associated with specific joints. The *primary motor region* of the cerebral cortex is primarily concerned with delicate voluntary movements, particularly of the facial and distal flexor muscles of the extremities.[95] Its left aspect controls the right side of the body, and its right aspect controls the left side. The *supplementary motor area* is concerned essentially with bilateral synergic movements. The *premotor area*, the cortical extrapyramidal center, is involved in the devel-

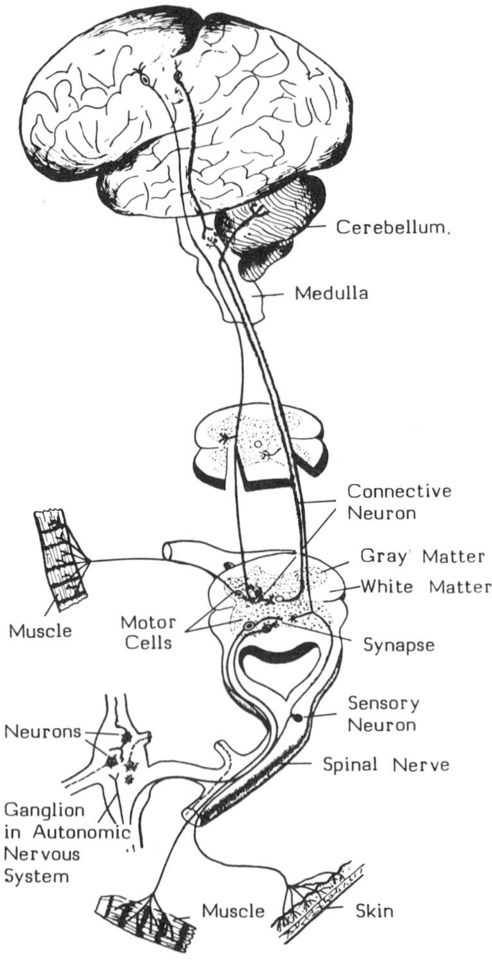

Figure 5.12. Schematic showing sensory and motor circuits of the brain and spinal cord.

opment of motor skills, and its fibers are linked to the cerebellum via thalamic nuclei.

The Descending Cerebral Motor Pathways

The brain dominates spinal reflexes. Skeletal activity is the net result of the influences upon *alpha* and *gamma* motor neurons of the spinal cord and upon the motor components of the cranial nerve nuclei. Such activity is essentially controlled by several descending motor pathways that directly or indirectly are under the management of the cerebral cortex, certain brain stem nuclei, the basal ganglia, and the cerebellum. These structures are termed as a whole the *suprasegmental motor system*[96] (Fig. 5.13).

The motor pathways originating in the cerebral cortex include five basic systems or tracts: corticospinal, corticobulbar, corticotectal, corticorubrospinal, and corticoreticulospinal. In the brain stem, the descending corticospinal tracts are joined by tracts from the midbrain, pons, medulla, and vestibular apparatus.[97]

In general, the pathways that pass through the anterior horn of the spinal cord to the anterior aspect of the gray matter tend to facilitate extensor activity and inhibit flexor activity. Conversely, the pathways that synapse in the posterior aspect of the gray matter tend to facilitate flexor and inhibit extensor neurons. The arrangement of the white tracts and the columns of gray matter are illustrated in Figure 5.14.

Basal Ganglia Influences

The cerebrum exerts its control over lower motor neuron activity either directly through the corticospinal and corticobulbar (pyramidal) tracts or indirectly through the polysynaptic extrapyramidal pathways such as the corticoreticulospinal and corticorubrospinal tracts. The many circuits and feedback loops within and between the structures related to the basal ganglia of the hemispheric subsubstance and rostral part of the brain stem interact with the cerebral cortex and cerebellum to indirectly affect the activity of the lower motor neuron reflex centers via thalamic circuits and midbrain nuclei.[98, 99]

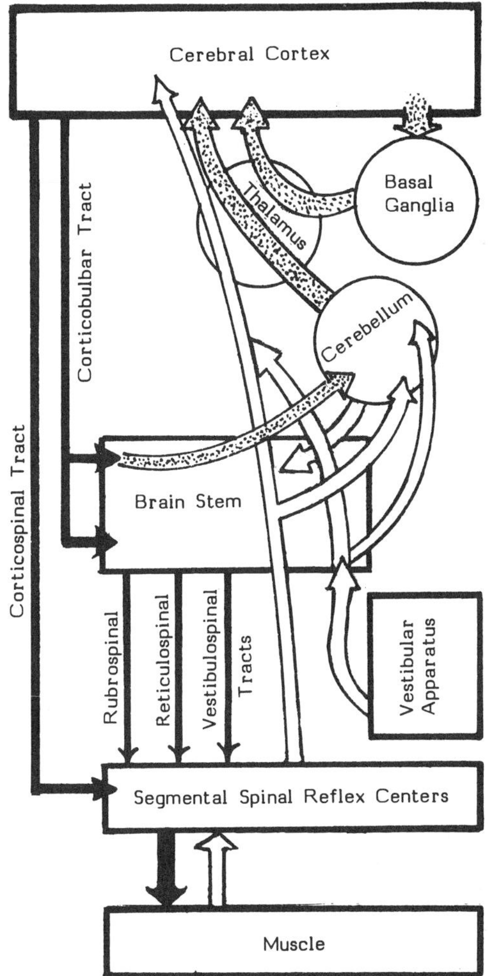

Figure 5.13. Diagram of the relationships between the major components of the suprasegmental motor system and the segmental spinal reflex centers. Main descending efferent tracts are shown in *black*, ascending afferents in *white*, and interconnectors by *stippled* areas.

Cerebellar Influences

The cerebellum is the director of somatic synergy throughout the body. It coordinates the activity of muscle groups spatially and times contractions so that motion will be smooth and accurate. In spite of the fact that the cerebellum receives an abundance of afferent fibers, its efferent fibers do not give rise to consciousness of sensation in the cerebellum, nor are these sensations perceived elsewhere in the brain. Cerebellar input is derived essentially from the cerebral cortex, the vestibular apparatus, the vestib-

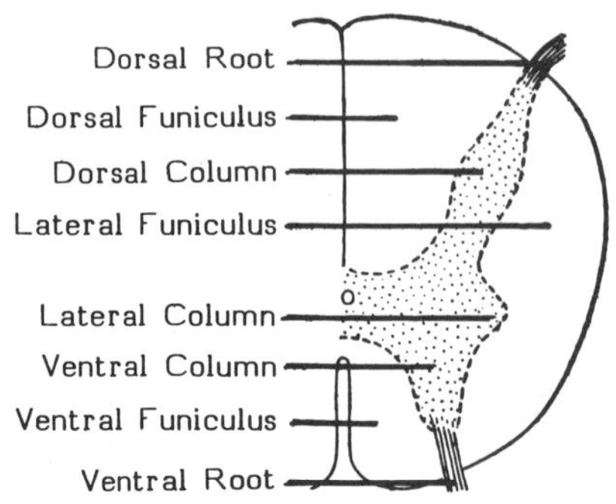

Figure 5.14. Cross section through the spinal cord to illustrate the arrangement of the funiculi of white matter and the columns of gray matter.

ular nuclei of the brain stem, muscle spindle stretch receptors, Golgi tendon organs, and joint and periarticular proprioceptive afferents.[100]

Cerebellar efferents transmit impulses to the vestibular mechanism, the cerebrum, and/or the spinal cord via complex circuits. In contrast to the cerebrum, cerebellar influence on movement is ipsilateral. Voluntary movement and its power, intellectual faculties, and sensory perception can be achieved without cerebellar assistance, but the motions will be awkward and disorganized such as typified in the inaccuracy and intention tremor of asynergia, and cerebellar ataxia.[101]

The Limbic System

The superior aspect of the brain stem contains the *reticular activating system*, which then merges into that part of the brain called the limbic system. The main part of the limbic system is the U-shaped hippocampus, which processes messages from short- and long-term memory so vital for learning. Lateral to the hippocampus is the amygdala and above is the hypothalamus, which together generate sex drives, thirst, hunger, heightened emotions, and altered states of consciousness. The hypothalamus is responsible for both the sympathetic fight-or-flight response and the parasympathetic relaxation response.[102]

Sustaining Mechanisms

Reflexes such as stretch reflexes, inverse myotatic reflexes, and deep tendon reflexes are self-limiting mechanisms whereby sensory impulses from muscle are transmitted to the same muscle via the afferent-cord-efferent reflex cycle. This type of activity, however, does not explain sustained activity such as is seen in voluntary phasic movements. Voluntary activity is initiated and controlled by brain centers. It does not depend upon sensory stimulation, but it does include the segmental reflex centers, especially the stretch reflex circuits. Volitionary action involves loop coactivation of γ- and α-efferents.

Control of Locomotion Patterns[103, 104]

In repetitive activities such as gait, muscle flexor and extensor groups must be fired and depressed at the proper time to afford smooth reciprocal actions, body part coordination, and adjustments to speed and external forces and conditions. During moderate gait, conscious control is only primary when gait is started, stopped, or during fatigue. This requires various sustaining excitatory and inhibitory spinal cord mechanisms acting on ipsilateral and contralateral muscle groups.

A pair of genetically determined *pattern generators* in the cervical spinal cord for the upper extremities and a pair in the lumbosacral cord for the lower extremities are believed to control action by exciting or inhibiting α- and γ-motor neurons in proper sequence. The activity level of the patterns are thought to be set by the midbrain. The generators receive specific and nonspecific input from the periphery, especially specific prompters from hip and shoulder capsules, and are also modified by the descending tracts and spinal reflexes to adapt to load and balance changes.

PROPRIOCEPTION MECHANISMS[105–112]

Proprioception refers to the inborn kinesthetic awareness of body posture, position, movement, weight, pressure, tension, changes in equilibrium, resistance of external objects, and associated stereotyped response patterns. This awareness is the result of impulses generated in afferent receptors located within muscles, tendons, joints, skin, middle ears, viscera, and eyes. The responsive reflex patterns consist of highly coordinated movements of numerous muscle groups and several joints that must be precisely regulated and timed as to sequence, speed, intensity, and duration.

Hirschy describes five types of sensory receptors: (1) *mechanoreceptors,* which detect mechanical deformation of the receptors or cells adjacent to the receptors; (2) *chemoreceptors,* which detect tastes, odors, arterial oxygen levels, osmolarity of body fluids, CO_2 concentrations, and other factors that make up body chemistry; (3) *thermoreceptors,* which detect changes in temperature, with some receptors detecting cold and others warmth; (4) *electromagnetic receptors,* which detect light on the retina; and last but not least, (5) *nociceptors,* which detect painful damage in the tissues, whether it be of a physical or chemical nature.[113] These sensory receptors initiate impulses from their sites to the spinal cord via Type A, B, and C afferent fibers.

Pain signals are essentially transmitted centrally by Type A fibers at velocities between 3 and 10 m/sec and by Type C fibers at velocities between 0.5 and 2 m/sec. Guyton states that these latter fibers constitute over two-thirds of all fibers within the peripheral nervous system.[114]

Upon entering the spinal cord at the dorsal roots, pain and temperature impulses enter the tract of Lissauer where they are transmitted up or down 1–3 segments and then terminate with second-order neurons in the gray matter of the posterior horns of the cord. From here, fibers pass through the anterior commissure to the opposite side of the cord where they form the lateral spinothalamic tract, whose impulses eventually terminate in the intralaminar nuclei of the thalamus, medulla, pons, and mesencephalon. Communication with the cerebral cortex is made via third-order neurons from the thalamus and intralaminar nuclei.

Muscle and Tendon Receptors[115, 116]

From 40–60% of nerve fibers entering a muscle are sensory in function. Some of these afferent fibers are concerned with pain, but most are concerned with proprioception to register muscle fiber contraction or stretch. This is invariably an *unconscious* process, yet it plays a vital part in controlling muscular force and timing.

The complete process is a combined effect from afferent fibers from muscles, tendons, and joints. These sensory muscle fibers originate from sites on perimysium, endomysium, or capillaries, or in interstitial fat. Other sensory fibers originate from receptors concerned purely with pressure. These are abundant in joint tissues and offer *conscious* information as to limb position.

Neuromuscular Spindles and the Stretch Reflex

The complex muscle spindles, interspersed among skeletal muscle fibers, offer the most important sensory feedback from muscles (Fig. 5.15). One large sensory annulospiral nerve fiber has branches that entwine around each muscle spindle, while other secondary flower-spray endings are sited near the extremities of the spindle (Fig. 5.16). Because they communicate messages about muscle fiber length (contraction magnitude), they are termed *stretch receptors.* In addition, they also communicate information about the speed of fiber length changes (velocity). The afferent receptors have a relatively low threshold to stretch and their impulses excite a feedback *stretch reflex* that produces contraction of the same muscle.[117]

When a muscle is passively stretched by a load, the lengthening of its fibers compresses the spindles, the afferent annulospiral terminals become depolarized, and asynchronous impulses are relayed to the spinal cord via the sensory afferents. The heavier the load, the greater the stretching and the more powerful the contraction to unload the spindles. Another mechanism occurs when, concurrent with voluntary muscle contraction, the midfiber zone of the fiber is stretched by contraction of the fiber's two polar segments.

The large muscle afferents from muscle spindles synapse directly with motor neurons without assistance from cord interneurons. This always excitatory and always unilateral monosynaptic reflex arc serves as the basis of the stretch reflex that is restricted to the segments at the level of sensory input.

Golgi Tendon Organs[118, 119]

The less complex Golgi organs offer the most important sensory feedback from tendons. These structures, unique to musculotendinous tissue, sense tension from either

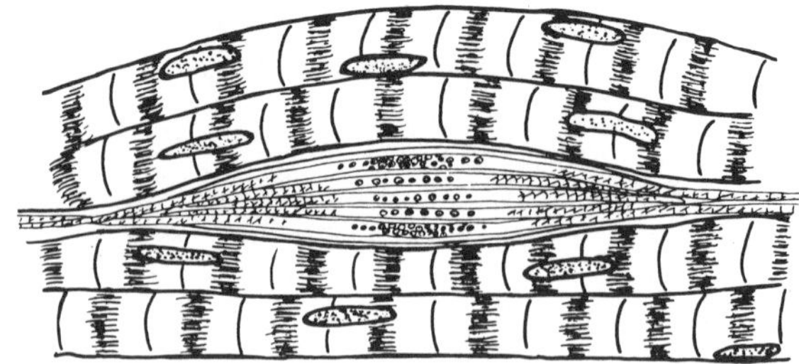

Figure 5.15. Longitudinal section representation of a neuromuscular spindle capsule lying parallel with contractile muscle fibers.

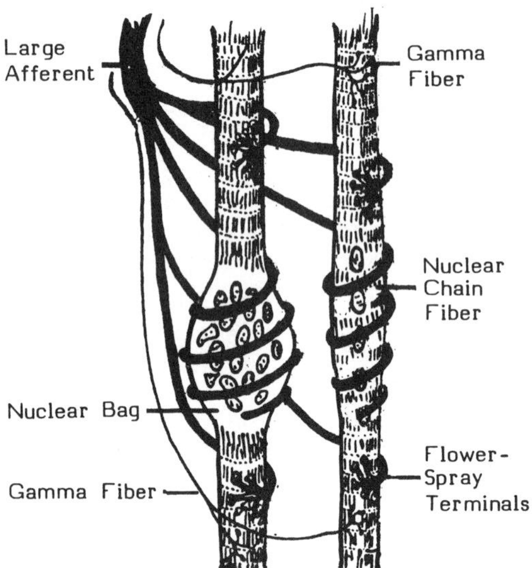

Figure 5.16. Diagram of a muscle spindle showing one nuclear bag (*left*) and one nuclear chain fiber (*right*). The large afferent nerve fibers (*black*) end in annulospiral endings around the midzone of the muscle fibers. The smaller afferent fibers end in flower-spray terminals. Much smaller efferent γ-fibers supply both types of intrafusal fibers, as shown at the *top* and *bottom* of the diagram.

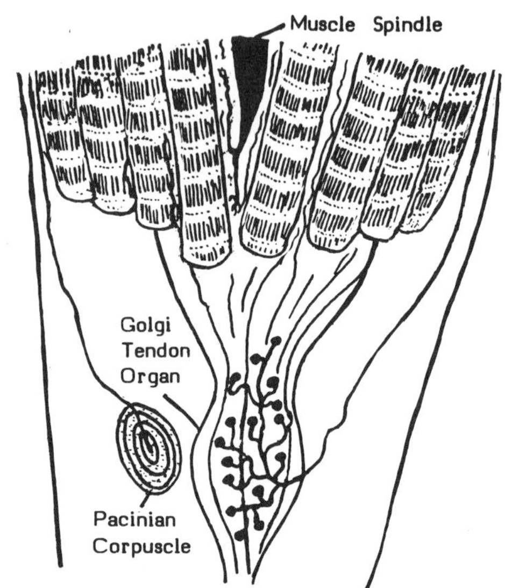

Figure 5.17. Site of a Golgi tendon organ at a musculotendinous junction.

muscle contraction or extreme stretching. They have a much higher threshold to stretch than stretch receptors. In contrast to stretch receptors, Golgi organ impulses reflexly *inhibit* contraction of the muscle of origin and its synergists.

Golgi tendon organs are embedded in the musculotendinous area, essentially to protect against overstretch (Fig. 5.17). Each Golgi organ is penetrated by one or two terminal sensory fibers, and each communicates in series with several muscle fibers belonging to different motor units.

Sensory input from Golgi tendon organs, pain receptors, and spindle flower-spray terminals to the spinal cord are transmitted to motor neurons by way of one or several interneurons and synpases which may have either an excitatory or inhibitory function. Through these multisynaptic routes, afferent impulses can be transmitted ipsilaterally, contralaterally, and inferiorly or superiorly to adjacent segments to excite accessory muscle groups or inhibit antagonists. Thus, each motor neuron is subject to numerous segmental influences as well as influences from higher centers transmitted via the descending pathways.

Joint Receptors[120-123]

Capsule and associated ligament and connective tissue afferent fibers originate from tiny areas of encapsulated collagen fasciculi (Fig. 5.18). They are readily subject to move-

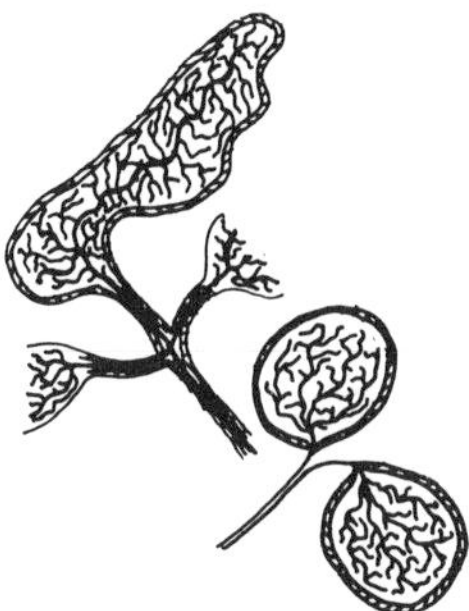

Figure 5.18. Two types of sensory receptor end organs. *Left*, a flower-spray Ruffini end organ. These slowly responding receptors located in joint capsules and the midlayer of skin signal messages of joint position and possibly of heat. *Right*, a Golgi-Mazzoni corpuscle, a small flower-spray pressure-sensitive organ containing an afferent neuron. They are found near joint capsules.

ment, compression, depolarization, and firing when the tendon is stretched from muscle contraction. If the minute muscle fibers terminating in the collagen fasciculi at the musculotendinous junction are actively tensed, the Golgi organs increase their discharge of afferent impulses. Passive stretching, however, does not increase the discharge unless it is extreme.

A few joint-related receptors are insensitive to movement but discharge in proportion to the joint angle. There is no position in which all joint receptors are silent.

Skin Receptors[124–126]

Most cutaneous receptors consist of a soft cellular core containing a nerve ending that is surrounded by a lamellated connective tissue capsule (Fig. 5.19), and their design varies somewhat according to function. Those concerned with touch, pressure, or pain function as both somesthetic exteroceptors and as proprioceptors. Skin receptors initiate many of the basic inborn protective reflexes such as grasp reflexes, withdrawal reflexes, and placement reactions.[127]

Labyrinthine Receptors[128–130]

Inner ear sensory organs contribute stimuli to postural tone through impulses arising when the neck is moved. Small particles of calcium (otoliths) are suspended within the fluid of the semicircular canals. When the head is tilted, the otoliths drift from one part of the canal's wall to another. As these

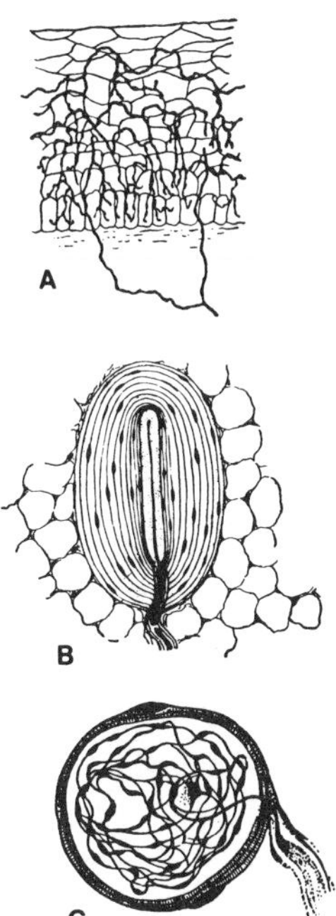

Figure 5.19. *A*, an end organ with diffuse sensory nerve fiber terminations in stratified squamous epithelium. Two types of surface receptors composed of a lamellated capsule enclosing a sensory nerve twig are shown. *B*, a Pacinian corpuscle, a rapidly responding receptor sited in the deep layer of skin and near tendons and joints. They are highly sensitive to movement, pressure, and vibration stimuli. *C*, a Meissner corpuscle, involving many terminals, found just beneath the dermis. They send patterned signals of touch necessary for precise discrimination and integrative processing.

floating otoliths touch the sides of the canal's walls, they press against a few of the many hair-like sensory nerve receptors which line the canal's walls. This slight pressure stimulates impulses to arise that ultimately produce a sensation of position and a reflex righting of the head relative to gravitational pull (Fig. 5.20).

Only slight stimulation is necessary to evoke the reflexes necessary to maintain the body erect. Equilibrium reflexes evoked by stimulation of the semicircular canals dominate all other righting reflexes. Once these reflexes are lost (eg, pathology), one must rely solely on muscle and tendon proprioceptors, visual stimuli, and cutaneous touch and pressure to maintain an erect position.

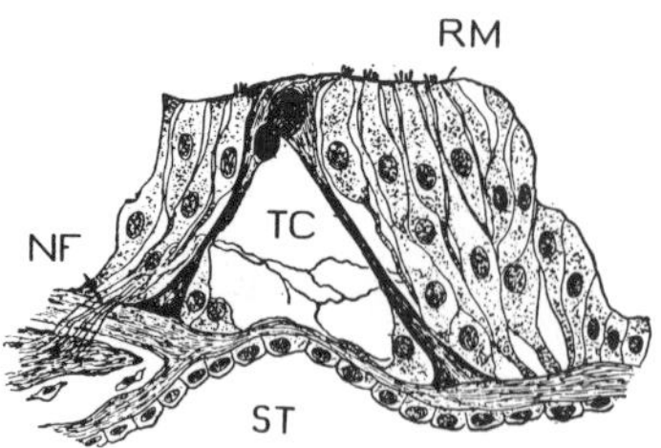

Figure 5.20. Schematic section of the organ of Corti. *TC*, tunnel of Corti; *ST*, scala tympani; *RM*, reticular movement; *NF*, nerve fibers.

Cervical Receptors[131, 132]

With the head erect, the labyrinths are placed in an optimum position to act synergically with the neck reflexes, and these in turn react with other existing proprioceptive and exteroceptive impulses to supply a symmetrical distribution of tone in proper quantities to postural muscles. Specifically, neck-righting reflexes are evoked from impulses arising in joint receptors of the neck to produce contraction to align the body with the head. A typical spinal proprioception pathway is shown in Figure 5.21.

The cervical muscles are richly supplied with proprioceptors, and the atlanto-occipital and atlantoaxial joints are especially endowed with receptors. These facts, in addition to the proprioception receptors of the inner ear, make head position important in maintaining structural balance. Almost all movements are started with a head movement in the direction desired, and only slight poorly directed head movement during a complicated movement is necessary to throw the entire body out of alignment. In contrast, cervical reflexes appear to be dominant on the upper limbs, while labyrinthine reflexes appear to be dominant on the lower limbs.

It is not unlikely that proprioceptive impulses combined with the interacting postural reflexes of good body mechanics play a role in the maintenance of good health and optimal performance. Conversely, the maladjustment of nervous impulses within the central nervous system as a result of pressure, irritation, or poor posture may be a causative factor in the production of poor health and hindered performance by contributing to dysfunction from the subtle yet persistent stress involved.

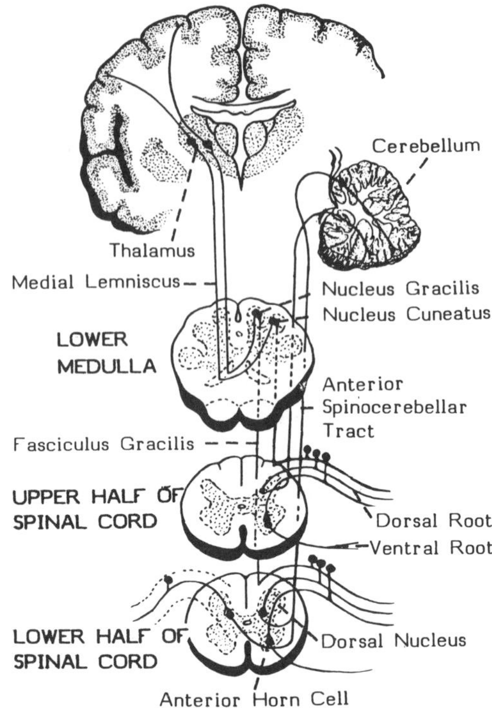

Figure 5.21. A typical proprioception pathway.

Balance Recovery

Besides those mechanisms involved in maintaining the erect posture against gravity, there are other postural mechanisms concerned with maintaining body equilibrium. These are vital to keep the body in the correct position during complex motor activities.[133, 134] For example, when the body is thrown off balance (eg, from a stumble or blow), compensatory movements beyond conscious control are made to restore normal posture. These reflex movements receive their sensory input from inner-ear proprioceptors, stretch receptors of the cervical musculature, other joint and muscle proprioceptors, the sensory organs of touch (especially of the plantar surfaces of the feet), and visual stimulation. Orientating visual impressions are important in maintaining erect posture by establishing relationships to objects about the individual.

Postural Equilibrium

Irregularities of postural control can be expected to result in deviations from normal standing values. Within normal parameters, healthy people have a slightly variable mean speed of sway and range of movement in the sagittal and coronal planes. Vision also affects these values significantly, as shown in differences between eyes-open and eyes-closed tests. In studies of normal subjects and amputees, it has been shown that postural sway increases with age, but the visual dependence for the control of sway is unaffected by age.[135]

Seliktar and associates devised a ballistic monitoring technique to establish criteria for postural disorders in the standing position. They found that each of the monitored parameters demonstrated three modes of oscillation which they called (1) tremor, (2) ataxia, and (3) sway, and that normal subjects, post-CVA (cerebrovascular accident) hemiplegics, and brain-injured subjects showed distinctly different patterns.[136]

While the mechanical oscillations of man's physiologic gravicenter have long been known, only recently has instrumentation been developed that can automatically evaluate an individual's sway parameters in terms of amplitude and frequency of body oscillations. Terekhov accomplished this by constructing a platform that translates body oscillations into electrical signals that are displayed immediately in numerical forms.[137]

TRAINING AND REHABILITATIVE CONSIDERATIONS[138, 139]

Doctors of today must ask and seek answers to many questions concerning human dynamics, for it is impossible to separate structure from function. This requires knowledge of how the nervous system integrates proprioceptive input and coordinates activity of the musculoskeletal system so that each unit involved will contribute its function properly. Thus, a primary concern within health care in its quest to maintain physical fitness is the integration of neurophysiologic and biomechanical information.

Physical Fitness[140]

Most studies used to evaluate physical performance have been in the field of athletics, but we can use this specialized information by applying it to the nonathletic patient's daily activities. While the principles remain the same, our only concerns are to keep in mind that (1) the demands of the nonathlete are much less, and (2) the factors considered in physical fitness are not equal in all people who could be judged highly fit.

The degree of vascularity of the capillary network between skeletal muscle fibers and in associated tissues depends greatly upon the type of exercise. The quantity of interstitial fat, most marked in atrophied muscle, is also determined by the degree of exercise. Lymph vessels are not found in voluntary muscle.

Strength[141–143]

The average ratio between muscle strength and an individual's weight has been computed to be about 26:6. Thus, the aggregate strength of the muscles of a 150-lb male is about 4000 lb. Since only a portion of all muscles can be employed for a specific task, only a small part of one's total strength can be utilized effectively for a particular task.[144]

In discussing strength, terminology is often confusing. The phrase "isometric (equal in length) strength" refers to muscle activity occurring without muscle shortening. "Isotonic (equal in tone) strength" means muscle activity with shortening of the muscle. Both of these general terms are physiologic misnomers: there *is* a degree of length change in isometrics due to tendon stretching, and in isotonics, normal tone *is* influenced by the altered mechanical advantage and resistance.[145–147]

Many feel that strength is the only training variable in enhancing the speed of muscle contraction and that tissue viscosity is relatively constant. This is only true, however, when strengthening actions mimic movements used in the activity desired.

Classifications of Strength

For discussion, strength can be divided into dynamic (isotonic), explosive, and static (isometric) types.[148]

Dynamic Strength. This is one's ability to lift, move, and support body weight, calling upon endurance when such functions are strenuously repeated; ie, explosive movements repeated in rapid succession (Fig. 5.22). Limits are imposed by speed-

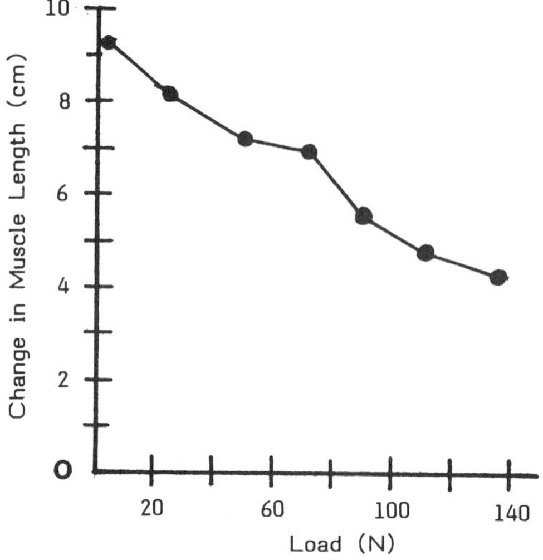

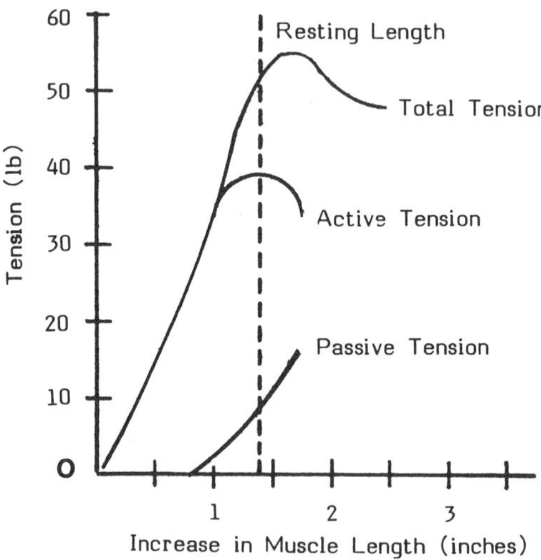

Figure 5.22. *Top*, chart of the ability of a typical muscle to shorten from a given initial length under successive applications of increasing load. *Bottom*, in contrast to ligaments or metals, muscle tissue displays both active and passive bahavior. The sum tensile reaction force of muscle is shown in the Blix curve displayed. The maximum tension that a muscle fiber can produce is determined by its length relative to its resting length, and it is generated at a relative displacement (1.2:1). Unlike metal, a muscle's reaction force is quite time-dependent because the higher the active component, the shorter the maintenance time.

resisting factors and the quantity and quality of energy-exchange factors.[149,150]

Explosive Strength. Explosive strength refers to the ability to release maximum power (energy) in the shortest possible time. Single violent efforts are commonly seen in activities in which speed factors are combined with the force and velocity features of active muscles. Response is determined by mechanical leverage (influenced by body type), immediate energy resources from tissue chemical coupling (influenced by glycogen and mineral ion levels), the quantity of actin and myosin filaments per fiber (influenced by training hypertrophy), and the number of fibers activated (influenced by learning experiences). The performance result of these forces is determined largely by the degree of dynamic viscosity.[151,152]

Static Strength. This refers to the exertion of a maximum force for a brief period against a fairly immovable object, such as is brought out in weight lifting. Such strength is dependent on the number of active muscle fibers involved in a specific activity; ie, the functional cross section (gross muscle less fat and connective tissue) of the muscle tissue exerting the force, with some assistance from the type of contraction and mechanical advantage in play. Lessening of central inhibition and greater relaxation of antagonists also play a part in the performance effect. Limits are imposed by exhaustion, motivation, Valsalva effects, pain, and quickly diminishing endurance. Muscles required to contract against increasing resistance become progressively stronger and usually, but not inevitably, hypertrophy; thus, women should have no fear that weight lifting with proper form will cause overdevelopment.[153,154]

Fatigue[155,156]

Either progressing central or local fatigue adversely affects skill: diminished skill is commonly associated with approaching exhaustion. As muscle perfusion is greater in a strong muscle than in a weak muscle, fatigue is to a great extent due to inadequate perfusion. However, the overt signs of pallor and the energy-wasting poor coordination, confusion, and staggering gait are to be blamed on inadequate blood flow to the posture-regulating center. Strength also has an effect on recovery: it tends to minimize the microtrauma secondary to oxygen lack and local weakness.

Strength Development[157]

Strength is developed in three manners: (1) *isotonically* by exercises against resistance in such a manner that body movements are allowed; (2) *isometrically* by exercises against resistance in such a manner that body movements are restricted—sometimes offering a shortcut to goals of equivalent repetitive drudgery; (3) *isokinetically* by exercises of a constant velocity against resistance which adapt to the angle of a joint. Isokinetic exercises are employed primarily to rehabilitate up to the point of normal strength at which other forms of exercise are used.[158,159]

At the tissue level, the value of strength training includes: (1) an increased proportion of active fibers because of the improved neuropathways and impulse transmission—in contrast to a well-conditioned muscle that has 90% activity, a poorly conditioned muscle may have as few as 60% active fibers; (2) an increase in thickness (hypertrophy) of specific slow-twitch and fast-twitch muscle fibers, the greatest reaction occurring in the pale fast-twitch fibers; (3) an increase in the threshold of contraction inhibitory mechanisms (eg, the Golgi sensory receptors); (4) an increase in contraction power and speed; and (5) a decrease of interfiber and muscle surface fat.

Muscle Power. Body power is determined by the rate at which energy can be released within muscle tissue: power = work/time. While the type of contraction, resistance, duration, quantity of repetitions, and number of exercise bouts are important in any exercise program, the most important factor appears to be that the contraction force developed by a muscle must be close to maximum if improved change is to be expected. It has been well established that low-repetition high-resistance exercises develop power; high-repetition low-resistance exercises develop endurance.[160–162]

Isometric Therapy. It has been shown that from 1–3 isometric contractions of 40–60% of maximum held for 3–5 seconds each day result in the maximum possible increase of muscular strength.[163] Others have determined that the maximum contraction of a muscle, held for a matter of seconds, will cause the muscle to grow in strength at an average of 4% per week. The claim is that the maximum contraction of a muscle is all that is necessary to strengthen slackened muscles. Such exercise, performed once each day to muscles of the body in the sedentary individual will increase strength 50% in 12 weeks according to the research conducted. Thus, evidence of disuse atrophy as seen clinically indicates a severe lack of activity of a muscle group. One disadvantage of purely isometric exercises is that benefits are confined to a range of motion of only 20° to either side of the training angle at which contraction is performed.[164,165]

Endurance[166]

Endurance, a manifestation of cardiovascular and respiratory function (both aerobic and anerobic capacity), manifests itself in a variety of physical activities. It is the capacity to maintain strenuous activity of a large number of muscle groups for a duration sufficient to demand prolonged resistance to fatigue. Endurance is basically limited by individual strength, amount of body fat in addition to external load, and by the amount of oxygen debt that can be tolerated during physical activity.[167,168]

In biomechanics, the term *endurance* is generally used to denote the ability of skeletal muscle to continue contractions relative to contraction length (time), contraction quantity (per unit of time), and contraction quality (force). During vigorous muscular effort, the endurance factor is determined by the initial glycogen content of muscle fibers and this is influenced by diet and training.[169]

Speed

Body speed is highly correlated with muscle power and is difficult to isolate.[170] Speed (fastness) can refer to locomotion time or reaction time. It can refer to the legs of a racer, the fists of a boxer, the arms of a goalie, the eyes of a skeet shooter. Reaction speed is determined by the interval between when stimuli are received by receptor organs and when the muscles react.[171,172]

As inertia is proportional to mass, total speed has three aspects: (1) time/distance in initiating body movement (explosive force of active muscles); (2) time/distance at a rate of acceleration to maximum; and (3) time/distance during loss of acceleration as the event is prolonged. During the end of a run, the reducing metabolic energy must cope with continuing resistances in air flow, tissue viscosity, surface friction, and other energy losses.

Because it is difficult for a bulky frame to accelerate quickly to a maximum speed, the ideal physique of a runner would be one with powerful legs and little weight elsewhere.[173] Performance is enhanced by a preliminary warm-up that raises intramuscular temperature; a slight increase in temperature enhances muscle-tissue viscosity and utilization of energy resources within the muscles that influence muscle contraction.

Motor Skills[174–177]

Skill enables a performer to accomplish more work with less effort. A lack of skill is exhibited in great effort and awkward movements, indicating poor impulse selection and neural adjustments. The basic factors that limit skill development are body type, weight, height, timing, coordination, integration of reflex actions, accuracy of movement, specificity of training, learning ability, individuality of coordinated movements, sense of feeling, motivation, and age (maturation of the nervous system).

As muscle activity patterns are dependent on the integrity of the nervous system, muscle education involves training nervous system patterns. This may involve the development of new patterns and other muscles to compensate for specific weaknesses. Keep in mind that antagonist relaxation is just as important as primer mover action during movement.

The Development of Motor Skills[178,179]

Motor skill development is a complex process of adjustment in which constant attention must be concentrated on the component spatial movements, the power and extent of movements, and the correlation of visual and proprioceptive input. At this early stage, performance is under the control of the motor area of the cerebral cortex.

With practice, the proper sequence of movements is "learned" and control is transferred to the premotor cerebral area at which point constant attention is no longer necessary. Concurrently, visual and proprioceptive data have been so correlated that the action can be carried out blindfolded and guided solely by proprioceptive input.

Development Potential

While performance assessment is often studied in an isolated compartmentalized fashion (eg, strength, endurance, aerobic-anerobic capacity, etc) by the physiologist, care must be taken clinically to avoid oversimplified specific-muscle training which does not enhance overall performance. For example, the development of isometric strength does not assure an improvement in dynamic performance. Because every physical activity demands a different combination of structural and physiologic capabilities, an individual's fitness must be adequate for the task at hand.[180]

Effects of Physical Training

Physical training increases the bulk of muscle fibers and increases muscle interstitial vascularity. Both of these factors have an influence upon the effects of acute muscle strain: an untrained muscle is more apt to bleed and form a hematoma than a trained muscle, and the physiologic mechanisms necessary to absorb extravasated fluid are more efficient in a trained muscle than in an untrained muscle.

Keep in mind that the quantity of muscle fibers does not increase after birth.[181] Exercise increases muscle quality, not quantity; it allows muscles to become larger, stronger, and better developed.[182] Also, muscle fibers that have been destroyed and replaced by fibrous tissue cannot be restored. The goal of muscle training is to increase the *quality* of fibers present.

Structural and Functional Variables

The development of physical performance during youth is greatly determined by body size, body type, the degree of maturation of the nervous system, and the degree of sexual maturation (more important in males than females).[183] Added to this, under conditions of good nutrition, the body of both the immature and the mature thrives on use, and use encourages adaptation to maintain a functional reserve of about 25% greater than demand.

There is a close correlation between one's degree of strength and endurance and one's degree of health because of the relationship to a greater capacity for physical work and a smaller functional response to the challenges of stress. The absence of signs of disease does not indicate health.

In addition to the variations among individuals of different ages, sex, race, and body type, there are also physiologic and psychologic variations within a single individual from instant to instant and day to day. These variants prevent any one set of kinesiologic data collected from an individual under one condition from being used to accurately predict performance in a second trial or to predict the performance of others.

Genetic Influences

In spite of neuromuscular integrity, little can be done to modify body type because many of the variables found in body build and its individual physiology are genetically determined. This is especially true for oxygen intake. While motor skills have an influence on efficiency, body type places a finite limit on biomechanic achievement goals.[184] In organized sports, a great deal of practice time is allotted to the development of physical skills, but many aspects of skill are also inherited (eg, receptor organ sensitivity).[185] The potential athletic "superstar" probably starts life with a peculiar biomechanical and/or neuromuscular physiologic advantage.

SELECTED CLINICAL CONSIDERATIONS

In terms of those neuromuscular factors that commonly affect human biomechanics, the most important aspects are muscle mass, tone, reflexes, fatigue, weakness, trauma, trigger points, and nerve and cord lesions.

Muscle Atrophy

Palpation and mensuration are used to determine muscle volume. On palpation, there should be a mass that is symmetrical bilaterally. A decrease in limb size is indicative of atrophy and usually associated with some degree of hypotonicity. The affected muscle becomes somewhat shrunken, poor in tone, and weak in strength.[186–188]

With the possible exception of noxious spinal influences, disuse atrophy is the most common cause of local muscle weakness. It may be the result of immobilization, an occupational lack of use of a particular muscle group, or disuse as a result of painful injury, nerve disease, or muscle disease. The examiner should take age, sex, occupation, and righthandedness or lefthandedness into consideration. Atrophy is especially difficult to evaluate in the aged or malnourished individual.

Atrophy is demonstrated in evaluations of muscle strength as well as of decrease in bulk.[189] Because of this decrease in mass, bilaterally compared circumferential measurements of limbs are helpful in evaluation. In situations of atrophy, it is important to keep in mind those features which distinguish disuse atrophy from denervation atrophy.

Disuse Atrophy. Features include moderate reduction in visible muscle size, mild to moderate diminished muscle strength (with paralysis in upper motor neuron lesions), normal tendon reflexes (hyperactive after initial shock in cases of upper motor neuron lesions), normal response to direct muscle stimulation, and mild and slowly progressing atrophy. Note that Pottenger showed that visceral malfunction can also produce these symptoms.[190]

Denervation Atrophy. Rapid reduction in visible muscle size, zero voluntary muscle strength, absent tendon reflexes, no response to direct brief muscle stimulation, and rapidly progressing atrophy are characteristic.[191]

Muscle Tone and Related Reflexes[192]

Myotonicity

Healthy muscle possesses a small amount of firm, palpable tension even at complete rest. It feels firm and resilient rather than flabby. In evaluating muscle tone, age, sex, body structure, occupation, physical avocations, and nutritional status of the patient must be considered.

Tone is most pronounced in those muscles which prevent the body from sagging from its erect position from the force of gravity such as at the ankle, knee, hip, spine, neck, and jaw. Thus, the erectors are referred to as the antigravity muscles.

During passive manipulation of a joint, a slight degree of resistance is encountered in the muscle, which is not part of a conscious effort on the part of the patient. Thus, the chief characteristics of normal muscle tone are subdued activity during relaxation and an involuntary reaction opposing mechanical stretch.

The clinical assessment of muscle tone is essentially the assessment of the *stretch reflex*. The stretch (myotatic) reflexes that control muscle tone are tested by (1) the tendon reflexes, and (2) slow sustained passive flexion and extension to activate the stretch reflex and note the resistance.

The chief difference between ergotropic and trophotropic action as far as the somatic system is concerned lies in the degree of muscle tone. The gamma system plays a decisive although not exclusive role in the regulation of muscle tone; ie, gamma fibers set spindle tone.[193]

Diagnostic Tendon Reflexes[194,195]

While a diagnosis of a neurologic disorder cannot be determined by reflexes alone, they are important aids in establishing the type and location of a lesion. Deep reflexes vary in direct proportion to muscle tone. A superficial reflex is any reflex phenomenon that may be induced by a light stimulus such as stroking the skin with a wisp of cotton, resulting in horripilation (gooseflesh) or muscle contraction. The afferent, center, and efferent aspects of superficial and deep reflexes are outlined in Table 5.1.

Note that: (1) In upper motor neuron or pyramidal fiber lesions, the deep tendon reflexes are exaggerated, but the superficial skin reflexes are decreased or absent. (2) In lesions of a lower motor neuron or the motor fibers from the anterior horn cells of the cord, both the deep and the superficial reflexes are decreased or absent.

A tendon jerk after percussion (Fig. 5.23) is a variation of the stretch reflex. The sharp blow causes a large number of spindle receptors to become depolarized simultaneously and a volley of synchronous, rather than asynchronous, impulses are transmitted to the effectors via the spinal cord. This has clinical significance, but it is of little importance as far as normal body posture and motion are concerned.

The tendon reflex evaluates the integrity of all components of the circuit from the muscle spindles to the muscle fibers. This includes the sensory receptors, the afferent nerves, the spinal cord segment(s) involved,

Table 5.1.
Superficial and Deep Reflexes

	Afferent	Center	Efferent
Superficial Reflexes			
Corneal	V	Pons	VII
Consensual	II	Midbrain	III
Accommodation	II	Occipital	III
Oculocardiac	V	Medulla	X
Carotid sinus	IX	Medulla	X
Uvular	IX	Medulla	X
Ciliospinal	Sensory nerve	T1–T2	Cervical sympathetics
Upper abdominal	T7–T10	Cord level	T7–T10
Lower abdominal	T10–T12	Cord level	T10–T12
Cremasteric	Femoral	L1	Genitofemoral
Plantar	Tibial	S1–S2	Tibial
Anal	Pudendal	S4–S5	Pudendal
Deep Reflexes			
Jaw jerk	Trigeminal	Pons	Trigeminal
Biceps	Musculocutaneous	C5–C6	C5–C6
Triceps	Radial	C6–C7	C6–C7
Radial	Radial	C6–C8	C6–C8
Patellar	Femoral	L2–L4	L2–L4
Achilles	Tibial	S1–S2	S1–S2

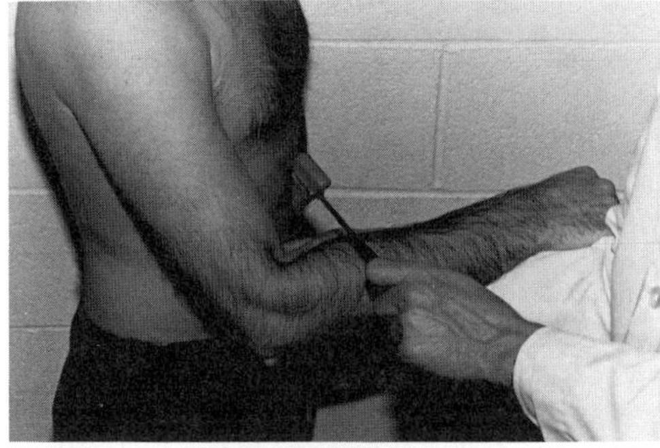

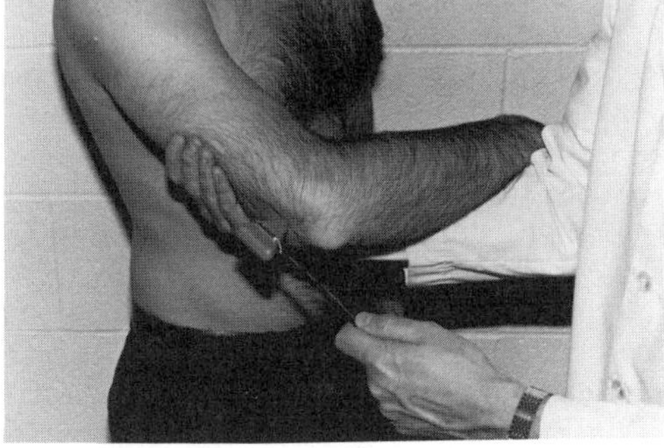

Figure 5.23. *Top*, testing the biceps reflex; *bottom*, testing the triceps reflex.

the alpha motor neurons and their axons, the apparatus at the neuromuscular junction, and the muscle fibers. The speed and magnitude of the reaction also gives clues as to adjacent segment and higher control center influence on the efferent neurons (ie, an exaggerated response when the inhibitory influences of the descending tracts are lacking). A grading system for deep reflexes is offered in Table 5.2.

Muscle Fatigue and Cramps

Weakness that occurs upon exertion and is progressive with muscular effort is called fatigability. A cramp is a painful muscular contraction. The term *fatigue cramp* refers to any painful muscular contraction associated with fatigue.

Background

When physical activity is conducted under highly warm/humid conditions, precautions must be taken to avoid dehydration fatigue, heat cramps, exhaustion, and stroke.[196] Under such conditions, muscle cramps result from electrolytic depletion and are temporarily disabling.

Table 5.2.
Grades of Deep Reflexes

Grade	Description
Grade 0	Reflex cannot be elicited.
Grade −3	Reflex is absent except on reinforcement.
Grade −2	Reflex is markedly decreased.
Grade 1	Reflex is weak.
Grade N	Reflex is normal.
Grade +1	Reflex is slightly hyperactive.
Grade +2	Reflex is markedly increased and often associated with unsustained clonus.
Grade +3	Reflex is markedly increased and often associated with sustained clonus.

An excised rested muscle tests alkaline with litmus paper, while a fatigued muscle tests acid because muscle contraction consumes nutrients and oxygen and produces acids and is the body's major source of heat. Acids accumulating as a result of continued activity tend to contribute to fatigue.

Clinical Implications

Fatigue, weakness, nervousness, pain, tenderness, paralysis, sensory loss, paresthesia, and abnormalities of muscle mass or tone are the most common signs and symptoms noted in neural disorders. Fatigue, weakness, and nervousness are frequently presented together, and they can usually be attributed to functional disorders or appear as a complication in organic disease.[197] Fatigue may be the only early symptom in the myopathies.

Fatigue Spasm[198]

More neuromuscular energy is expended in human postural, locomotive, occupational, and recreational efforts than is expended in any other vertebrate. Fatigue therefore intrudes itself upon most clinical profiles. A characteristic of all erector muscles of the axial skeleton is that when they experience postural and stress fatigue, they go into a splinting-type painful spasm. When such a provoked muscle tires and goes into fatigue spasm as a compensatory necessity, the muscle becomes painful because the spasm impinges upon the neurotendinous and neuromuscular receptors, and trigger mechanisms are created.[199] This pain is usually asymmetrical and of a distorting, compressing nature.

If there is a pre-existing defect, the asymmetrical fatigue spasm may be the burden that triggers a subliminal situation into an acute syndrome or may become the provocative factor in a nagging chronic discomfort that is stubborn to relieve. On the other hand, muscles get stronger with use. The only time a used muscle gets chronically weaker is when its nutrition is absent or reduced. This can be the product of noxious neurologic reflexes of inhibition or the result of disuse.[200]

Painful Splinting

Striated muscles, especially the erectors, can readily go into a painful splinting spasm when fatigued. The result is overt muscular dysfunction. In time, trophic changes occur and tone is lost.

Muscle splinting is typically seen as active, often involuntary, muscle contraction that immobilizes the part. It differs from muscle spasm in that relaxation of the affected muscles occurs at rest. Prolonged pain from bone, muscle, tendon, and joint lesions with resultant long-term muscle splinting or pseudoparalysis may lead to eventual osteoporosis in affected and possibly adjacent bones. Joint contractures may also develop. This is another example, similar to a psychic conversion symptom, wherein a sensory symptom may lead to definite structural changes.

Joint Motion Reflections

Johnson emphasizes that the skilled use of palpation within a format of simple passive gross motion tests for evaluating the intensity and direction of asymmetrical regional response to motion (eg, cervical rotation) will uncover early signs of somatic dysfunction.[201] In total patient management, such signs will provide evidence of disturbed somatosomatic and viscerosomatic reflex activities. Thus, the examiner should be alert to possible postural problems within the soma so that major segmental dysfunctions may be analyzed. Johnson also shows that different examiners will be in basic agreement on their findings when such tests are carried out in a standardized, uniform manner.

Muscle Weakness[202]

Inequality in muscle balance may be initiated by trauma, postural distortion phenomena, biochemical reactions, psychomotor responses, paralytic effects, or somatic and visceral responses. Weakness in the absence of further symptoms or signs is indicative of an emotional problem (eg, depression). However, weakness may be the only symptom of an early systemic disease such as Guillain-Barré syndrome.

Symptoms and Signs

Weakness is characterized by feelings of lassitude, tiredness, weariness, depletion, exhaustion, malaise, and loss of energy and motivation. It may be general or local. If local, the weakness may be described in lower or upper extremities, either distal or proximal. It may be localized in the trunk or head, or in respiration. It is also important to analyze weakness in terms of body segments because weakness always follows a neuroanatomic distribution in organic disease. A rule of thumb is that proximal weakness is the result of a myopathy, while a distal weakness is caused by a neuropathy.

Trauma

Frank trauma may cause inflammation, degeneration, etc, and particularly the muscular splinting reaction that muscles produce when their surrounding tissues are injured. This alters the position and motion of the structural tissues that are related. Sustained microtrauma, though of a less acute nature, may cause a slow continual irritation and eventually create degenerative changes which similarly alter muscular reaction.

The obvious trauma of a fall or blow that surprises a joint with the intrinsic muscles unprepared will cause a joint sprain with ligament injury, and a sudden slip during a lift is equally damaging to the unprepared or weak joint. However, the slower trauma of occupational strain is not as easy to visualize. Holding a baseball bat at arm's length to the side for 2 minutes will cause the shoulder to ache within 1 minute; but the big "catch" will be at the lumbosacral level in the ensuing hours and days.[203]

Postural Distortion Phenomena

Postural compensations for either mechanical activity or structural changes in the skeleton itself are referred to as postural distortion phenomena. These changes, as well as other causes of subluxation, often result in a series or combination of minor mechanical errors in the spine which together may be termed scoliosis, kyphosis, lordosis, distortion, or a similar term.

Such a distortion phenomenon depends on the ability of the spine to adjust to any interference in the body's vestibular, visual, or proprioceptive adaptation that is incompatible with the normal balance of the musculoskeletal system to gravity. Whether this structural imbalance creates disturbances or appears asymptomatic depends on the neurologic irritation developing within the tissues affected. The structural imbalance may not elicit overt disturbance at a given time; rather, disturbances may appear at a later date when they overcome the adaptative resistance of the individual.

Psychomotor Responses

These reponses refer to the reaction of musculature to emotional effects on the nervous system as the body depicts its psychologic stresses. They may be environmentally, socially, or intrinsically initiated.[204]

Somatic and Visceral Responses

Disorders in the neuromusculoskeletal system may often be a factor in visceral disorders and disease, and various somatovisceral and viscerosomatic reflexes can frequently be related to specific disorders. Somatic and visceral reflex responses refer to those secondary reactions of the muscular system to somatic or visceral sensory irritation that may develop elsewhere in a given neurologic segment. Our embryologic nature is such that the various components of a given spinal segment and its ramifications or neuromere may be influenced by sensory stimuli that arise from any tissue supplied by these components.[205,206] A simple reflex cycle is shown in Figure 5.24.

The somatic or visceral sensory impulses that enter into a given neurologic segment may cause a similar response throughout the various ramifications of that segment.

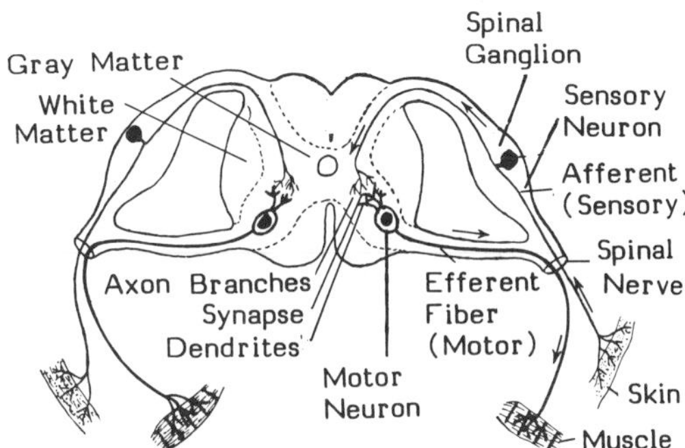

Figure 5.24. Cross section of the spinal cord with a pair of spinal nerves illustrating the relation of the neurons and the mechanism of a simple reflex cycle. *Arrows* indicate the path of a nerve impulse.

This, of course, depends upon certain states of sensitivity or facilitation, upon certain convergencies or divergencies within the nervous system, and particularly upon the intensity and duration of the initiating stimulation. Therefore, there could well be a visceral sensory irritation in the intestinal tract or other viscus that is causing motor changes not only in the internal organs, but also in the vascularity and the musculature of the body. These changes may result in motor alterations in the tone of muscles, consequently resulting in a spastic condition. If they are long-standing, degenerative changes, atony from atrophy, contractures, or other pathologic changes within the musculature may develop that can influence the mechanics of the vertebral or extravertebral segment(s) involved.[207]

When an average threshold stimulus is applied to a somatic receptor (eg, the skin), visceral function is influenced by way of the central connection in the gray matter of the spinal cord. If the sympathetic nervous system is involved, the activation occurs in the cells of the mediolateral column in the thoracolumbar area. Since the sympathetic axons terminate in the contractile mechanism of vascular smooth muscle fibers, the end result could be vasoconstriction.

Another factor should be considered. External pressure applied against the belly of a muscle activates primary afferents. For example, the elderly or weak often take unconscious advantage of this reflex by applying firm pressure on the ventral surface of their thighs when arising from a chair.

This increases the contractile force of the quadriceps and assists extension to the upright position.

Pathologic Weakness[208,209]

Primary disease of the neuromuscular system itself (eg, paralytic disease) affects musculoskeletal tone and strength, thus affecting position and quality of motion. Typical causes of pathologic muscle weakness and spasm are atrophy, muscle rupture, spastic paralysis, flaccid paralysis, myopathy, myasthenia gravis, periodic paralysis, root or nerve disease, upper and lower motor neuron syndromes, parkinsonism, and cerebellar disease. (See Table 5.3.)

Weakness Evaluated with Its Anatomic Origin

Weakness originating from a lesion at a particular anatomic site offers peculiar clinical findings. Six types of concern.[210]

Involvement of the Corticospinal Pathway. The stretch reflexes are hyperactive, and there is increased resistance to passive motion. There are abnormal reflexes and sensory perceptions. Weakness is usually more pronounced than atrophy.

Involvement of the Anterior Horn Cells. The stretch reflexes are absent or hypoactive. The weakness is generalized, but occasionally distal only. Weakness parallels the atrophy present.

Involvement of the Peripheral Nerves. The stretch reflexes are absent or hypoactive. Weakness is usually distal but sometimes generally distributed. Weakness parallels the atrophy present. Muscle fasciculations are sometimes seen. Paresthesia and sensory changes are usually present.

Involvement of the Myoneural Junction. Stretch reflexes are normal. Fatigue is greater than the weakness, and strength returns quickly with rest after exertion. Muscle fasciculations are rarely present. The disorder is usually seen first in the extraocular muscles, progressing in a variable, fluctuating course.

Involvement of the Muscle Fibers. Stretch reflexes are absent or hypoactive,

Table 5.3.
Common Causes of Neuromuscular Weakness and Paralysis

Site of involvement	Location	Clinical state
Upper motor neurons	Brain	Infarction Hemorrhage Neoplasm
	Brain stem	Infection Progressive pseudobulbar palsy Neoplasm
	Spinal cord	Demyelinating diseases Neoplasm Primary lateral sclerosis
Lower motor neurons	Brain stem	Progressive bulbar palsy Syringobulbia Poliomyelitis
	Spinal cord	Progressive muscular atrophy Syringomyelia Poliomyelitis
Nerve roots	Nerve roots	Intervertebral disc herniation Metabolic radiculopathies
Peripheral nerves	Peripheral nerves	Metabolic disorders Inflammatory disorders Trauma
Myoneural junction	Muscle	Myasthenia gravis Botulism
Muscle	Muscle	Polymyositis Muscular dystrophies

but the distal reflexes are usually normal. Weakness is proximal and parallels the atrophy present. Muscle fasciculations are rarely present.

Involvement of Function. Stretch reflexes are normal, and there are no muscle fasciculations or atrophy. Cogwheel responses and slowness of motion are present. There is a distinct overflow of activity and inconsistency in responses.

Weakness Evaluated by Its Site

The site of weakness may be symmetrical, asymmetrical, distal, or proximal in distribution.[211]

Symmetrical (Generalized) Weakness. This may result from a fault in the anterior horn cells, a fault at the myoneural junction, muscles, or may be of unknown origin.

Asymmetrical Weakness. This results from a fault in anterior horn cells, a fault in the peripheral nerves, a fault at the myoneural junction, muscles, or may be of unknown origin.

Essentially Distal Weakness. This condition results from a fault in the anterior horn cells, a fault in the peripheral nerves, a fault at the myoneural junction, muscles, or may be of unknown origin.

Essentially Proximal Weakness. This state results from a fault in anterior horn cells, a fault at the myoneural junction, muscles, or may be of unknown origin.

Types of Paralysis[212,213]

True paralysis is the complete inability to control a muscle or group of muscles. *Spastic paralysis* is commonly seen in lesions of upper motor neurons. *Flaccid paralysis* occurs in the peripheral type of nerve lesions affecting the lower motor neurons of the anterior horn cells. *Peripheral nerve paralyses* are especially apt to be accompanied by sensory symptoms, electrical changes, and wasting. *Brain-originating paralyses* have relatively few sensory symptoms (sometimes paresthesias) and relatively slight wasting, with mental changes, coma, or convulsions often preceding or following. *Cord paralyses* may or may not show these associations but are often accompanied by disorders of the bladder and rectum.

Muscle Injury[214–216]

Muscles are often injured by strain, contusion, laceration, indirect trauma, rupture, hernia, and occasionally by disease.

A muscle in traumatic or reflex spasm will become slightly inflamed. This may produce some transudation precipitation of fibrin, collagen, and mineral salt deposition, and, if extended, may result in a chronic myositis and myofibrosis. The myofascial planes usually become inflamed at the points of major stress, wherein transudation and fibrin formation produce myofascial plane adhesions.

Pain and Faulty Body Mechanics

Depending upon the constancy involved, postural and mechanical faults may cause severe pain in what appears to be mild postural defects or produce little or no pain in obvious cases of severe postural deficit. Minor postural deficits are often associated with considerable joint stiffness, and a quite faulty posture may be seen in a most flexible subject whose body positions change readily. Accumulative effects of constant or repeated small stresses over a long period can give rise to the same difficulties as severe sudden stress.[217]

Determination of the lesion site is often aided by noting the distribution of pain along the course of the involved nerve and the areas of cutaneous sensory disturbance. The pain may be localized below the site of involvement or it may be widespread as a result of referred or reflex pain.[218]

Excessive motor fiber stimulation results in pathologic, involuntary, and painful muscle spasm. This may be the result of toxic irritation of the anterior horn cells; encroachment irritation of the nerve root; irritation, stretching, or pressure upon a nerve trunk or plexus; irritation or pressure upon peripheral nerve branches; spasm secondary to trauma of an adjacent structure; primary spasm from direct irritation or trauma; or it may be of psychogenic origin.

Muscle and Tendon Strains

The general aspects of this subject have been discussed in Chapter 1. As mentioned, a strain is structural damage to a muscle or tendon resulting from overuse or excessive stretching, direct trauma, and/or overcontraction against resistance. It can involve anything from a minor irritation of muscle fibers to an actual separation of the tendon from the bone structure.

The exact cause of muscle fiber tears is unknown. Some feel that they are the result of technique error, some unknown circulating toxin, or a postural fault in which an activator muscle is jerked into action before the prime fixers are ready. Regardless of the cause, the mechanism appears to be a breakdown in coordination of the reflex inhibition necessary for synchronous contraction of antagonist muscle groups or a failure of the inverse myotatic reflex. For example, fatigue, weakness, and straining are known to cause a cortical bombardment of the spinal centers.[219]

The Stretch Reflex. It should be noted that the myotatic stretch reflex uses a single sensory neuron and is initiated by elongation of the muscle spindle's annulospiral receptors. The effect is a protective contraction designed to protect against further stretch so that the muscle may maintain a constant length. This reflex action is many times more severe if initiated by a sudden stretch (eg, dynamic thrust) than by a slow stretch. In addition, inhibitory impulses are transmitted to the motor neurons of the antagonists (reciprocal inhibition) and facilitating impulses are transmitted to the synergists—both of which enhance the physical response. The stretch reflex is not normally initiated by voluntary contraction. If there is spasm present after trauma, the irritating focus can usually be attributed to irritating ischemia initially and blood debris later.

The Inverse Myotatic Reflex. The more muscle fibers are passively stretched, the more powerful will be their contraction by the stretch reflex. However, this alert action by the low-threshold spindles is limited by the higher treshold Golgi tendon receptors that guard against an injurious reaction.[220] If a spastic muscle is stretched to the threshold of the Golgi tendon organs, the muscle will suddenly give way (clasp-knife reflex). This reflex restraint is termed *autogenic inhibition* and has an important therapeutic application in relaxing functionally spastic (splinting) muscles.[221]

Muscle Soreness and Stiffness

Muscle soreness may occur shortly after activity and pass quickly, or it may not appear until up to 48 hours after exercise and persist for several days. Stiffness, a sign of poor physical fitness in the weekend athlete or of unusual stress in the trained athlete, may be confused with minor strain, because both stiffness and strain produce pain due to increased intramuscular pressure. The stiffness syndrome features gradually increasing pain, swelling, and restricted motion.[222]

Most authorities today feel that stiffness is not due to the local accumulation of lactic acid. Rather, it is thought to result from the accumulation of extracellular muscle fluid due to increased capillary filtration pressure in an unconditioned muscle with a vascular bed that is unable to keep up with the necessary vascular return.[223] The dispersal of the accumulating extracellular fluid is also delayed because of the lack of lymphatics within voluntary muscle.

Muscle Cramps and Spasms[224,225]

Normally, many motor units rest while others are firing; but in the cramp phenomenon, all motor units fire and cause the spasm. Why this happens is not clear, but impaired fluid intake, electrolytic balance, and blood flow are often involved. Cramps are characterized by spontaneous prolonged, painful muscle contraction, usually occurring in voluntary weight-bearing flexor muscles. They often develop during sleep or soon after violent exertion and may vary from slight contractions to violent spasms.

Musculoskeletal disorders are frequently characterized by associated muscle cramps or spasms. These are powerful involuntary muscular contractions that shorten the flexor muscles and result in extreme, often incapacitating, pains stimulated by ischemia and hypoxia of muscle tissue. They are commonly associated with myositic, fibrositic, and articular disorders.

It has been estimated that 50–60% of the pains and discomforts that the average ambulatory patient has are the direct or indirect result of involuntary muscle contraction. Thus, the physician is compelled to consider the relationship of muscle contraction to pain symptoms in both diagnosis and therapy.

Neuromechanisms. Muscle spasm is an involuntary and aberrant contraction of a muscle part or whole as a result of some excessive motor fiber stimulation, such as irritation of (1) the anterior horn cells by the toxic elements of catabolic debris, accumulations consequent to faulty elimination, and circulatory disturbances; (2) an encroached nerve root from subluxation, paraforaminal congestion, herniated disc, and/or ligamentous thickening; (3) a nerve trunk or plexus, eg, piriformis, psoas major, scalenus anticus contraction; (4) peripheral nerve branches, eg, common peroneus by contracted tensor fascia lata, or occipital nerve by suboccipital spasm. Spasm may also occur as splinting secondary to injury as in sprain, avulsion fracture, and compression; within a muscle as the result of direct injury or irritation, often resulting from toxic accumulation, eg, toxic lumbago; or consequent to psychic stress.

Etiology. The primary causes of muscle spasm are postural and occupational fatigue, electrolyte imbalance, stress, trauma, derangement, emotional tension, psychic conversion syndromes, referred irritation from visceral involvements, and nerve root irritations associated with interosseous derangements.[226,227] When a synovial articulation is subjected to such stresses or toxic insult, the muscles that move the joint are reflexly provoked into spasm because of the irritation of the articular sensory bed. This spasm, often asymmetrical, will frequently force the joint into greater derangement or compression and thus set up the inimical phenomenon of circulus vitiosus. In cases of pathologic spasm, the patient's history may show that muscles in painful spasm may be relaxed at times if the muscles are provided a position of physiologic rest and an appropriate therapy is applied. Heat cramps are often caused by excessive salt loss. However, other factors may be involved such as muscle anoxia, cold, a blow or strain, or some yet unexplained reason. Violent exercise too soon after a meal increases the danger of active extremity cramps because much of the general circulation is diverted to the abdomen for absorption purposes. Hormonal factors may be involved in the female athlete, especially during the menstrual period. Cramps frequently follow drinking ice water or other cold drinks too quickly or in too large a quantity after exercise.[228]

Stretch Reflex Effects in Spasticity. A spastic resistance is essentially a stretch reflex activity whose receptors are the muscle spindles that are scattered in parallel with the muscle fibers. In common spasticity disorders, spastic muscles relax when the part is comfortably rested with support and become spastic with volitional movements, tendon tapping, vibration, or even startling noises. Three hypotheses have been put forward to explain the hyperactive stretch reflexes that occur in spasticity:[229]

1. Loss of corticospinal inhibition leaves the alpha motor neurons with a lower firing threshold so that they readily fire in response to any impinging sensory input, including that from stretch receptors.
2. A hyperactive gamma efferent system puts muscle spindles in a contracted state so that there is an abnormal response to stretch stimuli.
3. Spinal motor neurons normally exert a primarily inhibiting presynaptic modulating influence on afferent connections just proximal to the alpha motor neurons. Damage to or dysfunction of the corticospinal pathways weaken this influence so that afferent impulses from stretch or other sensory receptors are more likely to increase the firing rate of alpha motor neurons, even if the muscle spindles are not contracted.

Management. Relief can be provided biomechanically by passively stretching the affected muscle slowly with a sustained stretch within its normal range after intermittent cold applications, then applying firm pressure kneading. Leg spasms, invariably of the flexors, can be readily relieved by applying a strong active contraction in antagonist extensor muscles. The compressed spindles in the antagonists will evoke a reflex *reciprocal inhibition* of the affected spastic muscles (Fig. 5.25). Relaxation and warmth of the affected muscles usually offers further relief, and it sometimes helps to massage the spastic area toward the periphery.

In severe muscle tightness, cold is often

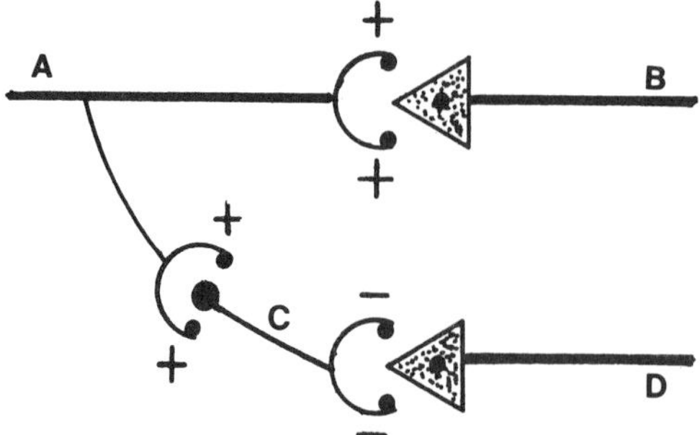

Figure 5.25. Simple inhibitory circuit in which a neuron, *A*, synapses with a motor neuron, *B*, and a short inhibitory interneuron, *C*. Although both synapses of *A* are excitatory, an inhibitory substance is secreted at the terminals of the interneuron synapse that prohibits motor neuron *D* from firing.

effective when combined with passive exercise. Have the patient flex or extend the limb against manual resistance in the direction of tightness and in the range where limitation occurs; follow this with voluntary relaxation. This should be done while cold applications are being applied. As the part begins to relax, the joint should be passively put through its normal range of motion. Probably one of the most effective adjunctive techniques is that of "spray and stretch" vapocoolant therapy.

Spasm can be treated by a number of therapies. Several authorities show how chiropractic adjustments, heat, cold, massage, isotonic exercise, and correction of systemic acidosis all tend to relieve spasm. They also explain how sustained manual pressure, meridian therapy, vibration, high-voltage current, interferential currents, transcutaneous electrical nerve stimulation (TENS), passive stretch, traction, joint manipulation, or inhibition of the gamma system by moderately increasing body temperature or by biofeedback will tend to reduce spasm and relieve the associated pain.[230–238]

After the most acute stage of pain has passed (usually after 48 hours), electrotherapy can be directed at relaxing muscle spasm. A tetanizing current is frequently recommended. High-voltage and interferential units appear to be best for this purpose, although several low-voltage modalities are often effective. The ideal situation, presently, is to alternately tetanize and then relax those muscle groups involved in an effort to break the spasm. After modulation of the pain has been achieved, therapy should be directed toward those procedures that relax muscle tissue and promote healing. Any modality that will produce controlled heat in specific muscle groups can be utilized.[239]

In stubbornly chronic states of spasticity, three innovative adjunctive therapies have been reported to be quite successful: (1) EMG biofeedback,[240–242] which returns pattern function through training; (2) acupuncture,[243–247] which appears to stimulate specific endorphins that function as natural (nonaddictive) opiates; (3) therapeutic distraction (tension) therapy, which is a form of manual traction or traction applied by certain braces.[248–252] Actually, the term *distraction* should not be used with manual tension-extension therapy because it is most unlikely that manual force would be sufficient to overcome the tensile strength of joint ligaments to the degree that an appreciable separation of joint surfaces would occur.

The incidence of cramps can be reduced by adequate warmup, salt, water, and protective clothing to prevent contusion. Muscle fatigue is frequently averted by sympathetic stimulation effecting an adrenaline reaction, as well as by correcting postural faults, neural and circulatory impairment, and actions which enhance respiratory efficiency.

Muscle Rupture[253–255]

A muscle action not balanced by reciprocal inhibition of the antagonistic muscle (eg, blow, unexpected force) may result in muscle rupture by sudden contraction or in a less common injury to its antagonist by overstretching. Muscles previously weakened by fatigue or disease are more apt to rupture. The asymptomatic ripple pattern (ladder muscle) seen in some athletes on passive stretch is not of traumatic origin but considered to be an effect of banding by overlying fascia.

If a complete tear occurs, the lesion is usually at the tendinous attachment to the muscle belly. Examination presents a locally spastic and tender muscle with swelling. Normal continuity is broken and quite obvious on palpation until obliterated by hemorrhage and swelling. Function is lost in proportion to the degree of tear. Direct evidence is gained by testing function with gravity eliminated. A bulge in a muscle's long axis on only vigorous contraction points to rupture.

In youth, muscle ruptures occur when a muscle is suddenly stressed beyond its tensile strength and the muscle fails. Such rupture is characterized by painful, knife-like, voluntary contraction followed by a sensation of extreme local weakness, ecchymosis at an area of local tenderness, swelling, edema, and hemorrhage. The onset is acute with searing pain that rapidly fades into a dull ache. Pain is increased on movement, especially against gravity. Weakness is not commonly associated. Contraction against resistance and passive stretching produce pain relative to the degree of hematoma. After the acute stage, persistent weakness remains and there is an increase in muscle bulk proximal to the rupture site upon contraction. In the late stage, extensive skin discoloration is common and often appears some distance from the site of injury. Subacute and/or chronic strains may result in myofascitis and/or myofibrositis.

In the elderly, muscle rupture occurs under minimal loads as a result of degeneration within the muscle's tendon. These ruptures are featured by less pain, swelling, tenderness, and ecchymosis; however, they do present the later persistent weakness and increased bulk upon contraction that is seen during youth.

Muscle Hernia, Dislocation, or Separation[253]

Complete muscle rupture is rare, but a split in a muscle sheath due to weakness or a break may allow the muscle tissue to herniate during contraction. It may follow injury or be a surgical complication. The sheath opening may be large or small. A soft mass is noted at the site of the opening during palpation that disappears when the muscle is contracted and reappears on relaxation. Weakness may be a complaint. Permanent correction can only be made by surgery.

In the event of trauma, the entire muscle or tendon may not tear loose or rupture. Most commonly, only a limited number of fasciculi are involved. This is known as *fascicular separation* and is commonly associated with "whiplash" cervical sprains and lumbar stress. In frequent sequelae, the structure is repaired with low-grade fibrosis and invaded by mineral salt deposits which interfere with normal function and mechanics.

Muscle Contractures[256]

Because of neural control, muscle fibers tend to adjust their lengths just long enough to produce the range of movement usually required. A muscle must be stretched and made to contract over the required range of movement if it is to retain its normal length. Contractures, highly resistant to passive stretching, result from fibrosis, circulation interference, tourniquet use, immobilization, or paralysis.

If during prolonged immobilization (eg, cast, support) a limb is flexed so that the muscles need only contract for a portion of the full range of motion, the muscles restricted will tend to adapt to this shortened length and later will be difficult to stretch to their original length (Fig. 5.26). The same effect of immobilization is seen in paralysis where unaffected antagonists draw the part into a shortened angle.

To prevent permanent contractures, the unparalyzed muscles must be passively stretched. During complete paralysis or in such conditions as the acute stage of poliomyelitis, disability will result if passive stretch is not used to reverse the effects of collagen depletion in ligaments, tendons, and joints.

Myalgia and Its Differential Diagnosis

Muscle pain has its peculiar characteristics. The pain that arises from an injury to muscle tissue may be elicited by making the muscle contract against resistance without allowing it to shorten; ie, preventing movement of adjacent joints. This test, although it may be of help in differentiating myalgia from the pain of other etiologies, is not absolute because it is not always possible, even with great care, to avoid some indirect pressure or tension on adjacent structures. In addition, pain that arises from a chronic contraction of muscle is not increased by contracting the muscle further.

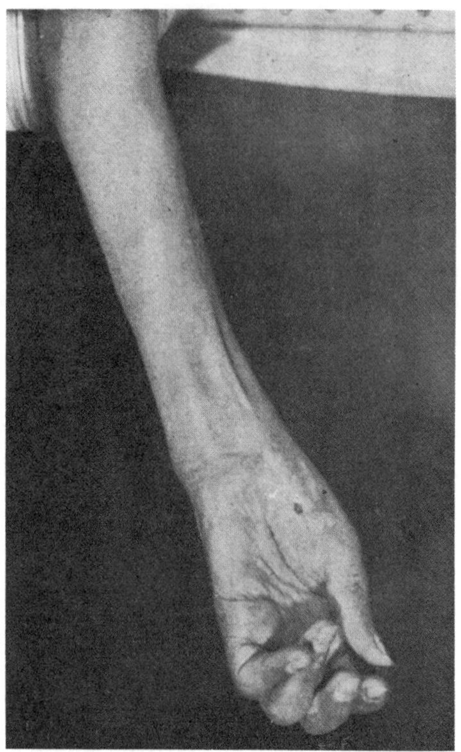

Figure 5.26. Volkmann's contracture: pronation and flexion of the hand with atrophy of forearm muscles, the result of circulatory impairment due to external pressure or radial artery damage.

Acute pain syndromes with a history of overexertion are often muscular in origin. This overexertion may be from (1) continuous contractions of long duration in a normal physiologic state, (2) vigorous jerky movements of short duration, or (3) a combination of stretch reflex and relaxation reactions if fibers have been stretched to an abnormal length. It has been shown that repeated stress can produce more soreness if a short rest interval is allowed between movements (eg, shoveling).

Myalgia

Pain that is due to sustained muscular contraction is ischemic in character. Lewis, a prominent researcher in the neurophysiology of pain, has shown that pain develops if exercise is carried out when local circulation is occluded; as soon as the circulatory flow is restored, the pain will disappear. Apparently, some "P" substance forms in the muscle and this is oxidized by the blood when the circulation to the area is restored. During sustained contraction, relative ischemia develops because, as a rule, blood flows freely only during relaxation. Sustained contraction impedes the blood flow so that P substances (amino-acid peptides) form and pain ensues. This is the probable explanation for the pain of myofibrositis in which some fibers are in a chronic state of contraction.[239]

Muscle Enlargement

Hypertrophy and spasm must be differentiated from the muscular enlargement that follows exercise. The increase in muscle bulk following exercise is caused by two factors: (1) the opening of capillaries during activity that are closed during rest; and (2) prolonged activity, which appears to increase the size of individual muscle fibers. This latter point is thought to be from an increase in sarcoplasm. A few authorities believe that even the quantity of myofibrils may increase during increased exercise over several weeks, although it has long been thought that the quantity of muscle fibers does not increase after birth.

Muscular Pain from Lymph Dysfunction

Pain of muscular origin is often a complex problem. Although skeletal muscle tissue lacks an intrinsic lymph supply, a muscle's connective-tissue sheath and tendons are richly endowed with lymphatic vessels. During the normal physiologic exchange of fluids through capillary walls, the quantity of fluid leaving the capillary is usually greater than that entering the venule. The related lymphatic network takes up this excess and eventually delivers it to the venous system. When normal, it is this process that allows a continuous exchange of tissue fluids and maintains a constant pressure of interstitial fluid.

The flow of lymph is increased during activity, as is capillary circulation, but this flow can be restricted by excessive pressure exerted by a constantly hypertonic or phasic contracted muscle. De Sterno shows that inhibited lymph drainage contributes to muscular pain during prolonged activity by (1) causing a buildup of interstitial fluids, which increases hydrostatic pressure, and (2) encouraging the accumulation of metabolic waste products that would normally be drained by the lymphatics and venules.[257]

Tendon Pain

Pain in damaged tendons usually arises when the attached muscle is contracted. The tendon fibers that are torn will usually not cause pain when the muscle is relaxed, but with the least muscle shortening, pain ensues. The pain of true tendonitis is often superficial, resulting from a tenosynovitis. It can be evoked by passively moving the tendon to and fro within its sheath.

Ligamentous Pain

Pain is elicited from irritable ligaments by stretching and deep pressure. Para-articular ligaments, and even deeper ones, can be stretched by passive movements of the related joint to the limit of the range of motion. When accessible to palpation, an irritated ligament will be tender; if it can be squeezed, pain will be evoked. For example, when inflamed interspinous ligaments are squeezed between palpating fingers, pain will be produced.

Trigger Points

A trigger point, sometimes called a myodysneuria, is a small, deep, hypersensitive area in a myofascial structure from which high-intensity impulses bombard the central nervous system and give rise to a deep-aching, sharply demarcated area of referred pain—in contrast to the ischemic compression nerve pain of prickling, tingling, and numbing that follows the segmental distribution of an entrapped peripheral nerve.

An irritable trigger point in or near a muscle is often a little-recognized cause of spasm and myofascial pain. Many cases of torticollis, shoulder pain, tennis elbow, substernal aches, lumbago, sciatica, hip pain, knee pain, and ankle pain can be traced to trigger-point mechanisms. Such conditions are frequently misdiagnosed as myalgia, myofascitis, nonarticular rheumatism, and sometimes as muscle strain or joint sprain. This is especially true when symptoms persist long after precipitating events.

Background[258-260]

Trigger areas may be produced by direct trauma to muscle or joint, chronic muscular stress, chilling of fatigued muscles, acute myositis, nerve root trauma, visceral ischemia or dyskinesia, arthritis, and hysteria. Long-term myofascial pain following activation of a trigger area is believed to be a reflex pain cycle sustained by the trigger area. The opposite is also true; ie, somatovisceral reflexes from trigger points may reinforce and perpetuate a visceral disorder such as ectopic cardiac rhythm, for one example.

A predisposing influence may be any factor that leads to chronic stress and fatigue. Nerve root compression, chronic visceral dysfunction, remote joint lesions, chronic infection, heavy alcohol consumption, a low metabolic rate with creatinuria, diminished serum potassium or calcium levels, diminished vitamin C or B levels, estrogen deficiency, and hypothyroidism are frequent factors that contribute to noxious feedback and perpetuate trigger points.

Impulse discharges from a trigger area may be related to vasoconstriction and other autonomic effects that are limited to a more or less predictable reference zone of pain. This is true for both visceral disease and the myofascial structures. One must distinguish between the site of pain (the reference zone) and the source of pain (the trigger area). Thus, it is important to differentiate true somatic pain from the somatic pain component of visceral pain. Although the somatic component of such pain syndromes may be relieved and indicated for this use, the visceral cause of the pain complex must never be overlooked by casual therapy for temporary relief of a trigger area.

Reference Zones[261,262]

Muscle pain exists in recognizable patterns in correspondence with a trigger point, but these pain patterns are often obscure or distant from the trigger point itself. That is, the site where the patient feels pain and the place where the pain originates are not usually the same. However, not all trigger areas are widely removed from their reference zones. The reference of pain may at times even circumscribe the trigger area. It may or may not follow the distribution of dermatomes, sclerotomes, peripheral nerves, or acupuncture meridians.

The referred pain is initiated or the site is found whenever the trigger site is stimulated by deep pressure, a small blunt probe, ultrasound, needling, extreme heat or cold, or stretching motions of the structure containing the trigger area. The resistance to stretching produces shortening of the affected muscle which limits motion and causes some weakness without atrophy. Trigger areas in myofascial structures can maintain pain cycles indefinitely; ie, the pain cycle may continue long after the precipitating cause has vanished because the mechanism that set the pain cycle in motion initially is not necessarily the same as that which keeps it going.

Common Sites[263, 264]

Trigger points are primarily found in the "stress sites" of the myofascial planes of the erector muscles, giving rise to a consistent distribution of referred pain which varies only slightly from person to person. This indicates that the impulses follow fixed pathways. These pathways are similar to those of visceral pain, which is referred in predictable patterns, but do not follow a simple segmental distribution. Once the pain reference pattern of a trigger point is known, it can be used to locate the muscle that is the source of the pain.

In time, a chain reaction is often seen in which satellite trigger points eventually develop. For example, scalene trigger points near the sternoclavicular junction, which refer pain to the upper chest and arm, are sometimes associated with satellites in the pectoralis minor or major. These in turn refer deep pain in the chest and medial arm, often leading to the incorrect assumption of angina or mastalgia (Fig. 5.27).

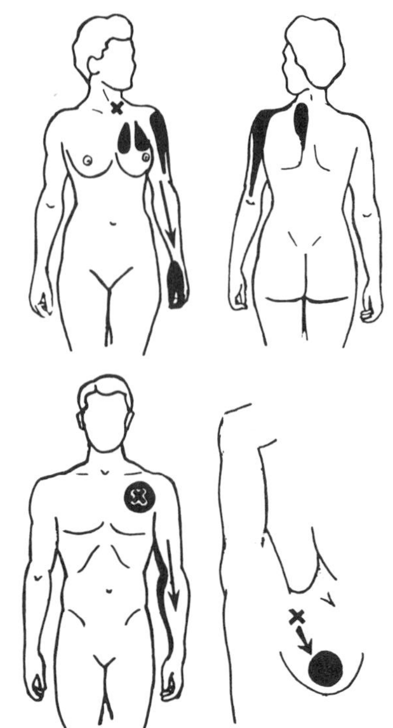

Figure 5.27. *Top, left* and *right*: scalene trigger point. *X*, common site. *Blackened areas* indicate typical sites of referred pain. *Bottom*, pectoralis minor trigger point shown on *left* and pectoralis major trigger point shown on *right*.

Nerve and Spinal Cord Lesions[265–267]

Any lesion producing an interruption of connections between the motor cortex or subcortical levels and the motor axons found in the anterior horn of the spinal cord is considered to be an upper motor neuron lesion. Such a lesion may interrupt corticospinal fibers or extrapyramidal fibers or both, since the pyramidal and extrapyramidal systems are so closely associated that lesions involving one will invariably encompass both. On the other hand, any damage to motor neurons whose axons reach skeletal muscle fibers produces a lower motor neuron lesion, whether the destruction is in the anterior horn, ventral roots, or peripheral nerves (See Table 5.4.)

Upper Motor Neuron Lesion Characteristics[268, 269]

Lesions of the upper motor neurons may occur anywhere along their course and may be the result of hemorrhage, thrombosis, trauma, inflammation, neoplasm, or a degenerative process. The classic clinical picture of an upper motor neuron lesion is portrayed as follows:

• Spastic type of paralysis or paresis on the opposite side of the body and below the level of the lesion if the lesion is at or above the medullary pyramid. Weakness is especially pronounced in the muscles of the limbs, and there is great difficulty with movements of the hands. Increased muscle

Table 5.4.
Differentiation of Upper and Lower Motor Neuron Lesions

Consideration	Upper motor neuron lesion	Lower motor neuron lesion
Site	Cerebral cortex or pyramidal tract	Anterior horn or peripheral motor neuron
Distribution	Diffuse or patchy	Segmental (number)
Reflexes		
Superficial	Absent	Absent
Deep	Exaggerated	Absent or hypotonic
Atrophy	Disuse, not prominent	Rapid extension, trophic
Trophic lesions	Minimal	Intense and extensive
Pathologic signs and reflexes	Present	Absent
Fasciculations	Not present	Present
Paralysis		
Type	Spastic and rigid	Flaccid
Location	Contralateral hemiparesis	Paresis limited to specific muscles

tone is expressed as firmness and stiffness, especially in the arm flexors and the leg extensors.

• There is minimal or no atrophy of the muscles involved, but there will be a later disuse atrophy. After a few days or a few weeks, stretch reflexes return in the involved muscles and usually become more active than usual. Muscle resistance to passive movements is exaggerated, often strong at the beginning of movement, then collapsing in a peculiar "clasp-knife" method as more force is applied.

• The superficial reflexes are abolished (Fig. 5.28). There is an increase of deep reflexes since the normal operation of gravity against the weight of the body may initiate stretch reflexes. Reflex contractions are exaggerated due to a loss of the inhibitory mechanism from the higher central level. The combination of this effect with contraction resulting from continuous discharge of brain stem excitatory mechanisms leads to a hypertonic state.

• The flexor nociceptive reflex and the Babinski sign can be observed. The nociceptive reflex evokes withdrawal of a body part by action of flexor muscles at one or several joints, depending on severity of stimulus, in response to injurious stimuli such as pricking, pinching, or burning. In a patient with a pyramidal tract lesion, the Babinski reflex is positive.

• No reaction of degeneration will be present in an upper motor neuron lesion. If the peripheral nerve resonds to electrical stimulation, it can be assumed that the lesion is in an upper motor neuron.

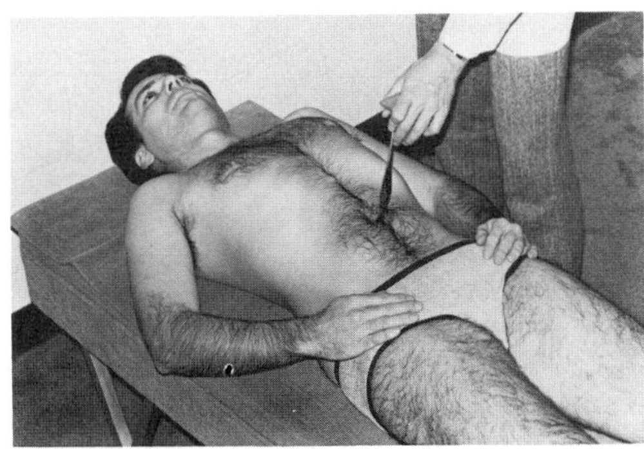

Figure 5.28. Testing the abdominal reflex. Contractions above the navel on sharp downward friction of the abdominal wall indicate normal activity of the spinal cord from the 5th to the 12th thoracic nerves. An absent reflex could indicate the following defective arc: upper quadrant reflex absent, T5–T8; midquadrant reflex absent, T9–T11; lower quadrant reflex absent, T11–T12; all sites diminished or absent, suspect upper motor neuron involvement. Abdominal reflexes are normally diminished or absent in the obese and the elderly.

Lower Motor Neuron Lesion Characteristics[268, 270]

Lesions of the lower motor neurons result from fractures, trauma, infection, toxins, vascular disorders, tumors, congenital malformation, and degenerative processes. Lesions involving spinal nerves or peripheral nerves induce both motor and sensory losses. In this type of lesion, the neuronal impulse from the upper central level or from the anterior gray horn of the spinal cord cannot reach the appropriate muscle fibers. The characteristic clinical picture is as follows:

- There is a loss of both superficial and deep reflexes. The stretch and tendon reflexes are abolished, thus producing a hypotonic state. No classic pathologic reflexes are present.
- Fibrillations and fasciculations are present only in the early stage during which muscles are undergoing atrophic changes.
- Flaccid paralysis is seen if there is no regeneration, the muscles involved eventually shrink and possibly are replaced by connective and adipose tissues. Muscle tone no longer exists because the peripheral nerve is unable to maintain it. The muscles become limp. Severe atrophy of muscles is observed within a few weeks (due to a lack of efferent impulses) that results in a degeneration of muscle fibers.
- Reaction of degeneration is seen from 10–14 days after the injury. The nerve is unable to conduct the electric current because of structural alterations.

Nerve Pinch and Stretch Syndromes[271]

Nerve "pinch" or "stretch" syndromes are often seen in trauma with the neck in flexion, but these syndromes can appear throughout the cranium, spine, pelvis, and extremities in many accidents. Hardly any peripheral nerve is exempt.

A *nerve stretch syndrome* is commonly associated with sprains, lateral cervical flexion with shoulder depression, or dislocations. Nerve fibers may be stretched, partially torn, or ruptured almost anywhere in the nervous system from the cord to peripheral nerve terminals.

A *nerve pinch syndrome* may be due to direct trauma, subluxation, a protruded disc which results in nerve compression, or fracture (callus formation and associated post-traumatic adhesions). Any telescoping, hyperflexion, hyperextension, or hyper-rotational force to the spine may result in a nerve "pinch" syndrome in which pain may be local or extend distally. Nerve pinch syndromes are less common than nerve stretch syndromes but more serious.

Nerve Fiber Degeneration and Regeneration Changes[272]

When a nerve fiber is destroyed by either disease or trauma, the part separated from the nerve cell body loses its myelin sheath and completely degenerates. The cell body is also affected in that the chromophilic substance of the cell body undergoes chromatolysis for several weeks in which extranuclear granules of RNA dissolve in the adjacent cytoplasm.

After injury, an injured peripheral nerve has some capability of repair. Schwann cells from the isolated strump proliferate in an attempt to bridge the gap to the severed axon. At the same time, the distal end of the axon begins to sprout in random directions. If some of these meet the proliferating stump of the isolated segment by chance, some twigs may enter neurolemmal tubes and lead to a peripheral sensory receptor or motor end plate, at a growth rate of 7–14 mm/week.

The Perplexing Reflexes[239]

The human body exhibits an astonishingly complex array of neural circuitry. Although the study of reflex communication between tissues under "voluntary" control and tissues under "autonomic" control (and their excitatory and inhibitory effect on one another) is still in its infancy, the answers to why so many visceral disorders mimic musculoskeletal disorders and why so many musculoskeletal disorders mimic visceral disorders appear to be on the horizon. Hypotheses are also being presented that help to explain the progressive reaction spread of some disorders that fail to respond to conventional therapies.

These reflexes can be classified into four broad categories: those communicating (1) from a site on the body wall, cranium, or limb to another site on the body wall, cranium, or limb (somatosomatic reflex); (2) from a site on the body wall, cranium, or limb (cutaneous, subcutaneous, musculoskeletal) to an internal organ or gland (somatovisceral reflex); (3) from an internal organ or gland to a site on the body wall, cranium, or limb (viscerosomatic reflex); and (4) from an internal organ or gland to another internal organ or gland (viscerovisceral reflex). It must also be kept in mind that these reflexes usually have segmental, propriospinal, and/or suprasegmental implications.

Inasmuch as many reflexes are modulated within the spinal cord, their potentional inter-relationship with a subluxation complex, and vice versa, cannot be ignored when we consider that a vertebral lesion can be a focus for either neuronal hyperexcitability or hypoexcitability. Thus all structures receiving efferent fibers via the IVF and all afferent fibers entering the IVF are potentially exposed to excessive stimulation or inhibition by some factor producing irritation, pressure, or tension at this vulnerable gateway.

Somatosomatic Reflexes

A somatosomatic reflex develops when a sensory receptor in the skin, subcutaneous tissue, fascia, striated muscle, tendon, ligament, or joint is stimulated to trigger a volley of reflex impulses to another anatomical location of this type via efferent sensory, motor, or autonomic fibers. Therapeutically, these reflexes are commonly evoked by gross manipulation, dynamic adjustments, light touch techniques, superficial heat or cold, electrotherapy, meridian therapy, hydrotherapy, traction, compression, vibration, percussion, and massage.

Somatovisceral Reflexes

A somatovisceral reflex develops when a sensory receptor in the skin, subcutaneous tissue, fascia, striated muscle, tendon, ligament, or joint is stimulated to trigger a volley of reflex impulses to viscera. Body wall stimulation produces both segmental organ responses and suprasegmental responses. Different forms of stimulation may produce similar organ responses and may produce different brain center responses affecting the body. The type of response, prolonged beyond stimulus termination, depends on the state of the organ and the body as a whole (ie, active, resting).[193] Therapeutically, these reflexes are commonly evoked by manipulation, superficial heat or cold, electrotherapy, meridian therapy (possibly, hydrotherapy, traction, compression, vibration, percussion, and massage.

Viscerosomatic Reflexes

A viscerosomatic reflex develops when a sensory receptor in an internal organ, a gland, or a vessel is stimulated to trigger a volley of reflex impulses to the skin, subcutaneous tissue, fascia, striated muscle, a tendon, a ligament, or a joint. It essentially operates through motor or sensory efferents (eg, the abdominal spasm overlying peritonitis, angina pectoris). Therapeutically, these reflexes are commonly evoked by spinal manipulation, spondylotherapy, spinal traction or compression, and biofeedback training.

Various researchers have attempted to show that visceral problems may refer to the skin or subcutaneous tissues and give rise to trigger points, acupuncture points, and/or other disorders.[273] Diagnostically, certain superficial areas have long been known to relate to an underlying visceral condition, such as pain in the right shoulder in gallbladder disease. It is often noted clinically that a disease in an internal organ will produce pain, tenderness, hyperesthesia, or hypesthesia, etc, in some area of skin. Such a viscerocutaneous reflex is thought by many to be mediated by unknown pathways of the sympathetic chain.

The Head-McKenzie sensory zone concept, as described by Judovich and Bates, shows how visceral pain can radiate to certain parts of the skin. A familiar example is cardiac ischemia with radiating pain to the left arm.[274] Wernoe found that a visceral problem can exhibit in a specific dermatomal segment via a viscerocutaneous reflex, and that the stimulation of the skin can have a distinct effect on a related visceral area via a cutaneovisceral reflex.[275]

Balduc points out that these reflexes are intensity-oriented (ie, the reflex response is proportional to the intensity of the visceral input), mediated by gamma fibers (excitation of flexor motor neurons, inhibition of extensor motor neurons), converge on the spine in a spatial gradient, converge on the head and neck or the pelvis, and produce both spinal and extraspinal effects. It is postulated that increased visceral activity influences a neurologic "gate" in the affected spinal cord segment. As the visceral gate opens, the somatic gate closes. The visceral impulses spread from the posterior to the anterior horn of the spinal cord and then to supraspinal centers that control the integrity of the reflex response, which is prolonged beyond stimulation termination.[193] The difference between somatovisceral and viscerosomatic reflexes appears to be only quantitative and to be accounted for by the lesser density of the nocicepetive receptors in the viscera.

Viscerovisceral Reflexes

A viscerovisceral reflex develops when a sensory receptor in an internal organ, gland, or vessel is stimulated to trigger a volley of reflex impulses to another anatomical location of this type via efferents of the autonomic nervous system. Rarely, however, does this reflex exist alone; ie, it usually has a segmental somatic component. Therapeutically, these reflexes are commonly evoked by spinal manipulation, deep heat, and hypnosis or other forms of psychotherapy.

Evaluating the Motor System[268, 276, 277]

Any sign of muscle weakness, atrophy, paralysis, or inco-ordination is significant. The muscular aspect of the motor system should be checked for tone, strength, and muscle volume, while nerve integrity is judged by the deep and superficial reflexes. Motor disorders may be caused by the same processes as sensory disturbances, such as by direct nerve injury, pathology, reflexes from visceral organs, and particularly nerve root involvement or upper motor neuron lesions.

Motor nerve root involvement is characterized by deep muscular pain in the muscles innervated. Early hypertonicity or muscular spasm is evident. Later or in chronic conditions, loss of tendon reflexes, muscular weakness, atrophy, and even trophic changes in the overlying skin may be present. Motor disturbances from upper motor lesions may also be a factor (hyper-reflexia). Abnormal reflexes, particularly if bilateral or similar in other reflexes, may be normal for a particular person. All signs must be correlated.

The extent of the symptomatology frequently offers a clue to the location of the disorder. In most chronic pyramidal tract lesions, especially when the trauma has been sudden but not insidious, a partial recovery of control is expected. This occurs mostly in the large proximal muscles of the shoulder and hip. Disorders of the pyramidal tract commonly produce defects that are more conspicuous in the upper limb. This is possibly because highly skilled movements are more prevalent there in comparison to mass contractions.

After nerve trauma, painstaking examination is required because multiple nerve injury, related tendon or other soft-tissue damage, and fractures may complicate the picture. The immediate site of injury would be first investigated, followed by the part's general appearance, voluntary motion, reflexes, and vasomotor changes. In addition to sensory and motor loss, the response to electric stimulation should be evaluated.

Muscle Testing[278, 279]

Muscle testing demands attention to detail and a good working knowledge of anatomy, muscle function, joint motion, muscle origin and insertion, muscle antagonistic and agonistic action, and their role in fixation. It is a procedure that depends greatly upon the skill, knowledge, and experience of the examiner.[280]

Many neuromuscular and musculoskeletal disorders show evidence of disturbed muscle tone such as weakness or spasm, but weakness is the predominating pattern found in muscle testing. This is often depicted as a compensatory hypertonicity in the antagonistic muscle. Both muscle testing and inspection may disclose a weakness in the absence of palpable or measurable atrophy. This type of muscle weakness that is relative to its antagonist is often associated with a palpable trigger point at the origin and/or insertion of affected muscles.

Muscle power should be evaluated when there is (1) a complaint of weakness or incoordination or (2) a need for an aid in subluxation analysis and in evaluating correction. The customary criteria for grading muscle strength are shown in Table 5.5.[281]

The development of tension against resistance is the most obvious property of muscle. The ability to develop tension and perform mechanical work is greatly affected by the length of the muscle at the moment of action. The two most common means to

Table 5.5.
Grades of Muscle Strength

Grade	Degree (title)	Description
Grade 5	100% (normal)	Complete range of motion against gravity with full resistance.
Grade 4	75% (good)	Complete range of motion against gravity with some resistance.
Grade 3	50% (fair)	Complete range of motion against gravity with no resistance.
Grade 2	25% (poor)	Complete range of motion against gravity eliminated.
Grade 1	10% (trace)	Evidence of slight contractility, but no joint motion.
Grade 0	0% (zero)	No evidence of contractility.

measure such tension are the maximum tension readout on a tensiometer (strain gauge) and the amount of load (eg, manual resistance) that can be moved.

Evaluating Strength Subjectively[282–284]

Astute gross observation, regional inspection, palpation, bilateral comparison, and correct positioning are essential before manual muscle testing is attempted to assure valid evaluation. When unilateral muscle weakness is suspected, it is always best to test the contralateral muscle first for resistance comparison. Pressure against action should be applied in a direction that is opposite to the line of the tested muscle's pull and at the distal aspect of the segment on which it inserts.

The "break" point in muscle testing, when the patient can no longer meet the resistance, is undoubtedly due to the Golgi tendon organ response. The loss of power is usually abrupt. This suggests that maximum strength depends a great deal on how efficiently an individual can cortically oppose the inhibition of his own Golgi tendon organ reflex.

The examiner should strive to evaluate one muscle at a time; thus the subject should be requested not to recruit allied muscles during resistance. The testing of individual muscles rather than muscle groups is essential in neuromuscular diagnosis and to determine the neurologic level. It is less important in gross biomechanical evaluation. In either case, extreme caution must be used during resistance to avoid creating cramps, stretch injuries, or excessive fatigue of the patient.

Common Pitfalls. The trouble with manual methods is that evaluation rests a great deal upon the subjective skill of the examiner, and some patients are more willing to exert maximum effort than others. Care must be taken that the direction and amount of pressure is controlled and consistent. The degree of strength can be determined only if pressure is applied *gradually* after the patient has "set" the muscle being tested against resistance. Also, the length of lever arms varies with patients and this affects relative strength, as does age, joint angle, bulk of body parts, and sex differences. Muscles often test difficulty in various positions such as prone, supine, and weight bearing. It also is important that the same examiner conduct and record initial and follow-up evaluations of the degree of "resistance."

Stabilization. To obtain maximum contraction, one segment (usually the site of origin) must be stabilized manually if not by muscle tension, body weight, or gravity, because a muscle exerts as much pull on its origin as it does on its insertion (Fig. 5.29). Poor stabilization results in erroneous conclusions.

Substitution. Possible substitution (eg, in dystrophy) and synergism must be eliminated by careful positioning and stabilization. If a muscle is called into action only in assistance when unusual force is necessary, it is referred to as an emergency mover or an accessory muscle. When the action of a muscle is to prevent the action of undesired contraction of another muscle, it is referred to as a neutralizing muscle. The action of emergency and neutralizing muscles must

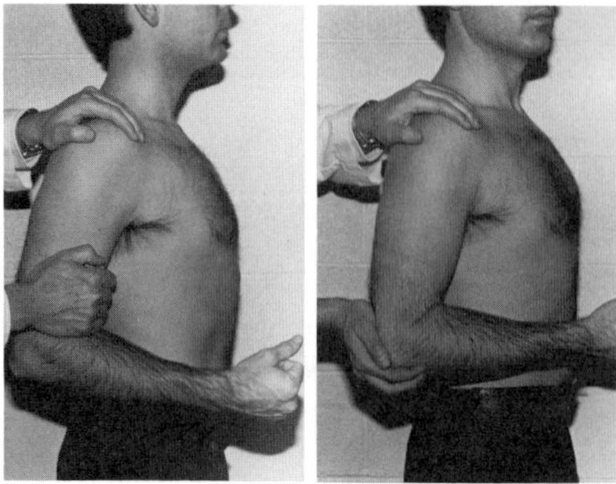

Figure 5.29. Testing the flexion (*left*) and extension (*right*) strength of the shoulder against resistance.

be carefully considered during clinical muscle testing to avoid erroneus conclusions. In addition, care must be taken that antagonistic muscles are relaxed.

Force vs Duration Factors. To determine whether it is the amount or the duration of the manual force, or both, that determines the examiner's perception of strength during muscle tests, Nicholas and associates designed an electromechanical device that was placed between the tester's hand and the patient's limb. The study measured the angular position of the limb during the test, the time interval during which the force was applied, and the force applied to the limb in 240 tests. It was found statistically that the impulse (ie, duration of examiner's effort multiplied by the average applied force) was the factor that most influenced the tester in determining the rating for patient muscle strength.[285]

Muscle Innervation. Another point to be considered is that several large muscles such as the pectoralis major, trapezius, deltoid, latissimus dorsi, triceps brachii, and quadriceps femoris are so constructed and innervated that portions of each muscle may function separately as well as together. The actions of different muscle parts may be palpated during function or recorded with greater accuracy by electromyography.

Evaluating Strength Objectively

The hand dynamometer and electromyograph are the typical objective clinical instruments available to record the force of muscular contraction.

The simple hand dynamometer gives the examiner four measurements: (1) strength of grip muscles, (2) fatigue rate of grip muscles, (3) recovery rate of these muscles, and (4) a bilateral comparison of the muscles of both hands. While initial readings are helpful in diagnosis, subsequent readings are helpful in determining the patient's rate of recovery. In dynamometry, three readings are usually taken on each hand in sequence to show strength, fatigue, and recovery rates.[286]

Electromyography is based on the fact that a relaxed muscle has (relatively) no associated electrical activity, while an active muscle has an action potential that can be measured by electrodes placed within or on the skin over a muscle (the latter is the usual practice). When the electrodes are connected to an oscilloscope, action potentials of muscles and specific parts of muscles may be viewed.

Spector feels that surface electromyography is one of the best means to assess the reliability of innovative as well as standard methods in the management of musculoskeletal disorders, thus decreasing the possibility of misdiagnosis and/or improper treatment.[287]

Electromyographic Feedback

Electromyographic feedback, used alone or in conjunction with other procedures, has attracted increasing interest in recent years as an adjunctive procedure in the care of many neuromusculoskeletal disorders. For example, Flor and associates treated patients suffering from chronic rheumatic back pain with EMG biofeedback, along with a control group, and showed that such therapy gave significant improvements in the duration, intensity, and severity of back pain complaints.[288] Kotses and Weiner evaluated the influence of home practice exercises on EMG levels after biofeedback training and found that participants who engaged in home practice exercises, regardless of their muscle training history, exhibited lower EMG levels during a no-feedback session than did individuals who did not practice their exercises at home.[289]

Such a technique has strong limitations, however. In comparing EMG feedback (auditory and visual display) with physical therapy for its relative effectiveness in training motor activity in hemiplegic patients, a study showed that while the feedback technique was effective in improving EMG activity it was not efficient in improving an active range of motion. In comparison, physical therapy (using tactile, proprioceptive, visual, and communicative modalities) enhanced a greater number of motor units.[290] It appears that EMG feedback works well for training individual muscles, reasonably well for muscle groups such as the knee or elbow extensors, but poorly for direct training of controlled limb movements that involve numerous muscles.[291]

Pressure Monitoring

A few years ago, Zatek Industries developed a small hand-held instrument called the Model 212 Pressure Monitor which is designed to measure resistive forces of 0–99.9 lbs and offers a digital readout display. A "Hold Peak" and "Memory Display" are also incorporated. In addition to the obvious purpose of objectively measuring the strength of active motion, it can be used to measure the response strength of tendon reflexes.[292]

Muscular Analysis during Gait[293–298]

After a muscle has been stretched, it is in its optimal state to offer maximum contraction force with a minimal energy cost. This is one of the advantages of the sustained backswing in throwing and batting.

Several muscle actions of the lower extremity offer excellent examples of contraction lengthening during gait. Most of these muscles are most active during the beginning and end of the stance and swing phases to accelerate and decelerate the angular moments of the lower extremities (Fig. 5.30). This point is important diagnostically, since it is at these periods of gait that specific muscular disorders will become most apparent. Activity is minimal during midstance and midswing, even though this is the period of most obvious movement.

Stance Actions. Immediately after heelstrike, the *gluteus maximus* is first elongated before its maximal contraction to assure the development of considerable tensile force to the hip. Also during early stance at a moderate speed, the *quadriceps* becomes elongated and active when the knee is flexed, to smooth flexion up to the point at which the center of mass moves anterior to the knee. During rapid gait, the quadriceps contracts to inhibit knee flexion and begin extension after toeoff.

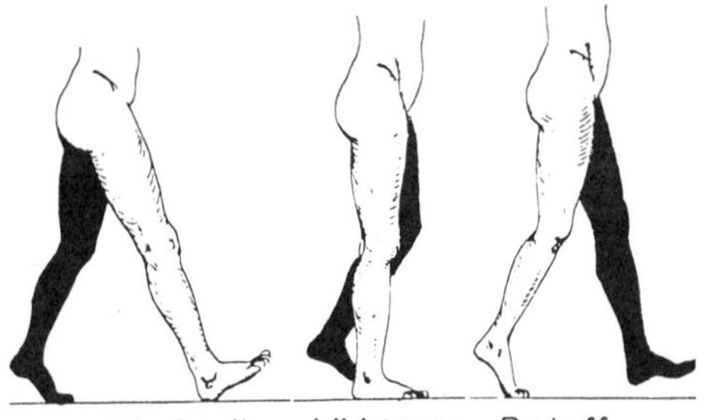

Figure 5.30. The heelstrike, midstance, and pushoff positions of gait.

During the stance phase, the *gluteus medius* and *minimus* (hip abductors) are in active lengthening contraction when the pelvis is drooping on the swing side and the femur is being slightly adducted. This helps to stabilize the pelvis. The *tibialis anterior* and *toe extensors* rest during midstance, but just after heelstrike they elongate and achieve their maximum contraction to dorsiflex the foot. At the end of stance, the *iliacus* is elongated as the hip extends and shortens as the swing phase begins to start hip flexion.

At the time of toeoff, there is slight action by the elongated *hamstrings*, which increases with walking speed, to increase knee flexion. The initially stretched *triceps surae* contract when the ankle is in 0° flexion, just long enough to achieve heel flexion.

Swing Actions. The *tensor fascia lata* contracts twice during a single cycle: (1) Its maximum contraction is when the swing phase is initiated, simultaneous with iliopsoas contraction, as an aid in hip flexion. At this point in gait, the band is elongated prior to activation. (2) It also contracts at the end of swing and at the start of stance. This is simultaneous with gluteus maximus contraction and resists posterior dislocation of the iliotibial tract where much of the gluteus maximus is inserted.

The *thigh adductors* are in a state of lengthening contraction at the beginning and during the end of the swing phase. At the end of the swing phase, the *hamstrings* become elongated and are active into early stance to aid hip extension by the gluteus maximus.

Importance of Normal Findings

In nerve, muscle, or gross static and dynamic analyses or any other diagnostic procedure, a clinician may use a normal finding to eliminate certain disorders during differential diagnosis. When properly interpreted, however, a normal value may also aid in differentiating among possible diagnoses that yield normal values with different frequencies of occurrence. Gorry and associates suggest a simple method by which the examiner estimates the probability of various diagnoses and combines these estimates with the anticipated frequency of negative results for each disorder under consideration.[299] Thus, from a clinical standpoint, and apart from the medicolegal factor involved, the recording and appraisal of a normal finding can be just as important as that of an abnormal finding.

Cortical Hemispheric Dominance[300, 301]

It is said that the brain (Fig. 5.31) has three levels corresponding to its evolutionary ancestry: (1) the brain stem from the reptilian period, (2) the limbic system from the mammalian level plus the cerebellum added to the brain stem, and (3) the higher cortex. The later levels are further divided into right and left hemispheres, and the whole brain has certain preferred communication paths. The brain stem is linked through the limbic levels to the cortex, and there are massive communication links between the two halves of the cortex.

The structurally ideal biped would be ambidextrous, but most people present a hemispheric dominance as expressed, for example, in right- or left-handedness, as well as in a dominant eye, ear, and foot. About 90% of the population has a genetically dominant right side that becomes firmly established about the age of 8 years. Attempts in maturity to acquire balanced bilateral motor activity interferes with normal speed, rhythm, and endurance.

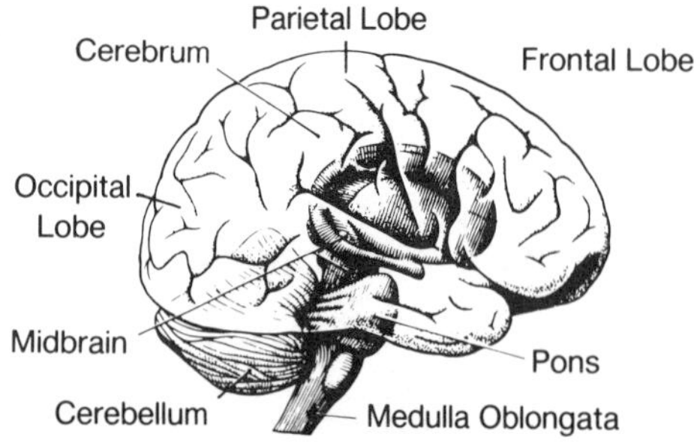

Figure 5.31. Lateral aspect of the brain.

Primary consciousness resides in the dominant hemisphere, and this side is responsible for such operations as logical thought, time-sequential analysis, categorizing, and speech. The nondominant side is responsible for such abilities as recognizing familiar people, places, and things; understanding maps and other abstractions; appreciating art and music; and perceiving holistic concepts.

The Reticular Activating System

Our ability to think, to perceive, and to respond to a stimulus with anything beyond a simple reflex is due to the cerebral cortex. But the cortex cannot function adequately unless it is aroused or awake, and the cortex cannot awaken itself from the sleep state. The *reticular activating system* (RAS), at the level of the brain stem, is extremely important in arousing the awareness level of the cerebral cortex (Fig. 5.32). Without it, consciousness is impossible.

In addition to arousing the cortex from a sleep state, the RAS monitors and regulates all muscular activity and sensory perceptions, switches on the cortex during sleep to produce vivid dreams, and inhibits the whole spinal cord to prevent sleepwalking. Stimulating some areas of the RAS with an electric current causes all muscular efforts and sensory perceptions to become exaggerated, as if the impulses themselves were stronger. Stimulating other areas of the RAS causes muscles and sensory perceptions to become weaker.

The cortex and the reticular system operate in a feedback mode in an attempt to maintain an optimum level of stimulation. Impulses reaching the cerebral cortex are fed back to the RAS. If the activity level becomes too high, the RAS sends inhibitory signals to the cortex to reduce the level of excitation, or vice versa if need be. It can thus be postulated that many spastic/anxi-

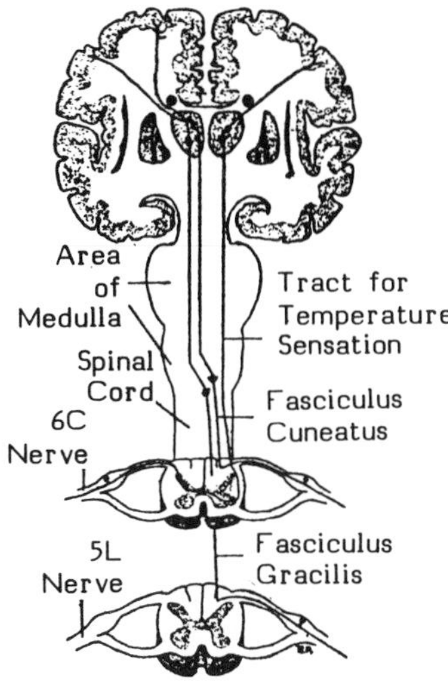

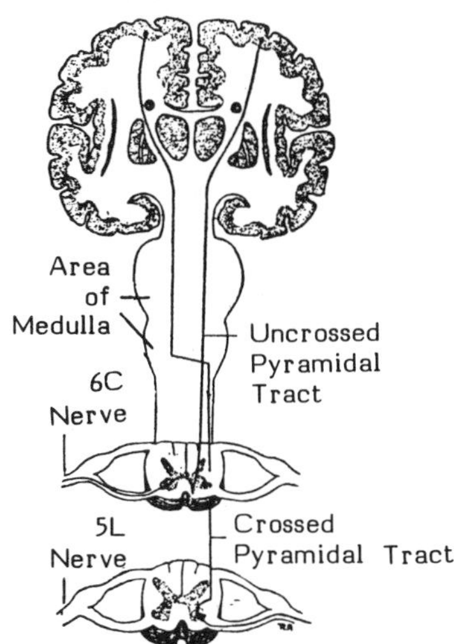

Figure 5.32. Schematic of the cerebral hemispheres and major tracts.

ety disorders or subtonic states can be attributed to a failure of the inhibitory or excitatory function of the RAS to maintain control within optimum levels.

Clinical Significance[302, 303]

When faced with stress (functional, physical, or emotional), it appears that the dominant hemisphere, via the RAS, delegates automatic chores to the less dominant and less competent side for temporary control. When the stress level is reduced, control is "switched back" to the finely organized dominant side. For some reason, this "switch back" may fail, and the result is abnormal neuromuscular effects. Frequently reversing requested directions, mirror writing, and other "switched" reactions are associated overt signs.

Unilateral neuromuscular disorders (eg, torticollis or low back pain) are frequently related to contralateral cerebral hemisphere dominance. Examination will invariably reveal specific muscle hypotonicity with contralateral hypertonicity. In such disorders, Goodheart notes that if the head of a supine patient is turned contralaterally toward the side of hypotonicity and the patient goes through the active motions of cross-crawling 10–12 times, a reduction in the tone of the spastic muscle will result. This effect can be reversed by having the patient move the arm and leg in unison on the side of hypertonicity, with the head again turned toward the weak muscle.

REFERENCES

1. Rosse C: Muscle action and its control. In Rosse C, Clawson DK (eds): *The Musculoskeletal System in Health and Disease*. Hagerstown, Md, Harper & Row, 1980, pp 57–59.
2. Morehouse LE, Cooper JM: *Kinesiology*. St. Louis, C.V. Mosby, 1950, pp 19–20.
3. Barham JN, Wooten EP: *Structural Kinesiology*. New York, Macmillan, 1973, pp 65–66.
4. Lay EM: The osteopathic management of temporomandibular joint dysfunction. In Gelb H (ed): *Clinical Management of Head, Neck and TMJ Pain and Dysfunction*. Philadelphia, W.B. Saunders, 1977, pp 514–519.
5. Gowitzke BA, Milner M: *Understanding the Scientific Basis of Human Movement*, ed 2. Baltimore, Williams & Wilkins, 1980, pp 85–93, 188–198.
6. Jokl P: Muscle. In Albright JA, Brand RA (eds): *The Scientific Basis of Orthopaedics*. New York, Appleton-Century-Crofts, 1979, pp 367–383.
7. Fowler WM Jr, Taylor RG: Differential diagnosis of muscle disease. In D'Ambrosia RD: *Musculoskeletal Disorders: Regional Examination and Differential Diagnosis*. Philadelphia, J.B. Lippincott, 1977, pp 93–95.
8. Basmajian JV: *Primary Anatomy*, ed 5. Baltimore, Williams & Wilkins, 1964.
9. Inman VT, Ralston HJ, Todd F: *Human Walking*. Baltimore, Williams & Wilkins, 1981, p 89.
10. Hollingshead WH, Jenkins DB: *Functional Anatomy of the Limbs and Back*. Philadelphia, W.B. Saunders, 1981, pp 15–16.
11. Gordon AM, Rosse C: Skeletal muscle. In Rosse C, Clawson DK (eds): *The Musculoskeletal System in Health and Disease*. Hagerstown, Md, Harper & Row, 1980, pp 33–39.
12. Morehouse LE, Cooper JM: *Kinesiology*. St. Louis, C.V. Mosby, 1950, pp 186–187.
13. Ishiko T: The organism and muscular work. In

Larson LA (ed): *Fitness, Health, and Work Capacity*. New York, Macmillan, 1974, p 59.
14. Williams JGP, Sperryn PN (eds): *Sports Medicine*, ed 2. Baltimore, Williams & Wilkins, 1976, p 293.
15. VanderWiel CJ, Hooker CW: Histology and biochemistry of muscle. In Wilson FC (ed): *The Musculoskeletal System: Basic Processes and Disorders*, ed 2. Philadelphia, J.B. Lippincott, 1983, pp 172–173.
16. Basmajian JV (ed): *Grant's Method of Anatomy*, ed 9. Baltimore, Williams & Wilkins, 1975, p 27.
17. Morehouse LE, Miller AT Jr: *Physiology of Exercise*. St. Louis, C.V. Mosby, 1948, pp 20–21.
18. Carlson FD, Wilkie DR: *Muscle Physiology*. Englewood Cliffs, NJ, Prentice-Hall, 1974.
19. Barham JN, Wooten EP: *Structural Kinesiology*. New York, Macmillan, 1973, pp 64–65.
20. Hollingshead WH, Jenkins DB: *Functional Anatomy of the Limbs and Back*. Philadelphia, W.B. Saunders, 1981, pp 17–19, 38–42.
21. Morehouse LE, Cooper JM: *Kinesiology*. St. Louis, C.V. Mosby, 1950, p 31.
22. Coers C, Woolf AL: *Innervation of Muscle*. Springfield, Ill, Charles C Thomas, 1959.
23. Basmajian JV (ed): *Grant's Method of Anatomy*, ed 9. Baltimore, Williams & Wilkins, 1975, pp 27–28.
24. Berthold CH: Morphology of normal peripheral axons. In Waxman SG (ed): *Physiology and Pathobiology of Axons*. New York, Raven Press, 1978.
25. Karvinen E, Komi PV: Neuromuscular performance. In Larson LA (ed): *Fitness, Health, and Work Capacity*. New York, Macmillan, 1974, pp 73–75.
26. Jokl P: Muscle. In Albright JA, Brand RA (eds): *The Scientific Basis of Orthopaedics*. New York, Appleton-Century-Crofts, 1979, p 382.
27. Gowitzke BA, Milner M: *Understanding the Scientific Basis of Human Movement*, ed. 2. Baltimore, Williams & Wilkins, 1980, pp 265–271.
28. Inman VT, Ralston HJ, Todd F: *Human Walking*. Baltimore, Williams & Wilkins, 1981, pp 89–92.
29. Hollingshead WH, Jenkins DB: *Functional Anatomy of the Limbs and Back*. Philadelphia, W.B. Saunders, 1981, pp 16–17, 42–45.
30. Huxley HE: The mechanism of muscular contraction. *Scientific American* 213(6):18, 1965.
31. Brash JC (ed): *Cunningham's Manual of Practical Anatomy*, ed 11. New York, Oxford University Press, 1948.
32. Gowitzke BA, Milner M: *Understanding the Scientific Basis of Human Movement*, ed 2. Baltimore, Williams & Wilkins, 1980, pp 198–211, 214–225.
33. Morehouse LE, Miller AT Jr: *Physiology of Exercise*. St. Louis, C.V. Mosby, 1948, p 18.
34. Moore KL: *Clinically Oriented Anatomy*. Baltimore, Williams & Wilkins, 1980, p 1xi.
35. Gordon AM, Rosse C: Skeletal muscle. In Rosse C, Clawson DK (eds): *The Musculoskeletal System in Health and Disease*. Hagerstown, Md, Harper & Row, 1980, pp 39–42.
36. Barham JN, Wooten EP: *Structural Kinesiology*. New York, Macmillan, 1973, pp 63–64.
37. VanderWiel CJ, Hooker CW: Histology and biochemistry of muscle. In Wilson FC (ed): *The Musculoskeletal System: Basic Processes and Disorders*, ed 2. Philadelphia, J.B. Lippincott, 1983, pp 174–175.
38. Ishiko T: The organism and muscular work. In Larson LA (ed): *Fitness, Health, and Work Capacity*. New York, Macmillan, 1974, p 57.
39. Prichard JW: Nerve. In Albright JA, Brand RA (eds): *The Scientific Basis of Orthopaedics*. New York, Appleton-Century-Crofts, 1979, pp 399–400.
40. Taylor RG, Fowler WM Jr: Electrodiagnosis of musculoskeletal disorders. In D'Ambrosia RD: *Musculoskeletal Disorders: Regional Examination and Differential Diagnosis*. Philadelphia, J.B. Lippincott, 1977, p 61.
41. Shambes GM: The influence of the muscle spindle on posture and movement. *Journal of the American Physical Therapy Association* 48:1094, 1968.
42. Jokl P: Muscle. In Albright JA, Brand RA (eds): *The Scientific Basis of Orthopaedics*. New York, Appleton-Century-Crofts, 1979, pp 380–381.
43. Karvonen MJ: Work and activity classifications. In Larson LA (ed): *Fitness, Health, and Work Capacity*. New York, Macmillan, 1974, p 43.
44. Walker SM, Schrodt GR: Contraction of skeletal muscle. *American Journal of Physical Medicine* 46:151, 1967.
45. MacDonald ML, Stanish WD: Neuromuscular system. In Scott WN, Nisonson B, Nicholas JA: *Principles of Sports Medicine*. Baltimore, Williams & Wilkins, 1984, pp 15–24.
46. Hill AV: The Design of Muscle. *British Medical Bulletin* 12:165–166, 1956.
47. Morehouse LE, Cooper JM: *Kinesiology*. St. Louis, C.V. Mosby, 1950, pp 196–198.
48. Gordon AM, Rosse C: Skeletal muscle. In Rosse C, Clawson DK (eds): *The Musculoskeletal System in Health and Disease*. Hagerstown, Md, Harper & Row, 1980, pp 47–48.
49. Gowitzke BA, Milner M: *Understanding the Scientific Basis of Human Movement*, ed 2. Baltimore, Williams & Wilkins, 1980, pp 97–99.
50. Morehouse LE, Miller AT Jr: *Physiology of Exercise*. St. Louis, C.V. Mosby, 1948, pp 23–24.
51. Gollnick PD, King DW: Energy release in the muscle cell. *Medical Science in Sports* 1:23, 1969.
52. Gibbs CL, Ricchiuti NV: Activation heat in muscle: Method of determination. *Science* 147:162, 1965.
53. Morehouse LE, Miller AT Jr: *Physiology of Exercise*. St. Louis, C.V. Mosby, 1948, pp 44–45.
54. Prichard JW: Nerve. In Albright JA, Brand RA (eds): *The Scientific Basis of Orthopaedics*. New York, Appleton-Century-Crofts, 1979, pp 388–390.
55. Clark RG: *Manter and Gatz's Essentials of Clinical Neuroanatomy and Neurophysiology*, ed 5. Philadelphia, F.A. Davis, 1975, pp 1–3, 10–12.
56. Daube JR, Sandok BA: *Medical Neurosciences*. Boston, Little, Brown, 1978, pp 48–51.
57. Eccles JC: The synapse. *Scientific American* 212(1):56, 1965.

58. Bullock TH: The neuron doctrine and electrophysiology. *Science* 129:17, 1959.
59. Mumenthaler M: *Neurology*. Chicago, Year Book Medical, 1977.
60. Jokl P: Muscle. In Albright JA, Brand RA (eds): *The Scientific Basis of Orthopaedics*. New York, Appleton-Century Crofts, 1979, pp 379–380.
61. Brazier MAB: *Electrical Activity of the Nervous System*, ed 4. Baltimore, Williams & Wilkins, 1977, pp 27–30.
62. Prichard JW: Nerve. In Albright JA, Brand RA (eds): *The Scientific Basis of Orthopaedics*. New York, Appleton-Century-Crofts, 1979, pp 396–399.
63. Curtis DR, Eccles JC: Synaptic action during and after repetitive stimulation. *Journal of Physiology (Cambridge)*, 150:374, 1960.
64. Gowitzke BA, Milner M: *Understanding the Scientific Basis of Human Movement*, ed 2. Baltimore, Williams & Wilkins, 1980, pp 225–239.
65. Hollingshead WH, Jenkins DB: *Functional Anatomy of the Limbs and Back*. Philadelphia, W.B. Saunders, 1981, pp 47–48.
66. Katz B: *Nerve, Muscle, and Synapse*. New York, McGraw-Hill, 1966.
67. McLennon H: *Synaptic Transmission*. Philadelphia, W.B. Saunders, 1963.
68. Daube JR, Sandok BA: *Medical Neurosciences*. Boston, Little, Brown, 1978, pp 82–86.
69. Brazier MAB: *Electrical Activity of the Nervous System*, ed 4. Baltimore, Williams & Wilkins, 1977, pp 75–90.
70. Taylor RG, Fowler WM Jr: Electrodiagnosis of musculoskeletal disorders. In D'Ambrosia RD: *Musculoskeletal Disorders: Regional Examination and Differential Diagnosis*. Philadelphia, J.B. Lippincott, 1977, pp 84–85.
71. Hall CD, Taft TN: Physiology of muscle. In Wilson FC (ed): *The Musculoskeletal System: Basic Processes and Disorders*, ed 2. Philadelphia, J.B. Lippincott, 1983, pp 185–187.
72. Kuffler SW, Nichols JG: *From Neuron to Brain*. Sunderland, Mass, Sinauer Associates, 1976.
73. Goodheart GL: *Collected Published Articles and Reprints*. Montpellier, Ohio, Williams County Publishing, 1969, pp 23–24.
74. Karpovich PV, Sinning WE: *Physiology of Muscular Activity*. Philadelphia, W.B. Saunders, 1971.
75. Roberts TDM: *The Neurophysiology of Postural Mechanisms*. New York, Plenum, 1967.
76. Daube JR, Sandok BA: *Medical Neurosciences*. Boston, Little, Brown, 1978, pp 308–311.
77. DeBacher G: Biofeedback in spasticity. In Basmajian JV (ed): *Biofeedback: Principles and Practice for Clinicians*. Baltimore, Williams & Wilkins, 1979, p 61.
78. Karvinen E, Komi PV: Neuromuscular performance. In Larson LA (ed): *Fitness, Health, and Work Capacity*. New York, Macmillan, 1974, pp 85–86.
79. Morehouse LE, Miller AT Jr: *Physiology of Exercise*. St. Louis, C.V. Mosby, 1948, p 30.
80. Clark RG: *Manter and Gatz's Essentials of Clinical Neuroanatomy and Neurophysiology*, ed 5. Philadelphia, F.A. Davis, 1975, pp 14–16.
81. Best CH, Taylor NB: *The Human Body*, ed 4. New York, Holt, Rinehart & Winston, 1963.
82. Rosse C: Muscle action and its control. In Rosse C, Clawson DK (eds): *The Musculoskeletal System in Health and Disease*. Hagerstown, Md, Harper & Row, 1980, p 75.
83. Inman VT, Ralston HJ, Todd F: *Human Walking*. Baltimore, Williams & Wilkins, 1981, p 100.
84. Morehouse LE, Miller AT Jr: *Physiology of Exercise*. St. Louis, C.V. Mosby, 1948, pp 37–38.
85. Guyton AC: *Textbook of Medical Physiology*, ed 3. Philadelphia, W.B. Saunders, 1966.
86. Morehouse LE, Miller AT Jr: *Physiology of Exercise*. St. Louis, C.V. Mosby, 1948, pp 35–37.
87. Clark RG: *Manter and Gatz's Essentials of Clinical Neuroanatomy and Neurophysiology*, ed 5. Philadelphia, F.A. Davis, 1975, p 15.
88. Hoyle G: How is muscle turned on and off? *Scientific American* 222(4):84, 1970.
89. Karvinen E, Komi PV: Neuromuscular performance. In Larson La (ed): *Fitness, Health, and Work Capacity*. New York, Macmillan, 1974, p 81.
90. Rosse C: Muscle action and its control. In Rosse C, Clawson DK (eds): *The Musculoskeletal System in Health and Disease*. Hagerstown, Md, Harper & Row, 1980, p 69.
91. Gowitzke BA, Milner M: *Understanding the Scientific Basis of Human Movement*, ed 2. Baltimore, Williams & Wilkins, 1980, pp 241–243, 250–254.
92. Karvinen E, Komi PV: Neuromuscular performance. In Larson LA (ed): *Fitness, Health, and Work Capacity*. New York, Macmillan, 1974, pp 81–83.
93. Patton HD et al: *Introduction to Basic Neurology*. Philadelphia, W.B. Saunders, 1976.
94. Chusid JG: *Correlative Neuroanatomy and Functional Neurology*, ed 17. Los Altos, Cal, Lange Medical Publications, 1979.
95. Clark RG: *Manter and Gatz's Essentials of Clinical Neuroanatomy and Neurophysiology*, ed 5. Philadelphia, F.A. Davis, 1975, p 147.
96. Rosse C: Muscle action and its control. In Rosse C, Clawson DK (eds): *The Musculoskeletal System in Health and Disease*. Hagerstown, Md, Harper & Row, 1980, p 70.
97. Clark RG: *Manter and Gatz's Essentials of Clinical Neuroanatomy and Neurophysiology*, ed 5. Philadelphia, F.A. Davis, 1975, pp 18–23.
98. Clark RG: *Manter and Gatz's Essentials of Clinical Neuroanatomy and Neurophysiology*, ed 5. Philadelphia, F.A. Davis, 1975, pp 160–166.
99. Rosse C: Muscle action and its control. In Rosse C, Clawson DK (eds): *The Musculoskeletal System in Health and Disease*. Hagerstown, Md, Harper & Row, 1980, p 73.
100. Clark RG: *Manter and Gatz's Essentials of Clinical Neuroanatomy and Neurophysiology*, ed 5. Philadelphia, F.A. Davis, 1975, pp 97–103.
101. Rosse C: Muscle action and its control. In Rosse C, Clawson DK (eds): *The Musculoskeletal System in Health and Disease*. Hagerstown, Md, Harper & Row, 1980, pp 73–74.
102. Clark RG: *Manter and Gatz's Essentials of Clinical Neuroanatomy and Neurophysiology*, ed 5. Philadelphia, F.A. Davis, 1975, pp 127–133.

103. Morton DJ, Fuller DD: *Human Locomotion and Body Form: A Study of Gravity and Man.* Baltimore, Williams & Wilkins, 1952.
104. Granit R: *The Basis of Motor Control.* New York, Academic Press, 1970.
105. Daube JR, Sandok BA: *Medical Neurosciences.* Boston, Little, Brown, 1978, pp 114–127.
106. Gowitzke BA, Milner M: *Understanding the Scientific Basis of Human Movement,* ed 2. Baltimore, Williams & Wilkins, 1980, pp 254–256, 257–265, 277–303.
107. Clark RG: *Manter and Gatz's Essentials of Clinical Neuroanatomy and Neurophysiology,* ed 5. Philadelphia, F.A. Davis, 1975, pp 31–34.
108. Davis H: Some principles of sensory receptor action. *Physiological Reviews* 41:391, 1961.
109. Adrian ED: Sensory mechanisms: Introduction. In Field J, Magoun HW (eds): *Handbook of Physiology.* Washington, DC, American Physiological Society, vol 1, 1959.
110. Knott M, Voss DE: *Proprioceptive Neuromuscular Facilitation.* New York, Harper & Row, 1968.
111. Everett NB: *Functional Neuroanatomy,* ed 6. Philadelphia, Lea & Febiger, 1971.
112. Adams RD, Victor M: *Principles of Neurology,* ed 2. New York, McGraw-Hill, 1981.
113. Hirschy LD: Utilization of TENS in conjunction with chiropractic methodology in the treatment of acute and chronic pain. *Ortho-Briefs, ACA Council on Orthopedics* April 1984, pp 23–29.
114. Guyton AC: *Medical Physiology,* ed 4. Philadelphia, W.B. Saunders, 1971, p 557.
115. Karvinen E, Komi PV: Neuromuscular performance. In Larson LA (ed): *Fitness, Health, and Work Capacity.* New York, Macmillan, 1974, pp 76–78.
116. Peele TL: *The Neuroanatomic Basis for Clinical Neurology,* ed 2. New York, McGraw-Hill, 1961.
117. Rosse C: Muscle action and its control. In Rosse C, Clawson DK (eds): *The Musculoskeletal System in Health and Disease.* Hagerstown, Md, Harper & Row, 1980, pp 61, 64–65.
118. Houk J, Hanneman E: Response of Golgi tendon organs to active contraction of the soleus muscle of the cat. *Journal of Neurophysiology* 30:466, 1967.
119. Clark RG: *Manter and Gatz's Essentials of Clinical Neuroanatomy and Neurophysiology,* ed 5. Philadelphia, F.A. Davis, 1975, p 16.
120. Gowtizke BA, Milner N: *Understanding the Scientific Basis of Human Movement,* ed 2. Baltimore, Williams & Wilkins, 1980, pp 303–306.
121. Wyke BD: Neurology of low back pain. In Jayson MIV (ed): *The Lumbar Spine and Back Pain,* ed 2. London, Pitman, 1980, p 265.
122. Wyke BD: Articular neurology and manipulative therapy. In *Aspects of Manipulative Therapy.* Proceedings of Multidisciplinary International Conference on Manipulative Therapy. Melbourne, Lincoln Institute of Health Sciences, Carlton, Victoria, August 1979, pp 67–72.
123. Dee R: Articular neurology. In Sokoloff L (ed): *The Joints and Synovial Fluid.* New York, Academic Press, 1978, p 177.
124. Gowitzke BA, Milner M: *Understanding the Scientific Basis of Human Movement,* ed 2. Baltimore, Williams & Wilkins, 1980, pp 306–308.
125. Granit R: *Receptors and Sensory Perception.* New Haven, Yale University Press, 1955.
126. Rose JE, Mountcastle VB: Touch and kinesthesis. Field J, Magoun HW (eds): *Handbook of Physiology.* Washington, DC, American Physiological Society, vol 1, 1959.
127. Clark RG: *Manter and Gatz's Essentials of Clinical Neuroanatomy and Neurophysiology,* ed 5. Philadelphia, F.A. Davis, 1975, pp 36–38.
128. Gowitzke BA, Milner M: *Understanding the Scientific Basis of Human Movement,* ed 2. Baltimore, Williams & Wilkins, 1980, pp 309–315.
129. Gernandt BE: Vestibular mechanisms. In Field J, Magoun HW (eds): *Handbook of Physiology.* Washington, DC, American Physiological Society, vol 1, 1959.
130. de Reuck AVS, Knight J (eds): *Myotactic, Kinesthetic, and Vestibular Mechanisms.* Ciba Foundation Symposium. Boston, Little, Brown, 1967.
131. Gowitzke BA, Milner M: *Understanding the Scientific Basis of Human Movement,* ed 2. Baltimore, Williams & Wilkins, 1980, pp 315–317.
132. Phillips RB: The irritable reflex mechanism. *ACA Journal of Chiropractic* January 1974.
133. Morehouse LE, Cooper JM: *Kinesiology.* St. Louis, C.V. Mosby, 1950, pp 134–138, 168, 295.
134. Morehouse LE, Miller AT Jr: *Physiology of Exercise.* St. Louis, C.V. Mosby, 1948, pp 36–37.
135. Fernie GR, Holliday PJ: Postural sway in amputees and normal subjects. *Journal of Bone and Joint Surgery* 60A:895–898, 1978.
136. Seliktar R et al: Dynamic features of standing and their correlation with neurological disorders. *Scandinavian Journal of Rehabilitation Medicine* 10:59–64, 1978.
137. Terekhov YV: Instrumentation for automatic measurement and real-time evaluation of man's postural equilibrium. *Journal of Medical Engineering* 2:182–186, 1978.
138. Hackett GS: *Ligament and Tendon Relaxation,* ed 3. Springfield, Ill, Charles C. Thomas, 1956.
139. Clarke HH: *The Application of Measurement to Health and Physical Education.* Englewood Cliffs, NJ, Prentice-Hall, 1945.
140. Morehouse LE, Rash PJ: *Sports Medicine for Trainers,* ed 2. Philadelphia, W.B. Saunders, 1963.
141. Hunsicker P: Human performance factors. In Larson LA (ed): *Fitness, Health, and Work Capacity.* New York, Macmillan, 1974, pp 350–352.
142. Knuttgen HG: Potentials for development. In Larson LA (ed): *Fitness, Health, and Work Capacity.* New York, Macmillan, 1974, pp 422–423.
143. Asmussen E: Muscular performance. In Rodahl K, Horvath SM (eds): *Muscle as a Tissue.* New York, McGraw-Hill, 1962.
144. Hebbelinck M, Ross WD: Body type and performance. In Larson LA (ed): *Fitness, Health, and Work Capacity.* New York, Macmillan, 1974, pp 266–267.
145. Craig TT: *Comments in Sports Medicine.* Chicago, American Medical Association, p 146.
146. Gowitzke BA, Milner M: *Understanding the Sci-*

entific Basis of Human Movement, ed 2. Baltimore, Williams & Wilkins, 1980, pp 94–95.
147. Singh M, Karpovich PV: Isotonic and isometric forces of forearm flexors and extensors. *Journal of Applied Physiology* 21:1435, 1966.
148. Schafer RC: *Chiropractic Management of Sports and Recreational Injuries*. Baltimore, Williams & Wilkins, 1982, p 102.
149. Simri U: Assessment procedures for human performance. In Larson LA (ed): *Fitness, Health, and Work Capacity*. New York, Macmillan, 1974, pp 364–365.
150. Williams JGP, Sperryn PN (eds): *Sports Medicine*, ed 2. Baltimore, Williams & Wilkins, 1976, pp 14–15.
151. Simri U: Assessment procedures for human performance. In Larson LA (ed): *Fitness, Health, and Work Capacity*. New York, Macmillan, 1974, pp 367–369.
152. Williams JGP, Sperryn PN (eds): *Sports Medicine*, ed 2. Baltimore, Williams & Wilkins, 1976, p 14.
153. Simri U: Assessment procedures for human performance. In Larson LA (ed): *Fitness, Health, and Work Capacity*. New York, Macmillan, 1974, pp 369–370.
154. Williams JGP, Sperryn PN (eds): *Sports Medicine*, ed 2. Baltimore, Williams & Wilkins, 1976, p 16.
155. Hall CD, Taft TN: Physiology of muscle. In Wilson FC (ed): *The Musculoskeletal System: Basic Processes and Disorders*, ed 2. Philadelphia, J.B. Lippincott, 1983, p 189.
156. Morehouse LE, Miller AT Jr: *Physiology of Exercise*. St. Louis, C.V. Mosby, 1948, pp 30, 32.
157. Guthrie-Smith, OF: *Rehabilitation, Re-education, and Remedial Exercises*. Baltimore, Williams & Wilkins 1943.
158. Schafer RC: *Chiropractic Management of Sports and Recreational Injuries*. Baltimore, Williams & Wilkins, 1982, p 106.
159. Ishiko T: The organism and muscular work. In Larson LA (ed): *Fitness, Health, and Work Capacity*. New York, Macmillan, 1974, pp 59, 62–63, 68–70.
160. Travers PR, Campbell WR: The organism and speed and power. In Larson LA (ed): *Fitness, Health, and Work Capacity*. New York, Macmillan, 1974, pp 99–101.
161. Knuttgen HG: Potentials for development. In Larson LA (ed): *Fitness, Health, and Work Capacity*. New York, Macmillan, 1974, pp 423–429.
162. Gordon AM, Rosse C: Skeletal muscle. In Rosse C, Clawson DK (eds): *The Musculoskeletal System in Health and Disease*. Hagerstown, Md, Harper & Row, 1980, p 54.
163. Muller EA: The regulation of muscular strength. *Journal of Association of Physical Medicine and Rehabilitation* 112:41, 1957.
164. Williams JGP, Sperryn PN (eds): *Sports Medicine*, ed 2. Baltimore, Williams & Wilkins, 1976, pp 65–66.
165. Craig TT: *Comments in Sports Medicine*. Chicago, American Medical Association, pp 146–148.
166. Knuttgen HG: Potentials for development. In Larson LA (ed): *Fitness, Health, and Work Capacity*. New York, Macmillan, 1974, pp 429–432.
167. Hunsicker P: Human performance factors. In Larson LA (ed): *Fitness, Health, and Work Capacity*. New York, Macmillan, 1974, p 352.
168. Williams JGP, Sperryn PN (eds): *Sports Medicine*, ed 2. Baltimore, Williams & Wilkins, 1976, pp 68–69.
169. Cerretelli P: Exercise and endurance. In Larson LA (ed): *Fitness, Health, and Work Capacity*. New York, Macmillan, 1974, pp 137–138.
170. Simri U: Assessment procedures for human performance. In Larson LA (ed): *Fitness, Health, and Work Capacity*. New York, Macmillan, 1974, p 370.
171. Schafer RC: *Chiropractic Management of Sports and Recreational Injuries*. Baltimore, Williams & Wilkins, 1982, p 103.
172. Williams JGP, Sperryn PN (eds): *Sports Medicine*, ed 2. Baltimore, Williams & Wilkins, 1976, pp 9–10.
173. Travers PR, Campbell WR: The organism and speed and power. In Larson LA (ed): *Fitness, Health, and Work Capacity*. New York, Macmillan, 1974, pp 105–106.
174. Gardner EM: Proprioceptive reflexes and their participation in motor skills. *Quest* 12:1, 1969.
175. Gowitzke BA, Milner M: *Understanding the Scientific Basis of Human Movement*, ed 2. Baltimore, Williams & Wilkins, 1980, pp 301–302, 308–309, 316–320.
176. Morehouse LE, Cooper JM: *Kinesiology*. St. Louis, C.V. Mosby, 1950, pp 207, 211–213.
177. Palmer ML, Toms JE: *Manual for Functional Training*. Philadelphia, F.A. Davis, 1980.
178. Schafer RC: *Chiropractic Management of Sports and Recreational Injuries*. Baltimore, Williams & Wilkins, 1982, p 104.
179. Gowitzke BA, Milner M: *Understanding the Scientific Basis of Human Movement*, ed 2. Baltimore, Williams & Wilkins, 1980, pp 106–109.
180. Gardner EB: The neurophysiological basis of motor learning: A review. *Journal of the American Physical Therapy Association* 47:1115, 1967.
181. Morehouse LE, Cooper JM: *Kinesiology*. St. Louis, C.V. Mosby, 1950, p 26.
182. Hollingshead WH, Jenkins DB: *Functional Anatomy of the Limbs and Back*. Philadelphia, W.B. Saunders, 1981, p 45.
183. Asmussen E: Development patterns in physical performance capacity. In Larson LA (ed): *Fitness, Health, and Work Capacity*. New York, Macmillan, 1974, pp 446–448.
184. Hebbelinck M, Ross WD: Body type and performance. In Larson LA (ed): *Fitness, Health, and Work Capacity*. New York, Macmillan, 1974, pp 277–280.
185. Williams JGP, Sperryn PN (eds): *Sports Medicine*, ed 2. Baltimore, Williams & Wilkins, 1976, pp 12–13.
186. Schafer RC: *Chiropractic Management of Sports and Recreational Injuries*. Baltimore, Williams & Wilkins, 1982, p 259.
187. Daube JR, Sandok BA: *Medical Neurosciences*. Boston, Little, Brown, 1978, p 168.
188. Jokl P: Muscle. In Albright JA, Brand RA (eds): *The Scientific Basis of Orthopaedics*. New York, Appleton-Century-Crofts, 1979, pp 374–375.
189. American Orthopaedic Association: *Manual of*

Orthopaedic Surgery. American Orthopaedic Association, 1972, pp 32–34.
190. Schafer RC: *Chiropractic Physical and Spinal Diagnosis*. Oklahoma City, Associated Chiropractic Academic Press, 1980, p IV-19.
191. Hall CD, Taft TN: Physiology of muscle. In Wilson FC (ed): *The Musculoskeletal System: Basic Processes and Disorders*, ed 2. Philadelphia, J.B. Lippincott, 1983, p 190.
192. Kuntz A: *The Autonomic Nervous System*. Philadelphia, Lea & Febiger, 1953.
193. Balduc HA: Overview of contemporary chiropractic science for the Chiropractic Association of Oklahoma. Convention notes. Northwestern College of Chiropractic, April 24, 1983.
194. Daube JR, Sandok BA: *Medical Neurosciences*. Boston, Little, Brown, 1978, p 190.
195. Walker HK: Deep tendon reflexes. In Walker HK, Hall WD, Hurst JW: *Clinical Methods*. Woburn, Mass, Butterworths, 1976, pp 832–839.
196. Schafer RC: *Chiropractic Management of Sports and Recreational Injuries*. Baltimore, Williams & Wilkins, 1982, p 112.
197. MacBryde CM, Blacklow RS: *Signs and Symptoms*, ed 5. Philadelphia, J.B. Lippincott, 1970, p 632.
198. Dorpat TL, Holmes TH: Mechanisms of skeletal muscle pain and fatigue. *Archives of Neurology and Psychiatry (AMA)* 74:528–540, December 1955.
199. Ufberg SH: Muscular nociception. *ACA Journal of Chiropractic* 14:93–96, September 1980.
200. Nelson W, personal correspondence, calling attention to the work of T.J. Bennett, 1980.
201. Johnson WI: Passive gross motion testing, parts I, II, and III. *Journal of the American Osteopathic Association* 81:298–303; 304–308; 309–13, 1982.
202. Heilman KM, Watson RT, Greer M: *Handbook for Differential Diagnosis of Neurologic Signs and Symptoms*. New York, Appleton-Century-Crofts, 1977, pp 17–20.
203. Watkins RJ: Monitoring subluxation inter-relationships. *Journal of Clinical Chiropractic* date unknown.
204. Borg G: Psychological aspects of physical activities. In Larson LA (ed): *Fitness, Health, and Work Capacity*. New York, Macmillan, 1974, pp 159–160.
205. Poole PB: Considerations of neurogenic pain. *Ortho-Briefs, Council on Chiropractic Orthopedics of the American Chiropractic Association* Fall 1982.
206. Sandoz R: Some reflex phenomena associated with spinal derangements and adjustments. *Annals of the Swiss Chiropractic Association* 7:45, 1981.
207. Sato A: The somatosympathetic reflexes. In Goldstein M (ed): *The Research Status of Spinal Manipulative Therapy*. NINCDS Monograph, No. 15, DHEW Publication No. (NIH) 76-998, Stock No. 017-049-00060-7, Washington, DC, U.S. Government Printing Office, 1975.
208. Adams RD (ed): *Diseases of Muscle*, ed 3. Hagerstown, Md, Harper & Row, 1975.
209. Schafer RC: *Chiropractic Physical and Spinal Diagnosis*. Oklahoma City, Associated Chiropractic Academic Press, 1980, pp IV-18–IV-19.
210. Fowler WM Jr, Taylor RG: Differential diagnosis of muscle disease. In D'Ambrosia RD: *Musculoskeletal Disorders: Regional Examination and Differential Diagnosis*. Philadelphia, J.B. Lippincott, 1977, p 103.
211. Fowler WM Jr, Taylor RG: Differential diagnosis of muscle disease. In D'Ambrosia RD: *Musculoskeletal Disorders: Regional Examination and Differential Diagnosis*. Philadelphia, J.B. Lippincott, 1977, p 118.
212. Clark RG: *Manter and Gatz's Essentials of Clinical Neuroanatomy and Neurophysiology*, ed 5. Philadelphia, F.A. Davis, 1975, pp 40–42.
213. Baker AB (ed): *Clinical Neurology*, ed 2. New York, Harper & Brothers, Hoeber Medical Division, 1962.
214. Kendall HO, Kendall FP, Boyton DA: *Posture and Pain*. Huntington, NY, Robert E. Krieger, 1977, pp 103–107.
215. Jacobson E: *Tension in Medicine*. Springfield, Ill, Charles C Thomas, 1967.
216. Joseph J: *Man's Posture: Electromyographic Studies*. Springfield, Ill, Charles C Thomas, 1960.
217. Pitkin HC, Pheasant HC: Sacroarthrogenetic tekalgia: A study of referred pain. *Journal of Bone and Joint Surgery*, vol 18, 1936.
218. Kellgren JH: Observations on referred pain arising from muscle. *Clinical Science* 3:175, 1938.
219. Schafer RC: *Chiropractic Management of Sports and Recreational Injuries*. Baltimore, Williams & Wilkins, 1982, p 244.
220. Wood KW: Myospasm, myosprain and myalgia. *The Digest of Chiropractic Economics* May/June 1985, pp 126–127.
221. Ng SY: Skeletal muscle spasm: Various methods to relieve it. *ACA Journal* 14:23, February 1980.
222. Morehouse LE, Miller AT Jr: *Physiology of Exercise*. St. Louis, C.V. Mosby, 1948, pp 32–33.
223. Williams JGP, Sperryn PN (eds): *Sports Medicine*, ed 2. Baltimore, Williams & Wilkins, 1976, p 301.
224. DeBacher G: Biofeedback in spasticity. In Basmajian JV (ed): *Biofeedback: Principles and Practice for Clinicians*. Baltimore, Williams & Wilkins, 1979, pp 61–62.
225. Andreoli G: Neurological implications of sports injuries. *New England Journal of Chiropractic* Winter 1979.
226. Kirkaldy-Willis WH: The pathology and pathogenesis of low back pain. In Kirkaldy-Willis WH (ed): *Managing Low Back Pain*. New York, Churchill Livingstone, 1983, p 24.
227. Bernie TS: The case for biofeedback as an integral part of chiropractic, Parts I, II, and III. *The Digest of Chiropractic Economics* September/October 1984, pp 69–70, 72, 130, 132; November/December 1984, pp 74, 76, 77, 79–80; January/February 1985, pp 32, 36.
228. Schafer RC: *Chiropractic Management of Sports and Recreational Injuries*. Baltimore, Williams & Wilkins, 1982, p 241.
229. DeBacher G: Biofeedback in spasticity. In Basmajian JV (ed): *Biofeedback: Principles and Practice for Clinicians*. Baltimore, Williams & Wilkins, 1979, p 61.
230. Ng SY: Skeletal muscle spasm: various methods

to relieve it. *ACA Journal of Chiropractic* 14:16–26, February 1980.
231. Karel L: The needle effect in the relief of myofascial pain. *Pain* 6:83–90, 1979.
232. Lowe JC: *Spasm*. Houston, McDowell Publishing, 1983, pp 83–118.
233. Mayer DJ, and Price DD: Central nervous system mechanisms of analgesia. *Pain* 2:279–404, 1976.
234. Melzack R, Stillwell DM, Fox EJ: Trigger points and acupuncture points for pain: correlations and implications. *Pain* 3:3–23, 1977.
235. Melzack R, Wall P: Pain mechanisms: A new theory. *Science* 150:971, 1975.
236. Wall PD: Gate control theory of pain mechanisms: A re-examination and restatement. *Brain* 101:1–18, 1978.
237. Siegele D: The gate control theory. *American Journal of Nursing* March 1974.
238. Sola AE: Myofascial trigger point therapy. *Medical Times* January 1982, pp 70–77.
239. Jaskoviack PA, Schafer RC: *Applied Physiotherapy*. Arlington, Va, American Chiropractic Association, to be published in 1986.
240. Baker M et al: Developing strategies for biofeedback: Applications in neurologically handicapped patients. *Physical Therapy* 57:402–408, 1977.
241. Basmajian JV, Regenos E, Baker M: Rehabilitating stroke patients with biofeedback. *Geriatrics* 32:85–88, 1977.
242. Brudny J et al: EMG feedback therapy: Review of treatment of 114 patients. *Archives of Physical Medicine and Rehabilitation* 57:55–61, 1976.
243. Ene EE, Odia GI: Effect of acupuncture on disorders of musculoskeletal system in Nigerians. *American Journal of Chinese Medicine* 11:106–111, 1983.
244. Hoang D: Acupuncture for paralysis due to stroke and multiple sclerosis. *American Journal of Acupuncture* 9:129–138, 1981.
245. Shibutani K, Kubal K: Similarities of prolonged pain relief produced by nerve block and acupuncture in patients with chronic pain. *Acupuncture and Electrotherapeutic Research* 4:9–16, 1979.
246. Yue S: Acupuncture for chronic back and neck pain. *Acupuncture and Electrotherapeutic Research* 3:323–324, 1978.
247. Wen HL: Acute central cervical spinal cord syndrome treated by acupuncture and electrical stimulation (AES). *Comparative Medicine East and West* 6:131–135, 1978.
248. Cox JM: *Low Back Pain*, ed 4. Baltimore, Williams & Wilkins, 1985, pp 196–199.
249. Markey LP: Markey distraction technique: New protocol for doctor and patient safety; a pragmatic approach. *Digest of Chiropractic Economics* July/August 1985, part I, pp 66, 68–69, 118.
250. Parry CBW: Stretching. In Basmajian JV (ed): *Manipulation, Traction, and Massage*, ed 3. Baltimore, Williams & Wilkins, 1985, pp 161–162.
251. Gonzna ER, Harrington IJ: *Biomechanics of Musculoskeletal Injury*. Baltimore, Williams & Wilkins, 1982, pp 170, 212, 217.
252. White AA III, Panjabi MM: *Clinical Biomechanics of the Spine*. Philadelphia, J.B. Lippincott, 1978, pp 353–354, 436–437.
253. Schafer RC: *Chiropractic Management of Sports and Recreational Injuries*. Baltimore, Williams & Wilkins, 1982, p 243.
254. Williams JGP, Sperryn PN (eds): *Sports Medicine*, ed 2. Baltimore, Williams & Wilkins, 1976, pp 294–295, 299–300.
255. American Orthopaedic Association: *Manual of Orthopaedic Surgery*. American Orthopaedic Association, 1972, p 34.
256. Salter RB: *Textbook of Disorders and Injuries of the Musculoskeletal System*. Baltimore, Williams & Wilkins, 1981, p 25.
257. De Sterno CV: The pathophysiology of TMJ dysfunction and related pain. In Gelb H (ed): *Clinical Management of Head, Neck and TMJ Pain*. Philadelphia, W.B. Saunders, 1977.
258. Wax M: Procedures in elimination of trigger points in myofascial pain syndromes. *ACA Journal of Chiropractic* October 1962.
259. Travell JG, Simons DG: *Myofascial Pain and Dysfunction: The Trigger Point Manual*. Baltimore, Williams & Wilkins, 1983, pp 5–37.
260. Gemmell HA: Myofascial pain syndrome. *Journal of the Chiropractic Association of Oklahoma* 3(3):10, 1984.
261. Schafer RC: *Chiropractic Management of Sports and Recreational Injuries*. Baltimore, Williams & Wilkins, 1982, p 256.
262. Berges PU: Myofascial pain syndromes. *Postgraduate Medicine* 53:161–168, 1973.
263. Brown BR: Diagnosis and therapy of common myofascial syndromes. *Journal of the American Medical Association* 239:646–648, 1978.
264. Cailliet R: *Soft Tissue Pain and Disability*. Philadelphia, F.A. Davis, 1980, pp 32–35.
265. Tran TA: Clinical correlations of the pyramidal system. *The Chirogram, LACC*, November 1976.
266. Heilman KM, Watson RT, Greer M: *Handbook for Differential Diagnosis of Neurologic Signs and Symptoms*. New York, Appleton-Century-Crofts, 1977, pp 21–22.
267. Haymaker W (ed): *Bing's Local Diagnosis in Neurological Diseases*, ed 14. St. Louis, C.V. Mosby, 1956.
268. Tran TA: The motor system: A general look at its components and their clinical correlation. *The Chirogram, LACC*, October 1976.
269. Taylor RG, Fowler WM Jr: Electrodiagnosis of musculoskeletal disorders. In D'Ambrosia RD: *Musculoskeletal Disorders: Regional Examination and Differential Diagnosis*. Philadelphia, J.B. Lippincott, 1977, pp 78–79.
270. Taylor RG, Fowler WM Jr: Electrodiagnosis of musculoskeletal disorders. In D'Ambrosia RD: *Musculoskeletal Disorders: Regional Examination and Differential Diagnosis*. Philadelphia, J.B. Lippincott, 1977, pp 79–80.
271. Craig TT: *Comments in Sports Medicine*. Chicago, American Medical Association, pp 22–23.
272. Prichard JW: Nerve. In Albright JA, Brand RA (eds): *The Scientific Basis of Orthopaedics*. New York, Appleton-Century-Crofts, 1979, pp 405–408.
273. De Sterno CV: The pathophysiology of TMJ dysfunction and related pain. In Gelb, H (ed): *Clinical Management of Head, Neck and TMJ Pain*

and Dysfunction. Philadelphia, W.B. Saunders, 1977.

274. Hart FD (ed): *The Treatment of Chronic Pain*. Philadelphia, F.A. Davis, 1974, p 8.
275. Gaensler EA: *Journal of Clinical Investigation* 30:406, 1951.
276. Hall CD, Greene WB: Disorders of Muscle. In Wilson FC (ed): *The Musculoskeletal System: Basic Processes and Disorders*, ed 2. Philadelphia, J.B. Lippincott, 1983, pp 194–195.
277. Herman RM et al (eds): *Neural Control of Locomotion*. New York, Plenum Press, 1976.
278. Daube JR, Sandok BA: *Medical Neurosciences*. Boston, Little, Brown, 1978, pp 188–190.
279. Walther DS: *Applied Kinesiology*. Pueblo, Col, Systems DC, 1981, 1981, vol 1, pp 244–246, 250–253.
280. Schafer RC: *Chiropractic Management of Sports and Recreational Injuries*. Baltimore, Williams & Wilkins, 1982, p 89.
281. Schafer RC: *Chiropractic Management of Sports and Recreational Injuries*. Baltimore, Williams & Wilkins, 1982, pp 89–90.
282. Daniels L, Worthingham C: *Muscle Testing*, ed 4. Philadelphia, W.B. Saunders, 1980, pp 3–6.
283. Kendall HO, Kendall FP, Wadsworth GE: *Muscles: Testing and Function*, ed 2. Baltimore, Williams & Wilkins, 1971, pp 3–10.
284. American Orthopaedic Association: *Manual of Orthopaedic Surgery*. American Orthopaedic Association, 1972, pp 27–31.
285. Nicholas JA et al: Factors influencing manual muscle tests in physical therapy. *Journal of Bone and Joint Surgery* 60A:186–190, 1978.
286. Kirby JD: *Essentials of Physical Diagnosis*. North Hollywood, Cal, Chiropractic Business Services, 1978, pp 25–26.
287. Spector B: Surface electromyography as a model for the development of standardized procedures and reliability testing. *Journal of Manipulative and Physiological Therapeutics* 2:214–222, 1979.
288. Flor H et al: Efficacy of EMG biofeedback, pseudotherapy, and conventional medical treatment for chronic rheumatic back pain. *Pain* 17:21–31, 1983.
289. Kotses H, Weiner H: Effects of home practice exercises on EMG activity subsequent to biofeedback training. *American Journal of Clinical Biofeedback* 5:103–109, 1982.
290. Mroczek N, Halpren D, McHugh R: Electromyographic feedback and physical therapy for neuromuscular retraining in hemiplegia. *Archives of Physical Medicine and Rehabilitation* 59:258–267, 1978.
291. DeBacher G: Biofeedback in spasticity. In Basmajian JV (ed): *Biofeedback: Principles and Practice for Clinicians*. Baltimore, Williams & Wilkins, 1979, p 62.
292. Laufenberg PC: New dimensions in neurologic evaluation. *The Digest of Chiropractic Economics* May/June 1979, pp 10–12, 105–106.
293. Inman VT, Ralston HJ, Todd F: *Human Walking*. Baltimore, Williams & Wilkins, 1981, pp 103–104, 116–117
294. Stolov WC: Normal and pathologic ambulation. In Rosse C, Clawson DK (eds): *The Musculoskeletal System in Health and Disease*. Hagerstown, Md, Harper & Row, 1980, pp 321–323.
295. Daniels L, Worthingham C: *Muscle Testing*, ed 4. Philadelphia, W.B. Saunders, 1980, pp 167–177.
296. Hoppenfeld S: *Physical Examination of the Spine and Extremities*. New York, Appleton-Century-Crofts, 1976, pp 133–141.
297. Eftman H: The function of muscles in locomotion. *American Journal of Physiology* 125:357, 1939.
298. Kelley DL: *Kinesiology: Fundamentals of Motion Descriptions*. Englewood Cliffs, NJ, Prentice-Hall, 1971.
299. Gorry GA, Pauker SG, Schwartz WB: The diagnostic importance of the normal finding. *New England Journal of Medicine* 298:486–489, 1978.
300. Goodheart GL: *Collected Published Articles and Reprints*. Montpellier, Ohio, Williams County Publishing, 1969, pp 28–30.
301. Morehouse LE, Cooper JM: *Kinesiology*. St. Louis, C.V. Mosby, 1950, pp 218–219.
302. Stoner F: *The Eclectic Approach to Chiropractic*. Las Vegas, FLS Publishing, 1975, pp 341–342.
303. Walther DS: *Applied Kinesiology*. Pueblo, Col, Systems DC, 1981, 1981, vol 1, pp 121–129.

SUGGESTED READINGS

Aarons MW et al: Applied kinesiology, pressure point, and pain control technics. Lombard, Ill, National College of Chiropractic, National-Lincoln School of Postgraduate Chiropractic Education, 1974.

Afifi AK, Bergmann RA: *Basic Neuroscience*. Baltimore, Urban & Schwarzenberg, 1980.

Ansari MS, Faruqui SR: Effects of nutrition on neurotransmitters. In Coyle BA, Martinez DP (eds): *Proceedings of the Second Conference on Current Topics in Chiropractic: Reviews of the Literature*, May 4–5, 1985. Sunnyvale, Cal, Palmer College of Chiropractic—West, 1985, section D4.

Bishop B: Pain: Its physiology and rationale for management. Part I, neuroanatomical substrate of pain. Part II, analgesic systems of the CNS. *Physical Therapy* 60:18–20; 21–23, 1980.

Dyson GHG: *Mechanics of Athletics*. London, Hodder and Stoughton, 1977.

Goss CM (ed): *Gray's Anatomy of the Human Body*, ed 29. Philadelphia, Lea & Febiger, 1973.

Hall MC: *The Locomotor System: Functional Anatomy*. Springfield, Ill, Charles C. Thomas, Publishers, 1965.

Jewett DL, Rayner MD: *Basic Concepts of Neuronal Function*. Boston, Little, Brown, 1983.

Keele CA, Smith R (eds): *The Assessment of Pain in Man and Animals*. London, Livingstone, 1962.

Knapik JJ, Ramos MU: Isokinetic and isometric torque relationships in the human body. *Archives of Physical Medicine and Rehabilitation* 61:64–67, 1980.

Noback CR, Demarest RJ: *The Nervous System: Introduction and Review*. New York, McGraw-Hill, 1972.

Noordenbos W: *Pain: Problems Pertaining to the Transmission of Nerve Impulses Which Give Rise to Pain*. New York, Elsevier, 1959, pp 95–96, 182.

Rosquist WLM: *Encyclopedia of the Spinal Touch Treatment*. Salt Lake City, German Therapology, 1975.

Schafer RC: *Symptomatology and Differential Diagnosis*.

Arlington, Va, American Chiropractic Association, to be published in 1986.

Schmorl G, Junghanns H: *The Human Spine in Health and Disease*, ed 2. New York, Grune & Stratton, 1971.

Scott MG: *Analysis of Human Motion: A Textbook in Kinesiology*. New York, Appleton-Century-Crofts, 1963.

Speransky AD: *A Basis for the Theory of Medicine*. New York, International Publishers, 1943.

Steindler A: *Kinesiology of the Human Body*. Springfield, Ill, Charles C Thomas, 1973.

Tran TA: Essentials of the neurological examination: Tests for cerebral function. *The Chirogram, LACC*, July 1975.

Wallis C: Unlocking pain's secrets. *Time* June 11, 1984, pp 58–66.

Ward LE: *The Dynamics of Spinal Stress*. Long Beach, Cal, SSS Press, 1980.

Wells KF, Luttgens K: *Kinesiology: Scientific Basis of Human Motion*. Philadelphia, W.B. Saunders, 1976.

Yamshon LJ, Bierman W: Kinesiologic electromyography. *Archives of Physical Medicine* 3:286–289, May 1949.

Part 2

CLINICAL BIOMECHANICS OF THE SPINE AND PELVIS

CHAPTER 6
General Spinal Biomechanics

CHAPTER 7
Basic Clinical Considerations in Treating the Neck and Back

CHAPTER 8
The Cervical Region

CHAPTER 9
Selected Clinical Problems of the Cervical Spine and Temporomandibular Joint

CHAPTER 10
The Thoracic Region and Related Clinical Problems

CHAPTER 11
The Lumbar Spine and Pelvis

CHAPTER 12
Selected Disorders of the Lumbar Spine and Pelvis

CHAPTER 13
Scoliosis

CHAPTER 6

General Spinal Biomechanics

This chapter discusses the vertebral column as a whole and serves as a foundation for the following chapters that consider the regional aspects of the spine and pelvis. Emphasis here is on gross structure, function, spinal kinematics, and other general biomechanical implications.

BACKGROUND

The vertebral column is a mechanical marvel in that it must afford both rigidity and flexibility.

The Spine as a Whole[1-5]

The segmental design of the vertebral column allows adequate motion among the head, trunk, and pelvis; affords protection of the spinal cord; transfers weight forces and bending moments of the upper body to the pelvis; offers a shock-absorbing apparatus; and serves as a pivot for the head. Without stabilization from the spine, the head and upper limbs could not move evenly or smoothly, or support the loads imposed upon them (Fig. 6.1).

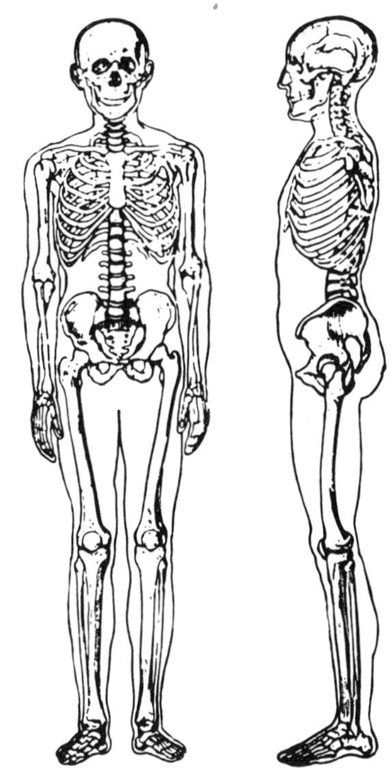

Figure 6.1. The relationship of the spine to total body habitus.

Essentially because of its various adult curvatures, the bony spine is anatomically divided into the 7 cervical vertebrae, the 12 thoracic vertebrae, the 5 lumbar vertebrae, and the ossified 5 sacral and 4 coccygeal segments. From C1 to S1, the articulating parts of these vertebrae are the vertebral bodies, which are separated by intervertebral discs (IVDs) and the posterior facet joints. The IVDs tend to be static weight-bearing joints, while the facets function as dynamic sliding and gliding joints.

Weight Distribution

The flexible vertebral column is balanced upon its base, the sacrum. In the erect position, weight is transferred across the sacroiliac joints to the ilia, then to the hips, and then to the lower extremities. In the sitting position, weight is transferred from the sacroiliac joints to the ilia, and then to the ischial tuberosities.

Spinal Length

About 75% of spinal length is contributed by the vertebral bodies, while 25% of its length is composed of disc material.[6] The contribution by the discs, however, is not spread evenly throughout the spine. About 20% of cervical and thoracic length is from disc height, while approximately 30% of lumbar length is from disc height. In all regions, the contribution by the discs diminishes with age.

Topographic Landmarks[7-10]

The approximately topographic landmarks in relation to the anatomy of the vertebral column and pelvis are as follows:

Inion: Prominence, midline of occipital base
C1: About ½ inch inferior and slightly anterior of the mastoid process
C2: First prominent spinous process below the inion
C4: Hyoid bone
C6: Cricoid cartilage
C7: Second prominent spinous process below the inion
T1: Most prominent spinous process in the region
T2: Jugular notch
T5: Angle of Louis
T7: Inferior angle of the scapula, third prominent spinous process below the inion
T10: Xiphoid process
L1: Transpyloric plane
L3: Umbilicus
L4: Iliac crests
L5: Transtubular plane
S2: Level with posterior-superior iliac spines (PSISs)
Sciatic notch: about 2 inches inferior and 1 inch lateral to the PSIS
Ischial tuberosity: about 2 inches inferior to apex of coccyx, on a vertical line through the PSIS

Development of the Spine[11–15]

In brief, development occurs in three stages: mesenchymal, chondrification, and ossification.

Mesenchymal and Chondrification Origins

Just prior to the 4th week of embryonic development, a vertebral segment begins to develop as paired condensations of mesenchyme (somites) around the longitudinal notochord and dorsal neural tube. One or usually two chondrification centers appear (6 weeks) in the centrum and begin to form a cartilaginous model surrounded by anterior and posterior longitudinal ligaments which are complete by 7–8 weeks. Chondrification centers also form in the neural arches and costal processes. A thick ring of nonchrondrous cells establishes the model IVD around the longitudinal string of beaded notochordal segments (Fig. 6.2).

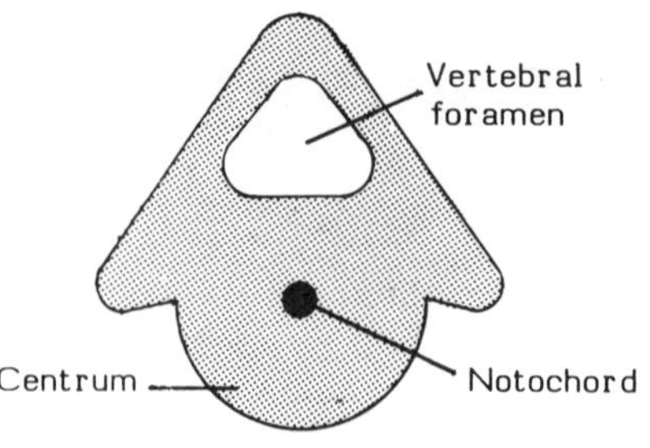

Vertebral arch
Costal process
CHONDRIFICATION STAGE

Figure 6.2. Schematic illustrations of the mesenchymal and chondrification stages of vertebral development.

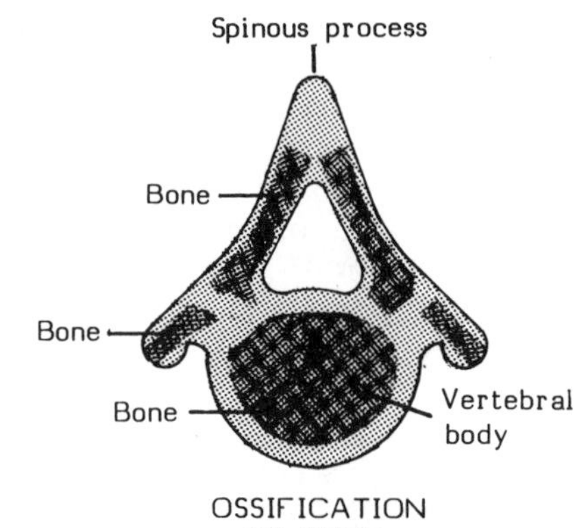

Figure 6.3. The early stages of vertebral ossification.

Ossification

A vertebra at term is in three primary ossifying centers: the oval centrum and the two aspects of the neural arch. However, the ossification process is well under way by the 16th week of gestation. Each of the three parts are united by hyaline cartilage. A cartilaginous ring develops around the anterior and lateral periphery of the centrum-disc interface, which firmly anchors the anulus to the centrum (Fig. 6.3). The two halves of the arch ossify posteriorly by appositional growth, during the first year in the cervical region, with complete ossification in the lumbar region by the age of 8 years. The progression is from above downward. The centrum, which ossifies endochrondrally, joins the arch during the 3rd to the 6th year in the lumbar area and firmly fuses between the 5th and 8th year in the cervical region. In contrast, the progression is from below upward. During development, the superior and inferior cortex of the centrum thickens in the middle, and, with a cartilaginous plate that is thicker at the periphery, forms the vertebral plateau.

Secondary Epiphyses

Scale-like traction epiphyses on the tips of the spinous and transverse processes and ring-like pressure epiphyses on the superior and inferior aspects of the vertebral body appear obvious shortly after puberty (age 13–16 years) and fuse prior to the age of 25 years to form a thickened periphery (Fig. 6.4). When ossified, this ring receives Sharpey's fibers of a disc's anulus laminations. Abnormal ossification leads to Scheuermann's disease.

Normal Spinal Movements[16–18]

Planes of Motion

Normal movements of a vertebral segment relative to its supporting structure below may be described in accordance with its ability to laterally flex on the coronal plane, rotate on the transverse plane, and anteroflex and retroextend on the sagittal plane (Fig. 6.5). To some degree, all vertebrae are able to function in all three dimensions; however, the magnitude of such movements varies to some degree in the different regions as well as in the transitional areas.

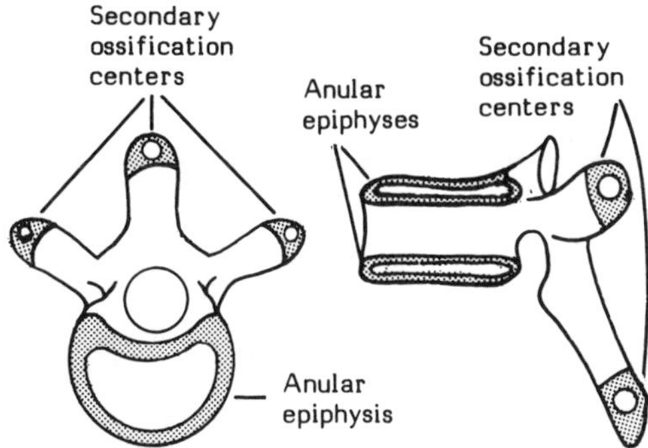

Figure 6.4. Anular and secondary vertebral ossification centers.

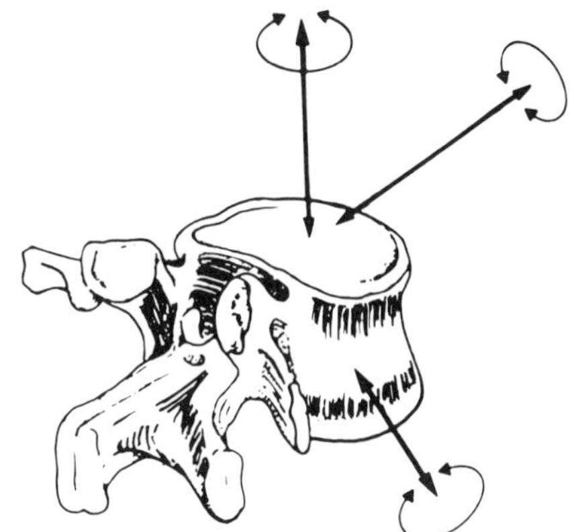

Figure 6.5. The six degrees of freedom involved in spinal kinematics.

As the spine is normally curved in its A-P aspect, few spinal motion units move on a horizontal plane because few discs are parallel to the ground. Horizontal motion occurs only at the centers of the curves such as near the C5, T6, and L3 disc areas (Fig. 6.6).

Extent of Motion

In the A-P direction, male mobility usually exceeds female mobility. On the other hand, female mobility usually exceeds male mobility in lateral flexion.

Spinal motion between vertebrae takes place essentially at the fibrocartilaginous IVD and the zygapophyseal joints formed by the inferior facets of the superior vertebra and the superior facets of the inferior vertebra. Movement is also governed by the flexibility of the disc and the slope of the articulating facets. All spinal motions require free gliding of the articular facets. While motion of any one vertebra is quite minimal, the sum motion of the 24 vertebral segments is considerable.

The IVDs are relatively large in the cervical area in comparison to the size of their bodies. The inferior cervical bodies are concave and the superior bodies are convex in their A-P and lateral aspects to allow overlapping during quite free flexion, extension, and lateral bending. In the thoracic area, the IVDs are relatively smaller, flatter, and

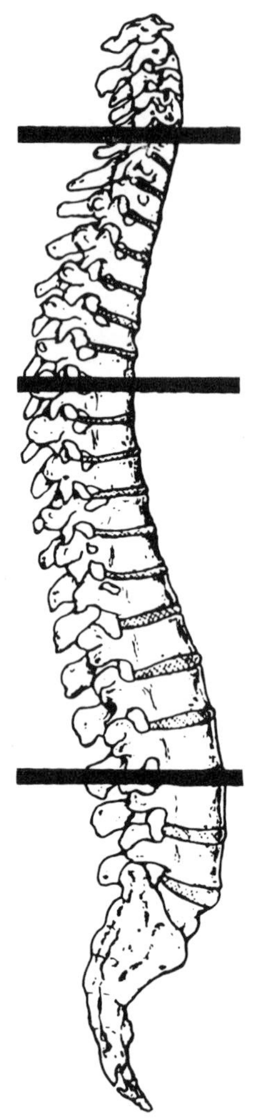

Figure 6.6. The only three areas (approximate) where the spine is able to move on a horizontal plane.

wedge-shaped compared to their bodies. The discs are quite large in the lumbar area.

The anterior convexity of the cervical and lumbar regions decreases during flexion, and it is not uncommon for the cervical curvature to slightly reverse during complete flexion.

Flexion is the most pronounced spinal motion. About 75% of all spinal flexion below the neck occurs in the lumbar spine, and about 70% of all lumbar flexion occurs at the lumbosacral joint. Normally, the degree of lumbar flexion is up to and only slightly over the flattening normal lordosis, thus total possible flexion must be achieved by hip rotation. In fact, some people can bend forward to touch the floor with little change in the spinal curves (Fig. 6.7).

Action and Brake Mechanisms

Flexion. During flexion, the IVD tends to compress at its anterior aspect, the anterior set of articular facets glide anteriosuperiorly upon the mating set of superior facets of the vertebra below, and the range of motion is checked by the posterior anulus of the disc, the posterior longitudinal ligament, the intertransverse ligaments, the supraspinous ligament, the extensor muscles, and the dorsolumbar aponeurotic sheet of fascia.

Extension. Extension has a much lower magnitude than flexion. The IVD tends to compress at its posterior aspect, and the inferior set of articular facets glide posterioinferiorly upon the mating superior facets below. The motion is checked by the anterior anulus of the disc, the anterior longitudinal ligament, all the anterior and lateral muscles that contribute to flexion, the anterior fascia and visceral attachments, and

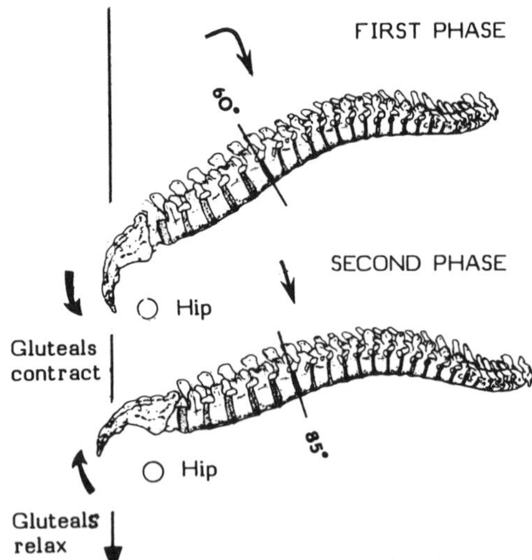

Figure 6.7. Forward flexion takes place in two phases. *Top*, in the first 60° of flexion, the pelvis is locked by the posterior pelvic muscles. About 70% of this motion occurs at the lumbosacral joint, 20% between L5 and L4, and 10% between the L1 and L3 vertebrae. *Bottom*, in the second phase, 60–85°, the hip releases and the pelvis rotates forward. The return extension occurs in reverse order of these two phases.

probably spinous process and/or lamina jamming at maximum extension.

Rotation. Spinal rotation is limited by the planes of the articular facets, the thickness of the associated IVDs, and the resistance offered by the fibers of the disc's anulus and the vertebral ligaments under torsion.

Lateral Bending. Sideward abduction involves a degree of tilting of vertebral bodies on their discs. The anterior aspect of the vertebral bodies in the upper spine also rotates toward the side of convexity, the posterior aspect swings in the opposite direction, and the facets tend to slide open on the convex side and override on the concave side. The motion is checked by the intertransverse ligaments and intercostal tissues on the convex side, behind the fulcrum, and the apposition of ribs on the concave side in the thoracic region.

Coupling and Related Effects. Some motions restrict other motions and enhance still others. For example, flexion and extension restrict rotation and lateral bending ranges. Rotation decreases A-P motion and is accompanied by a degree of lateral flexion. Lateral flexion inhibits A-P motion, and it enhances cervical rotation toward the concave side and lumbar rotation toward the convex side.

THE VERTEBRAE AND PERTINENT OSTEOLOGY[19-21]

When viewed as a whole, the entire vertebral column can be thought of as three segmented rods: a major pillar of anteriorly stacked vertebral bodies and discs, and two minor pillars of posteriorly stacked bilateral articular processes (Fig. 6.8) These tripod-arranged pillars progressively increase in size from C1 to L5 as a mechanical adaption to increasingly progressive load to which the vertebrae are subjected in the erect position. Likewise, the compression strength of the vertebrae progressively increases from C1 to L5.

Functional Anatomy[22]

A vertebra consists of a main body located anteriorly and a bony arch located posteriorly. The vertebral arch is composed of two bilateral, short, stout pedicles which

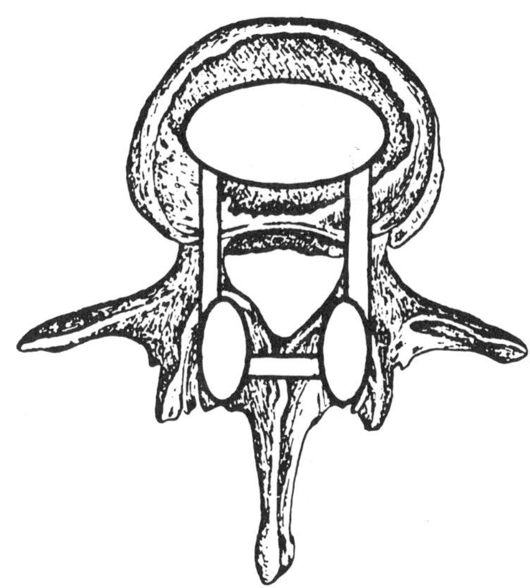

Figure 6.8. When viewed from above, the weight-bearing architecture of the spine resembles a large ovoid anterior pillar (vertebral body), joined to two interconnected smaller ovoid pillars (articular processes) by the horizontal pedicles.

join the arch to the vertebral body and two plate-like laminae which span the pedicles. In addition to their posterior articulating surfaces, each pedicle has superior and inferior rounded grooves which form the intervertebral foramina (IVFs) through which the spinal nerves pass. The arch supports two transverse, one spinous, and four articular processes.

Each aspect of a vertebra has a major function. The vertebral body serves as the weight-bearing aspect, the bilateral superior and inferior processes determine the direction of motion and restrict abnormal movement, the vertebral arch encases the spinal cord and its coverings, and the spinous and transverse processes serve as bony levers for muscle and ligament attachment.

Basic Regional Differences[23-28]

In addition to the differences in size, the 1st, 2nd, and 7th cervical vertebrae are atypical; the wedge-shaped thoracic vertebrae have articular facets for the ribs; and the lumbar spine has mammary processes. There are also significant regional differences in the spinous processes, laminae, and transverse processes. Figures 6.9, 6.10 and 6.11 exhibit the major structures.

It is important to keep in mind that as

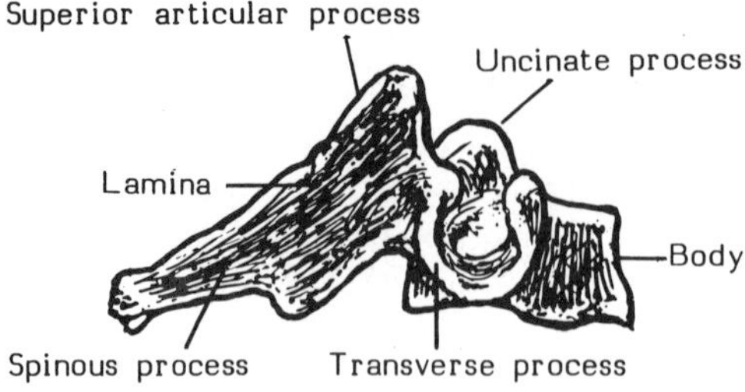

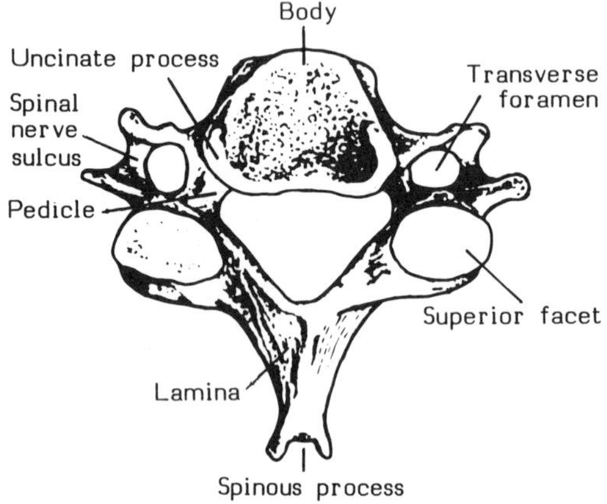

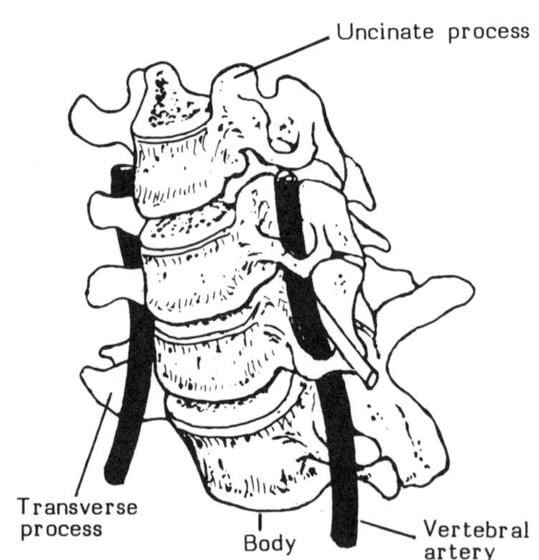

Figure 6.9. *Top*, lateral view of a 4th cervical vertebra; *center*, view from above; *bottom*, oblique view of the lower cervical vertebrae.

much as one-third of a typical human spine shows some variation from the textbook "normal." This is often reflected in an increase or decrease in the number of vertebrae or ribs, malformed unions, abnormal facet facings and unilateral differences, and differences in curvature arcs.

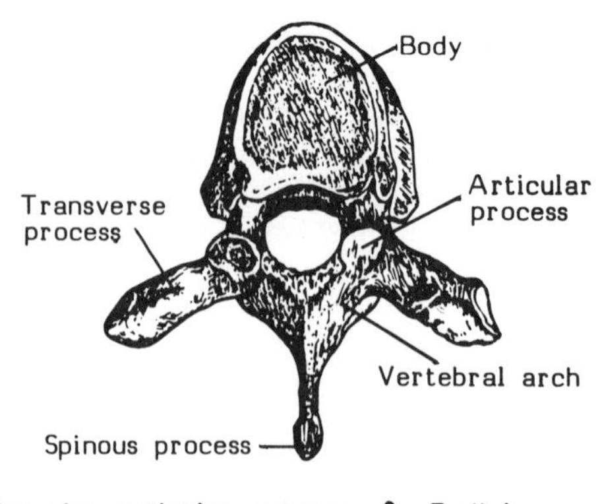

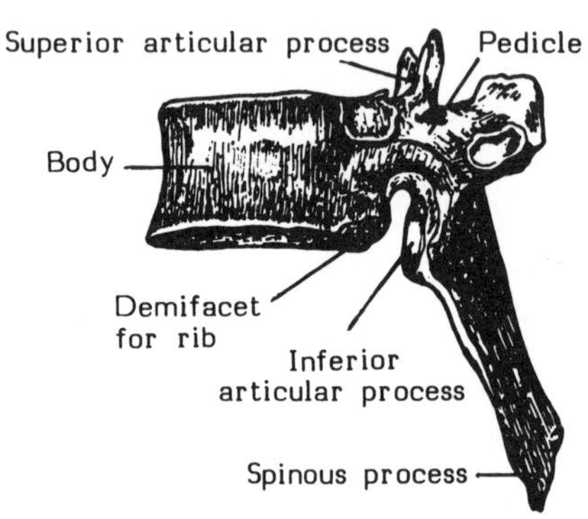

Figure 6.10. *Top*, view from the superior of a 6th thoracic vertebra; *bottom*, view from the lateral.

Spinous Processes

In the cervical and lumbar regions, the spinous processes project fairly posteriorly except for a posterior tubercle that replaces the spinous process of the atlas. Cervical processes are usually bifid and of equal length in Caucasians but nonbifid in Negroes. The process of C7 is called the vertebrae prominens, but it is sometimes shorter than that of T1. In the thoracic region, the spinous processes are bifid, often of unequal length, and turned downward and overlap like shingles. This is most pronounced in the T2–T10 area. Consequently, extension is severely limited there, and A-P movements are made much more freely in the cervical and lumbar regions. The spinous processes of the lumbar spine resemble thick, relatively large, quadrilateral plates. The L5 segment has the smallest lumbar process.

Laminae

The laminae overlap slightly in the cervical spine, overlap severely in the thoracic

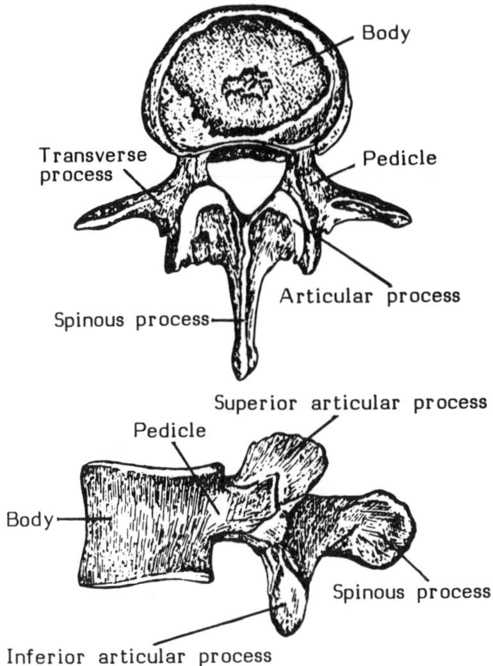

Figure 6.11. *Top*, view from the superior of a second lumbar vertebra; *bottom*, view from the lateral.

spine, and do not overlap at all in the lumbar region. When overlap is absent, bony protection is diminished. Similar gaps are also seen at the atlanto-occipital, atlantoaxial, lumbosacral, and sacrococcygeal juntions.

Transverse Processes

The cervical vertebrae contain foramina within their transverse processes for passage of the vertebral vessels. All channel the vertebral artery, vein, and sympathetic fibers, except for the smaller C7 foramina which do not transmit the artery and are occasionally absent. With the exception of the wide transverse processes of the atlas and C7, the horizontal processes of C2–C6 are relatively small, fairly equal in width, located anterior to the facet joints, and turn inferior-anteriorly to overlap the IVFs. If a transverse process of C7 is as wide as or wider than that of T1, a cervical rib is often associated. The wide, thick, strong transverse processes of the thoracic spine arise posterior to the IVFs and articular processes, sit further posteriorly than those of the cervical or lumbar regions, serve as fulcra for the ribs (T1–T10) at their specialized transverse process facets, and act as lever arms for muscles and ligaments. The widths of the thoracic transverse processes progressively decrease caudally, while those of the lumbar region increase to L3 and then slightly decrease at L4 and L5. The transverse processes of the lumbar spine project as thin plates that extend dorsolaterally in the upper region and progressively become more anterolateral as L5 is approached.

Joints of Luschka

Near the posterolateral aspect of the adult cervical IVDs, small, bilateral, oblique cavities often appear that can be mistaken for true synovial joints. These uncovertebral articular modifications (Luschka's joints) are located between the superior surfaces of the uncinate processes and the corresponding lateral tips of the articular surface below. They are evident around 8–10 years of age in only some people; thus, several authorities feel they represent degenerative changes in accommodation to stress.[29]

The Vertebral Motion Unit[30–34]

Because it serves as the axial support of the trunk, the erect spinal column is a primary concern in static postural equilibrium. Since the body is never actually in a static state in life but exists in a state of "quiet dynamics" in the static postural attitude and a state of "active dynamics" in movement, the kinetic aspects of normal spinal biomechanics are an important consideration. Total spinal function is the sum of its individual component units.

An intervertebral "motion unit" consists of two vertebrae and their contiguous structures forming a set of articulations at one intervertebral level, thus conferring a quality and quantity of motion to the relationship of two vertebrae (Fig. 6.12). These units are firmly interconnected by the IVD and restraining ligaments and are activated by muscles that respond to both sensory and motor innervation.[35]

The biomechanical efficiency of any one of the 25 vertebral motion units from atlas to sacrum can be described as that condition (individually and collectively) in which each gravitationally dependent segment above is

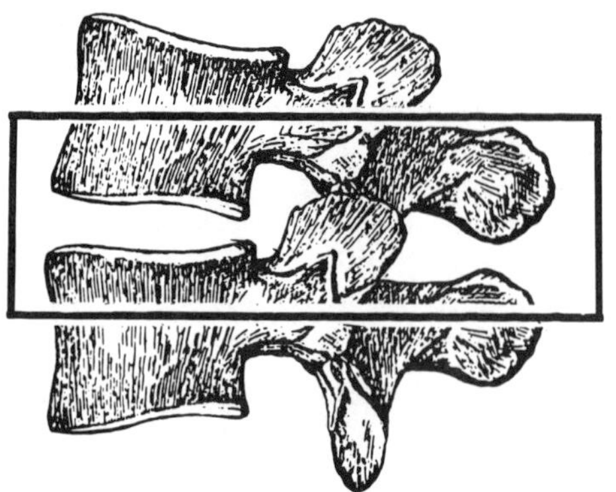

Figure 6.12. Functional area of an intervertebral motion unit.

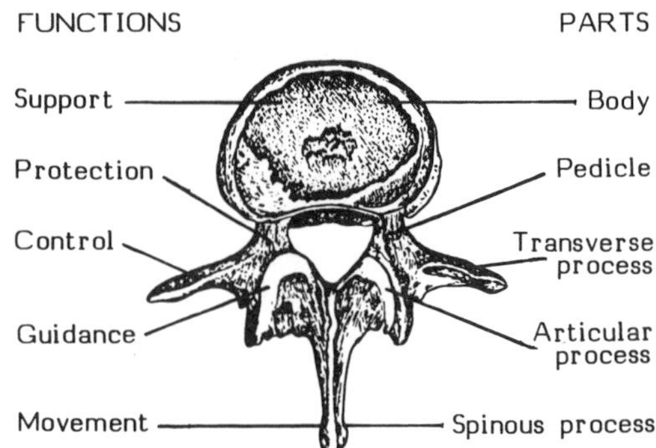

Figure 6.13. The primary parts related to major functions of a thoracic vertebra, as viewed from above.

(1) free to seek its normal resting position in relation to its supporting structure below, (2) free to move efficiently through its normal ranges of motion, and (3) free to return to its normal resting position after movement.

The Anterior Portion

The anterior portion of the motion unit includes the roughly cylindrical vertebral bodies, the hydraulic IVD, the anterior and posterior longitudinal ligaments, and the other associated soft tissues. This anterior portion is weight bearing, shock absorbing, and supportive, and it plays an essentially static role. At the slightly concave superior and inferior aspects of the vertebral body are the vertebral end plates. The anterior portion of the unit has very little sensory innervation. Changes or pathology affecting these structures, even though they may be quite spectacular in appearance on an x-ray film and may alter biomechanics and spinal mobility significantly, are seldom accompanied by much pain or other subjective discomfort in the local area.

The Posterior Portion

The non-weight-bearing, tuning-fork-shaped, posterior aspect of a motion unit consists of the two pedicles, two laminae, neural foramina, articular processes and apophyseal articulations, the ligamenta flava and those that encapsulate the articulation, the spinous and transverse processes, the interspinous and supraspinous ligaments, and all the muscles and other attached soft-tissue structures (Fig. 6.13). The posterior portion of the motion units, which plays an essentially dynamic role, is rich in sensory and proprioceptive nerves. Thus, problems that affect these structures are usually painful.

The Vertebral Body

The vertebral body can be considered as a miniature long bone in structure; ie, a hard shell surrounding a spongy interior containing an array of crisscrossing trabeculae and red marrow. However, the cancellous portion of a vertebra is much thinner than that seen in a long bone.

Vertebral Body Loading[36–41]

Although some axial load is carried by the vertebral facets, the majority of compression load is borne by the vertebral bodies. Load upon a superior end-plate is directed to the inferior end-plate via the cancellous core and the cortical shell. Not only does the cancellous core share load distribution with the cortical shell, but during loading (especially at high rates) it serves as the main resistor of dynamic peak loads via its energy-absorbing trabeculae and marrow.

Core Strength. The cancellous core of the vertebral body provides 55% of its vertebral strength, and the cortical shell provides 45% of its strength up to the age of 40 years. This core strength sharply decreases after the age of 40 years to about 35%, with 65% provided by the cortex. Beyond 60 years, however, this decrease in core strength is much more gradual.[42, 43] Bone strength appears to be directly related to mineral content, and a small loss of osseous tissue has a profound effect on bone strength. A 25% loss of osseous tissue decreases bone strength 50%. Comparative values of healthy vertebral bodies are offered in Figure 6.14.[44]

Core Deformation. The cancellous core of a vertebral body can undergo up to 9.5% deformation prior to fracture, compared to only 2% for the cortical shell. Thus, it is unlikely to have compression fractures of the core without fractures of the shell. Figure 6.15 depicts failure with and without a healthy disc.

Considerations in Interspinal Postures[45]

The vertebral body deserves special consideration in evaluating interspinal posture because even if we usually think of its function as forming the anterior boundary of the neural canal and a slight contribution to the boundary of the foramen, almost any change in its size, shape, or position will alter these boundaries. Second, the vertebral body must be considered in its function as a contributor to the vertebral articulation, for limited or excessive movement of this articulation influences the neural canal and the intervertebral foramen. In some instances, it is difficult to separate the change of the vertebral bodies from that of the IVDs.

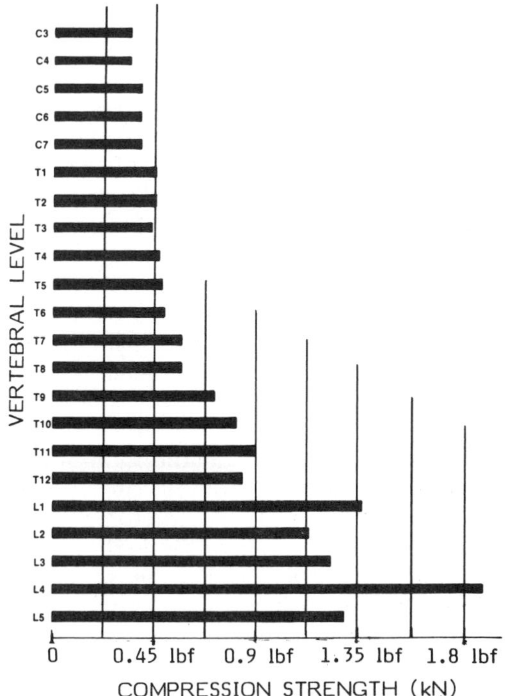

Figure 6.14. A chart of comparative vertebral body compression strength from C3 to L5.

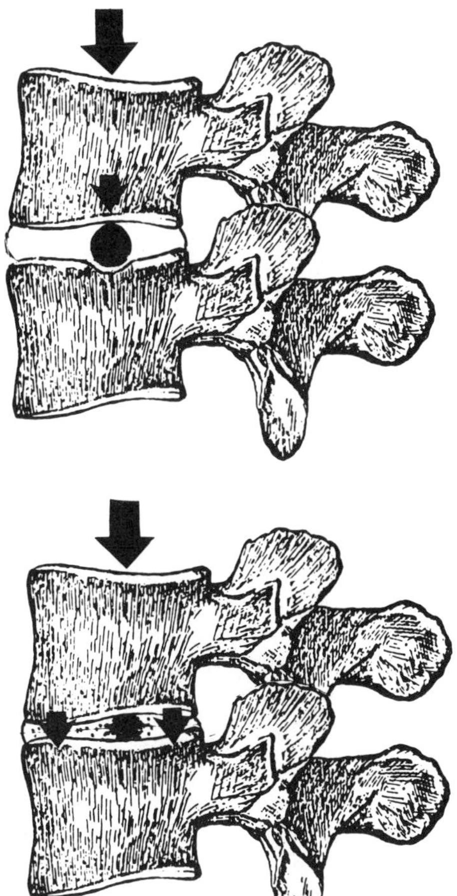

Figure 6.15. *Top*, vertebral body failure from excessive compression of a healthy disc when the greatest stress is central. Note compression node at the superior aspect of the inferior vertebra. *Bottom*, failure from compression of a degenerative disc, when the greatest forces are peripheral (from lack of central resistance) rather than central.

Changes Relevant to Interspinal Posture. Changes of the medullary substance that influence interspinal posture include (1) loss of substance, (2) collapse, (3) comminuted fragmentation, (4) scalloping of margins, (5) wedging that may be triangular, quadrilateral, or trapezoid in shape, (6) biconcave deformity (cupping), (7) serrated formations, (8) irregular cartilaginous plates such as in osteochrondrosis or underdevelopment of the secondary ossification centers, (9) Schmorl's nodes, and (10) osteophytes.

Changes Usually Irrelevant to Interspinal Posture. The internal structure or medullary portion of the vertebral body undergoes a number of changes that do not *necessarily* influence spinal posture. These include (1) lack of substance, (2) sclerosis, (3) condensation, (4) eburnation, (5) fasciculation, (6) osteoporosis, and (7) compression. Changes in the vertebral body that do not appreciably alter the A-P curve, neural canal, or foramina, but do denote limitation of movement or fixation, include marginal sclerosis or endplate sclerosis which may be in the form of lipping or spurring. Exostosis or marginal vertebral hypertrophy occurs following trauma or chronic abnormal weight-bearing changes, in much the same fashion as that which develops on the margin of the articular facet. These overgrowths may or may not produce encroachment of the spinal canal or foramina, depending upon location.

Other factors influencing size, shape, and position of the vertebral bodies include a long list of congenital anomalies such as hemivertebrae, osteochondrodystrophy, achondroplasia, and dyschondroplasia.

Planes of Articulation[46, 47]

Paired diarthrodial articular processes (zygapophyses) project from the vertebral arches. The superior processes (prezygapophyses) of the inferior vertebra contain articulating facets, which face somewhat posteriorly. They mate with the inferior processes (postzygapophyses) of the vertebra above, which face somewhat anteriorly. Each articular facet is covered by a thin layer of hyaline cartilage which faces the synovial joint. Vertebrae facet angulation varies with the level of the spine.

Fisk states that these joints are more prone to osteoarthritic changes than any other joint in the body: "Evidence of disc degeneration precedes this arthritis in the lumbar spine, but there is no such relationship in the cervical spine."[48] However, most authorities agree with Grieve that the presence of arthrotic changes in the facet planes does not, of itself, necessarily have any effect upon ranges of movement, neither does the presence of osteophytosis.[49]

The Cervical Area

The plane of articulation is about perpendicular to the sagittal plane and inclined about 45° to the vertical plane in the cervical region.[50] The lateral cervical gravity line extends from the apex of the odontoid process through the anterior aspect of T2. The relatively stable base between T1 and T2 progressively changes upward so that the planes of articulation tend to be forced inferior, posterior, but not medial as in the thoracic and lumbar regions of the spine.

A horizontal locking-type base of support at the atlantoaxial articulation is quite similar to that found at the lumbrosacral area. The inferior articular surfaces of the atlas offer a bilateral, medial, and inferior slant which forces the atlas to move inward toward the odontoid to allow rotary movements of the head. Excessive A-P movement is stabilized by the anterior and posterior rings and check ligaments. The posteromedially slanted cup-like superior articular surfaces of the atlas help stabilize the occipital articulating surfaces. These concave facets allow free rocking for A-P nodding.

From C3 to C7, the almost flat and thus freely mobile articular processes are found at the junction of the pedicles and laminae. The inferior facets face downward and forward and glide on the superior facets of the vertebra below, which face upward and backward (Fig. 6.16). Maximum cervical A-P movement usually takes place between C5 and C6, and it is almost impossible to actively flex the neck without causing some flexion in the upper thoracic region.

The Thoracic Area

In the thoracic spine, the direction of the superior articulations is posterolateral, and the inferior processes face anteromedially. This slant comes closer to the vertical axis as the thoracic spine progresses caudally. The facets are inclined about 60° to the vertical plane in the midthoracic spine. The articular planes of the thoracic vertebrae allow greater rotation but less flexion and extension than that seen in the more horizontal articular planes of the lumbar verte-

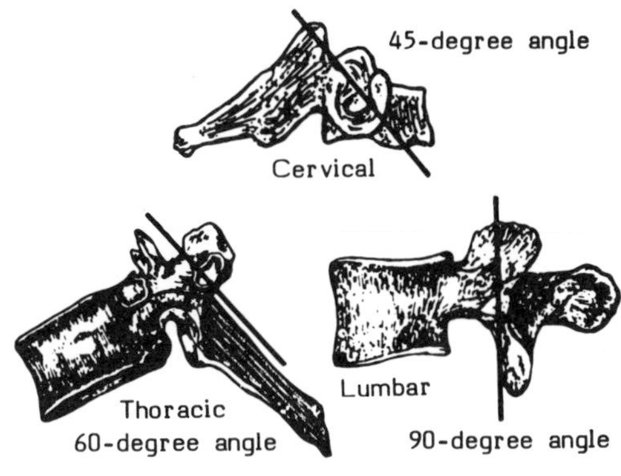

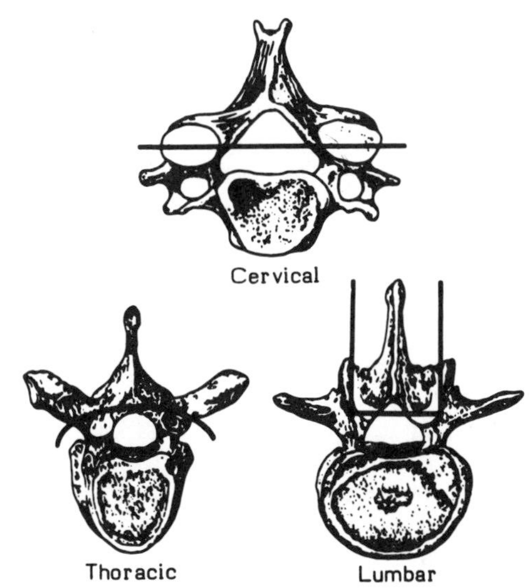

Figure 6.16. *Top*, a comparison of typical cervical, thoracic, and lumbar facet orientations, as viewed laterally. *Bottom*, views from above.

bra. Thoracic movement is restricted in all directions because of the attached rib cage. Gravitational forces fall upon the articular surfaces in such a manner as to direct each vertebra more inferior, posterior, and medial until gravity brings the curve back toward the centered balance point.

The Lumbar Area

The facets in the lumbar region describe moderately sloped surfaces rather than a single-plane angle as seen in the cervical and thoracic area and are fairly parallel to the vertical plane. The convex inferior facets mate with concave superior facets. L1 to L5, the plane of the articular facets changes from mediolateral to anteroposterior and lies, for the most part, in the sagittal plane.

From the middle of the anterior surface of T12, the body's gravity line extends downward to the anterior aspect of the sacral base. Weight distribution in the lumbar region is governed chiefly by the inclination of each vertebral body articulation. The lumbosacral articulations are slightly more horizontal than those above them. This allows greater A-P and lateral motion but affords less joint locking than in the vertebrae above.

The horizontal inclination of L5, spreading out toward the coronal plane, becomes progressively more vertical from L4 to L1 as the dorsolumbar articulation is approached. These changes in articular planes allow the lower back to bend and twist to accommodate gravitational force during movement. The upper lumbar joints are J-shaped when viewed laterally, thus their anterior aspect resists forward displacement.

The lateral center line of gravity falls upon the spinal points because of gradual changes in the angles of the inclined planes of the various articular surfaces. Van Dusen points out that this tends to force each lumbar vertebra more inferior, medial, and anterior or posterior until gravity brings the apex of the curve back toward the balancing point.[51]

Body weight is borne ultimately in the lower back essentially by the L5 disc, sacral base, and sacroiliac joints. This weight is forced slightly anterior on the load surfaces to place the lateral pelvic gravity line at the anteroinferior aspect of S2. Gravitational weight during development wedges the sacrum between the innominates because of their peculiar laterally inclined planes that allow the sacrum to move inferiorly, anteriorly, and medially, coupled with the anteroinferior angulation of the sacral base.

Many of the abnormal orientations found in the lower spine can be attributed to the fact that the lumbar facet joints are not determined until the secondary curves are developed in the erect position. The stresses imposed during the development stage can easily lead to the high incidence of asymmetry.

Facet Angle Variations

An important influence of interspinal posture is that of the facet facing of each posterior intervertebral joint, with the alterations of the facings most commonly occurring in the lumbar and lower cervical regions. The facings are more frequently altered between L4 and L5 than at any other level in the vertebral column.

Symmetric facets glide with production of little friction. However, if the facets deviate in their direction of movement, the unparallel articulating surfaces "scrub" upon one another. Articular variances of the processes and facets over a period of time even in the absence of injury at the level of abnormality, will present thickening of the covering of the facet, referred to as marginal sclerosis. This hardening process is usually followed by hypertrophy or exostosis and produces an appearance of an irregular articular surface when the facet is viewed in profile in roentgenography. Coexistent with this finding, the interarticular spaces gradually become narrowed, hazy, obscured, and even obliterated on x-ray films.

Since these various facet and interarticular manifestations are due to either chronic abnormal weight-bearing or specific trauma, the term arthrosis is used rather than posterior intervertebral osteoarthritis. It seems a more reasonable descriptor because of the implications of the suffix "-itis." Although there may not be evidence of direct bony encroachment from the process of arthrosis directly into the intervertebral foramina, one must consider that the process of arthrosis does produce a general narrowing of the diameters of the intervertebral foramina and hence produces interference with the normal expression of nerve impulse transmission.

Normal articular angles described in any text are approximations. There is considerable variation from one person to another and from the transition of one region to another. For example, the transitional vertebra between the thoracic and lumbar regions is usually given as T12, but it might be any vertebra from T9 to L1, according to White and Panjabi.[52]

Facet Strength

Torsional Strength. The articulating processes and their capsular ligaments provide up to 45% of torsional strength of a vertebral motion unit, in contrast to 45% by the disc and longitudinal ligaments and 10% by the interspinous ligaments. These percentages will vary with different postures.[53]

Compression Strength. The facets normally carry about 18% of a vertebra's total axial load but can contribute up to 33% of its compression strength, depending upon posture.[54] The facets of a lower lordotic curve (C5–C7, L3–L5) carry more weight than those of other areas.

The Intervertebral Foramina[55, 56]

Generally, an intervertebral foramen is bounded above by the inferior pedicle notch of the superior vertebra, below by the superior pedicle notch of the inferior vertebra, anteriorly by the IVD and parts of the two vertebral bodies, and posteriorly by the superior and inferior articular processes.

Vertebrae move in the planes of their articulations, and it is at the level of the posterior intervertebral articulations along with their facets that most subluxations occur and influence the IVFs far more than any other articulations of the spinal column. Changes in the diameter of normal IVFs result in an abnormal joint formation, which predisposes to subluxation as well as being a direct factor in altering the curves of the particular region of the spine in which this structural defect is found.

Size and Shape

When viewed laterally, an IVF is generally elliptical in shape, with the diameter of its vertical axis about double its A-P dimension. Because of this, there is usually adequate space for changes in vertical dimension (eg, dynamic axial traction or compression, disc flattening) without injury to the IVF contents as long as there is adequate fat and fluid present. However, reduction of an already short transverse diameter can produce a number of noxious effects. For this reason, complete disc collapse vertically is often asymptomatic, while a slight posterolateral herniation may protrude upon the IVF and produce severe symptoms.

The Cervical Area. In the cervical region, the foramina are more in the shape of rounded gutters than orifices, averaging 1 cm in length. There is no IVF between the atlas and the occiput or between the atlas and the axis. The C1 nerve exits over the superior aspect of the posterior arch of the atlas in the vertebral artery sulcus. The C2 nerve exists between the inferior aspect of the posterior arch of the atlas and the superior aspect of pedicle of the axis. It then dangerously transverses the lateral atlantoaxial joint, anterior to the ligamentum flava. The C3–C8 nerves exit through short oval canals, which increase in size as they progress caudally. Cervical nerves, especially, fill the transverse diameter of the their IVFs. Thus, any disorder that reduces this dimension (eg, subluxation, osteophytes, disc herniation, edema) will undoubtedly compromise the integrity of the IVF contents (Fig. 6.17).

The Thoracic Area. In the thoracic region, the pedicle notch of the vertebra above is quite deep, while that of the vertebra below is relatively shallow. The result is a pear-shaped canal with sharp bony edges that predisposes to fibrotic changes from chronic irritation. The vertebral body and the disc of the superior vertebra form most of the IVF's anterior boundary.

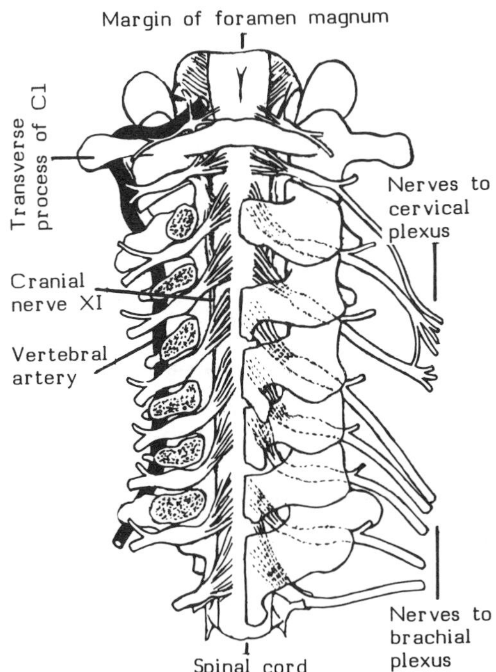

Figure 6.17. Posterior view of the cervical region. *Left*, laminae have been removed to expose the precarious position of the interforaminal contents.

The Lumbar Area. In the lumbar region, an IVF is shaped like a kidney bean. It takes considerable posterolateral disc protrusion to encroach the nerve exiting at the same level, because the lumbar IVFs are relatively large. When herniation does cause trouble, it is usually due to pressure on the laterally placed nerve root on the vertebra above. Sunderland stresses the fact that the passage of the medial branch of the lumbar dorsal ramus and its accompanying vessels through the osseofibrous tunnel and the intimate relationship of the neurovascular bundle to the capsule of the apophyseal joint represents a potential site of fixation and entrapment following pathologic changes involving the joint.[57]

Contents

Each foramen is dynamic, widening and expanding with spinal motion, serving as a channel for nerve and vascular egress and ingress, and allowing compression and expansion of the lipoareolar bed. From one-third to one-half of the foraminal opening is occupied by the spinal nerve root and its sheath, with the remaining portion filled essentially by fat, connective tissue, and various vessels.

The following specific structures are found in the IVF: the anterior nerve root, the posterior nerve root, a part of the dorsal nerve root ganglion, a bilaminar sleeve of dura and arachnoid membrane to the ganglion, a short continuation of the subarachnoid space with cerebrospinal fluid which ends just after the ganglion, the recurrent meningeal nerve, the spinal ramus artery, the intervertebral vein, and lymphatic vessels.

Size Alterations

Factors That Change the Diameter. The typical factors modifying the diameters of the IVFs are (1) the disrelation of facet subluxation, (2) changes in the normal static curves of the spine, (3) the presence of induced abnormal curves of the spine, (4) degenerative thinning, bulging, or extrusion of the related IVD, (5) swelling and sclerosing of the capsular ligaments and the interbody articulation, and (6) marginal proliferations of the vertebral bodies and articulations.

Consequences of Diameter Alteration. The above factors insult the viable contents of the IVF and subject its contents to physiologic compromise that results in nerve root pressure, traction, or torque; constriction of the spinal blood vessels; intraforaminal and paraforaminal edema; induration and sclerosing of the periarticular ligaments with incarcerating insult upon the contained receptors; forcing of the foraminal contents into protracted constriction and altered position; and other such consequences. Nerve tissue tolerates slow compression quite well without offering obvious symptoms. Acute phenomena are usually the result of friction, severe or repeated trauma, and encroachment from degenerative thickening or exostosis.

Congenital Anomalies and Deformities of the Neck and Back[58–60]

We speak of a functional norm, yet in clinical practice we usually find variations. Simon[61] was referring to dental anomalies when he stated that "all we ever find are variations; an exact ideal normal does not exist, cannot exist. And this is our enigma; in theory we will never find the normal, in practice we forever feel its need and apply it constantly." This same precept can be applied to the spine, to any structure.

A large variety of overt spinal malformations may be witnessed on occasion. Their brief descriptions are listed below:

- *Anomalous formation of the spinous process*: when two touch, the condition is called Bastrup's disease.
- *Basilar invagination or impression*: elevation and softening of the posterior cerebellar fossa with the atlas protruding above Chamberlain's line (a line across the hard palate to the posterior margin of the foramen magnum).
- *Cervical rib*: rib or portion of rib from C7 or another cervical vertebra.
- *Failure of fusion*: occurring at an articular process, a spinous process, transverse process, or epiphyseal plate (limbus bone).
- *Hemivertebra*: failure of differentiation of an individual vertebra; failure of one half of a vertebral body to develop, leaving the other half in a parasagittal position.
- *Lumbarization*: growth of S1 as a separate lumbar segment; may be pseudo or true, bilateral or unilateral.
- *Occipital vertebra*: a morphologic structure resembling a vertebral segment which surrounds the foramen magnum.
- *Os odontoideum*: congenital nonunion of the odontoid with the body of the axis.
- *Ossiculum terminale*: nonunion of the secondary ossification center at the tip of the dens.
- *Overdevelopment or elongation of the transverse process*: usually of L5 or C7, and may cause a bursa to form and give rise to bursitis.
- *Paramastoid process*: bony column arising from the transverse process of the atlas which articulates with the base of the skull at the jugular process.
- *Platybasia*: flattening of the basilar angle to an excess of 150° (135° is normal) without invagination of the posterior cranial fossa; a softening of the anterior cerebellar fossa with an increase in Martin's basilar angle (a line drawn from the root of the nares, to the anterior clinoid process, to the anterior border of the foramen magnum).
- *Ponticulus lateralis*: a bony arch extending from the superior articulating surface of the atlas to its transverse process.
- *Ponticulus posticus*: ossification of the posterior portion of the atlanto-occipital ligament.
- *Sacralization*: growth of L5 to S1, may be pseudo or true, bilateral or unilateral (Fig. 6.18).
- *Sagittal clefted vertebrae*: bifid vertebrae; failure of unification of the laterally placed primary ossification centers of the vertebral bodies.
- *Spina bifida occulta*: failure of the neural arch to close in the posterior midline without protrusion of elements of the spinal canal and often associated with tropism. It is the most common developmental abnormality of a vertebra, usually located at the L5 or S1 level, and often associated with a patch of hair overlying the defect. The defect is seen to some degree in 10% of the population. If several vertebrae are involved, the defect is termed rachischisis and is frequently associated with a variable degree of neurologic disorder.
- *Spondylolysis*: defect in the pars inter-

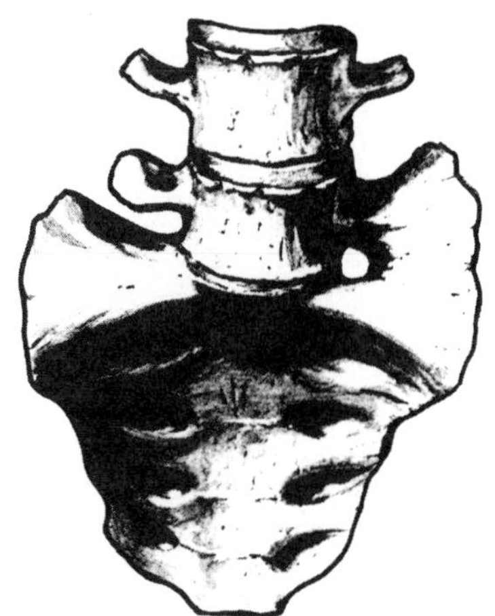

Figure 6.18. True unilateral sacralization of the 5th lumbar vertebra.

articularis that usually leads to anterior displacement of the vertebral body (spondylolisthesis) later in life.

- *Spondyloschisis*: separation of the pars interarticularis; isthmus separation in which the pars interarticularis fails to ossify. Most consider it to be a failure of ossification of a fatigue fracture. It may be bilateral or unilateral, with or without spondylolisthesis.
- *Sprengel's deformity*: congenital elevation of the scapula with adduction and downward rotation of the scapula attended by kyphoscoliosis of the brachiocervical spine.
- *Supernumerary vertebral segments*: congenital development of additional vertebral segments.
- *Third condyle*: an arch on the anterior margin of the foramen magnum, which articulates with the odontoid in cases of an occipital vertebra.
- *Tropism*: asymmetrical or anomalous development of a zygapophysis, usually seen as a sagittal disposition of the lumbosacral facets.
- *Vertebral fusion*: examples include (1) Klippel-Feil syndrome, a synostosis (growing together) of vertebrae of the cervical spine, characterized by a short neck, low hairline, and limited neck movement, and sometimes by scoliosis, spinal bifida, and Sprengel's deformity; (2) block vertebra, congenital synostosis of other vertebrae such as the thoracics or lumbars; (3) atlanto-occipital fusion (occipitalization) of the atlas with the base of the skull; (4) paraoccipital process, a bony connection between the occiput and the first transverse process, lying close to the condyle.

THE SPINAL JOINTS AND PERTINENT ARTHROLOGY

Each vertebral segment articulates with adjacent vertebrae and ribs through a complex system of joints, ligaments, and levers. The stability of the spine and pelvis is not due to its inherent ligamentous stability, which is meager as a whole, but arises through its dynamic neuromuscular structures and control system.

The Vertebral Joints[62–66]

As many as 97 true synovial diarthroses and an even greater number of amphiarthroses are involved in spinal movement. All these diarthroses are the gliding type except for the odontoid pivot joint on the atlas. Synarthroses are found only during development.

The dynamic functions of the spine are dependent upon seven articulations: (1) posterior intervertebral (synovial), (2) vertebral bodies and IVDs (nonsynovial), (3) costovertebral (synovial), (4) uncovertebral joints of Luschka (synovial?), (5) sacroiliac (nonsynovial), (6) symphysis pubis (nonsynovial), and (7) iliofemoral (synovial).

The fact that some of these joints are synovial and some are nonsynovial accounts for the expression of localized pain witnessed clinically in the synovial joints and the absence of pain in the nonsynovial types of articulation. The other contributing factor of pain elicitation is found in the sensory nerves of the periosteum or perichondrium. The posterior intervertebral articulations contain both synovial membrane and perichondrium, whereas the anterior vertebral body articulation contains neither of these two connective tissues.

The spine exhibits two main areas of articulation: at the vertebral body and at the vertebral arch. Two forms of nonsynovial amphiarthroses connect adjacent vertebral bodies: the IVDs represent symphyses, and the anterior and posterior longitudinal ligaments form syndesmoses. The articulations of the vertebral arches involve the apophyseal joints, the ligamentum flava, and the interspinous and intertransverse ligaments.

The Intervertebral Disc Area[67–71]

The elasticity of the IVDs is diminished throughout the day as an individual remains in the upright position and the discs are subjected to compression forces producing dehydration. Thus, the length of the spine is gradually diminished so that a person is shorter at night than in the morning. In senility or from a premature breakdown in the disc's gel, disc thickness and elasticity are diminished, thus disc flexibility and resistance to jarring are lessened.

The IVDs are numbered by the vertebra above; spinal nerves, by the vertebra below. Thus, for example, a posterolaterally herniated C6 disc may affect the C7 nerve.

Functional Anatomy[72–74]

There is no true disc between the occiput and atlas or between the atlas and the axis. The L5 disc is considered the last disc, but rudimentary discs are sometimes present between the sacral segments, sacrococcygeal junction, and the coccygeal segments.

The joints between C3 and S1 vertebral bodies are unique symphyses formed by the apposing vertebral plateaus and the IVD. Each disc unit consists of three distinct parts: the endplates, anulus fibrosus, and nucleus pulposus.

The Endplates. These are thin sheets of cortical bone and relatively tough hyaline cartilage that separate the disc from the vertebral body above and below. They tend to prevent herniation of the nucleus into the adjacent vertebral bodies (Fig. 6.19).

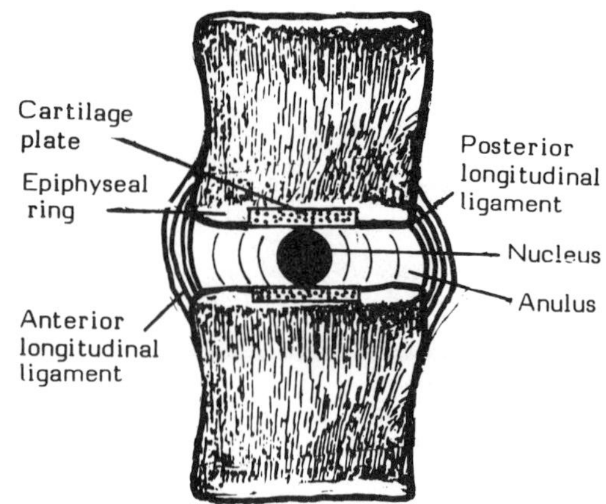

Figure 6.19. Relation of endplates to the intervertebral disc and longitudinal ligaments.

The Anulus Fibrosus. The peripheral part of the disc is composed of laminated bands of concentric fibers. The apposing layers of fibers are angled (±30°) in opposite oblique direction (crisscrossed). The fibers become angled less obliquely toward the periphery so that they are nearly vertical at the edge of the disc and almost horizontal near the core. In this manner, the anular fibers extending from one endplate to the other serve as coiled springs that tend to hold the adjacent vertebral bodies together against the pressure of the nucleus. The anular fibers are loosely attached to the vertebral endplates centrally but strongly fixed to bone at the periphery (Sharpey's fibers). Fibers near the circumference blend into the posterior and anterior longitudinal ligaments.

The number of lamellae in the anulus is the same at all points around the disc. However, these fibers are distorted and compressed by the effect of posture on the secondary curve in the lumbar region, resulting in thickening of the anterior portion of the anulus.

The Anulus and Loading. The outer disc carries 25% of vertical compression forces. It is best designed to carry tension forces, while the nucleus is better constructed to carry compression loads. Anulus fibers are usually stouter and stronger anteriorly and centrally, thus contributing to the higher incidence of posterolateral herniation.

The Nucleus Pulposus. The central part of the disc is surrounded laterally by the central ring of the anulus and above and below by the vertebral plateaus (Fig. 6.20). It resembles a small, transparent, mucopolysaccharide gelatinous sphere (80–90% water) under both internal and external pressure that gives it considerable elastic rebound, and it is devoid of nerve fibers and blood vessels. Its shape allows motion in all directions. There is *no* definite structural interface between the nucleus and the anulus in the *adult*; ie, the tissues blend rather than appose. The nucleus is a remnant of the beaded string of intervertebral notochordal cells that did not degenerate.

The Nucleus and Loading. The ability

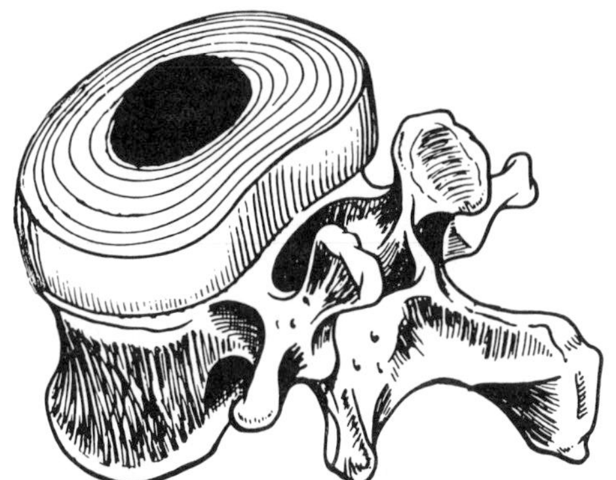

Figure 6.20. Drawing of a vertebra showing its superior disc. The nucleus pulposus is depicted in *black*, surrounded by the rings of the anulus.

of the nucleus to absorb and retain water under high imbibition pressure is unique to living tissue. As a ball bearing between two relatively flat surfaces, the nucleus allows six degrees of freedom.[75] However, the extent of motion at any particular disc is limited by the various ligaments and facet planes. The nucleus, highly resistant to compression, carries or distributes the majority of axial compression forces. It transmits some forces horizontally to the anulus, and the amount increases when the spine is flexed and the load is increased as in lifting. Actual displacement of the nucleus occurs most often in severe scoliosis as a result of disc degeneration and the abnormal distribution of forces on the disc.

Regional Variables. Disc *thickness* varies in the different spinal regions as the result of the degree of curvature, load, vertebral body size, and hydrophilic capacity. Discs are thinnest in the cervical region and progressively thicken as the spine progresses caudally (Fig. 6.21). However, it is the *ratio* of disc thickness to vertebral body thickness that governs segmental mobility. This ratio is greatest in the cervical region and least in the thoracic area. The *surface area* of the nucleus (nucleus/anulus ratio) relative to the overall disc, and the *position* of the nucleus relative to the midline also vary slightly according to spinal region (Fig. 6.22). Data from Kapandji and others in this regard are summarized in Table 6.1.[76,77]

These facts are important because it has been shown that the IVD functions optimally, has the greatest resistance to stress,

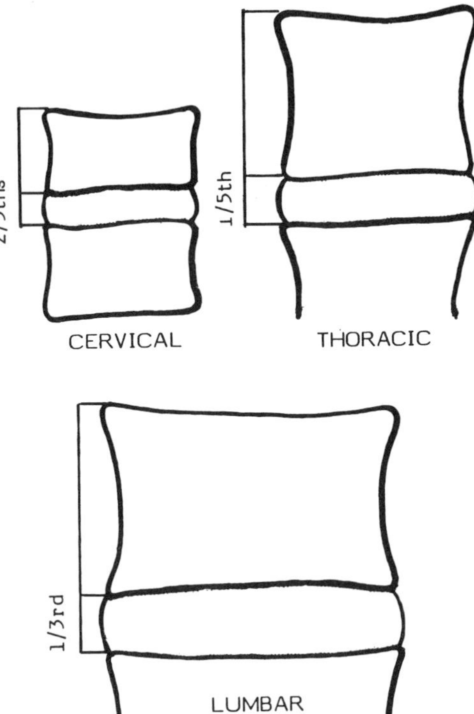

Figure 6.21. The average ratio of cervical, thoracic, and lumbar discs to vertebral body heights.

and allows optimum mobility when (1) the nucleus is located near the center of the disc, (2) the height of the disc is of normal proportions, (3) its dimensions are symmetrical, and (4) the disc is well hydrated.

Biomechanical Reactions[78–85]

The disc is subjected to a variety of loads: compression by gravity and pushing; traction by being pulled; tensile stress by flexion, extension, and lateral bending; torsion and shear by axial rotation; and various multiple combinations of each. Since the back muscles use the spine as a lever in maintaining balance, the forces upon the IVDs and vertebrae are much greater than the forces of the body weight above.

Disc Bulge. During spinal movement, the peripheral anulus bulges slightly posteriorly during extension, anteriorly during flexion, and toward the side of lateral bending. This is opposite to what some might think. Concurrent with bulging is disc contraction on the contralateral side (Poisson effect). The healthy nucleus remains near

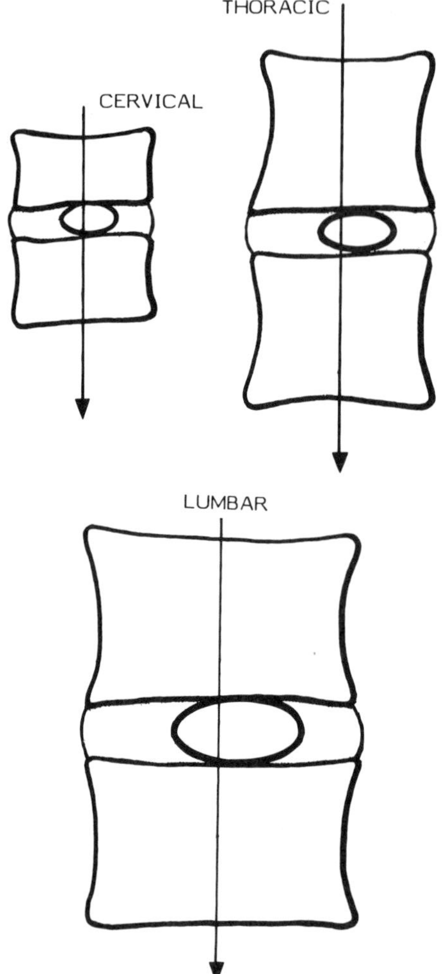

Figure 6.22. The position of the weight-bearing nucleus pulposus varies in relation to the vertical midline in the various regions of the spine. It also varies in relative surface area size to that of the anulus.

its normal position with only slight movement toward the anular bulge.

Preloading. Because the nucleus is strongly hydrophilic and encased, its pressure is never zero, even if completely unloaded.[86] This "preloaded" factor offers an inherent tension that offers greater resistance to compression and lateral flexion forces. The "swollen" state of the nucleus also creates a constant pressure directed peripherally to the fibers of the anulus (Fig. 6.23). The hydrophilic character of the nucleus decreases during constant load and advanced age, and this contributes to the reduction of spinal flexibility. The preload pressure of the nucleus is enhanced by about 30 lb of inherent pressure exerted by the anulus and intervertebral ligaments.

Loading. In the static position, the load on a disc is much greater than the superimposed body weight. This is the result of the center of gravity being anterior to the disc causing a bending moment that must be resisted by posterior muscle action that increases the compression force. During forward flexion, the L3 disc is subjected to about double the body weight above. If a 45-lb external load is added (eg, a child being lifted) the disc carries a force three times the superimposed body weight. These pressures are substantially increased in the sitting position. During erect dynamic activities, disc forces rise to double static forces without the addition of external load.

Reaction of Axial Tension. When a vertebral motion unit is subjected to elongation (eg, during vertical stretching, A-P and lateral bending, rotation while flexed, mechanical traction, or hanging from a horizontal bar), the vertebral bodies tend to separate, the disc thickens, nuclear pressure reduces, and vertical anular fiber tension toward the periphery of the disc increases. Tensile loads produce perpendicular normal stresses that are readily absorbed by the crisscrossed anular layers and relatively larger parallel shear stress in the anulus that has little resistance. This is an early factor in most disc failures (Fig. 6.24).

Reaction to Axial Compression. When

Table 6.1.
Intervertebral Disc Regional Variables (Approximate)

Discs	Average thickness	Disc/Body ratio	Nucleus/Anulus ratio	Position to vertical axis
Cervical	3 mm	2:5	4:7 (57% nucleus)	Centered—posterior
Thoracic	5 mm	1:5	3:7 (43% nucleus)	Posterior
Lumbar	9 mm	1:3	4:6 (67% nucleus)	Centered—posterior

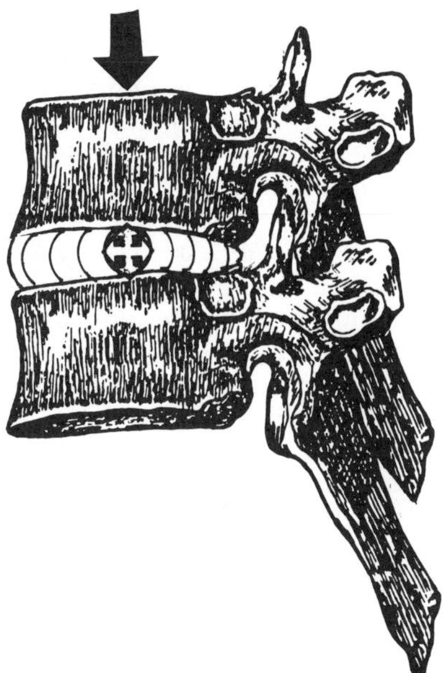

Figure 6.23. The preloaded nucleus pulposus exerts pressure in all directions in the neutral state.

a vertebral motion unit is under axial compression (eg, body weight, with or without external load), the vertebral bodies tend to approximate, the disc flattens, nuclear pressure increases, the endplates are subjected to greater pressure, and anular fiber tension increases from forces projected laterally from the nucleus.[87] Forces are normally transmitted evenly throughout the nucleus. The closed, pressurized container of the nucleus conforms to the law of Pascal, which states that "any external force exerted on a unit area of a confined liquid is transmitted undiminished to every unit area of the interior of the containing vessel." The anular fibers are stressed somewhat vertically (compressive) and horizontally (tensive) but greater in line with their obliqueness (tensile). A disc is stiffer under compression than tension because nuclear pressure is increased under compression.[88]

This centralized loading tends to deflect the endplates away from the disc at the periphery so that the dimension of the disc increases centrally and the center of the end-plate becomes deformed.[89] Such loading *cannot* produce disc rupture (unless the disc is burst by an unusually heavy and fast axial force) even if the disc is torn, but the disc does bulge (especially laterally and anteriorly) as it flattens. If excessive loading fractures an endplate centrally, the nucleus tends to be driven into the vertebral body (traumatic Schmorl's node).

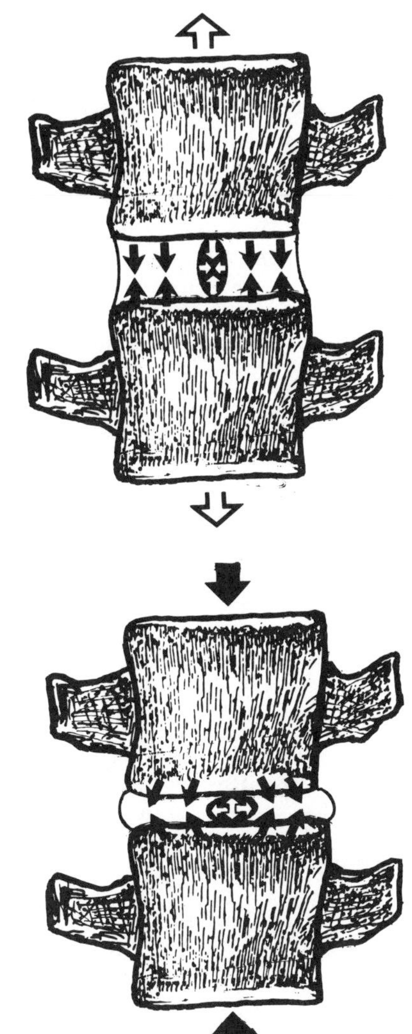

Figure 6.24. *Top*, in axial tension, nucleus pressure reduces and the anular fibers, especially at the periphery, offer tensile resistance. *Bottom*, in axial compression, pressure within the nucleus increases and tension within the anular fibers increases from forces projected horizontally from the nucleus.

When compression load to a motion unit becomes excessive, the unit fails with fracture of the endplate or vertebral body and little damage to the disc.[90] Bending and torsional stresses appear to be more dangerous to disc integrity than axial loads. However, once a disc becomes degenerated, the stress of compression load substantially increases. Central endplate fractures are more often associated with a healthy disc with a firm nucleus that generates maximum bending moments at the plate. In contrast, peripheral endplate fractures are commonly associated with a degenerated nucleus in which most forces are carried via the outer anulus.

Reactions to Asymmetrical Forces. When a disc is loaded unilaterally, the disc initially becomes wedge-shaped and the normally parallel vertebral plateaus form an angle (Fig. 6.25). This vertically stretches the anular fibers opposite to the weight-bearing side, but this action is quickly *counteracted by opposite forces transmitted laterally from the nucleus* to help the disc return to its normal shape. This self-stabilization factor is the product of a healthy nucleus and anulus working as a mechanical couple.[91]

Reaction to Oblique Forces. When a load is applied obliquely to the superior vertebra of a motion unit, the force is resolved into (1) a vertical force that tends to flatten the disc directly under the point of

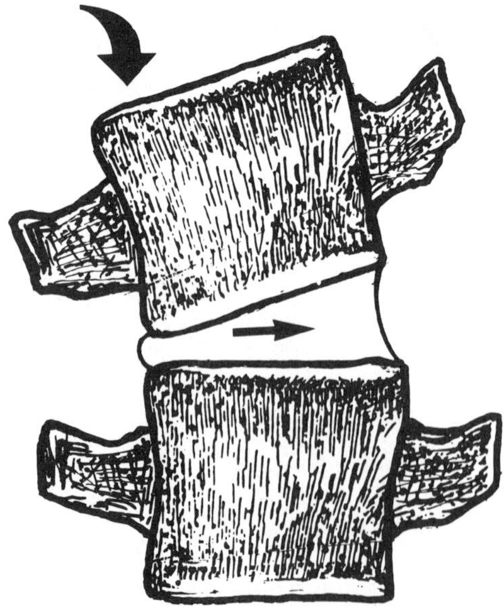

Figure 6.25. When a disc is loaded asymmetrically, the anulus bulges on the side of force and stretches on the side opposite the force. These compression and tensile forces tend to stabilize each other (rebound) with help from nuclear horizontal forces toward the opposite direction.

application and to approximate the vertebrae, and (2) a horizontal force parallel to the plateaus that tends to move the upper vertebra toward the direction of force. This motion stretches the anular fibers in the direction of force, which sets up a self-stabilizing couple effect.

Reaction to Flexion, Extension, and Lateral Forces. When the spine is subjected to bending loads during flexion, half of the disc on the convex side suffers tension, widening, and contraction, while the other half of the disc on the concave side suffers compression, thinning, and bulging (Fig. 6.26).[92] Concurrently, and in opposite fashion, the nucleus bulges on the side of tension and contracts on the side of compression, which increases tension on the adjacent anulus. As mentioned, this creates a self-stabilizing counteracting flexion force to the motion unit that aids a return to the resting position.[91] An opposite reaction is seen during spinal extension, when the nucleus bulges forward and tension is increased on the anterior anulus to establish a counterforce. During lateral flexion, the anulus and upper vertebra tilt toward the base on the side of abduction and the nucleus bulges away from the side of flexion.

Reaction to Rotary Forces. As mentioned, the apposing layers of anular fibers run alternately oblique in opposite directions. When a vertebra twists, the oblique fibers angled toward the direction of rotation become stretched, and the oblique fibers running against the direction of rotation tend to relax (Fig. 6.27). The greatest tension from stretch is seen centrally, where the fibers are nearly horizontal. This increases nuclear pressure by compression in proportion to the amount of rotation and is the most frequent mechanism of traumatic disc rupture. At the transitional areas of the spine, these forces are often magnified by one region rotating clockwise while the other is firmly fixed or rotating counterclockwise (eg, scoliosis, shoveling, sports injuries).

Farfan's cadaver studies showed that lumbar rotation is associated with a anterolateral tilt that increases the distance between the lateral margins of the vertebral bodies on the side of convexity.[93] This especially stretches the posterolateral anulus,

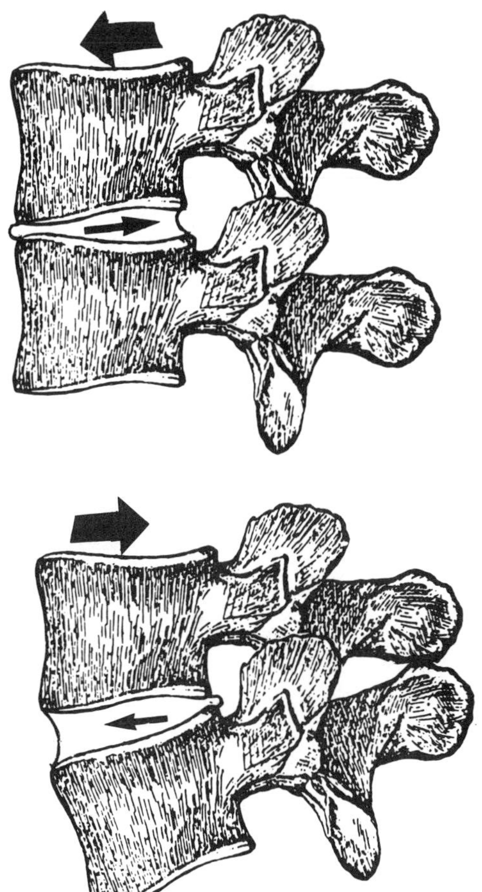

Figure 6.26. The hydraulic mechanism of the intervertebral disc. During flexion (*top*) the anterior anulus bulges from compression and the posterior anulus stretches from the tensile load. The nucleus follows this linear action by being shifted slightly posteriorly, but bulges and contracts in the opposite directions to the bulging and stretching of the anulus. During extension (*bottom*), the opposite processes occur.

and excessive rotation produces a bulging of part of the disc with a compensatory contraction of its contralateral aspect. The anular filaments may separate, causing the disc to lose some of its stiffness property and an inability of the vertebral segment to return to its normal position when the torsion stress is removed. If this were to happen in vivo, a chronic unstable rotational subluxation could be expected to result.

Reaction to Torsion and Shear. Several studies indicate that torsional stress is the type of stress most damaging to discs. Torsion forces in a disc produce horizontal and vertical shear stresses of equal magnitude that vary relative to the instantaneous axis of rotation. The most damaging shear forces are those perpendicular to fiber direction.

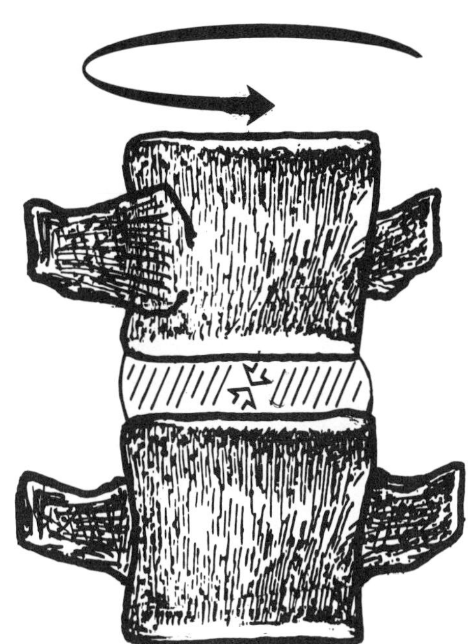

Figure 6.27. During spinal rotation, the oblique fibers of the anulus angled in the direction of movement become tensile loaded. Those fibers angled opposite to the direction of movement relax.

Resistance to torsion is offered essentially by the discs and facet joints, in almost equal proportion. Farfan points out that discs in the lumbar spine are not equally sensitive to torsional stress.[94] The upper lumbar discs, which are fairly round, are more resistant to torsion than the lower kidney-shaped discs. An L5 that is deeply seated in the pelvis, has a large lumbosacral angle, or has short iliotransverse ligaments is quite protective against torsion. However, these same factors that protect against torsion will subject the area to greater axial forces (Fig. 6.28).

The shear stresses resulting from torsional loading are fairly concentrated along the periphery of the anulus with a much smaller amount located centrally. A disc has a high stiffness resistance to shear in the horizontal plane; thus it is rare that a nucleus would fail from shear load alone.

Creep and Relaxation Behavior. The *viscoelastic* properties of the disc offer it

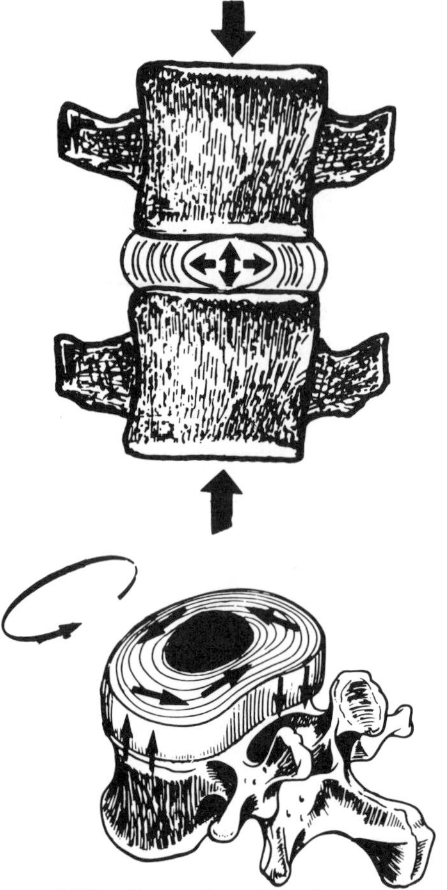

Figure 6.28. *Top*, schematic of compression meeting nuclear pressure. The anulus is bulged outward, and the endplates are depressed. *Bottom*, torsional forces produce great horizontal as well as axial shear stress.

creep and *relaxation* behavior. The greater the load, the greater the deformation and the faster the rate of creep. A degenerated disc exhibits less viscoelasticity, less creep, and less capability of attenuating shocks and vibrations uniformly over the full surfaces of the endplates.[95]

Fatigue and Hysteresis Properties. The viscoelastic nature of a disc offers other time-dependent properties such as *fatigue* and *hysteresis*, which vary in reaction depending upon whether the load is applied quickly with high amplitude (jerk) or slowly with a low magnitude (pressure fatigue failure). As the repair and regeneration capabilities of the avascular disc are low, the fatigue life of a disc is quite low when subjected to repetitive loading. On failure, the result is radial and circumferential tears. When a disc is subjected to repetitive cycles of load and unload (eg, hopping), the shock waves directed from the feet to the head are substantially absorbed by disc hysteresis. This effect is minimal in the T9–L2 area. It decreases when the load-unload cycle is prolonged (eg, constant bumping) and during old age when viscoelasticity is low.[96]

The Apophyseal Joints[97–99]

The articulating processes have synovial joint capsules that are strengthened by two strong anterior and posterior ligaments, with fibers running perpendicular to the facet plane. They attach just beyond the margin of the facets. They are quite loose and elastic in the cervical region to allow greater mobility without capsule stretch. They are tighter and stronger in the thoracic and lumbar regions.

Functional Considerations

The faces of the articular facets are covered by tough hyaline cartilage and separated by meniscus-like tabs of synovium that originate from the synovial lining. These tabs glide in and out of the joint during motion, but are rarely nipped during joint jamming. The tabs appear to allow a degree of extra shock-absorbing and pressure-absorbing protection for the articular cartilage.

Vertebral tilting as seen in subluxations with disc wedging alters the relationship of apposing articular surfaces to produce a change in the direction of compressive forces on these joints. In contrast, severe rotation produces a jamming compression on ipsilateral facets and contralateral facet opening. When continuous compression is applied to any active and mobile joint, cartilaginous erosion followed by arthritis can be expected.

Possible pain-provoking mechanisms at the facet joints include capsular ligament sprain, facet jamming or fixation by subluxation, pinching of a synovial fringe, entrapment of a loose cartilaginous body in the joint, and cervical or lumbar meniscoid entrapment.

Contribution to Stability

It has long been thought that the posterior ligaments provide the majority of joint stability to the spine. Studies on the lumbar spine, however, have shown that the apophyseal joints provide a greater restraint to flexion and extension movements than do the lumbar ligaments.[100] These researchers also found that the age changes that most severely influence movement in the elderly occur in the IVDs rather than in the posterior elements.

Changes within a Subluxation Complex

The posterior articular facets of the spine possess the histological capability to account for many of the various phenomena found in the subluxation syndrome. Their close proximity to the IVF is of special interest because both structural and functional changes in these facets have been shown to affect the nerve root.

In writing of experimental investigations of the apophyseal joints, especially of normal joint structures and their reaction to injury, Reiter describes an anatomical study of 75 postmortem spines that revealed significant changes, many of which would not be visible on x-ray.[99] The capsular changes included edema, granular ossification, calcification, and adhesion between the capsule and the meningeal covering of the nerve root adjacent to it. The intra-articular changes included hypertrophy of the menisci up to four times normal size, occasional chondrification and ossification of the menisci, detached bodies, ulcerated areas of denuded hyaline cartilage, cartilage thinning, fibrillation, and osteophytic marginal proliferation.

The Spinal Ligaments and Pertinent Syndesmology[101,102]

In the spine, as in the extremities, the purpose of a ligament is to limit or modify joint movement. The articulation between the adjacent vertebral bodies is supported by the anterior and posterior longitudinal ligaments. During dynamic actions, the resiliency of these ligaments offers a cushioning effect that does much to relieve stress on the anulus. The articulations of the vertebral arches are essentially supported by the ligamenta flava and the supraspinous, interspinous, and intertransverse ligaments.

Functional Anatomy[103,104]

Groups of unaxial fibrous ligaments link together vertebral segments, commonly check axial tensile forces, and infrequently buckle under axial compression (Fig. 6.29). They must be elastic enough to allow physiologic motion, be strong enough to resist excessive motion, exhibit some pretension in the neutral state to provide some stability, and be damping and ductile enough to absorb shock energy without permanent deformation.

The anterior and posterior longitudinal ligaments have intimate attachment to the vertebral bodies and disc spaces, exhibit

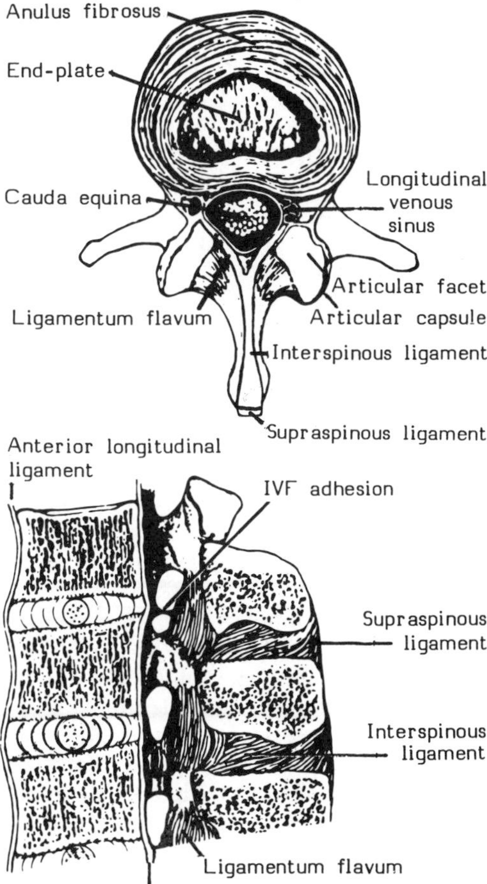

Figure 6.29. *Top*, view from above the major spinal ligaments; *bottom*, lateral view of a midsagittal spinal section.

slight in situ pretension, readily stretch with disc bulge, and lose much of their viscoelastic properties in old age. They extend from the base of the occiput to the sacrum, are strong against A-P stress, but may be sprained by excessive rotation.

Anterior Longitudinal Ligament. This ligament narrows at its origin at the occiput, widens as it descends, and is firmly attached to the atlas and the anterolateral surfaces of the vertebrae periosteum. It narrows slightly at disc intervals and lightly attaches to the anterior surfaces of the IVDs. It is especially thick and narrow in the thoracic region, with some fibers extending over four or more vertebrae. Chronic traction of this ligament is believed to be the cause of anterior lipping of the vertebral body. In hyperextension (whiplash) injuries of the neck, the anterior ligaments become severely stretched.

Posterior Longitudinal Ligament. The posterior ligament covers the transverse ligament of the odontoid, the body of the axis, and the posterior surface of the vertebral bodies and discs, and finally attaches to the coccyx. It is firmly attached to the IVDs but separated from the vertebral bodies by the venous plexuses. It is also thicker in the thoracic region but widens rather than narrows at the disc level. As this ligament descends to the lumbar region, it begins to narrow so that at the S1 level it has only half its original width and offers a structural weakness to the disc posterolaterally. This is mechanically unfortunate because the discs at the lumbar area must carry severe loading forces, and this weakness contributes to a high incidence of posterolateral disc herniation at the lower lumbar area (Fig. 6.30).

Ligamentum Flava. This short, strong, yellow, highly elastic ligament covers the interlaminar spaces, spanning between the anterior surface of the lower lamina and the superoposterior surface of the higher vertebra, and serves as the posterior boundary of the spinal cord from C2 to S1. The heavy flat bands are separated at intervals in the midline by veins of the external and internal vertebral plexuses. The ligamentum flava readily stretches (35–45%) with spinal flexion, contracts (10%) without buckling in extension, and exhibits substantial in situ pretension (15%) in the neutral position,

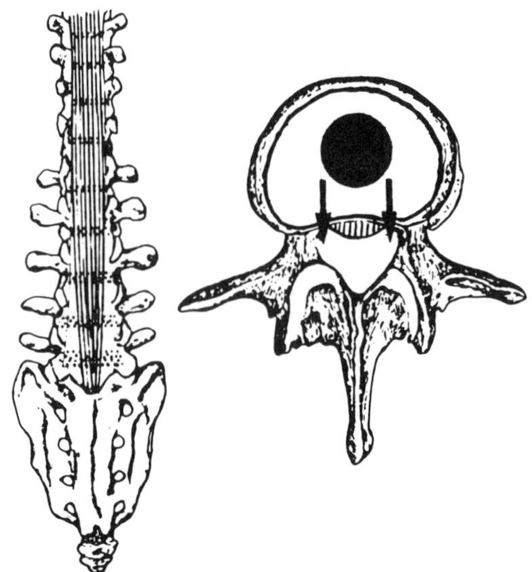

Figure 6.30. *Left*, schematic of the posterior longitudinal ligament. Note how it narrows as it descends the lumbar region, where forces tend to be unrestricted by the strap. The posterior arch of the spine has been removed in the drawing. *Right*, view from above. *Arrows* show posterolateral areas of disc weakness, where the ligament protects only centrally.

which contributes to disc pretension. This ligamentous pretension prohibits buckling upon neutral relaxation but not upon spinal extension. With aging, some of the elastic fibers (highest proportion in the body) are replaced with fibrous tissue.

Interspinous and Supraspinous Ligaments. Tough posterior interspinous and supraspinous (supraspinal) ligaments join the posterior aspects of the spinous processes from the cervical to the sacral area and reach their maximum tension when the spine is flexed. Bursal formation between the interspinous and supraspinous ligaments is quite common. The *interspinous ligaments* are poorly developed in the cervical region, thin and narrow in the thoracic region, and relatively broad and thick in the lumbar area. They connect the root and apex of each process during most of life but frequently degenerate in the later years of life. The *supraspinous ligaments,* composed of thin fibrous bundles, extend down the tips of the spinous processes as a slender band. They are well developed in the cervical region and blend with interspinous fibers to be called the *ligamentum nuchae.*

Considerable low-back shear forces are witnessed in the erect position because of the lumbar lordosis. These forces are checked somewhat by a meager supraspinous ligament which passes posteriorly to the vertebral facets. However, neither the supraspinous ligament nor the facets have any effect upon compression forces.

Intertransverse Ligament. This thin ligament attaches between the horizontal surfaces of each transverse process, serving as a biomechanical long lever when tensed. The fibers are extremely sparse in the cervical and lumbar regions but well developed in the thoracic area where the fibers are closely intertwined with the deep layer of spinal muscles.

THE VERTEBRAL CANAL AND RELATED TISSUES[46, 105, 106]

The spinal cord, continuous with the medulla oblongata at the foramen magnum, is protected within the spine anteriorly by the posterior aspect of the vertebral body, posteriorly by the bony laminae, and laterally by the pedicles. Further protection and stability are provided by the cord's three membranes, the two fluid-filled spaces, the ligamentum flava and dentate ligaments, and the nerve roots. To accommodate necessary innervation for the limbs, the spinal cord is enlarged at the cervical segments (C4–T1), essentially to supply the brachial plexus, and at the lumbosacral segments (L2–S3), essentially to supply the lumbar and sacral plexuses (Fig. 6.31). The average sagittal diameter of the adult cervical vertebral canal is 18 mm.

Cord-Canal Relationships[107]

In reference to the origin of the 31 pairs of spinal nerves, a spinal cord "segment" does not necessarily correspond in height or location to its corresponding numbered vertebra and disc and spinal nerve, or the level of the spinous process. The cervical spine contains 8 cord segments; the thoracic spine, about 20 segments; and the lumbar spine, probably only some sacral and the coccygeal segments. The adult spinal cord can generally be considered to occupy only the upper two-thirds of the vertebral canal.

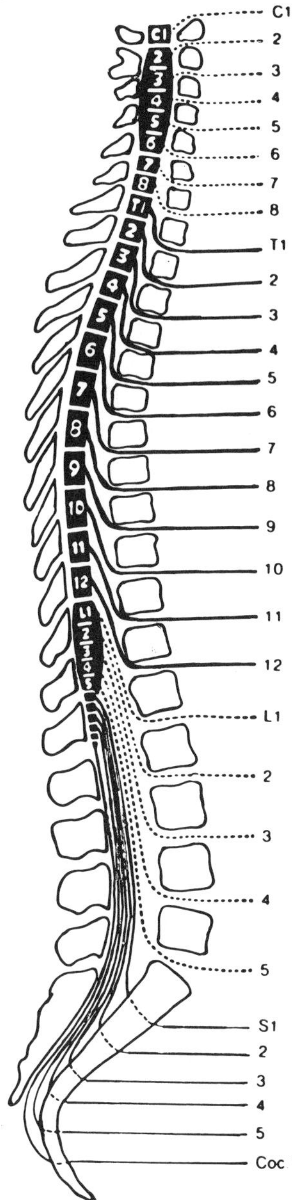

Figure 6.31. The lateral relation of spinal segments to vertebral level.

In the embryo, the spinal cord and vertebral canal are about equal in length until about the 10th week. Because the vertebral column grows faster than the spinal cord, this relationship does not persist. The cord terminates near the level of S1 at 24 weeks, the L3 disc at birth, the L2 disc at age 5 years, and higher in the adult. This is usually near the level of the L1 disc. Occasionally, it is seen during surgery to terminate in the adult as high as T12 or as low as L3.

As the lower third of the vertebral column is approached, the length and obliquity of the nerve roots must progressively increase to reach their respective IVFs.

In the adult, the average linear measurements for the cord and canal are: spinal cord in males, 45 cm, and in females, 42 cm; spinal canal in males, 70 cm, and in females, 60 cm.

The vertebral canal increases in length during spinal flexion and lateral bending, and decreases in length during extension. This is considerably reduced because of the flexion-rotation coupling that occurs. Because of its substantial degree of flexibility, the cord easily adapts to the normal lengthening and shortening of the canal during movements.[108]

Functional Anatomy[109–111]

The Meninges

The spinal cord is sheathed by three cylindrical membranes that extend from the foramen magnum to the midsacral region: the internal pia mater, the middle arachnoid, and the exterior dura mater (Fig. 6.32).

The Pia Mater. The highly vascular pia membrane covers the spinal cord proper. Its outer layer is composed essentially of a loose network of collagenous fibers, and its inner layer consists of a meshwork abundant with elastic fibers. Between these two layers is a fine network of blood vessels.

The Arachnoid. The delicate, transparent, web-like, avascular, elastic fibrous arachnoid parallels the dura mater and pia mater. It is separated from the dura membrane by a serous fluid-filled potentially subdural space that contains threads of connecting subdural trabeculae. It is separated from the pia membrane by a cerebrospinal fluid-filled subarachnoid space that contains tiny venous plexuses and threads of connecting arachnoid trabeculae that become continuous with the outer collagenous pia membrane. When considered together, the pia mater and arachnoid are called the leptomeninges.

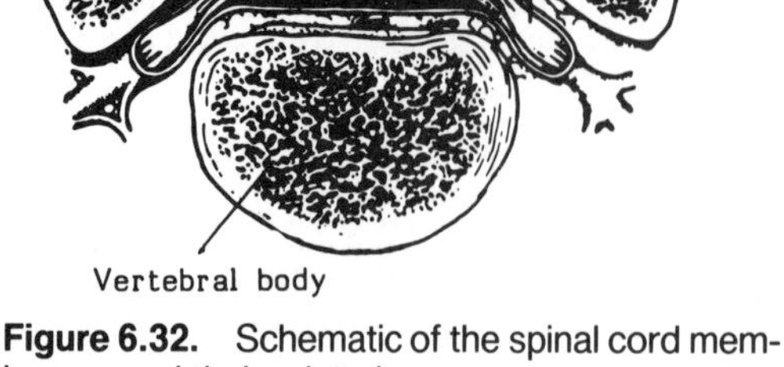

Figure 6.32. Schematic of the spinal cord membranes and their related spaces.

The Biodynamical Aspects of Cerebrospinal Fluid. It is widely accepted that a primary function of cerebrospinal fluid (CSF) is to provide lymphatic drainage for the central nervous system (CNS), that this fluid has one of the smallest time constants of any body fluid, and that stagnant or altered CSF flow has an adverse influence on CNS function. Freedman makes a good case that biomechanical aberrations of the spinal column may adversely affect CSF flow and CNS function. It is hypothesized that this cause-effect relationship may be a common physiologic denominator within various (seemingly different but often equally effective) chiropractic adjustment techniques.[112]

The Dura Mater. The tough, dense, outer connective tissue dura mater is separated from the bony canal by a potential space filled with fat and veins, which helps to reduce friction and contributes to the absorption of shock energy. However, the dura is firmly attached at the foramen magnum, at the bodies of C2 and C3, and in the remaining spine by bridging trabeculae. As well as enclosing the spinal cord, the dura also envelops the spinal roots, nerve, and ganglia as it passes through the IVF and becomes continuous with the epineurium.

The dura, arachnoid, and pia membranes tightly invest the spinal roots as well as the spinal cord, and their extensions surround the cauda equina and fuse at the external terminal filum.

The Dentate Ligaments

The 20–21 dentate (sawtoothed) ligaments derive from thickened pia mater. They are inferiorly inclined and extend bilaterally between the anterior and posterior nerve roots from the foramen magnum to the T12–L1 area, penetrate the arachnoid and its fluid-filled spaces, and fix to the inner surface of the dura membrane (Fig. 6.33). They provide a unique pretensed suspension system against sudden jars.[113] It is because of the dentate ligaments that the spinal cord and nerve roots, but not the rootlets, are put under tension during spinal movements.

The Spinal Cord Proper

Cord Flexibility. Although dentate ligaments help to stabilize the spinal cord in a central position in the canal and help to protect against undue stretch, the cord is still flexible enough (10% of length) under small loads to move as much as ⅜ inch. The cord is quite elastic when deformed axially, but prone to severe damage if a vertebra is displaced horizontally.

A space-occupying sclerotic or fibrotic lesion will restrict the cord's mobility and extensibility and thus increase tensile, torsion, and compression stresses. The symptoms thus produced can be alleviated if the cord can be relaxed.

Grieve implies that if a biomechanical evaluation could be routinely conducted at the microscopic level in clinical practice, many neurologic disorders in which no mechanical component is suspected would be shown to have their origin in tension of nervous and vascular microtissues producing a reduction of conduit diameter that interferes with function.[114] We should be reminded here that D. D. Palmer stated before the turn of the century that "chiropractic as a science is founded on tone."[115]

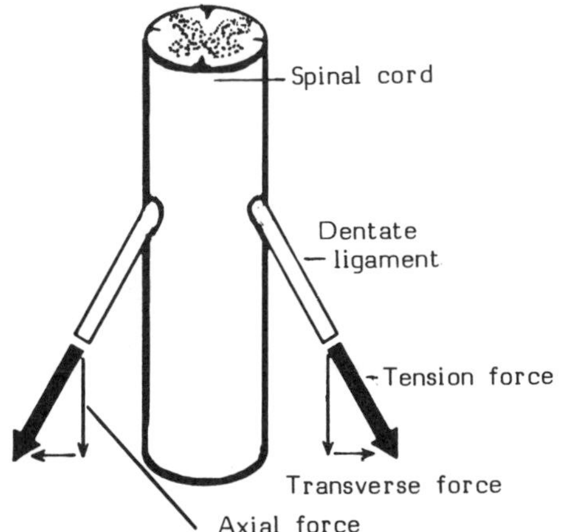

Figure 6.33. A unilateral diagonal dentate ligament would provide the spinal cord with axial and transverse pretension, but the bilateral pair offers the added benefit of resistance against axial tension.

Cord Folds. In its neutral state, the cord possesses accordion-like folds that flatten on stretch (flexion) and increase on relaxation (extension). This folding and unfolding mechanism is responsible for about three-quarters of the cord's change in length from full flexion to full extension. Once these folds have flattened during spinal flexion, the cord is subjected to direct tensile forces. Like a rubber band, the diameter of the cord then reduces on stretch and increases on relaxation.

The Cervical Cord. Inasmuch as maximum cervical movement is located at the C5–C6 level and the spinal cord snugly fills the cervical canal, degenerative arthritic changes and disc herniations in this area may encroach upon the canal contents. As the cervical cord is at its maximum width at this level, injury may readily lead to neurologic damage.

The Lumbar Cord. The spinal cord ends near the L1 disc. Below this, the elements of the cauda equina are within the vertebral canal of the lumbar spine. The mobility of the cauda equina roots in the relatively large canal provides a safety factor not found in the cervical or thoracic regions. This safety factor, however, is minimized in spinal stenosis.

The Spinal Nerves[116, 117]

A single spinal nerve trunk is a mixture of several posterior sensory (afferent) and anterior motor (efferent) rootlets. The anterior fibers arise from cell bodies in the spinal cord's ventral gray horn, while the posterior fibers are from cell bodies in the spinal dorsal root ganglia that lie outside the cord and partially within the IVF. A ganglion usually rests against the pedicle. Except for C1 and C2, which do not have IVFs, the common trunk forms just outside the IVF, where it quickly divides into anterior and posterior rami (Fig. 6.34).

The posterior rami turn sharply backward to supply the spinal muscles and skin of the back. Sunderland feels that the passage of

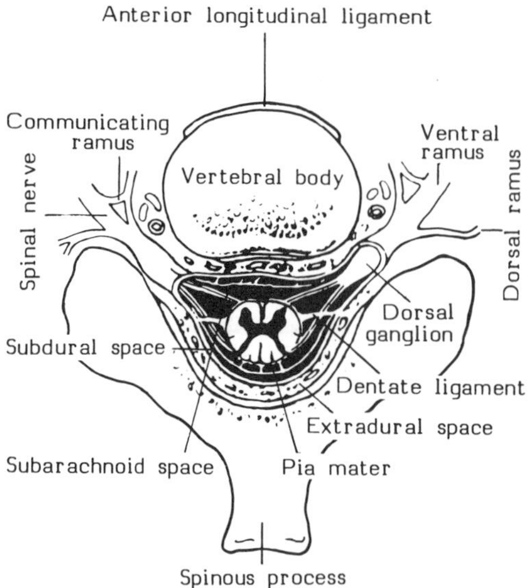

Figure 6.34. The relationship of the major contents of the vertebral canal as viewed from above.

the cutaneous branches through the muscles and fascia of the back should not be overlooked as potential sites of entrapment.[118] Such entrapment most frequently occurs of the greater occipital nerve and the cutaneous branches of the posterior rami of L1–L3 nerves.

A few posterior rami intermix branches but most remain segmental. The anterior rami run anterior and laterally, and most enter into plexuses or connect with sympathetic fibers by way of the rami communicantes, whereafter their specific identity is impossible to determine. In the fused sacral region, the anterior and posterior rami exit the bony canal through the anterior and posterior foramina, respectively.

The nerve roots are not normally firmly attached to the margins of the IVFs, and thus are able to move about quite freely during spinal motions. However, fibrotic changes following the granulation tissue of irritation, especially in the lower cervical region, frequently fix the sleeve at one or more points which contributes to traction on the sheath and its contents during movements. These attachments increase in strength with aging and other degenerative changes.

Position

Position in Foramina. In the cervical spine, the nerve root is anterior and inferior to the facets; in the thoracic spine, directly anterior to the facets (Fig. 6.35); and in the lumbar spine, anterior and superior to the facets, under the pedicles.

Foraminal Compression. The nerve root is often compressed in the IVF by a subluxated articular facet and less often by a herniated disc or a spur from the posterior aspect of the vertebral body. These disorders can be worsened by a state of spinal stenosis which narrows the vertebral canal and the tunnels by which the nerve roots must pass as they exit the IVFs.

Sensory Manifestations[119–121]

Segmental Sensory Supply. The area of a vertebral motion unit derives high-threshold sensory fibers from:

1. The (usually) two fine branches of the recurrent (sinuvertebral) meningeal nerve, running anterior to the spinal nerve in the IVF. An autonomic branch from the paravertebral plexus accompanies the recurrent spinal nerve, usually within the same sheath. These supply the anterior dura, the blood vessels of the spinal canal, the posterior longitudinal ligament, the cortex of the vertebral bodies, and the surface of the

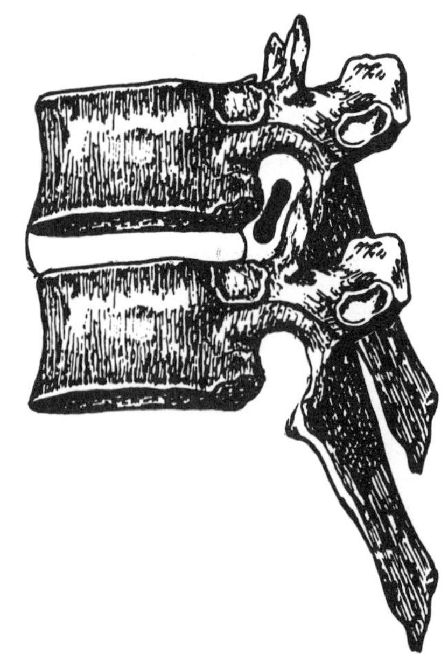

Figure 6.35. The position of the nerve root within the thoracic region is directly anterior to the facets. Most nerve roots occupy about 50% of the ovoid foraminal space.

posterior anulus. No fibers, or extremely few fibers, enter the central disc. Communicating and linking branches extend across, up, and down at least one segment, and frequently produce radiating or referred symptoms.

2. The medial branch of the posterior primary ramus. These fibers supply the ligaments and muscles of the posterior aspect of the vertebral unit. As in all synovial joints, the capsules of the articular processes, their fat pads, and their intrinsic and extrinsic ligaments are richly endowed with pain and proprioception fibers. This nerve also sends communicating and linking branches across, up, and down at least a segment. Figure 6.36 depicts most pain-sensitive and nonsensitive areas of a vertebral motion unit.

From this we can see that the vertebral joint itself receives innervation from rostral and caudal segments in addition to those from the local segment. This means that a segmentally arranged nerve supply (with its specific dermatomes, muscles, and reflexes) is not available to evaluate a particular vertebral motion unit with certainty.

Nerve Fiber Proportions. There are about three times more sensory fibers than motor fibers in the cervical area, one and a half more in the thoracic region, and twice as many in the lumbar area.

Pain Distribution. When the anterior root is irritated, pain is felt in the muscles supplied and often becomes self-perpetuating from the focal spasm produced (ie, a trigger point syndrome) with myotomal distribution. When the posterior root is irritated, pain is felt in its dermatomal distribution.

The Autonomics

Because the autonomic nerve pathways innervating musculoskeletal tissues are intimately connected with the spinal nerves, one can appreciate that these systems do not operate in isolation[122,123] (Fig. 6.37). Structural disorders in the spine frequently cause, contribute to, or mimic such "functional" disorders as Ménière's disease, causalgia, shoulder-hand syndrome, asthma, sphincter spasms, cluster headaches, angina, and a large variety of referred pains.

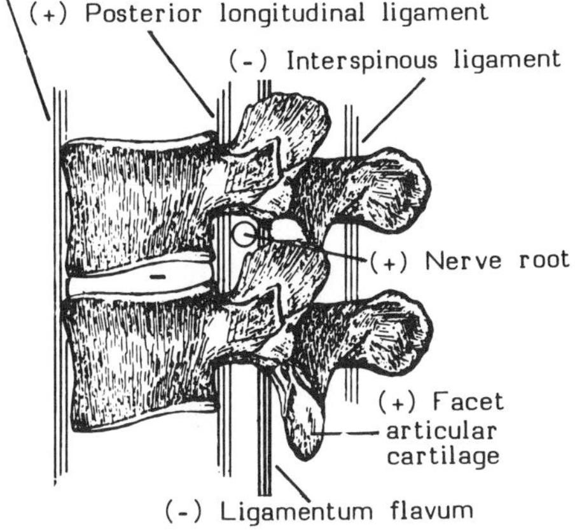

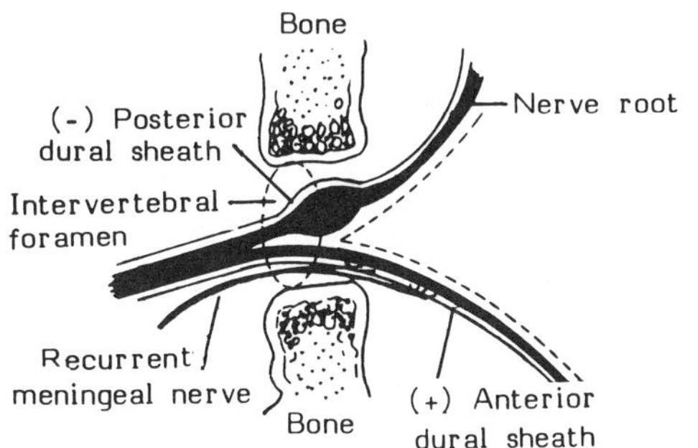

Figure 6.36. *Top*, the posterior and anterior longitudinal ligaments, nerve root, facet articular cartilage and capsule, paravertebral muscles and fascia, walls of the arteries and veins, and periosteum of the vertebral body are pain-sensitive tissues (+). The deep and anterolateral aspects of the IVD, the ligamentum flavum, and the interspinous ligament are considered nonsensitive (−) because they are devoid of sensory fibers, but their exterior surfaces are usually innervated. *Bottom*, in addition to the above, the posterior dural sheath of the nerve root is not pain sensitive, but the anterior portion of the sheath is supplied by the recurrent meningeal nerve and is pain sensitive.

SPINAL CIRCULATION AND PERTINENT ANGIOLOGY[124–126]

All skeletal muscles have a rich blood supply consisting of an intricate network of capillaries. The arrangement of the capillary network is such that each muscle fiber is placed in relation to several (4 or 5) capillary vessels. Many of these capillaries are closed during rest, opening only on the demand of activity.

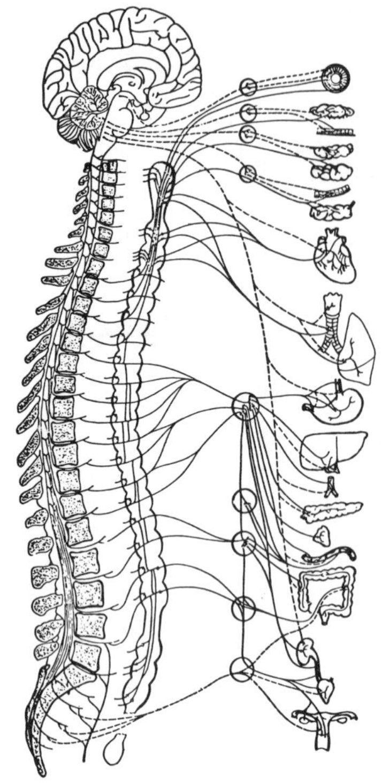

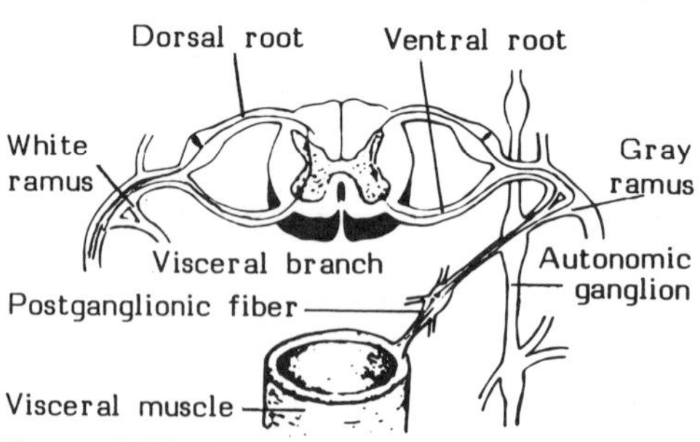

Figure 6.37. *Top*, the wide distribution of the autonomic nervous system and its relationship to the spinal nerves. *Bottom*, the relationship of the spinal cord to automatic ganglia and viscera.

The average body contains about 62,000 miles of capillaries whose surface area totals 6300 square miles. With these data in mind, it is understandable that strong muscular contractions can effect fatigue and soreness by obstructing capillary circulation to continuously working muscles.

Area Vasculature

The Arterial System

An anterior artery, descending in the ventral median sulcus, and two posterior arteries, descending along the posterolateral sulcus, supply the spine (Fig. 6.38). The latter arise from either the vertebral arteries or the posteroinferior cerebellar arteries. These anterior and posterior axial conduits are often small, irregular, and must be reinforced at intervals by radicular arteries that branch from nearby spinal arteries arising outside the vertebral column.[127]

In the cervical area, the vertebral artery runs in the foramen transversarium of the transverse processes of C2–C6 and offers branches to each segment. Similar arteries arise from the intercostal and lumbar arteries branching from the aorta. The lateral sacral arteries give branches to the sacral segments. In each instance, the segmental artery offers several anterior twigs to the front and sides of the vertebral body and posterior branches to the spinal muscles and IVF. After the latter branch passes through the IVF, it enters the vertebral canal and divides into three branches: (1) an anterior branch, which (*a*) supplies the posterior aspect of the vertebral body to anastomose with the lateral and anterior twigs of that part of the artery that did not enter the IVF, and (*b*) gives off ascending and descending twigs; (2) an intermediate branch, which supplies the nerve root and spinal dura; and (3) a posterior branch, which supplies the vertebral arch, extradural contents, and dura.

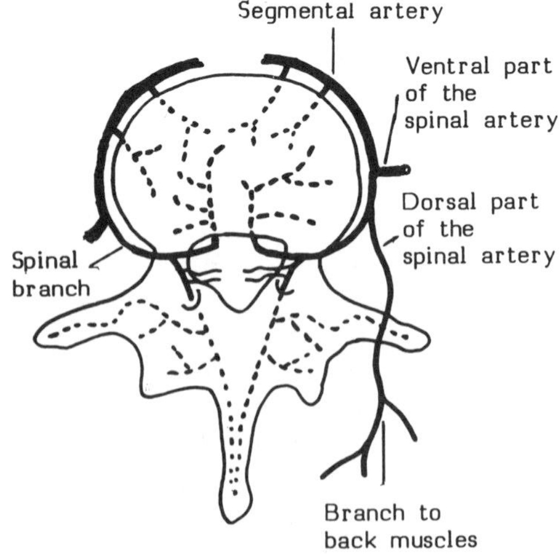

Figure 6.38. Schematic of the arterial supply of the vertebral area, as viewed from above.

The Venous System

The venous system of the spine (Batson's plexus) is a valveless plexus separate from that of the thoracoabdominal cavities. It is derived from the veins of the extremities, body wall, neck, and head. Any increase in intrathoracic or intra-abdominal pressure (eg, Valsalva maneuver) shunts venous blood to the vertebral system. This contributes to the spinal pain of many patients with structural spinal faults. The close tie between spinous venous pressure and neurologic integrity is clearly exhibited when the jugular compression test elicits paresthesia in the lower extremities.

Cord Circulation[128, 129]

Arterial Supply

Each cervical vertebral artery offers a branch at the brain stem to form a single anterior spinal artery which runs the length of the cord lying over the median fissure. It tapers as it courses downward in the thoracic cord and gives off central branches at intervals of about 2 mm which, in turn, branch both peripherally and centrally. The anterior spinal artery supplies all the cord with the exception of the posterior columns and posterior horns.

In addition, the vertebral arteries contribute a branch to unilateral posterior spinal arteries that form longitudinal plexiform channels as they progress caudally to supply the posterior columns and horns. The anterior spinal artery appears to be the main source of blood supply to the posterior arteries below the upper thoracic level.

Radicular Support

The arterial system of the cord does not have extensive collateral circulation. It relies heavily on extraspinal radicular artery sources. Any interruption of these (eg, IVF encroachment) can produce serious neurologic damage. The superior portion of the anterior spinal artery is assisted by radicular arteries that enter through the IVFs of the midcervical, lower cervical, and upper thoracic levels. A large radicular artery (great spinal) enters between the T9 and L3 levels and is believed to be responsible for one-fourth to one-half the blood supply of the cord below this level. A severe drop in blood pressure for 3–5 minutes can so compromise radicular circulation that necrosis of the thoracic neurons occurs.

Venous Drainage

The abundant veins of the spinal cord drain into the intervertebral veins which communicate with other plexuses. The immediate part of the system involves the (1) internal plexuses, whose pia branches drain the contents of the vertebral canal, vertebral arch, and posterior vertebral body and leave through the IVF; and (2) external plexuses, which drain the anterior and lateral aspects of the vertebral body and its associated tissues (Fig. 6.39). If the prostate is cancerous, pelvic blood returning to the heart via the

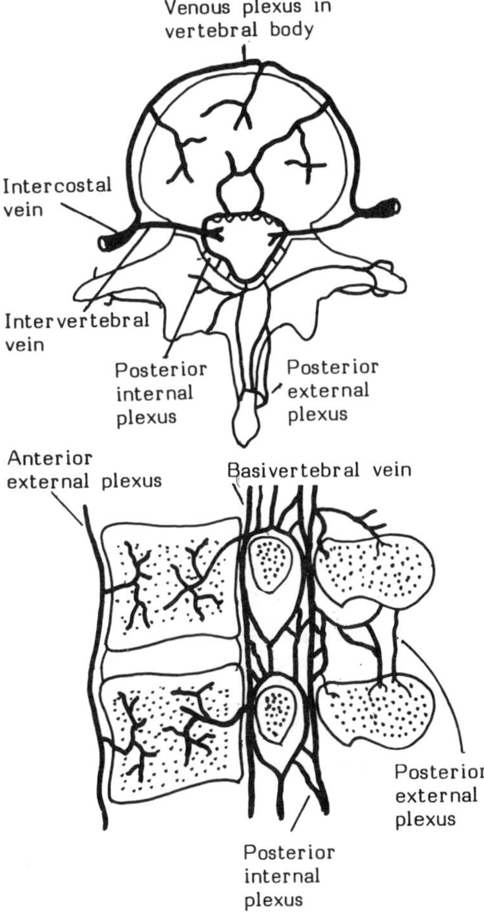

Figure 6.39. *Top*, schematic of the venous supply of the vertebral area, as viewed from above; *bottom*, a lateral midsagittal section of the area, showing the relationship of the major veins to the osseous structures and soft tissue areas.

vertebral plexuses rather than the inferior vena cava may initiate spinal metastasis.

Disc Nutrition[130, 131]

The IVD or at least the nucleus pulposus is primitive mesenchymal tissue. Only during early life does it have a blood supply, namely a twig of the spinal artery of the corresponding level. This artery, which arises bilaterally, penetrates at the posterolateral aspect of the disc. In the early months of fetal life, it involutes and atrophies. Thereafter, discs obtain nutrition by means of canaliculus seepage and imbibition of adjacent fluids through the endplates and anulus.[132] This does not mean that IVDs are biologically inert like cartilage. They have a high rate of metabolic activity that is dependent on the vascularity of the core of the vertebral bodies above and below (Fig. 6.40).

The Dynamic Craniospinal System

While the cranial sutures are immovable in cadavers and anatomic specimens, they are slightly movable in the living body, although it is often taught that they are not. The two uniting and five intervening layers between the edges of adjacent bones in the skull offer a strong bond of union but one which will permit definite but limited movement.[133] This movement is necessary for the tissue respiration of the brain and spinal

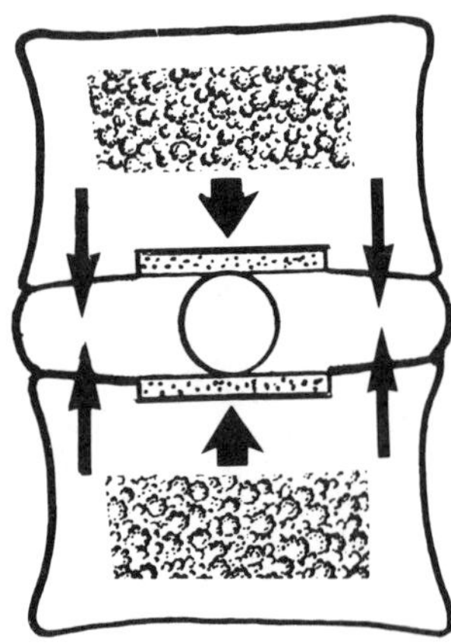

Figure 6.40. The transfer of nutrients occurs from the spongiosa marrow of the vertebral body through the endplates and the anulus. Glucose and oxygen pass via the central endplates; sulfate, to form anular fibers, passes via the peripheral anulus.

cord and is controlled by the following structures and motions: (1) the inherent motility of the brain and spinal cord, (2) the fluctuations of the cerebrospinal fluid, (3) the mobility of the intracranial and intraspinal membranes, (4) the articular mobility of the cranial bones, and (5) the involuntary mobility of the sacrum between the ilia. Lay and others report this based upon the separate research of Sutherland, Becker, and Retzlaff.[134]

Involuntary Cranial Motion

Every organ in the body exhibits a pulsation or inherent rhythmic action which features a slow, worm-like movement.[135] The brain and spinal cord are no exceptions to this, manifesting a slow, rhythmic coiling and uncoiling of the hemispheres and a longitudinal movement of the spinal cord within the spinal dura. This combined motility of the central nervous system and movement of the cerebrospinal fluid manifest as a hydrodynamic activity (pump) and a bioelectric interchange (dynamo). Upon very light palpation of the cranium, this pulsation can be felt to have a rate of about 10 to 14 cycles per minute. It is the result of the pull of the dural membranes, the fluctuating cerebrospinal fluid, and the inherent motility of the CNS.

The sphenobasilar symphysis appears to be the key cranial articulation. Prior to 25 years of age, it has a cartilaginous union; after this age, it has the resiliency of cancellous bone. Flexion of both the sphenoid and occiput increases the dorsal convexity and results in elevation of the phenobasilar symphysis toward the vertex. Extension does just the reverse. In other words, flexion of the midline bones appears as a slight increase in convexity; extension, a slight decrease in convexity. The occiput, sphenoid, ethmoid, and vomer are primarily involved. The paired bones move in synchronized internal and external rotation with the midline bones, especially the temporals, parietals, and maxillae.

Involuntary Sacral Motion

In addition to normal voluntary and postural motions of the sacrum, between the ilia, the sacrum responds to the inherent motility of the CNS, fluctuation of the cerebrospinal fluid, and pull of the intracranial and intraspinal membranes in a fashion similar to that of the cranial bones. Upon light palpation, it is felt as a slight rocking synchronized with cranial motions.

Since all voluntary and involuntary systems are encased in fascial envelopes connected directly or indirectly to the base of the skull through the cervical, thoracic, abdominal, pelvic, and appendicular fascial connections, all organs are subjected to this rhythm in addition to the rhythms of their particular voluntary or involuntary activity throughout life. The spine, pelvis, and extremities affect the head and dental occlusion via the temporals because there is a direct dura attachment of the sacrum to the cervical spine and occiput.

THE SPINAL MUSCLES AND PERTINENT MYOLOGY[136–142]

Viewed simply, the entire spine can be contrasted with a flexible mast of a sailing ship sitting on the S1 deck, with the shoulder girdle viewed as a transverse spar. For support, there are several major triangles and inverted triangles of muscular and ligamentous check "guys" that link the mast to bony supports. When the pelvis tilts laterally downward (eg, gait, short leg), the guys automatically become taut to assist body equilibrium (Fig. 6.41). This design makes the spine a first-class lever system in which loading has a considerable mechanical advantage.

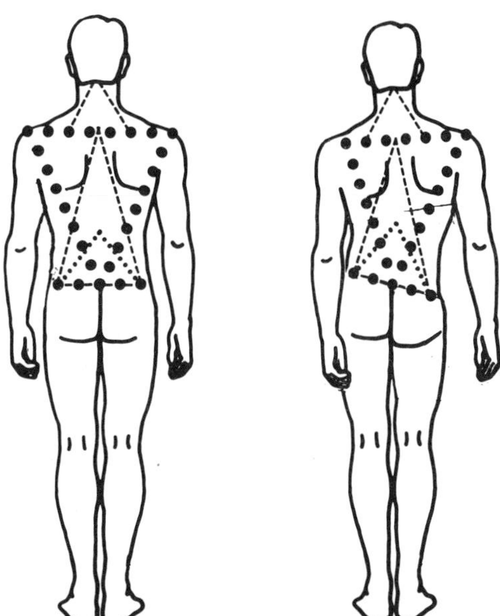

Figure 6.41. The triangular guy wire architecture of the larger spinal muscles.

The Postvertebral and Prevertebral Muscles

The spinal muscles consist of a large number of quite small muscles arranged in a complicated manner with converging and diverging fascicles. They are arbitrarily grouped by location or function, since they work in groups rather than individually, and only some of them have biomechanical significance in the spine.

The long muscles are placed superficially, the intermediate muscles lie deeper, and the short muscles occupy the deepest layer. The superficial and intermediate muscles are the extrinsic muscles of the back, concerned primarily with movements of the shoulder girdle, trunk, and respiration. The deep spinal muscles are the intrinsic muscles of the back, concerned primarily with segmental movements of the vertebral column.

The Deep Postvertebral Intrinsic Layer

These small, short, intersegmental muscles play an important role in specific segmental movement. They include the *interspinales*, connecting adjacent spinous processes; *intertransversarii*, connecting adjacent transverse processes; *rotatores*, connecting the transverse process below to the laminae above; *levatores costarum*, connecting transverse processes to the ribs; and, deep to the semispinalis, the *multifidi*, which occupy the groove on each side of the spinous processes from the sacrum to the axis. Under the trapezius and rhomboids in the neck lie the *splenius capitis* and *cervicis*, bandage-like muscles that arise medially from the C7–T6 spinous processes and ligamentum nuchae to attach laterally on the upper cervical transverse processes and the occiput.

Fisk believes that the deep and middle layers of spinal muscle especially are the site of "tennis elbow" type lesions, with all that this implies.[143]

The Intermediate Postvertebral Extrinsic Layer

These muscles arise from the transverse processes of each vertebra and attach to the spinous process of one or more vertebrae above. They consist of the *semispinalis capitis* in the occipital area, *semispinalis cervicis* in the cervical area, and *semispinalis thoracis* in the thoracic area. The serratus inferior, superior, and posterior are intermediate muscles usually discussed with the thorax rather than the spine.

The Superficial Postvertebral Extrinsic Layer

The outer layer of spinal muscles consists of the *iliocostalis* (lumborum, thoracis, cervicis) laterally, which inserts at the rib angles and lower cervical transverse processes; the *longissimus* (thoracis, cervicis, capitis), which inserts at thoracic transverse processes and ultimately reaches the skull (Fig. 6.42); and the underdeveloped flat *spinalis* (thoracis, cervicis, capitis) medially, which attaches its medial fibers at the thoracic spinous processes. These three muscle groups are collectively called the *erector spinae* and are involved in vertebral extension. The large lumbosacral portion of the erector spinae is frequently considered as one muscle, the *sacrospinalis.*

The superficial layer also includes the levator scapulae and rhomboids, which are primarily involved in movements of the shoulder girdle.

The lateral position of the erector spinae is called the *iliocostalis system,* composed of the iliocostalis cervicis, thoracis, and lumborum divisions. Their fibers arise from ribs and insert on higher ribs except in the cervical region where they attach to transverse processes of C4–C6.

The *longissimus system* also consists of cervis, thoracis, and lumborum divisions. Lower fibers arise from the common tendon of the erector spinae and insert into lower ribs and adjacent transverse processes. Middle fibers arise from upper thoracic transverse processes and attach at C2–C6 transverse processes. Capitis fibers arise on or near the articular processes of C4–C7 and insert at the mastoid area. The major role of the iliocostalis, longissimus, and serratus systems is played in respiration and not in spinal motion. The *serratus posterior, superior,* and *inferior* arise essentially from the upper and lower thoracic spinous processes and ligamentum nuchae and insert on upper and lower ribs.

The Prevertebral Muscles

These are the four relatively large muscles that encase the abdominal area: the *rectus abdominis,* running vertically at the anterior midline; *internal oblique*; *external oblique*; and *transverse abdominis* (Fig. 6.43).

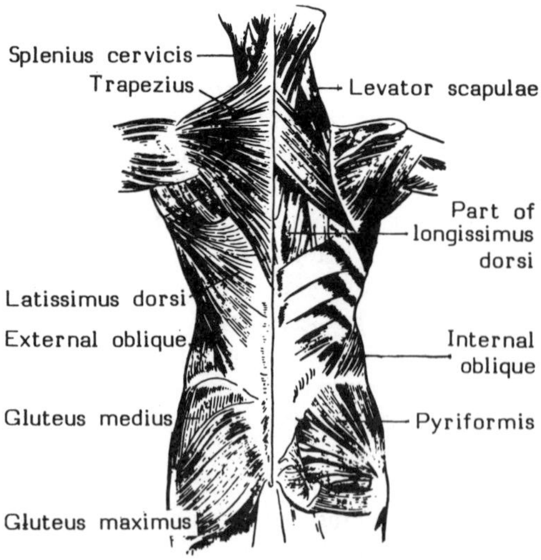

Figure 6.42. The posterior muscles of the back.

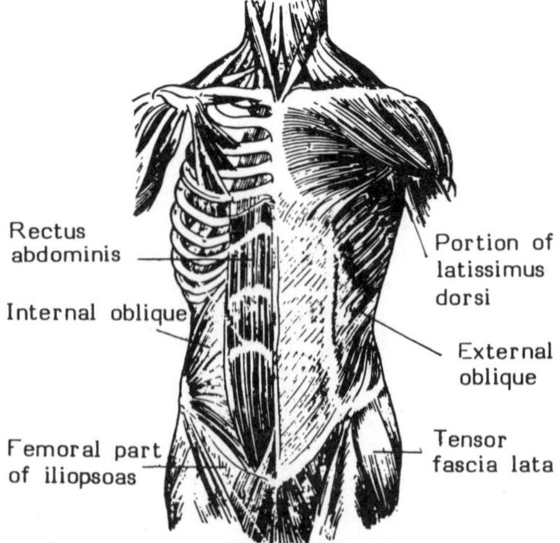

Figure 6.43. The anterior muscles of the trunk.

Spinal Movements[144–147]

The approximate degrees of spinal motions for various vertebral segments are shown in Figure 6.44, and the important movers are shown in Figure 6.45.

Spinal Extension

The spinal extensors span the entire length of the vertebral column, originating from the laminae, transverse processes, and ribs as diagonal strips and inserting as multiple tendon inserts on the spinous processes. This group of muscles, known collectively as the *erector spinae,* has the sole function of restoring the flexed spine to neutral and controlling flexion momentum as an antagonist guard. Bilateral action by the splenius capitis, cervicis, rotatores, interspinales, and multifidi is also involved in spinal extension.

The erector bundles are subdivided by innumerable connective tissue planes, and the entire group is enveloped by a strong fascia in the lumbar region that is strongly anchored to the transverse processes. This tends to spread a mechanical load over a large area.

As the erector spinae are the only muscles in the body supplied solely by the posterior rami of the spinal nerves, local pain, splinting, or unilateral weakness of this muscle group points to spinal nerve involvement.

General Stability. A spine devoid of its muscles but containing all its ligaments is most unstable. The majority of the stability of the spine can be attributed to the action of the spinal muscles. The guy-wire arrangement of the *erector spinae* provide ideal lateral stability for the spine. If defective, spinal deformity is the immediate result. This fact is readily confirmed when the unilateral loss of a few spinal nerves produces a severe scoliosis.

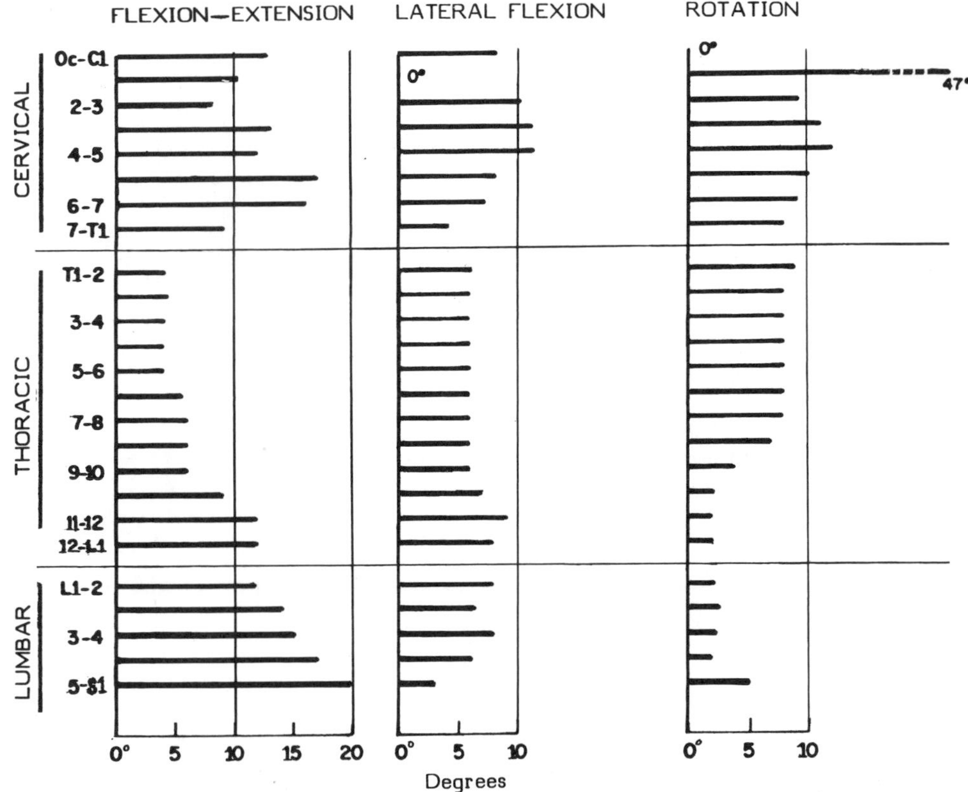

Figure 6.44. Compared approximate values of flexion-extension, lateral flexion, and rotation, in degrees, for various spinal levels, as redrawn from data of White and Panjabi. Other authorities differ somewhat from these figures.

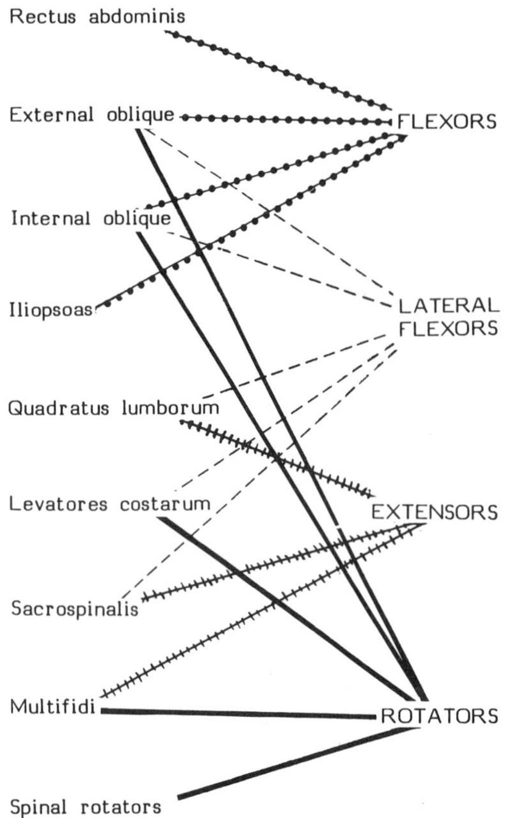

Figure 6.45. Movements of the spine and their related major movers.

Static Balance. The erector spinae do not assist in maintaining static neutral balance. They are myographically inactive during erect stance. When in static equilibrium, we normally rest primarily on weight-bearing joints against ligament resistance. With the exception of extremely slight and intermittent iliopsoas, longissimus dorsi, and rotatores muscle action, little spinal activity is required. There is slightly more activity in the sitting position than in the standing posture.

Spinal Flexion

The flexor muscles, developed most in the cervical and lumbar regions, are represented chiefly by the anterior *longus coli* and *scalene* muscles in the cervical area and the more lateral *sternomastoid* muscles, which are powerful assistants. In the lumbar region, the *psoas major* flexes the trunk on the thigh at the hip but has little effect on flexion of individual lumbar segments. The lumbar spine is essentially flexed by the anterior *rectus abdominis* with help from the lateral *external* and *internal obliques*. During typical flexion and extension, there is little change in the dorsal curve (Fig. 6.46).

The first 70° of forward bending is due to flexion of the lumbar segments; the pelvis is locked by strong contraction of the *gluteus maximus, medius,* and *hamstrings*. The following 25° of flexion takes place by hip release and pelvic rotation (Fig. 6.17).

Spinal Lateral Flexion

The *quadratus lumborum* and *intertransversarii* are probably the only purely lateral flexors of the spine. Additional lateral bending motion is achieved by unilateral contraction of the spinal flexors and extensors.

Spinal Rotation

Voluntary rotation is minimal in the lumbar region. The *sternomastoid* in the cervical

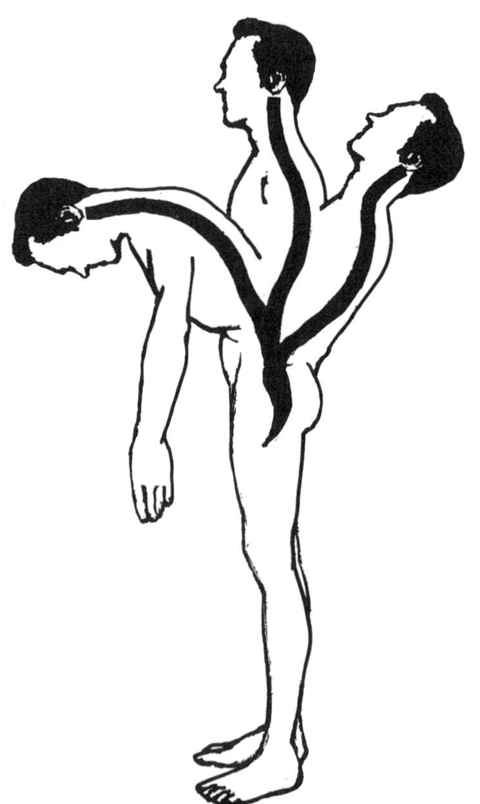

Figure 6.46. Note that in A-P spinal motion the lumbar curve flattens on flexion and slightly increases on extension, but the thoracic spine shows little alteration.

area and the *abdominal obliques* in the trunk are usually considered the most powerful rotators. However, myographic studies have shown that the most active spinal muscles during axial rotation are the *erector spinae* on the side moving posteriorly and the *musculi rotatores* and *multifidi* on the side moving anteriorly. There is also activity of the ipsilateral *splenius capitis, cervicis, gluteus medius*, and *tensor fascia lata*.

GENERAL ASPECTS OF VERTEBRAL SUBLUXATIONS

Abnormal spinal biomechanics clinically relates to the intervertebral subluxations and other spinal malfunctions that result in structural and physiologic inadequacies of the spinal column. This state is the condition of a vertebral motion unit that has lost its normal structural and/or functional integrity and is, therefore, unable to move from its normal resting position, to move properly through its normal range of motion, or to return to its normal resting position after movement.[148,149]

Types of Subluxations

There are numerous methods of classifying vertebral subluxations. Each has its own rationale and each has had certain validity that has been a contribution to our understanding of this complex phenomenon.

Clinical Classes of Subluxation

The seven commonly recognized clinical types of subluxation are: (1) *functional subluxation*, a functional and slight "off centering" with partial fixation in an otherwise normal articular bed; (2) *pathologic subluxation*, an "off centering" derangement in an articular bed that has become deformed as the result of degenerative changes; (3) *traumatic subluxation*; consequent to an extraneous or intrinsic force and the associated muscle spasm; (4) *reflex subluxation*, "off centering" induced by asymmetrical muscle contraction from aberrant visceral or somatic reflexes; (5) *defect subluxation*, subluxation of an anomalous or developmentally defective spinal or pelvic segment; (6) *fixation subluxation*, hypomobile fixation wherein a spinal or pelvic segment that is in a neutral position of mobility fails to fully participate in movement (Fig. 6.47); and (7) *hypermobile subluxation*, pathologic segmental increase in movement consequent to the loss of integrity of the retaining mechanism caused by trauma or degenerative pathology.

Terminology[150–156]

What is called a vertebral subluxation in chiropractic is the alteration of the normal dynamic, anatomical, or physiologic relationships of contiguous articular structures. The concept of an "off centered" and/or "fixated" vertebral or pelvic segment that has a unique effect upon the neuromuscular bed which may be the cause of, aggravation of, or "triggering" of certain syndromes is a major contribution to health science by the chiropractic profession. This contribution has undergone considerable refinement since its inception, but this is not unique in the health sciences.

The degree of derangement of a bony segment within its articular bed may vary from a microtrauma to one that is macroscopic and quite readily discernible. It is always attended to some degree by articular dysfunction, neurologic insult, and stressed muscles, tendons, and ligaments. Once produced, the lesion usually becomes a focus of sustained irritation from which a barrage of impulses stream into the spinal cord where internuncial neurons receive and relay them to motor pathways. The muscular contraction that provoked the subluxation originally is thereby reinforced, thus perpetuating both the subluxation and the pathologic process.

Confusion exists because the term chiropractic refers to both structural position (both static and dynamic) and related func-

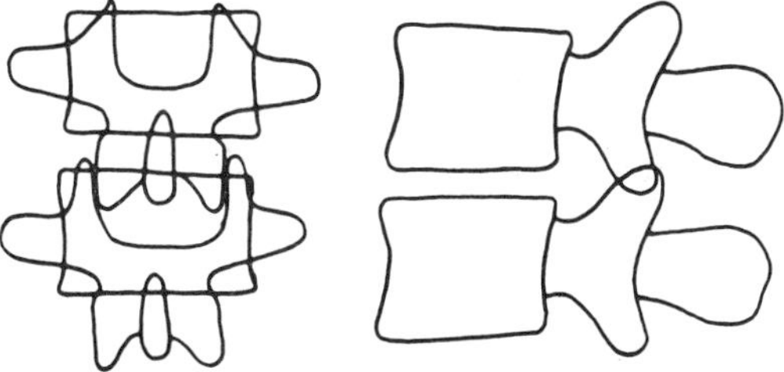

Figure 6.47. *Left*, schematic posterior view of the intervertebral motion unit in the normal position; *right*, lateral view of the intervertebral motion unit in the normal position.

tional abnormalities (both static and dynamic), and a defintion that serves one aspect does not necessarily serve another.[157] In the words of Gillet, "Vertebrae do not slip out of place. They are not displaced out of their physiological boundaries. They have not gone out of their limits of motion. When we adjust subluxations, we do not replace vertebrae."[158,159] As far back as the first chiropractic textbook published (1906), Smith and associates fought the idea of "a bone out of place."[160,161] They emphasized that "a simple subluxated vertebra differs from a normal vertebra only in its field of motion and the center of its field of motion," a concept valid today.

The "off centering" referred to is usually far less in extent than the "near dislocation" used by medical orthopedists. In chiropractic semantics, this "off centering" may not even exist in the static spine as seen in the "subluxation" of fixation that produces an abnormal pivot within the normal physiologic range of motion or in the hypermobile segment that returns to a centered position in the neutral position.[162] Conversely, an "off centered" vertebra that is not interfering with function is rarely considered a "subluxation" in clinical chiropractic.

To date, no one definition has been able to serve all that is implied in chiropractic. Osteopaths[163,164] have used the term "vertebral lesion," but this jargon implies a pathologic or traumatic discontinuity of tissue or loss of function that may or may not exist with a "subluxation." Hildebrandt[165] has used the term "dysarthria" in an attempt to imply the dynamic rather than the static "off centering" aspects of the motion unit, but even he realizes that this is often confused with the imperfect articulation of speech.

An accurate term could be devised, but this would require an extensive polysyllabic word that would be so cumbersome to use that it would be ignored by the mainstream of health science. Thus, until this dilemma is solved, the word "subluxation" will continue to be used.

Motion Unit Classes of Subluxations[33,166,167]

The biomechanical element of the vertebral motion unit subluxation is classified in accord with its static or kinetic aspects and with the number of vertebral motion units involved.

Static Vertebral Motion Unit Subluxation-Fixations

Flexion Subluxation. This is characterized by approximation of the vertebral bodies at the anterior and by separation of the vertebral bodies, facets, and spinous processes at the posterior. When found, it is indicative of irritative microtrauma to the anterior IVF; forced excursion of the nucleus pulposus and bulging of anular fibers; stretching of the posterior longitudinal, interspinal, and supraspinal ligaments; traction shearing stress of the synovia of the facet articulations; and biomechanical impropriety of the motion unit (Fig. 6.48).

Extension Subluxation. An extension subluxation features separation of the vertebral bodies at the anterior and approximation of the vertebral bodies, facets, and spinous processes at the posterior. Such a subluxation points toward irritative microtrauma at the posterior IVF, forced excursion of the nucleus pulposus and bulging of the anulus, stretching of the anterior longitudinal ligament, imbrication of the facet articulations with compressive shearing stress to the synovia of the facet articulations, and biomechanical insult of the vertebral motion unit.

Lateral Flexion Subluxation. This is characterized by approximation of the vertebral bodies and facets on the side of flexion and separation of the vertebral bodies and facets on the side of extension. This type of subluxation possibly indicates irritative microtrauma to the IVD on the side of flexion, imbrication of the facets and compressive shearing stress to the synovia on the side of flexion, forced excursion of

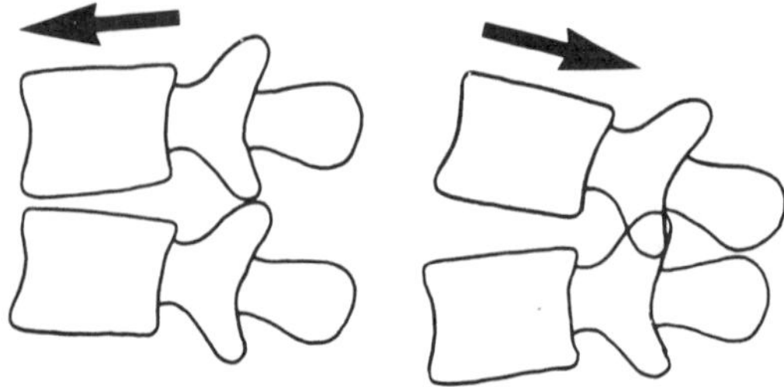

Figure 6.48. *Left*, flexion malposition; *right*, extension malposition.

the nucleus pulposus with bulging of the anulus, stretching of the anterior longitudinal ligament at its lateral aspect, and biomechanical impropriety of the vertebral motion unit (Fig. 6.49).

Rotational Subluxation. Such a subluxation features rotatory displacement of the vertebral bodies laterally and posteriorly on the side of rotation, with torsion of the facet articulations in the direction opposite to vertebral body rotation. This situation signifies torsion binding of the anulus, decreased resiliency of the IVD due to torque compression of the anular fibers, torsion stretching of the anterior and posterior longitudinal ligaments, rotatory imbrication of the facets with reverse shearing stress to the synovia, and biomechanical insult of the vertebral motion unit.

Anterolisthesis Subluxation without Spondylolysis. This is characterized by an anteroinferior excursion of the vertebral body at the anterior and by anterosuperior excursion of the vertebral body and facets at the posterior. It encourages irritative microtrauma at the anterior IVD, forward shearing stress to the anulus, stretching of the anterior and posterior longitudinal ligaments, imbrication of facets with forward shearing stress to the synovia, and biomechanical impropriety of the vertebral motion unit (Fig. 6.50).

Anterolisthesis Subluxation with Spondylolysis. This features anterior excursion of the vertebral body independent of the posterior division of the motor unit. The posterior division of the unit remains in position with the structure below because of separation of the pars. It is characterized by irritative microtrauma to the posterior aspect of the IVD, forced excursion of the nucleus pulposus with bulging of the anulus, forward shearing stress of anular fibers, stretching of the anterior longitudinal ligament, and biomechanical insult of the vertebral motion unit.

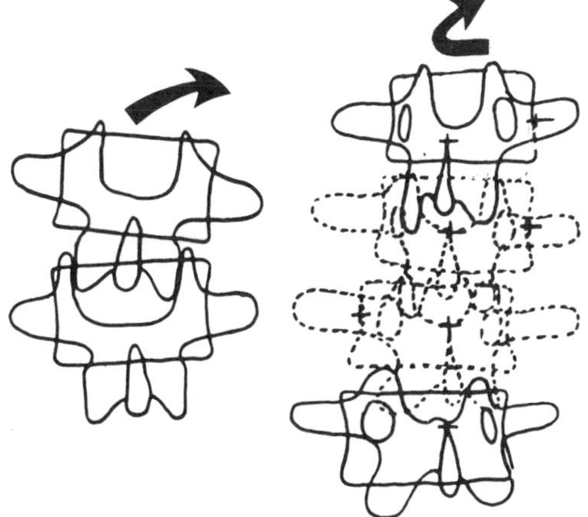

Figure 6.49. *Left*, lateral flexion malposition; *right*, rotational malposition.

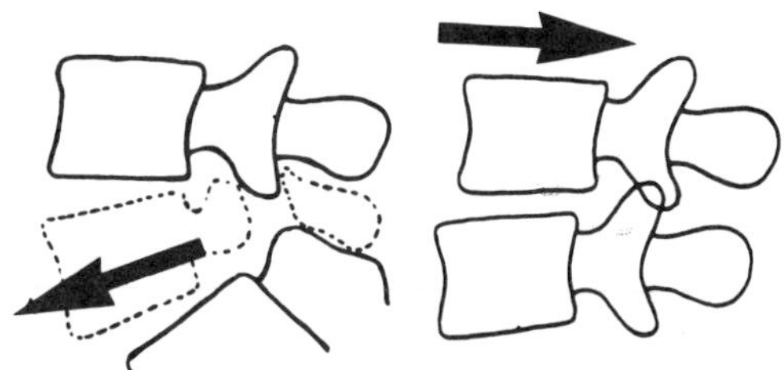

Figure 6.50. *Left*, anterolisthesis or spondylolisthesis; *right*, retrolisthesis.

Retrolisthesis Subluxation. Such a subluxation features posteroinferior excursion of the vertebral body and by posteroinferior excursion of the facets. This subluxation signifies irritative microtrauma to the posterior IVD, posterior shearing stress of the anulus, stretching of the anterior and posterior longitudinal ligaments, imbrication of the facets with posterior shearing stress to the synovia, and biomechanical impropriety of the vertebral motion unit.

Laterolisthesis Subluxation. This is characterized by lateral, superior, and posterior excursion of the vertebral body on the side of deviation and separation of the facets on the side of deviation with reverse torsion and approximation on the side opposite deviation. It suggests irritative microtrauma to the IVD on the side opposite deviation, lateral and posterior shearing stress to the anulus on the side of deviation, imbrication of facets and anterior shearing of the synovia on the side opposite deviation, and biomechanical insult to the vertebral motion unit (Fig. 6.51).

Decreased Interosseous Space Subluxation. This type of subluxation features narrowing of the vertical IVF space and inferior excursion of the facets. It is characterized by degeneration of the IVD with approximation of the vertebral bodies, traumatic compression of the IVD with possible

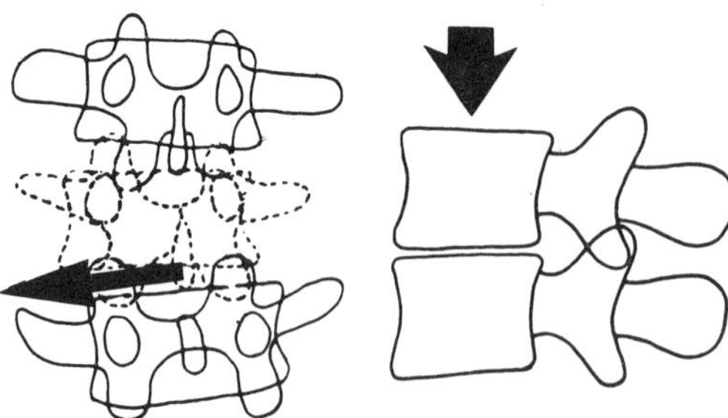

Figure 6.51. *Left*, laterolisthesis; *right*, decreased interosseous spacing.

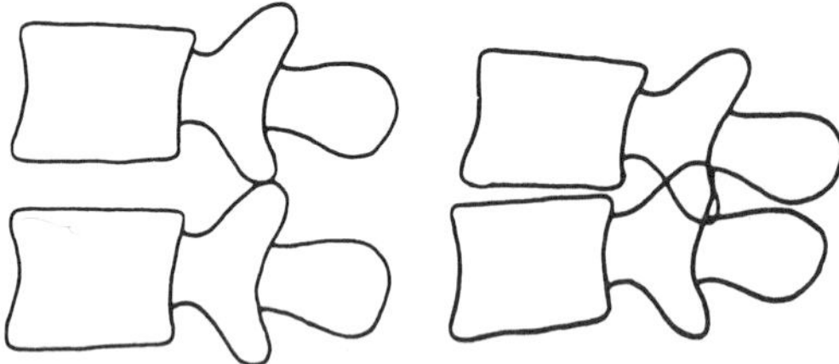

Figure 6.52. *Left*, increased interosseous spacing; *right*, foraminal occlusion.

herniation of the nucleus through an endplate, imbrication of the facets with compressive shearing stress to the synovia, compression of the contents of the IVF, and biomechanical impropriety of the vertebral motion unit.

Increased Interosseous Space Subluxation. This is characterized by superior excursion of the vertebral body and the facets. It results in inflammatory swelling or pathologic enlargement of the IVD, traction shearing stress to the anulus and the synovia of the facet articulations, stretching of the anterior and posterior longitudinal ligaments, and biomechanical insult to the vertebral motion unit (Fig. 6.52).

Foraminal Encroachment Subluxation. This features potential concomitant findings of other types of subluxations with a possible relationship to osteophytic IVF spurs in conjunction with other types of subluxations. It features associated micro- and macrotraumas to the vertebral motion unit; compression, irritation, and swelling of the foraminal contents; osseous and soft tissue primary degenerative processes of the vertebral motion unit structures; and interforaminal neurovascular insult initiating possibly disseminated secondary pathophysiologic processes.

Costovertebral-Costotransverse Subluxation. This disorder features misalignment of the costal processes in relation to the vertebral bodies and transverse processes independent of vertebral motion unit subluxation (ie, primary) or misalignment of the costal processes in relation to the vertebral bodies and transverse processes as a result of vertebral subluxation (ie, secondary). These disorders present painful, difficult, and/or restricted respiratory movements of the ribs, shearing stress to the capsular ligaments and synovia, and inducation of a vertebral motion unit subluxation, and/or contribute to a chronic subluxation, induction of spinal curvatures, aggravation of curvatures present, and irritations to the sympathetic ganglia and rami communicantes.

Sacroiliac Subluxation. This is characterized by misalignment of the sacrum in relation to the ilia independent of bilateral innominate involvement (ie, primary) or misalignment of the sacrum in relation to the ilia as a result of bilateral innominate involvement (ie, secondary). These situations encourage irritative microtrauma to the interarticular structures, and induction of a subluxation, and/or contribute to chronic subluxations, induction of spinal curvatures, aggravation of curvatures present, and biomechanical impropriety of the pelvis in static or dynamic postural accommodations.

Kinetic Vertebral Motion Unit Subluxation-Fixations

Hypomobility and/or Fixation Subluxation. This common subluxation is characterized by fixation of the vertebral motion unit in relation to the supporting structure below and compensatory hypermobility of the vertebral motion unit above the level of fixation (Fig. 6.53). The irritative, excessive function of the hypermobile vertebral motion unit results in micro- and macrotrauma to the IVD, anterior and posterior longitudinal ligaments, periosteum, etc; muscular irritation, spasticity, muscle trauma, fatigue, etc; neurologic insult within the confines of the neural canal and IVF; vascular insult to the paraspinal and interforaminal blood vessels; and biomechanical impropriety of all vertebral motion units involved.

Hypermobility Subluxation. This fea-

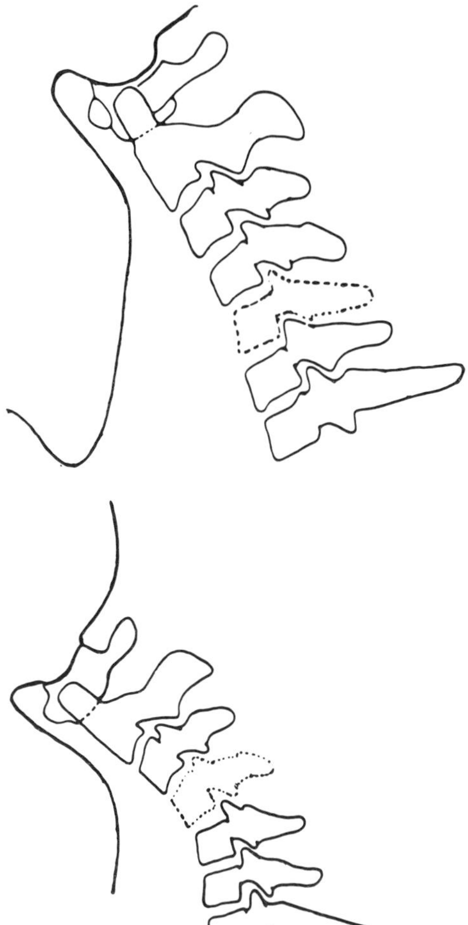

Figure 6.53. *Top*, vertebral hypomobility; *bottom*, vertebral hypermobility shown on stress-flexion film tracing.

tures a hypermobile vertebral motion unit in relation to a normally functioning or hypomobile motor unit below. It has the same features as that of a hypomobile and/or fixation subluxation except for a possible traumatically loosened vertebral motion unit as opposed to compensatory hypermobility of a vertebral motion unit within its normal range of motion.

Aberrant Movement Subluxation. This type of subluxation, frequently traumatic in origin, is characterized by movement of a vertebra "out of phase" with the segment above and below where two motion units are involved. It suggests microtrauma to both of the vertebral motion units involved, occlusion of the IVFs above and below the aberrant segment, shearing stress to the IVDs and synovia of both vertebral motion units, restriction of the neural canal, and biomechanical impropriety of both vertebral motion units (Fig. 6.54).

Gross Structural Alterations

Mechanical spinal disturbances can adversely affect the body in a number of ways such as (1) load stress on muscles leading to hypertrophy or atrophy and alterations of local muscle strength; (2) leverage stress at joints leading to weakness or sprain of ligaments, articular and intra-articular cartilage damage, and synovitis; and (3) compression stress or trauma on nerves leading to increase or decrease of normal conduction with consequent functional changes.

Compression stress on bone leads to sclerosis or alteration of its normal shape and internal architecture, and pressure stress on

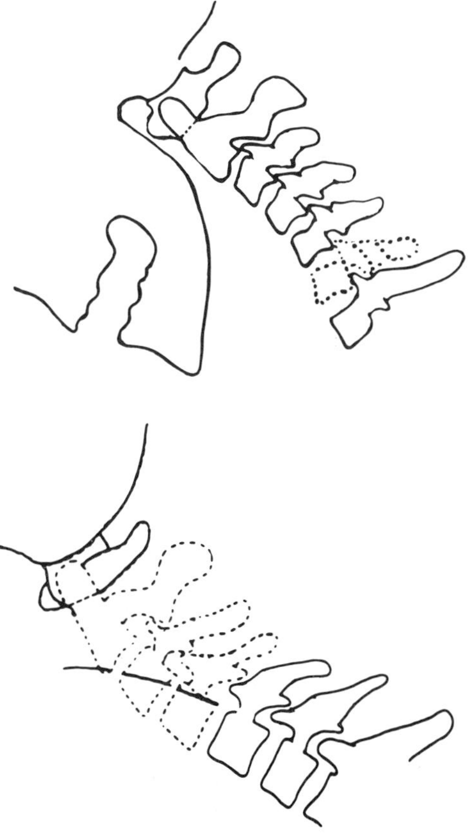

Figure 6.54. Stress film tracings. *Top*, aberrant mobility of a vertebra; *bottom*, abnormal motion of a cervical section.

connective tissues leads to thickening or thinning. Various combinations of factors influence cartilage degeneration, such as severe isolated or repeated minor trauma, chronic mechanical stress or tension, local circulatory excesses or deficiencies, idiopathic biochemical factors, developmental anomalies or malformations, nutritional factors, and the inherited cellular quality of the cartilage.

Structural Changes[168–170]

The primary physical and mechanical factors that often negatively influence the body are gravity, pressure, weight load, inertia, compression, elasticity, leverage, movement, stretch, expansion, and contraction. With these forces in mind, a vertebral subluxation may be grossly determined by its structural alterations and manifestations.

Palpable alterations of the normal anatomical relationships of one joint to another are frequently found. These mechanical changes may occur in the static recumbent, sitting, or standing positions, or in various ranges of motion as the segments and their supporting tissues are put through either active or passive ranges of motion. Subluxations are also evident by the presence of certain objective or subjective signs and symptoms when the joint and tissues are put through various orthopedic tests. Overstress at the area of the zygapophyses and the attending inflammatory reaction may give rise to a moderate radiculitis.

Mechanical errors in position or motion may be brought about by structural alterations in the supporting tissues of the joint itself. These in turn may be brought about by: (1) genetic and developmental abnormalities causing asymmetry of the vertebrae, cartilage, muscular structure, etc; (2) various acquired disease processes within the joint such as arthritic degeneration, avascular necrosis, or a neuropathic process that causes the cartilage, bone, ligaments, or musculature to be structurally altered; (3) the resolution of macro- or microtraumas, strains, sprains, or of other primary pathology may cause fibrosis, degeneration, or other retrograde changes of a structural nature within the joints themselves.[171]

These same processes not only develop within the vertebral column and its paravertebral tissues but also in the musculoskeletal tissues of the appendicular skeleton. Thus, similar lesions may exist remote from the spine which perpetuate neuropathic responses by their presence.[172] When the cause is within the structures of the spine, the effects are more evident because of the close anatomical proximities and the functional importance of normal motion unit activity or integrity to the various components of the nervous system.

Such structural faults are not, of course, the major criteria upon which a subluxation's presence and importance are based, for the body is able to adapt to many structural faults and diminish their influences upon it. Consequently, the signs and symptoms of neuropathic processes are more significant than structural alterations. The major clinical importance is not the positional relationship of the osseous segments, but the significance of the soft tissue and functional changes that are causing or are affected by the alteration. The position of the segment is important because it suggests or reflects changes in the neuromusculoskeletal and visceral systems.[173]

Postural Analysis

Posture can be defined as the relationship of each body structure to the entire structure (Fig. 6.55). Anatomists and neurologists no longer question the significance of the entire proprioceptive bed disposition in the ligamentous and myologic elements of the spine and pelvis.

Gravitational forces create subluxations and spinal distortions by the constant pull of body structures toward the center of the earth. Such distortions are increased by increasing the distance of the vertebrae from the center line of gravity and are decreased by decreasing the distance of the vertebrae from the center line of gravity. Thus, during spinal and pelvic anaysis, it is imperative that spinal mechanics and structural deviation are interpreted from the gravitational center line if the body is to be returned to its normally balanced position.[174]

Precipitating Factors of Spinal Subluxations[175,176]

A vertebral subluxation may be either a cause or an effect, and the immediate causes

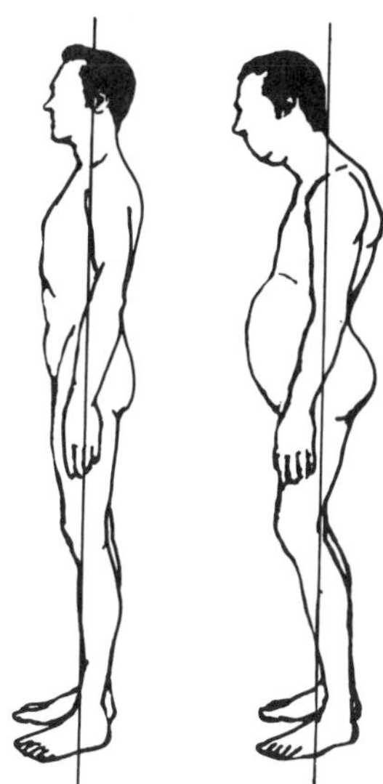

Figure 6.55. Good alignment is shown (*left*) when the lateral gravity line falls through the dens and shoulder tip, slightly behind the mid hip joint, and slightly in front of the knee and ankle joints' vertical axes. Poor posture (*right*) predisposes to spinal subluxations because of the abnormal load carriage.

may be divided into two major categories: the unequal or asymmetrical muscular effects upon the joint structures and the inequality in the supporting tissues of a particular joint such as the cartilage, IVD, ligaments, etc. Some form of internal or external stress is necessary to produce a subluxation to a degree sufficient to cause a state of dysfunction.[177]

As discussed in Chapter 5, inequality in muscular balance (ipsilateral weakness and compensatory contralateral contraction) may be initiated by (1) trauma, (2) postural distortion phenomena, (3) psychomotor responses, (4) somatic and visceral responses, and (5) paralytic effects. Two other causes not previously discussed are (6) biochemical reactions and (7) stress factors, both of which may or may not overtly manifest biomechanically.

Biochemical Reactions

Acute or chronic hypo- or hypertonicity of musculature may be due to various biochemical changes within related tissues.[178] This may be brought about by either local or general pathologies that may cause anoxia, ischemia, toxicity, etc; by foreign bodies; or by systemic fatigue-producing activities, nutritional deficiencies or excesses, caustic chemical exposure, ingestion of harmful chemicals, inhalation of noxious gases, microorganism toxins, abnormal glandular activity, excessive heat or cold, or electric shock affecting the chemical environment of cells histologically.

Stress Factors Resulting in Subluxation

Depending on the degree of stress produced, any internal or external stress factor involves the nervous system directly or indirectly, resulting in decreased mobility of the vertebra of the involved neuromere. This decreased mobility may be the result of (1) muscle splinting, especially on the side of greatest stimulation according to Pflüger's law or (2) abnormal weight distribution to the superior facets and other structures of the vertebrae involved.

Pflüger's law states that if a stimulus received by a sensory nerve extends to a motor nerve of the opposite side, contraction occurs only from corresponding muscles; and, if contraction is unequal bilaterally, the stronger contraction always takes place on the side that is stimulated.[179] When affecting one or more vertebrae, this state of decreased mobility of the motion unit encourages nerve dysfunction leading to pathologic processes in the areas supplied by the affected nerve root or neuromere, depending upon the degree and chronicity of involvement.

Effects of Spinal Subluxations[180–185]

Many spinal subluxations have more than one immediate cause and effect. Abnormality of development may be complicated by degenerative joint disease, retrograde changes, inflammation, and muscle splinting, for example. The effects may be directly upon blood vessels and nerves, reflex in nature, etc. Therefore, a complicated and far-reaching series of interacting and interdependent changes occurs which may be designated as a subluxation syndrome.

As a primary concept of chiropractic science, spinal subluxations may result in the development of disease states locally within the vertebral motion unit itself or throughout the body. These primary and secondary effects of subluxations may be divided into three major categories:

1. The mechanical effect, motion, and balance of the local segment, or the effect upon the skeleton elsewhere, due to compensatory distortions and alterations as proprioceptive mechanisms attempt to correct the mechanics in the presence of structural imbalance.

2. The effect of any localized condition occurring within the articulations due to interarticular stress and trauma (often microtrauma) such as irritation, inflammation, swelling, necrosis, and other degenerative changes.

3. The neurologic scope of subluxation effects may be grossly differentiated as nerve pressure, nerve stretch, nerve torsion, circulatory changes, meningeal irritations, cerebrospinal fluid flow alterations, alterations of proprioceptive responses and reflexes, or traumatic insult to the rami communicantes or sympathetic ganglia, among many others.

The neurologic effects are undoubtedly the more important of the three from a clinical aspect.

There are 115 diarthroses within the spine and pelvis vulnerable to the abnormal movement related to subluxation. Each of these articulations is a site of proprioceptive sensitivity which under articular strain is insulted and provoked to express pain. As mentioned, a working hypothesis regarding segmental malposition is that the displacement fixation causes adjacent areas of the spine to become hypermobile, resulting in stress of adjacent motion units. Neurologic feedback may cause the elicitation of adrenocorticotropic hormone (ACTH) and a resulting increase in the production of corticosteroids as an adaptive mechanism, according to the Hans Selye stress concept. This may also be reflected by possible blood sugar changes.

Events at the Intervertebral Foramina[186–191]

The normal cross-sectional area of an IVF leaves ample room for its neural contents. The IVF narrowing that occurs during spinal extension movements has little if any adverse effects. The channel contents are normally free to adjust to movements throughout the normal range of regional motion. Pathologic changes in and near the foramen may reduce its dimensions and lead to compression, but, as Sunderland points out, friction over osseofibrous irregularities or traction on a nerve or nerve roots fixed in the foramen by an adhesion is much more likely.[118]

When a vertebral motion unit is under constant stress, changes occur in adjacent IVDs, ligaments, membranes, muscles, and other associated tissues which produce some degree of fixation. The adjacent IVFs are altered in size. As a rule, two of them become smaller than normal, and the other two become larger than normal. Nerve roots and other contents of the affected IVFs are subjected to insult at the smaller foramina and stretching at the larger foramina (Fig. 6.56).

Effects of Microtrauma. Initially, the zygapophyseal articular complex of a subluxated vertebral motion bed is subjected to the stress of "off centering" and is attended by the following aspects of microtrauma: (1) minute hemorrhage, transudation, and arteriovenous stagnation from the sluggish circulatory flow resulting from the motion unit's decreased mobility and arterial backup; (2) para-articular and paraforaminal traumatic edema; (3) eccentric compression stress upon the IVD and the zygapophyseal cartilages; (4) possible separation of minute fasciculi of the retaining fibers of the anulus, joint capsule, dural root sleeve, and nerve root sheath; (5) stress insult of

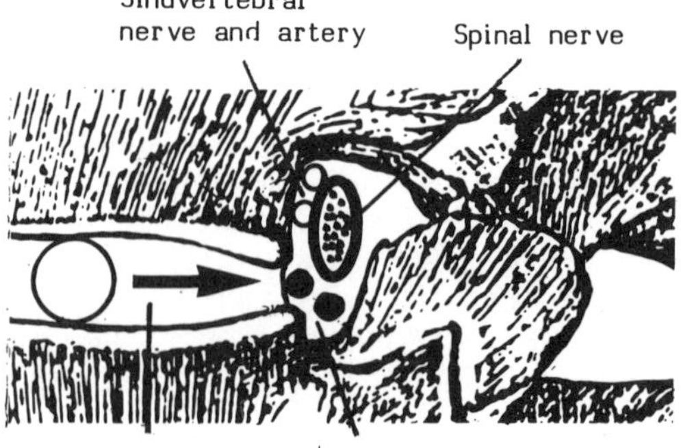

Figure 6.56. Posterolateral disc herniation can readily encroach upon the nerve root, the recurrent meningeal nerve and sinuvertebral artery passing anterior to the nerve root, the two veins passing inferior to the nerve root, and other structures within the intervertebral foramen.

the proprioceptive bed; (6) minute crushing of the periosteal margins with resultant proliferative irritation; and (7) minute tearing of the attachments of the dural root sleeves if they attach to the lining of the IVF.

Consequences. The following pathologic changes occur.

1. Extravasation and edema, along with the precipitation of fibrinogen into fibrin, result in interfascicular, foraminal, articular, and capsular thickening and adhesions that restrict fascicular glide, ingress and egress of the foraminal contents, and the competent movement of the vertebral segment within its articular bed.
2. Whenever there is extravasation, mineral salts are precipitated and infiltration and sclerosing result.
3. Binding adhesions may develop between the dural root sleeves and the nerve roots within the inter-radicular foramen and between the spinal nerve root sheath and the inner margins of the IVF.
4. When subjected to microtrauma, mesenchymal connective tissue undergoes a relatively rapid and extensive degenerative change with loss of functional integrity and substance.

Sensory Responses and Reflexes. Perhaps the most significant effect is that of proprioceptive irritation. The musculoskeletal tissues, and particularly the ligaments and paravertebral or intervertebral musculature of the spine, are richly endowed with proprioceptive receptors. First, when overly stimulated by stretching, these neurons interpret the stimuli as somatic sensory stimulation which may be perceived as pain. Second, they may also send reflexes to their motor components and cause muscular changes within the paravertebral muscles or elsewhere in the soma supplied by the segment.[192,193] Third, they may be interpreted as visceral sensory stimuli, whose visceromotor response alters circulatory changes, smooth muscle activity, glandular secretions, or trophic activity in the musculoskeletal tissues or viscera supplied by a given neurologic segment. It is this vast ability of the proprioceptive sensory beds to influence motor changes, of a somatomotor or visceromotor nature, that is perhaps the most universal effect of vertebral subluxation.

Direct Nerve Pressure. The nerve roots are normally well protected from trauma by the bony border of the IVF and the tough fibrous dura. However, Schaumburg shows that when distorted by degenerative bone and joint disease or a variety of space-occupying lesions, these same protective layers may damage the delicate neural structures.[194] Direct nerve pressure may come from the misaligned osseous segment itself or from the various soft-tissue pathologies causing or affected by the mechanical fault such as contractures, adhesions, inflammatory residues, atrophies, and cysts and tumors of related tissues. The direct physical nerve pressure may be responsible for motor alterations and sensory disturbances within this particular nerve and its innervated structures or may cause other ramifying reflexes.

Studies discussed by Sharpless show that the posterior nerve roots are about five times more susceptible to compression block than a peripheral nerve.[195] As little as 10 mm Hg pressure held for 15–30 minutes reduces the compound action potentials of posterior roots to about half their initial value. This effect is probably due to mechanical deformation rather than ischemia, since the larger fibers are blocked first. It is believed that anoxia affects the small fibers first.

Ganglion Irritation/Compression. Irritation/compression of a dorsal root ganglion may be a factor. The sensory dorsal root ganglion of each spinal nerve generally lies within the upper medial aspect of the IVF, a precarious position. Whenever the transverse diameter of the IVF is modified, the ganglion may be subject to compression and irritation. This is especially true at the cervical level where the ganglion tends to occupy the medial limits of the IVF and is thus vulnerable to and most likely to become invovled in any changes in IVF diameter on any event of trauma or the manifold tissue processes of discogenic spondylosis. For example, an acute whiplash-like mishap to the cervical spine, especially of the hyperextension type, may force the vagus and the superior cervical sympathetic ganglion against the transverse processes of the atlas and axis, provoking the bizarre autonomic reactions that not uncommonly attend this condition.

Intraneural Effects. It is probable that any interference with or abnormality of (1) the interstitital fluids in which the nerves lie and/or (2) the intracellular fluid of the nerve itself in the nerve axoplasm will cause a breakdown of the sodium pump mechanism that will prevent the normal flow of impulses along the nerve fibers concerned. These abnormal impulses refer to an overaction or underaction in the rate of impulse frequency along the nerve. Once a threshold stimulus has been reached, a nerve will fire in accordance with the all-or-none law.

Meningeal Irritations. Mechanical errors in motion and position may cause tractional effects upon the meningeal coverings of the cord or dural root sleeves that may produce mechanical pressure upon the neurons emanating from the cord itself. These may, therefore, cause the elicitation of abnormal neurologic motor effects or sensory interpretations.

Altered Nerve Root Level. Induced disrelation between position level and course direction of nerve root origin (spinal cord) and nerve root exit (IVF) is an important factor. Whenever there is subluxation, changes in normal curves, or the presence of abnormal curves, the relative levels of the points of nerve root origin and exit are altered and the nerve root becomes vulnerable to encroachment compression or irritation. This is because whenever the normal curves of the spine are grossly modified (eg, kyphotic deviation of the cervical spine; lordotic exaggeration of the lumbar spine; scoliotic deformity, especially at the cervicobrachial area and lumbosacral junction), the nerve root is forced to assume an unusual approximation to one or the other walls of the IVF. Thereafter, the least additional deviation may precipitate a nerve root irritation syndrome. In addition, a vertebral column affected with partial fixation of several segments when subjected to flexion, extension, and circumduction efforts will be attended by marked tension upon the dural root sleeves and the related spinal nerve radicles, especially the cauda equina (Fig. 6.57).

When for any reason one or more vertebral segments are embarrassed by abnormal motor action, added articular and proprioceptive responsibility is imposed upon the

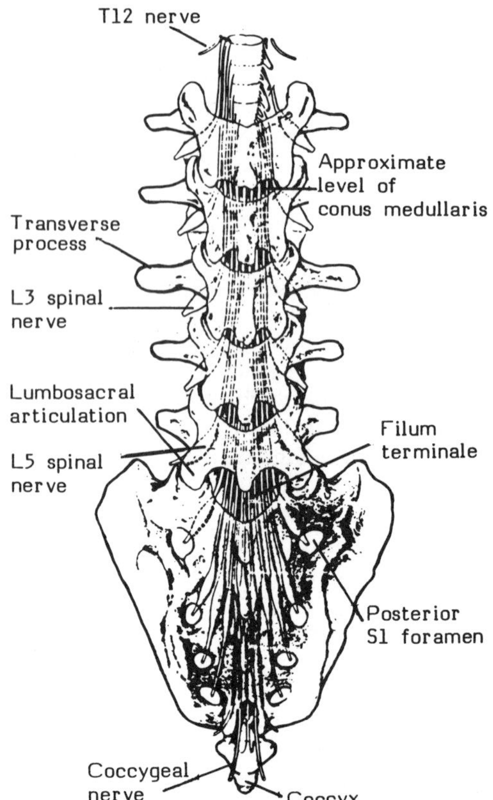

Figure 6.57. Dorsal view schematic of the lower spine showing the terminal part of the cord and caudal equina in the lumbosacral region. Swelling or adhesions within any intervertebral foramina would interfere with the normal freedom and function of the nerve roots during activity.

segments above and below the involved area. Thus there is an extension of harmful effects that may have noticeable complications. In addition, the phenomenon of bipedism neurologically necessitated the development of an ascending and descending reticular activating mechanism. It can be assumed that spinal and pelvic interosseous disrelation may over stimulate the ascending portion of the reticular activating mechanism. On the other hand, excessive attention stress may, by means of the descending portion, provoke overstimulation of the cellular elements in the anterior and lateral horns and provoke abnormal somatic and autonomic reactions.

Paraforaminal Adhesions. Paraforaminal adhesions as the result of stress and traumatic edema often result in a painful restriction of the normal back-and-forth glide (¼–⅓ inch) of the nerve root within the IVF. Symptoms simulate a low-grade radiculitis: increased pain on movement, straining, and stretching; pain on changing positions and when placing the involved part in extension.

Circulatory Changes. Decreased mobility (eg, vertebral fixation) of a motion unit within its normal physiologic range of movement may cause sluggish lymphatic or vascular circulation that is further influenced by mechanical pressure. This can cause chemical or physical changes within tissues, such as anoxia, toxicity, swelling, edema, etc, and the consequent derangement of normal function brought about by these disorders. Local irritation at the site of misalignment and a decreased ability to move produce an inflammatory reaction with edema leading to a disturbance in the normal exchange of nutrients and waste products between capillary and extracellular fluid. Added to this stasis is the probable factor of lactic acid buildup in the area as a result of acid leaking from the surrounding hypertonic muscles.

Local Toxicity Effects. The venous stagnation from arterial backup can produce local toxicity. While toxic metabolic end products (eg, urea, uric acid, creatinine, lactic acid) accumulate in the stagnant tissue and congested capillary beds, there is also a corresponding decrease in nutrient and oxygen concentration in these fluids. Thus, the nerves emanating from the involved area will be deficient in necessary nutrients and quite possibly hypoxic as well. The buildup of metabolic waste products in the area of the IVF may also alter the normal pH of local fluids causing a breakdown of the Krebs cycle, due to decreased oxygen and toxicity, which causes a partial breakdown of the sodium pump mechanism, resulting in an ionic imbalance. As the sodium pump can no longer maintain a normal ionic balance, the imbalance can result in a degree of erratic nerve conduction and edema in the tissues of the immediate area. This erratic nerve conduction may be exhibited in all nerves passing through the involved IVF and immediate area. When toxicity occurs in either the central or peripheral nervous systems, the formation of acetylcholine at the level of involvement will be interfered with and result in further disturbances due to increased nerve conduction impairment. This situation, along with the toxicity effects upon the nerve, may well result in abnormal membrane permeability leading to dysfunction.

Cerebrospinal Fluid Flow Alterations. These refer to the mechanical effect upon the flow of cerebrospinal fluid within the central nervous system and perhaps within the peripheral nerve origins themselves. Cerebrospinal fluid stagnation possibly occurs in association because of the intimate relationship between spinal fluid and venous blood, contributing to toxicity in the nerve root area. According to some researchers, minute pressure on meninges alters the flow of cerebrospinal fluid and interferes with its ability to remove wastes and provide nutritional substances to the cord and nervous system. This may be either the effect of direct mechanical pressure or impairment of motion necessary for proper inflow and outflow of this nutrient material.

Distal Neurologic Manifestations of Subluxations[196,197]

Because of the effects of the subluxation's microtrauma and the consequent pathologic changes involved, the neurologic insult may result in (1) modification of the basic chronaxie; (2) alteration of normal impulse amplitude, wave length, and force intensity; and/or (3) extension of the refractory period.

The neurologic manifestations of a subluxation are not always indicated by the response the nervous system makes to irritation not external to it (ie, discernible in its immediate area) but rather from within the body. Thus, it can be an intrinsic source of neurologic irritation. This altered state of the nerve fiber's threshold and the impulse proper leads to dysfunction of the sensory, motor, vasomotor, and spinovisceral responses.

Somatic Responses. Dysfunctions in the somatic-sensory field include varying degrees of discomfort and pain, tension, superficial and deep tenderness, muscular tone, periosteal tenderness, hyper- and hypoesthesia, haptic sensations, acroparesthesia, formication, flushing, numbness, coldness, and postural fatigue. Dysfunctions in the somatomotor field include painful, and especially proximal, muscle spasms; abnormal muscular tone (from hypotonicity to spasm), weakness, atrophy, or degeneration in long-standing cases; sluggish and uncoordinated movements; paralyses; fasciculations, tics, and tremors.

Visceral Motor Responses. Visceromotor responses of the nervous system may be exhibited in several ways. For example:

1. Dysfunction in the vasomotor field include local swellings, angioneurotic edema, flushing, blanching, mucous membrane congestion, urticaria, and dermatographia. Minor changes in the circulation of the skin can be measured by various heat-sensitive devices, thermography, galvanometers, or infrared photography. Such changes often parallel circulatory changes in the deeper tissues because they too are affected by similar vasomotor responses.
2. Changes in the ability of the skin to secrete oils or perspiration which can be measured by various electrical means.[198] These secretory errors may also be indicative of similar changes in deeper visceral tissues. Hyperhidrosis or dryness, as well as hyperesthesia or hypoesthesia, in a local area near the spine implies altered vasomotor activity in the subsequent spinal segment. Hyperesthesia and hyperhidrosis are usually associated with an increased flare (red response) to scratching and a decrease in electrical skin resistance.
3. Dysfunctions in the spinovisceral field include visceral musculature abnormalities, glandular and mucuous membrane secretory malfunctions, and sphincter spasms of the detrusor muscles and myocardium.[199]
4. Changes in the quality of tissue from trophic disturbances such as atrophies, degenerations, thinning or discoloration of the skin, or other changes that reflect viscerotrophic abnormalities.

Visceral Manifestations of Gross Postural Faults

Postural faults, which may be either the cause or result of vertebral subluxations, are readily visualized in postural analysis. Pressure or stretching stress of viscera and their supports leads to disturbed visceral function and abnormal reflexes.

Abnormal body mechanics affecting the thoracic and abdominal cavities interfere with normal function by (1) abnormal efferent visceral stimuli reaching organs from the facilitated segment, (2) abnormal tensions and stretching of visceral supports, nerves, blood and lymph vessels, (3) venous pooling as the result of inactivity, diaphragm dysfunction, organ displacement, and sustained postural stress, or (4) abnormal vasomotor impulses to blood vessels. Blocking stress or irritation of blood vessels leads to ischemia or congestion.

There are many general effects to the body as a whole besides these local effects because each abnormal stress results in abnormal discharges of afferent impulses to the central nervous system with consequent hormonal reactions that are systemic in character. Also considered must be the associated emotional stress as the result of the local stress, which contributes to the clinical picture.

BASIC BIOMECHANICAL CONSIDERATIONS IN EVALUATING SPINAL PAIN

The general public associates the management of "backache" with chiropractic probably more than any other disorder because of the profession's reputation for offering relatively rapid relief by conservative means. This has been a "dual-edged sword," for it has contributed to the public's difficulty in associating chiropractic care with disorders far removed from the spine.

Clinical Cautions

Mental "Boxes"

Tunnel Thinking. There is probably no other area in clinical practice in which the tendency is stronger to reduce patient profiles to conform to preconceived notions than that of spinal pain. Granted, patterns do occur, and we will present them in this book as a basis for thought, but the exceptions may outweigh their textbook descriptions.

The Evasive "Normal." When Earl Rich was head of the Roentgenology Department at Lincoln Chiropractic College, and after viewing thousands of spinal films, he felt that the typical adult spine contained about seven anomalies on the average. In clinical practice, we constantly search for the ideal normal and rarely find it.[200] It seems that all we ever find are variations. Yet, we often hold in our minds a visualization of a necessary "normal" that we strive to attain for an individual, which is often impossible. This creates an enigma.

This-for-That Concepts. Case failure is too often the result of "this-for-that" thinking in prejudiced diagnostics and therapeutics; eg, is this a "Type A" case, a "Class II" distortion, or a "routine" reaction? Orthopedists, especially, often assume that every pain goes with some musculoskeletal derangement similar in severity to the patient's complaint.[201] Such an iatrophysics approach completely ignores the body's holistic nature, adaptive ability, and individual normal variances from the preconceived "textbook norm."

Structural vs Functional Emphasis

From a purely mechanical viewpoint, we commonly think of movement being the result of the shape of the planes of articulation, assuming that a certain shape causes certain motions. This contributes to assumptions that structure always governs function and that function is always dependent on structure. This, like most clinical definites, is a half-truth, because movement occurs long before ossification establishes the osseous planes. And this does not consider the many severe bumps and jars suffered during childhood.

The science and art of chiropractic orthopedics are concerned with the postural relationships of articular surfaces, both normal and abnormal; the analysis of harmful influences on improper structural relationships; the diagnosis and correction as is possible of such abnormal relationships; and the management of prevention of disturbances resulting from such malrelationships.[202]

Pure orthopedics is not concerned with function to a great extent, but concentrates upon structure with function playing a platonic role. From this strict structural viewpoint, function is dependent on structure and is regarded as secondary. The major emphasis is on the position of rest rather than the dynamics of articulation. However, although movements of mature joints are influenced essentially by the design of the articular planes, these planes have attained their shape because of functional movements made during development. In addition, it is not rare to see a subluxation in which movement has *not* accurately followed the normal plane of movement.

During the clinical analysis of structure, Lieb offers three postulates worthy of consideration.[203] He points out quite accurately that (1) without structure there is no function, (2) without correct structure there is not correct function, and (3) incorrect function, however, may adversely affect not only correct structure, but also seriously affect developing structures. Thus, *structure can be the effect of function, and function can be the effect of structure.*[204] There is no need to divide into "chicken and egg" camps if we stay with reality, in the "now."

In chiropractic, we view so many static x-ray films, see so many static diagrams in books and professional papers, and palpate so many patients in the relaxed position that it is often very difficult to think of a subluxation in its dynamic sense. And when we do, our visualization often represents a series of static "stills."

Spinal Pain[205–208]

The doctor is misled who believes he can understand the patient's perception of pain. We can only seek to understand the patient's reaction to it. This is true whether the pain is isolated or generalized, local or referred. Although all pain does not have organic causes, there is no such thing as "imagined" pain.

Pain that can be purely isolated as a structural, functional, or an emotional effect is rare. More likely, all three are superimposed upon and interlaced with each other in various degrees of status. This is also true for neural, vascular, lymphatic, and hormonal mechanisms.

The four most common mechanisms producing spinal pain are IVD degeneration, posterior joint dysfunction, IVF pressure (compression or traction), and abnormal somatovisceral reflexes. It is important to differentiate local causes of spinal pain from diseases referring pain to the spinal area. Classes of selected vertebral causes of spinal pain are outlined in Table 6.2. Classes of

Table 6.2.
Classification of Selected Vertebral Causes of Spinal Pain

Traumatic
  Dislocation
  Fracture
  Sprain
  Strain
  Subluxation
	Inflammatory arthropathy
	  Ankylosing spondylitis
	  Collagen diseases
	  Fibrositis
	  Focal sepsis
	  Gouty rheumatism
	  Muscular rheumatism
	  Osteochondritis
	  Panniculitis
	  Psoriasis
	  Regional ileitis
	  Reiter's disease
	  Rheumatoid arthritis
	  Ulcerative colitis

Infection
  Brucella melitensis
  Escherichia coli
  Staphylococcal
  Tubercular
	Metabolic
	  Osteomalacia
	  Osteoporosis

Developmental
  Hypermobility
  Kyphosis
  Lordosis
  Scoliosis
  Spondylolisthesis
  Various anomalies
	Systemic
	  Secondary involvement of primary infection and general disease processes such as typhoid fever, brucellosis, actinomycosis, influenza, smallpox, gout, blood dyscrasias, alkaptonuria, and cancer

Degenerative
  Apophyseal osteoarthritis
  Cauda equina disorders
  Degenerative disc lesions
  Hyperostosis
  Joint instability
  Nerve root compression
  Spinal cord diseases
	Miscellaneous
	  Iatrogenic causes such as unskilled or ill-advised manipulation, myelography, surgery with subsequent adhesions, and poorly fitted or prolonged use of supports
	  Psychogenic conversion syndromes

Tumorous
  Myelomatosis
  Secondary carcinoma	

Idiopathic
  Paget's disease
  Rare bone diseases	

selected pathologies simulating spinal pain are shown in Table 6.3. Again, these tables are offered as "thought provokers," not as boundaries.

Prevalent Theories

Although there are many good theories, the actual cause of common neck or back pain remains unknown unless gross pathology can be demonstrated. There is no one type of subluxation picture or abnormality that is associated with all forms of spinal pain, nor does the presence of a subluxation or abnormality mean that the patient will have pain. Diagnosis must be approached with caution because of the many structural, functional, and psychologic mechanisms that may be involved (Fig. 6.58).

We know that mechanical pressure (traction or compression) on axons or nerve trunks *inhibits* rather than excites. This blocking effect would appear to contraindicate spinal manipulation whose aim is to relieve *pain* caused by a stretched or compressed IVF. However, rapid transient mechanical distortions (such as would be aggravated during normal motion) depolarize nerve trunks and mechanoreceptors and produce impulse bursts of short duration. Other explanations include (1) soft-tissue receptors as the source of pain impulses, (2) vascular pulsations offering repeated transient mechanical stimuli to tensed or compressed roots, or (3) inflammation foci responsible for sustained neural discharge rather than mechanical forces.[209]

Incidence

Spinal pain not associated with gross trauma or obvious pathology has been com-

Table 6.3.
Classification of Selected Pathologies Simulating Spinal Pain

Cervical pain
Malignant lymphadenopathy
Pancoast tumor
Subarachnoid hemorrhage
Vertebral artery syndrome
Thoracic pain
Aortic aneurysm
Bronchial carcinoma
Cardiac enlargement
Coronary artery disease
Gallbladder disease
Herpes zoster
Hiatus hernia
Pulmonary disease
Lumbar pain
Aortic obstruction
Colon carcinoma
Disseminated sclerosis
Endometriosis
Hip disease
Miscellaneous pelvic carcinoma
Obstruction of iliac arteries
Pancreatic carcinoma
Peptic ulcer
Rectal carcinoma
Renal disease
Short leg syndrome
Spinal cord tumor
Miscellaneous
Visceral diseases causing referred pain to the spine or pressure erosion
Central nervous system diseases such as meningitis, poliomyelitis, syringomyelia, tetanus, spinal subarachnoid hemorrhage
Psychogenic causes
Iatrogenic manifestations

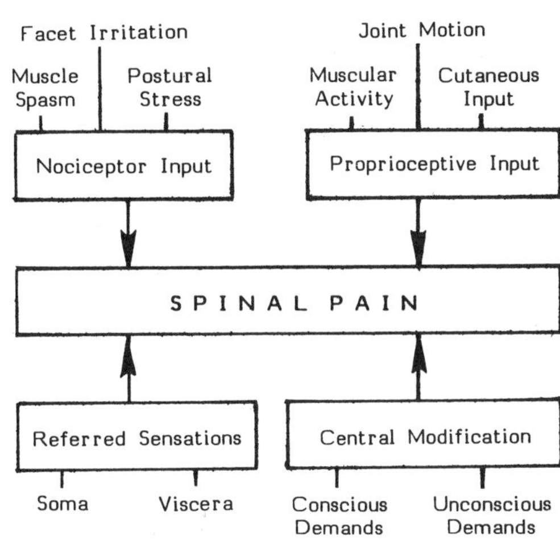

Figure 6.58. Common factors that influence spinal pain.

mon to mankind since the earliest civilizations. These common disorders have their highest incidence during middle age (30–50 years) and frequently originate near the more mobile areas of the spine (Oc–C1, L5–S1).

While the literature abounds with discussions on industrial and sports-related injuries, about 43% of musculoskeletal injuries occur in the home, 16% at work, 34% in public places and recreational areas, and 7% in automobiles. Regardless of the site of trauma, the common response includes inflammation and repair.

A relationship of the magnitude of loading and the degree of motion of the various spinal regions to the incidence of pain has been established. The cervical region, which has the second rank in pain incidence, has the highest degree of motion and the lowest weight load. In contrast, the lumbar region, which has the highest rank in pain incidence, has the second rank in mobility and the highest weight load. The relatively stiff thoracic region, which has the lowest rank in pain incidence, has the least range of mobility and the second rank of weight load.

General Aspects of Spinal Inspection and Palpation [210–214]

The art and science of spinal examination, analysis, and diagnosis mandate that the patient be examined in more than one postural stance or position. The discovery of the indication of subluxations depends upon the spine being observed in multiple positions because certain lesions are more obvious in one attitude than in another. The (1) Adams position, (2) anatomic position, (3) prone position, and (4) supine position are suggested for a complete spinal analysis.

It is assumed that, prior to mobilizing procedures, any indication of fracture, dislocation, advanced arteriosclerosis, hemorrhage, or cord injury has been considered.

Static Bony Palpation

The identification of the bony segments of the spine is done by palpating and counting. This requires the development of a refined tactile sense on the part of the examiner. It is important to count the vertebrae so as to correlate and document the involved segment neurologically.[215]

Since the 1890s, digital examination of the spinal column has been conducted within chiropractic for evidence to determine "incorrect positioning" of one vertebra relative to another.[216] For the most part today, static palpation seeks to determine only the probable locations of subluxations by the variations in muscular tonus, texture, and sensitivity because bone anomalies are far too frequent.

Soft-Tissue Palpation[217,218]

Healthy paravertebral tissue presents a normal texture, is not tender to moderate touch and has no lasting soreness following minor trauma. However, local hyperalgesia, abnormal soft-tissue tone, and lasting soreness are common findings associated with subluxations. Adjacent soft tissues will frequently feel boggy or thickened near rigid muscle. These two signs alone represent a disturbance in local homeostasis. This may be the pathophysiologic result of trauma or the effect of changes induced by functional (visceral or psychologic) or other disturbances by way of the controlling and communicating neural, vascular, lymphatic, or hormonal processes that determine homeostatic balance.

Resting muscle is electrically silent as shown by electromyography and relaxed as shown by palpation. Conversely, muscle tissue near a subluxation is often active as shown by electromyography and spastic as shown by palpation. Propping the patient in different positions with pillows often will decrease electromyographic activity, but it does not appear to reduce the palpable firmness. This would indicate that the increased tone is not necessarily due to muscle contraction from nociceptive input. However, it is well established that irritation of the posterior joints and ligaments readily leads to reflex spasm of the erector spinae and other extensors.

In the absence of muscle contraction, one hypothesis is that this change in texture is the result of local fibrositis; it has been shown that the cutaneous pain threshold is significantly reduced in fibrositis. Other theories attribute it to a neurogenic inflammatory process or an interference with normal axoplasmic flow resulting in normal neuron trophicity. Gillet feels it is a state of hypertonus of the autonomic mechanism, not far from normal, as there is often no pain (except on deep palpation) such as that exhibited in extremity muscle spasm.[219]

It is possible, with practice, to palpate the comparative tone of the spinal intrinsic muscle. The rotatores or multifidi are the most easily palpated and are helpful in evaluating subluxations. The intertransversarii (levator costae in the thoracic area) are more difficult to palpate but are quite helpful indicators.

Muscle tone evaluation requires precise knowledge of anatomy and much practice at the technique of gliding the fingertips transversely across the muscle fibers with the skin of the patient moving as part of the fingertip. For the rotatores, the glide is axially along the side of and very close to the spinous process at the muscle insertion. Also located here will often be hyperesthesia (or less frequently, paresthesia), which induces even further muscle contraction by reacting to the pressure of the palpating fingertips.

Gonstead advised to search for areas of edema in sites of poor tisssue tone which feel softer to the touch than normal areas. These areas are often found at or near the level of involvement.

An area of chronically indurated muscle tissue is often located adjacent to an area of muscle that has entered into a state of fatty degeneration. When found through palpation, this area should not be confused with that of a common lipoma (adipoma). Lipomata are soft benign fatty tumors, which are frequently multiple but not metastatic, varying in size from a pea to a large egg. While most lipomata are located just below the skin, those embedded between deep skeletal muscles tend to rise to the surface when the involved muscle is exercised and to recede during rest.

Since pain from nerve roots or pathways is referred toward the periphery, the entire nerve leading from the area should be explored where possible. In addition, tenderness, masses, spasms, local temperature, areas of excessive moisture or dryness, their size and character, and other points should be noted.

The Basic Factors Involved in Spinal Examination[220]

Whether spinal or extraspinal, musculoskeletal symptoms may be the first clues in the diagnosis of poor structural or stress adaptation. The most common musculoskeletal symptoms are joint stiffness, joint swelling, and joint pain. The nature of the damage usually depends on the direction of the applied force on bones and the manner in which these bones are attached to other structures.

Spinal Motions[221,222]

The examination of the musculoskeletal system is different for an acutely injured patient than for a patient presenting nontraumatic complaints. For instance, active and passive ranges of spinal motion should not be conducted until after roentgenograms have demonstrated the mechanical integrity of the joint. During spinal analysis, the major motions evaluated are flexion, extension, right and left lateral flexion, and right and left rotation. Motion of a superior segment is described in terms of the segment beneath it.

Although regional examination will be discussed in future chapters, certain basic points are appropriate here.

Normal Rotation. When the spine is in a neutral standing or sitting position, the anterior surface of a vertebral body in the lower spine will rotate to the side opposite the lateroflexion with the vertebral bodies tending to crawl out from under the load. This pattern of function usually takes place within multiple spinal segments, but dysfunction will occur when ligaments and muscles attached to and affecting the vertebral articulations are shortened or lengthened to effect restricted or excessive motion of one or more segments. When the neutral position is resumed, each spinal joint should return to its "normal" position.

Scoliotic Rotation. The direction of vertebral rotation is determined by inspection and dynamic palpation of the transverse processes, with one transverse process being more posterior on the side toward which the vertebra has rotated. If one or more segments are rotated to one side in the neutral position, lateroflexion will usually be noted on the side opposite the rotation. In spinal flexion, the segment rotated will be laterally flexed to the same side with a loss in its ability to bend forward. During spinal extension, the segment is rotated to the same side and is inhibited in bending backward.

Motion Restriction. Functional limitation may be the result of pain associated with movement (Fig. 6.59), joint instability, or restricted joint movement by muscular spasm or hypertonicity, ligamentous or capsular shortening, bony ankylosis, thickening or adhesions in the periarticular structures, or obstruction by bony overgrowths or gouty tophi.

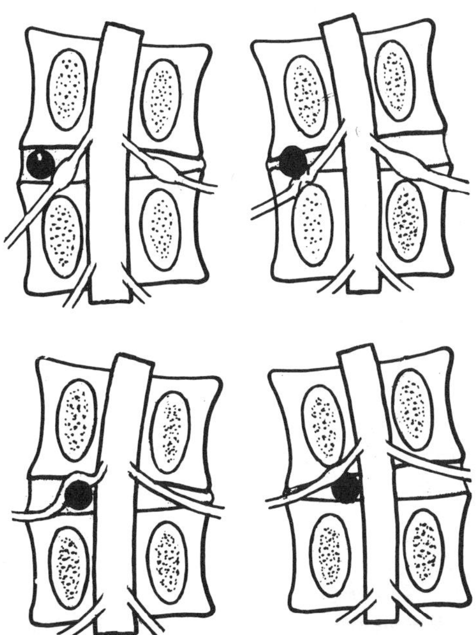

Figure 6.59. Spinal movements in the presence of disc herniation (shown in *black*) may offer distinct diagnostic clues. *Top*, when protrusion exists lateral to the nerve root, the patient obtains relief by bending away from the lesion and pain (*top left*). Pain is increased by bending toward the lesion when the root is caught between the hernia and the inferior pedicle (*top right*). *Bottom*, on the other hand, when a left protrusion exists medial to the nerve root, pain is increased by bending away from the side of pain because the hernia places an irritative traction on the nerve root (*bottom left*). The patient obtains relief by bending *toward* the side of pain (*bottom right*), which relaxes the tension on the nerve root.

Excessive Motion. Excessive motion such as in joint tears is recognized simply by contrast with the limits furnished us by our knowledge of anatomy and physiology of joint motion at different ages. These are extremely rare except in cases of severe trauma such as in athletic injuries, vehicular accidents, or falls from great heights. The more common cause in the spine is the hypermobility felt adjacent to an area of hypomobility.

Caution. Although a patient may actively move freely through all gross ranges of motion, this is not necessarily proof of segmental freedom. Such a conclusion is an error commonly made by general practitioners. Careful one-by-one static and dynamic palpation of the vertebral segments will often reveal extremely tender sites (previously unknown to the patient) and numerous segmental fixations in one or more planes.[223,224] With the exception of ankylosing spondylosis or some other generalized disorder of the spine, gross mobility evaluation of large regions of the spine have little clinical significance that can be applied to corrective therapy. Such evaluations are of more interest to insurance companies than to health science.

Evaluating Gross Joint Motion and Strength

The range of motion for any particular spinal area is usually recorded in degrees by a goniometer with comparable measurement of the opposite side noted. When asymmetry of motion range is observed, the examiner must determine whether the side with the greater movement is weak or the side with less motion is restricted. Testing of the strength of a group of muscles is made by carrying the spinal region to the extreme of allowed movement permitted by the antagonist muscles after which the examiner resists an active maximum effort by the patient to contract the muscles being tested. Strength is recorded bilaterally from Grade 5 to Grade 0.[225]

Case Management. No injury is static. It continues to produce harmful effects on the injured person until either the injury or the person is defeated. As these effects are systemic as well as local, the response to injury is also both systemic and local. For this reason, injuries and their effects must be evaluated from the standpoint that the *whole* person is injured and not from the view that an otherwise well person is afflicted with a local defect or that only a part of the individual is affected.

Since the effects of injury and the body's efforts to defeat them are constantly changing, the doctor cannot rely on infrequent observations or on one major symptom in evaluating the condition of the patient, especially one seriously disabled. Repeated observations must be made and indications of the patient's condition must be considered to obtain as clear a picture as possible of the patient's status and the treatment required at the moment the particular observation is made.

Rehabilitation. After acute symptoms subside, a gradual rehabilitation program can be initiated which encourages the inflammatory reaction of resolution to pass quickly and reduces fibrous thickening of tissues. A great deal of atrophy, muscle weakness, and fibrous induration can be eliminated by applying progressive rehabilitation as soon as possible. Naturally, timing must be coordinated with the type of injury; ie, bone injuries require longer support and rehabilitation procedures than do soft-tissue injuries.

Posttraumatic Functional Stiffness Prevention. We recognize that enforced inactivity following major surgery leaves an indurated scar of thick fibrous tissue that remains tight and uncomfortable for a considerable time after surgery. Likewise, severe joint injury inevitably results in overabundant scar tissue from necessary immobilization. Even minor disorders treated with long-term immobilization develop scar tissue which permanently restricts function. On the other hand, uncomplicated surgery, wounds, sprains followed by ambulation in a day or two result in a cicatrix which is not tight, but rather soft and pliable. This same principle applies to spinal joint injuries. It would appear to be a worthy objective, if not mandatory, to carefully control rehabilitation toward full return of function with minimal scar tissue and fixation.[226]

REFERENCES

1. Kapandji IA: *Physiology of the Joints: The Trunk and Vertebral Column*, ed 2. New York, Churchill Livingstone, 1981, vol 3, pp 12–13.

2. Moore KL: *Clinically Oriented Anatomy*. Baltimore, Williams & Wilkins, 1980, pp 605–607.
3. White AA, Panjabi MM: *Clinical Biomechanics of the Spine*. Philadelphia, J.B. Lippincott, 1978, p 1.
4. Barham JN, Wooten EP: *Structural Kinesiology*. New York, Macmillan, 1973, pp 239–241.
5. Morehouse LE, Cooper JM: *Kinesiology*. St. Louis, C.V. Mosby, 1950, pp 37, 41.
6. Basmajian JV (ed): *Grant's Method of Anatomy*, ed 9. Baltimore, Williams & Wilkins, 1975, pp 13–14.
7. States AZ: *Spinal and Pelvic Technics*, ed 2. Lombard, Ill, National College of Chiropractic, 1968, p 6.
8. Hollingshead WH, Jenkins DB: *Functional Anatomy of the Limbs and Back*. Philadelphia, W.B. Saunders, 1981, pp 196–197.
9. Firth JN: *Firth's Technic Notes*, revised ed by Baltzell LG, Mackey RH, 1967, pp 1–3. Publishing data not shown. Available from National College of Chiropractic.
10. Grieve GP: *Common Vertebral Joint Problems*. New York, Churchill Livingstone, 1981, pp 31–35.
11. Sensenig EC: The early development of the human vertebral column. *Contributions to Embryology*, 33:21–51, 1949.
12. Gehweiler JA Jr, Osborne RL Jr, Becker RF: *The Radiology of Vertebral Trauma*. Philadelphia, W.B. Saunders, 1980, pp 3–6, 47–55.
13. Parke WW: Development of the spine. In Rothman RH, Simeone FA (eds): *The Spine*. Philadelphia, W.B. Saunders, 1975, vol 1, pp 1–13.
14. Parke WW: Applied anatomy of the spine. In Rothman RH, Simeone FA (eds): *The Spine*. Philadelphia, W.B. Saunders, 1975, vol 1, pp 19–20.
15. Moore KL: *Clinically Oriented Anatomy*. Baltimore, Williams & Wilkins, 1980, pp 620–622.
16. White AA, Panjabi MM: The basic kinematics of the human spine: A review of past and current knowledge. *Spine* 3:12–20, 1978.
17. Cailliet R: *Low Back Pain Syndrome*, ed 3. Philadelphia, F.A. Davis, 1981, pp 37–41, 49–51.
18. Grieve GP: *Common Vertebral Joint Problems*. New York, Churchill Livingstone, 1981, pp 38–41.
19. Kapandji IA: *Physiology of the Joints: The Trunk and Vertebral Column*, ed 2. New York, Churchill Livingstone, 1981, vol 3, pp 18–19, 22–25.
20. Basmajian JV (ed): *Grant's Method of Anatomy*, ed 9. Baltimore, Williams & Wilkins, 1975, pp 11–13.
21. Roper N: *Man's Anatomy, Physiology, Health and Environment*, ed 5. New York, Churchill Livingstone, 1976, pp 55–57.
22. Moore KL: *Clinically Oriented Anatomy*. Baltimore, Williams & Wilkins, 1980, pp 610–620.
23. Gehweiler JA Jr, Osborne RL Jr, Becker RF: *The Radiology of Vertebral Trauma*. Philadelphia, W.B. Saunders, 1980, pp 7–32.
24. White AA, Panjabi MM: *Clinical Biomechanics of the Spine*. Philadelphia, J.B. Lippincott, 1978, pp 81–82.
25. Parke WW: Applied anatomy of the spine. In Rothman RH, Simeone FA (eds): *The Spine*. Philadelphia, W.B. Saunders, 1975, vol 1, pp 49–50.
26. Rosse C: The vertebral column. In Rosse C, Clawson DK (eds): *The Musculoskeletal System in Health and Disease*. Hagerstown, Md, Harper & Row, 1980, pp 124–130.
27. Hollingshead WH, Jenkins DB: *Functional Anatomy of the Limbs and Back*. Philadelphia, W.B. Saunders, 1981, pp 197–200.
28. Morehouse LE, Cooper JM: *Kinesiology*. St. Louis, C.V. Mosby, 1950, pp 37, 41, 43.
29. Gehweiler JA Jr, Osborne RL Jr, Becker RF: *The Radiology of Vertebral Trauma*. Philadelphia, W.B. Saunders, 1980, p 74.
30. Cailliet R: *Low Back Pain Syndrome*, ed 3. Philadelphia, F.A. Davis, 1981, pp 1–12.
31. Parke WW: Applied anatomy of the spine. In Rothman RH, Simeone FA (eds): *The Spine*. Philadelphia, W.B. Saunders, 1975, vol 1, p 38.
32. White AA, Panjabi MM: *Clinical Biomechanics of the Spine*. Philadelphia, J.B. Lippincott, 1978, pp 35–42, 56, 486.
33. Hildebrandt RW, Howe JW: *Spinal Biomechanics and Subluxation Classification*. Lombard, Ill, National College of Chiropractic, 1974.
34. Sandoz R: Newer trends in the pathogenesis of spinal disorders: a tentative classification of the functional disorders of the intervertebral motor unit. *Annals of the Swiss Chiropractors' Association* 5:93–180, 1971.
35. Drum DC: The vertebral motor unit and intervertebral foramen. *ACA Journal of Chiropractic* 10:25–30, March 1976.
36. Burstein AH et al: Failure characteristics of bone and bone tissue. In Kenedi RM (ed): *Perspectives in Biomedical Engineering*. New York, Macmillan, 1973.
37. McElhaney: Discussion: Anatomical and biomechanical studies. In Goldstein M (ed): *The Research Status of Spinal Manipulative Therapy*, NINCDS Monograph, No. 15, DHEW Publication No. (NIH) 76-998, Stock No. 017-049-0 0060-7, Washington, DC, U.S. Government Printing Office, 1975, pp 121–127.
38. White AA, Panjabi MM: *Clinical Biomechanics of the Spine*. Philadelphia, J.B. Lippincott, 1978, pp 25–30, 55–56.
39. Bartley MH et al: The relationship of bone strength and bone quality in health, disease, and aging. *Journal of Gerontology* 21:517, 1966.
40. Rockoff SD, Sweet E, Bleustein J: The relative contribution of trabecular and cortical bone to the strength of human lumbar vertebrae. *Calcified Tissue Research* 3:163, 1969.
41. Evans FG: *Stress and Strain in Bones*. Springfield, Ill, Charles C Thomas, 1957.
42. Bell GH et al: Variation in strength of vertebrae with age and their relation to osteoporosis. *Calcified Tissue Research* 1:75, 1967.
43. Weaver JK: Bone: Its strength and changes with aging and an evaluation of some methods for measuring its mineral content. *Journal of Bone and Joint Surgery* 41A:935, 1966.
44. White AA, Panjabi MM: *Clinical Biomechanics of the Spine*. Philadelphia, J.B. Lippincott, 1978, p 24.

45. Rich E: Subluxations: Their influence on posture. *ACA Journal of Chiropractic* February 1961, pp 37–38.
46. Gehweiler JA Jr, Osborne RL Jr, Becker RF: *The Radiology of Vertebral Trauma.* Philadelphia, W.B. Saunders, 1980, pp 58–68.
47. Kendall HO, Kendall FP, Wadsworth GE: *Muscles: Testing and Function,* ed 2. Baltimore, Williams & Wilkins, 1971, p 28.
48. Fisk JW: *The Painful Neck and Back.* Springfield, Ill, Charles C Thomas, 1977, p 28.
49. Grieve GP: *Common Vertebral Joint Problems.* New York, Churchill Livingstone, 1981, p 41.
50. White AA, Panjabi MM: *Clinical Biomechanics of the Spine.* Philadelphia, J.B. Lippincott, 1978, p 509.
51. Van Dusen LG: *Chiropractic Relationship to Gravitational Force.* Sodus, NY, 1968, p 8.
52. White AA, Panjabi MM: *Clinical Biomechanics of the Spine.* Phildelphia, J.B. Lippincott, 1978, pp 23, 25.
53. White AA, Panjabi MM: *Clinical Biomechanics of the Spine.* Philadelphia, J.B. Lippincott, 1978, p 33.
54. Nachemson A: Lumbar interdiscal pressure. *Acta Orthopaedica Scandinavica* Supplementum 43, 1960.
55. Grieve GP: *Common Vertebral Joint Problems.* New York, Churchill Livingstone, 1981, pp 53–55.
56. Drum DC: The vertebral motor unit and intervertebral foramen. In Goldstein M (ed): *The Research Status of Spinal Manipulative Therapy,* NINCDS Monograph, No. 15, DHEW Publication No. (NIH) 76-998, Stock No. 017-049-0 0060-7, Washington, DC, U.S. Government Printing Office, 1975, pp 65–68.
57. Sunderland S: Anatomical perivertebral influences on the intervertebral foramen. In Goldstein M (ed): *The Research Status of Spinal Manipulative Therapy,* NINCDS Monograph, No. 15, DHEW Publication No. (NIH) 76-998, Stock No. 017-049-0 0060-7, Washington, DC, U.S. Government Printing Office, 1975, p 139.
58. Rosse C: The vertebral column. In Rosse C, Clawson DK (eds): *The Musculoskeletal System in Health and Disease.* Hagerstown, Md, Harper & Row, 1980, pp 130–132.
59. Macnab I. *Backache.* Baltimore, Williams & Wilkins, 1977, pp 12–15.
60. Hensinger RN, MacEwen GD: Congenital anomalies of the spine. In Rothman RH, Simeone FA (eds): *The Spine.* Philadelphia, W.B. Saunders, 1975, vol 1, pp 157–158.
61. Lischer BE (trans): *Fundamental Principles of Systematic Diagnosis of Dental Anomalies.* Boston, Stratford Press, 1926.
62. Fisk JW: *The Painful Neck and Back.* Springfield, Ill, Charles C Thomas, 1977, pp 35–38.
63. Rosse C: The vertebral column. In Rosse C, Clawson DK (eds): *The Musculoskeletal System in Health and Disease.* Hagerstown, Md, Harper & Row, 1980, pp 122, 124.
64. Parke WW: Applied anatomy of the spine. In Rothman RH, Simeone FA (eds): *The Spine.* Philadelphia, W.B. Saunders, 1975, vol 1, pp 28–31.
65. Kapandji IA: *Physiology of the Joints: The Trunk and Vertebral Column,* ed 2. New York, Churchill Livingstone, 1981, vol 3, pp 26–27.
66. Barham JN, Wooten EP: *Structural Kinesiology.* New York, Macmillan, 1973, pp 243–244.
67. Coventry MB: Anatomy of the intervertebral disk. *Clinical Orthopaedics* 67:9, 1969.
68. Gehweiler JA Jr, Osborne RL Jr, Becker RF: *The Radiology of Vertebral Trauma.* Philadelphia, W.B. Saunders, 1980, pp 71–74.
69. Parke WW: Applied anatomy of the spine. In Rothman RH, Simeone FA (eds): *The Spine.* Philadelphia, W.B. Saunders, 1975, vol 1, pp 31–33, 50.
70. Rosse C: The vertebral column. In Rosse C, Clawson DK (eds): *The Musculoskeletal System in Health and Disease.* Hagerstown, Md, Harper & Row, 1980, p 122.
71. Hollingshead WH, Jenkins DB: *Functional Anatomy of the Limbs and Back.* Philadelphia, W.B. Saunders, 1981, pp 200–201, 203–204.
72. Macnab I: *Backache.* Baltimore, Williams & Wilkins, 1977, pp 1–12.
73. Kapandji IA: *Physiology of the Joints: The Trunk and Vertebral Column,* ed 2. New York, Churchill Livingstone, 1981, vol 3, pp 28–31.
74. White AA, Panjabi MM: *Clinical Biomechanics of the Spine.* Philadelphia, J.B. Lippincott, 1978, pp 2–4.
75. Kapandji IA: *Physiology of the Joints: The Trunk and Vertebral Column,* ed 2. New York, Churchill Livingstone, 1981, vol 3, p 34.
76. Kapandji IA: *Physiology of the Joints: The Trunk and Vertebral Column,* ed 2. New York, Churchill Livingstone, 1981, vol 3, pp 38–39.
77. Pope MH et al: Measurement of intervertebral disc space height. *Spine* 2:282–286, 1977.
78. Jensen GM: Biomechanics of the lumbar intervertebral disk: A review. *Physical Therapy* 60:765–773, 1980.
79. Jessen AR: The intervertebral discs: Shock absorbers or shock transmitters? *ACA Journal of Chiropractic* 9:121–127, October 1975.
80. Lin HS et al: Systems identification for material properties of the intervertebral joint. *Journal of Biomechanics* 11:1–14, 1978.
81. Morris JM: Biomechanics of the spine. *Archives of Surgery* 107:418–423, 1973.
82. Kapandji IA: *Physiology of the Joints: The Trunk and Vertebral Column,* ed 2. New York, Churchill Livingstone, 1981, vol 3, pp 36–37, 40–41.
83. White AA, Panjabi MM: *Clinical Biomechanics of the Spine.* Philadelphia, J.B. Lippincott, 1978, pp 4–17, 55.
84. Parke WW: Applied anatomy of the spine. In Rothman RH, Simeone FA (eds): *The Spine*: Philadelphia, W.B. Saunders, 1975, vol 1, pp 50–51.
85. Evans DC: Biomechanics of spinal injury. In Gonzna ER, Harrington IJ: *Biomechanics of Musculoskeletal Injury.* Baltimore, Williams & Wilkins, 1982, pp 163–172.
86. Kapandji IA: *Physiology of the Joints: The Trunk and Vertebral Column,* ed 2. New York, Churchill Livingstone, 1981, vol 3, pp 32–33.
87. Kapandji IA: *Physiology of the Joints: The Trunk*

and Vertebral Column, ed 2. New York, Churchill Livingstone, 1981, vol 3, p 40.
88. Broberg K: On the mechanical behavior of intervertebral discs. *Spine* 8:151–165, 1983.
89. Perry O: Fracture of the vertebral end-plate in the lumbar spine. *Acta Orthopaedica Scandinavica* Supplementum 25, 1957.
90. Hickey DS, Hukins DWL: Relation between the structure of the annulus fibrosus and the function and failure of the intervertebral disc. *Spine* 5:106–116, 1980.
91. Kapandji IA: *Physiology of the Joints: The Trunk and Vertebral Column*, ed 2. New York, Churchill Livingstone, 1981, vol 3, pp 32, 40.
92. White AA, Panjabi MM: *Clinical Biomechanics of the Spine*. Philadelphia, J.B. Lippincott, 1978, p 55.
93. Farfan HF, Sullivan JD: The relation of facet orientation to intervertebral disc failure. *Canadian Journal of Surgery* 10:179, 1967.
94. Farfan HF et al: The effects of torsion on the lumbar intervertebral joints: The role of torsion in the production of disc degeneration. *Journal of Bone and Joint Surgery* 52A:468, 1970.
95. Kaleps I, Kazarian LE: Analysis of compressive creep behavior of the vertebral unit subjected to a uniform axial loading using exact parametric solution equations of Kelvin-solid models. Parts I and II. *Journal of Biomechanics* 17:113–130; 131–136.
96. Kapandji IA: *Physiology of the Joints: The Trunk and Vertebral Column*, ed 2. New York, Churchill Livingstone, 1981, vol 3, pp 34–35.
97. Fisk JW: *The Painful Neck and Back*. Springfield, Ill, Charles C. Thomas, 1977, pp 28–34.
98. Parke WW: Applied anatomy of the spine. In Rothman RH, Simeone FA (eds): *The Spine*. Philadelphia, W.B. Saunders, 1975, vol 1, pp 28–29.
99. Reiter L: Apophyseal joint functional anatomy and experimental findings. *PCC Research Form* 1(2):49–52, Winter 1985.
100. Twomey LT, Taylor JR: Sagittal movements of the human lumbar vertebral column: A quantitative study of the role of the posterior vertebral elements. *Archives of Physical Medicine and Rehabilitation* 64:319–321, 1983.
101. White AA, Panjabi MM: *Clinical Biomechanics of the Spine*. Philadelphia, J.B. Lippincott, 1978, p 17–23, 55.
102. Parke WW: Applied anatomy of the spine. In Rothman RH, Simeone FA (eds): *The Spine*. Philadelphia, W.B. Saunders, 1975, vol 1, pp 33–35.
103. Hollingshead WH, Jenkins DB: *Functional Anatomy of the Limbs and Back*. Philadelphia, W.B. Saunders, 1981, pp 201–203.
104. Gehweiler JA Jr, Osborne RL Jr, Becker RF: *The Radiology of Vertebral Trauma*. Philadelphia, W.B. Saunders, 1980, pp 76–78.
105. White AA, Panjabi MM: *Clinical Biomechanics of the Spine*. Philadelphia, J.B. Lippincott, 1978, pp 51–55, 56, 119–123, 270.
106. Hollingshead WH, Jenkins DB: *Functional Anatomy of the Limbs and Back*. Philadelphia, W.B. Saunders, 1981, pp 216–224.
107. Burke DC, Murray DD: *Handbook of Spinal Cord Medicine*. London, Macmillan, 1975, pp 1–12.
108. Illi FW: *The Vertebral Column: Life-line of the Body*. Chicago, National College of Chiropractic, 1951, pp 33–39, 61–72.
109. Grieve GP: *Common Vertebral Joint Problems*. New York, Churchill Livingstone, 1981, pp 56–73.
110. Moore KL: *Clinically Oriented Anatomy*. Baltimore, Williams & Wilkins, 1980, pp 657–659.
111. Helfet AJ, Gruebel Lee DM: *Disorders of the Lumbar Spine*. Philadelphia, J.B. Lippincott, 1978, pp 26, 204–210.
112. Freedman BG: The biodynamical aspect of cerebrospinal fluid in disease and health. *Journal of Manipulative and Physiological Therapeutics* 2:79–84, 1979.
113. McAlpine JE: A discussion of the dentate ligament neural traction mechanism. *ICA Review* October–December 1980.
114. Grieve GP: *Common Vertebral Joint Problems*. New York, Churchill Livingstone, 1981, p 56.
115. Palmer DD: *The Science, Art and Philosophy of Chiropractic*. Portland, Oreg, Portland Printing House, 1910, p 7.
116. Parke WW: Applied anatomy of the spine. In Rothman RH, Simeone FA (eds): *The Spine*. Philadelphia, W.B. Saunders, 1975, vol 1, pp 35–37.
117. Moore KL: *Clinically Oriented Anatomy*. Baltimore, Williams & Wilkins, 1980, pp 649–651.
118. Sunderland S: Anatomical perivertebral influences on the intervertebral foramen. In Goldstein M (ed): *The Research Status of Spinal Manipulative Therapy*. NINCDS Monograph, No. 15, DHEW Publication No. (NIH) 76-998, Stock No. 017-049-00060-7, Washington, DC, U.S. Government Printing Office, 1975.
119. Fisk JW: *The Painful Neck and Back*. Springfield, Ill, Charles C. Thomas, 1977, pp 15–17.
120. Cailliet R: *Low Back Pain Syndrome*, ed 3. Philadelphia, F.A. Davis, 1981, pp 25–31.
121. Haldeman S: Spinal and paraspinal receptors. *ACA Journal of Chiropractic* 6:25–30, May 1972.
122. Grieve GP: *Common Vertebral Joint Problems*. New York, Churchill Livingstone, 1981, pp 64–65, 68–69.
123. Gandhavadi B, Rosen J, Addison R: Autonomic pain. *Postgraduate Medicine* 71(1):85–90, 1982.
124. Parke WW: Applied anatomy of the spine. In Rothman RH, Simeone FA (eds): *The Spine*. Philadelphia, W.B. Saunders, 1975, vol 1, pp 39–42, 46–48.
125. Fisk JW: *The Painful Neck and Back*. Springfield, Ill, Charles C Thomas, 1977, pp 44–45.
126. Gehweiler JA Jr, Osborne RL Jr, Becker RF: *The Radiology of Vertebral Trauma*. Philadelphia, W.B. Saunders, 1980, pp 45–47.
127. Burke DC, Murray DD: *Handbook of Spinal Cord Medicine*. London, Macmillan, 1975, pp 3–4.
128. Gehweiler JA Jr, Osborne RL Jr, Becker RF: *The Radiology of Vertebral Trauma*. Philadelphia, W.B. Saunders, 1980, pp 68–70.
129. Moore KL: *Clinically Oriented Anatomy*. Baltimore, Williams & Wilkins, 1980, pp 651–655.
130. Parke WW: Applied anatomy of the spine. In Rothman RH, Simeone FA (eds): *The Spine*. Philadelphia, W.B. Saunders, 1975, vol 1, pp 38–39.

131. Fisk JW: *The Painful Neck and Back*. Springfield, Ill, Charles C Thomas, 1977, pp 24–26.
132. Martino JA: The disc as a hydraulic system and possible clinical effects. *ACA Journal of Chiropractic* 4:29, May 1970.
133. Langmore L: Cranial and facial adjusting: The CSF circulation of the eye and ear. *ACA Journal of Chiropractic* 3:19–24, April 1969.
134. Lay EM: The osteopathic management of temporomandibular joint dysfunction. In Gelb H (ed): *Clinical Management of Head, Neck and TMJ Pain and Dysfunction*. Philadelphia, W.B. Saunders, 1977.
135. Ostroff C: The rhythmicity of living systems. *ACA Journal of Chiropractic* 10:38–42, April 1976.
136. Hollingshead WH, Jenkins DB: *Functional Anatomy of the Limbs and Back*. Philadelphia, W.B. Saunders, 1981, pp 210–216.
137. Fisk JW: *The Painful Neck and Back*. Springfield, Ill, Charles C Thomas, 1977, pp 39–43.
138. Kapandji IA: *Physiology of the Joints: The Trunk and Vertebral Column*, ed 2. New York, Churchill Livingstone, 1981, vol 3, pp 10–11.
139. White AA, Panjabi MM: *Clinical Biomechanics of the Spine*. Philadelphia, J.B. Lippincott, 1978, pp 47–51, 56.
140. Barham JN, Wooten EP: *Structural Kinesiology*. New York, Macmillan, 1973, pp 248–254.
141. Rosse C: The vertebral column. In Rosse C, Clawson DK (eds): *The Musculoskeletal System in Health and Disease*. Hagerstown, Md, Harper & Row, 1980, pp 133–137.
142. Moore KL: *Clinically Oriented Anatomy*. Baltimore, Williams & Wilkins, 1980, pp 638–644.
143. Fisk JW: *The Painful Neck and Back*. Springfield, Ill, Charles C. Thomas, 1977, p 40.
144. Kapandji IA: *Physiology of the Joints: The Trunk and Vertebral Column*, ed 2. New York, Churchill Livingstone, 1981, vol 3, pp 44–49.
145. Parke WW: Applied anatomy of the spine. In Rothman RH, Simeone FA (eds): *The Spine*. Philadelphia, W.B. Saunders, 1975, vol 1, pp 48–50.
146. White AA III, Panjabi MM: Spinal kinematics. In Goldstein M (ed): *The Research Status of Spinal Manipulative Therapy*, NINCDS Monograph, No. 15, DHEW Publication No. (NIH) 76-998, Stock No. 017-049-0 0060-7, Washington, DC, U.S. Government Printing Office, 1975, pp 96–97.
147. Carpenter SA et al: An investigation into the effect of organ irritation on muscle strength and spinal mobility. *Bulletin of the European Chiropractors Union* 25(2), 1977.
148. Howe JW: A contemporary perspective on chiropractic and the concept of subluxation. *ACA Journal of Chiropractic* 10:165–167, December 1976.
149. Taylor HH: Is a subluxation a lesion with a fixation causing joint dysfunction? *ACA Journal of Chiropractic* 15:29–30, March 1981.
150. Drum DC: The nature of the problem: A functional concept of vertebral subluxations. *The Kentucky Chirogram* 36:78.
151. Shephard WD: Subluxation: Compensation or strain? *The Texas Chiropractor* June 1975.
152. Higley HG: A modern interpretation of the principles of chiropractic: The subluxation is today universally recognized as being a clinical entity. *ACA Journal of Chiropractic* March 1962, pp 29–30.
153. Watkins RJ: Subluxation terminology since 1764. *ACA Journal of Chiropractic* 2:65–70, September 1968.
154. Brantingham JW: A survey of literature regarding the behavior, pathology, etiology, and nomenclature of the chiropractic lesion. *ACA Journal of Chiropractic* 19(8):65–68, August 1985.
155. Minkiewicz O: The definition of the vertebral subluxation. *The Digest of Chiropractic Economics* September/October 1985, p 145.
156. Beatty HG: *Anatomical Adjustive Technic*. ed 2. Denver, University of Natural Healing Arts, 1939, p 95.
157. Nelson WA: Function vs structure. *ACA Journal of Chiropractic* 4:7–8, February 1970.
158. Gillet H, Liekens M: *Belgian Chiropractic Research Notes*. Huntington Beach, Cal, Motion Palpation Institute, 1981, p ii.
159. Gillet H: A definition of the subluxation. *The Texas Chiropractor* February 1974.
160. Smith O: *Naprapathic Chartology*. Chicago, Chicago College of Naprapathy, 1917, p 17.
161. Langworthy SM, Smith O, Paxson MC: *Modernized Chiropractic*. Cedar Rapids, Ia, American School of Chiropractic, 1906.
162. Levine M: Remarks on the spinal subluxation. *ACA Journal of Chiropractic* August 1963, pp 33–34, 70.
163. McCole GM: *An Analysis of the Osteopathic Lesion*. Great Falls, Mont, published by the author, 1935.
164. Greenman PE: Manipulative therapy in relation to total health care. In Korr IM (ed): *The Neurobiologic Mechanisms in Manipulative Therapy*. New York, Plenum, 1978, p 44.
165. Hildebrandt RW: The scope of chiropractic as a clinical science and art: An introductory review of concepts. *Journal of Manipulative and Physiological Therapeutics* 1(1):10, 1978.
166. Schafer RC (ed): *Basic Chiropractic Procedural Manual*, ed 4. Arlington, Va, American Chiropractic Association, 1984, pp 233–240.
167. Haldeman S: The pathophysiology of the spinal subluxation. In Goldstein M (ed): *The Research Status of Spinal Manipulative Therapy*, NINCDS Monograph, No. 15, DHEW Publication No. (NIH) 76-998, Stock No. 017-049-0 0060-7, Washington, DC, U.S. Government Printing Office, 1975, pp 217–219.
168. Schafer RC: *Chiropractic Management of Sports and Recreational Injuries*. Baltimore, Williams & Wilkins, 1982, pp 282–283.
169. Sandoz R: Some physical mechanics and effects of spinal adjustments. *Annals of the Swiss Chiropractors' Association* 6:91–142, 1976.
170. Jessen AR: Spurs, stress, strain and subluxations. *ACA Journal of Chiropractic* 5:1–8; 9–10, January, February 1971.
171. Schafer RC (ed): *Basic Chiropractic Procedural Manual*, ed 4. Arlington, Va, American Chiropractic Association, 1984, p 3.
172. Kothheimer WJ: An integration of cranial distor-

tion patterns and atlas fixation complexes. *ACA Journal of Chiropractic* 4:30–32, May 1970.
173. Schafer RC (ed): *Basic Chiropractic Procedural Manual*, ed 4. Arlington, Va, American Chiropractic Association, 1984, pp 5–6.
174. Nilsson AV: The price man pays for being orthostatic. *ACA Journal of Chiropractic* 9:98–101, August 1975.
175. Schafer RC: *Chiropractic Management of Sports and Recreational Injuries*. Baltimore, Williams & Wilkins, 1982, pp 279–280.
176. De Jarnette MB: The chiropractic subluxation. *ACA Journal of Chiropractic* pp 8–11, 46, June 1965.
177. Gitelman R, Fitz-Ritson D: Somato-somatic reflexes. *ACA Journal of Chiropractic* 18(1):8–11, January 1984.
178. Ridler RE: Myodynamic identification of vertebral subluxation. *ACA Journal of Chiropractic* 5:70–72, September 1971.
179. Stone M: The varied effects of structural alignment by muscle contraction. *ACA Journal of Chiropractic* April 1961, pp 31–32.
180. Brunarski DJ: Functional considerations of spinal manipulative therapy. *ACA Journal of Chiropractic* May 1980.
181. Keller JJ: Spinal extension. *Annals of the Swiss Chiropractors' Association* 6:187–206, 1976.
182. Singarajah KV: Neurophysiological evidence for manipulative therapeutic principles: Involvement of synaptic interactions. *Annals of the Swiss Chiropractors' Association* 6:143–160, 1976.
183. Droz JM: Indications and contraindications of vertebral manipulation. *Annals of the Swiss Chiropractic Association* 5:81, 1971.
184. Johnson J: Manipulative body mechanics therapy. *Journal of the American Osteopathic Association* 60, June 1961.
185. Leach RA: The chiropractic theories. *ACA Journal of Chiropractic* 15:19–22, March 1981.
186. Janse J: *Principles and Practice of Chiropractic*. Lombard, Ill, National College of Chiropractic, 1976, pp 48–50.
187. Neff SD: The neuroanatomy of vertebral subluxations. *ACA Journal of Chiropractic* 14:55–56, April 1980.
188. Grieve GP: *Common Vertebral Joint Problems*. New York, Churchill Livingstone, 1981, pp 94–100.
189. Steer JC, Horney FD: Evidence for passage of cerebrospinal fluid along spinal nerves. *Journal of the Canadian Medical Association* 98:71–74, 1968.
190. Christiansen MC: Chiropractic philosophy: The application of pertinent pathological concepts. *ACA Journal of Chiropractic* September 1963, pp 27–28, 65–66.
191. Pleasure D: Nerve root compression: effects on neural chemistry and metabolism. In Goldstein M (ed): *The Research Status of Spinal Manipulative Therapy*, NINCDS Monograph, No. 15, DHEW Publication No. (NIH) 76-998, Stock No. 017-049-00060-7, Washington, DC, U.S. Government Printing Office, 1975, pp 197–202.
192. Ebel JN: Reflex relationships of paravertebral muscles. *American Journal of Physiology* 200(5), May 1961.
193. Haldeman S: Interactions between the somatic and visceral nervous systems. *ACA Journal of Chiropractic* 5:57–64, August 1971.
194. Schaumberg HH, Spencer PS: Pathology of spinal root compression. In Goldstein M (ed): *The Research Status of Spinal Manipulative Therapy*. NINCDS Monograph, No. 15, DHEW Publication No. (NIH) 76-998, Stock No. 017-049-00060-7, Washington, DC, U.S. Government Printing Office, 1975.
195. Sharpless SK: Susceptibility of spinal roots to compression block. In Goldstein M (ed): *The Research Status of Spinal Manipulative Therapy*. NINCDS Monograph, No. 15, DHEW Publication No. (NIH) 76-998, Stock No. 017-049-00060-7, Washington, DC, U.S. Government Printing Office, 1975.
196. Schafer RC: *Chiropractic Management of Sports and Recreational Injuries*. Baltimore, Williams & Wilkins, 1982, p 286.
197. Watkins RJ: Some clinical hypotheses. *ACA Journal of Chiropractic* December 1964, pp 25, 62.
198. Schafer RC (ed): *Basic Chiropractic Procedural Manual*, ed 4. Arlington, Va, American Chiropractic Association, 1984, p 5.
199. Gitelman R, Fitz-Ritson D: Somatovisceral reflexes. *ACA Journal of Chiropractic* 18(4):38–42, April 1984.
200. Gehweiler JA Jr, Osborne RL Jr, Becker RF: *The Radiology of Vertebral Trauma*. Philadelphia, W.B. Saunders, 1980, pp 33–34.
201. Hubbard JH: The management of chronic pain of spinal origin. In Rothman RH, Simeone FA (eds): *The Spine*. Philadelphia, W.B. Saunders, 1975, vol 2, p 840.
202. Homewood AE: Visceral vs musculoskeletal. *The Digest of Chiropractic Economics* March/April 1983, pp 46, 137.
203. Lieb MM: Oral Orthopedics. In Gelb H (ed): *Clinical Management of Head, Neck and TMJ Pain and Dysfunction*. Philadelphia, W.B. Saunders, 1977.
204. Nelson WA: Function vs structure. *ACA Journal of Chiropractic* 4:7–8, February 1970.
205. Hubbard JH: The management of chronic pain of spinal origin. In Rothman RH, Simeone FA (eds): *The Spine*. Philadelphia, W.B. Saunders, 1975, vol 2, pp 837–839.
206. Harner RN, Wienir MA: Differential diagnosis of spinal disorders. In Rothman RH, Simeone FA (eds): *The Spine*. Philadelphia, W.B. Saunders, 1975, vol 1, pp 53–54, 55–57.
207. Blumer D: Psychiatric considerations in pain. In Rothman RH, Simeone FA (eds): *The Spine*. Philadelphia, W.B. Saunders, 1975, vol 2, pp 871–874, 904–905.
208. Fisk JW: *The Painful Neck and Back*. Springfield, Ill, Charles C. Thomas, 1977, p 27.
209. Haldeman S, Hammerich K: The evolution of neurology and the concept of chiropractic. *ACA Journal of Chiropractic* 7:57–63, August 1973.
210. Johnston WL: The role of static and motion palpation in structural diagnosis. In Goldstein M (ed): *The Research Status of Spinal Manipulative*

Therapy. NINCDS Monograph, No. 15, DHEW Publication No. (NIH) 76-998, Stock No. 017-049-000607, Washington, DC, U.S. Government Printing Office, 1975.

211. Johnson AC: *Palpation of Spine, Internal Organs, Muscles, Muscle Testing in Diagnosis*. Palm Springs, Cal, published by the author, 1980, pp 1–20.
212. Johnson AC: *Postural Correction*. Los Angeles, Chiropractic Educational Extension Bureau, undated (1950s), pp 8, 11–14.
213. Hoppenfeld S: *Physical Examination of the Spine and Extremities*. New York, Appleton-Century-Crofts, 1976, pp 106–114, 238–246.
214. Grove AB: *Chiropractic Technique: A procedure of Adjusting*. Madison, Wisc, published by the author, 1979, pp 39–40.
215. Reinert OC: *Fundamentals of Chiropractic Techniques and Practice Procedures*. Chesterfield, Mo, Marian Press, 1983, pp 107–128.
216. Palmer DD: *The Science, Art and Philosophy of Chiropractic*. Portland, Oreg, Portland Printing House, 1910.
217. Stoddard A: *Manual of Osteopathic Practice*. New York, Harper & Row, 1969, pp 85–92.
218. Grieve GP: *Common Vertebral Joint Problems*. New York, Churchill Livingstone, 1981, pp 196–199.
219. Gillet H, Liekens M: *Belgian Chiropractic Research Notes*. Huntington Beach, Cal, Motion Palpation Institute, 1981.
220. McRae R: *Clinical Orthopaedic Examination*, ed 2. New York, Churchill Livingstone, 1984, pp 13–21, 71–96.
221. Kapandji IA: *Physiology of the Joints: The Trunk and Vertebral Column*, ed 2. New York, Churchill Livingstone, 1981, vol 3, pp 42–43.
222. McAndrews JF: Spinal motion examination. *ACA Journal of Chiropractic* 3:38–40, May 1969.
223. Alley JR: The clinical value of motion palpation as a diagnostic tool: A review. *Journal of the Canadian Chiropractic Association* 27:97–100, 1983.
224. Johnston W et al: Interexaminer study of palpation in detecting location of spinal segmental dysfunction. *Journal of the American Osteopathic Association* 82:839–845, 1983.
225. Schafer RC: *Chiropractic Management of Sports and Recreational Injuries*. Baltimore, Williams & Wilkins, 1982, pp 278–279.
226. Hirata I Jr: *The Doctor and The Athlete*. Philadelphia, J.B. Lippincott, 1974, pp 81–82.

SUGGESTED READINGS

Albright JA, Brand RA: *The Scientific Basis of Orthopaedics*. New York, Appleton-Century-Crofts, 1979.

Breathnach AS: *Frazer's Anatomy of the Human Skeleton*, ed 5. London, England, J & A Churchill, 1958.

Dolan JP, Holladay LJ: *First-Aid Management: Athletics, Physical Education, Recreation*, ed 4. Danville, NY, Interstate Printers & Publishers, 1974.

Howe JW: The role of x-ray findings in structural diagnosis. In Goldstein M (ed): *The Research Status of Spinal Manipulative Therapy*. NINCDS Monograph, No. 15, DHEW Publication No. (NIH) 76-998, Stock No. 017-049-00060-7, Washington, DC, U.S. Government Printing Office, 1975.

Mills KLG: *Guide to Orthopaedics*. New York, Churchill Livingstone, 1981.

Salter RB: *Textbook of Disorders and Injuries of the Musculoskeletal System*. Baltimore, Williams & Wilkins, 1981.

Stagnara P et al: Reciprocal angulation of vertebral bodies in a sagittal plane: Approach to references for the evaluation of kykphosis and lordosis. *Spine* 7:335–342, 1982.

Suh CH: Biomechanical aspects of subluxation. In Goldstein M (ed): *The Research Status of Spinal Manipulative Therapy*. NINCDS Monograph, No. 15, DHEW Publication No. (NIH) 76-998, Stock No. 017-049-00060-7, Washington, DC, U.S. Government Printing Office, 1975.

Turek SL: *Orthopaedics: Principles and Their Application*, ed 3. Philadelphia, J.B. Lippincott, 1977.

Williams JGP, Sperryn PN (eds): *Sports Medicine*, ed 2. Baltimore, Williams & Wilkins, 1976.

Wilson FC (ed): *The Musculoskeletal System: Basic Proccesses and Disorders*. Philadelphia, J.B. Lippincott, 1983.

Woodburne RT: *Essentials of Human Anatomy*, ed 4. New York, Oxford University Press, 1968.

CHAPTER 7

Basic Clinical Considerations in Treating the Neck and Back

This chapter delineates the common factors involved in treating common neuromusculoskeletal disorders of the spine and related tissues such as strains, sprains, trigger-point development, and the general aspects of bone and joint disorders. The basic factors involved in disc degeneration, referred syndromes, and spinal fixations are also portrayed. The chapter concludes with a description of the basic neurobiomechanics involved in conservative spinal therapeutics and common adjunctive therapies frequently utilized.

GENERAL ASPECTS OF MUSCULOSKELETAL INJURY

The initial treatment of acute spinal injury does not differ greatly from that of other musculoskeletal injuries except for special concern for the nerve roots, pathways, and spinal cord.[1]

The Stages of Healing

After any severe strain or sprain, there is undoubtedly a degree of soft-tissue microhemorrhage. Resolution begins after bleeding stops to organize minute thrombi to form the richly vasculated granulation tissue which allows:[2]

1. The *inflammatory stage* in which the white blood cells dissolve extravasated blood elements and tissue debris, characterized by swelling and local tenderness.

2. The *reparative stage* in which the network of fibrin and the fibroblasts begin the reparative process, characterized by local heat, redness, and diffuse tenderness.

3. The *toughening stage* of fibrous deposition and chronic inflammatory reaction, characterized by palpable thickening and induration in the area of reaction, with tenderness progressively diminishing.

These stages may occur after any strain or sprain. Thus, such a process can readily be set up in the apophyseal facets as the result of degenerative disc-space narrowing or trauma. As intervertebral discs lose height, the posterior joints override and subluxate, and the repeated damage to the posterior joints, especially when associated with subluxation, leads to degenerative changes (see Fig. 7.1).

Care during the Healing Process

After displacement has been corrected or a fixation has been released, nothing should be done during the complicated healing stage that might disrupt the natural process. Firth[4] continually reminded his students that "there is too much fiddling with the spine." The injury itself is all the local stimulation necessary for maximum response. Direct massage, heat, hydrocollators, whirlpool baths, ultrasonics, enzymes, etc, are usually contraindicated because they only add additional stimulation to an already maximally stimulated area.[2] However, acupuncture is often helpful in draining excessive energy away from the area.

The best procedure is to anticipate each step in the healing process and provide the opportunity for natural processes to express themselves. This is not to say that if a variation is seen at one of the normal stages of

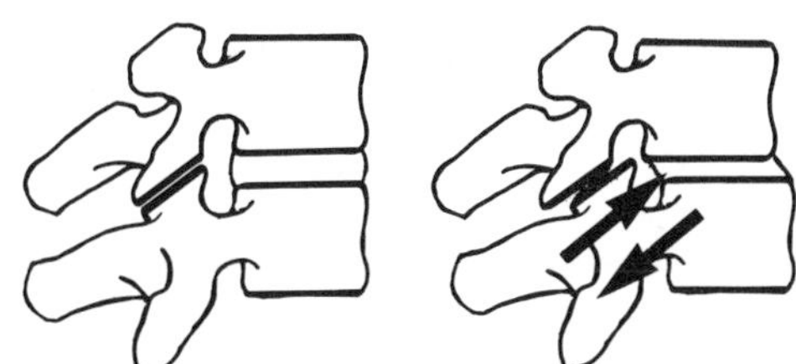

Figure 7.1. *Left*, normal motion unit relationships. *Right*, during abnormal facet motions (eg, thinned disc), a scrubbing action can take place at the posterior facets that sets up the various stages of inflammation, repair, and adhesions that can lead to sites of fixation.

healing that treatment should not be varied accordingly.

Good care during healing requires repeated inspection and sometimes external support. Periodic and regular appraisal can usually be made simply through inspection and palpation. When dealing with many injuries, one becomes astute in seeing and feeling the various stages of healing. Continuous support during the resolution stage may be provided by external measures without impairing the natural healing process.

SPINAL STRAINS AND SPRAINS

Healthy muscle function includes contraction for power production to overcome intrinsic and extrinsic loading. Equally important is a muscle's capability to relax contraction (physiologic elasticity) and yield to passive stretch (physical elasticity). Coordination is the result of strength and physiologic elasticity in proper relation, interplay, and sensory regulation. Muscle function, dysfunction, and rehabilitative therapy are shown in Table 7.1, adapted basically from Kraus's data.[5]

Spasms and Spasticity

General spasm of the spinal muscles guarding motion in the vertebral joints can be viewed by watching body attitude (eg, stiff carriage) and by efforts to bend the spine forward, backward, and to the sides. If we are familiar with the average range of motility in each direction and at different ages, this test is usually easy and rapid. Isolated segmental spasms, however, cannot be determined by such screening tests.

When muscles become acutely spastic or chronically indurated, normal movement is impaired and foci for referred pain are established. Even with proper conditioning and warmup procedures, myalgic syndromes are commonly seen when treating athletes because they habitually ignore the warning signals of pain. The degree of impairment is essentially determined by the severity of spasm, the amount of induration, and the extent of functional disability.

Both spastic and indurated muscles are characterized by circulatory stasis, which is essentially the effect of compressed vessels. This leads to poor local nutrition and the accumulation of metabolic debris. Palpation will often reveal tender areas that feel taut, gristly, ropy, or nodular.

Management

Treatment should be directed to normalize the continuous motor firing, dislodge collections of metabolic debris, and improve nutrition and drainage. Regardless of the modality used, its intensity should be maintained below the threshold of pain to prevent a protective contraction of the involved musculature. Heat (superficial or deep), high-voltage current, negative galvanism, sine-wave stimulation, interferential currents, fluidotherapy, ultrasound, ice massage, deep friction massage, and other types of massage have all proved effective.

When deep manual or mechanical massage or vibration is used, several clinicians

Table 7.1.
Basic Muscle Function, Dysfunction, and Rehabilitative Therapy

Function	Dysfunction	Therapy
Strength	Weakness	Exercises against resistance
Physiologic elasticity	Spasticity	Relaxing exercises, autosuggestion, biofeedback therapy, postural correction
	Spasm	Pain relief, "gate" blockage techniques, relaxing exercises
	Tension	Relaxing exercises, psychotherapy, hypnotherapy, hydrotherapy
Physical elasticity	Contracture	Stretching exercises, joint mobilization
Coordination	Incoordination	Strengthening and relaxation exercises, coordination training and practice

believe that pressure across muscle fibers tends to release accumulated metabolic by-products, while pressure parallel to muscles fibers (directed to the heart) enhances drainage.[6] When spastic areas to not release adequately or when conventional methods only offer temporary relief, a nutritional evaluation should be made. Calcium, vitamin D, and/or magnesium deficiency may be contributing factors.[7]

Strains[8, 9]

Spinal strains are afflictions of the young and healthy in whom strong back muscles guard the segments. When stressed, the pain and tenderness will exhibit away from the midline unless the erector spinae are involved. Older people with a degree of disc degeneration will inevitably manifest symptoms of posterior joint stress rather than muscle injury.

Tendinitis is not as common in the spine as it is in the extremities, but it does occur with strenuous effort. As the result of the vascular reaction and local edema, point tenderness is found at the musculotendinous junction or at the attachment to bone.

Gelb[10] points out that "restoring muscles to their physiologic resting length is a *three-dimensional concept*; it entails placing the origin and insertion of the muscles in correct three-dimensional relationship."

Management

The management of strains and sprains, whether they involve the spine or extraspinal structures, is essentially identical. Initially, concern must be given to the acute inflammatory process involved, for which emphasis would be on rest and support of the injured tissues, reduction of edema, pain control, protection, and healing enhancement.

The adjunctive therapies commonly used are cryotherapy, interferential currents, high-voltage therapy, meridian therapy, mechanical support, and possibly padding. Once this stage has passed (eg, 72 hours), any procedure or modality that promotes restoration of normal tissue flexibility, elasticity, relaxation during rest, and strength during action or normal stress will be of benefit. Typical examples of rehabilitative therapy are periodic adjustments to correct a muscular or ligamentous fixation with or without malposition, goading/massage, vibration/percussion, stretching exercises, fluidotherapy, electrotherapy, diathermy, ultrasound, intermittent traction, underwater exercise, and carefully monitored progressively increasing active exercise against resistance.

Sprains[11, 12]

During the range of normal physiologic movement, the vertebrae move quite freely. Once the range of motion is approached, the spinal ligaments provide important protection by resisting forces and absorbing energy before they fail. When either a spinal or an extremity segment is subjected to excessive tensile load, failure is at either the bone or the ligament (Fig. 7.2). (*Note*: Usually, bone fails first with loading at a slow rate, and ligaments fail first with loading at a rapid rate.)

Sprung Spine. The final degrees of spinal flexion are checked essentially by the posterior fibers of the anulus and the posterior capsules. If the disc is dehydrated (degenerated), an abnormal degree of flexion is allowed. A sudden, forceful spinal flexion when the pelvis is fixed may rupture one or more supraspinous ligament fibers (eg, buttock falls). Pain is localized and rarely radiates.[13]

Spinal Instability[14, 15]

The term *spinal instability* refers to that state of a vertebral segment which cannot maintain its normal relationships with its contiguous structures under normal loading conditions for the individual. The results are

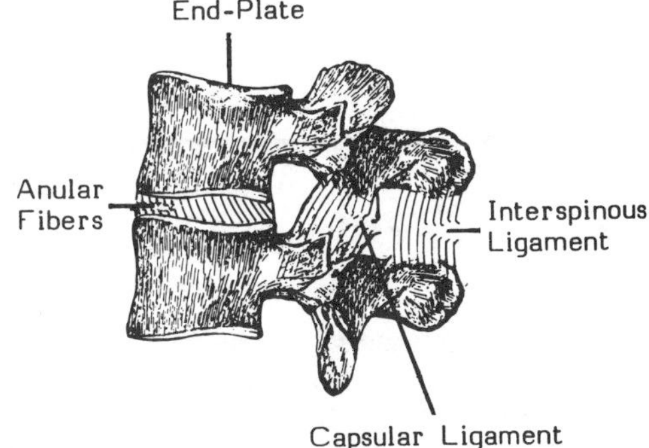

Figure 7.2. Common sites of vertebral motion-unit sprain.

possible irritation of the nerve, root, or cord; intolerable pain; and degenerative structural alterations. The cause can be traumatic, pathogenic, or iatrogenic from misapplied surgery or manipulation.

Several authorities feel that the first sign of disc disease is that of abnormal motion on flexion. Macnab attributes most pain associated with disc lesions to repetitive ligamentous strain due to chronic hyperextension of the posterior vertebral joints and the resulting arthritis. Farfan believes that the more advanced changes found in disc disease (eg, marginal osteophytes, degenerated facets, pseudospondylolisthesis) are also due to mechanical stresses. Both Macnab and Farfan consider these changes to be the result of segmental instability.

Hypermobile Subluxations

Hypermobility is permitted by ligamentous laxity, disc degeneration, and remolding of the posterior articulations (Fig. 7.3). It may be primary (ie, localized trauma or pathology limited to one or more motion units) or secondary. The secondary factors include those resulting from a primary problem often far removed from the spine, such as lower limb asymmetries, eccentric weight bearing, misuse or overuse of spinal tissues associated with postural-occupational stresses, and system-oriented disorders such as hypoglycemia that may increase the degree of spinal curvatures through chronic fatigue.

As segmental instability requires stabilization, the primary question in diagnosis is locating and determining the primary problem or maladaption that is overloading and chronically stretching the involved motion unit. A hypermobile unit is not tightened by spinal adjustment.

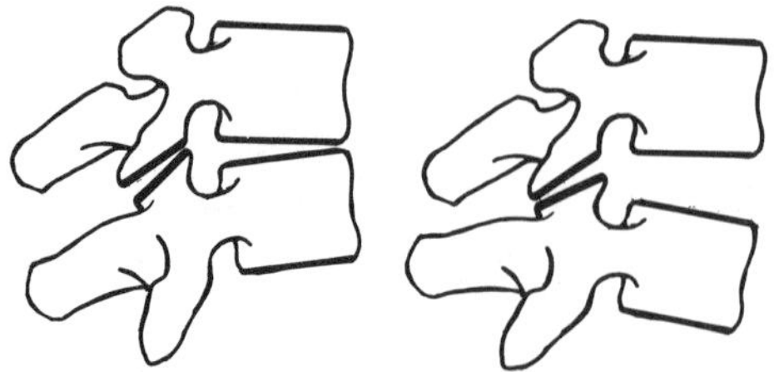

Figure 7.3. Mechanical instability of the intervertebral disc allows considerable abnormal flexion and extension at the posterior joints rather than the normal gliding movements. This state, exaggerated in the drawings, can readily lead to acute subluxation and degenerative changes.

Hypermobility is the variant of subluxation that is most apparent in roentgenography. The overt signs include traction spurs, interruption of Hadley's "S" curve, excessive A-P body shift at extremes of flexion and extension, abnormal opening and closing of disc space during lateral bending, appearance of segmental hyperextension on neutral lateral films, change in articular relations to the joint-body line, reactive spondylosis and arthrosis, etc.

A hypermobile subluxation indicates laxity of the holding elements—a positional relationship of two vertebrae in which their bodies or apophyseal joint surfaces or both are in a position that they could never occupy during any phase of a normal physiologic movement. It is particularly obvious in spondylolisthesis, laterolisthesis, and retrolisthesis, and in excessive disc space gapping in the sagittal or frontal plane. Instability in these cases becomes even more obvious at the extremes of movement, hence the value of carefully conducted stress films if they are not contraindicated.

On top of and/or below such a subluxation, a fixation subluxation in one or more particular arcs of movement (eg, forward flexion from an internal disc derangement) may be exhibited. Thus, this subluxation, which is often not roentgenographically demonstrable, is a dysfunction clinically discernible through motion and muscle palpation.

It has been a widely held view that the overly stretched ligaments and weakened cartilage of a joint (as seen in a hypermobile subluxation complex) could not be regenerated once they had deteriorated. Pennell, however, points out that controlled studies on rabbits conducted by Salter showed almost complete regeneration of hyaline-like cartilage and functional recovery when passive motion was utilized. The injured synovial joints of the two control groups, which either had immobilized joints or had been allowed normal weight-bearing cage activity, showed relatively little or no improvement.[16]

All subluxations appear to follow a progression. For example, a spondylolisthetic vertebra may start off with essentially normal mechanics, then slowly become hypermobile with middle age. An evident subluxation must be viewed in the context of the entire clinical picture.

Posterior Joint Injuries

The stability of the posterior synovial joints of the spine is primarily established by action of surrounding musculature. Excessive joint stress results in strained muscles and sprained ligaments. When stress is chronic, degenerative changes occur. Joints anywhere in the body are usually injured from a direct stress leading to connective tissue contusion and a possible degree of intra-articular fracture. The force is often an unexpected one for which protective mechanisms have not been put in force, or it may be so excessive that protective mechanisms fail.[17]

Synovial lining is slightly phagocytic, regenerative if damaged, and secretes synovial fluid, which is a nutritive lubricant that has bacteriostatic and anticoagulant characteristics.[18] This anticoagulant effect may result in poor repair for an intra-articular fracture in which the fracture line is exposed to synovial fluid (eg, apophyseal facets).

Spinal Joint Locking or Blocking

Good defines spinal joint blocking within a subluxation syndrome as an actively maintained, reversible, biomechanical phenomenon in which paravertebral spasm (especially unilateral multifidus and rotatore contraction) physiologically locks one or more motion segments, causing a shift of the axes of motion toward an apophyseal joint to the degree that the unsynchronized segment is unable to articulate about the new axis.[19] Thus, any method that assists relocation (normalization) of the axes of movement, which releases the nociceptor feedback, or that relaxes the unisegmental spasm will be effective in reducing acute joint hypomobility whose initial origin was that of strain.

MYALGIA (FIBROSITIS)[20, 21]

Myalgia or muscular rheumatism is a generalized term referring to aching muscles associated with stiffness, tenderness, and varying degrees of disability increased by active motion. Rare is the person who has not suffered some form of stiff neck, dorsodynia, lumbago, or sore extremity muscles after unusual exertion or chilling. It appears to be the most common form of persistently recurring pain other than headaches.

Background

Fibrositis is a better term than myalgia since the nonspecific inflammatory changes occur chiefly in the white fibrous connective tissue of tendons, muscles, nerve sheaths, fascia, periosteum, joint capsule, and ligaments. These changes include hypothermic edema and proliferation of white fibrous connective tissue as a result of chilling, toxic influences, acute trauma, chronic strain, or physical fatigue.

Thermal and barometric changes, vitamin B deficiency, chemical intoxication, metabolic imbalances, as well as dampness and respiratory infection are important precipitating factors. Focal infection is often an important factor as is a malfunctioning colon. Regardless, the mode factor is via the capillary circulation and the nervous system.

The early state is one of effusion with a localized inflammatory serofibrinous exudate causing puffy swelling. The exudate may be absorbed or organized by fibroblast invasion and proliferation of fibrous tissue. In the latter stage of fibrous thickening, fibrous bands and nodules sometimes form in the muscles and fascia as adhesions and press on arterioles and nerve filaments producing contracture and atrophy.

Such a condition is undoubtedly a part of the arthritic syndrome which has a wide variety of manifestations; for example, intramuscular fibrositis (myositis, myofascitis, muscular rheumatism), bursal fibrositis (bursitis), perineural fibrositis or interstitial neuritis (eg, sciatica), periarticular fibrositis (capsulitis, capsular rheumatism), tendinous fibrositis (Dupuytren's fibrositis), or subcutaneous fibrositis (panniculitis).

Common Causes[22]

While any disease that primarily affects joints may cause an associated poorly localized aching in a muscle or muscles, the following conditions are those that usually present muscle pain with minimal or no articular involvement.

Infection

The patient reports an acute onset associated with fever and other signs of infection.

Tendinitis, Peritendinitis, and Capsulitis

The history commonly presents an acute or insidious onset associated with trauma to or excessive strain of the involved region. Some investigators, however, dispute this, feeling that many times there is no overt trauma involved. Bennett contends that visceral irritation produces local skeletal vasoconstriction which sets up spasm, joint irritation, etc.[23] Thus, a joint or tendon may become painful without trauma, either overt or covert. The course is self-limiting, but joint deformity may result. There is local tenderness over the tendon insertion and around the joint. Motion limitation is common.

Psychogenic Rheumatism

The history presents poorly localized muscle pain, more commonly reported by females. The course is chronic, nonprogressive, and nondeforming. There are diffuse or localized areas of muscle tenderness.

Drug-Induced Myalgia

There is a history of administration of steroids, diuretics, anticonvulsants, etc; often remissions can be associated with not taking the drug. Physical findings are usually negative, but there may be some pulmonary involvement.

Other causes include rheumatoid arthritis, polymyalgia rheumatica, dermatomyositis, scleroderma, systemic lupus erythematosus, and various connective tissue diseases.

Combined Weakness and Tension

Muscle inactivity produces weakness and stiffness that lead to a large variety of muscle problems (eg, atrophy), and irritation leads to emotional imbalance and spinal tension syndromes. Kraus[24] feels that "if both underexercise and over-irritation coincide, and if the physical response to stimuli is inhibited or prevented, the chronic, repeated inhibitions of the fight-or-flight response contribute to disease."

The normal response to excessive stimulation (eg, pain, fear) is an increase in epinephrine release, an increase in muscular tension, heart beat, blood pressure, and respiratory rate, and a shifting of blood volume peripherally. If this normal response is inhibited over a prolonged period, this, according to Kraus, enhances hypokinetic disease.

In normal relaxed attitudes, the tonic muscles contract only to the degree necessary for the posture desired, and the phasic muscles relax. During chronic stress, many phasic muscles remain in a constant state of residual tension as a guard against some psychic perception of danger. If this contraction becomes severe, pain results which produces increased contraction and a noxious cycle of spasm-pain-spasm occurs. Prolonged spasm leads to contracture because the muscle's physical elastic property diminishes, resulting in restricted yield to stretch and possible fiber tearing under heavy loading.

Management

Whenever possible, the underlying cause must be found and eliminated, and treatment is often a challenge. The first concern should be to remove neural and circulatory interference. As adjunctive therapies, relaxation, heat, electrotherapy, dietary supplementation, low salt intake, support of the affected part, contrast baths, exercise, counterirritation, acupuncture, and massage all help somewhat but not always completely.

MYOFASCIAL TRIGGER POINTS IN THE NECK AND BACK

Visceral or somatic trigger-point irritation can produce a degree of spasm of the paravertebral muscles ipsilaterally in 2–3 segments on the same side as the entering afferent. However, if the irritation is severe, this effect will spread up, down, and contralaterally (eg, as in renal colic). In this regard, Stoddard reminds us that the sharp "textbook" demarcation made between the somatic and autonomic nervous systems is erroneous.[25]

Common Sites

Although one or more trigger points may occur in any muscle, they usually form in clusters, and certain muscles and muscle groups (eg, the antigravity muscles) appear to be more liable than others (Table 7.2).

Trigger point pain may be localized in one muscle or group, or it may also involve remote muscles or groups. Primary trigger points in the gluteus medius, for example, are commonly related to secondary trigger points in the neck and shoulder girdle. Thus, while trigger points in the neck and upper thoracic muscles may be found to be responsible for or contributing to tension headaches, a group of "mother" trigger points should be sought on the dorsal aspect of the ilia.

Predisposing Factors

Myofascial pain may be the most common pain problem faced by most physicians.[26] It may present as a primary complaint or as a crippling adjunct to any number of other problems (eg, unequal leg lengths, disuse, immobilization, chronic strains, poor posture, gait disturbances, connective-tissue diseases, arthritides). Trigger-point syndromes often appear related to a lack of appropriate (but not excessive) exercise; thus, they are less common (but not absent) in athletes and laborers than they are in sedentary workers.

The major conditions that appear to predispose to myofascial trigger mechanisms near the spine include chronic strain as the result of prolonged repetitive movement, subluxation, fatigue, tension, infection, neural lesions, nutritional deficiencies, syndromes of the menopause or male climacteric, and hypometabolism with creatinuria.

Precipitating Factors

A trigger point can be demonstrated much more easily than it can be defined. Clinicians for many years have found highly localized, exquisitely sensitive areas within or near a painful region. When pressure is placed on the sensitive spot (trigger point), local pain, referred pain, or both may be initiated. Besides deep pressure, an appli-

Table 7.2.
Common Trigger Point Syndromes[a]

Location	Primary reference zone or symptoms[b]
Upper Body	
Infraspinatus	Posterior and lateral aspects of the shoulder
Intercostal muscles	Thoracodynia, especially during inspiration
Levator scapulae	Posterior neck, scalp, around the ear
Pectoralis major	Anteromedial shoulder, arm
Pectoralis minor	Muscle origin or insertion
Quadratus lumborum	Anterior abdominal wall, 12th rib, iliac crest
Rectus abdominis	Anterior abdominal wall
Semispinalis capitis	Headache, facial pain, dizziness
Splenius cervicis	Headache, facial pain, dizziness
Sternocleidomastoideus	Headache, dizziness, neck pain, ipsilateral ptosis, lacrimation, conjunctival reddening, earache, facial and forehead pain
Trapezius	Lower neck and upper thoracic pain, headache
Lower Body	
Anterior tibialis	Anterior leg and posterior ankle
Gastrocnemius/soleus	Posterior leg, from popliteal space to heel. These trigger points may be involved in intermittent claudication.
Gluteus medius	Quadratus lumborum, tensor fasciae latae, gluteus maximus and minimus, sacroiliac joints, hip, groin, posterior thigh and calf, cervical extensors, upper thoracic muscles
Tensor fasciae latae	Lateral aspect of the thigh, from ilium to knee

[a] Adapted from Sola,[27] with slight modification.

[b] Reference patterns vary considerably according to the severity and chronicity of the trigger point phenomenon involved.

cation of heat, cold, electrical stimulation, needling, or some other stimulus may evoke a painful trigger-point reaction. The power of such a reaction appears to be moderated by a number of general factors (eg, conditioning, genetic predisposition, hormonal balance, scar tissue from previous injury, and prolonged emotional stress).

Trigger points are generally considered to be "weak" points within myofascial tissue that are particularly sensitive to stress-induced change. That is, they may remain quiescent until a certain stress (mechanical or metabolic) triggers a syndrome that involves a number of positive feedback cycles such as sensory and motor reflexes, sympathicotonia, vascular responses, and, possibly, extracellular fluid changes, which eventually lead to hypertonia, fatigue, and endogenous pain or the intensification of traumatic pain.

The most common precipitating factor is thought to be motion that produces stretching of the tissue containing the focal spot.[27] This ignites a self-perpetuating cycle of pain–spasm–pain that may persist even after the precipitating cause has been removed (eg, subluxation). Other precipitating factors include acute trauma, an inflammatory process, unusual or excessive exercise, chills, IVD herniation producing nerve root pressure, immobilization, and severe anxiety.

Cycles of physiologic responses arising from trigger points typically involve (1) well-defined pathways (eg, motor reflexes, sensory changes), (2) anticipated autonomic feedback reflexes, and (3) hypothesized microscopic tissue changes. Motor and sensory reactions are usually exhibited in local and general muscle fatigue, hypertonia, weakness, possibly a fine tremor, hyperirritability, pain, and hypoesthesia. The autonomic concomitants are similar to those seen with meridian acupoints.[28] Travell believes that these autonomic reactions are frequently expressed as decreased skin resistance, increased pilomotor reaction in the reference area, vasodilation (possibly with dermatographia), and skin temperature changes (coolness). In the typical myofascial syndrome, laboratory analyses and roentgenography fail to show significant bone, joint, or metabolic changes.

Etiologic Hypotheses

Kraus states that the frequent result of chronic muscle tension and spasm is trigger-point development.[24] The effect can be referred pain on application of pressure over the trigger area, hyperalgesia, joint stiffness, movement limitation, weakness, and autonomic dysfunction occurring in the area of reference (target area). Once one muscle has been affected by trigger points, its whole system of related antagonists and synergists is affected. This muscular dysfunction leads to episodes of tension, spasm, radiating pain, and more trigger points unless proper therapy is offered.

Several other hypotheses are described below, and many facets of each overlap.

A Myochemical Explanation

Sandman states that the focus of pain appears to arise from exercise of an ischemic muscle and/or from chemoreceptor and mechanoreceptor stimulation resulting from pressure by accumulated metabolic debris or irritation by released acetylcholine, blood serum, bradykinin, histamine, inflammatory exudates, substance P, and/or 5-hydroxytryptamine.[29] He believes that the amount of degeneration or pathologic alteration created may relate directly to the length of time these conditions are allowed to exist within a muscle.

Neurophysiologic Explanations

Although the exact physiologic mechanisms of trigger-point pain are unknown, Sola offers a rational neurophysiologic explanation.[26] He believes that, because of physiologic defense mechanisms such as splinting and bracing of muscles, vasomotor changes, increased sympathetic discharge, and hormonal and other humoral changes in plasma and extracellular fluids, the spastic muscle or its fascia (which is probably more sensitive than surrounding tissue because of previous injury or a genetic weakness) fatigues and signals its distress to the central nervous system. A number of responses may result. For example, various muscles associated with the trigger point may become more tense and begin to fatigue because of motor reflexes. Sympathetic responses lead to vasomotor changes within and around the trigger point.

Zimmermann reports that local ischemia following vasoconstriction or increased vascular permeability following vasodilation may lead to changes in the extracellular environment of the cells involved, release of algesic agents (eg, bradykinins, prostaglandins), osmotic changes, and pH changes—all of which may increase the sensitivity or activity of nociceptors in the area.[30] The sympathetic hyperactivity may also cause smooth muscle contraction in the vicinity of nociceptors, thus increasing their activity. This increased nociceptor input may then contribute to the cycle by increasing motor and sympathetic activity, which, in turn, leads to increased pain. This pain may be shadowed by growing fatigue that adds an overall mood of distress to the patient's status and feeds back to the cycle.

Sola believes that, as tense muscles in the affected area begin to fatigue in an environment of sympathicotonia and local biochemical change, latent trigger points within the involved muscles may also begin to fire—thus adding to the positive feedback cycle and spreading the pain to these muscles or muscle groups.[26] Finally, the stress of pain and fatigue, coupled with both increased muscle tension and sympathicotonia throughout the body (conceivably with ipsilateral emphasis through the sympathetic chain), may lead to focal exacerbations or trigger points in other muscles that are far removed from the initial area of pain.

A Neurochemical Explanation

On the other hand, Simons offers a neurochemical explanation of trigger-point development that also deserves consideration. He believes that a traumatically induced tear in the sarcoplasmic reticulum initially causes the release of calcium, which acts in conjunction with adenosine triphosphate (ATP) to continuously stimulate local contractile activity.[31] This uncontrolled contraction shortens and tenses fibers within the involved muscle bundle(s). Such increased physiologic activity can initiate a subsequent increase in sustained, uncontrolled, localized metabolic activity by the muscles, which is capable of producing substances that cause a hypersensitivity of involved sensory nerve fibers and, possibly, stimulate localized reflex vasoconstriction to help control what otherwise might be a rapidly increasing metabolic activity. The result is local tenderness, referred pain, and decreased blood flow within the involved muscle area.

Once the local energy and nutrient supply becomes restricted in this manner, ATP stores become depleted. When this occurs, the local physiologic contracture of muscle fibers is converted to an energy-deficient contraction. Thus, the sarcoplasmic reticulum of the muscle must be repaired. If sufficient energy is not available, the calcium pump (which is the most energy-sensitive step in the contractile mechanism) will respond with continued muscle contraction, creating an even greater energy depletion.

It is hypothesized that normal function may be restored by stretching the locked actin and myosin filaments far enough apart to eliminate contraction (eg, deep friction massage). Simons believes that enough ATP will then accumulate to restore a normal sarcoplasmic reticulum, which would allow the inhibited circulation to slowly remove the accumulation of metabolic by-products.

Trigger Point Therapy

A large variety of therapies have been used to successfully treat trigger-point syndromes. The more common means include goading, deep friction massage, mechanical percussion/vibration, spray-and-stretch, ultrasound, high-voltage current, and other forms of stimulating electrotherapy. It should be noted that deep pressure therapy (manual or mechanical) is contraindicated in any patient receiving anti-inflammatory drugs (eg, cortisone) because subcutaneous hemorrhage may result.

Any trigger point therapy is generally considered more effective if the involved area is placed in a position of relaxed passive stretch during treatment. In addition, regardless of the type of procedure utilized to treat trigger points, the intensity of the therapy must be kept just below the threshold of pain because pain will initiate a defensive reflex contraction, which would aggravate the disorder rather than alleviate it. Most authorities believe that, regardless of the therapy utilized, it should be concluded with some form of therapeutic heat that is followed by passive stretching movements in all ranges of motion within patient tolerance.

Trigger points are described throughout this book. For further information, please refer to the Index.

BONE INJURIES[32]

When subjected to weight-bearing, traumatic, or occupational stress, bone demineralizes and undergoes degenerative changes resulting in deformity of the articulating surfaces. Concurrently, the attending excoriation of the articular periosteal margins results in proliferative changes in the form of lipping, spur formation, or eburnation that may or may not restrict segmental mobility and function.

Bone Bruises

Certain simple contusions that involve subcutaneous tissues overlying bone and the periosteum are often referred to as "bone bruises." They are not common to the spine, expect to the spinous processes, because most of the osseous structures are well padded by muscle. Because the periosteum is richly endowed with nerves and vessels, severe bruises and fractures are quite painful despite lack of roentgenographic evidence.[33] When the periosteum is affected, tenderness will be present long after true soft-tissue tenderness has eased, sometimes for several months. Wherever the site, the individual is disabled or considerably hampered as long as tenderness exists. Pain from any cause produces a protective reflex spasm of the phasic muscles that restricts mobility.

Management

Various types of soft-tissue contusions and tears may be associated. Local cold, compression with an elastic bandage, rest and elevation, and pain control are the priorities in the acute stage (3–4 days). Any form of local heat, deep vibration, or deep massage must be avoided during this stage. Pain control and healing enhancement are efficiently achieved with electrotherapy (eg, interferential current, high-voltage current, acupoint stimulation, negative galvanism). External padding is often important to avoid aggravation of the injured tissues.

Spinal Fractures and Dislocations[34–36]

Generally, ligaments are stronger than bone against most forces. Bone is weakest in lines of tensile stress, second weakest in lines of shear, and strongest in lines of compression. Once healed, a fractured vertebra will often (50% of cases) be able to sustain equal or higher loads before failure.

Especially in the cervical spine, the anterosuperior or anteroinferior rim of a vertebral body, which is firmly anchored to the adjacent anulus, is readily fractured in either extension (tension) or flexion (shear) injuries. In compression overload, the endplate usually fails first (Fig. 7.4). Post-traumatic narrowing of an IVD interspace points to anulus failure and suggests a picture of shear or tensile stress.

The greatest torsional stiffness of the spine is found at the thoracic-lumbar transition, which is usually at the T12–L1 disc. The highest stress concentrations are found at these segments, as witnessed by the high incidence of fractures at this area.

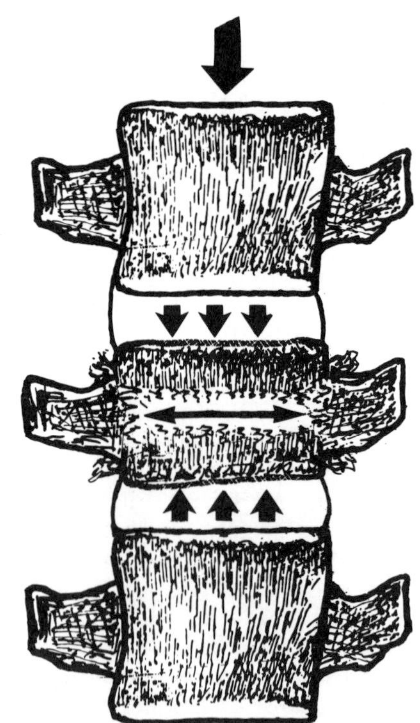

Figure 7.4. If severe compression forces are applied to a healthy spine, the discs will remain intact and cause a "bursting" pressure fracture of the weaker spongiosa caught between the hydraulic forces.

Common sites of spinal fractures and dislocations and their mechanisms of injury will be discussed in future chapters.

ARTHROTIC PATHOLOGY[37,38]

A discussion of spinal pathology is beyond the scope of this text except when these disorders have direct biomechanical implications in diagnosis or conservative therapy. This is not to say that biomechanical mechanisms may not be superimposed or involved as contributing factors in the clinical pictures of cord diseases, tumors, cysts, connective tissue diseases, infection, metabolic disturbances, birth defects, etc.

Certain pathologic processes, however, cannot be separated from their biomechanical implications; eg, bone damage, traumatic arthritis, disc degeneration and hernias, root compression, spinal stenosis, and structural deformities. These topics will be briefly discussed in this section and future chapters when appropriate.

Traumatic Arthritis

When trauma is the chief factor, an acute arthritis may be induced. The extent of the local reaction is relative to the severity of the injury and the resistance of the tissues. Repeated injuries from excessive joint stress may cause pathologic reactions or produce derangements within the joint. Or arthritis resulting from a single severe injury, especially if improperly treated, may be indefinitely prolonged and result in chronic symptoms and permanent disability (Fig. 7.5).

Acute traumatic arthritis presents signs of pain, possible ecchymosis, and soft-tissue swelling of periarticular tissue. Motion is usually limited because of pain, and there is joint instability if the force is strong enough to tear a tendon or joint capsule. Intra-articular fractures and fragments are infrequently associated. The prognosis is excellent in those receiving efficient treatment; however, a subacute arthritis may, at times, persist indefinitely.

Periostitis

Periostitis is infrequently associated with spinal joint injury. It is the result of violent muscle strain that damages the periosteum. If severe enough to detach a chip of periosteum, a degree of hematoma develops. The bruised area is extremely tender and movements are restricted. Physical examination makes one suspicious of fracture, but early roentgenographic findings are negative. Later, ossification of the hematoma is exhibited by induration of the swelling and new bone formation.

Periosteum does not cover the articular surfaces of synovial joints.[39] Thus, a true periostitis will not appear in the posterior joints of the spine.

"Kissing" Spinous Processes[11]

If the disc is well hydrated, the spinous processes do not touch on normal extension. However, if the disc is degenerated and thinned, chronic apposition of the spinous processes frequently produces bursal development in adaptation (Fig. 7.6). Chronic stress, usually at the center of lordotic curves, can lead to a picture of bursitis similar to that found in the extremities, but major symptoms are more likely to come from the disc or posterior articular proc-

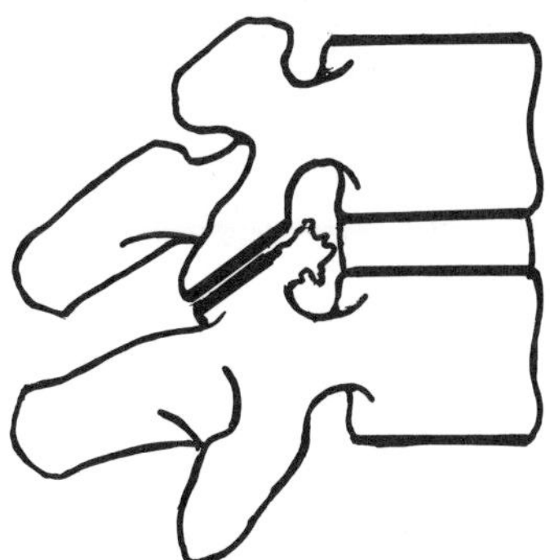

Figure 7.5. Arthritis on an inferior process resulting in an irritative encroachment of the contents of the intervertebral foramen.

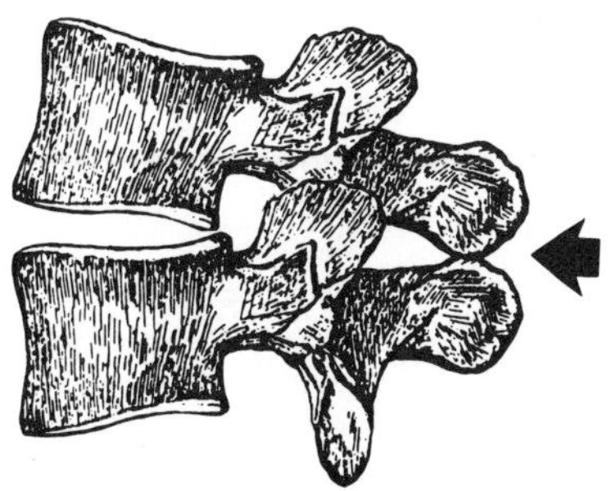

Figure 7.6. Posterior apposition from an unstable disc resulting in "kissing" spinous processes and possible bursa development.

esses. The bursal involvement is usually subclinical and imposes itself upon the total picture as a contributing factor.

We are referring here to a functional degenerative process. This should not be confused with an anomalous formation of spinous processes (Bastrup's disease) in which two or more spinous processes touch. Although the structural picture may be the same, the etiology is far different.

Infection[40,41]

The earliest symptoms and signs of acute bone or joint infection are local pain and tenderness in the periarticular region. The patient has extreme difficulty or refuses to move the area. The cardinal signs of infection may appear much later than pain and tenderness, and often never appear. Roentgenograms are of little help in arriving at an early diagnosis; when evidence is obvious, the disease is chronic. Sometimes comparative films exhibit slight soft-tissue evidence.

Joint infection may be the result of a rare penetrating wound, but it is commonly blood-borne. A degree of hematoma or hemarthrosis is an invitation to a subclinical blood-borne condition to manifest. Persistent pain following adequate treatment may indicate the presence of a secondary low-grade and asymptomatic infection or irritation in spite of blood reports to the contrary. In such cases, suspicion should be directed toward a distant focus of infection.

Metabolic Disturbances[42,43]

In the cancellous part of an osteoporotic vertebra, there is greater loss of horizontal trabeculae than vertical trabeculae. This factor, rarely viewed on roentgenographs, has a profound effect on vertebral strength.

Other primary metabolic considerations besides osteoporosis are shown in Table 7.3, along with other disorders that are associated with spinal pain.

DISC DEGENERATION, PROTRUSIONS, AND RUPTURES[44–46]

In the absence of severe trauma, disc height is a reflection of disc hydration. As dehydration increases with age and late degeneration, the nucleus tends to lose its turgor, and disc height can be used as an indication of these two factors. But this is not to say that advanced degeneration cannot be found in a disc of normal height. The tip of the superior articular facet should not reach a line extending backward from the undersurface of the vertebral body above (Macnab's[47] joint body line) if disc degeneration is absent.

The Phases of Vertebral Unit Degeneration

Kirkaldy-Willis[48] has divided the degenerative process into three phases (dysfunction, instability, and stabilization), which a patient may pass into, out of, and return to, depending upon various circumstances such as degeneration progression and recurrent trauma (intrinsic or extrinsic).

After injury, the phase of dysfunction exhibits relatively minor pathologic changes in the involved vertebra's disc and posterior facets, and there are few, if any, residual symptoms following recovery. The phase of instability features segmental hypermobility as the result of lax facet capsules and weakened anular structure. The phase of stabilization is characterized by a return of segmental stability as the result of area fibrosis, apophyseal osteophytes, and centrum osteophytes within the disc and at the disc's periphery. Table 7.4 presents a summary of the findings, with some modification, described by Kirkaldy-Willis.

The Degenerative Process[49–51]

The degenerative process usually begins in the nuclear substance and then extends into the anulus and the endplate. When this degenerative process begins, abnormal movements result. This weakening process eventually involves the retaining fibers of Sharpey, the interbody articulations of Luschka, and the crisscrossing intertwining fibroelastic fasciculi comprising the laminae of the anulus (Fig. 7.7). From here, the process extends into the periosteal articular margins from traction strain, resulting in proliferative changes that end in eburnation, lipping, and even osteophytosis (traction spur type).

This entire conglomerate of events may be referred to as a degenerative proliferative arthrosis of the spine or discogenic spon-

Table 7.3.
Typical Disorders Associated with Spinal Pain (Acute/Chronic)

Type	Examples	
Degenerative process	Apophyseal osteoarthritis Cauda equina disorders Disc degeneration Hyperostosis Joint instability	Nerve root compression Spinal cord disease Spinal stenosis Spondylolisthesis Spondylosis
Developmental deficit	Bastrup's disease Hypermobility Kyphosis Lordosis Scoliosis	Short-leg syndrome Spondylolisthesis Various anomalies (eg, hemivertebrae)
Iatrogenic origin	Ill-advised manipulation Misplaced spinal tap Myelography	Poorly fitted support Postsurgical adhesions Prolonged use of support
Infective arthropathy or neuropathy	Actinomycosis Brucellosis Icterohemorrhagica Influenza Leptospirosis Meningitis Osteomyelitis Paratyphoid fever Poliomyelitis	Smallpox Staphylococcal infection Subarachnoid hemorrhage Syphilis Syringomyelia Tetanus Tuberculosis Typhoid fever
Inflammatory arthropathy	Ankylosing spondylitis Fibrositis Focal sepsis Muscular rheumatism Osteochondritis Panniculitis Polyarteritis nodosa Polymyalgia arteritica	Psoriasis Regional ileitis Rheumatoid arthritis Reiter's disease Secondary spondylitis Systemic lupus erythematosus Ulcerative colitis
Metabolic deficit	Gouty rheumatism Hyperparathyroidism Osteomalacia	Osteoporosis Paget's disease of the spine
Spinal tumors	Aneurysmal bone cysts Hodgkin's sarcoma Myelomatosis	Neurofibroma Secondary carcinoma
Trauma	Disc protrusion Dislocation Facet syndrome Fracture Obesity Postural fault	Short-leg syndrome Spondylolisthesis Sprain Strain Subluxation

dylosis. The following consequences to this process may be listed:

1. Detachment of a segment of the end-plate and a weakening of the anulus fibrosis. This disrupts the integrity of the confining ring of the anulus, most frequently at one of the posterolateral aspects with possible prolapse or even frank nuclear herniation between the vertebral body and the displaced piece of hyaline cartilage (Fig. 7.8).

2. A loosening of the retaining mechanism of the IVD as well as the entire motion unit, resulting in disc prolapse and the hyperkinesis of the vertebral segment from an undue gravitational weight-bearing patho-

Table 7.4.
Phases of Vertebral Unit Degeneration

Features	Dysfunction	Instability	Stabilization
History	Strain/sprain	Strain/sprain with likely history of previous injury	Chronic episodes of pain
Signs and symptoms	Perivertebral muscle splinting; pain (usually local, unilateral) that is aggravated by certain movements (eg, "catches"); tenderness of hypertonic erectors; lateral flexion unilaterally restricted; painful extension from flexion; antalgic scoliosis with muscle contraction on concave side of lateral bending	Similar to those of dysfunction, except feelings of weakness and periodic tendency toward collapse are usually reported; a segmental shift may be seen during extension from flexion	Radicular pain; area stiffness; incapacitating attacks after minor trauma; muscle weakness
Biomechanics	Rotation or compressive overstress leading to subluxation	Hypermobile joint motion with frequent subluxation; facets probably open and malpositioned	Hypomobile joint motion
Pathology	Small anular disc tears; possible disc bulging or herniation; possible nuclear displacement; synovitis leading to facet fixation due to intra-articular adhesion and/or articular cartilage degeneration; probable facet displacement (subluxation)	Lax anulus and posterior joint capsules; coalesced disc tears; degenerated nucleus with probable displacement; circumference bulging of disc at periphery; probable abrupt change in pedicle height; possible A-P shift of unit during flexion and extension; possible tilt of unit on rotation; possible nipping of a synovial fold	Fibrosis; loss of nuclear substance; severe disc-space thinning; apophyseal osteophytes; centrum osteophytes; possible ankylosis; probable root entrapment

logic interosseous disrelationship (eg, subluxation). Because weight is now imposed through the displaced plate onto the vascular spongiosa, a zone of necrosis occurs and the nucleus dips into the vertebral body (Schmorl node).

3. An undue traumatic stress upon the ligamentous retaining mechanism with

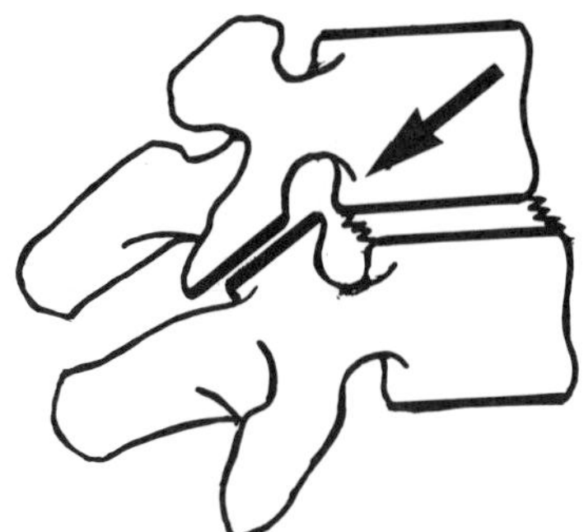

Figure 7.7. Anterosuperior subluxation of a superior process into the intervertebral foramen as the result of weakened or stretched intervertebral disc fibers.

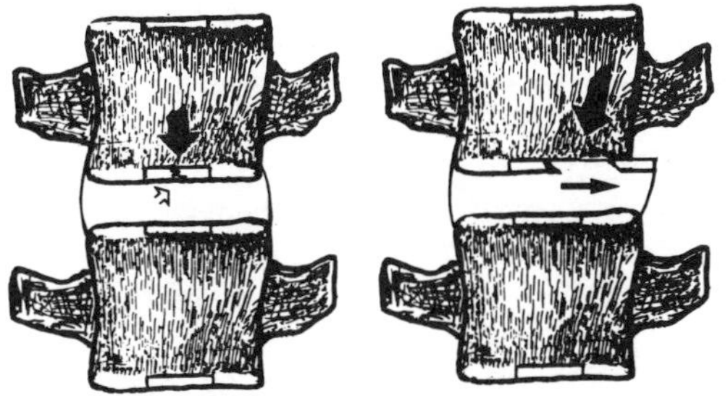

Figure 7.8. *Left*, endplate fracture is often the first stage of disc rupture. *Right*, a severe subsequent force can displace a fragment toward the periphery.

traumatic insult inflicted upon the proprioceptive bed. This usually occurs posterolaterally where the anuluar fibers are weakest and support by the posterior longitudinal ligament is deficient. Such insult results in nagging pain and asymmetrical reflex spasm of those muscles that relate to the vertebral segment of the motor bed involved.

Biochemical Factors

Interference with normal anular fiber synthesis results in increased polymerization. This and the associated increased fluid pressure of the nucleus increase intradisc tension, leading to nuclear degeneration, prolapse, and anular herniation.[52]

Immunologic Factors

It is hypothesized that during the degenerative process, destroyed tissue stimulates an autoimmune inflammatory response which may or may not involve the nerve roots. This may account for episodes of pain exacerbations and remissions. Inflammation, granulation, and fibrosis are part of the resulting picture.[53]

Disc Protrusions and Ruptures[54]

Inasmuch as the IVD has sensory fibers only at its posterior superficial aspect, most exacerbating and remitting spinal pain cannot be attributed to the disc itself. Rather, involvement of the sensitive articular facets and IVF contents is much more likely.

Types of Intervertebral Disc Pathology

The consequences of the degenerative process have been discussed. To gain a broader viewpoint, another method of classifying the various types of IVD pathology is to review Charnley's seven types:[55]

Type I: acute sprain, usually from unexpected loading (see Fig. 7.2). There are usually severe pain and muscle spasm. Nonsciatic referred pain is commonly associated. There may be rupture of some of the peripheral or central anular fibers, slight endplate fracture, and stress to the capsular or interspinous ligaments and posterior arch muscle fibers. Lasègue's straight-leg raising test is negative.

Type II: a nontraumatic, idiopathic, sudden intake of fluid by the nucleus pulposus, causing irritation of the peripheral anular fibers because of the nuclear pressure being transmitted horizontally. There are back pain and muscle spasm without referred pain or sciatica. Lasègue's test is negative.

Type III: slight abnormal bulging of some of the posterolateral fibers with slight IVF encroachment. In addition to local back pain, pain may be referred into the sacroiliac area, buttocks, hip, and posterior thigh. There is no neuromuscular deficit, and Lasègue sign is negative (Fig. 7.9).

Type IV: herniation of part of the nucleus into the peripheral anulus which, in turn, bulges into the vertebral canal. There is local back pain increased with Valsalva's straining maneuvers, true sciatica, and a positive Lasègue test. These are signs of irritation of a nerve root (Fig. 7.10).

Type V: floating nuclear fragment. This chronic condition is sometimes associated with disc degeneration. There are episodes of back pain, with or without sciatica, de-

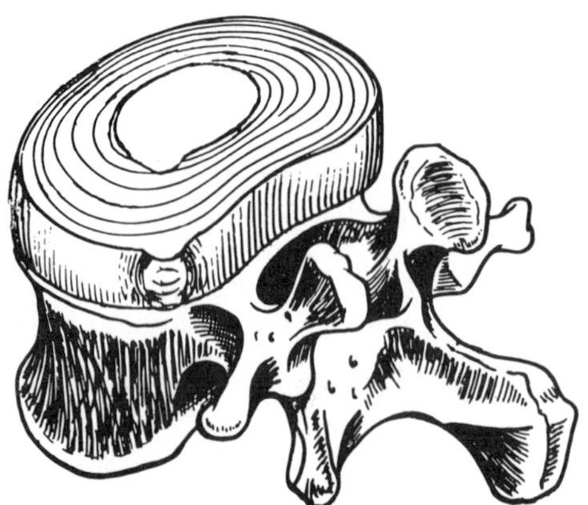

Figure 7.9. Type III intervertebral disc disruption exhibiting a slight protrusion. Referred hip and thigh pain is common in this type of lesion.

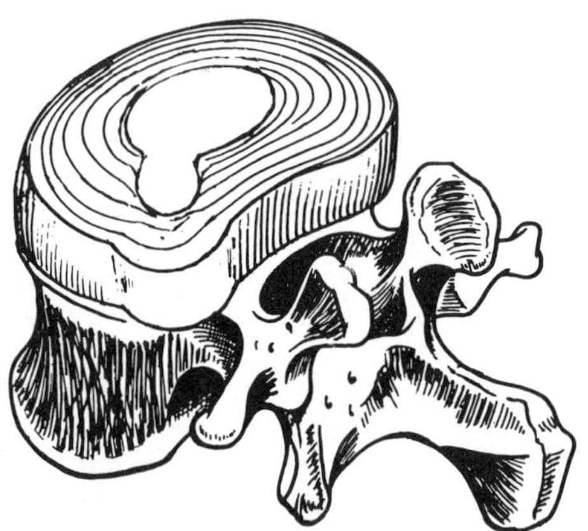

Figure 7.10. Type IV anular bulge. Nerve root irritation frequently exhibits sciatica.

pending upon the position of the fragment and the magnitude of stress (Fig. 7.11).

Type VI: anchored nuclear fragment. This is often the aftermath of Type V in which the nucleus is fixed within the peripheral anulus or vertebral canal with probable IVF encroachment. The nerve root becomes chronically irritated from mechanical pressure, chemical irritation, autoimmune response, or a combination of these factors. There is true sciatica with a positive Lasègue sign. A narrowing of the IVD space is usually associated (Fig. 7.12).

Type VII: advanced disc degeneration. When a disc is not well hydrated and nourished, it is unable to serve its hydraulic function. Disc narrowing and arthritic processes of the vertebral bodies are invariably associated (Fig. 7.13). Symptoms vary

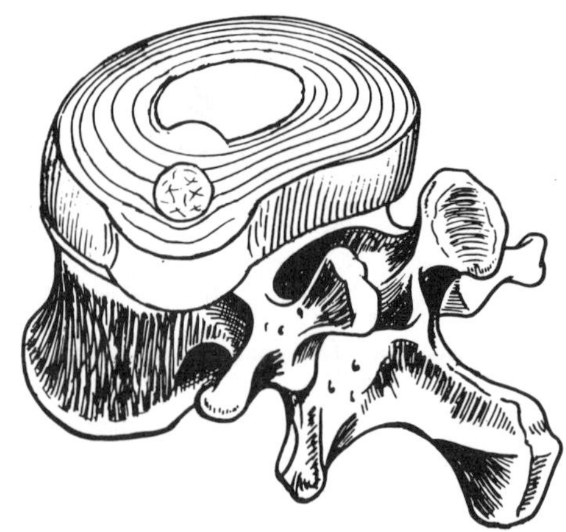

Figure 7.11. Type V disc disruption with a floating, isolated nuclear fragment. Pain usually exacerbated by an increase in intra-abdominal pressure or certain movements.

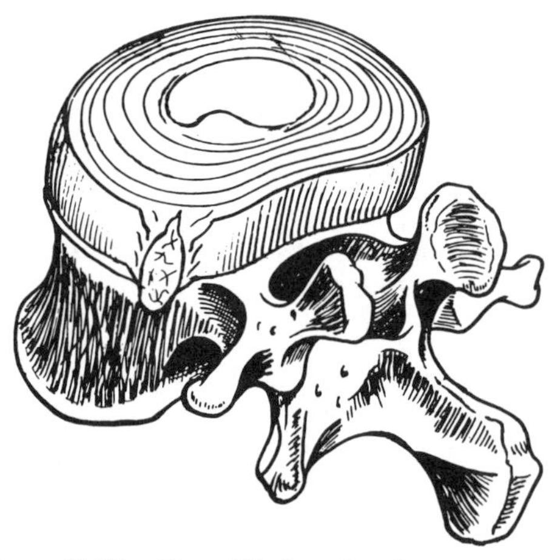

Figure 7.12. Type VI disc showing a ruptured sequestration. The nuclear fragment may or may not be anchored at some point.

from severe to none, and they may be chronic or intermittent.

Management

In Type I, II, or III disorders, correction of related articular subluxation-fixation, rest without immobilization, and relief of pain are usually all that are necessary for acute-stage resolution. Bed rest should be on a firm mattress to minimize bending moments; in the side position, a soft pillow should be used between the knees to reduce torsion. Traction and careful mobilization are often helpful additional adjuncts with Type IV disorders. If rest and adjustments

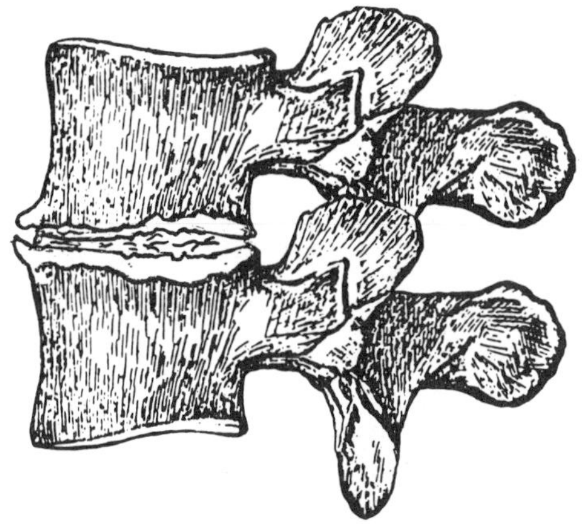

Figure 7.13. Type VII advanced degenerated disc with arthritic manifestations. The cause may be either traumatic or pathologic.

do not move the fragment into a nonsensitive position in Type V conditions, referral for surgical excision may be necessary. Because of the anchored position of Type VI disorders, conservative measures such as manipulation and traction often fail unless the fixation can be released and replaced in a nonsensitive position with a force that does not injure other tissues.[56] If pain is severe in Type VII disorders and does not respond to conservative measures, referral may be the only alternative.

Occupational Considerations in Disc Disorders

With the exception of nursing, most occupations associated with heavy lifting, carrying, pushing, or pulling do not appear to be directly associated with acute disc disorders. When failure does occur, it is usually associated with an unexpected exertion. Golf, bowling, or baseball accidents are sometimes associated with disc failure, but disc disorders are not common to most sports. On the contrary, women in late pregnancy and people over 5 years in a sedentary occupation (eg, executives, typists) have a high incidence of trouble. Race or body weight does not seem to be a factor. Traveling salesmen and tractor, truck, and other motor equipment drivers have a high incidence of disc herniations. This is probably attributed to several factors: IVD pressure increases in the sitting position, driving subjects the spine to constant "thumping" and vibrations (ie, load fatigue), the extended position of the lower extremities, and the lack of postural variation. An increased spinal intraosseous blood pressure is commonly associated with complaints of low back pain.

Root Compression[57–61]

When a patient fails to find relief from customary therapy, misguided extended pursuit is often justified on the basis of explanations currently in vogue. These often include facet impingement on the nerve root, motion unit instability, IVF encroachment by a disc fragment, pedicular kinking, nerve root fibrositis, or pseudoarthrosis. Such conditions may in fact exist, but they should not justify failure to seek other causes (eg, referred pain). Chronic root compression with its signs of functional loss is not a common syndrome when compared to symptoms of acute or subacute inflammatory irritation.

Foraminal Encroachment

During their exit from the IVF, the nerve roots often lie fairly close to the inner edge of the superior facet. In subluxation, the superior process can override the surface of the inferior process and produce direct irritation of the root by the inferior process, with or without compression, during motion. Direct compression can also result from the root's being caught between the inferior process and the body of the superior vertebra or caught between a hypertrophied inferior process and the superior body.[62,63]

Pedicular Kinking

This is associated with chronic IVD degeneration in which the disc space is quite thin and the vertebral bodies approximate each other asymmetrically from either lateral disc collapse or a laterally tilted vertebral body (eg, scoliosis). As the superior vertebral body descends, it may impose its pedicle on the exiting nerve root. Macnab feels that the most common mechanism is that the nerve root becomes entrapped in the gutter formed by a wide lateral protrusion of the disc and the superior pedicle[64] (Fig. 7.14).

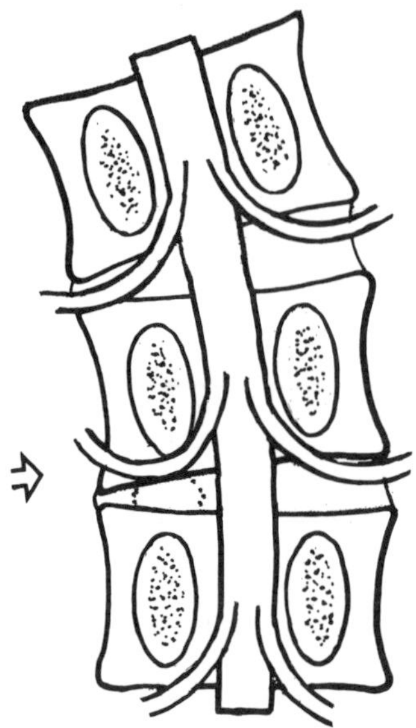

Figure 7.14. During lateral bending under load or in asymmetrical collapse of the disc laterally, the tilt leads to the nerve root being kinked between the adjacent pedicle and a bulging disc, giving rise to root irritation/compression symptoms.

Subarticular Entrapment

This type of compression usually occurs from arthritic hypertrophy of the superior articular facet. The bony mass compresses the nerve root which exits beneath the medial border of the superior articular facet. The root is caught between the posterior aspect of the vertebral body and the facet.

Axial Compression

Axial compression is never a problem with a healthy, wellhydrated disc. If the disc space narrows considerably, the spinal canal can be narrowed in the midline by several mechanisms. Typically, these include posterior subluxation of the superior vertebra, anterior subluxation of the inferior vertebra, a diffuse posterior anular protrusion or rupture, kinking of the ligamentum flavum and thickened capsules from laminae shingling, arthritic hypertrophy of the superior processes, or a combination of these factors.

It should be kept in mind, however, that the IVF is usually quite roomy. There can be complete disc collapse without any degree of compression. Also, there can be considerable compression on a root without any overt signs of malfunction if the pressure develops slowly. Entrapment, from whatever cause, can be encouraged by a transforaminal ligament, an adhesion, or an overgrowth, especially in the lumbar region, which restricts the normal mobility of the root in the IVF.[65]

Spinal Stenosis

Spinal stenosis can present a bony root entrapment syndrome. Narrowing of the spinal canal can occur either laterally or in the midline of the canal. If it occurs laterally, compression of the nerve roots can result from foraminal impingement, pedicular kinking, or subarticular entrapment. If it occurs in the midline, compression of the cord or cauda equina can result.[66–68]

REFERRED PAIN AND REFLEXES[69–74]

Todd has stated: "In holding up its own weights, the body may exert muscular effort far beyond what is really called for; and it can continue to do this because of its reservoir of energy. But in so doing, if the parts are held out of alignment and away from the axis of gravity, peculiar strains are put upon the spinal structure, which may give way with results of a quite unforeseen and disastrous nature. Sometimes the end results are remote from the site of strain; and, moreover, symptoms may be misleading because of the nature of referred and reflected pain."[75]

Pain in one region of the body may indicate disease elsewhere because nerve supply often overlaps; eg, pain associated with the ureter can result in reflex spasm of the lumbar muscles (see Table 7.5).[76] Such pain radiates to distant parts of the body depending upon the intensity of the stimulus, amplitude of the afferent impulse, and excitatory state of the spinal cord at the level into which the noxious impulses enter.

Visceral disease or dysfunction frequently refers pain to the spinal segments supplying the involved viscera and also alters the function of other viscera sharing the same nerve supply.[77] In addition, the probability of somatic dysfunction occurring in segmentally involved areas causing visceral dysfunction

Table 7.5.
Typical Referred Syndromes Associated with Spinal Pain

Origin	Examples	
Psychic focus	Anxiety Camptocormia Compensation neurosis	Depression Hysteria Malingering
Cranial focus	Encephalitis Hematoma Meningitis	Skull fracture (basilar) TMJ dysfunction Tumor
Neck focus	Malignant lymphadenopathy Postpharyngeal abscess	Subarachnoid hemorrhage Vertebral artery deficit
Thoracic focus	Aortic aneurysm Bronchial carcinoma Cardiac enlargement Coronary artery disease Esophageal carcinoma Gallbladder disease	Herpes zoster Hiatus hernia Malignant lymphadenopathy Mediastinal mass Pancoast tumor Pulmonary disease
Abdominal focus	Abdominal sphincter spasm or obstruction Ascites Enteritis (chronic) Malignant lymphadenopathy	Pancreatic carcinoma Pancreatitis (chronic) Peptic ulcer(s) Pyelonephritis Renal carcinoma
Pelvic focus	Aortic obstruction Colon cancer Disseminated sclerosis Ectopic pregnancy Endometriosis Endometritis Ileocecal stenosis	Iliac artery obstruction Malignant lymphadenopathy Ovarian cyst/tumor Prostate carcinoma Prostatitis Rectal carcinoma Uterine carcinoma
Lower extremity focus	Ankle/foot dysfunction Hip disorder	Postural stress (eg, somatosomatic reflexes)

or of other somatic structures sharing the same nerve supply should be considered.[78] The nervous system is not a one-way street: somatosomatic, somatovisceral, viscerovisceral, and viscerosomatic reflexes must be considered. For example, Lieb shows a number of before-and-after full spine roentgenographs in which severe spinal scoliosis, lordosis, and kyphosis have been greatly reduced solely through the correction of dental occlusion.[79]

Headaches

Headaches, the most frequent symptom in America today, are usually attributed to tension, migraine, abnormal sinus, tumor, vascular disorders, or hysteria. Often neglected causes are overall postural strain and trauma to the cervical spine. Headaches caused by viscerosomatic reflexes from the gallbladder, stomach, and duodenum are much more common than suspected. Nausea or vomiting with headaches is usually considered to have a neurologic basis of a vascular nature; however, a vagal disturbance due to upper cervical function may be the offender.

Cervical Reflexes

Cervical reflexes can be easily overlooked. Vertigo makes basilar insufficiency or Ménière's syndrome suspect, but vertebral artery ischemia due to upper cervical dysfunction or an atlanto-occipital subluxation secondary to scoliosis may be the reason. In blackout spells of an unexplained nature, epilepsy and arterial occlusive disease are suspect, but cervical somatic dysfunction involving the cervical ganglia may be the cause. Numbness or tingling in the hands is seen in a number of neuropathies. However, the cause may be musculoskeletal in origin such as degenerative disc disease or somatic dysfunction of the cervical spine, brachial plexus entrapment due to clavicular and upper rib abnormality, or carpal tunnel syndrome. In a lower cervical motion-unit dysfunction resulting in brachial distribution symptoms, there are somatosomatic reflexes that have afferents from and efferents to the soma.

Shoulder Symptoms

Gallbladder disease associated with referred pain near the right scapular tips is an example of viscerosomatic reflexes having afferents from a viscus and efferents to a somatic area. Frequently overlooked is the gallbladder reflex causing cardiac arrhythmia. However, several diseases may refer pain to the back, shoulder, or arm other than the gallbladder; for example, coronary artery disease, empyema, pneumothorax, pericarditis, mediastinal lesions, peptic ulcer, diaphragmatic hernia, perisplenitis, and subphrenic abscess. In coronary occulsion associated with nausea and vomiting, there are viscerovisceral reflexes that have afferents from a viscus and efferents to a viscus. Pain radiating to the arm may also be a reflex from brachial neuropathy caused by dysfunction or degenerative disease of the cervical spine or a trigger point.

Chest Symptoms

Several common chest symptoms may indicate visceral disease or, as often, referred musculoskeletal problems. Ventilatory impairment is usually suspected in dyspnea, but it may be the result of rib cage dysfunction, spondylitis, or paravertebral muscle spasm and pain. Air hunger at rest is a cardinal sign of anxiety and often seen in chronic obstructive pulmonary disease; it is, however, also a reflex sign of rib cage dysfunction of a musculoskeletal nature. Chest pain points to coronary insufficiency, dissecting aneurysm, or may be of esophageal or pleural origin; but chest pain may also be the result of somatic rib cage dysfunction, tirgger points of the thorax, costochondral or costovertebral strain, or be referred pain from the gallbladder, stomach, duodenum, or pancreas.

In chest pains associated with a cough, pulmonary infections, pneumonia, lung abscess, and bronchitis are usually suspected, along with pleuritis and lung or pleural tumors. Reflex considerations would include costovertebral dysfunction, costochondral dysfunction or separation, or rib fracture. In cough with chest pain, one normally thinks of acute or chronic infection, chronic bronchitis, bronchial tumor, pulmonary embolism, broncholith, bronchiectasis, postnasal discharge, or the inhalation of irritants. However, reflexes from clavicular strain affecting recurrent laryngeal nerves, cervical subluxation, or cerumen impaction should not be overlooked.

Referred Pain and Tenderness

Both somatic and visceral afferents are capable of acting on common pools of spinal cord neurons that are subject to summation, enhancing, and inhibiting effects.

Irritation from either pathologic or traumatic processes can refer pain and/or tenderness locally, distally, or both. Because tenderness can be referred, some examiners are misled into believing that the site of irritation must be at the site of palpable tenderness. *This often leads to misdiagnosis.* The richly innervated posterior joint facets especially may send signals above, below, and outward from the focal site of irritation.

In some cases, a paravertebral inflammatory reaction need not be a result of infection but of irritation from malfunction in a part of the gastrointestinal tract that reflexly produces vasospasm in the joint, and hence, pain. We must be aware that irritation produced by malfunction of a viscus can produce many symptoms difficult to diagnose.

Zones of hyperalgesia, often associated with cutaneous vasoconstriction and hypermyotonia, are more commonly associated with acute and subacute visceral disease than are chronic disorders. The afferent fibers occupying the pre- and postganglionic pathways of the autonomic system from soma and viscera have a general segmental arrangement. The segmental distribution of referred pain and tenderness in soma and visceral dysfunction is usually listed as shown in Table 7.6.[80–84]

Other Common Reflex Irritations

Many sensory disturbances can be caused by reflex irritation of somatic musculoskel-

Table 7.6.
Classic Locations of Segmental Pain

Priority suspect nerve(s)	Area of localized pain	Priority suspect nerve(s)	Area of localized pain
Trigeminal	Anterior head and face	T5–12	Peritoneum
C1–2, T7–12	Occiput	T6–10	Pancreas, spleen
C2–3	Forehead	T7–9	Ascending colon
C3, T1–5	Neck	T8–9	Gallbladder
C3–4, T1–3	Aortic arch	T9–10	Small intestines
C3–4, T1–5	Heart	T9–11	Transverse colon
C3–4, T1–8	Head and face	T10–11	Umbilical area, ovary, testicle
C3–4, T3–5	Lungs		
C3–4, T6–7	Stomach, cardiac aspect	T10–12	Crown of head, scrotum, lower limbs
C3–4, T8–10	Stomach, pyloric aspect		
C3–4, T7–9	Liver	T10–12, S1–3	Prostate
C4	Shoulder girdle, temple area	T10–L1	Kidney, uterine body
		T11–L1	Urethra, epididymis
C5	Deltoid area	T11–L2	Bladder neck, descending colon
C6	Thumb		
C7	First or index finger	T11–L1	Suprarenal area
C8	Fourth finger	T12–L1, S1–4	Uterine neck
T1	Fifth finger	T12–L2	Ureter
T1–4	Thorax	L1	Groin
T2	Nipple area	L1–3, S1–4	Bladder body, rectum, genital organs
T2–4	Bronchi		
T2–5	Upper limbs	L3	Knee, medial aspect
T2–12	Pleura	L5	Great toe
T4–5	Mammae bodies	S1	Fifth toe
T4–7	Thoracic aorta	S2	Thigh, posterior aspect
T5–8	Esophagus (caudal)	S2–4	Cervix

Note: Authorities differ somewhat as to exact levels, and variances of a segment above or below are commonly given by different authorities. The above data are a composite of the findings from several sources (courtesy of Associated Chiropractic Academic Press).

etal tissues in addition to nerve root involvements and/or peripheral irritations. These symptoms lack the typical features of nerve root involvement such as are observed in cervical compression tests and usually do not create significant motor changes. They often arise from inflammatory tissues or fibrotic muscles, tendons, or ligaments which characteristically act as trigger areas. That is, their stimulation (eg, with deep pressure) initiates the reflex pain.

Some of the typical reflex neuralgias are listed in the following examples:[85]

- Marked hypertonicity and tenderness of the occipital musculature and the consequent C1 or C2 neuralgia associated with upper cervical subluxation.
- Hypertonicity and tenderness of the muscles and tendons of the rotator cuff consequent to rotator cuff tendinitis and associated with referred pain into the posterolateral arm. These manifestations are often aggravated by cervical subluxation and spondyloarthrosis.
- Hypertonicity and tenderness of the musculature around the scapula common to the scapulocostal syndrome. These areas often cause reflex pain down the ulnar side of the upper extremity and are often aggravated by sectional thoracic scoliosis and thoracocostal subluxations or duodenal malfunction.
- Hypertonicity and tenderness of the piriformis, which may cause a posterior sciatic reflex neuralgia and even peripheral nerve pressure. This is common to many sacral

subluxations or gonadal irritation and malfunction.

• Hypertonicity and tenderness of the gluteal musculature and sacroiliac ligaments, which may reflect pain over the sciatic trajectory. Such disorders are often caused or affected by sacroiliac subluxations or reflexes from pelvic congestion.

• Hypertonicity and tenderness of the tensor fascia latae and the consequent reflex pain down the lateral thigh associated with iliofemoral tendinitis and innominate subluxation.

SPINAL FIXATIONS[86–92]

A spinal articulation may be fixed, totally or partially, in its neutral position, or it may be fixed anywhere within its range of A-P, lateral flexion, or rotational motion. Thus, a fixation is not synonymous with a subluxation but is a state superimposed upon a subluxation. *If an articular subluxation is not fixed, it undoubtedly would reduce itself automatically in most cases during normal spinal motions.*

In compensation to a local area of fixation, adjacent joints are forced to assume roles of increased mobility (hyperkinesia) leading to clinical instability. Also, when an unilateral articulation is partially fixated, its contralateral partner is forced to assume the role of both through pivotal hypermobility about an abnormal axis. Invariably, it will be the site of excessive mobility that is symptomatic rather than the site of the cause of the abnormal movement. Gillet believes that one exception to this is the suboccipital area, which he feels is often involved in a multimuscular state of fixation.

Total fixation is most frequently found at the atlanto-occipital, lower thoracic, and sacroiliac articulations. In most instances, however, mobility is not restricted in all directions. The earlier a fixation is corrected, the less chance there is for chronic degenerative changes to occur and the greatest change in mobility can be noted after adjustment.

Cause-and-Effect Relationships

Both spinal and extraspinal subluxations and fixations can be primary causes or secondary effects of each other.[93]

Subluxation as the Primary Entity

In a situation of trauma, a vertebra can be forced out of its normal alignment and jammed into an abnormal position of unrest. Trauma inevitably is associated with severe, protective, phasic muscular spasm. In time, the related muscles will become hypertonic by postural reflexes in their effort to correct the situation, even when the phasic fibers relax. The related paravertebral ligaments will shorten to accommodate their restricted need for mobility. Here, fixation is secondary to the subluxation. Its state is usually acute and unilateral.

This same type of subluxation is seen secondary to peripheral irritation (eg, visceral irritation), when the subluxation is sustained through sensory or autonomic input to the efferent neurons via cord interneurons. Since the nervous system is not a one-way street, it is often difficult to determine if the subluxation here is a contributing cause or a complicating effect.

Fixation as the Primary Entity

Severe muscular contraction, from whatever stimuli, can lock a segment or pull a vertebra out of its position of rest. This site of primary fixation is, in turn, usually an adaptive mechanism secondary to a vertebral anomaly or asymmetry, a unilateral short leg (structural or functional), a remote adaptive mechanism to an acute subluxation that has been corrected, habitual postural imbalance (eg, occupational or otherwise), or unilateral overdevelopment. Here, the associated subluxation is secondary to the fixation. It is usually chronic and bilateral.

We can therefore appreciate that a subluxation or fixation can be locally primary or secondary. One type can be found at one site and the other type at another site, and one type can be superimposed upon the other at the same site.

Types of Fixation

Four major mechanisms are involved in articular fixation: muscular, ligamentous, intra-articular, and osseous. These mechanisms may occur singularly but more often they occur in combination, and they may occur in one motion unit or several.

The mechanisms that hold a vertebra in

subluxation are varied and often controversial. Smith[94] held that the cause was a muscular or ligamentous fixation. In 1923, Downing described the osteopathic lesion in similar terms.[95] Other causes have been attributed to bony impingement (Palmer), trigger points (Travell), viscerosomatic reflexes (Bennett), articular adhesions (Stoddard), capsular adhesions (Mennell), disc displacement (Cyriax), nuclear displacements (Barge), meniscoid fragments (Schmorl and Junghans), synovial tabs (Haddley), acquired apophyseal asymmetry (Caplans), and various combinations of these factors.

Each region of the spine appears to have its peculiar characteristics in regard to fixation development. Certain muscles have a greater tendency to hypertonicity, and certain ligaments have a greater tendency to shortening. These characteristics, which depend upon the muscles' physical properties and functional roles, will be discussed in future chapters. Obviously, the type of fixation and degree of degeneration present, among other factors, determine the magnitude of adjustment force necessary for freeing the fixation.

Muscular Mechanisms

Contracted musculature will fixate a vertebral segment. To appreciate the mechanisms involved, two points should be kept in mind that have been previously discussed:

1. Muscles receive dual efferent innervation: (1) via the large phasic high-threshold neurons that provide intermittent voluntary or reflex impulses of short duration and fast velocity for movement, and (2) via the smaller postural lower-threshold neurons that provide reflex impulses of longer duration and slower conduction to maintain constant muscle tone. Activity of the latter is essentially sustained by the stretch reflex.

2. Phasic unilateral muscle contraction produces an automatic relaxation of its antagonists and a temporary abolition of the antagonists' postural tone via reciprocal inhibition.

A dynamic chiropractic adjustment, utilizing a high velocity and low amplitude, that is designed to increase the distance between muscle origin and insertion would quickly elongate the contracted muscle fibers and encourage relaxation via the *Golgi tendon organ reflex*. On the other hand, slow intermittent manipulation or traction would encourage resistance via the *stretch reflex*.

Muscular fixations in the spine are the most numerous, the most symptomatic, the most liable to be unilateral, and the most visible in terms of "displacement." Fortunately, they are the easiest to correct by either direct or indirect means. Unfortunately, they are the most liable to return. A long-standing state of hypertonicity will lead to fibrotic degenerative changes. Thus, for practical purposes, such a muscle or muscle group acts and responds to treatment as would ligamentous tissue.

Acute reflex muscular fixations are usually the product of another site of chronic fixation-generating noxious reflexes. Thus, they often disappear immediately when the primary site is normalized. They are also the most likely to exhibit a predictable specific pattern in response to a primary remote site of chronic fixation. The hypertonicity is usually restricted to the short muscles, but the long muscles are occasionally involved.

No technique or modality will substantially strengthen a muscle or permanently shorten a lax muscle. Only exercise will do that. Various techniques and modalities may be applied to relax spasticity, but only active and passive stretching exercises will (in time) lengthen shortened connective-tissue fibers.

Paravertebral Ligamentous Mechanisms

Shortened ligamentous tissue will fixate a vertebral segment. It is the nature of ligamentous tissue to adapt (shorten) itself to the range of motion used by the individual. While muscle contraction may be unilateral or bilateral, ligamentous shortening not occurring in the midline is almost always bilateral, with one side usually shorter than the other. Ligamentous fixations invariably produce a degree of torsion, and only a slight increase in mobility is appreciated immediately after adjustment.

Intra-articular Mechanisms

Chronic hypomobile fixation of any diarthrodial joint results in para-articular ligamentous shortening and eventual joint cartilage degeneration. This degenerative process is usually initiated by a readily correctable state, poorly defined as joint "glueing" and similar to the early adhesive state of "frozen shoulder" capsulitis. Early proper adjustment breaks the seal and encourages a rapid return of mobility.

Shortening of capsular ligaments tends to restrict motions other than rotation, but the effect of capsular shortening is much more pronounced in the extraspinal joints than in the spine. Because body joints are coupled in kinematic chains, the effects of extraspinal fixations may be referred to the spine.

Osseous-Fibrous Mechanisms

Bony ankylosis is the ultimate mechanism of fixation. Since it is usually the result of advanced pathologic processes and adaptive in nature, it does not fall into the realm of correctable fixation. Freeing a pure ankylosis will generally cause more harm than good and thus is contraindicated (eg, rheumatoid arthritis).

Fibrous ankylosis, common to thoracic degenerative changes, does not contraindicate manipulation. However, fibrous tissues adapt slowly and correction requires frequent care utilizing many different types of therapy over many months, if not years, to see an appreciable structural change.

Motion Palpation

Since manipulative therapy introduces motion into the spine, it appears logical that it should be applied at the joint site where motion is restricted or lacking.[96] Essentially, the diagnostic process involves seeking palpatory sites of motion restriction[97] or a lack of joint play[98] while the joint is put through maximum ranges of passive motion. Another approach is to seek radiographic evidence of restricted joint motion on stress films.[99]

Joint play is described as that motion which can be elicited passively at the end of active motion. Although joint play is necessary for normal joint function, it is not influenced by a patient's volition. In other words, total joint motion is the sum of the voluntary range of movement plus or minus the joint play exhibited.[100] Bergmann points out that joint play cannot be isolated or produced by the action of voluntary muscles, but normal voluntary action depends on normal joint end-play. Pain and spasm occur when a joint is forced (actively or passively) in the direction in which normal joint end-play is lacking. Once normal joint play is restored by manipulation, the associated pain and spasm subside. Specific techniques for determining segmental motion and end-play will be described in future chapters.

BASIC NEUROBIOMECHANICS IN CONSERVATIVE SPINAL THERAPEUTICS

The doctor of chiropractic should consider each individual as an integrated being and give special attention to spinal mechanics and neurologic, muscular, and vascular relationships.[101] In regard to health maintenance, the practitioner should view a patient as a dynamic, complex being having an innate intelligence that provides a marked capacity for self-healing,[100] when factors interfering with the body's recuperative powers can be reduced.

With respect to chiropractic treatment and patient management, typical examples of the basic procedures that may be used in accordance with the chiropractic physician's clinical judgment include spinal adjusting, manipulation, physical modalities, rehabilitation, nutritional and psychologic counseling, supportive appliances, and emergency first aid.[102] The general aspects of those procedures having the greatest biomechanical impact will be described in this and the following section. Specific applications will be described in following chapters.

Therapeutic Objectives

The aims of therapy naturally change with the needs of the individual patient. The general objectives of therapeutic clinical biomechanics include the relief of pain, the reduction of muscular hypertonicity and spasm, the improvement of mobility, the improvement of soft-tissue pliability, the improvement of stabilization, the improvement of segmental structural alignment, and the improvement of overall body balance. These objectives imply the normalization of neural, vascular, lymphatic, and hormonal mechanisms for proper metabolic homeostasis.

Basic Considerations in Adjustive Therapy

The most specialized and significant therapy employed by the chiropractor involves the adjustment of the articulations of the human body, especially of the spinal column, manually or mechanically, actively or passively, for the purpose of restoring normal articular relationship and function, restoring neurologic integrity, and influencing physiologic processes.[100]

Basic Considerations

There is a recent trend by some to lump what a chiropractor does during "an adjustment" under the general category of spinal manipulative therapy (SMT). This author is often uncomfortable with such a generalization because what a chiropractor attempts to do is far removed from those general "mobilization" and gross "manipulation" procedures conducted by physiotherapists and many osteopaths, which typically are attempts to increase a restricted range of movement of a joint by stretching contractures.

Although the chiropractic "adjustment" is at the foundation of chiropractic therapeutics, few have tried to define it. Sandoz states that it is a passive manual maneuver during which the three-joint complex (IVD and apophyseal joints) is suddently carried beyond the normal physiologic range of movement without exceeding the boundaries of anatomical integrity.[103,104] Swezey, an allopath, refers to a dynamic chiropractic adjustment as the high-velocity short-arc–induced passive movement of one articulating surface over another.[105] Few would strongly object to either of these attempts to define the purely structural effect induced, if the objective is solely to mobilize a fixation or realign a subluxation. Unfortunately, such purely mechanical concepts are limited; eg, they fail to consider the induced stimulation upon the cord, root, and mechanoreceptors of the area and the local and remote "spillover" effects of such stimuli.

More than 20 years ago, Levine[106] had the foresight to warn those who defined the chiropractic adjustment solely in structural terms without considering the neurologic overtones involved:

In discussing chiropractic techniques, it is only proper to note that chiropractic holds no monopoly on manipulation. Manipulation for the purpose of setting and replacing displaced bones and joints, including spinal articulations, is one of the oldest therapeutic methods known. It has been and still is an integral part of the armamentarium of healers of all times and cultures.

What differentiates chiropractic adjusting from orthopedic manipulations, osteopathic maneuvers, massage, zone therapy, etc? In one sentence, it is *the dynamic thrust!* The use of the dynamic thrust is singularly chiropractic. And it is the identifying feature of chiropractic techniques.

However, chiropractic's rationale is hardly based on the fact that its adjustive techniques are applied with a sudden impulse of force. It is the reasons why these techniques are applied, and why they are applied in a certain manner, that distinguish chiropractic from other healing disciplines, manipulative or not. In fact, some chiropractic techniques of recent vintage are *not* characterized by sudden application. We are thinking of those techniques which have been named "non-force," though strictly speaking, the term is a misnomer. What makes them also part of chiropractic is that they are designed to serve the same purpose as the dynamic thrust, though whether they are equally efficient is a moot question.

Manipulation and Motion Barriers[107–110]

All types of joint manipulation impose static and dynamic forces across joint surfaces.

Within its anatomic range of motion, a normal vertebra exhibits (1) a voluntary active range, (2) an involuntary passive range, and (3) a slight paraphysiologic motion at the end of the passive range which is determined by ligamentous laxity and elasticity. These ranges, depicted in Figure 7.15, are utilized in therapeutic exercise, mobilization, and adjustive techniques.

To appreciate this, an understanding of the barrier concept is necessary. When a joint is passively tested for range of motion, the examiner will note increasing resistance to motion referred to as a "bind" or the physiologic motion barrier.[111] When the joint is carried past this point, the added motion becomes painful to the patient. This point is referred to as the anatomical motion barrier. In evaluating the degrees of passive motion, joints should be moved near the elastic motion barrier. Thus, joint motion

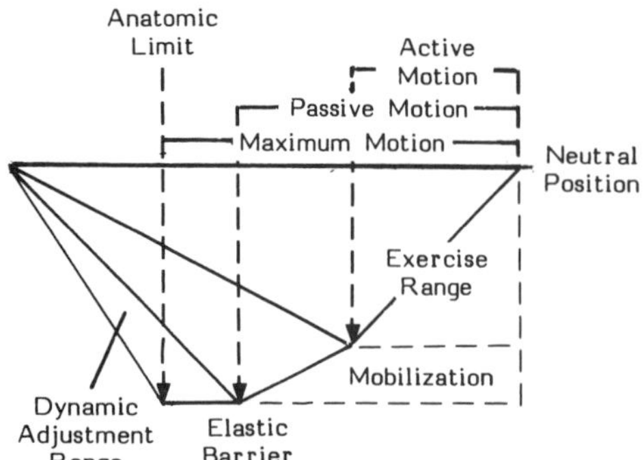

Figure 7.15. Comparative ranges of movement during exercise, mobilization, and dynamic adjustive techniques.

evaluation is accomplished by passively carrying the joint(s) through a range of motion until the elastic barrier is encountered, and then recording the degrees of movement allowed.

Active motion usually exists from the neutral position to the point of tissue resistance, while passive motion extends past this to near the elastic barrier. The usual objective of mobilization techniques is to restore the normal range of passive joint motion from the neutral position to the normal elastic barrier.[112] Thus, it is longer in range than that of active motion and to the maximum point of passive motion. Most osteopathic "leverage" techniques are conducted within this range, as are many chiropractic extremity techniques. In contrast, dynamic specific chiropractic spinal adjustments are usually carried a step further into the paraphysiologic range, often to the anatomical limit, but the duration of the application of force is only a fraction of a second.

Specific Chiropractic Adjustments[113–117]

The biomechanical objective here is to restore mobility throughout the active, passive, and paraphysiologic range of motion. Because of the dynamic forces involved, such techniques must carefully consider the exact geometric plane of articulation (normal or abnormal), asymmetry, the force magnitude to be applied, the direction of force, torque, coupling mechanisms, the state of the holding elements (eg, spastic muscles, articular fixations, stiffness and damping factors), the integrity of the check ligaments (eg, stretched, shortened), and any underlying pathologic processes (eg, sclerotic, arthrotic, osteoporotic) of the structures directly or indirectly involved. As local temperature, trabeculae arrangement, density, nutrition, etc, are variables that affect the material properties of tissues, these factors must also be considered.

Skilled spinal adjustments often involve the breaking of the synovial seal of the posterior joints which results in an audible "snap." While some feel this is of little significance, most authorities feel that breaking the joint seal permits an increase in mobility (particularly that not under voluntary control) for 15–20 minutes—allowing the segment to normalize its position and mobility.[118–120]

Unsuccessful manipulations that result in increased pain rarely present an audible joint release, while successful adjustments usually result in an immediate sense of relief even though pain and spasm are still present, a reduction in palpable hypertonicity, and an improvement in joint motion, and are followed by a gradual reduction in symptoms.

In view of our previous discussions on compensatory patterns, adaptive biomechanical responses, and reflex spasms, Gillet warns: *Never readjust subluxations that already have been corrected without searching for the causes of their recurrence.*[97] If a correction must be made several times within a period of several days, it can usually be assumed that this site is secondary to a more primary area somewhere else in the body. Granted some positive influence can be made on this side of the neural cycle, but it cannot be considered good clinical judgment if treatment is limited to this site.

Upper Cervical Techniques

While most adjustive techniques are applied at the focal site of symptom expression, others might apply the stimulus to a remote location to correct abnormal biomechanics affecting the spinal cord and local proprioceptive receptors.[121–131] This is seen in several occipital condyle and upper cervical specific techniques such as:

- Craton's technique
- Gregory's atlas subluxation complex technique
- Grostic technique

- Life upper cervical technique
- Mears' technique
- Palmer upper cervical technique
- Sweat's upper cervical technique

Such remote effects are also witnessed with various cutaneous, subcutaneous, fascial, and muscle reflex techniques. It should be kept in mind that advocates of specific upper cervical techniques and Logan Basic technique, and even dentists by correcting TMJ dysfunction, have demonstrated the reduction of scoliosis and remote symptoms by reflex effects. While the complex neurologic and/or biochemical mechanisms involved in these effects have not as yet been definitively determined, the empirical results achieved in many cases cannot be denied. An open mind on this subject should be maintained until many more of the mysteries of human physiology have been solved.

The Role of Joint Receptors[132–134]

When manipulation is applied to any joint, changes in muscle, tendon, capsule, and ligamentous tension stimulate mechanoreceptors embedded within the affected stretched tissues.

Types and Function

The apophyseal joints of the spine contain three of the four types of sensory mechanoreceptors that are stimulated by tissue tension. The four types are:

Type I: These are globular corpuscles, thinly encapsulated, embedded in three-dimensional grape-like clusters of 3–8 corpuscles. They are found in the outer layers of joint capsules, originating from small myelinated nerve fibers. These very low-threshold, slowly adapting biologic transducers are stimulated by slight increases in both static and dynamic local tissue stretching. They readily respond during active and passive manipulation. Their firing frequency, occurring even during joint rest and immobilization from static tension, is increased during capsule tension and decreased during capsule relaxation. Thus, their degree of activity is proportional to and signals the velocity, direction, and amplitude of joint movement (ie, tissue stretch).

Type II: These consist of conical receptors, thickly encapsulated, found individually or in clusters of 2–4 corpuscles. They are located in the deep subsynovial layers of joint capsules and articular fat pads, originating from medium-size myelinated nerve fibers. They have a low threshold, as do Type I receptors, but adapt readily to dynamic tension changes and do not fire during joint rest. These receptors signal that joint motion has been initiated, but offer no information as to joint velocity, direction, or amplitude of movement. During the ipsilateral tissue stretch of activity, they produce only short bursts of impulses that blend into Type I impulses; simultaneously, impulses from the contralateral relaxed ligamentous fibers are greatly reduced in the Type I tonic nerve fibers. During axial traction, however, Type I discharges remain proportional to the tension force.

Type III: These are relatively large fusiform receptors, thinly encapsulated, found individually or in clusters of 2–3 corpuscles. They are sited at the surface of extremity joint ligaments, collaterally and intrinsically, originating from large myelinated nerve fibers. These high-threshold receptors are *absent* in intrinsic vertebral ligaments but are affected indirectly within the extremities during spinal motion. They adapt slowly to dynamic changes in tissue tone but fire continuously when activated by severe dynamic changes of tissue tone.

Type IV: These are the nociceptive receptors, and they have two subtypes:

1. One subtype is the three-dimensional plexuses of unmyelinated nerve fibers found embedded in joint capsules, articular fat pads, and the outer coat of joint blood vessels, but absent in menisci and discs, synovial tissue, and articular cartilage. They comprise the articular nociceptive system that is normally inactive during joint rest but activated during joint motion or chemical irritation (eg, inflammation), thus providing the major source of joint pain.

2. The other subtype is the free unmyelinated nerve endings found weaving between collateral and intrinsic joint ligament fibers of both axial and appendicular joints.

Both forms originate from tiny myelinated and unmyelinated nerve fibers, are extremely high-threshold receptors, nonadapting, highly sensitive to abnormal tissue metabolites, and have an intimate morphologic relationship with the other types of joint receptors.

Central Effects

The afferent discharges from Type I and II capsule receptors especially offer important effects during professional manipulation or traction. Wyke describes reflex, pain suppression, and position perception effects.

Reflex Effects. The afferent nerve fibers of articular receptors transmit polysynaptically with fusiform motor neurons within the central nervous system. Connection with α-neurons is absent. The circuits contribute to the activity messages produced at the fusiform muscle spindle receptors, thus affecting muscle tone and the stretch reflexes of voluntary muscle. Specific joint manipulation affects muscle activity both locally (ipsilateral and contralateral) and remotely because the afferent nerve fibers from the mechanoreceptors involved give off collateral branches that are distributed both segmentally and intersegmentally. Thus, joint manipulation and traction produce reflex muscle tone changes (via motor unit facilitation and inhibition) so often seen in clinical application of various techniques.

Pain Suppression Effects. If Type IV receptors are involved in a joint disorder involving the capsule or ligaments, polysynaptic afferent impulses are transmitted to α-fibers of the local muscle motor pools to produce abnormal reflex activity. Pain is simultaneously manifested by neural synapses within the basal nucleus of the spinal cord's gray matter to ascending tracts to the limbic areas of the cerebral cortex. This spinal "gate" can regulate the central flow of nociceptive transmission if affected by inhibitory peripheral receptor impulses. Type I, II, and III receptors offer fibers within the dorsal roots that enter the posterior horns of the cord. They synapse with neurons of the apical spinal nucleus that connect with presynaptic terminals of the nociceptive afferent fibers located in basal nuclei. Because the apical interneurons release an inhibitory transmitter substance at the synapse, nociceptive impulses are inhibited. Thus, muscle stretching and joint manipulation (as well as compression, cold, acumassage, and deep vibration) produce peripheral receptor stimulation that creates presynaptic inhibition of nociceptive activity in the basal nucleus to dampen the central perception of pain. These pathways are more active during youth than old age, and this possibly explains why certain manipulative techniques are more effective in the young than in the elderly. Regardless, the relief of pain through reflexogenic mechanisms provides an important therapy in nonmedical case management by utilizing manipulative and cutaneous electronic stimulation techniques.

Positional Effects. Messages from Type I receptors make a significant contribution to postural and kinesthetic perception. They arise from the dorsal and dorsolateral columns of the spinal cord and finally are relayed through complex synaptic relays to the parietal and paracentral regions of the cerebral cortex. It is for this reason that loss of Type I receptor activity (spinal or extraspinal) from traumatic, inflammatory, or degenerative joint processes manifests in abnormalities of posture, gait, and specific joint movement because of inhibited kinesthetic perception.

Effects on Vertebrogenic Pain and Dysfunction

Since there has been a realization for many years that the basis of chiropractic therapy cannot rest on empirical results alone, controlled research studies have been encouraged through such organizations as the Foundation for Chiropractic Education and Research (FCER). The osteopathic profession and more recently the allopathic profession, as well as the scientific community in general, have also increased their investigation of why corrective manipulative therapy, especially that of the spine, exerts its influence on somatic and visceral functions.

It is a basic premise of chiropractic that a relationship exists between dysfunction of the nervous system and disease. It is also fundamental that some aberration within the spinal column produces the nerve dysfunction, or more specifically, that a malpositioned vertebra is at fault.[100] Bergmann reminds us that, in addition to this malposition, it must be clearly understood that the nerve dysfunction results from more than the structural misalignment. There are neuropathophysiologic, kinesiopathologic, myopathologic, histopathologic, biochemical, and possibly somatopsychic effects involved. Correction of the subluxation/fixation tends to restore normal physiologic processes, and the pathologic processes involved subside to the degree that they are reversible.

It is likely that several overlapping processes are involved in the typical subluxation complex and its reduction by adjustive and manipulative therapy. Individually, the three most popular hypotheses currently being investigated to determine the effects of chiropractic primary therapy are:

1. *The impulse-related theory*; eg, improving the transmission or expression of neurologic impulses.[135–141]

2. *The nonimpulse-related theory*; eg, improving the transmission of axonal transport mechanisms.[142–146]

3. *The biochemical theory*; eg, decreasing the local sensitivity of joint afferents and discouraging the production of metabolic debris, including bradykinin, and/or stimulating the production of CNS endorphins.[120,147–151]

Reflex and Peripheral Stimulation Techniques

It has long been recognized that peripheral stimulation has an influence on somatic and visceral pathways.[152–156] A number of topographic techniques being utilized with light or heavy pressure are based on the premise that cutaneous, subcutaneous, fascial, and/or muscle stimulation tend to "balance" abnormal neurocyclic foci or enhance normal physiologic processes. Several such techniques (primary and ancillary) currently being investigated are listed below:[116,151,157–174]

- Activator methods
- Acupressure
- Acupuncture (needle, needle/electrical)
- Applied kinesiology
- Arnholz's spastic muscle technique
- Auriculotherapy
- Bennett's neurovascular reflexes
- Bioenergetic synchronization
- Chapman's neurolymphatic reflexes
- Craniopathy methods
- Cyriax's transverse friction technique
- DeJarnette's sacro-occipital technique
- Directional nonforce technique
- Electrical acupoint stimulation (non-needle)
- Endonasal and allied techniques
- Logan basic technique
- Perianal reflexes
- Rosquist's spinal touch system
- Spondylotherapy
- Sutherland's cranial technique
- The Toftness system
- Travell's trigger point therapy

ADJUNCTIVE THERAPIES

To assist primary chiropractic therapy, a large number of ancillary procedures are frequently utilized for their preparatory and complementary influence upon adjustment effectiveness and their support of the healing process.[100,151,164,166,175] Common, but not inclusive, applications are shown in Table 7.7. All such modalities can have a direct or indirect therapeutic influence on the biomechanics of the body through their action on circulation (arterial, venous, lymphatic); musculoskeletal, nerve, and glandular tissues; and the psychic centers.

Specific applications of many of these modalities and procedures in the treatment of biomechanical disorders will be presented in future chapters. However, some general principles that are pertinent to all regions of the body will be described in the following sections of this chapter.

Therapeutic Exercise[176–179]

Most patients in pain follow instructions to the letter. Once pain diminishes, a functional "deafness" often appears in the patient. This is especially witnessed in the areas of preventive counseling and ergonomic advice. Rare is the practitioner who is not frequently exasperated by such a patient. Nevertheless, properly supervised stretching exercises will do much to rehabilitate the patient with areas of spinal stress associated with hypertonic muscles and shortened ligaments.

Although strength-developing exercises would be beneficial to strengthen the spine, the typical nonathletic patient will not follow them to the length of time necessary, and possibly their benefit has been over-

Table 7.7.
Common Adjunctive Procedures Used in Chiropractic

Counseling	Orthotics
Activities	Aircasts and stirrups
Exercise	Back rests
Hygiene	Bandages and belts
Nutrition	Braces and casts
Posture	Corsets and collars
Rest	Foot stabilizers
Safety	Orthopedic pillows
Cryotherapy	Shoe lifts
Cold packs	Slings
Ice massage	Taping/strapping
Vapocoolant sprays	Percussion/vibration
Electrotherapy	Psychotherapy
High-voltage current	Biofeedback
Interferential currents	Hypnosis and suggestion
Low-voltage current	Reality therapy
Magnetic current	Segmental mobilization
Exercise	Manual
Isometric	Mechanical
Isotonic	Soft-tissue manipulation or massage
Mechanical	Deep friction massage
Muscle re-education	Receptor-tonus method
First aid procedures	Rolfing and allied techniques
Hydrotherapy	Spastic muscle techniques
Colon therapy and lavage	Therapeutic heat
Therapeutic baths	Deep-heat modalities
Intermittent compression	Fluidotherapy
Meridian therapy	Superficial-heat modalities
Acupuncture	Traction and stretching
Ryodoraku	Manual
Nutrition	Mechanical
Diets	Ultrasound
Supplementation	Ultraviolet radiation

emphasized in the literature. In fact, the flexion exercises recommended by some writers apply the same forces as those seen in improper lifting. One can hardly think of an isotonic exercise that would not increase intradisc pressure.

Isometric exercise would appear to be the most beneficial during the postacute state. Such exercise has the least effect upon the large sensory receptors that provoke spasm. This subject will be discussed further in the next chapter.

The general objectives of any therapeutic exercise program should be to (1) relieve pain and improve function, (2) relax unnecessary musculature, (3) increase strength to that necessary for the individual's lifestyle, (4) obtain flexibility within the required ranges of movement, (5) remove metabolic waste accumulations by improving circulation, (6) gain smooth, efficient, coordinated motion, and (7) develop the kinesthetic sense of good alignment.

Home Exercise Prescriptions

Comprehensive therapy cannot be restricted to the office environment. Nutritional counseling and prescribed home exercises, for example, have been shown to be of extreme benefit in both musculoskeletal and visceral disorders.[180,181] Obviously, to be effective in enhancing a patient's rehabilitation, exercise must be conducted with sufficient warmup, frequency, duration, and intensity, and these factors must be based upon the individual patient's current functional and biomechanical status. Thus, explicit, motivational instruction and patient compliance are often basic factors in arriving at a successful outcome.

Pain Control[182–184]

If the gate theory of pain is correct, heat, massage, and transcutaneous sensory overload applied by any means are effective temporary methods in inhibiting the transmission of painful stimuli (see Table 7.8).[151] This seems especially true if the pain is initiated by an inflammatory or reflex condition.[185,186] The involved muscles should not be actively moved during therapy because this would stimulate the large receptors and provoke spasm.[187] Even if the gate theory is not absolute, we do know by experience that the reduction of muscle spasm is comforting to the patient and tends to reduce acute distortion.

Melzack and associates showed that transcutaneous electrical nerve stimulation (TENS) as adjunctive therapy, is more effective than gentle, mechanically administered massage in the treatment for low-back pain.[188] TENS has also been shown to be effective in cases of severe trauma associated with spinal cord damage (eg, fracture) or with soft-tissue injury.[189]

In comparing electroacupuncture with selected physical therapy modalities such as moist heat, ultrasound, traction, and electrical stimulation, Santiesteban found that electroacupuncture was far superior in increasing range of motion, increasing degree of straight leg raising, and decreasing pain in cases of acute spinal pain.[190] These results support the work of others who have found significant benefits of acupuncture in the treatment of sciatica.[191–194] Not all studies have agreed with these conclusions, however.[195]

Traction[196–198]

Traction is one of the oldest methods used in the treatment of spinal distress and deformities (Fig. 7.16).[199] Besides providing structural realignment, it has been shown that traction (manual or mechanical) owes some of its benefits to the same mechanisms applied in deep massage (ie, intermittent stretching).[200] However, as is true of all therapeutics, there are indications and contraindications for its application. Typical indications are shown in Table 7.9.[201]

Traction has been shown to increase disc height in normal spines,[202,203] but it is controversial whether this occurs in advanced IVD disease.[204,205] In addition, traction may

Table 7.8.
Typical Pain Syndromes That Are Usually Relieved by TENS Analgesia

Systemic Pain	Head and Neck	Abdomen
Bursitis	Cluster headaches	Bladder pain
Cancer	Dental disorders	Bowel stasis
Causalgia	Migraine	Diverticulosis
Multiple sclerosis	Spondylosis	Dysmenorrhea
Neuralgia	Sprains/strains	Labor
Osteoarthritis	Suboccipital headaches	Postoperative pain
Phantom limb syndrome	TMJ syndrome	
Raynaud's syndrome	Tic douloureux	
Rheumatoid arthritis	Torticollis	
Synovitis	Trigeminal neuralgia	
	Whiplash	
Back Pain	**Lower Extremities**	**Upper Extremities**
Coccydynia	Angle pain	Epicondylitis
Facet syndrome	Foot pain	Frozen shoulder
Intercostal neuralgia	Fractures	Hand pain
IVD syndrome	Ischialgia	Peripheral nerve injury
Lumbago	Joint mobilization	Sprains/strains
Lumbosacral pain	Knee pain	Subdeltoid bursitis
Radiculitis	Passive stretch pain	Wrist pain
Sprains/strains	Sciatica	
Thoracodynia	Sprains/strains	
Whole-back pain	Tendinitis	
	Thrombophlebitis	

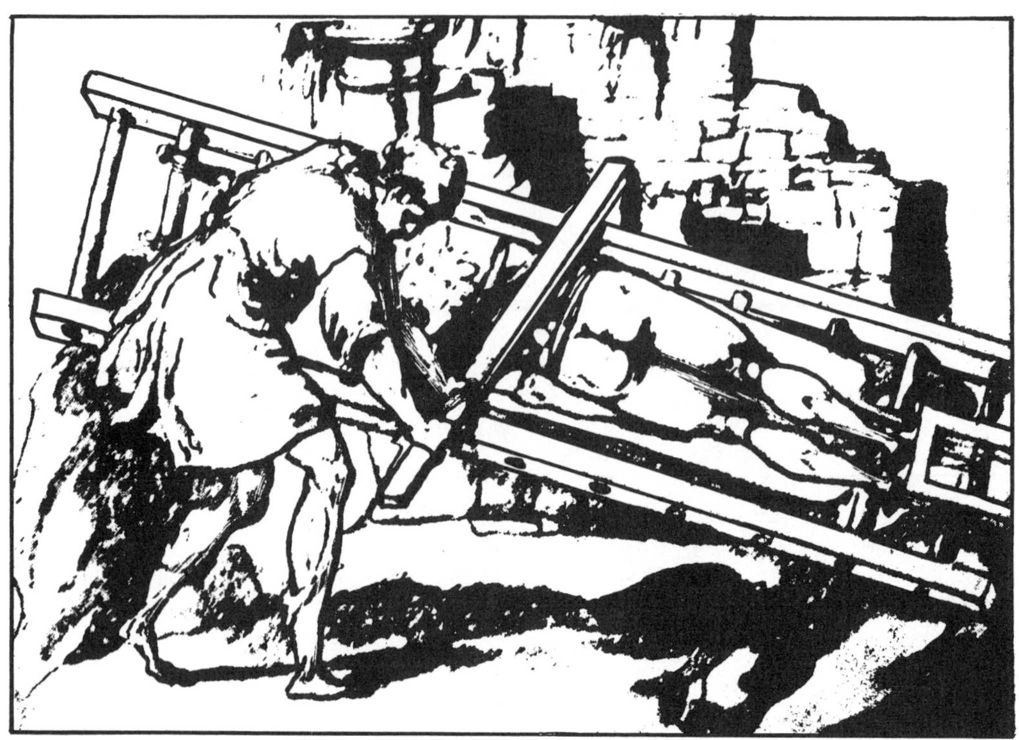

Figure 7.16. Demonstration of a crude method of reducing a spinal distortion by using traction and leverage pressure, as described by Hippocrates in *Articulation*, XLVII. The individual was strapped to a ladder, traction was applied to the upper body, and a board was used as a lever to force the spine into better alignment.

tend to relieve or irritate a disc protrusion, depending upon the relationship of the hernia to the nerve root (Fig. 7.17). If precautions are taken, however, bulging discs have been shown to recede and remain receded with traction.[204,206]

Biomechanical Supports[207–209]

Immobilization supports provide a distinct advantage in therapeutics, but they should never be applied without careful consideration of the biomechanical and physiologic objectives involved (Fig. 7.18). Their primary purposes are to afford rest, support, balance, and corrective mechanical forces. Braces are not a panacea but neither should they be avoided because of some ill-founded dogma.

What is the pathologic state of the spine? What mechanical alterations are to be achieved by the support? What type of forces are necessary and how are they to be applied? Where is the greatest force to be applied? Which motions should be restricted, and which should be allowed freedom? These questions must be answered, along with a prognosis of the residual effect and psychologic impact the support will have on the patient.

Transverse Friction Massage

The transverse friction technique (TFT) consists of precise, deep, sweeping massage that is directed against (transverse to) the scar-like fibrotic fibers (microscopic adhesions) in musculotendinous or fascial tissue, which invariably form after soft-tissue trauma[210] but may also be the result of soft-tissue degenerative processes.

Cyriax, who developed this technique, and others point out the following technique criteria:[211,212]

1. The precise focal spot must be located, and normal tissues must be avoided, when possible, during the treatment.

2. To avoid blistering the skin during

Table 7.9.
General Indications in the Use of Traction

CONTINUOUS TRACTION	
Articular jamming	Scalenus anticus syndrome
Brachial neuritis	Scoliosis
Compression fractures	Spasticity
Degenerative disc disease	Spinal nerve root impingement
IVD syndrome (early stages)	Spondylolisthesis
IVF narrowing	Sprains (splinting effect)
Joint hypomobility	Steinbrocker's syndrome
Kyphosis	Stimulation of mechanoreceptors
Lordosis	Torticollis (subacute)
Occipital neuralgia	Vertebral subluxation (subacute, chronic)
Osteoarthritis	Whiplash syndrome (uncomplicated)
Perivertebral adhesions, contractures and fixations	
INTERMITTENT TRACTION	
Deficient IVD hydration	Perivertebral congestion
Joint hypomobility	Perivertebral hypotonicity
Kyphosis (chronic)	Post-traumatic edema
Lordosis (chronic)	Scoliosis (chronic)
Occipital neuralgia	Stimulation of mechanoreceptors
Osteoarthritis	Vascular and lymphatic stasis
Perivertebral adhesions, contractures and fixations	Vertebral subluxation (chronic)

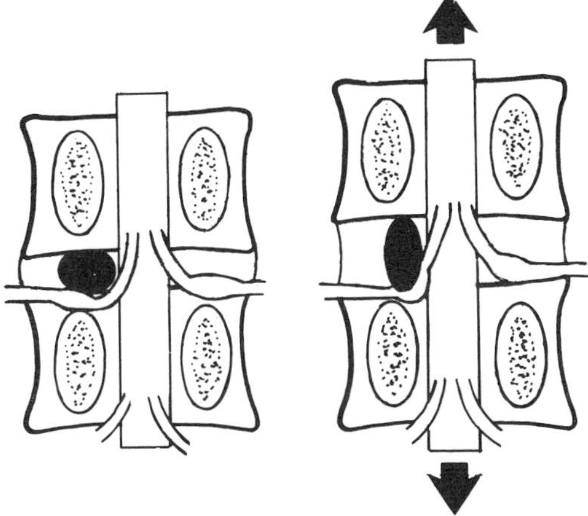

Figure 7.17. *Left*, diagram of a left disc protrusion (in *black*). *Right*, during traction, severe tensile stress is applied to the nerve root as movement of the root is restricted within the vertebral canal. This is most often seen in the patient who lists toward the side of pain.

therapy, the therapist's rigid fingers and the patient's skin must move as one.

3. The therapist's whole hand should move during the therapy, not just the fingers. Even then, various finger positions are often used to avoid finger fatigue when applying TFT.* Examples include using two fingertips, opposed thumb and any finger, the middle finger crossed over index finger, or the index finger crossed over the middle finger, and the hands may be alternated.

4. The to-and-fro sweeping pressure must be made *across* the fibers of the involved structure. The deep friction element (often painful) of the massage is essential.

5. The muscles must be maintained in a position of relaxation throughout the treatment, but involved tendons with a sheath must be kept taut so that the friction will smooth the roughened inner and outer surfaces of the tendon.

6. Care must be taken to differentiate the

* Because it usually takes several minutes of TFT to be effective, we have often substituted the use of a rubber-tipped T-bar (as used in Nimmo's receptor-tonus technique) or a Novafon unit with a small ball-type massage head and have found the use of these instruments to be less tiring and equally effective. The Novafon is a relatively inexpensive intrasound-vibration modality (between infrasound and ultrasound) that emits mixed frequencies of 100–10,000 Hz, and can reportedly penetrate to a depth of 2¼ inches. Tissue heat is not produced in this range of audible sound waves (see Fig. 7.19).

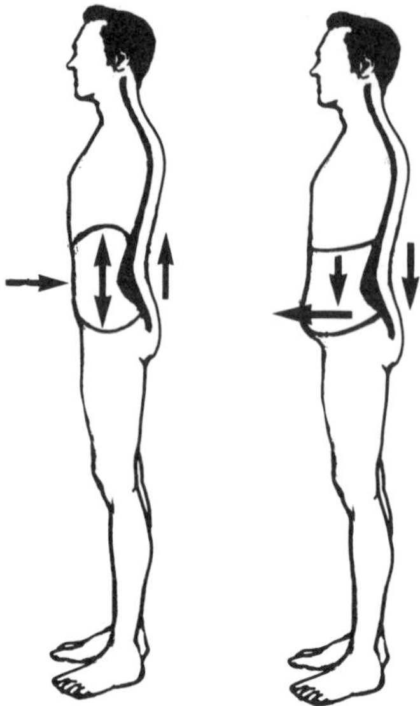

Figure 7.18. *Left*, the abdominal cavity serves as a hydraulic sac. Firm abdominal muscles tend to keep the diaphragm up, the pelvic floor down, and to elongate the lumbar spine. This tends to reduce added stress to the weight-bearing lumbar vertebral segments by seating the weight of the viscera within the pelvic basin. *Right*, conversely, weakened abdominal muscles allow the diaphragm to descend, the viscera to protrude anteriorly, and the lumbar curve to increase anteriorly. This adds to lumbar stress and hypertonicity of the posterior musculature. Most back pain is exacerbated not by a weak back, but by a weak abdomen.

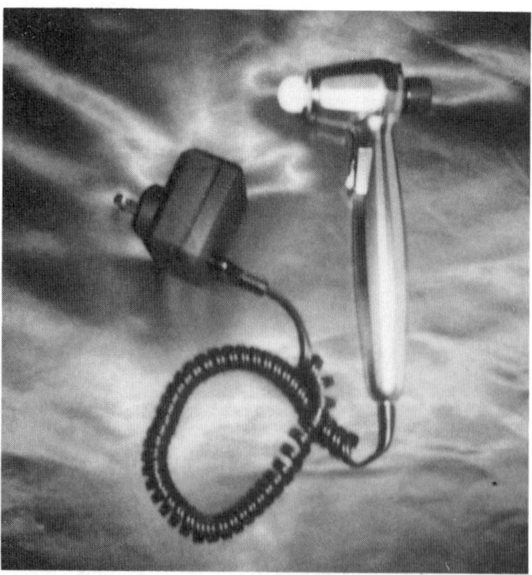

Figure 7.19. A Novafon intrasound unit.

pain associated with the patient's complaint and the tenderness arising from the TFT. The therapy should be discontinued immediately when the patient's pain ceases, even though tenderness initiated by the therapy may persist. This can be determined by testing involved muscles against resistance and involved ligaments by stretching.

Common examples of fibrotic development are seen following strains, sprains, tendinitis, capsulitis, IVD lesions, facet syndromes, and arthritis (traumatic or degenerative). They may also occur secondary to malignant disease, fracture, and dislocations.[158] Focal tenderness, a restricted range of motion (fixation), and muscle wasting are invariably associated. Paresthesia, referred pain, and structural deformity may or may not be related.

Nash offers the following adjunctive protocol:[213]

1. When the site is extremely tender, TFT should be preceded with 15 minutes of cryotherapy, such as an ice pack over a slightly moistened towel.

2. After TFT, the use of pulsed ultrasound or negative galvanism over the site treated is recommended. The more acute the pain, the higher the pulse rate of the current, but without exceeding the manufacturer's prescriptive mandates. As both ultrasound and negative galvanism have the effect of softening fibrotic deposits, any modality that has a similar effect may be substituted. Care must be taken not to elevate tissue temperature since that may encouarge a hardening reaction by denaturing protein at the site. The typical treatment parameters are 15 minutes at 0.5–1.0 ma/in^2 of electrode surface. If iontophoresis is utilized with galvanism, soaking the negative pad in a 1.5% solution of potassium chloride prior to the 15-minute application may be considered. Nash suggests that the patient be scheduled on alternate days since residual post-therapy tenderness would prohibit TFT on successive days. He reports that results can be expected in 2–3 weeks in the average case.

3. The chronic condition will often exhibit associated motor weakness. Thus, rehabilitative therapy must be instituted. The proper time to begin exercises for toning the involved musculature is when the patient

demonstrates a range of motion of at least 75% of that of the noninvolved contralateral extremity. The exercise must be specific to the muscle; therefore the "form" must be demonstrated to the patient. This form includes body position, rate of performance, duration, intensity of resistance, proper movement of the part during the workout, and, finally, the rest period between exercise sets. After demonstration, the patient should be asked to perform the instructions under the supervision of the doctor to insure that the form of the exercise is proper. After this, the patient should be given written instructions as to how the program is to be performed. The number of repetitions in each set, how many sets constitute a routine, and how many routines are to be performed each day should be noted in the written prescription. For example:

Exercise for 30 repetitions/minute.
Rest for 30 seconds.
Repeat exercise for 30 repetitions.
Rest for 30 seconds.
Repeat exercise for 30 repetitions.

This routine must be performed three times each day until your next office visit. Caution: perform the exercises in proper form, and rest as indicated. If there is any uncomfortable reaction, call the office for instructions.

When the patient returns to the office, he or she should demonstrate the the exercise so that the doctor can evaluate the form being used and correct any errors. If a dynamometer or some other objective type of strength measuring device is available, the doctor can have an original figure against which to judge improvement of the weakness.

Rehabilitation following Spinal Distress[214–217]

After acute stress or during recuperation of a chronic disorder, stretched ligaments make one or more vertebral motion units relatively unstable. Until the restricting ligaments accommodate, and most are slow to adapt to a new range of motion, there is always predisposition to reinjury. This may or may not require temporary support and/or a regimen of therapeutic exercise. Keep in mind that much of spinal stability is provided by musculature (Fig. 7.20). In most spinal disorders, there is unilateral weakness or hypertonicity present that provides a constant tendency towards segmental rotation until bilateral balance is relatively permanent.

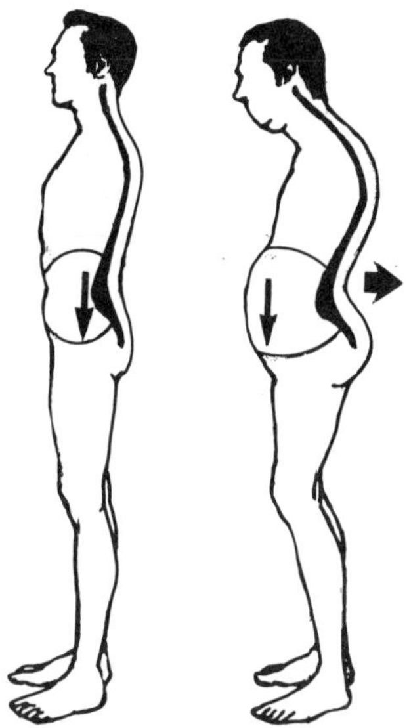

Figure 7.20. *Left*, in good posture and weight balance, gravitational forces fall slightly anterior to the sacrum. *Right*, in obesity with weak abdominal muscles, the center of mass is shifted anteriorly, causing an increase in the sacral angle and hyperextension of the lumbodorsal area. This posture associated with chronic back pain can be benefited by a corset that would afford good abdominal support and by weight loss and the development of the abdominal muscles.

The patient must be thoroughly counseled in the efficient biomechanics of normal living; eg, stance and sitting posture, arising from the sitting and recumbent positions, rest, sleeping positions, proper pillow and mattress use, driving position, entering and leaving an automobile, working postures, ideal pushing and pulling techniques (Fig. 7.21), lifting and bending procedures, proper footwear, appropriate therapeutic exercises, home therapies, etc, and what activities should be avoided. Case management cannot be restricted to the few minutes at the doctor's office.

Just because an ideal adjustment has been made, it is no indication that the vertebra will hold this new position without assistance. Except for those seen following a severe accident, most subluxations seen in practice are not new occurrences. They are acute mani-

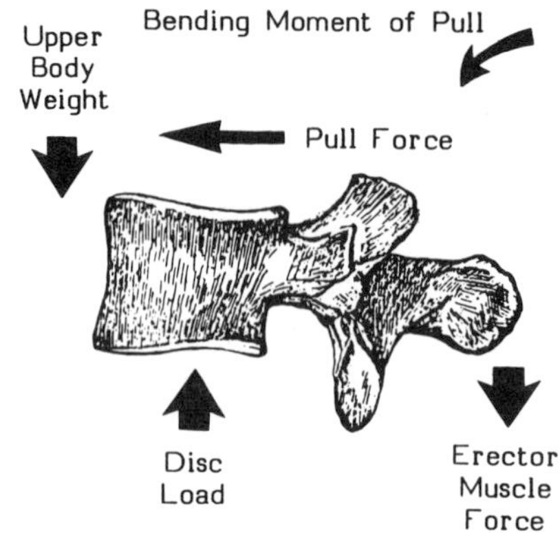

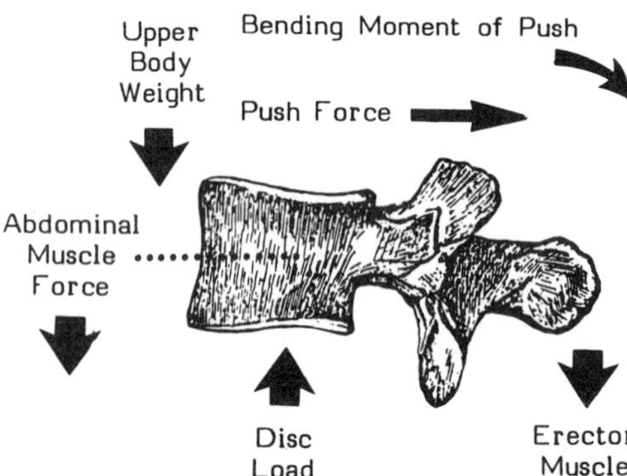

Figure 7.21. The bending moments involved in pulling and pushing. During a pull, the spinal erectors resist the bending moments created by the horizontal forces. During a push, the anterior abdominal muscles resist the bending moments. Less effort is required by the rectus abdomini during pushing than the erector spinae during pulling because the anterior muscles have a much longer lever arm.

festations of a chronic problem; often soft tissues have shortened unilaterally and stretched contralaterally. A degree of ligamentous stretching must accompany any degree of stress or any form of corrective mobilization or there would be no separation of the fixation. Several minutes of rest following adjustment will at least allow the elastic fibers to accommodate. During this time of postadjustment rest, warmth can often be used effectively to help reduce associated muscular spasm and hypertonicity and to bring nutrients to the area and remove metabolic ash.[218] To adjust a patient and send him rapidly on his way, only to repeat the process visit after visit, is not professional case management. It smacks of quackery.

REFERENCES

1. Jefferson G: Discussion of spinal injuries. *Proceedings of the Royal Society of Medicine* 21:625, 1928.
2. Hirata I Jr: *The Doctor and the Athlete,* ed 2. Philadelphia, J.B. Lippincott, 1974, p 77.
3. Macnab I: *Backache.* Baltimore, Williams & Wilkins, 1977, pp 86–87.
4. Firth JN: Lecture to students regarding chiropractic case management, Lincoln Chiropractic College, Indianapolis, 1949.
5. Kraus H: *Therapeutic Exercise.* Springfield, Ill, Charles C Thomas, 1963.
6. Jaskoviak P, Schafer RC: *Applied Physiotherapy.* Arlington, Va, American Chiropractic Association. To be published in 1986.
7. Lowe JC: Calcium, magnesium, and muscle spasms. *The Chiropractic Family Physician* ACA Council on Diagnosis and Internal Disorders 3(6):18, 20–21, September 1981.
8. Macnab I: *Backache.* Baltimore, Williams & Wilkins, 1977, p 80.
9. Clawson DK: Musculoskeletal trauma. In Rosse C, Clawson DK (eds): *The Musculoskeletal System in Health and Disease.* Hagerstown, Md, Harper & Row, 1980, p 418.
10. Gelb H: Patient evaluation. In Gelb H (ed): *Clinical Management of Head, Neck and TMJ Pain and Dysfunction.* Philadelphia, W.B. Saunders, 1977.
11. Macnab I: *Backache.* Baltimore, Williams & Wilkins, 1977, pp 83–84.
12. Clawson DK: Musculoskeletal trauma. In Rosse C, Clawson DK (eds): *The Musculoskeletal System in Health and Disease.* Hagerstown, Md, Harper & Row, 1980, pp 416–417
13. Newman PH: Sprung back. *Journal of Bone and Joint Surgery* 34B:30, 1952.
14. Macnab I: *Backache.* Baltimore, Williams & Wilkins, 1977, pp 144–154.
15. Farfan HF: *Mechanical Disorders of the Low Back.* Philadelphia, Lea & Febiger, 1973.
16. Pennell RJ: Passive motion therapy and automatic priority adjusting. *The Digest of Chiropractic Economics* March/April 1983, p 12.
17. Mennell JMcM: *Joint Pain.* Boston, Little, Brown, 1964, pp 12–13.
18. Williams JGP, Sperryn PN (eds): *Sports Medicine,* ed 2. Baltimore, Williams & Wilkins, 1976, pp 271, 273.
19. Good AB: Spinal joint blocking. *Journal of Manipulative and Physiological Therapeutics* 6(1):1–7, March 1985.
20. Schafer RC: *Chiropractic Management of Sports and Recreational Injuries.* Baltimore, Williams & Wilkins, 1982, pp 248–249.
21. Kehl EW: Myalgia. *ACA Journal of Chiropractic* 2:49–52, July 1968.
22. Macnab I: *Backache.* Baltimore, Williams & Wilkins, 1977, pp 82–83.
23. Bennett TJ: *A New Clinical Basis for the Correction*

of Abnormal Physiology. Burlingame, Cal, published by the author, 1960.

24. Kraus H: Muscular aspects of oral dysfunction. In Gelb H (ed): *Clinical Management of Head, Neck and TMJ Pain and Dysfunction*. Philadelphia, W.B. Saunders, 1977.
25. Stoddard A: *Manual of Osteopathic Technique*, ed 2. London, Hutchinson, 1962.
26. Sola AE: Myofascial trigger point therapy. *Medical Times* January 1982, pp 70–77.
27. Travell J: Myofascial trigger points: Clinical view. In Bonica JJ, Albe-Fessard D (eds): *Advances in Pain Research and Therapy*. New York, Raven Press, 1976.
28. Travell J: Referred pain from skeletal muscle. *New York State Journal of Medicine* February 1, 1955.
29. Sandman KB: Myofascial pain syndromes: Their mechanism, diagnosis and treatment. *Journal of Manipulative and Physiological Therapeutics* 4(3):135–139, September 1981.
30. Zimmermann M: Physiological mechanisms in chronic pain. In *Pain and Society*, report of Dahlem Workshop, Berlin, November 1979. Deerfield Park, Fla, Basle, 1980, pp 283–298.
31. Simons DG: Myofascial triggerpoints: A need for understanding. *Archives of Physical Medicine and Rehabilitation* 62, March 1981.
32. Clawson DK: Musculoskeletal trauma. In Rosse C, Clawson DK (eds): *The Musculoskeletal System in Health and Disease*. Hagerstown, Md, Harper & Row, 1980, p 407.
33. Hirata I Jr: *The Doctor and the Athlete*. Philadelphia, J.B. Lippincott, 1974, pp 116–117.
34. Norrell HA: Fractures and dislocations of the spine. In Rothman RH, Simeone FA (eds): *The Spine*. Philadelphia, W.B. Saunders, 1975, vol 2, pp 529–535.
35. Keene JS, Goletz TH, Lilleas F: Diagnosis of vertebral fractures. *Journal of Bone and Joint Surgery* 64:586–585, 1982.
36. Clawson DK: Musculoskeletal trauma. In Rosse C, Clawson DK (eds): *The Musculoskeletal System in Health and Disease*. Hagerstown, Md, Harper & Row, 1980, pp 407–416.
37. White AA, Panjabi MM: *Clinical Biomechanics of the Spine*. Philadelphia, J.B. Lippincott, 1978, pp 85–86.
38. Macnab I: *Backache*. Baltimore, Williams & Wilkins, 1977, pp 24–25.
39. Williams JGP, Sperryn PN (eds): *Sports Medicine*, ed 2. Baltimore, Williams & Wilkins, 1976, pp 252–253.
40. Hodgson AR: Infectious disease of the spine. In Rothman RH, Simeone FA (eds): *The Spine*. Philadelphia, W.B. Saunders, 1975, vol 2, pp 567–572.
41. Macnab I: *Backache*. Baltimore, Williams & Wilkins, 1977, pp 28–30.
42. Parfitt AM, Duncan H: Metabolic bone disease affecting the spine. In Rothman RH, Simeone FA (eds): *The Spine*. Philadelphia, W.B. Saunders, 1975, vol 2, pp 599–600.
43. Macnab I: *Backache*. Baltimore, Williams & Wilkins, 1977, pp 38–43.
44. White AA, Panjabi MM: *Clinical Biomechanics of the Spine*. Philadelphia, J.B. Lippincott, 1978, pp 284–293.
45. Farfan HH: Symptomatology in terms of the pathomechanics of low-back pain and sciatica. In Haldeman S (ed): *Modern Developments in the Principles and Practice of Chiropractic*. New York, Appleton-Century-Crofts, 1980, pp 171–184.
46. Grieve GP: *Common Vertebral Joint Problems*. New York, Churchill Livingtone, 1981, pp 90–92.
47. Macnab I: *Backache*. Baltimore, Williams & Wilkins, 1977, p 200.
48. Kirkaldy-Willis WH: The three phases of the spectrum of degenerative disease. In Kirkaldy-Willis WH (ed): *Managing Low Back Pain*. New York, Churchill Livingstone, 1983, pp 24–25, 73–89.
49. Macnab I: *Backache*. Baltimore, Williams & Wilkins, 1977, pp 84–91.
50. Haldeman S: The pathophysiology of the spinal subluxation. In Goldstein M (ed): *The Research Status of Spinal Manipulative Therapy*, NINCDS Monograph, No. 15, DHEW Publication No. (NIH) 76-998, Stock No. 017-049-0 0060-7, Washington, DC, U.S. Government Printing Office, 1975, pp 221–222.
51. Rothman RH, Simeone FA: Lumbar disc disease. In Rothman RH, Simeone FA (eds): *The Spine*. Philadelphia, W.B. Saunders, 1975, vol 2, pp 446–448.
52. Simeone FA, Rothman RH: Cervical disc disease. In Rothman RH, Simeone FA (eds): *The Spine*. Philadelphia, W.B. Saunders, 1975, vol 1, pp 388, 390–391.
53. Simeone FA, Rothman RH: Cervical disc disease. In Rothman RH, Simeone FA (eds): *The Spine*. Philadelphia, W.B. Saunders, 1975, vol 1, pp 390–391.
54. Macnab I: *Backache*. Baltimore, Williams & Wilkins, 1977, pp 91–96.
55. Charnley J: Acute lumbago and sciatica. *British Medical Journal* 1:344, 1955.
56. White AA, Panjabi MM: *Clinical Biomechanics of the Spine*. Philadelphia, J.B. Lippincott, 1978, pp 303–320, 337–338.
57. Macnab I: *Backache*. Baltimore, Williams & Wilkins, 1977, pp 97–104.
58. Sunderland S: The anatomy of the intervertebral foramen and the mechanisms of compression and stretch of nerve roots. In Haldeman S (ed): *Modern Developments in the Principles and Practice of Chiropractic*. New York, Appleton-Century-Crofts, 1980, pp 45–64.
59. Luttges MW, Gerren RA: Compression physiology: Nerves and roots. In Haldeman S (ed): *Modern Developments in the Principles and Practice of Chiropractic*. New York, Appleton-Century-Crofts, 1980, pp 65–89.
60. Drum DC: The vertebral motor unit and intervertebral foramen. In Goldstein M (ed): *The Research Status of Spinal Manipulative Therapy*. NINCDS Monograph, No. 15, DHEW Publication No. (NIH) 76-998, Stock No. 017-049-00060-7, Washington, DC, U.S. Government Printing Office, 1975, pp 63–70.
61. Sharpless SK: Susceptibility of spinal roots to

compression block. In Goldstein M (ed): *The Research Status of Spinal Manipulative Therapy.* NINCDS Monograph, No. 15, DHEW Publication No. (NIH) 76-998, Stock No. 017-049-00060-7, Washington, DC, U.S. Government Printing Office, 1975, pp 155–160.
62. Parke WW: Applied anatomy of the spine. In Rothman RH, Simeone FA (eds): *The Spine.* Philadelphia, W.B. Saunders, 1975, vol 1, pp 35–36.
63. Sunderland S: Anatomical perivertebral influences on the intervertebral foramen. In Goldstein M (ed): *The Research Status of Spinal Manipulative Therapy,* NINCDS Monograph, No. 15, DHEW Publication No. (NIH) 76-998, Stock No. 017-049-0-0060-7, Washington, DC, U.S. Government Printing Office, 1975, pp 129–139.
64. Macnab I: *Backache.* Baltimore, Williams & Wilkins, 1977, p 101.
65. Schaumberg HH, Spencer PS: Pathology of spinal root compression. In Goldstein M (ed): *The Research Status of Spinal Manipulative Therapy,* NINCDS Monograph, No. 15, DHEW Publication No. (NIH) 76-998, Stock No. 017-049-0-0060-7, Washington, DC, U.S. Government Printing Office, 1975, pp 141–147.
66. Wedge JH, Kirkaldy-Willis WH, Kinnard P: Lumbar spinal stenosis. In Helfet AJ, Gruebel Lee DM (eds): *Disorders of the Lumbar Spine.* Philadelphia, J.B. Lippincott, 1978, pp 51–61.
67. Benson DR: The back: Thoracic and lumbar spine. In D'Ambrosia RD (ed): *Musculoskeletal Disorders.* Philadelphia, J.B. Lippincott, 1977, pp 285–287.
68. Porter RW, Wicks M, Ottewell D: Measurement of the spinal cord by diagnostic ultrasound. *Journal of Bone and Joint Surgery* 60B:481–484, 1979.
69. Schafer RC: *Chiropractic Management of Sports and Recreational Injuries.* Baltimore, Williams & Wilkins, 1982, pp 263–264.
70. Grieve GP: *Common Vertebral Joint Problems.* New York, Churchill Livingstone, 1981, pp 176–196.
71. Korr IM: The spinal cord as organizer of disease processes: Some preliminary perspectives. *Journal of the American Osteopathic Association* September 1976.
72. Stonebrink RD: Neurological features of the chiropractic philosophy. *ACA Journal of Chiropractic* 2:S33–S40, May 1968.
73. Haldeman S: The neurophysiologic mechanisms of pain. *ACA Journal of Chiropractic* 10:53–63, June 1976.
74. Cassidy JD, Kirkaldy-Willis WH, McGregor M: Spinal manipulation for the treatment of chronic low back and leg pain: An observational study. In Buerger AA, Greenman PE (eds): *Empirical Approaches to the Validation of Spinal Manipulation.* Springfield, Ill, Charles C Thomas, 1985, pp 133–134, 141, 144, 146.
75. Todd M: *The Thinking Body.* New York, Dance Horizons, 1968.
76. Schafer RC: *Symptomatology and Differential Diagnosis.* Arlington, Va, American Chiropractic Association. To be published in 1986.
77. Martin RJ: Autonomic nerve control and neurovascular dynamics. *ACA Journal of Chiropractic* 3:65–72, October 1969.
78. Sittinger R: Central nervous system allergy: Chemical and mechanical aspects of visceral syndromes. *ACA Journal of Chiropractic* 9:131–134, November 1975.
79. Lieb MM: Oral orthopedics. In Gelb H (ed): *Clinical Management of Head, Neck and TMJ Pain and Dysfunction.* Philadelphia, W.B. Saunders, 1977, pp 32–71.
80. Hildebrandt RW (ed): *J. Janse: Principles and Practice of Chiropractic.* Lombard, Ill, National College of Chiropractic, 1976, pp 106–109.
81. Janse J, Houser RH, Wells BF: *Chiropractic Principles and Technic.* Chicago, National College of Chiropractic, 1978, pp 516–518.
82. Houser RH: *Visceral Innervation.* Des Moines, Ia, Foundation for Chiropractic Education and Research, 1968.
83. Johnson AC: *Chiropractic Physiological Therapeutics,* ed 5. Palm Springs, Cal, published by the author, 1977, pp 44–45.
84. Johnson AC: *Palpation of Spine, Internal Organs, Muscles, Muscle Testing in Diagnosis.* Palm Springs, Cal, published by the author, 1980, pp 25–27.
85. Schafer RC (ed): *Basic Chiropractic Procedural Manual,* ed 4. Arlington, Va, American Chiropractic Association, 1984, p 79.
86. Gillet H, Liekens M: *Belgian Chiropractic Research Notes.* Huntington Beach, Cal, Motion Palpation Institute, 1981, pp 11–39, 61–69, 71, 79–80, 92–100, 104–106.
87. Stierwalt DD: *Fundamentals of Motion Palpation.* Davenport, Ia, published by the author, 1977, pp 1–2.
88. Goodheart GL: *Collected Published Articles and Reprints.* Montpellier, O, Williams County Publishing, 1969, pp 61–62.
89. Gillet H, Liekens M: A further study of spinal fixations. *Annals of the Swiss Chiropractic Association,* 4:41, 1967.
90. Gillet H: The anatomy and physiology of spinal fixation. *Journal of the National Chiropractic Association* December 1963.
91. Gillet H: Evolution of a chiropractor. *National Chiropractic Journal* November 1945, December 1946, November 1947, January 1949, December 1949, January 1951.
92. Vladef T, Hardy M: The theory of fixation points. *National Chiropractic Journal* June 1945.
93. Stonebrink RD: Palpation for vertebral motoricity. *ACA Journal of Chiropractic* 3:11–14, February 1969.
94. Smith O: *Naprapathic Chartology.* Chicago, Chicago College of Naprapathy, 1917, p 17.
95. Downing C: *Osteopathic Principles in Disease.* San Francisco, R.J. Orozco, 1923.
96. Cassidy JD, Kirkaldy-Willis, McGregor M: Spinal manipulation for the treatment of chronic low back and leg pain: an observational study. In Buerger AA, Greenman PE (eds): *Empirical Approaches to the Validation of Spinal Manipulation.* Springfield, Ill, Charles C Thomas, 1985, p 125.
97. Gillet H, Liekens M: *Belgian Chiropractic Research*

Notes. Huntington Beach, Cal, Motion Palpation Institute, 1981.

98. Mennell JMcM: *Back Pain.* Boston, Little, Brown, 1960.
99. Maurer EL: *Practical Applied Roentgenology.* Baltimore, Williams & Wilkins, 1983, pp 14, 17, 30.
100. Bergmann T: Integrated chiropractic methods. Compilation of notes presented to the convention of the Oklahoma Chiropractic Association, April 23, 1983. In cooperation with Northwestern College of Chiropractic.
101. American Chiropractic Association: *Chiropractic State of the Art.* Arlington, Va, American Chiropractic Association, 1984, pp 4, 8.
102. Counsel on Chiropractic Education: Position/Policy Paper, adopted January 21, 1978.
103. Sandoz R: Some reflex phenomena associated with spinal derangements and adjustments. *Annals of the Swiss Chiropractors Association* 7:45, 1981.
104. Sandoz R: Some physical mechanisms and effects of spinal adjustments. *Annals of the Swiss Chiropractors Association* 6:91, 1976.
105. Swezey RL: The modern thrust of manipulation and traction therapy. *Seminars in Arthritis and Rheumatism* 12(3):326, 1983.
106. Levine M: *The Structural Approach to Chiropractic.* New York, Comet Press, 1964, p 85.
107. Cassidy JD, Kirkaldy-Willis WH, McGregor M: Spinal manipulation for the treatment of chronic low back and leg pain: an observational study. In Buerger AA, Greenman PE (eds): *Empirical Approaches to the Validation of Spinal Manipulation.* Springfield, Ill, Charles C Thomas, 1985, pp 123–127.
108. Kirkaldy-Willis WH: Manipulation. In Kirkaldy-Willis WH (ed): *Managing Low Back Pain.* New York, Churchill Livingstone, 1983, pp 175–177.
109. Schafer RC: *Chiropractic Management of Sports and Recreational Injuries.* Baltimore, Williams & Wilkins, 1982, p 278.
110. Molloy RD: A correlation between muscle testing and chiropractic treatment. Thesis, Anglo-European College of Chiropractic, 1976.
111. Will TE: Hypothetical considerations with regard to the biochemical basis of manipulative therapy. *ACA Journal of Chiropractic* 13:119–123, December 1979.
112. Grice AS: A biomechanical approach to cervical and dorsal adjusting. In Haldeman S (ed): *Modern Developments in the Principles and Practice of Chiropractic.* New York, Appleton-Century-Crofts, 1980, pp 338–339.
113. Grice AS: A biomechanical approach to cervical and dorsal adjusting. In Haldeman S (ed): *Modern Developments in the Principles and Practice of Chiropractic.* New York, Appleton-Century Crofts, 1980, pp 338–340.
114. Sandoz R: Some physical mechanisms and effects of spinal adjustments. *Annals of the Swiss Chiropractors Association* 6:91–92, 1976.
115. Gitelman R: The treatment of pain by spinal manipulation. In Goldstein M (ed): *The Research Status of Spinal Manipulative Therapy,* NINCDS Monograph, No. 15, DHEW Publication No. (NIH) 76-998, Stock No. 017-049-0 0060-7, Washington, DC, U.S. Government Printing Office, 1975, pp 277–281.
116. Baltzell LG, Mackey RH (eds): *Firth's Technic Notes.* Publishing data not shown. Available from National Chiropractic College, 1967.
117. Pettibon Bio-Mechanics Institute. *Pettibon Spinal Bio-Mechanics: Theory and Implications,* ed 2. Vancouver, Wash, Pettibon Bio-Mechanics, 1978, pp 84–87.
118. Kirkaldy-Willis WH: Manipulation. In Kirkaldy-Willis WH (ed): *Managing Low Back Pain.* New York, Churchill Livingstone, 1983, pp 176–177.
119. Sandoz R: The significance of the manipulative crack and of other articular noises. *Annals of the Swiss Chiropractors Association* 4:47, 1969.
120. Will TE: The biomechanical basis of manipulative therapeutics: Hypothetical considerations. *Journal of Manipulative and Physiological Therapeutics* 1(3):153–156, September 1978.
121. Kfoury PW (ed): *Catalog of Chiropractic Techniques.* Chesterfield, Mo, Logan College of Chiropractic, 1977.
122. Kale M: The upper cervical specific. Parts one and two. *Today's Chiropractic* July/August 1984, pp 28–29; September/October 1984, pp 27–30.
123. McAlpine JE: A discussion of the dentate ligament neural traction mechanism. *International Review of Chiropractic* October/December 1980, pp 35–39.
124. Craton EF: Condyle—paraglenoid ligament. Parts 1 and 2. *Today's Chiropractic* November/December 1984, p 46; July/August 1985, pp 25–27.
125. Mears DB Sr: *The Mears Technique.* St. Albans, Vt, published by the author, 1976.
126. Gregory RR: A kinesiological basis for the C-1 adjustment. Parts I and II. *The Digest of Chiropractic Economics* January/February 1983; March/April 1983.
127. Craton EF: Occipital-atlantal articulation redefined. *The Texas Chiropractor* February 1978.
128. Homewood AE: Micro-manipulation. Part 1. *The Digest of Chiropractic Economics* September/October 1985, pp 45–46.
129. Barvinchack E: Upper cervical superstress in the blocked pelvis. *The Digest of Chiropractic Economics* September/October 1985, p 63.
130. Lieb MM: Oral orthopedics. In Gelb H (ed): *Clinical Management of Head, Neck and TMJ Pain and Dysfunction.* Philadelphia, W.B. Saunders, 1977, pp 56–71.
131. Sweat RW: Miscellaneous articles appearing in *Today's Chiropractic,* 1978–1985.
132. Wyke BD: Articular neurology and manipulative therapy. In *Aspects of Manipulative Therapy.* Proceedings of Multidisciplinary International Conference on Manipulative Therapy, Melbourne, Lincoln Institute of Health Science, Carlton, Victoria, Australia, August 1979, pp 67–72.
133. Grieve GP: *Common Vertebral Joint Problems.* New York, Churchill Livingstone, 1981, pp 163–170.
134. Spengler DM: *Low Back Pain: Assessment and Management.* New York, Grune & Stratton, 1982, pp 1–8.
135. Canadian Memorial Chiropractic College: *Seg-*

mental Neuropathy. Toronto, Canadian Memorial Chiropractic College (undated; early 1980s?).
136. Zolli F: *Chiropractic Concepts in Healing*. Old Brookville, NY, New York Chiropractic College, 1984.
137. Homewood AE: *The Neurodynamics of the Vertebral Subluxation*, ed 3. City of publication not shown, published by the author, 1981.
138. Leach RA: *The Chiropractic Theories*. Mississippi State, Mid-South Scientific Publishers, 1980.
139. Verner JR: *The Science and Logic of Chiropractic*. Englewood, NJ, published by the author, 1941.
140. Stephenson RW: *Chiropractic Textbook*. Davenport, Ia, published by the author, 1927.
141. Palmer DD: *The Science, Art, and Philosophy of Chiropractic*. Portland, Oreg, Portland Printing House, 1910.
142. Korr IM (ed): Nonimpulse-based mechanisms. In *The Neurobiologic Mechanisms in Manipulative Therapy*. New York, Plenum Press, 1978, pp 291–358.
143. Brazier MAB: *Electrical Activity of the Nervous System*, ed 4. Baltimore, Williams & Wilkins, 1977, pp 14–25.
144. Ochs S: A brief review of material transport in nerve fibers. In Goldstein M (ed): *The Research Status of Spinal Manipulative Therapy*, NINCDS Monograph, No. 15, DHEW Publication No. (NIH) 76-998, Stock No. 017-049-0-0060-7, Washington, DC, U.S. Government Printing Office, 1975, pp 189–194.
145. Ochs S: Axoplasmic transport. In Tower DB (ed): *The Basic Neurosciences*. New York, Raven Press, 1975, vol 1, pp 137–146.
146. Ochs S: Axoplasmic flow in neurons. In Gaito J (ed): *Macromolecules and Behavior*. New York, Appleton-Century-Crofts, 1966.
147. Berger PA et al: Behavioral pharmacology of the endorphins. *Annual Review of Medicine* 33:397–415, 1982.
148. Guillemin R et al: The endorphins, novel peptides of brain and hypophyseal origin, with opiate like activity: Biochemical and biologic studies. *Annals of the New York Academy of Science* 197:131–157, 1979.
149. Wei LY: Scientific advance in acupunture. In Kao FF, Kao JJ (eds): *Recent Advances in Acupuncture Research*. Garden City, NY, Institute for Advanced Research in Asian Science and Medicine, 1979, pp 49–71.
150. Fields A: Acupuncture and endorphins. *International Journal of Chinese Medicine* 1(2):10, June 1984.
151. Jaskoviak P, Schafer RC: Pain suppression in the twentieth century. In *Applied Physiotherapy*. Arlington, Va, American Chiropractic Association. To be published in 1986.
152. Dittmar E: Cutaneo-visceral neural pathways. *British Journal of Physical Medicine* 15:208, 1952.
153. Kuntz A: Anatomic and physiologic properties of cutaneo-visceral vasomotor reflex arcs. *Journal of Neurophysiology* 8:421–429, 1943.
154. Richins CA, Brizzee K: Effect of localized cutaneous stimulation on circulation in duodenal arterioles and capillary beds. *Journal of Neurophysiology* 12:131–136, 1949.
155. Kuntz A, Hazelwood LA: Circulatory reactions in the gastrointestinal tract elicited by local cutaneous stimulation. *American Heart Journal* 20:743–749, 1940.
156. Dale RA: The principles and systems of microacupuncture. *International Journal of Chinese Medicine*, 1(4):15–42, December 1984.
157. Kfoury PW (ed): *Catalog of Chiropractic Techniques*. Chesterfield, Mo, Logan College of Chiropractic, 1977.
158. Cyriax J: *Textbook of Orthopaedic Medicine: Treatment by Manipulation, Massage and Injection*, ed 11. London, Bailliere Tindall, 1984, vol 2.
159. Walther DS: *Applied Kinesiology, Volume II, Head, Neck, and Jaw Pain and Dysfunction—The Stomatognathic System*. Pueblo, Colo, Systems DC, 1983.
160. Travell JG, Simons DG: *Myofascial Pain and Dysfunction: The Trigger Point Manual*. Baltimore, Williams & Wilkins, 1983.
161. Walther DS: *Applied Kinesiology, Volume I, Basic Procedures and Muscle Testing*. Pueblo, Colo, Systems DC, 1981.
162. Hains G: *Post-Traumatic Neuritis*. Trois-Rivieres, Quebec, published by the author, 1978.
163. Gelb H (ed): *Clinical Management of Head, Neck and TMJ Pain and Dysfunction*. Philadelphia, W. B. Saunders, 1977.
164. Johnson AC: *Chiropractic Physiological Therapeutics*. Palm Springs, Cal, published by author, 1977.
165. DeJarnette MB: *Sacro Occipital Technic*. Nebraska City, published by the author, privately distributed, 1976.
166. Janse J: *Principles and Practice of Chiropractic*. Lombard, Ill, National College of Chiropractic, 1976.
167. Stoner F: *The Eclectic Approach to Chiropractic*. Las Vegas, FLS Publishing, 1975.
168. Rosqest WLM: *Encyclopedia of the Spinal Touch Treatment*. Salt Lake City, German Therapology Inc, 1975.
169. Harper WD: *Anything Can Cause Anything*, ed 3. Seabrook, Tex, published by the author, 1974.
170. Wales AL: The work of William Garner Sutherland. *Journal of the American Osteopathic Association* 71:788–793, 1972.
171. Reinert OC: *Chiropractic Procedure and Practice*, ed 3. Florissant, Mo, Marian Press, 1972.
172. Goodheart GL: *Collected Published Articles and Reprints*. Montpellier, O, Williams County Publishing, 1969.
173. Magoun HI: *Osteopathy in the Cranial Field*, ed 2. Kirksville, Mo, Journal Printing Company, 1966.
174. Arnholz WW: *Chiropractic and The Arnholz Adjustment of Muscle Spasm Textbook*, ed 6. West Los Angeles, published by the author, 1977.
175. American Chiropractic Association: *Chiropractic State of the Art*. Arlington, Va, 1984, pp 4–7, 11.
176. Daniels L, Worthingham C: *Therapeutic Exercise for Body Alignment and Function*, ed 2. Philadelphia, W. B. Saunders, 1977, pp 37–43.
177. Lee M, Wagner MM: *Fundamentals of Body Mechanics and Conditioning*. Philadelphia, W.B Saunders, 1949.

178. Licht S (ed): *Therapeutic Exercise.* New Haven, Conn, E. Licht Publisher, 1961.
179. Spengler DM: *Low Back Pain.* New York, Grune & Stratton, 1982, pp 105–106, 111–112.
180. Payne FE: A practical approach to effective exercise. *American Family Physician,* 19:76–81, 1979.
181. Kotses H, Weiner H: Effects of home practice exercises on EMG activity subsequent to biofeedback training. *American Journal of Clinical Biofeedback* 5:103–109, 1982.
182. Hubbard JH: The managment of chronic pain of spinal origin. In Rothman RH, Simeone FA (eds): *The Spine.* Philadelphia, W.B. Saunders, 1975, vol 2, pp 845–846, 848–849, 856–861.
183. White AA, Panjabi MM: *Clinical Biomechanics of the Spine.* Philadelphia, J.B. Lippincott, 1978, pp 278, 309.
184. Hart FD: *The Treatment of Chronic Pain.* Philadelphia, F.A. Davis, 1974.
185. Wolf SL: Perspectives on central nervous system responsiveness to transcutaneous electrical nerve stimulation. *Physical Therapy* 58:1443–1449, 1978.
186. Melzack R, Stillwell DM, Fox EJ: Trigger points and acupuncture points for pain: Correlations and implications. *Pain* 3:3–23, 1977.
187. Fisk JW: *The Painful Neck and Back.* Springfield, Ill, Charles C Thomas, 1977, p 154.
188. Melzack R, Vetere P, Finch L: Transcutaneous electrical nerve stimulation for low back pain. *Physical Therapy* 63:489–493, 1983.
189. Gersh MR, Wolf SL: Applications of transcutaneous electrical stimulation in the management of patients with pain. *Physical Therapy* 65:314–321, 1985.
190. Santiesteban AJ: Comparison of electroacupuncture and selected physical therapy for acute spinal pain. *American Journal of Acupuncture* 12:257–262, 1984.
191. Lewith GT, Turner G, Machin D: Effects of acupuncture on low back pain and sciatica. *American Journal of Acupuncture* 12:21–32, 1984.
192. Pontinen PJ: Acupuncture in the treatment of low back pain and sciatica. *Acupuncture and Electro-Therapeutics* 4:53–57, 1979.
193. Berman DA: Pain relief and acupuncture: The if, why and how. *American Journal of Acupuncture* 7:31–41, 1979.
194. Debreceni L: On the possible specific role of acupuncture loci in therapeutics. *Comparative Medicine, East and West* 5:177–179, 1977.
195. Mendelson G et al: Acupuncture treatment of chronic back pain. *American Journal of Medicine* 74:49–55, 1983.
196. Voss DE et al: Traction and approximation. *Proprioceptive Neuromuscular Facilitation: Patterns and Techniques,* ed 3. Philadelphia, Harper & Row, 1985.
197. Saunders HD: *Orthopaedic Physical Therapy: Evaluation and Treatment of Musculoskeletal Disorders.* Minneapolis, published by the author, 1982.
198. Lawson GA, Godfrey CM: A report on studies of spinal traction. *Journal of Medical Services* (Canada) 14:762–771, 1958.
199. Schafer RC: *Chiropractic Health Care,* ed 3. Des Moines, Ia, The Foundation for Chiropractic Education and Research, 1979, p 67.
200. Wood EC: *Beard's Massage Principles and Techniques,* ed 2. Philadelphia, W.B. Saunders, 1974.
201. Jaskoviak P, Schafer RC: Traction, stretching, vibration, and bracing. In *Applied Physiotherapy.* Arlington, Va, American Chiropractic Association. To be published in 1986.
202. Basmajian JV (ed): *Manipulation, Traction and Massage,* ed 3. Baltimore, Williams & Wilkins, 1985, pp 172–206.
203. Harris R: Traction. In Licht S (ed): *Massage, Manipulation, and Traction.* New Haven, Elizabeth Licht, 1960, pp 223–251.
204. Gupta RC, Ramarao SV: Epidurography in reduction of lumbar disc prolapse by traction. *Archives of Physical Medicine and Rehabilitation* 59:322–327, 1978.
205. Swezey RL: *Arthritis: Rational Therapy and Rehabilitation.* Philadelphia, W.B. Saunders, 1978, pp 139–142.
206. Hood LB, Chrisman D: Intermittent pelvic traction in the treatment of the ruptured intervertebral disc. *Physical Therapy* 48:21–30, 1968.
207. White AA, Panjabi MM: *Clinical Biomechanics of the Spine.* Philadelphia, J.B. Lippincott, 1978, pp 345–351, 372.
208. Macnab I: *Backache.* Baltimore, Williams & Wilkins, 1977, pp 142–144.
209. Goldthwait JE et al: *The Essentials of Body Mechanics in Health and Disease,* ed 5. Philadelphia, J.B. Lippincott, 1952.
210. Sterns ML: Studies on development of connective tissue in transparent chambers in rabbit's ear. *American Journal of Anatomy* 67:55, 1940.
211. Cyriax J: *Textbook of Orthopaedic Medicine: Diagnosis of Soft Tissue Lesions,* ed 8. London, Bailliere Tindall, 1982, vol 1, pp 13–18.
212. Chamberlain GJ: Cyriax's friction massage: A review. *Journal of Orthopedics and Sports* 4:16–22, 1982.
213. Nash JM: Personal communication.
214. Nickel VL (ed): *Orthopedic Rehabilitation.* New York, Churchill Livingstone, 1981.
215. Jacobs MD: Preventive spinal hygiene and the human machine. *ACA Journal of Chiropractic* August 1980.
216. Kelley TA Jr: Rehabilitation of the spinal cord injured patient. In Rothman RH, Simeone FA (eds): *The Spine.* Philadelphia, W.B. Saunders, 1975, vol 2, pp 907–912, 916–921.
217. Hirschberg GG, Lewis L, Thomas D: *Rehabilitation.* Philadelphia, J.B. Lippincott, 1964.
218. Stillwell KG: Therapeutic heat and cold. In Krusen FH (ed): *Handbook of Physical Medicine and Rehabilitation,* ed 2. Philadelphia, W.B. Saunders, 1971, p 259–261.

SUGGESTED READINGS

Aegerter E, Kirkpatrick JA: *Orthopedic Diseases,* ed 3. Philadelphia, W.B. Saunders, 1968.

Burns L, Chandler LC, Rice RW: *Pathogenesis of Visceral Disease Following Vertebral Lesions.* Chicago, American Osteopathic Association, 1948.

Denslow JS: Pathophysiologic evidence of the osteopathic lesion. Data on what is known, what is not known, and what is controversial. In Goldstein M (ed): *The Research Status of Spinal Manipulative Therapy,* NINCDS Monograph, No. 15, DHEW Publication No. (NIH) 76-998, Stock No. 017-049-00060-7, Washington, DC, U.S. Government Printing Office, 1975, pp 227–234.

Grice AS: Muscle tonus change following manipulation. *Journal of the Canadian Chiropractic Association* December 1974.

Hadler NM: *Medical Management of the Regional Musculoskeletal Diseases.* New York, Grune & Stratton, 1984.

Hardy AG, Elson R: *Practical Management of Spinal Injuries,* ed 2. New York, Churchill Livingstone, 1976.

Jones CL: Damaging effects of a misaligned musculoskeletal system. *Journal of the American Podiatry Association* October 1971.

Kane WJ (ed): *Current Orthopaedic Management.* New York, Churchill Livingstone, 1980.

Larson LA (ed): *Encyclopedia of Sport Sciences and Medicine.* London, Collier-Macmillan, 1971.

Maigne R: *Orthopedic Medicine.* Springfield, Ill, Charles C Thomas, 1976.

Mills KLG: *Guide to Orthopaedics.* New York, Churchill Livingstone, 1981.

Perkins G: *Ruminations of an Orthopaedic Surgeon.* London, Butterworths, 1970.

Ruge D, Wiltse LL (eds): *Spinal Disorders: Diagnosis and Treatment.* Philadelphia, Lea & Febiger, 1977.

Troup JDG: Biomechanics of the spine. In Murdoch G (ed): *Advances in Orthotics.* London, Edward Arnold, 1976.

CHAPTER 8

The Cervical Region

This chapter considers those factors that are of biomechanical and related clinical interest imperative to the satisfactory evaluation of common or not infrequent cervical syndromes. The kinesiology and kinematics of the neck and the effects and mechanisms of cervical trauma are discussed that are pertinent to the diagnosis and management of muscoloskeletal disorders of the neck.

BACKGROUND[1-4]

The viscera of the neck serve as a channel for vital vessels and nerves, the trachea, esophagus, and spinal cord, and as a site for lymph and endocrine glands. The cervical spine provides musculoskeletal stability and support for the cranium, and a flexible and protective column for movement, balance adaptation, and housing of the spinal cord and vertebral artery. When the head is in balance, a line drawn through the nasal spine and the superior border of the external auditory meatus will be perpendicular to the ground.

Cervical subluxations may be reflected in total body habitus, and insults can manifest themselves throughout the motor, sensory, and autonomic nervous systems. Many peripheral nerve symptoms in the shoulder, arm, and hand will find their origin in the cervical spine. Nowhere in the spine is the relationship between the osseous structures and the surrounding neurologic and vascular beds as intimate or subject to disturbance as it is in the cervical region.[5]

Many of the skeletal landmarks readily observed in the thin individual are frequently obscured in the obese (Fig. 8.1). Except for the manatee and some sloths, all mammals have seven cervical vertebrae.

KINESIOLOGY OF THE NECK[6-9]

The cervical spine is a miracle in design and structure because it moves in various planes. It must support the head, and it must move the eyes and the ears for various sensory orientations.

Mechanically, the head teeters on the atlanto-occipital joints, shaped like cupped palms tipped slightly medially. Because the line of gravity falls anterior to these articulations, a force must be constantly provided in the upright posture by the posterior neck muscles to hold the head erect. Added to this gravitational stress is the action of the anterior muscles of the neck, essentially the masticatory, suprahyoid, and infrahyoid groups, which as a chain join the anterior cranium to the shoulder girdle.

Flexion, extension, rotation, lateral flexion, and circumduction are the basic movements of the cervical region. Movements of the head on the neck are generally confined to the occiput-atlas-axis complex and can be

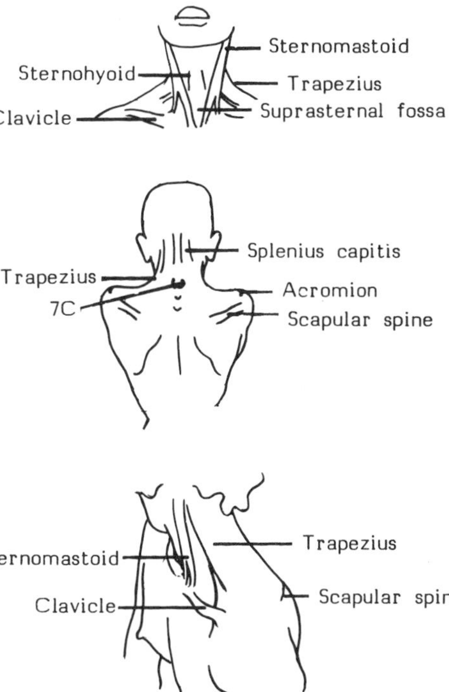

Figure 8.1. Landmarks of the surface anatomy of the neck.

described separately from movements of the neck on the trunk. The prime movers and accessories involved in neck motion are listed in Table 8.1.

Cervical motions are usually tested with the patient seated, unless the patient is unable to hold his head erect. Passive motion should never be attempted if spinal fracture, dislocation, advanced arteriosclerosis, or severe instability is suspected.

Evaluating Gross Muscle Strength of the Neck[10–19]

Muscle strength is recorded on a scale of 5 to 0 or in a percentage and compared bilaterally whenever possible. Grading has been previously described. The major muscles of the neck, their primary functions, and their innervation are listed in Table 8.2.

Flexion

Flexion of the neck as a whole is conducted primarily by the sternocleidomastoideus, the longus group, and the rectus capitis anterior and lateralis, with secondary assistance from the scalenes (Fig. 8.2) and hyoid muscles. Extension is controlled by the upper trapezius, splenius group, the semispinalis group, and the erector spinae, forming the paravertebral extensor mass. Secondary assistance is provided by several small intrinsic neck muscles and the levator scapulae.

The position to test strength of the cervical flexors is taken by stabilizing the patient's sternum with one hand to prevent thoracic flexion and placing the plam of the other hand against the patient's forehead. Strength is evaluated by having the patient slowly attempt to flex his neck against this resistance.

Extension

The strength of the many extensors is evaluated by placing the stabilizing hand in the patient's upper dorsal area to prevent thoracic extension and the palm of the resisting hand over the occiput of the patient. Strength is measured by having the patient slowly extend his neck against this resistance. The stabilizing hand may be placed on the superior aspect of the trapezius between the neck and the humerus to palpate muscle contraction at the same time.

Phillips points out the necessity of normally lax ligaments at the atlantoaxial joints to allow for normal articular gliding, thus making tonic muscle action the only means by which head stability is maintained.[20] Goodheart feels that the splenius (Fig. 8.3) is responsible for maintaining head level more than any other muscle, and that occip-

Table 8.1.
Neck Motion

Joint motion	Prime movers	Accessories
Flexion	Sternocleidomastoid Longus colli Longus capitis Rectus capitis anterior Rectus capitis lateralis	Scalenes Hyoid muscles
Extension	Trapezius, upper Splenius capitis Splenius cervicis Semispinalis capitis Semispinalis cervicis Erector spinae capitis Erector spinae cervicis	Transversospinalis group Levator scapulae
Rotation	Sternocleidomastoid Trapezius, upper Splenius capitis Splenius cervicis	Scalenes Transversospinalis group
Lateral flexion	Scalenes Levator scapulae	Transversospinalis group Rectus capitis lateralis

Table 8.2.
Major Muscles of the Neck

Muscle	Major function	Spinal segment
Erector spinae, upper	Extension, rotation	C1–T1
Longus colli	Flexion	C2–C6
Longus capitis	Flexion	C1–C3
Rectus capitis anterior	Flexion	C1–C2
Rectus capitis lateral	Flexion	C1–C2
Scalenes	Flexion, rotation	C4–C8
Semispinalis capitis	Extension, rotation	C1–T1
Semispinalis cervicis	Extension, rotation	C1–T1
Splenius capitis	Extension, rotation	C1–C8
Splenius cervicis	Extension, rotation	C1–C8
Sternocleidomastoid	Flexion, rotation	C2, XI
Trapezius, upper	Extension, rotation	C3–C4

Spinal innervation varies somewhat in different people. The spinal nerves listed here are averages and may differ in a particular patient; thus, an allowance of a segment above and below those listed in most text tables should be considered.

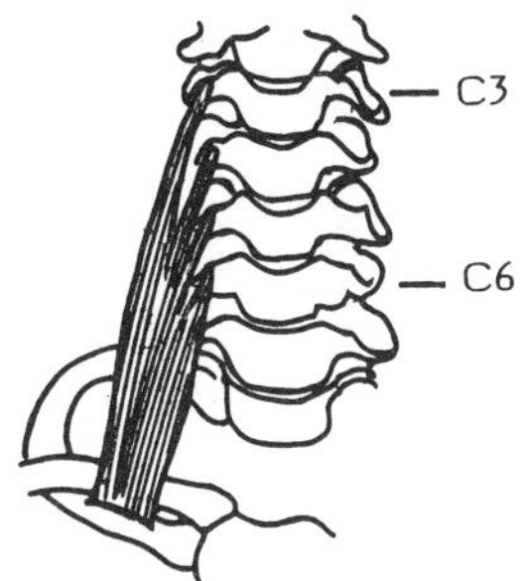

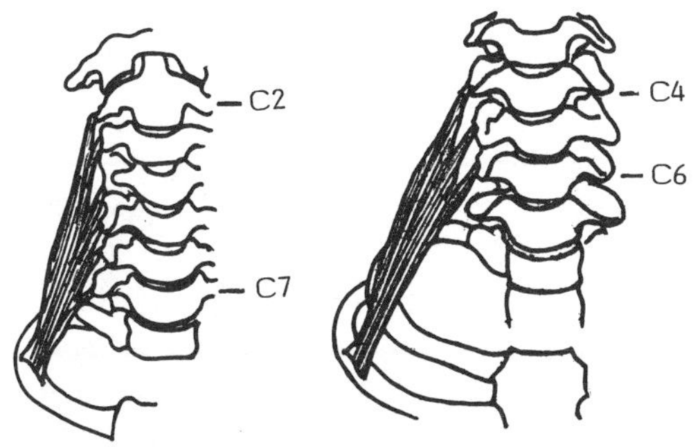

Figure 8.2. The scalene muscle group. The scalenus anterior is shown in the *top* diagram, scalenus medius in the *bottom left* diagram, and scalenus posterior in the *bottom right* diagram.

ital sideslip and jamming frequently are associated here.[21]

Rotation

The primary muscles involved in cervical rotation are the sternocleidomastoideus, upper trapezius, and splenius group, with some assistance provided by the scalenes and intrinsics.

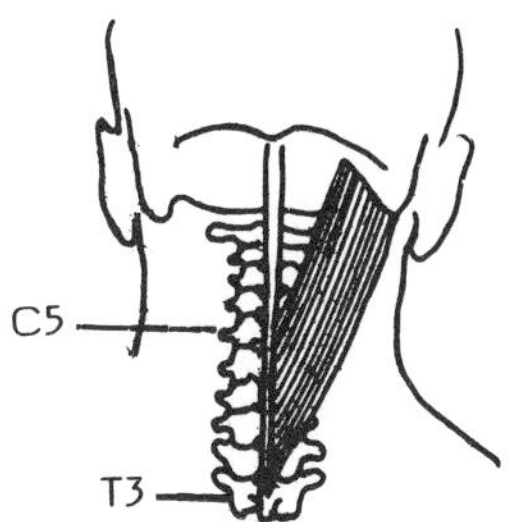

Figure 8.3. The splenius capitis.

Muscle strength of the cervical rotators is tested by standing in front of the patient and placing the stabilizing hand on the patient's left shoulder and the resisting palm against the patient's right cheek when right rotation is being measured. The examiner's hand positions are switched for testing left rotation strength. Rotational strength is evaluated by having the patient attempt to slowly rotate his head against this resistance for each side.

Lateral Flexion

Lateral flexion is accomplished by the scalenus anticus, medius, posticus, and the levator scapulae (Fig. 8.4). Secondary assistance is provided by the small lateral intrinsic muscles of the neck.

Muscle strength of the lateral flexors is tested by standing at the side of the patient and placing the stabilizing hand on the patient's shoulder to prevent thoracic move-

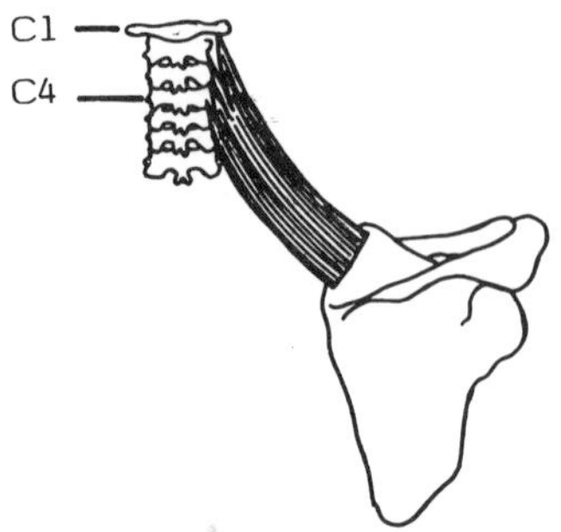

Figure 8.4. The levator scapula muscle.

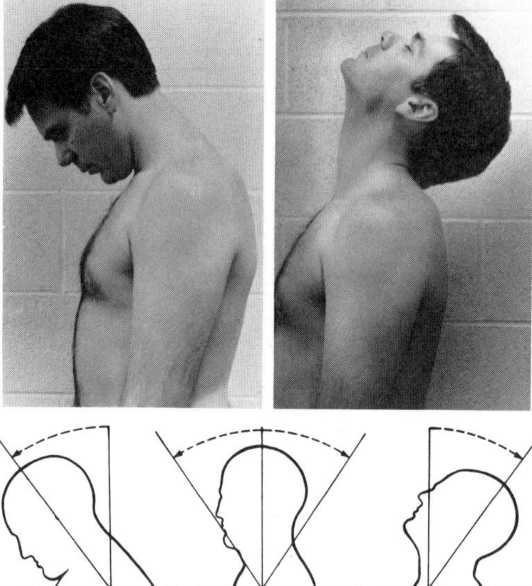

Figure 8.5. Evaluating active neck flexion and extension.

ment and the resisting palm on the patient's skull above the ear. Muscle strength is evaluated by having the patient slowly flex his neck laterally against this resistance.

Evaluating Gross Joint Motion of the Neck[22-30]

Gross joint motion is roughly screened by inspection during active motions (Figs. 8.5, 8.6, and 8.7). When a record is helpful, it is usually measured by goniometry. The patient is placed in the neutral position, with the goniometer centered with its base on line with the superior border of the larynx and the goniometer arm along the mastoid process. The neutral reading, flexion, extension, rotation, and lateral flexion are recorded.

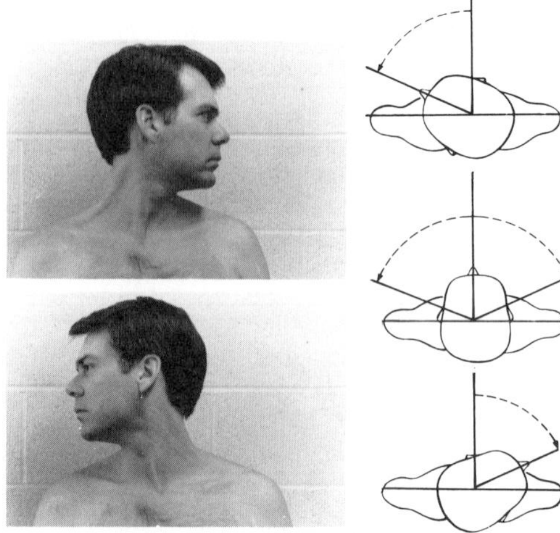

Figure 8.6. Evaluating active neck rotation.

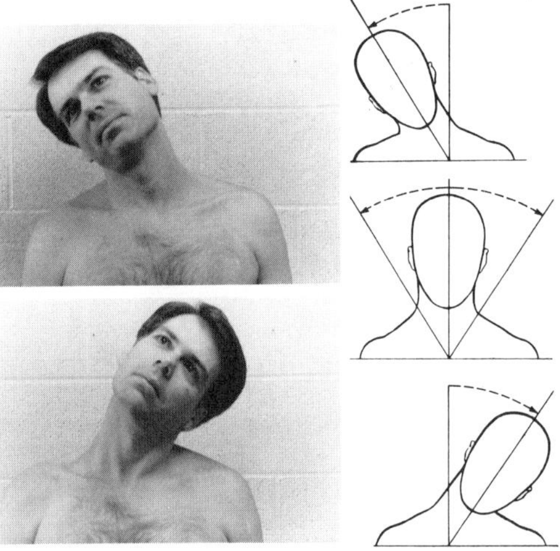

Figure 8.7. Evaluating active neck lateral flexion.

Flexion and Extension

The patient flexes his head as far forward as possible, keeping the goniometer arm along the mastoid process. The end of the flexion motion is recorded. Then, starting from the neutral position, the patient extends his head as far back as possible, keeping the goniometer arm along the mastoid process. The end of neck extension is recorded. In cases of ankylosis, the goniometer is placed to measure the neutral position, and the deviation from this point is recorded.

Rotation

The patient is placed in the neutral position, and the patient's shoulders are steadied with the hands. The patient rotates his head as far to the right and left as possible. The arc of motion is estimated separately for right and left motion by the position of the patient's chin in relation to his shoulder. The goniometer is not necessary for this evaluation. In situtations of ankylosis, the angle at which the cervical region is fixed is estimated by noting the position of the patient's chin and the angle is recorded.

Lateral Flexion

The patient is placed in the neutral position with his arms abducted to steady the shoulders. The goniometer is centered over the back of the neck with the base on the C7 spinous process, and the goniometer arm is extended along the midline of the neck. The neutral reading is recorded. Then the reading is recorded after the patient has bent his neck as far to the left as possible, the reading being taken after the end of lateral flexion. The reading for the right side is recorded in the same manner. In cases of ankylosis, deviations are recorded from the neutral position.

CLINICAL BIOMECHANICS OF THE CERVICAL CANAL[31-33]

The tips of the cervical spinous processes correspond to the level of the succeeding cord segment; eg, the C5 spinous process is approximately on a level with the C6 segment of the cord.

Structural Considerations

The highly mobile cervical spine is unique in that it must provide flexibility and yet protect highly complex neurologic centers within; ie, the lower portion of the medulla oblongata and the portion of the spinal cord that emits the cervical and brachial plexus.

The Structural Pillars

In addition to providing flexibility for sensory orientation (vision, hearing, smell), the cervical spine must provide support for the weight of the cranium. The pillars that must support the weight of the head are (1) initially, the two pillars (lateral masses) of the atlas, and (2) caudally, the anterior and posterolateral aspects of the motion segments below; ie, the vertebral bodies and their discs, and the apophyseal joints, respectively. This distribution of weight is rarely divided evenly, being greater on the anterior aspect during upright relaxation with good posture and greater posteriorly during movements away from the central line of gravity.

Cranial weight is distributed from a two-column mechanism at the occipitoatlantal junction to a three-column mechanism at the atlantoaxial junction, resulting in a pyramidal distribution of forces between the center of mass of the head and the three weight-bearing points on the superior aspect of the axis—a level that is the most mobile point of the spinal column.

The Suspension System

The spinal cord in tethered within the dura by the dentate ligaments. Grieve points out that the upper dentates are the strongest and are attached to the dura inside the posterior cranial fossa, behind the canal for the 12th cranial nerve. Because these intraspinal ligaments, which are under tension, project inferiorly and the nerve roots are angled superiorly, the tensile forces on the cord are relatively balanced during spinal motion. This allows the cord to maintain its relatively central position within the vertebral canal—a position that provides maximum protection. Further protection is provided by cerebrospinal fluid, epidural and extradural fat, and the longitudinal ligaments of the canal.

Nerve Root Relationships

Within the canal, the nerve roots and their sleeves of dura and arachnoid tissue are *loosely attached* to the cervical IVFs. These attachments increase in strength during degenerative processes and with advancing age.[34] At their exit from the foramen, however, the lower roots (C4–C7) are *strongly attached* in the gutter of the transverse process by the epineurial sheath, extensions from the prevertebral fascia, and other connective tissue fibers of the area.[35]

Dynamics of the Cervical Cord

The length of the spinal canal shortens during extension and lengthens during flexion (forward and lateral),[36] and the spinal cord must do likewise to avoid injury during flexion. This is accomplished by the cord's being pleated in an accordion-like fashion during rest and unfolding during any lengthening process.

Changes during Flexion

During flexion, the slack in the cord and its neurons, the dura, and the roots progresses to tension.[37] Because the cord is attached to the coccyx, any tension arising in the cervical area will be transmitted as far caudally as the lower sacral roots.[35]

As in any elastic bar, the cross-section of the cord increases or decreases whenever the cord shortens or lengthens, respectively.[38] Although the spinal cord has a high stretch coefficient when tension is applied slowly, elastic deformation is only necessary at the extremes of spinal motion.[39] Only about 2 or 3 mm of segment-level movement occurs in the cervical spine. The meninges, which have more white fibers than elastic fibers, are not as elastic. They become taut when their length approaches a 5% increase. Thus, while the cord and dura are both under tension during spinal motion, the tension of the dura results from its structural properties and extradural attachments plus root tension, and that of the cord results from the rubber-like dentate bands.[40] This process also mandates that any tension applied to the cord will be rapidly transmitted to the dura and roots, and vice versa.

Changes during Extension

The spinal cord and the roots slacken during extension and slightly gravitate because of gravitational pull. The "free space" of the canal is decreased by three factors during extension: (1) posterior bulging of the IVD, (2) buckling of the relaxed dura, and (3) anterior bulging of the ligamentum flavum.[34,44]

Changes during Rotation and Lateral Flexion

Ipsilateral anterior roots relax and the dorsal roots become stretched during rotation. During lateral flexion, the IVFs narrow in height ipsilaterally and elongate contralaterally. Undue tension can be placed on the contralateral dentate bands and IVF contents, and compressive forces can be applied to the contents of the ipsilateral IVF. This is especially true if degenerative changes have occurred.

Points of Common Injury

The two most vulnerable points of cord injury in the cervical spine are at the odontoid and the C5–C6 interface.

Because the atlas-odontoid serves as a pivot for the cranial mass it is highly vulnerable to injury. If the odontoid fractures, which is not uncommon in severe head and neck injuries, the atlas becomes unstable and can readily cause the freed peg to compress or lacerate the medulla. Even without fracture, a torn transverse ligament (uncommon) will allow the atlas to dislocate anteriorly so that the odontoid will stab the medulla.

The C5–C6 interface is the apex of the "normal" cervical lordosis, and thus serves as the point of maximum functional activity and overstress. If C5 dislocates anteriorly, as happens frequently when a severe axial compression force is applied to the extended neck, the inferior C5 facets override the superior C6 facets and become locked, compressing the spinal cord between the arch of C6 and the posterosuperior aspect of its centrum. This is one reason why the neck of a patient suffering a severe head-neck blow should never be flexed or extended (eg, to insert an airtube) until the possibility of fracture-dislocation has been eliminated.

Effects of Pathologic Changes on the Cord

Several other factors besides fracture and dislocation may produce cord compression (static or dynamic) or reduce cord flexibility (increasing cord tension). Some common examples are space-occupying lesions (eg, tumor, hemorrhage, edema), central stenosis, IVD protrusion, end-plate fracture, ligamentous hypertrophy, soft-tissue sclerosis, CSF disorders, root-sleeve fibrosis or swelling, ischemia consequences, glial scars from demyelinating disease, and postinflammatory adhesions; the most common cause is osteophytes extending from the uncovertebral joints, according to Kapandji.

Breig feels that it is *increased cord tension* (regardless of cause), with its histologic and microcirculatory effects that produce conductivity and circulatory impairment, that accounts for most of the motor, sensory, and autonomic dysfunction associated with cervical cord syndromes.[42,43]

Clinical Implications in Chiropractic

It can be postulated that the same tension mechanisms that occur in the cord, dura, and roots during normal physiologic flexion will occur chronically in the relaxed state when the cervical curve or a single motion unit is hypolordotic. In addition, normal consequences will be compounded whenever a stretched (bow-string) cord is applied against any space-occupying lesion (spondylotic ridge, IVD protrusion, tumor).[44] In time, this condition will result in actual flattening of the cord at this point and in ischemic degeneration from pressure on the anterior spinal artery, the radicular arteries, and/or their capillary beds.[45–47] Likewise, it can be projected that the same factors that narrow the canal during normal extension will occur chronically in the relaxed state when the cervical curve or a single motion unit is hyperlordotic.

GENERAL ASPECTS OF CERVICAL TRAUMA

Blows to the head or neck may result in unconsciousness, but most blows do not. Rather, the effect is a "subconcussive" or "punch drunk" effect for a few moments. This state may be the effect of a severe blow to the head or the cumulative effects of many blows.[48,49] It is assumed that the reader is well acquainted with the proper emergency procedures involved in head and neck trauma.

The anterior and lateral aspects of the neck contain a wide variety of vital structures that have no bony protection. Partial protection is provided by the cervical muscles, the mandible, and the shoulder girdle. After spinal injury, a careful neurologic evaluation must be conducted. Note any signs of impaired consciousness, inequality of pupils, or nystagmus. Do outstretched arms drift unilaterally when the eyes are closed? Standard coordination tests such as finger-to-nose, heel-to-toe, and heel-to-knee, and the test for Romberg's sign should be conducted, along with superficial and tendon reflex tests. For reference, the segmental functions of the cervical nerves are listed in Table 8.3.

Cervical spine injuries can be classified as (1) *mild* (eg, contusions, strains); (2) *moderate* (eg, subluxations, sprains, occult fractures, nerve contusions, neurapraxias); (3) *severe* (eg, axonotmesis, dislocation, stable fracture without neurologic deficit); and (4) *dangerous* (eg, unstable fracture-dislocation, spinal cord or nerve root injury).

Injury Incidence[50–55]

Because of its great mobility and relatively small structures, the cervical spine is the most frequent site of severe spinal nerve injury and subluxations. A wide variety of cervical contusions, Grade 1–3 strains and sprains, subluxations, disc syndromes, dislocations, and fractures will be seen as the result of trauma. The peak incidence of cervical injury occurs in the 3rd decade, with the vast majority of the accidents occurring in males. Body build does not appear to be a major factor. High-speed activities have the highest injury rate.[56]

Considerable cervical spine injury can be attributed to the small, curved vertebral bodies, the wide range of movement in many planes, and the more laterally placed intervertebral articulations which require the nerve roots to leave the spinal canal in an anterolateral direction. There is greater space within the cervical canal than below, but this space is occupied by cord enlargement.

The axis and C6 are the most vulnerable to injury according to accident statistics. The atlas is the least involved of all cervical vertebrae. In terms of segmental structure, the vertebral arch (50%), vertebral body (30%), and intervertebral disc (30%) are most commonly involved in severe cervical trauma. While the anterior ligaments are only involved in 2% of injuries, the posterior ligaments are involved in 16% of injuries.

Basic Posttraumatic Roentgenographic Considerations of the Neck[57–60]

A well-founded appreciation of normal variations, epiphyseal architecture, developmental defects, and congenital anomalies is a distinct aid in evaluating injuries of the cervical area. After the age of 8 years, the

Table 8.3.
Segmental Function of Cervical Nerves

Segment	Function
Cervical plexus (C1–C4)	
C1	Motor to head and neck extensors, infrahyoid, rectus capitis anterior and lateral, and longus capitis
C2	Sensory to lateral occiput and submandibular area; motor, same as C1 plus longus colli
C3	Sensory to lateral occiput and lateral neck, overlapping C2 area; motor to head and neck extensors, infrahyoid, longus capitus, longus colli, levator scapulae, scaleni, and trapezius
C4	Sensory to lower lateral neck and medial shoulder area; motor to head and neck extensors, longus colli levator scapulae, scaleni, trapezius, and diaphragm
Brachial plexus (C5–T1)	
C5	Sensory to clavicle level and lateral arm (axillary nerve); motor to deltoid, biceps; biceps tendon reflex; primary root in shoulder abduction, exits between C4 and C5 discs
C6	Sensory to lateral forearm, thumb, index and half of 2nd finger (sensory branches of musculocutaneous nerve); motor to biceps, wrist extensors; brachioradialis tendon reflex; primary root in wrist extension, exits between C5 and C6 discs
C7	Sensory to second finger; motor to wrist flexors, finger extensors, triceps; triceps tendon reflex; primary root in finger extension, exits between C6 and C7 discs
C8	Sensory to medial forearm (medial antebrachial nerve), ring and little fingers (ulnar nerve); motor to finger flexors, interossei; no reflex applicable; primary root in finger flexion, exits between C7 and T1 discs
T1	Sensory to medial arm (medial brachial cutaneous nerve); motor to interossei; no reflex applicable; primary root in finger abduction, exits between T1 and T2 discs

neck, with few exceptions, attains an adult form in which growth plates present few diagnostic problems.

On the standard lateral and anteroposterior (A-P) views, the anterior and posterior soft tissues deserve careful inspection. Signs of widened retrotracheal space, widened retropharyngeal space, displacement of the prevertebral fat stripe, laryngeal dislocation, or tracheal displacement should be sought. Abnormal vertebral alignment may be exhibited by a loss of the normal lordotic curve or even an acute kyphotic hyperangulation, vertebral body displacement, abnormal dens position, widened interspinous space, or rotation of the vertebral bodies. Abnormal joints may portray unusual IVD space symmetry or widening of an apophyseal joint space. It is easy to miss lower cervical fractures inasmuch as they are often obscured on lateral views by the subject's shoulders if proper precautions are not taken.[63]

Force Effects in Severe Cervical Trauma[62,63]

Compression Forces

Excessive compression forces on the neck commonly lead to facet jamming and fixation, isolated or multiple fractures of the atlantal ring, or vertical, oblique, or bursting fractures of the lower cervical bodies.

Hyperflexion Forces

Excessive anterior bending forces may produce hyperflexion sprain of the posterior ligaments, compressive wedging of the anterior anulus and vertebral body, anterior subluxation, anterior bilateral or unilateral dislocation with locked facets, and spinous process avulsion. Abnormal widening of a spinous interspace on a lateral roentgenograph should arouse suspicion of ruptured posterior ligaments.

Hyperextension Forces

The effects of posterior bending moments may include hyperflexion sprain of the anterior ligaments, wedging of the posterior anulus and vertebral body, posterior subluxation, horizontal fracture of the anterior arch of the atlas, fracture of the anteroinferior margin of a vertebral body, compression of the posterior arch and associated structures, posterior bilateral or unilateral dislocation, spinous process fracture, and traumatic spondylolisthesis.

Hyperrotary Forces

Excessive segmental rotation about the longitudinal axis produces anterior or posterior ligament torsion overstress, rotary subluxation, spiral loosening of the nucleus pulposus, and unilateral or bilateral atlas-axis dislocation. The traumatic moments involved invariably include shear forces.

Shear Forces

Excessive shearing forces create disruption of the anterior or posterior ligaments, endplate displacement, anterior or posterior subluxation or dislocation, anterior or posterior fracture displacement of the dens, and anterior compressive fracture of the anterior ring of the atlas or a vertebral body.

Lateral Hyperflexion Forces

The effects of excessive lateral bending include transverse process fracture, uncinate process failure, lateral dislocation-fracture of the odontoid process, lateral wedging of the anulus and vertebral body, and brachial plexus trauma.

Soft-Tissue Injuries of the Posterolateral Neck

Cervical Contusions

Contusions in the neck are similar to those in other areas. They often occur in the cervical muscles or spinous processes. Painful bruising and tender swelling will be found without difficulty, especially if the neck is flexed. They present little biomechanical significance unless severe scarring occurs.[64]

Direct Nerve Trauma[65,66]

Nerve trauma occurs from contusion, crushing, or laceration.

Neurapraxia. Recovery of nerve contusion usually occurs within 6 weeks. Nerve contusion may be the result of either a single blow or persistent compression. Fractures and blunt trauma are often associated with nerve contusion and crush. Peripheral nerve contusions exhibit early symptoms when produced by falls or blows. Late symptoms arise from pressure by callus, scars, or supports. Mild cases produce pain, tingling, and numbness, with some degree of paresthesia. Moderate cases manifest these same symptoms with some degree of motor and/or sensory paralysis and atrophy.

Axonotmesis. After nerve crush, recovery rate is about an inch per month between the site of trauma and the next innervated muscle. If innervation is delayed from this schedule or if the distance is more than a few inches, surgical exploration should be considered.

Neurotmesis. Laceration from sharp or penetrating wounds is less frequently seen than tears from a fractured bone's fragments. Surgery is usually required. Stretching injury typically features several sites of laceration along the nerve and is usually limited to the brachial plexus.

General Aspects of Strains and Sprains[67,68]

Anterior injuries are more common to the head and chest which project further anteriorly, but a blunt blow from the front to the head or chest may result in an indirect extension or flexion injury of the cervical spine. In any spinal injury, rarely is the trauma the product of a single force. For example, while extension, flexion, and lateral flexion injuries are often described separately in this chapter, rotational, compressive, tensile, and shearing forces are invariably part of the picture.

Incidence. (Grades 1–3) or indirect muscle injuries are common, frequently involving the erectors. Flexion and extension cervical sprains are also common (Grades 1–3) and usually involve the anterior or posterior longitudinal ligaments, but the capsular ligaments may be involved. In the neck especially, strain and sprain may coexist. Severity varies considerably from mild to dangerous. The C1 and C2 nerves are especially vulnerable because they do not enjoy the protection of an intervertebral foramen (IVF).

Typical Signs and Symptoms. Cervical sprain and disc rupture are often associated with severe pain and muscle spasm and are more common in adults because of the reduced elasticity of supporting tissues. Pain is often referred when the brachial plexus is involved. Cervical stiffness, muscle spasm, spinous process tenderness, and restricted motion are common. When pain is present, it is often poorly localized and referred to the occiput, shoulder, between the scapulae, arm, or forearm (lower cervical lesion), and may be accompanied by paresthesia. Radicular symptoms are rarely evident unless a herniation is present. Spasm of the sternocleidomastoideus and trapezius may be due to strain or irritation of the sensory fibers of the spinal accessory nerve as they exist with the C2–C4 spinal nerves.

Case Management. Diagnosis and treatment are similar to that for any muscle strainsprain, but concern must be given to induced subluxations during the initial strain. This point has been reported in numerous chiropractic papers as well as in allopathic studies.[69] Palpation will reveal tenderness and spasm of specific muscles. In acute scalene strain, both tenderness and swelling will usually be found. When the longissimus capitis or the trapezius are strained, they stand out like stiff bands.

Prognosis. Many cervical strains heal spontaneously but may leave a degree of fibrous thickening or trigger points within the injured muscle tissue. Residual joint restriction following acute care is more common in traditional medical care than under mobilizing chiropractic management.

Extension Strain/Sprain and Whiplash[70–75]

The head may be flexed forward so that the chin strikes the sternum or thrown sideward so that the ear strikes the shoulder and the neck can still be within the normal range of motion. It is most rare, however, that the occiput strikes the back and does not exceed normal cervical extension.

Mechanisms. Other than those in automobile accidents, the forces in whiplash are usually administered from below upward; eg, an uppercut blow to the chin or a blow to the forehead while running forward. This is in contrast to the compressive type of hyperextension or hyperflexion injury in which the force is usually from above downward. Thus, knowing the direction of force, even if the magnitude is unknown, is important in analyzing the effects. A facial injury usually suggests an accompanying extension injury of the cervical spine as the head is forced backward.

Kinematics. In whiplash resulting from a mild automobile collision, the cervical trauma is due to indirect trauma from acceleration-deceleration forces. If the head does not strike anything, the injury is produced solely by inertia forces (Fig. 8.8). The body is moving as a whole at the same speed as the automobile. If the automobile is struck from the rear, the unrestrained head is whipped backward because it is not restrained by the seat, and then rebounds forward. If the automobile is struck from the front or hits a relatively immovable object, the head is thrown forward and then rebounds backward. Thus, the inertia force displaces the head in the direction opposite to the automobile's acceleration. The first movement is that of translation which produces a shearing force at the base of the neck because the bending movement is greatest at that point.[76,77]

The rebound is caused by several factors. In a front-end collison, for example, there is an initial flexion *elongation* of the cervical spine after impact that is followed by a rebound extension. The rebound is produced by the rapid deceleration of the automobile, the impact from the seat, and the stretch reflex produced within the stretched neck and upper dorsal muscles. This reflex can be quite severe, and because it occurs when the neck is at its full range of move-

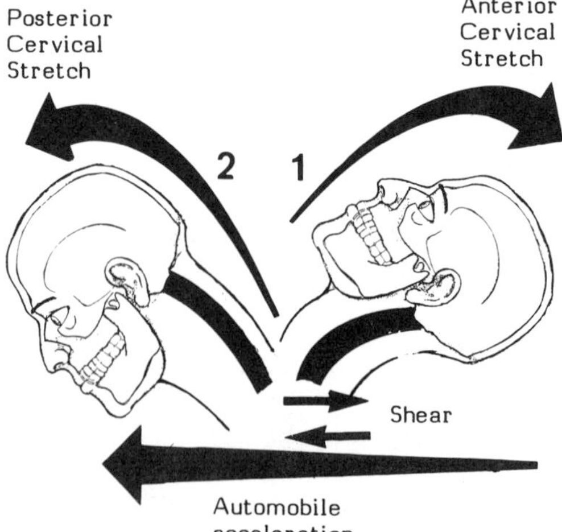

Figure 8.8. Basic kinematic mechanisms involved in a rear-end collision, showing initial and following movement sequences.

ment, the pull generates considerable *compression* as well as extension.

Effects. When the head is violently thrown backward (eg, whiplash), the damage may vary from minor to severe tearing of the anterior and posterior longitudinal ligaments.[78] This flattens the cervical curve in about 80% of cases, and a degree of facet injury must exist even if not evident on film. Stretching to the point of hematoma may occur in the sternocleidomastoideus, longus capitis, longus cervicis, and scalene muscles[79] (Fig. 8.9). Severe cord damage can occur that is usually attributed to momentary pressure by the dura, ligamentum flavum, and laminae posteriorly, even without roentgenographic evidence. Even without any cord deficit, severe damage to the nerve roots may occur as the facets jam together and close upon the IVF, especially if fracture occurs.[80] Incidence is highest at the C4–C6 area. Severe stretching of the vertebral arteries and sympathetic trunk to some degree is inevitable.

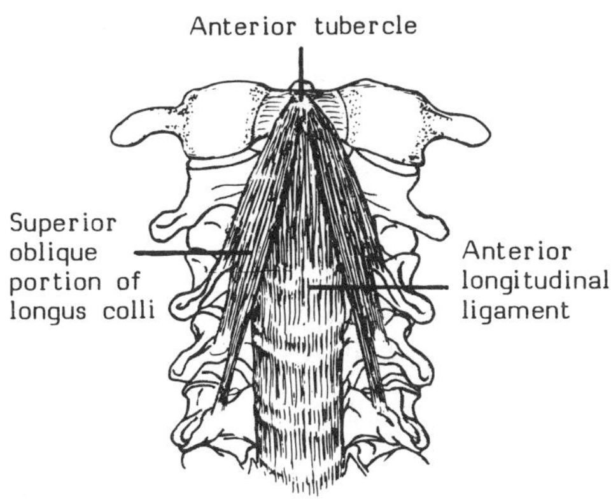

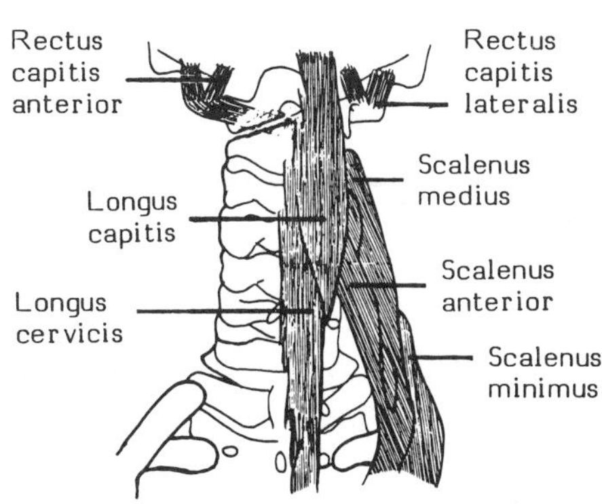

Figure 8.9. *Top*, the major prevertebral ligaments; *bottom*, the major prevertebral muscles.

Cailliet[81] points out that it is difficult to visualize a sprain causing rupture of the ligaments of a joint without causing some derangement of the opposing joint surfaces, which by definition is an orthopedic subluxation. If a whiplash injury is considered a severe sprain, an orthopedic subluxation injury must be assumed to have occurred even if it has been spontaneously reduced. Such subluxations may occur during the initial movement and/or the rebound movement, and it is not unusual to have manifestations of a flexion sprain superimposed upon manifestations of an extension sprain. In the typical whiplash injury, whether it be from hyperextension or hyperflexion or both, the effects of traumatic elongation and compression are compounded by underlying fixations, arteriosclerosis, spondylosis, ankylosing spondylitis, etc.

Signs and Symptoms. Severe sprain can be assumed if cervical pain arises immediately after the accident or shortly thereafter. Difficulty in opening the mouth points to severely strained suprahyoid muscles.[82] If severe muscle splinting of the neck is accompanied by pain in the mastoid-mandible area, the possibility of fracture (probably odontoid or midcervical) must be eliminated immediately. Severe pain and spasm not arising until the following day suggest severe strain of one or more posterior cervical muscle groups. Specific involvement depends on the position of the head and neck during impact. Pain, spasm, and related neurologic focal signs generally suggest either cord damage or root injury from associated lateral hyperflexion or dislocation that may have been spontaneously reduced.

Besides neck pain, a wide variety of usually overlapping features may be exhibited after an extension injury. For example, expressions may be seen in:

1. Neuropathy (radiculitis, cerebral concussion, IVD fault, hoarseness, dysphagia, headache, visual disturbances, nystagmus).[83–85]
2. Vasomotor disturbances (vertebral artery injury).[86]
3. Musculoskeletal impairment (overt hypermobility and hypomobility at different segments, and extensive trigger-point development).[87]

4. Audiovestibular faults (deafness, vertigo).[88–90]
5. Deficits of memory (cerebral concussion amnesia).[91]

This discussion has concerned itself with whiplash strains and sprains of varying degrees of severity that can usually be treated conservatively. Similar mechanisms with greater force factors that result in fracture, locked dislocation, and grossly torn tissues will be described later in this chapter.

Case Management. Treatment of mild or moderate injuries not exhibiting severe neurologic trauma requires reduction of subluxation, physiotherapeutic remedial aid, a custom-fitted supporting collar for several weeks depending upon the clinical symptoms and signs, and graduated therapeutic exercises beginning with isometric contractions. Continuous traction, which reduces the cervical lordosis, may be helpful in extension injuries after the acute stage, but it would usually be contraindicated when the cervical curve has reversed (eg, flexion strain).

Flexion Strain/Sprain[92–94]

Slight anterior subluxation is usually not serious, but neurologic symptoms may appear locally or extend down th arm.

Mechanisms. An occipital injury usually suggests an accompanying flexion injury of the anterior cervical spine and posterior soft tissues as the skull is forced forward (Fig. 8.10). Flexion injury may also be a part of whiplash, superimposed upon an extension injury.

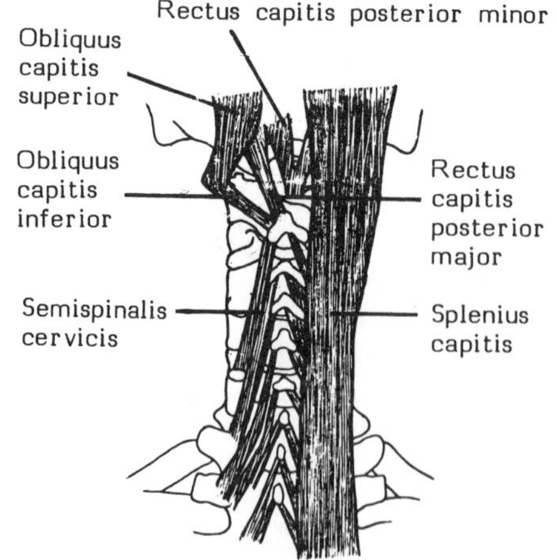

Figure 8.10. Some major posterior cervical muscles.

Effects. The posterior paraspinal tissues are overstretched, the facets are sprung open, and the process of bleeding, edema, fibrosis, and adhesions is initiated. Fractures of endplates may be difficult to assess early. Disc degeneration and posttraumatic osteoarthritis may follow, which lead to spondylosis.

Case Management. Management is similar to that of extension injuries, except that the period of necessary immobilization is often shorter (6–8 weeks).

Lateral Flexion Strain/Sprain[95–97]

Traumatic brachial plexus traction syndromes will be discussed later in this chapter. These usually occur when the neck is not only severely flexed sideward but also flexed forward and down so that the head is anterior to the shoulder.

Trigger Points[98]

The cervical and suprascapular areas of the trapezius, usually a few inches lateral to C7, frequently refer pain and deep tenderness to the lateral neck (especially the submastoid area), temple area, and angle of the jaw (Fig. 8.11). The sternal division of the sternocleidomastoideus refers pain chiefly to the eyebrown, cheek, tongue, chin, pharynx, throat, and sternum. The clavicular division refers pain mainly to the forehead (bilaterally), back of and/or deep within the ear, and rarely to the teeth. Other common trigger points involved in "stiff neck" are in the levator scapulae, the splenius cervicus lateral to the C4–C6 spinous processes, and the splenius capitis over the C1–C2 laminae (Fig. 8.12). These points are often not found unless the cervical muscles are relaxed during palpation.

Adjunctive Therapies[99, 100]

The reduction of spasm is often necessary prior to structural correction and to maintain a corrected position after adjustment. Case management of soft-tissue injuries in the cervical region will be described in the next chapter. However, a few points deserve mention here.

Passive Stretch. Mild passive stretch is an excellent method of reducing spasm in the long muscles. Heavy passive stretch, however, destroys the beneficial reflexes. One technique, for example, is to place the patient prone on an adjusting table of which the headpiece has been slightly lowered. The patient's head is turned toward the side of the spastic muscle. With head weight alone serving as the stretching tensile force, the spasm should relax within 2–3 minutes. Thumb pressure, placed on a trigger area, is then directed toward the muscle's attachment and held for a few moments until relaxation is complete.

Therapeutic Heat or Cold. Heat is also helpful, but cold and vapocoolant sprays have proved to be more effective in acute cases.

Therapeutic Exercise. Mild isotonic exercises are useful for improving circulation and inducing the stretch reflex, especially in the cervical extensors. These exercises should be done supine to reduce exteroceptive influences on the central nervous system. In chronic cases, relaxation training with biofeedback is helpful.

Traction.[101] The effects of cervical traction are often dramatic but sometimes short-lived if a herniated disc is involved. Extreme care must be taken in post-traumatic cases to eliminate the possibility of instability prior to traction. For example, the use of traction following traumatic spondylolisthesis in which the anterior longitudinal ligament has been separated can produce severe displacement with catastrophic effects (Fig. 8.13).

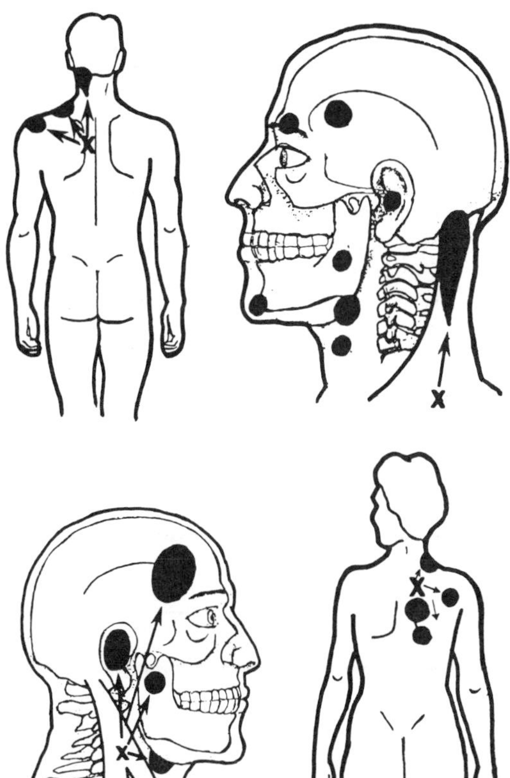

Figure 8.11. *Top*, trapezius trigger point; *X*, common site. *Blackened areas* indicate typical sites of referred pain. *Bottom left*, sternocleidomastoid trigger point. *Bottom right*, levator scapulae trigger point.

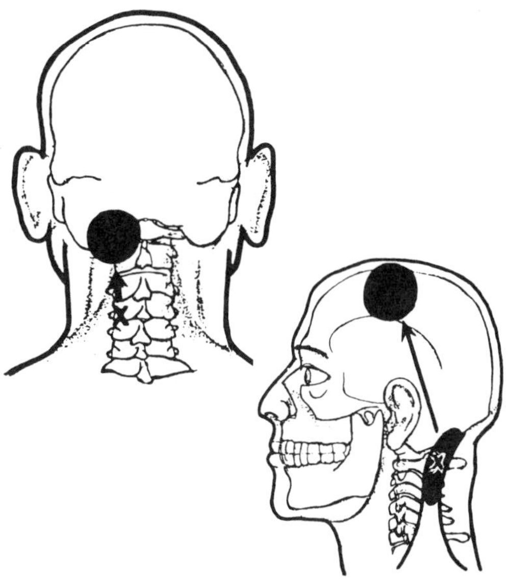

Figure 8.12. *Top left*, splenius cervicis trigger point; *X*, common site. *Blackened areas* indicate typical sites of referred pain. *Bottom right*, splenius capitis trigger point.

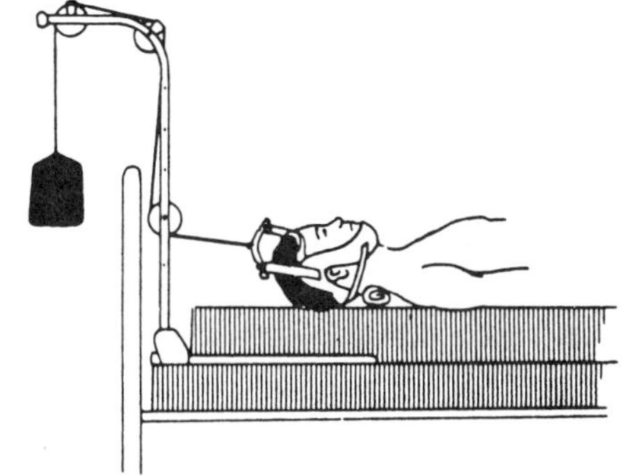

Figure 8.13. Simple cervical traction apparatus.

In any vertebral, occipital, or pelvic subluxation, physiotherapy, traction, muscle relaxants, gross manipulations, muscle stretching, injections, or other methods will not offer much relief by themselves unless the fixated articulation is correctly adjusted so that intrinsic function can be normalized.

CLINICAL BIOMECHANICS OF THE UPPER CERVICAL SPINE

For study, it is best to divide the cervical spine into upper and lower regions because of its anatomical design and functional arrangement. The upper spine is composed of the occipital condyles, the atlas, and the axis. It is different morphologically and functionally from the lower cervical spine that is made up of vertebrae C3–C7. The axis is thus a transitional vertebra in that its superior aspect is part of the upper complex and its inferior aspect is part of the lower complex.

Regional Structural Characteristics[102–109]

The spinal canal of the upper cervical region is relatively large to accommodate the cervical enlargement of the cord. The pedicles, apophyseal joints, uncinate processes, and transverse processes have characteristics peculiar and specific to the cervical spine.

The Occipital Condyles

The occipitoatlantal junctions are typically described as ball-and-socket–type joints, in which the condyle "ball" is elipsoid and its axis is transverse, which permits flexion-extension and a slight amount of rotation and lateral flexion.[110] Rude, however, has shown that the occipital condyles vary greatly in shape and the specific design of the facets determines their movement.[111] While typically convex, many have been found to be square, rhomboidal, rectangular, flat, prismatic, or concave (rare), and some have split forms. Flattened and prismatic (angular) condyle facets allow great slipping and tipping during motion. A convex condyle facet allows only rotary slippage if the corresponding atlantoid facet has a similar radius.

Craton also found that differences in area size of the two condyle-glenoid groove surfaces resulted in different articular mobility.[112] The least mobile articulation exhibited the least erosion of the cartilage plates, and he suggests that a condyle sideslip with a counterclockwise rotation was the cause of the variable erosion and size.

The Atlas[113,114]

In several anatomical respects, the atlas can be considered a sesamoid between the occiput and axis that serves as a biomechanical washer or bearing between the occipital condyles and the axis (Fig. 8.14). The atlas is an elongated bony ring with right and left lateral masses, an anterior arch, a posterior arch, and bilateral transverse processes that extend from each lateral mass. The absent body of the atlas is represented by its anterior arch and the dens of the axis. The inner aspect of the anterior arch contains a facet for the dens. An IVD does not exist between the occiput and the atlas, nor does the atlas exhibit IVFs or a distinct spinous process.

The Lateral Masses and Articular Processes. The lateral masses are oval in shape with an oblique anteromedial articulation. They must support the weight of the head, which comprises about 7% of body weight. The articular surfaces on the superior side of the lateral masses are biconcave to allow for the seating and movement of the biconvex occipital condyles and are relatively large to dissipate the weight of the head. The inferior articulating facets of the atlas have an inferomedial articulation with anteroposterior convexity to fit the articulation of the superior facets of the axis. These inferior facets of the atlas lie directly underneath the superior facets, unlike those of

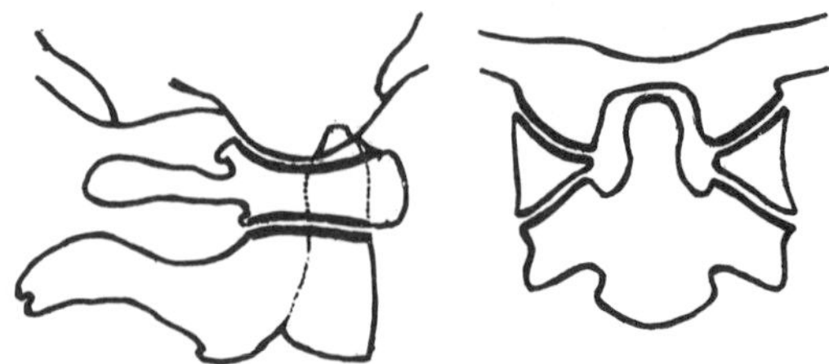

Figure 8.14. The atlanto-occipital joints. *Left*, lateral view; *right*, A-P view. As the plane of articulation is less in the sagittal plane than in the frontal plane, traumatic A-P occipital subluxation or dislocation is more likely than lateral displacement.

subjacent apophyseal joints whose inferior facets lie posterior to the superior facets.

The Posterior Arch. The posterior arch of the atlas thickens posteriorly to where it forms the posterior tubercle (Fig. 8.15). The posterior arch is grooved to offer some bony protection for the vertebral artery which runs just behind the lateral mass. This groove is a frequent fracture site.

The Transverse Processes. Only the lumbar vertebrae have transverse processes that extend further from the midline than the atlas. This great width increases the leverage of the muscles that insert at the transverse processes. Unlike other cervical vertebrae, the transverse processes of the atlas are not grooved to allow egress of a nerve root. The transverse processes of the atlas, as other cervical vertebrae, contain a conduit (foramen transversarium) for the vertebral artery.

The Axis[115,116]

The inferior facets of the atlas fit the superior facets of the axis like epaulets on sloping shoulders (Fig. 8.16). The plane is about 110° to the vertical. To allow maximum rotation of the upper cervical complex without stress to the contents of the vertebral canal, the instantaneous axis of rotation

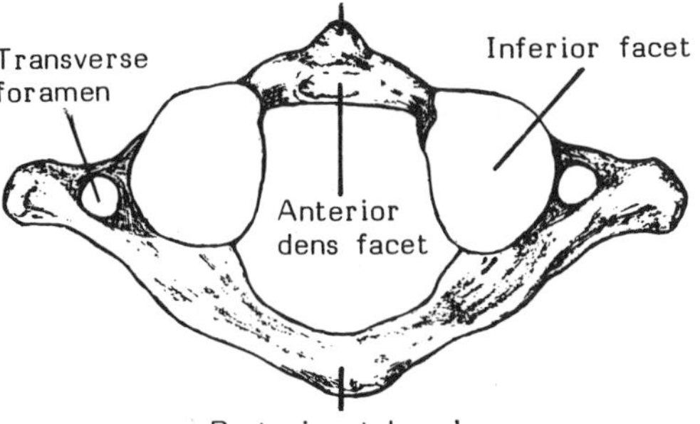

Figure 8.15. The atlas, *top*, viewed from above; *center*, viewed from the superolateral; *bottom*, viewed from below.

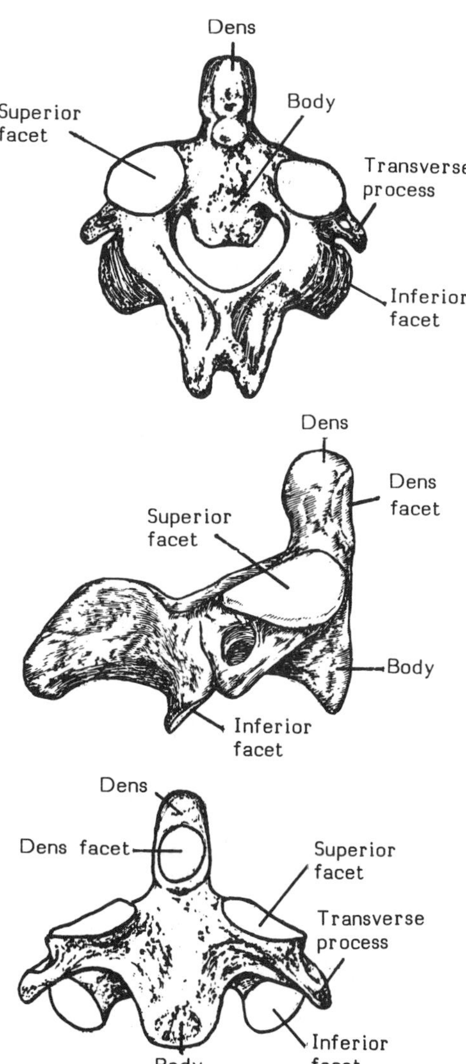

Figure 8.16. The axis, *top*, viewed from the superoposterior; *center*, viewed laterally; *bottom*, viewed from the anterior.

is placed close to the spinal cord (ie, near the atlanto-odontoid articulation).

The Anterior Arch. The C1–C2 joint is an unusual joint in that the inner anterior arch of C1 has a small facet that is in contact with the odontoid process of C2, separated only by a small synovial cavity. A small synovial bursa also separates the posterior aspect of the odontoid from the cruciate ligament (Fig. 8.17). The osseous and ligament complex of this area allows great rotation and some flexion and extension. The anterior arch of C1 normally remains 1 mm from the odontoid in flexion and extension. If there is widening of this space to greater than 3 mm in the adult or 44 mm in the child, damage to the transverse ligament of the atlas can be suspected.

Rotational Restriction. Rotation of C2 on C3 is limited by a mechanical blocking mechanism that protects the vertebral artery from excessive torsion. The anterior tip of the superior articular process of C3 impinges on the lateral margin of the foramen transversarium of C2. This same blocking mechanism is also found in the subjacent cervical vertebrae (Fig. 8.18).

The Occipitocervical Ligaments[117–121]

The cross-shaped *cruciate ligament* completely secures the odontoid process. Its main portion is the triangular bilateral transverse ligament, which passes posteriorly on the dens and connects to the lateral masses of the atlas, crossing in front of the spinal cord. Its main function is to restrict anterior

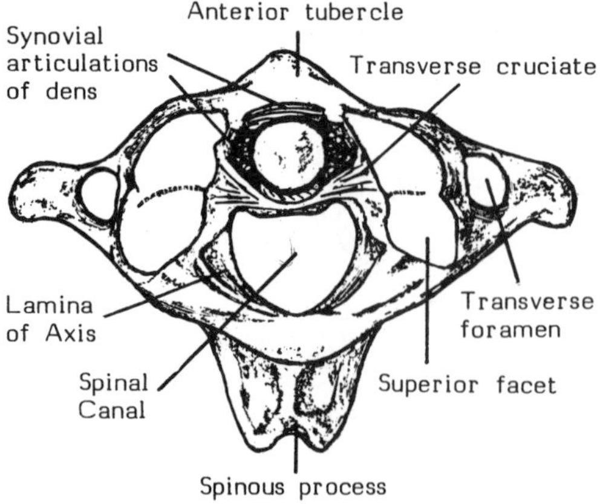

Figure 8.17. The atlanto-odontoid articulation as viewed from above.

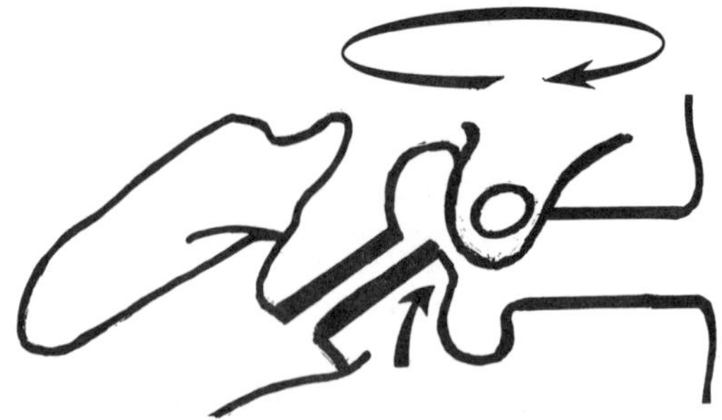

Figure 8.18. The A-P translation of C2 on C3 is limited by mechanical blocking when the antero-superior top of the articular process of C3 strikes the bony ring of the transverse foramen of C2.

translation of the atlas. There are also two vertical bands. One rides from the dens up to the basiocciput, and the other extends from the dens posteriorly down to the body of the axis. Because these ligaments are often tough, the odontoid will usually fracture prior to ligament failure. In addition, accessory atlantoaxial ligaments extent superiorly and laterally from the base of the inferior vertical cruciate and join the base of the dens with the inferomedial aspect of the lateral mass of C1.

Anterior to the upper arm of the cruciate lie the apical and alar ligaments. The thin, elastic *apical ligament* connects the tip of the dens to the anterior margin of the foramen magnum, and the stronger lateral *alar ligaments* connect the medial aspect of the occipital condyles obliquely with the superolateral aspect of the odontoid (Fig. 8.19). These three guy-wire ligaments, collectively called the dentate ligaments of the dens, tend to limit rotation and lateral bending, but their capabilities are quite limited.

The *atlantoepistrophic ligament* runs between the anterior body of the axis and the inferior aspect of the anterior ring of the atlas, and the *atlanto-occipital ligament* connects the superior aspect of the anterior ring of the atlas and the occipital tubercle.

The posterior longitudinal ligament terminates upward as the strong, broad, fan-shaped *membrana tectoria* which extends superiorly from the base of the odontoid, over the posterior dens, then obliquely angles forward to blend with the dura and the clivus of the basiocciput periosteum at the anterior aspect of the foramen magnum. Its most posterior aspect joins the occiput to

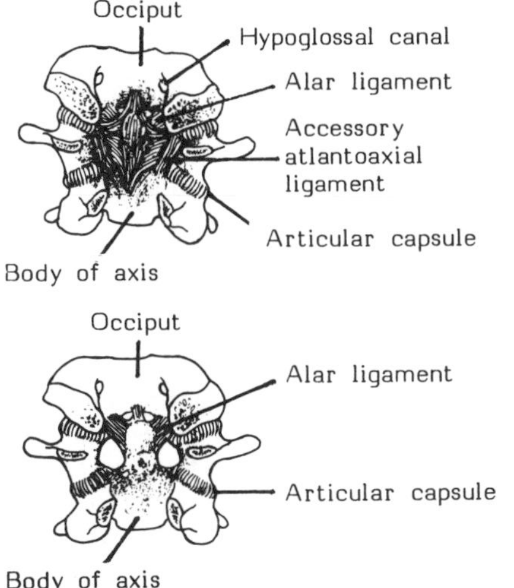

Figure 8.19. Ligaments of the odontoid process.

the posterior ring of the atlas, and it serves to check excessive A-P motion. Its deep lateral part connects the posterior body of C2 with the anterolateral ring of the atlas.

The broad, dense, anterior longitudinal ligament blends posteriorly with the anterior *atlanto-occipital membrane* which extends superiorly from the upper body of the axis to connect the anterior tubercle of the atlas with the margin of the foramen magnum. It blends laterally with the facet capsules.

The ligamentum flavum terminates superiorly as the *posterior atlantoaxial membrane* that joins the posterior arch of the axis to the posterior ring of the atlas. It then arches over the vertebral artery above the atlas and attaches to the foramen magnum as the *atlanto-occipital membrane* to join the atlas with the occiput (Fig. 8.20).

Short, thin *capsular ligaments* surround the atlanto-occipital diarthrotic articulations; and short, thick, loose capsular ligaments surround the C1–C2 diarthrosis. Their fibers lie perpendicular to the facet planes, and they are remarkably lax when the articulations are in a position of rest. The capsules are reinforced laterally by the atlanto-occipital fibers extending from the jugular process of the occiput to the lateral masses of the atlas and the transverse processes of the axis. The capsular and lateral ligaments are normally loose enough in the A-P plane to allow nodding, but taut

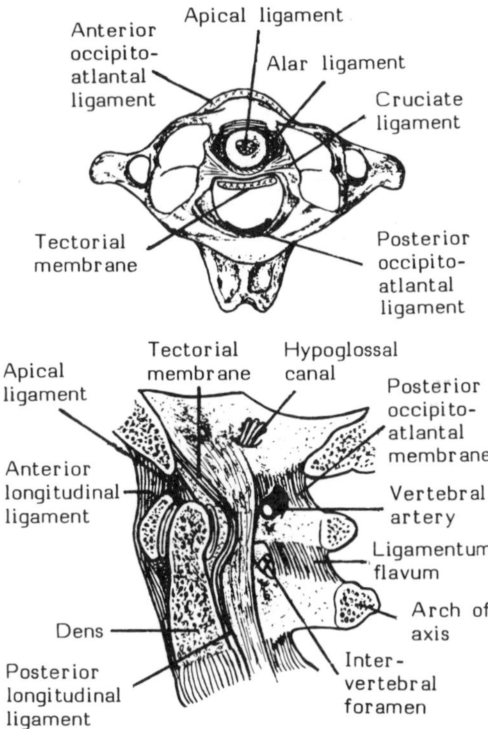

Figure 8.20. Upper cervical ligaments, *top*, as viewed from above; *bottom*, sagittal section.

enough lateally so that the occiput and atlas move as a unit during moderate rotation and lateral flexion of the neck (Fig. 8.21).

The triangular *nuchal ligament band* runs in the midline from the posterior border of the occiput to the posterior tubercle of the atlas and the C2–C7 spinous processes, dividing the posterior aspect of the neck into right and left halves. It is not unusual to find evidence on a lateral roentgenograph of nuchial ossification, indicating an old spinous process fracture.

Kinematics of the Upper Cervical Spine[122–128]

An understanding of the basic kinematics of the cervical spine is vital to accurate clinical diagnosis and therapeutic applications. All movements in the cervical spine are relatively free because of the saddle-like joints. The cervical spine is most flexible in flexion and rotation. The latter occurs most freely in the upper cervical area and is progressively restricted on moving downward through the cervical area.

Note: The specific range of cervical motion

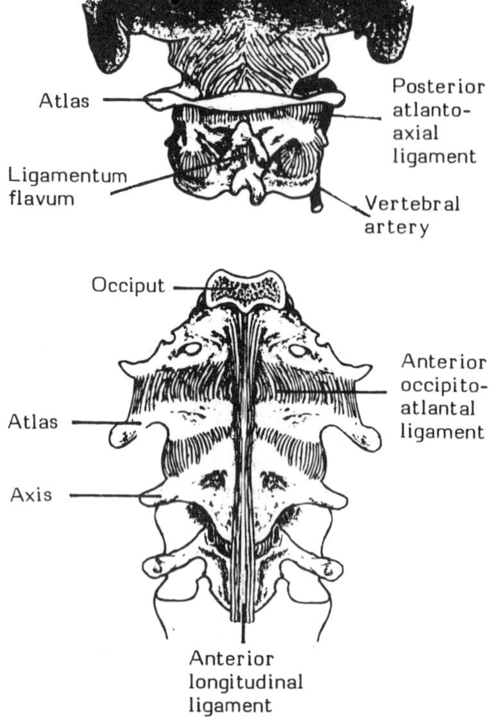

Figure 8.21. *Top*, the major postvertebral ligaments of the upper cervical area; *bottom*, the major prevertebral ligaments.

differs quite widely among so many authorities that any range offered here should be considered hypothetical, depending on individual planes of articulation, other variances in structural design (eg, congenital, aging degeneration, posttraumatic), and soft-tissue integrity. This wide variance in opinion also holds for the centers of motion described.

Biomechanical Upper Cervical Instability[129,130]

Moderately strong soft-tissue connections exist within the occiput-atlas-axis complex. Osseous, muscle, tendon, ligament, and lymph node abnormalities tend to restrict motion, while tissue tears and lax ligaments without associated muscle spasm allow too much motion.

Stability is provided the C1–C2 joint by paravertebral ligaments and muscle attachments. When weakening of these supports occurs (eg, rheumatoid arthritis, trauma, postural stress), a dangerous state of instability can arise. Each infant presents a considerable degree of cervical instability because of the relatively large head weight superimposed on the small underdeveloped spine.

Flexion and Extension[131–133]

A great deal of cervical motion is concentrated in specific spinal areas. About half of flexion and extension occurs at the atlanto-occipital joints, with the other half distributed among the remaining cervical joints. Inasmuch as the nucleus of the disc is nearer the anterior of a *complete* cervical vertebra, A-P motion is more discrenible at the spinous process than at the anterior aspect of the vertebral body.

In the cervical spine, flexion and extension occur around a horizontal axis that lies in the body of the vertebra below. For C2, it is located in the posteroinferior aspect of the body of C3 and progressively moves anteriorly and superiorly for each segment caudally.[134]

Flexion Range. Without any neck participation, the head can be moved 10° in flexion between the occiput and atlas, according to Cailliet[135] (Fig. 8.22). During strict upper neck flexion, the condyles roll backward and slide slightly posterior on the atlas while the atlas rolls anteriorly and somewhat superiorly, taking the odontoid with it so that the dens slightly approaches the clivus of the basiocciput. As the atlas slides anteriorly in relation to the condyles, the posterior arch of the atlas and occiput separate only slightly, but this is exaggerated if movement is virtually isolated at the atlanto-occipital joint (eg, ankylosing spondylitis). Also during flexion, the inferior lateral masses of the atlas roll upward poste-

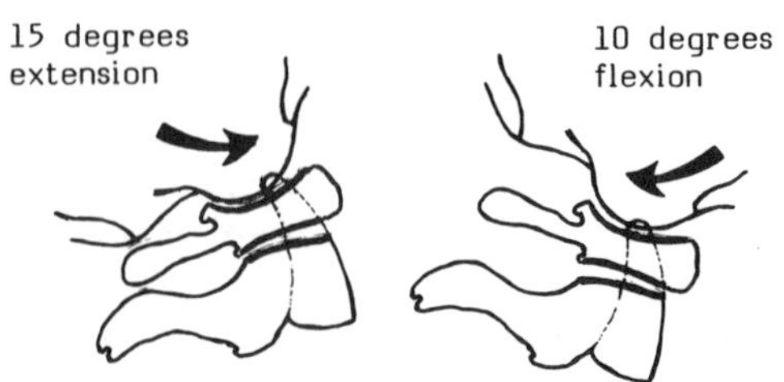

Figure 8.22. Atlanto-occipital flexion and extension.

riorly and slide backward on the superior facets of the axis for about 5°. Opening of the superior aspect of the atlanto-odontoid space is not appreciably restricted by the delicate cruciate ligament. Movement is restricted mainly by the apophyseal capsules, the ligamentum flavum, the interspinous ligament, the posterior nuchal muscles, and impact of the chin against the sternum.

Extension Range. The skull can be extended on the atlas for about 15° without any participation by other cervical vertebrae. During normal extension of the neck, the condyles slide anteriorly on the atlas; the atlas rolls upward so that its posterior arch approximates the occiput. Slight opening of the inferior aspect of the atlanto-odontoid space occurs, but it is limited by the tectorial membrane. Similarly, the posterior arches of the atlas and axis also approximate. The range of extension of C1 on C2 is usually given as 10°. During forced extension, the posterior arch of the atlas is caught as in a vise between the occiput and axis.

Active Motion. Regional active cervical flexion and extension motions are tested by having the patient raise and lower the chin as far as possible without moving the shoulders. Note the smoothness of motion and degree of limitation bilaterally.

Passive Motion. Passive cervical flexion and extension are examined by placing the hands on the sides of the patient's skull and rolling the skull anteroinferiorly so that the chin approximates the sternum and posterosuperiorly so that the nose is perpendicular to the ceiling.

Occipitoatlantal Motion during Flexion. This is a remarkable two-phase process. During the first phase, the occiput anteflexes on the atlas. During the second phase of flexion, however, the occiput retroflexes relative to the atlas and axis.[136]

Rotation[137,138]

Approximately half of rotational movement takes place at the atlantoaxial joints about the odontoid process, with the remaining half distributed faily evenly among the other cervical joints. During rotation, the odontoid represents a peg encased within a fairly enclosed ring or a stake surrounded by a horseshoe.

Range. During rotation, the occipital condyles and the atlas initially move as one unit on the axis (Fig. 8.23). Approaching the end of the range of motion, the condyles can rotate several degrees (8–10°) upon the atlas in the direction of movement. Only a few authorities contest this fact. C1 rotation occurs about the dens of C2 which serves as a pivot. As mentioned, 50% of total neck rotation occurs between C1 and C2 (capable of 80–100° rotation) before any rotation is noted from C2 to C7 or at the atlanto-occipital joint. After about 30° of atlas rotation on the dens, the body of the axis begins to rotate, followed by progressively diminishing rotation in the remaining cervical segments. Because the atlanto-occipital and atlantoaxial apophyseal articulations are not horizontal, rotation must be accompanied by a degree of coupled tilting.

Active Rotation. Regional active rotary motion is tested by having the patient move his nose as far as possible to the left and right without moving his shoulders. Note the snoothness of motion and degree of limitation bilaterally.

Passive Rotation. Passive rotation is examined by placing the hands on the patient's skull and turning the head first to one side and then to the other so that the chin is in line with the shoulder.

If a complete fixation occurs between C1 and C2, the remaining cervical segments tend to become more mobile in compensation. Thus, gross inspection of neck rotation (or other motions) should never be used to evaluate the function of individual segments.

Lateral Flexion[139–141]

Cervical lateral flexion is essentially performed by the unilateral contraction of the neck flexors and extensors with motion occurring in the coronal plane. Such flexion is accompanied by rotational torsion below C2, distributed fairly equally in the normal cervical joints. This is, when the cervical spine as a whole bends laterally, it also tends to rotate anteriorly on the side of the concavity so that the vertebral bodies arc further laterally than the spinous processes.

Range. Normally, about a 45° tilt can be observed between the skull and the shoulder. About 5° of this occurs at the atlanto-occipital joint (Fig. 8.24), following

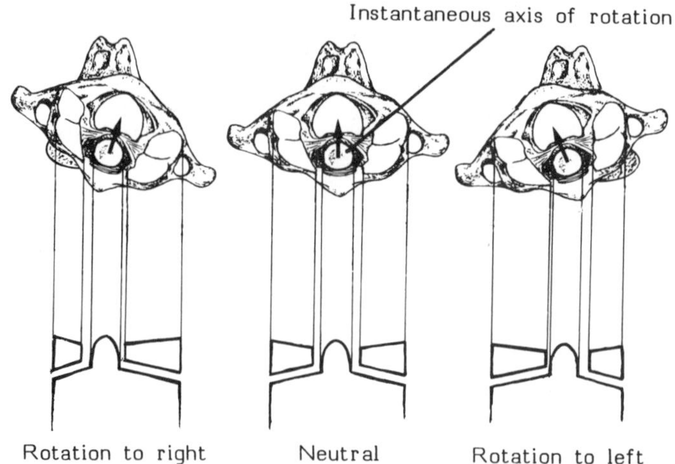

Figure 8.23. Rotation of the atlas (*top*) and its representation on an A-P film (*bottom*).

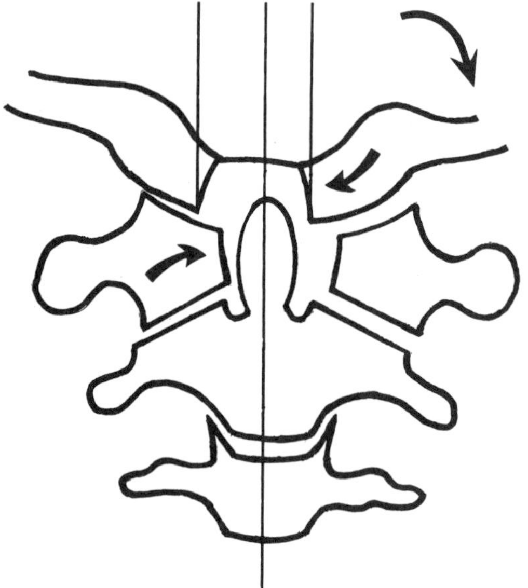

Figure 8.24. Atlanto-occipital and atlantoaxial lateral flexion. During lateral bending, only 5° of motion are exhibited at the atlanto-occipital and 6° at the atlantoaxial articulations. However, the occiput slips toward the convexity and the atlas slips toward the concavity. This creates shear forces at the superior articulations of the atlas and distortion of the odontoid space.

the arc of the condyles on the superior facets of the atlas; and 6° occurs at the atlantoaxial joint, following the arc of the inferior facets of the atlas on the superior facets of the axis. As the occiput and atlas shift laterally as one unit toward the concavity during lateral bending, the space between the dens and lateral mass of the atlas widens on the concave side. At the same time, the occipital condyles translate slightly laterally on the superior facets of the atlas toward the convexity and the atlas slips slightly toward the side of concavity. These movements are quite slight unless there is a degree of instability involved. If the atlanto-occipital capsular ligaments are weakened, the condyle on the side of lateral bending may strike the tip of the odontoid. The body of the axis tends to rotate toward the concavity while its spinous process shifts toward the convexity because of the coupling mechanism.

Active Lateral Flexion. Regional active side bending is tested by having the patient attempt to touch each ear on the respective shoulder without moving the shoulders.

Passive Lateral Flexion. Passive side bending is tested by placing the hands on the patient's skull and bending the head sideward toward the patient's fixed shoulder on each side.

Occipitoatlantal Movement[142, 143]

The oblique cup-and-saucer atlanto-occipital joints are designed essentially for a limited range of A-P nodding movement. Translatory movements are slight; most action is a rolling movement. The long axes of the joints are obliquely set, but a slight curve in the coronal plane allows a few degrees of lateral tilt.

Flexion/Extension. The prime mover of atlanto-occipital flexion is the rectus capitis anterior, aided by the longus capitis. The range is limited essentially by the elasticity of the posterior ligaments and by the tip of the dens meeting the bursa below the anterior rim of the foramen magnum. Extension is powered by the rectus capitis posterior group. Extension and lateral tilt of the upper cervical region is restricted by tension of the tectorial membrane and the posterior arch of the atlas becoming trapped between the occiput and the axis.

Lateral Flexion. Lateral bending is produced by the rectus capitis lateralis, with assistance by the semispinalis, splenius capitis, sternomastoideus, and trapezius. The range is limited essentially by the alar ligaments. In mild coronal lateral flexion and transverse rotation of the head and neck, the occiput and atlas move as a unit because of the planes of the articular facets. Close observation will show that the occiput specifically abducts from the atlas without rotation about a vertical axis. Thus, the atlas is caught between trying to follow the motion of the occiput or of the axis. This stress, according to Gillet, forces a slight amount of rotation of the occiput on the atlas even though the design of the condyles is not conducive to such rotation.[144]

Atlantoaxial Movement[145,146]

The loose articular capsules of the C1–C2 joint probably allow the greatest degree of inherent instability present in the cervical spine.

Flexion/Extension. In addition to the rolling motion of the atlas on the occiput, the atlas is capable of some tilting in which the anterior ring of the atlas moves upward on the odontoid and the posterior arch rides downward, or vice versa (Fig. 8.25). During severe flexion, there could be considerable separation of the anterior arch of the atlas from the odontoid, but it is checked by the weak transverse arms of the cruciate and by tension of the stronger tectorial membrane. Extension is more readily resisted when the anterior arch meets the odontoid and the interarticular tissues compress.

Rotation. During normal movement, the occiput and atlas move as one about the odontoid process of the axis. Keep in mind that the odontoid of the axis is usually quite firmly attached to the occiput by the ligament complex. These ligaments (especially the alar ligaments, transverse cruciate, and

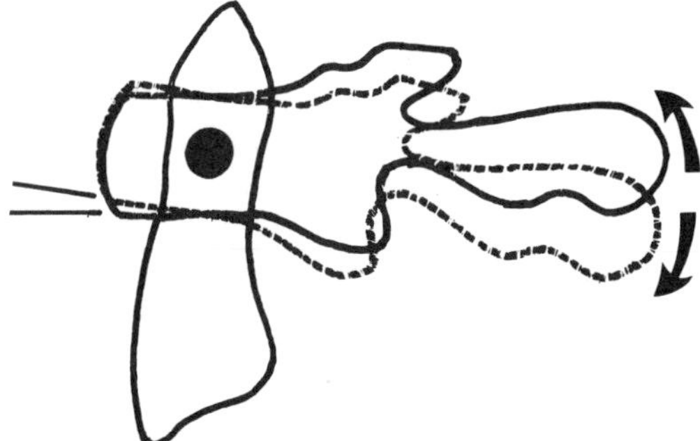

Figure 8.25. During atlantoaxial flexion and extension, the atlas slides up and down on the odontoid in relation to the instantaneous axis of rotation (*black dot*). The longer lever arm behind produces more noticeable motion posteriorly than anteriorly.

the apophyseal capsules of the axis) tend to restrict axial rotation to 45°, compared to a 90° range by the atlas. Although the inferior facets of the atlas and the superior facets of the axis may be concave, their articular cartilages offer a biconvex design. Atlantoaxial rotation is powered by the obliquus capitis and rectus capitis posterior major, with assistance offered by the ipsilateral splenius capitis and the contralateral sternocleidomastoid. During maximum atlantoaxial rotation in a supple spine, there is considerable kinking or stretching of the contralateral vertebral artery.

Lateral Flexion. When lateral flexion is fairly restricted to the upper cervical area, the articulating facet spaces open on the side of convexity and compress on the side of concavity. However, when lateral flexion is fairly generalized throughout the cervical region, the lateral masses of the atlas sideslip toward the side of concavity so that the space between the lateral mass and the odontoid increases on the side of the concavity. Naturally, this is limited by the size of the bony crescent about the dens, unless the cruciate is torn.

Upper Cervical Trauma[147–155]

Any severe movement of the cervical spine may result in unconsciousness and possible death. The result of severe movement may be fracture or dislocation that injures the spinal cord, often fatally if it occurs within the upper cervical area. Even mild spinal cord trauma may result in sensory and motor paralysis. Neck hyperextension injuries may cause compression injury to the vertebral arteries, causing a temporary oxygen loss to the brain that may result in unconsciousness, if not greater damage through rupture. The nerve function of the cervical plexus is shown in Table 8.4.

Disturbances in this area usually arise from muscular spasm of one or more of the six muscle bundles that have attachments on the occiput, atlas, or axis. Unequal tension and ultimate fibrotic changes within the paravertebral structures can readily influence the delicate nerve fibers and vascular flow. The vertebral artery is frequently involved by compression of the overlying muscles in the suboccipital triangle. In fact, West points out that the vertebral artery has been completely occluded by turning the head backward and to the opposite side during postmortem studies.[156] Even without a degree of arteriosclerosis, the vertebral artery can be considered a quite firm tube in the adult that responds poorly to twisting and pressure.

Background[157–160]

Neurologic disturbances may result from muscular and fibrotic changes along the cranial nerve pathways which exit from the skull and pass intimately between and under suboccipital fasciculi. Five of the cranial nerves are thus vulnerable: the facial, glossopharyngeal, vagus, spinal accessory, and hypoglossal. In addition, circulatory impairment of major and minor nerves of the neck may alter the function of those cranial nerves that do not exit from the skull proper, such as the olfactory, optic, oculomotor, trochlear, trigeminal, abducens, and auditory, but which are contained within the cranium and remote from vertebral subluxation encroachment effects.[161] We should not overlook the fact that it is essentially muscle that produces and maintains the subluxation. Attention must be paid to the reasons why the subluxation has been produced and is maintained.[162]

A careful study of most clinical subluxations will reveal that they are infrequently "unusual" positions. Commonly, they are *normal positions in a state of fixation*. In the neutral position, for example, an inferior atlas subluxation-fixation exhibits the posterior arch of the atlas approximating the spinous process of the axis-the *normal* position of the atlas during extension. The same is true of superior, posterior, and lateral listings: all are normal positions if found in flexion, rotation, or lateral bending, but abnormal if found in other positions.[163–165]

In a discussion of spinal motion of any region or segment complex, it should be constantly kept in mind that minor pathologic changes and individual variances from the "norm" considerably alter the biodynamics involved. Neither static position on roentgenography nor dynamic palpation alone can be used as the basis to determine the need for or the results of adjustive therapy. Static palpation is often grossly in error because of the many anomalies in asymmetry found in the typical spine. The whole clinical picture must be utilized.

Common Occipital Subluxations[166–172]

Inasmuch as all freely moveable articulations are subject to subluxation, the atlanto-

Table 8.4.
Nerve Function of the Cervical Plexus (C1–C4)

Nerve	Function
Lesser occipital	Sensory to skin behind ear and mastoid process
Greater auricular	Sensory to skin over parotid, jaw angle, ear lobe, and front of mastoid process
Cervical cutaneous	Sensory to skin over anterolateral portion of neck
Supraclaviculars	Sensory to skin over medial infraclavicular area, pectoralis major and deltoid
Muscular branches	Motor to capitus anterior and lateralis, longus capitus, longus colli, hyoid muscles, sternocleidomastoideus, trapezius, levator scapulae, scalenus medius
Phrenic	Sensory to costal and mediastinal pleura and pericardium; motor to diaphragm

occipital diarthrosis is no exception. The stress at this point is unusual when one considers that the total weight of the cranium is supported by the ring of the atlas, about one-twentieth the circumference of the skull, and a variety of spinal muscles, subject to spasm and hypertonicity, have their attachments on the occiput.

Being near the end of a kinematic chain, the atlanto-occipital joints are subject to numerous degrees of subluxation in flexion, extension, rotation, and laterality. Rotary subluxation is not uncommon, especially if the atlantal cups are shallow. Excessive rotation is allowed by the lax check ligaments and capsules. Head weight, the angle of force, the planes of articulation, and the integrity of the para-articular tissues determine the stability present.

Right/Left Condyle Inferior or Superior. A unilateral suboccipital muscle spasm causes the affected condyle to be pulled deep into the articulating concavity of the atlantal lateral mass on one side (sunken condyle). This may not be attended by a degree of rotation. Inspection from the back shows a low, medially inclined mastoid process on the side of involvement (Fig. 8.26). Palpation discloses the mastoid riding close to the transverse process of the atlas, tension and tenderness in the groove between the mastoid and the lower jaw, and fullness in the groove between the occiput and the posterior ring of the atlas on the side of involvement. A right or left condyle superior may be considered the converse aspect of a right or left condyle inferior. That is, as one condyle is pulled inferiorly and anteriorly, the other condyle presents a superior and posterior picture, or vice versa. There are certain situations, however, that indicate a unilateral abnormality without converse adaptation. This latter condition usually follows a blow to the vertex downward when the head is somewhat laterally flexed and the condyle on the side of the concavity is jammed into the lateral mass of the atlas (eg, spearing tackle).

Right/Left Condyle Inferior with Associated Anterior Rotation. All atlanto-occipital movements tend to be associated with a degree of rotation because the occipital condyles and the articulating surfaces of the lateral masses of the atlas approximate each other more at the anterior than the posterior. Thus, most sunken condyles will be associated with a relative amount of rotation. On the side of involvement, inspection from the back reveals a medial head tilt. Palpation reveals approximation of the mastoid and transverse process of the atlas and approximation of the inferior nuchal ridge and the posterior arch of the atlas on the involved side. These points are widened on the opposite side. A right or left superior condyle with associated posterior rotation is often considered the contralateral aspect of a right or left inferior condyle attended by an anterior rotation. Illi feels it is always attended by a degree of arthritis and determines the primary subluxation roentgenographically by the side showing the greatest degree of degenerative articular alteration.

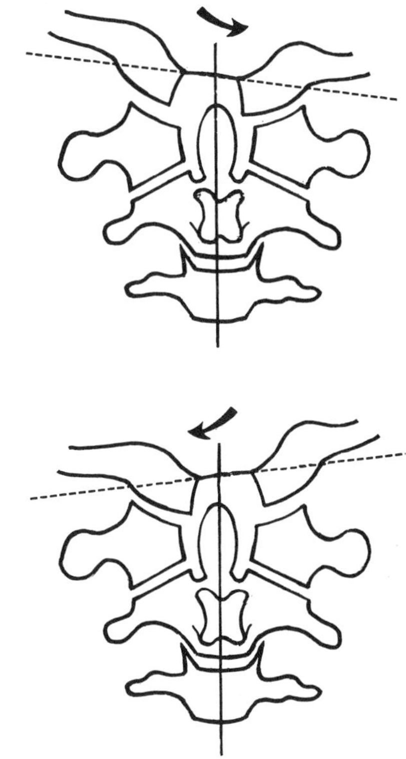

Figure 8.26. *Top*, right condyle inferior subluxation; *bottom*, left condyle inferior subluxation.

Right/Left Condyle Inferior with Associated Posterior Rotation. This type of subluxation or its contralateral representation is less common than that associated with anterior rotation. It usually results from vigorous twisting trauma such as an athletic contact activities. On the side of involvement: (1) inspection from the back shows the head held in a stiff inferior position with some posterior deviation; and (2) palpation discloses a mastoid that is inferior and posterior in relation to the transverse process of the atlas, and the inferior nuchal ridge approximating the posterior arch of the atlas.

Suboccipital Jamming. This common subluxation, usually of a trigeminal (ophthalmic division) reflex nature, is often seen in people under severe visual or mental stress. Irritative impulses cause contraction of suboccipital muscles that pull the occiput upon the posterior arch of the atlas, creating a painful bilateral condylar jamming (Fig. 8.27). A compressive vertex blow is a rare cause. Palpation reveals suboccipital spasm, tenderness, nodular swellings, and a closing of the inferior nuchal ridge on the posterior arch of the atlas. Although the condition is usually bilateral, one side may be affected more than the other.

Common Atlas Subluxations[173–179]

Right or Left Lateral Atlas. An atlantal sideslip between the atlas and axis articulations is usually attended by a degree of superiority and anteriority on the side of laterality because of the inclination of the articulating surfaces. Only in cases of severe twisting trauma will this not be the case. Ipsilaterally, palpation will reveal the transverse process of the atlas to be more lateral and slightly superior and anterior than its counterpart.

Bilateral Superior or Inferior Atlas. In this type of subluxation, the atlas tilts up or down bilaterally in its transverse plane without an attending sideslip. Deep palpation may reveal the posterior arch of the atlas either approximating the occiput with a gap between the posterior tubercle of the atlas and the spinous process of the axis or approximating the spinous process of the axis with a gap between the atlas's posterior tubercle and the occiput (Fig. 8.28).

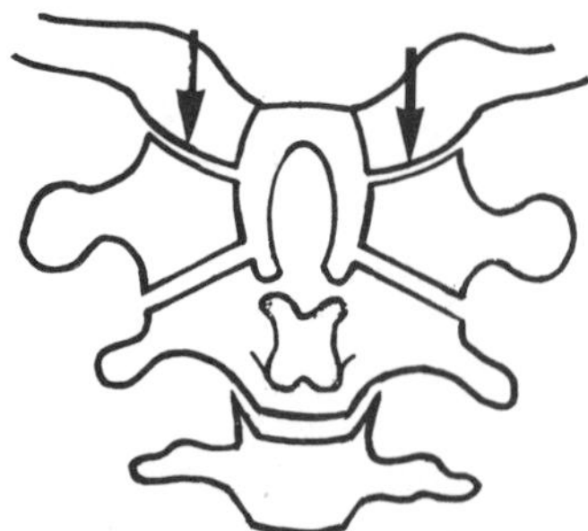

Figure 8.27. Suboccipital jamming.

Right or Left Fixed Anterior Rotation of the Atlas. These subluxations are often associated with vagal syndromes because the anteriorly rotated transverse of the atlas may easily cause pressure on the vagus nerve. In such a rotary state, the counterpart of an atlas listed right anteriorly would be left posterior. On the side of involvement, inspection from the back reveals suboccipital fullness. Bilateral palpation of the posterior ring of the atlas reveals a prominence on the side of posteriority, with the transverse process of the atlas being closer to the mastoid and its counterpart closer to the mandible.

A clinical test, suggested by Goodheart, is

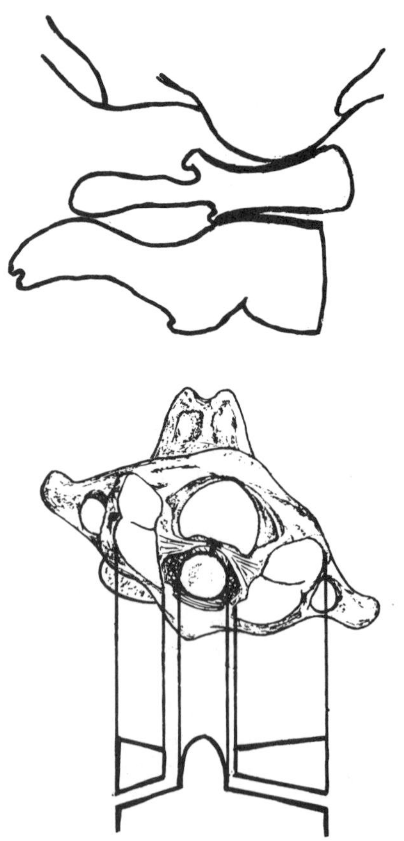

Figure 8.28. *Top*, lateral view of bilateral inferior atlas; *bottom*, left fixed anterior rotation of the atlas.

to have the patient lying supine, then to passively rotate the head right and left. If an anterior atlas subluxation exists on the left, the atlas has already turned to the right so that the patient's head will turn much further to the right. But when it is turned from right to left, the atlas cannot come out of its fixed anterior position on the left, thus motion is relatively restricted. This test is a valid indication only in the absence of muscular spasm or some other type of motion barrier restricting rotation (eg, lower cervical unilateral fixation).

Common Axis Subluxations[180–184]

With the possible exception of L5, no other vertebra is subluxated more frequently than the transitional C2. The C2–C3 apophyseal joints are the most mobile and least stable of any in the vertebral column with the exception of the C1–C2 joints. The most common symptom is a unilateral suboccipital neuralgia on the side of rotational posteriority. On this side, palpation discloses a tender prominence over the articulating process and a deviation of the spinous process away from the midline (Fig. 8.29). Posterior axial subluxations are sometimes misdiagnosed as anterior atlantal subluxations.

Rotary subluxations of the axis are common structural causes of cervical migraine. This cervical neuralgia is invariably unilateral, beginning in the upper neck and extending over the skull into the temporal and possibly the orbital areas. The greater occipital nerve (C2) is affected (Fig. 8.30).

Rotary subluxations of one or more of the upper three vertebrae (particularly the axis) may cause pressure upon the superior cervical ganglion. The autonomic syndrome produced may incorporate excessive facial and forehead perspiration, dry mouth and nasal mucous membranes, dryness and tightness of the throat, dilated pupils, tending toward exophthalmos, pseudomigrainous attacks due to unilateral angioneurotic edema, facial vasomotor disturbances with possible angioneurotic swelling, and moderate tachycardia with functional arrythmias.

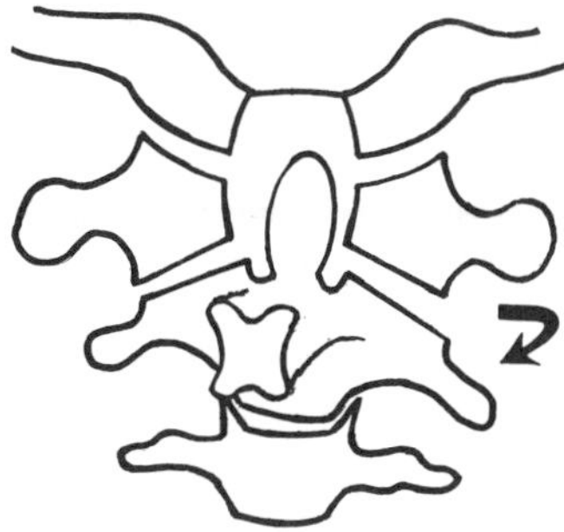

Figure 8.29. Rotary subluxation of the axis, right transverse posterior. The axis slips posteroinferiorly on the right and anterosuperiorly on the left, in accordance with the planes of articulation.

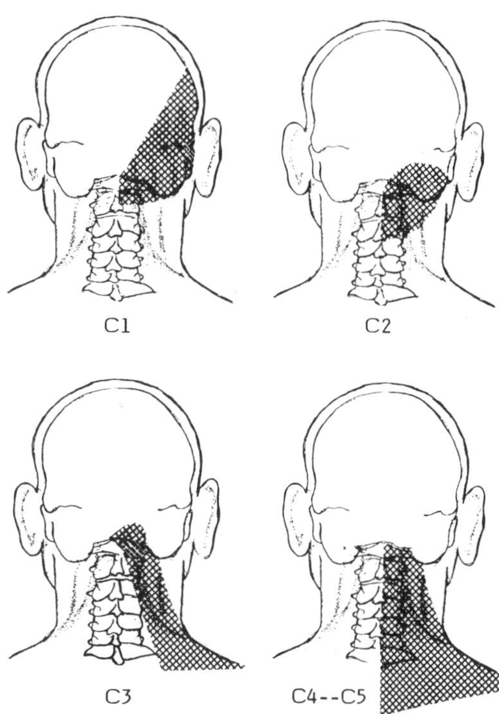

Figure 8.30. Areas of referred pain from C1–C5 nerve root irritation.

The Occipito-Atlanto-Axial Complex

The occipital condyles, atlas, and axis function as a unit with unique characteristics. The normally ball-and-socket-type articulations at the occipitoatlantal joint allow flexion, extension, and slight rotation and lateral flexion. The facets of the atlas and axis are both convex, which allows considerable rotation and minimal lateral flexion, and their loose capsules and ligamentous straps allow significant flexion and extension. The axis, however, has more ligamentous attachments with the skull than does the atlas.[110] Many of these attachments bypass the atlas, as does the spinal dura. The muscles that attach to the axis extend widely—to the skull and atlas above, and to all the lower cervicals, the upper five thoracics, the first rib, and the scapulae below.

During any type of lumbopelvic distortion in which the sacral base has assumed an unnatural position, cervical compensation normally occurs to maintain the eyes horizontally forward and near the midline. However, because the occipito-atlanto-axial complex allows only slight lateral bending, scoliotic compensation must occur *below* the axis. If this does not occur in habitually maintaining the axis on the horizontal plane, stress on the dural membranous structures above will be produced. Thus, it can be appreciated that any problem from above or below that interferes with the role of the axis will produce widespread problems because of the extensive myofascial relationships. For this reason, Dove recommends that the function of the axis be checked in each and every case for which problems manifest in the head, cervical area, upper thoracic area, and shoulder girdle.

Condyle Fracture, Dislocation, and Instability

Fractures of an occipital condyle are extremely rare, but they do occur and the possibility must always be eliminated in cases of trauma to the head and neck.[185] Because cord damage can be assumed, traumatic occipitoatlantal dislocation is generally considered incompatible with life. A few cases have survived after such trauma, with unexpectedly minimal neurologic deficits.[186] The characteristic film signs are an abnormal basion-odontoid alignment, posterior displacement of the atlas, and marked retropharyngeal soft-tissue swelling.

Although occipitoatlantal instability is rarely seen, Finney and Roberts describe a case that was diagnosed from flexion and extension stress views.[187] The patient reported neck pain and transient episodes of visual-field impairment followed by unconsciousness when he hyperextended his neck. These symptoms disappeared after surgical fusion of the occipito-atlanto-axial complex. This example draws attention to the possible relationship of the occipitoatlantal level to visual symptoms and transient ischemic attacks.

Fractures and Dislocations of the Atlas[188–195]

Atlanto-occipital dislocations, often bilateral, are usually quickly incompatible with life. Any severe orthopedic subluxation in the upper cervical area can lead to quadriplegia or death, often with little warning and few symptoms to differentiate it initially from a mild strain. Thus, it is always better to be extra cautious (and to be accused of being overly concerned in mild injuries) to insure against a possible disaster.[196] Signs and symptoms vary from subtle to severe pain and gross motor involvement. Tenderness may be acute over the posterior atlas, aggravated by mild rotation and extension. Invariably, the C2 nerve roots, which exit below the atlas, will be involved. Loss of occipital sensation to a pin prick should verify this.[197]

These severe disorders are presented here for two reasons. First, an acute patient may enter the office after suffering an accident. Second, an untreated fracture and spontaneously reduced dislocation may have healed without adequate professional care and reflect symptoms many months or years later.

Classes. The atlas may be fractured at its posterior arch, ring, or anterior arch. There are six common types of severe injury, all of which are serious. Keep in mind that nontraumatic dislocations of the upper cervical complex are more common than traumatic dislocations (eg, congenital anomalies, arthritis, infection), and their possibility should never be overlooked.

1. *Atlanto-occipital dislocation.* This usually, but not always, anterior displacement of the occiput on the atlas results from a severe horizontal force from behind that shears the skull across the atlas, rupturing the articular capsules and damaging the medulla. This rare occurrence can often be accurately evaluated by computing Powers ratio on a lateral roentgenograph (Fig. 8.31).

In 33 cases of traumatic atlantoaxial trauma, Maiman and Cusick[198] found seven examples of dislocation without an associ-

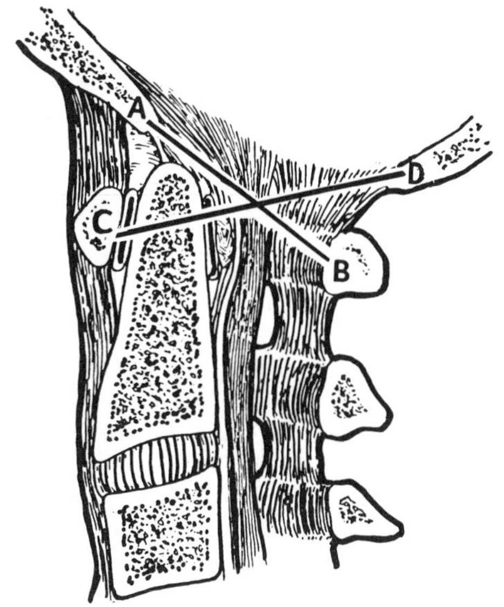

Figure 8.31. Powers ratio in determining possible anterior atlanto-occipital dislocation. If the ratio between line *AB* and *CD* is greater than 1, an anterior dislocation exists. This is true even if a fracture or an atlantoaxial dislocation coexists. Point *A* is at the midline anterior margin of the foramen magnum, found where the inner and outer basiocciput tables meet. Point *B* is at the midpoint of the arch-canal line of the atlas, where the posterior arch of the atlas joins the posterior tubercle. Point *C* is at the midpoint of the posterior surface of the anterior arch of the atlas. Point *D* is at the midline posterior margin of the foramen magnum, found on a lateral roentgenograph by following the inner table of the occiput down and forward.

ated fracture of the odontoid process. While some of the cases (five) had a history of cranial trauma, others only reported a wide variety of subjective complaints (eg, cervical pain, headache) and varying neurologic deficits. This emphasizes the need for detailed roentgenographic analysis in all cases presenting with cervical signs and/or symptoms.

2. *Atlas dislocation with fractured dens.* The atlas may displace anteriorly on the asis or the occiput may displace posteriorly on the atlas and fracture the odontoid process if the ligaments hold. The force may be hyperextensive or hyperflexive. The patient may survive if extreme care is taken in transportation to the hospital. If the transverse ligament is avulsed from the atlas, a small fragment of bone may lie between the odontoid and the cord. If the odontoid is displaced posteriorly, the situation is usually fatal because of injury to the cord. Post-traumatic spontaneous fusion of C1 to the occiput is always a potential complication if the patient survives.

3. *Fractured posterior arch of the atlas.* This usually occurs from a severe vertical compression force during extension in which the lateral masses are fixed between the condyles and the pillars of the axis, and the posterior ring fractures and displaces outward. A base fracture of the odontoid is often associated. If a fracture line is not evident on lateral roentgenography (differentiated from congenital clefts), headache, suboccipital pain, stiffness, acute suboccipital jamming, and subtle signs of basilar insufficiency from compression of the vertebral artery should still stimulate suspicions.

Of all atlantoid fractures, according to most literature, those of the posterior arch are the most common yet easily overlooked because the displacement is usually mild. The common site is at the narrowest portion just posterior to each lateral mass, usually at the groove for the vertebral artery. Retropharyngeal swelling is usually absent, and oblique views are often necessary for demonstration.

4. *Jefferson fracture.* A more severe vertical compression blow may split the atlas and burst the lateral masses outward, disrupting both the anterior and posterior rings into several fragments[199] (Fig. 8.32). Ring fractures are frequently produced by blows on top of the head in which vertical forces are dispersed laterally. Keep in mind that if a severe axial force is produced through the skull downward, the inclined condyles of the occiput serve as a mechanical wedge upon the atlas. This is usually evident in an open-mouth x-ray view. Overhang of the atlantal lateral masses and widening of the paraodontoid space will be associated. Severity depends upon fragment displacement relative to the cord and other vital tissues. That is, if the ligaments do not retain these fragments, death from cord damage will be likely.

Another point to consider is that the cervical spine has a natural lordosis which normally dissipates axial forces. However,

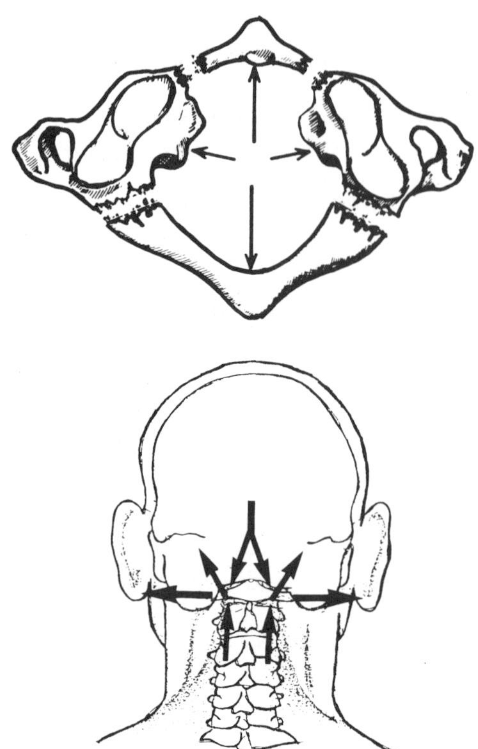

Figure 8.32. Jefferson fracture of the atlas. *Top*, separation of the ring of the atlas at four common sites, viewed from above; *bottom*, direction of forces, viewed from the posterior.

as the neck moves from the extended to the flexed position, a position is reached where the vertebrae are fairly aligned vertically. A rapid compression overload in this position is most likely to result in an exploding-type fracture.

Most authorities state that fractures of the anterior arch are rare, minimally displaced, usually comminuted, and frequently require tomography to be detected. However, Iversen and Clawson[200] feel that fractures to the anterior arch are quite common and found either in the midline or just lateral to the midline.

A few cases have been reported in which compressive forces have caused the atlas to spread without fracture.[201] While compression fracture of the atlas without fracture is not common, this possibility should not be overlooked during roentgenographic analyses.

5. *Atlas-axis displacement.* In C1–C2 A-P dislocations, C1 most often displaces anteriorly relative to C2. If a force comes from the back, undoubtedly the muscle will be unprepared and the force will meet minimum resistance. Yet anterior dislocation is rare, and posterior displacement is even more infrequently seen. Forward dislocation widens the predental space and alters a roentgenographic line connecting the cortices of the anterior parts of the spinous processes from C1 to C7, unless the process of C2 is fused or congenitally short. If this is suspected, careful flexion-extension views or a C1–C2 tomogram are recommended. The mechanism of injury is usually hyperflexion or hyperextension; and even in moderate cases, signs of trauma to the occipital nerve should be evident. In rare instances where there are sufficient traction forces to rupture the anterior longitudinal ligament, the anterior ring of the atlas may be lifted up and over the dens so that an intact odontoid is seen anterior to the anterior ring.

6. *Orthopedic rotary subluxation of the atlas on the axis.* Forced rotation of the upper neck may produce a locked rotary displacement of a lateral mass of the atlas on the subjacent superior facet of the axis. This requires atlantal rotation in excess of 45° on the axis. A neurologic deficit is not commonly involved. The patient will appear with this head rotated to one side and cocked away from the side of rotation ("cock robin" position). Care must be taken to differentiate this sign which is also so common in acute torticollis.

Fractures and Dislocations of the Axis[202–208]

Odontoid fractures are often produced by severe forces directed to the head, and the direction of force usually determines the direction of displacement. Suboccipital tenderness may be present. A severe extension force may fracture the odontoid at its base, with possible odontoid posterior displacement. The danger of cord pressure is great.

Open-mouth and careful flexion-extension standard roentgenographic views or tomography may be necessary for accurate determination. The atlantal-dens interval should not exceed 2–3 mm in adults even during cervical flexion. The interval is slightly more (eg, as much as 4–5 mm during flexion) in children under the age of 8 years.

Types. The classic order of Anderson and D'Alonzo[209] is applicable:

Type I: Avulsion of the upper part of the odontoid. This is rare.

Type II: Fracture through the base of the odontoid at or below the level of the superior articular facets of the axis. This is the most common type of axial fracture, and the cruciate ligaments may remain intact. Occasionally the odontoid will not be displaced but be slightly tipped as a result of a toggle effect shown on flexion-extension films. This type of fracture is usually quite unstable and leads to nonunion.

Besides being the most common type of fracture in the upper cervical area, fractures at the base of the odontoid process are also the most liable to nonunion in the adult.[210] It should also be noted that odontoid fractures are not uncommon in children.[211] If they are discovered early and promptly treated by an orthopedic surgeon (often by noninvasive procedures), the outcome is usually favorable.

Care must be taken not to confuse odontoid nonunion with os odontoideum. In os odontoideum, the process is about 50% smaller than normal, round, and separated from the hypoplastic odontoid by a wide gap. The remnant hypoplastic odontoid appears as a hill forming upward from the slope of the superior articular facets. The fracture line in nonunion is narrow and at or below the level of the superior articular facets, and the process is normal in size and shape.[212-214]

Instability of an os odontoideum may readily damage the upper cervical cord and exhibit a variety of signs and symptoms. The common manifestations include post-traumatic neck pain, gradually appearing signs of medullary compression, atlantoaxial instability, interlaminar fusion between C1 and C2, or possibly, no overt signs at all.[215]

Type III: Fracture of the body of the axis. Displacement may not occur. A small bone chip separated from the anteroinferior rim of the axis at the point of rupture of the anterior longitudinal ligament (Fig. 8.33) may be a clue to hyperextension—associated with retropharyngeal soft-tissue swelling and/or dislocation of the prevertebral fat strip. About 36% of axial fractures occur

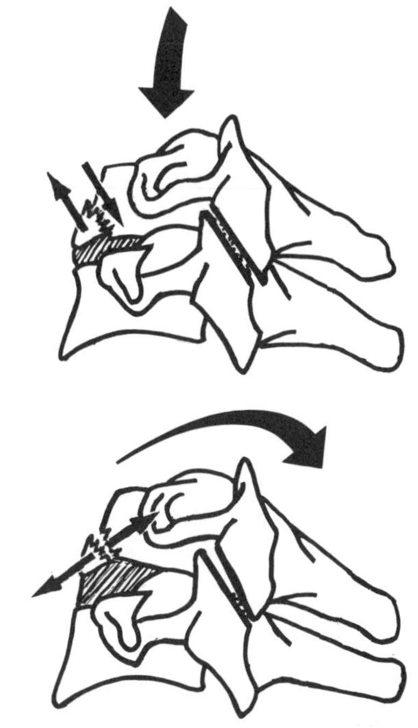

Figure 8.33. *Top*, anteroinferior bone chip as the result of compressive shear forces associated with axial overload; articular facets are jammed. *Bottom*, fragment at same site from extension tension stress; facets are jammed at the posterior.

through the cancellous bone of the body of the axis, are stable, and heal without difficulty. Endplate fracture and displacement are invariably associated.

Hangman's Fracture.[216-218] This traumatic spondylolisthetic injury by distraction and extension causes fracture of the C2 when the chin is fixed and the forehead is struck. The classic damage is a bilateral fracture through the lateral posterior arch and into the intervertebral notch.[219] The posterior elements of the axis dislocate in relation to C3, while the anterior elements dislocate in relation to the atlas and skull. Survival is not common, but when it occurs without overt spinal cord involvement, only minor complaints such as local pain, stiffness, and tenderness over the spinous process may be expressed.

Vertical Dislocation. This is usually a secondary effect of a pathologic process in which the odontoid enters the foramen magnum (eg, rheumatoid arthritis, spinal tuberculosis, osteogenesis imperfecta, or Paget's disease). The severity of neurologic involvement varies considerably from case to case regardless of roentgenographic findings.

CLINICAL BIOMECHANICS OF THE LOWER CERVICAL SPINE

Regional Structural Characteristics[220-223]

Nature has made many structural adaptations in the cervical region because of the small structures, the required range of motion, and the enlarged cord in this region in comparison to other spinal regions (Fig. 8.34). The laminae are slender and overlap, and this shingling increases with age. The osseous elevations on the posterolateral aspect that form the uncovertebral pseudojoints tend to protect the spinal canal from lateral IVD herniation, but hypertrophy of these joints added to IVD degeneration can readily lead to IVF encroachment.

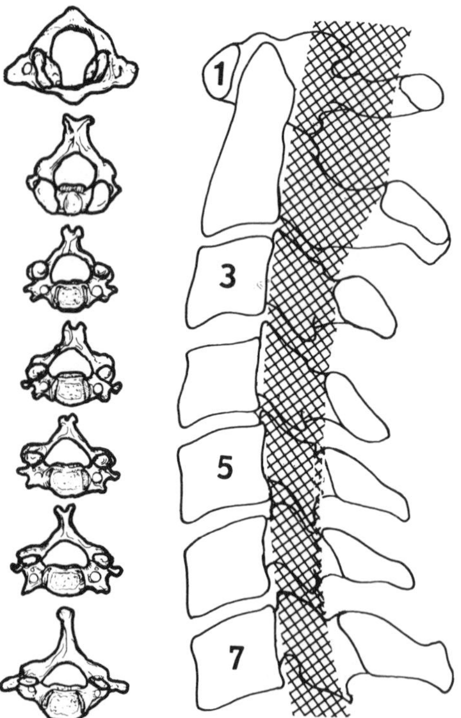

Figure 8.34. *Left*, comparison of cervical vertebrae as viewed from above. Note differences in design of the spinal canal, width of transverse processes, and length of spinous processes. *Right*, sagittal view of the cervical region showing space for the spinal cord within the cervical spine. Dimensions (A-P) are approximately 22 mm at the atlas, 20 mm at the axis, and 12 mm at C4–C7.

The IVDs are broader anteriorly than posteriorly to accommodate the cervical lordosis. Authorities differ as to the typical location of the nucleus pulposus in the cervical region. Kapandji places it centrally. Cailliet places it slightly posterior (further anterior than a lumbar nucleus), and Jeffreys says its is distinctly posterior from the midline.

The Intervertebral Foramen

The boundaries of the cervical IVFs are designed for motion rather than stability, in contrast to the dorsal and lumbar regions (Fig. 8.35). The greatest degree of functional IVF diameter narrowing occurs ipsilaterally in lateral bending with simultaneous extension.

The Facet Joints[224]

The ovoid and tear-drop-shaped articular processes incline medially in the coronal

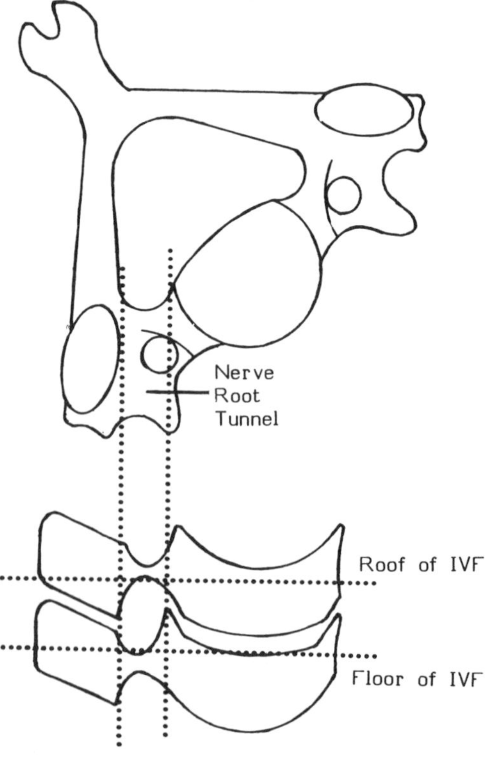

Figure 8.35. Schematic of the structural relationships of the intervertebral tunnel. *Top*, from above; *bottom*, sagittal section.

plane and obliquely in the sagittal plane so that they are at about a 45° angle to the vertical. Their bilateral articular surface area, which shares a good part of head weight with the vertebral body, is about 67% of that of the vertebral body.

The short, thick, dense *capsular ligaments* bind the articulating processes together, enclosing the articular cartilage and synovial tissue. Their fibers are firmly bound to the periosteum of the superior and inferior processes and are arranged at a 90° angle to the plane of the facet. This allows maximum laxity when the facets are in a position of rest. They normally allow no more than a few millimeters of movement from the neutral position per segment, and possibly provide more cervical stability than any other ligament. Capsulitis from overstretch in acute subluxation is common. The posterior joint capsules enjoy an abundance of nociceptors and mechanoreceptors, far more than any other area of the spine.

Within the capsule, small tongues of meniscus-like tissue flaps project from the articular surfaces into the synovial space. They are infrequently "nipped" in severe jarring at an unguarded moment during the end of extension, rotation, or lateral bending, establishing a site of apophyseal bursitis (Fig. 8.36).

The Uncovertebral Articulations

The joints (or fissures) of Luschka are located on the anterolateral surfaces of the vertebral body and act as tracts that guide the motion of coupled rotation and lateral flexion and limit sidebending. These saddle-like joints begin development between the ages of 6 and 9 years and are complete at 18 years.[225] Whether or not they are true synovial joints is highly controversial.[226] Gehweiler feels that they represent functional adaptation by the cervical IVDs to the increased mobility of the cervical vertebrae at the time that the uncinate processes are reaching their full height.

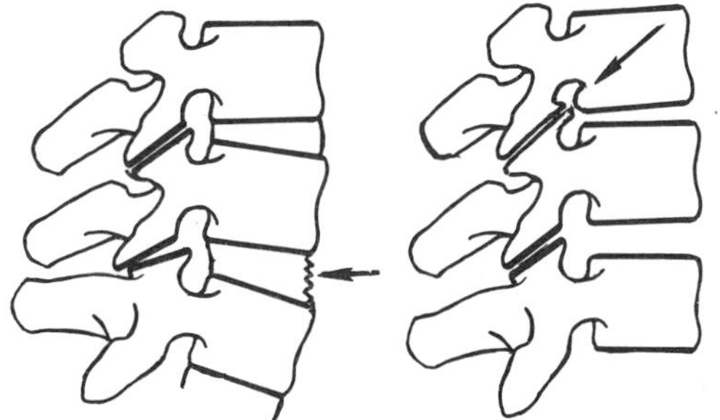

Figure 8.36. *Left*, extension subluxation encouraging impingement of the intervertebral foramen as the result of lax anterior fibers of the anulus. *Right*, x-ray film tracing showing osteophytic encroachment of the intervertebral foramen in the superior vertebra, compared to a normal foramen in the inferior segment.

The Lower Cervical Ligaments[227, 228]

The 5 lower, relatively similar, cervical vertebrae possess 8 intervertebral ligamentous tissues, 4 posterior and 4 anterior. The anterior ligaments are the anterior longitudinal ligament, the anulus fibrosus, the posterior longitudinal ligament, and the intertransverse ligament. The posterior ligaments are the ligamentum flavum, the capsular ligaments, and the interspinous and supraspinous ligaments.

The *anterior longitudinal ligament* rides close to the anterior vertebral bodies and blends with the anulus as it crosses the IVD space. It is quite thin, translucent, and thickest and widest over the anterior anulus. It tends to limit extension, as does the anulus.

The *posterior longitudinal ligament* is firmly attached to the IVD but separated from the vertebral bodies (except the lips) by the retrocorporeal nutrient vessels. By not following the concavity of the vertebral bodies, the posterior longitudinal ligament offers a smooth anterior wall for the spinal cord. However, thickening or ossification of this ligament can encroach upon the vertebral canal. It is much thicker than its anterior counterpart, but like its counterpart, it is widest as the disc level. It tends to limit flexion, as does the anulus.

The thin, fibrous, *intertransverse ligament* runs longitudinally between adjacent transverse processes, just anterior to the vertebral artery, joining the anteroinferior aspect of the transverse process above to the anterosuperior lip of the transverse process below. It serves to limit contralateral lateral bending and rotation.

The strong, thick, elastic *ligamentum flavum* connects the lamina of adjacent vertebrae, riding essentially within the vertebral canal. Its usually great elasticity prevents buckling that would impinge upon the contents of the spinal canal (Fig. 8.37).

The *interspinous ligament* and the *supraspinous ligament* are poorly developed in the upper cervical region. In the lower levels, the supraspinous ligament is continuous with the ligamentum nuchae posteriorly and continuous with the interspinalis ligaments anteriorly. The supraspinous ligaments overlap and obliquely cross the midline, attaching themselves to the cervical spinous processes. The interspinous and supraspinous ligaments tend to check flexion, rotation, and anterior displacement during flexion.

The inelastic *ligamentum nuchae* extends in the posterior midline from the vertebra prominens to the occiput, blending with the posterior edge of the interspinous ligament (Fig. 8.38). It is poorly developed in humans compared to most other mammals, yet it serves as a cervical strap that is a mechanism of defense against flexion injuries of the intrinsic muscles and structural displacement. When it degenerates (eg, old age), the head drops forward from the trunk and the cervical curve straightens.

Kinematics of the Lower Cervical Spine[229–234]

The IVDs contain an exceptional amount of elastin, which allows the IVDs to conform to the many possible planes of movement. Excessive flexion is limited by the ligamentous and muscular restraints on the separating posterior arches, and overextension is limited by bony apposition. Other factors include the resistance of the anular fibers to translation, the stiffness property of the anulus relative to its vertical height, and the physical barrier produced by the uncinate processes that are fully developed in late adolescence.

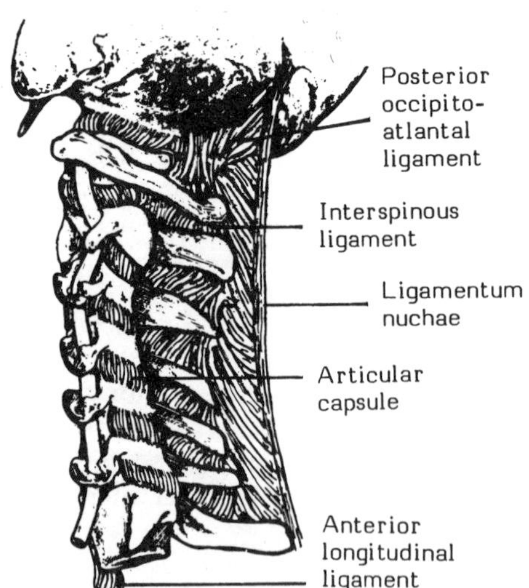

Figure 8.37. Posterolateral schematic of the ligaments of the cervical region.

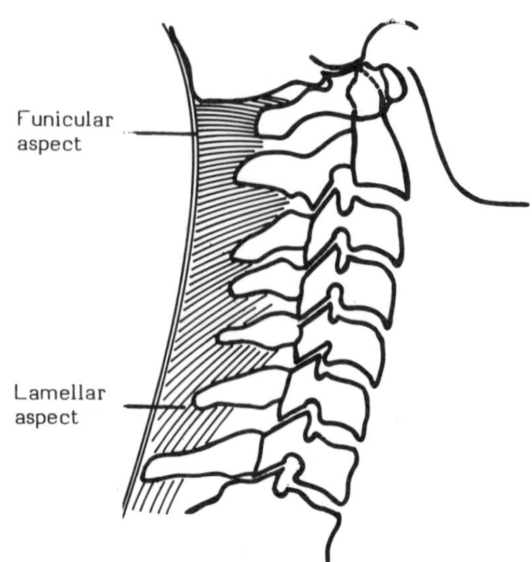

Figure 8.38. Nuchal ligament, as viewed laterally.

Biomechanical Lower Cervical Instability[235]

Traumatic cervical instability exists when the ligamentous straps are so severely disrupted that an attempt by the neck to actively support the head results in malalignment of one or more cervical motion units to the degree that nerve roots or the spinal cord become injured. In contact sports, such a Grade 3 sprain is typically caused by an axial compression force when the neck is in hyperflexion or hyperextension.

Subtle instability is rarely obvious in the ambulatory patient. The most important stabilizing agents in the middle and lower cervical spine are the anulus fibrosus, especially the anterior and posterior ligaments, and the muscles, which serve as important contributing stabilizers. Upon dynamic palpation, any segmental motion exceeding 3 mm should arouse suspicions of lack of ligament restraint.

Moderate Positional Instability. This

state is characterized by weakened support of the head, segmental hypermobility, a flattened cervical curve, sharp posterior pain on movement, mild neurologic deficits, potential subluxation or dislocation (if not immobilized), and, possibly, associated fracture (eg, clay shoveler's fracture, tear drop fracture).

Severe Positional Instability. This variety features complete loss of support of the head in certain positions, overt structural damage (ligamentous and/or skeletal), either anteriorly or posteriorly; severe neck pain and moderate to severe neurologic deficits; possible cord signs; and, possibly, associated facet dislocation or burst fracture.

The Weakened Link Syndrome. This is another clinical picture of potential catastrophy, in which previous injury or injuries have increased the vulnerability of the cervical spine to damage if further trauma is applied. Albright describes the situation as a neck that features mild compression fractures with angulation seen in flexion, inelastic posterior ligaments as the result of healed sprains, eroded and remolded facets that poorly restrict subluxation, and stiff IVDs that are thin and degenerated.[236] A silent hemangioma of a vertebral body may be present. The patient may be completely asymptomatic and sometimes roentgenographically negative, even under stress tests, until moderate trauma produces a dramatic collapse and probably death.

Segmental Angulation. Angulation of one vertebral segment (on a lateral roentgenograph) in excess of 11° greater than on adjacent vertebra that is not chronically compressed is also indicative of instability and pathologic displacement (Fig. 8.39). While conservative traction may reduce the associated displacement, it is doubtful that a normal resting position can be guaranteed without surgical fusion in severe cases.

Neurologic Deficit. There is a rough correlation between the degree of structural damage present and the extent of the neurologic deficit. This is more true in the lower cervical area than in the upper region where severe damage may appear without overt neurologic signs. In either case, however, it is doubtful that such a deficit would exhibit without an unstable situation existing. It is not unusual for a patient to exhibit a neurologic deficit without static displacement; ie, the vertebral segment has rebounded back into a normal position of rest.

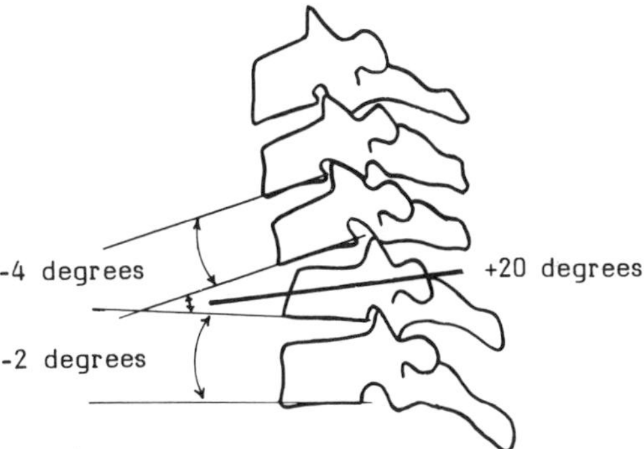

Figure 8.39. Abnormal segmental angulation. A difference of 11° or more between one vertebra and either of its adjacent vertebrae is considered evidence of clinical instability.

Facet Action[237]

In the middle and lower cervical area, A-P motion is a distinctly gliding translation because of the 45° facet planes and the A-P biconcave discs and vertebral bodies. During flexion and extension, the superior vertebra's inferior facets slide anterosuperiorly and posteroinferiorly on the inferior vertebra's superior facets. During full flexion, the facets may be almost if not completely separated. It is for this reason that an adjustment force is usually contraindicated in the fully flexed position. The center of motion is often described as being in the superior aspect of the body of the subjacent vertebra.

Some pivotal tilting of the superior facets, backward in extension and forward in flexion, is also normal near the end of the range of motion. The facets also tend to separate (open) on the contralateral side of rotation and lateral bending. They approximate (jam) during extension and on the ipsilateral side of rotation and lateral bending. Likewise, the foramina normally open on flexion, narrow on extension, and close on the concave side of lateral flexion. Because of the anterosuperior slant of the lower cervical facets, an inferior facet that moves downward must also slide posterior, and vice versa.

Any corrective adjustment must take into consideration the overall degree of the cervical lordosis, the *planes of articulation*, the *facet tilting* present, and the degree of *facet opening*, as well as any underlying pathologic process involved, and must apply just enough force to overcome the resistance of the fixation.

Coupling Patterns[238-240]

During lateral bending, the vertebral bodies tend to rotate toward the concavity while the spinous processes swing in a greater arc toward the convexity. Note that this is *exactly opposite to the coupling action in the lumbar spine*. During cervical bending to the right, for example, the right facet of the superior vertebra slides down the 45° plane toward the right and posterior and the left facet slides up the 45° incline toward the left and anterior. This coupling phenomenon is seen in circumstances in which an unusual ratio of axial rotation and lateral bending produces a subluxation or unilateral facet dislocation.

The amount of cervical rotation that is coupled with lateral flexion varies with the segmental level. At C2, there is 1° of rotation with every 1.5° of lateral flexion. This 2:3 ratio changes caudally so that the degree of coupled rotation decreases. For example, at C7, there is 1° of rotation for every 7.5° of lateral flexion, a 2:15 ratio.

Range of Motion[241-244]

All cervical vertebrae from C2 to C7 partake in flexion, extension, rotation, and lateral flexion, but some segments (eg, C5) are more active than others.

Flexion and Extension. In the C3–C7 area, flexion and extension occur as slight tipping and gliding translation of the upper on the lower facets, accompanied by disc distortion. During flexion, the upper facets ride over (but not beyond) the lower and produce a facet-interface gap posteriorly while the disc is compressed anteriorly and stretched posteriorly. During extension, the opposite effects occur; ie, the upper facets ride backward, producing a gapping anteriorly while the disc is compressed posteriorly and stretched anteriorly.

Flexion and extension occur around a horizontal axis that lies in the body of the vertebra below. The site of greatest movement in flexion is near the C4–C5 level (39°). This fact probably accounts for the high incidence of arthritis at the midcervical area. Segmental extension movement is fairly well diffused.

Lateral Flexion. Cervical sidebending is greatest near the C2–C3 level (20°), and influence diminishes caudally (15–17°). Motion is fairly restricted to the occipitoatlantal and atlantoaxial joints during the first 8° of lateral flexion. The arc of lateral motion is determined by the planes of the covertebral joints (Fig. 8.40).

Coupling. Lateral flexion in the cervical region is coupled with rotation so that the vertebral bodies rotate posteriorly to the side of lateral flexion and the spinous processes deviate to the side of convexity. This coupled motion forces the facets on the concave side to slide down and press together, while the facets on the convex side ride up and separate. The effect is the same for the uncovertebral articulations. During the first 15° of lateral flexion, this coupled rotation

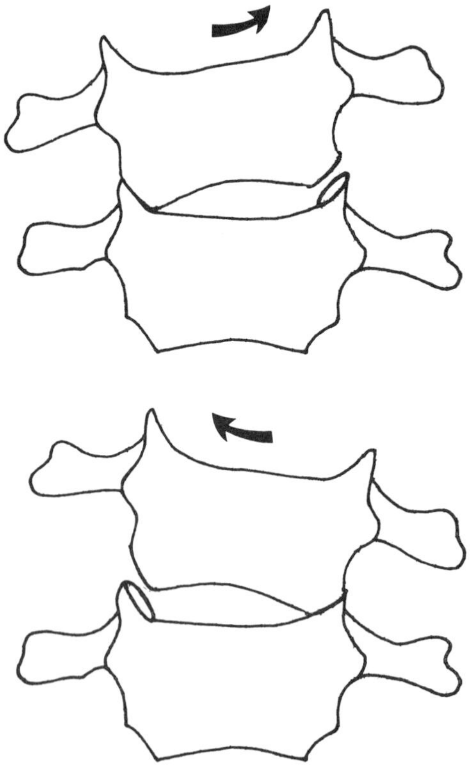

Figure 8.40. Coronal section of two midcervical vertebrae showing the motion of lateral flexion created by the planes of the covertebral joints.

takes place mainly at the axis. Beyond 15°, the remaining cervical segments rotate, with the least amount of rotation occurring in the lower segments.

Rotation. Rotation is greatest near the C5–C6 level (34°), slightly less above (26–28°) and considerably less below (13–15°). Just as lateral flexion is coupled with rotation, rotation is coupled with lateral flexion. The axis of rotation is located anterior to the body of C3 and moves posteriorly in the lower cervicals so that the axis of rotation for C7 lies in the anterior aspect of the centrum of C7.

Motion of the Transitional Cervicothoracic Area

In the cervicothoracic area, normal movement is somewhat similar to that in the lumbosacral area insofar as the type of stress (not magnitude of load) to which both areas are subjected is similar. L5 is relatively immobile on the sacrum and C7 is relatively immobile on T1, with the major amount of movement in the cervicothoracic junction being at C6–C7 and primarily that of rotation.

Reversal of the Normal Cervical Curve[245]

As opposed to the primary thoracic kyphosis which is a structural curve, the cervical and lumbar anterior curves are functional arcs produced by their wedge-shaped IVDs, and they normally flatten in the non-weight-bearing supine position. Likewise, they quickly adapt to changes involving the direction of force.

A pathologic straightening of the normal anterior curve of the cervical spine, as viewed in a lateral weight-bearing x-ray film, results in mechanical alteration of normal physiologic and structural integrity (Fig. 8.41). The normal vertical A-P line of gravity, as viewed laterally, falls approximately through the odontoid and touches the anterior border of T2. As the cervical spine tends to flatten in the erect position, the gravity line passes closer to the center of the cervical discs.

Incidence. Cervical kyphosis occurs most frequently after the age of 40 years, and the sexes appear equally affected. The cause is often the result of trauma-producing whiplash injury, herniated disc, subluxation, dislocation, fracture and/or ligamentous (especially posterior) injury. Torticollis, arthritis, malignancy, tuberculosis, osteomyelitis, and other pathologies may be involved.

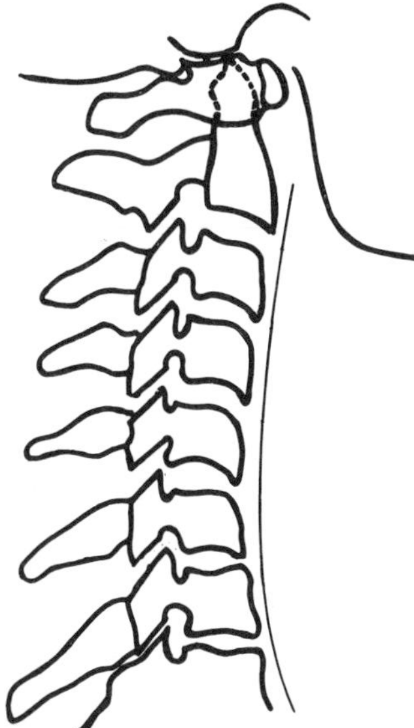

Figure 8.41. X-ray film tracing depicting a pathologic reversal of the normal cervical lordosis.

Etiology. While the cervical curve is the first secondary curve to develop in the infant, its maintenance in the erect posture is essentially determined by the integrity of the lumbar curve. A flattened cervical spine that is not compensatory to a flattened lumbar spine is usually the result of a local disorder such as a subluxation syndrome caused by posterior shifting of one or more disc nuclei, hypertonicity of anterior musculature, or anterior ligamentous shortening as the result of local overstress, inflammation, occupational posture, or congenital anomaly.

In a reduced curve (cervical hypolordosis), as Bergmann reminds us, more weight has to be borne on the vertebral bodies and discs; while in an increased curve (hyperlordosis), more weight must be borne by the facets. The shape of the vertebra and angles of the facet and disc determine the degree of lordosis. If through degenerative changes and/or stress responses these are altered, the "normal" arc of the curve will be changed. Numerous studies have been conducted relating ideas of what the normal curve should be, and all seem to be in agreement that the cervical lordosis extends down to T2, with C5 being the midpoint or stress vertebra.[246]

The force of gravity on the cervical lordosis normally falls just anterior to the support of the posterior cervical musculature. When the cervical curve flattens, a larger workload is placed on the musculature of the neck to maintain biomechanical integrity (Fig. 8.42).

In his monograph, Bergmann also mentions the radiographic studies of Jochumsen who measured the distance from the anterior body of C5 to a line running from the anterior arch of the atlas to the anterosuperior aspect of the body of C7 (Fig. 8.43). Jochumsen then set up a classification of cervical curves as follows:

1. Hyperlordosis – over +9 mm
2. Mean lordosis – +3 to +8 mm
3. Hypolordosis – +1 to +2 mm
4. Alordosis – +1 to −3 mm
5. Kyphosis – under −3 mm

Another approach used by some roentgenologists is to draw one line through the anterior and posterior tubercles of the atlas and another line through the inferior plate of C7. Secondary lines are then drawn at right angles from each of these base lines, and the angle created by the perpendicular lines is measured. An angle of 35–40° is considered normal, less than 35° indicates hypolordosis, and more than 40° indicates hyperlordosis.

Other methods can also be used. Pettibon[247] states that, mechanically, the strongest and most resilient curve is an arc with a radius of curvature equal to the chord across the arc, and he uses the Delmas index as depicted by Kapandji[248] (Fig. 8.44). As

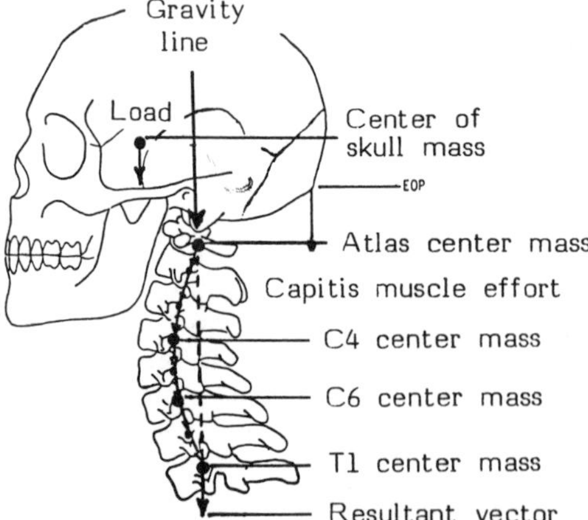

Figure 8.42. The force of gravity on the cervical curve falls just in front of the support of the posterior cervical muscles. Thus, a greater workload must be borne by the cervical extensors if the curve tends to flatten.

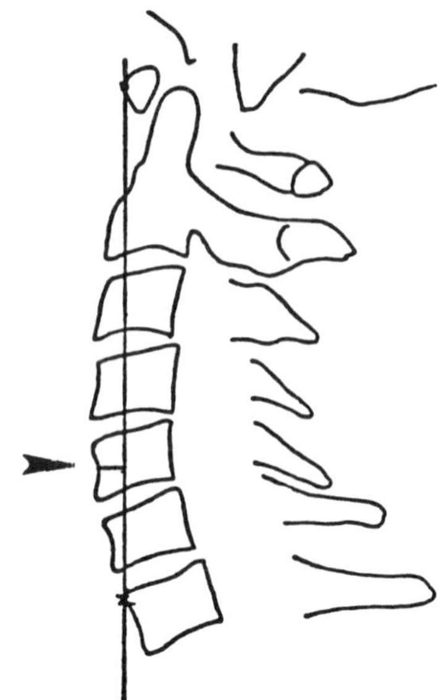

Figure 8.43. Jochumsen's system to measure the cervical curve. A measure is taken of the distance between the anterior body of C5 and a vertical line extended from the anterior arch of the atlas to the most anterior-superior point of the body of C7.

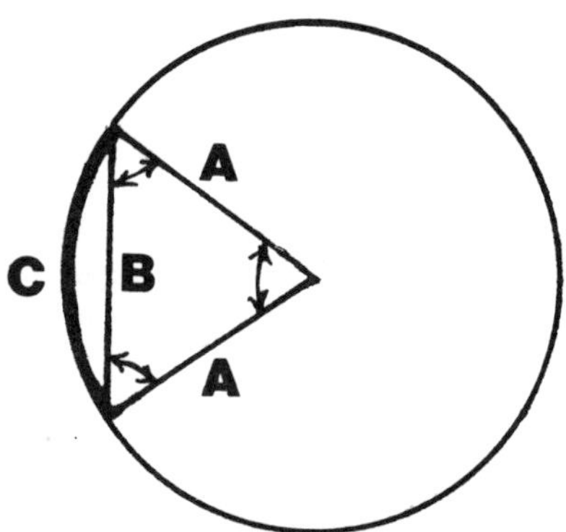

Figure 8.44. Mechanically, the strongest and most resilient curve is an arc that has a radius of curvature equal to the chord across the arc. In the above drawing, *A* represents the radius, *B* the chord (A = B), and *C* the arc of the curve. All angles are 60° in this example.

the radius increases, the curve increases (flattens, as in hypolordosis).

Effect of Atlas Position. It has been postulated by several authorities that the cervical curvature is directed by the position of the atlas; ie, a hyperlordotic cervical spine is compensated for by the atlas moving superiorly, and a flattened curve is compensated for by the atlas moving inferiorly.[249–251] After studying the lateral cervical films of 109 patients, however, Ng has shown statistically that subluxation of the atlas in the A-P plane does not necessarily accompany an alteration of cervical curvature.[252] No significant correlation could be found between the atlantopalatal angle and the degree of cervical curvature, thus indicating that an anterosuperior atlas does not accompany cervical hyperlordosis, or vice versa.

Symptoms and Signs. Cervical flattening is usually the result of paraspinal spasm secondary to an underlying injury, irritation, or inflammatory process. The acute clinical picture is one of torticollis. Other manifestations include headaches (occipital, occipital-frontal, supraorbital), vertigo, tenderness elicited on lateral C4–C6 nerve roots, neuritis involving branches of the brachial plexus because of nerve root pressure, hyperesthesia of one or more fingers, and loss or lessening of the biceps reflex on the same or contralateral side. In rare cases, the triceps reflex may be involved. One or more symptoms are frequently aggravated by an abnormal position of the head such as during reading in bed, an awkward sleeping position, or long-distance driving.

Roentgenographic Considerations.[253] Rehberger reports the typical radiographic findings to include loss of the normal lordotic curve by the straightened cervical spine (78% of cases), anterior and posterior subluxation on flexion and extension views, narrowing of IVD spaces at C4–C6 in 46% of cases, discopathy at the affected vertebral level as the injury progresses, and osteoarthritic changes which are often accompanied by foraminal spurring.

Biomechanics. A flattened cervical spine in the erect posture resembles a normal spine during flexion. To appreciate the mechanisms involved, it is well here to review the biomechanics involved. The nucleus of the disc serves as a fulcrum during flexion and return extension. When the spine is subjected to bending loads during flexion, half of the *disc* on the convex side suffers tension, widens, and contracts, while the other half of the disc on the concave side suffers compression, thins, and bulges. Concurrently, the *nucleus* bulges on the side of tension and contracts on the side of compression, which increases tension on the adjacent anulus.[254] This creates a self-stabilizing counteracting flexion force to the motion unit that aids a return to the resting position.

Case Management. Specific correction of offending vertebral subluxations should be accomplished. Adjunctive care includes massage and methods to reduce the chronic muscle spasm such as ultrasound, diathermy, hydrocollator packs, reflex spinal techniques, and a rolled towel placed under the neck in the supine position to increase the cervical curve. The individual should be instructed to sleep without a pillow. Cervical muscle re-education is quite helpful.

Prognosis. Rehberger[253] and Barge[255] report that the prognosis is excellent if the condition is treated early and the case is not complicated by fracture or dislocation, but guarded if the trauma is severe. In cases of minimal cervical discopathy, at least symptomatic relief can be expected. Prognosis is poor in advanced degenerative osteoarthritis.

Lower Cervical Trauma[256–258]

Fractures of the cervical spine are usually the result of blows, falls, or vehicular accidents. Most cervical fractures are characterized by neck pain that tends to radiate into the trapezius and upper extremities. Referred pain may radiate to the scalp, and upper extremity pain and paresthesias may be present. The neck is rigid because of protective splinting. Point tenderness, upper extremity motor and sensory disturbances, and easy fatigue of involved musculature are common. In many cases, however, the patient will be asymptomatic except for mild symptoms—thus, a potential disaster is waiting to happen.

Cervical fractures and dislocations are not common, except in the elderly when a degree of osteoporosis is evident. They are usually the result of severe trauma. Bruises on the face, scalp, and shoulders may offer clues as to the mechanism of injury. Signs of vertebral tenderness, limitation in movement, muscle spasm, and neurologic deficit should be sought. As in upper cervical damage, careful emergency management is necessary to avoid paralysis and death. Fracture and/or dislocation of any cervical vertebra require hospitalization for reduction, bone traction, and casting. Keep in mind that overdiagnosing instability of C2–C3 is a common pitfall.

Subluxations[259–269]

Because of the planes of normal articular processes, a straight horizontal subluxation is an anatomical impossibility unless there is a fracture of the articular processes. The body of any lower cervical vertebra follows the planes of the covertebral and posterior facets in movement. If a spinous process moves left, it does so by inscribing an arc toward the superior and anterior, while simultaneously the right transverse process moves inferiorly and somewhat posteriorly. It is thus impossible for an individual vertebra to be rotated straight right or left on its longitudinal axis, and irrational to make a listing of right or left. A vertebra cannot be subluxed without one of the articular processes moving either superiorly or inferiorly; thus it can be said that superiority or inferiority attends every posterior/anterior subluxation.

It should be kept in mind that the nerve root is anterior and inferior to the facets in the cervical spine. If subluxation of a vertebra occurs in a superior direction, the contents of the IVF become stretched because elongating and narrowing the vertical diameter of the IVF will cause traction upon the nerve trunk plus compression against the anterior portion of the foramen. If there is subluxation in an inferior direction, shortening and widening of the foramen occurs. Because the nerve sheath is often firmly anchored by tissues connecting it to the borders of the foramen in the adult, a stretching effect is exerted on the nerve sheath whenever its shape is altered. It can thus be appreciated that enlarging the IVF can cause as much trouble as a reduction in the size of the IVF. Also, it is impossible to subluxate a vertebra between C2 and L5 (inclusive) without changing the shape of its IVD in compensation.

A subluxation of one or more of the lower cervical vertebrae often involves the brachial plexus. Table 8.5 lists the nerves of the plexus and their functions.

Inasmuch as the distribution of the brachial plexus is so extensive, a multitude of abnormal reflections may be seen in its areas of distribution which can only be appreciated by knowledge of the pathophysiology involved. A few of the more common disturbances caused by lower cervical subluxations would include shoulder neuralgias, neuralgias along the medial arm and forearm or elbow, unclassified wrist drop and hand dystrophies, acroparesthesia, weak grip strength, and vague "rheumatic" wrist or hand complaints. A subluxation of one or more of the C3, C4, or C5 segments may involve the phrenic nerve and produce symptoms of severe chronic hiccup and other diaphragmatic disorders.

General Aspects of Fractures and Dislocations[57, 93, 147, 148, 155, 159, 160, 270–274]

Isolated fractures following trauma occur at all levels of the cervical spine. Vertebral body fractures, however, occur most frequently at C6 and C7 and least frequently at C4. The four common types of vertebral body fractures are anterior marginal fractures from A-P forces, comminuted fractures from axial forces, and lateral wedge fractures and uncinate process fractures from lateral stress. Vertical compression or flexion compression damage (Fig. 8.45) is sometimes seen, but extension injuries (eg, whiplash) are more common. Spinous process fractures usually occur at the C6 or C7 level after acute flexion or a blow to the flexed neck, producing ligamentous avulsion. There is immediate "hot" pain in the area of the spinous process which is increased by flexion. Any injury to C6–C7 is difficult to view on film because of overlapping structures.

Fractures of the articular processes are not readily exhibited on standard films. Woodring reports that 16 of 77 patients with cervical fractures demonstrated fractures of the articular process by multidirectional tomography, while only two demonstrated

Table 8.5.
Nerve Function of the Brachial Plexus (C5–T1)

Nerve	Function
Radial	Motor for wrist and thumb extension; sensory to dorsal web space between thumb and index finger
Ulnar	Motor for little finger abduction; sensory to distal ulnar aspect of little finger
Median	Motor for thumb apposition and abduction; sensory to distal radial aspect of index finger
Axillary	Motor to deltoid muscle; sensory to lateral arm and deltoid patch on upper arm
Musculocutaneous	Motor to biceps muscle; sensory to lateral forearm

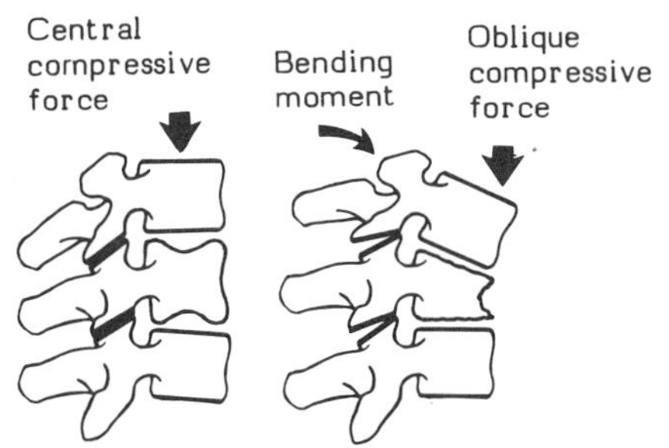

Figure 8.45. Vertebral body damage centrally as the result of excessive compression force directed vertically (*left*) and eccentrically (*right*) to produce a severe bending moment.

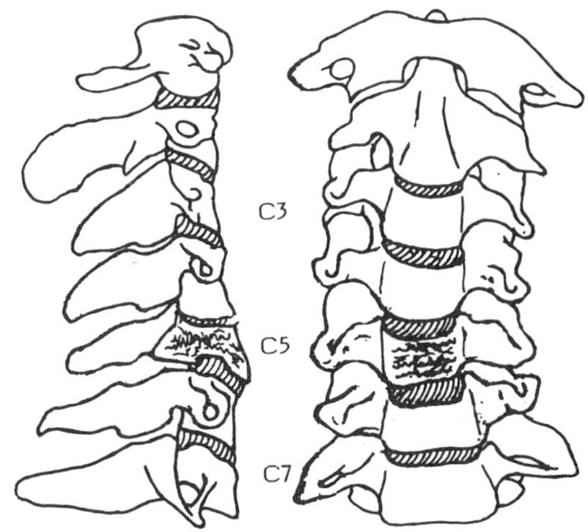

Figure 8.46. *Left*, schematic of bursting fracture of C5 vertebral body resulting from excessive compression. *Right*, lateral wedge compression fracture of C5 vertebral body.

such fractures on standard films.[275] The signs and symptoms varied from minimal to acute cervical radiculopathy, persistent neck pain, and sometimes unilateral or bilateral facet dislocation.

Compression Injuries.[276–278] Vertebral body crush fractures are rare, and less common in the cervical spine than elsewhere (Fig. 8.46). They are the result of a vertical force, often during flexion, such as that of a football "spearing tackle." Compression fractures of articular processes occur in extension injuries to the neck. They are not common, with the exception of those occurring from automobile "whiplash" injuries and diving into shallow water. They are not usually demonstrable on A-P or lateral films until deformity is severe, but oblique views will often demonstrate them. They are best seen on "pillar" views. The pillar view is taken with the trunk A-P and the head turned 45° to the side. These views, to be taken bilaterally, will show the articular pillar in profile. Apophyseal fractures are frequently quite apparent when present in pillar views.

It is most difficult to conceive of a vertebral compression fracture not being secondary to severe endplate fracture, even if roentgenographic evidence of endplate failure is not seen. Invariably, the endplate must fail first in a healthy vertebra subjected to extreme vertical and/or bending forces.

Flexion Injuries.[92, 279–282] In a blow to the occiput directed upward, the posterior elements receive the greatest trauma because of the shear component in the hyperflexion force. During forceful cervical flexion, a unilateral facet dislocation and/or fracture may occur with the contralateral side remaining intact, especially if the force is oblique (Fig. 8.47). Bilateral dislocation or fracture-dislocation may occur if the facets are forced to override without rotation.[283] Unilateral dis-

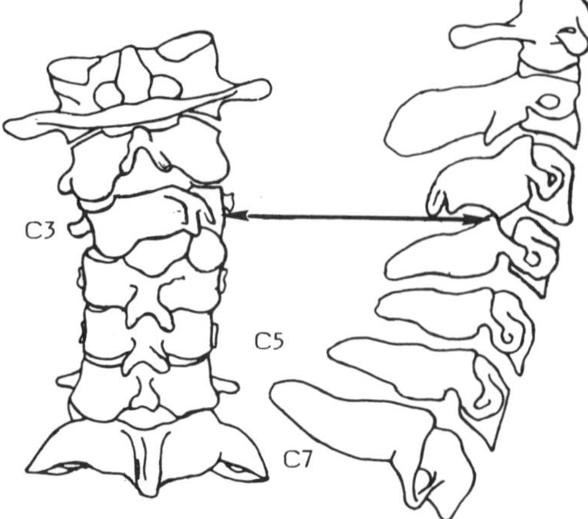

Figure 8.47. Schematic of unilateral locked facet of C3 resulting from hyperflexion with rotation.

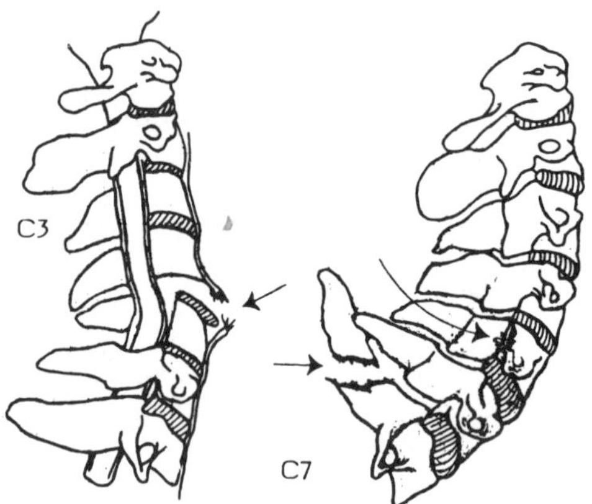

Figure 8.48. *Left*, severe hyperextension sprain of C4–C5 with rupture of the anterior longitudinal ligament and avulsion. *Right*, hyperextension fracture of the posterior arch of C5 and fracture of the spinous process of C7.

location is more common in the lower cervical area than in the upper area.

Extension Injuries.[73,74,76,284-288] Forceful extension can produce tearing of the anterior longitudinal ligament and anterior anulus which may coexist with an avulsion fracture at the lips of the anterior vertebral body (Fig. 8.48). If rupture occurs, further force is absorbed by the articular processes, spinous processes, laminae, and pedicles, in that order. About 50% of all cervical fractures are of the vertebral arch. If the articular processes fracture and the posterior arch fails, the vertebral body will inevitably be displaced anteriorly. Transverse pedicle fracture or severe posterior subluxation may also occur. Keep in mind that the articular pillars of the C3–C7 vetebrae are not designed like the lateral masses of the atlas. These pillars project laterally on each side at the junction of the lamina and pedicle.

Tenderness will usually be shown along the lateral musculature. Upper extremity pain or numbness and restricted cervical motion at one or more interspaces during flexion and extension may be exhibited. Neurologic symptoms may be severe and prolonged without demonstrable roentgenorgraphic evidence. Cord damage without apparent structural damage may result from a bulge created by a buckled degenerated (nonelastic) ligamentum flavum at the posterior of the spinal canal (Fig. 8.49). The

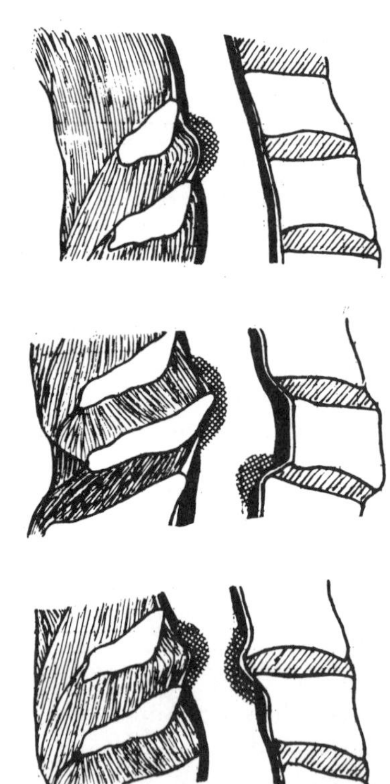

Figure 8.49. *Top*, spinal cord encroachment by thickening of the yellow ligament. *Center*, "pincher phenomenon" produced by posterior arch of the middle vertebra which has slipped anteriorly and the superior edge of the body of the subjacent vertebra. *Bottom*, pincher encroachment posteriorly by ligament hypertrophy and anteriorly by a bulging disc and spur on the superior lip of the subjacent vertebra.

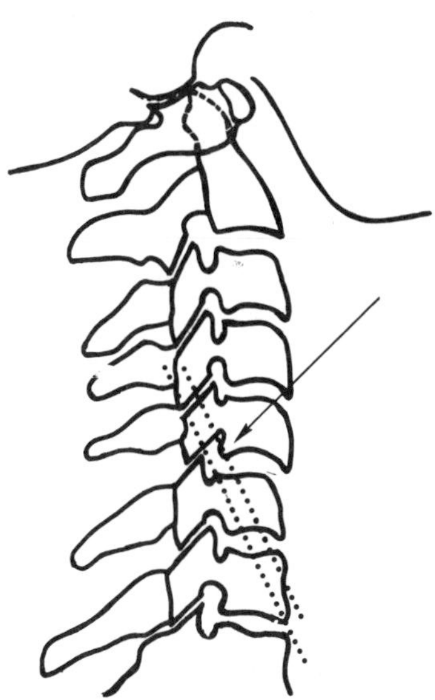

Figure 8.50. Enlargement of an intervertebral foramen resulting from ligament instability following hyper-rotation. Translatory displacement at the area in question is measured by drawing parallel lines from the posteroinferior angle of the vertebral body above and the posterosuperior angle of the vertebral body below on a lateral x-ray film. A distance of 3.5 mm or more suggests clinical instability.

cord may also be pinched between the posteroinferior edge of the superior vertebral body and the laminae of the inferior segment.

Lateral Flexion Injuries.[95,96,275,289] When the head is forced to severely tilt laterally, there is always a coupled component of rotation involved. Compression wedging of structures on the concave side occurs, and tension on the structures on the convex side is produced. There are four typical severe traumatic effects throughout the cervical area: (1) the dens will fracture and displace laterally; (2) a unilateral compression fracture of the vertebral body will occur; (3) there will be fracture of the uncinate or transverse process, or fracture and/or dislocation of the articular process ipsilaterally with ligamentous rupture contralaterally; (4) there will be brachial plexus avulsion, possibly associated with a cervical and/or thoracic fracture.

Rotary Injuries.[290] These are often found combined with flexion, extension, and lateral flexion injuries.[291] Keep in mind that while the cervical ligaments are quite resistant to pure flexion and extension stress, they are far less resistant to shear stress (Fig. 8.50). It is for this reason that (1) the anterior longitudinal ligament is often torn when the neck is overextended and rotated and (2) the posterior ligaments, posterior joint capsules, and posterior longitudinal ligament (in that order) rupture when the neck is overflexed and rotated.

REFERENCES

1. D'Ambrosia RD: *Musculoskeletal Disorders: Regional Examination and Differential Diagnosis.* Philadelphia, J.B. Lippincott, 1977, pp 178–186.
2. Hoppenfeld S: *Physical Examination of the Spine and Extremities.* New York, Appleton-Century-Crofts, 1976, pp 106–111.
3. Hollingshead WH, Jenkins DB: *Functional Anatomy of the Limbs and Back.* Philadelphia, W.B. Saunders, 1981, pp 354–364.
4. Schafer RC: *Chiropractic Physical and Spinal Diagnosis.* Oklahoma City, Associated Chiropractic Academic Press, 1980, p VIII-1.
5. Janse J: *Principles and Practice of Chiropractic.* Lombard, Ill, National College of Chiropractic, 1976, p 205.
6. Bowen WP, Stone HA: *Applied Anatomy and Kinesiology: The Mechanism of Muscular Movement,* ed 6. Philadelphia, Lea & Febiger, 1949.
7. D'Ambrosia RD: *Musculoskeletal Disorders: Regional Examination and Differential Diagnosis.* Philadelphia, J.B. Lippincott, 1977, pp 178–179, 190–192.
8. Moorehouse LE, Cooper JM: *Kinesiology.* St. Louis, C.V. Mosby, 1950, pp 49–50.
9. Hoppenfeld S: *Physical Examination of the Spine and Extremities.* New York, Appleton-Century-Crofts, 1976, p 114.
10. Johnson RM, Southwick WO: Surgical approaches to the spine. In Rothman RH, Simeone FA (eds): *The Spine.* Philadelphia, W.B. Saunders, 1975, vol 1, pp 76–78, 87–88.
11. Barham JN, Wooten EP: *Structural Kinesiology.* New York, Macmillan, 1973, pp 263–265.
12. Esch D, Lepley M: *Musculoskeletal Function: An Anatomy and Kinesiology Laboratory Manual.* Minneapolis, University of Minnesota Press, 1974, pp 18–19, 45–48.
13. Kendall HO, Kendall FP, Wadsworth GE: *Muscles: Testing and Function,* ed 2. Baltimore, Williams & Wilkins, 1971, pp 207, 264–267, 270.
14. Goodheart GL: *Collected Published Articles and Reprints.* Montpellier, O, Williams County Publishing, 1969, pp 17–19.
15. Schafer RC: *Chiropractic Physical and Spinal Diagnosis.* Oklahoma City, Associated Chiropractic Academic Press, 1980, p VIII-14.
16. Daniels L, Worthingham C: *Muscle Testing: Techniques of Manual Examination,* ed 4. Philadelphia, W.B. Saunders, 1980, pp 16–20.
17. Fisk JW: *The Painful Neck and Back.* Springfield, Ill, Charles C Thomas, 1977, 39–40.

18. Royce J: *Surface Anatomy*, Philadelphia, F.A. Davis, 1965.
19. Cohen RL: Minimal exam of cervical spine. *Journal of the Chiropractic Association of Oklahoma* 3(3):8–9, 1984.
20. Phillips RB: Upper cervical biomechanics. *ACA Journal of Chiropractic* 10:127–134, October 1976.
21. Goodheart GL: *Collected Published Articles and Reprints*. Montpellier, O, Williams County Publishing, 1969, p 16.
22. Ferlic D: The range of motion of the "normal" cervical spine. *Bulletin of Johns Hopkins Hospital* 110:59, 1962.
23. Grice AS: Preliminary evaluation of 50 sagittal cervical motion radiographic examinations. *Journal of the Canadian Chiropractic Association* 2(1), 1977.
24. Kapandji IA: *Physiology of the Joints: The Trunk and Vertebral Column*, ed 2. New York, Churchill Livingstone, 1980, vol 3, pp 170, 246.
25. Schafer RC (ed): *Basic Chiropractic Procedural Manual*, ed 4. Arlington, Va, American Chiropractic Association, 1984, pp 287–289.
26. Schafer RC: *Chiropractic Physical and Spinal Diagnosis*. Oklahoma City, Associated Chiropractic Academic Press, 1980, p VIII-12.
27. Hoppenfeld S: *Physical Examination of the Spine and Extremities*. New York, Appleton-Century-Crofts, 1976, pp 115–117.
28. Evans DC: Biomechanics of spinal injury. In Gonzna ER, Harrington IJ: *Biomechanics of Musculoskeletal Injury*. Baltimore, Williams & Wilkins, 1982, p 172.
29. Johnson RM, Southwick WO: Surgical approaches to the spine. In Rothman RH, Simeone FA (eds): *The Spine*. Philadelphia. W.B. Saunders, 1975, vol 1, pp 69–72.
30. Fisk JW: *The Painful Neck and Back*. Springfield, Ill, Charles C Thomas, 1977, pp 81–84.
31. Kapandji IA: *Physiology of the Joints: The Trunk and Vertebral Column*, ed 2. New York, Churchill Livingstone, 1980, vol 3, pp 248–250.
32. White AA, Panjabi MM: *Clinical Biomechanics of the Spine*. Philadelphia, J.B. Lippincott, 1978, pp 54–55.
33. Grieve GP: *Common Vertebral Joint Problems*. New York, Churchill Livingstone, 1981, pp 32–33, 56–59.
34. Brain, Lord, Wilkinson (eds): *Cervical Spondylosis*. London, Heinemann, 1967.
35. Sutherland S: Anatomical perivertebral influences on the intervertebral foramen. In Goldstein M (ed): *The Research Status of Spinal Manipulative Therapy*, NINCDS Monograph, No. 15, DHEW Publication No. (NIH) 76-998, Stock No. 017-049-0-0060-7, Washington, DC, U.S. Government Printing Office, 1975, p 129.
36. Breig A: *Biomechanics of the Central Nervous System: Some Basic Normal and Pathological Phenomena*. Stockholm, Almquist & Wiksell, 1960.
37. Brodal A: *Neurological Anatomy in Relation to Clinical Medicine*, ed 2. London, Oxford University Press, 1969.
38. Breig A, Turnbull I, Hassler O: Effects of mechanical stress on the spinal cord in cervical spondylosis. *Journal of Neurosurgery* 15:45, 1966.
39. Goddard MD, Reid JD: Movements induced by straight leg raising inthe lumbo-sacral roots, nerves, and plexus, and in the intra-pelvic portion of the sciatic nerve. *Journal of Neurology, Neurosurgery and Psychiatry* (London) 28:12, 1965.
40. Penning L: *Functional Pathology of the Cervical Spine*. Amsterdam, Excerpta Medical Foundation, 1968.
41. Reid JD: Effects of flexion-extension movements of the head and spine upon the spinal cord and nerve roots. *Journal of Neurology, Neurosurgery and Psychiatry* (London) 23:214. 1960.
42. Breig A: *Adverse Mechanical Tension in the Central Nervous System*. Stockholm, Almquist & Wikell, 1978.
43. Breig A: Overstretching of, and circumscribed pathological tension in, the spinal cord—a basic cause of symptoms in cord disorders. *Journal of Biomechanics* 3:7, 1970.
44. Brodal A: *Neurological Anatomy in Relation to Clinical Medicine*, ed 2. London, Oxford University Press, 1969.
45. Fried LC, Doppman JL, Chiro G: Direction of blood flow in the primate cervical spinal cord. *Journal of Neurosurgery* 33:325, 1970.
46. Hoff J et al: The role of ischemia in the pathogenesis of cervical spondylotic myelopathy. *Spine* 2:100, 1977.
47. Breig A, Turnbull I, Hassler O: Effects of mechanical stress on the spinal cord in cervical spondylosis. *Journal of Neurosurgery* 15:45, 1966.
48. Schafer RC: *Chiropractic Management of Sports and Recreational Injuries*. Baltimore, Williams & Wilkins, 1982, pp 331–333.
49. Palo J: I love boxing, but .... *ACA Journal of Chiropractic* November 1983, pp 56, 59.
50. Jeffreys E: *Disorders of the Cervical Spine*. London, Butterworths, 1980, pp 48–49.
51. Williams JGP, Sperryn PN (eds): *Sports Medicine*, ed 2. Baltimore, Williams & Wilkins, 1976, pp 352–353.
52. Balkany TJ, Jafek BW, Rutherford RB: The management of neck injuries. In Zuidema GD, Rutherford RB, Ballinger WF (eds): *The Management of Trauma*, ed 3. Philadelphia, W.B. Saunders, 1979, p 342.
53. Yashon D: *Spinal Injury*. New York, Appleton-Century-Crofts, 1978, pp 6–9.
54. Haycock CE (ed): *Sports Medicine for the Athletic Female*, Oradell, NJ, Medical Economics, 1980, pp 298–303.
55. Larcher AC: The making of a football field physician. Transcription of a tape cassette; no resource data shown.
56. Schafer RC: *Chiropractic Management of Sports and Recreational Injuries*. Baltimore, Williams & Wilkins, 1982, pp 327, 329–330.
57. Fielding JW: Dynamic anatomy and cineradiography of the cervical spine. In Bailey RW (ed): *The Cervical Spine*. Philadelphia, Lea & Febiger, 1974.
58. McCall I, Park WM, McSweeney T: The radio-

logical demonstration of lower cervical injury. *Clinical Radiology* 34:235–240, 1973.
59. Bowerman JW: *Radiology and Injury in Sport.* New York, Appleton-Century-Crofts, 1977, pp 35–51.
60. Jeffreys E: *Disorders of the Cervical Spine.* London, Butterworths, 1980, pp 17–23, 81.
61. Schafer RC: *Chiropractic Management of Sports and Recreational Injuries.* Baltimore, Williams & Wilkins, 1982, p 330.
62. Babcock JL: Cervical spine injuries. *Archives of Surgery* 111:646–651, 1976.
63. Evans DC: Biomechanics of spinal injury. In Gonzna ER, Harrington IJ: *Biomechanics of Musculoskeletal Injury.* Baltimore, Williams & Wilkins, 1982, p 165–172.
64. Schafer RC: *Chiropractic Management of Sports and Recreational Injuries.* Baltimore, Williams Wilkins, 1982, p 333.
65. Iverson LD, Clawson DK: *Manual of Acute Orthopaedic Therapeutics.* Boston, Little, Brown, 1977, p 17.
66. Schafer RC: *Chiropractic Management of Sports and Recreational Injuries.* Baltimore, Williams & Wilkins, 1982, pp 265–266.
67. Clark WM, Gehweiler JA, Leib R: Significant signs of cervical spine trauma. *Skeletal Radiology* 3:201, 1979.
68. Inman OB (ed): *Chiropractic Manual of the Traumatized Cervical Spine.* Atlanta, Georgia Chiropractic Association, 1978, pp 28–29.
69. Lehman JJ: Manual therapy in upper cervical spinal dysfunction: A clinical study. *Physiotherapy Canada* 30:302–304, 1978.
70. Erhardt R: Whiplash injury of the cervical spine and the cervical syndrome. In Inman OB (ed): *Chiropractic Manual of the Traumatized Cervical Spine.* Atlanta, Georgia Chiropractic Association, 1978, pp 3–6.
71. Jeffreys E: *Disorders of the Cervical Spine.* London, Butterworths, 1980, pp 82–86.
72. McKenzie JA: The dynamic behavior of the head and cervical spine during "whiplash." *Journal of Biomechanics* 4:477–490, 1971.
73. Forsyth HF: Extension injuries of the cervical spine. *Journal of Bone and Joint Surgery* 46A:1792, 1964.
74. Martinez JL, Garcia DJ: A model for whiplash. *Journal of Biomechanics* 1:23–32, 1968.
75. Janse J: *Principles and Practice of Chiropractic.* Lombard, Ill, National College of Chiropractic, 1976, pp 219–221.
76. Janecki CJ Jr, Lipke JM: Whiplash syndrome. *American Family Physician* 17(4):144–151.
77. Bailey RW: *The Cervical Spine.* Philadelphia, Lea & Febiger, 1974, pp 91–97.
78. Gay JR, Abbott KH: Common whiplash injuries of the neck. *Journal of the American Medical Association* 152:1698, 1953.
79. Macnab MB: Acceleration-extension injuries of the cervical spine. *Symposium on the Spine.* St. Louis, C. V. Mosby, 1969, pp 19–17,
80. Gershon-Cohen J, Budin E, Glauser F: Whiplash fractures of cervicodorsal spinous processes. *Journal of the American Medical Association* 155:560, 1954.
81. Cailliet R: *Neck and Arm Pain.* Philadelphia, F.A. Davis, 1974, p 61.
82. Gitelman R, Fitz-Ritson D: Acceleration/deceleration injuries (whiplash). *ACA Journal of Chiropractic* 17:68, April 1983.
83. Macnab I: Acceleration injuries of the cervical spine. *Journal of Bone and Joint Surgery* 46A:1797–1799, 1964.
84. Ommaya A: *Lawyer's Medical Journal* 6(4):379–401, 1971.
85. Roca P: *Annals of Ophthalmology* 1972, pp 63–73.
86. Seletz E: *Journal of the American Medical Association* 168:1750–1755, 1958.
87. Gukenberger M: *Scandinavian Journal of Rehabilitation Medicine* 4:150–153, 1972.
88. Braaf M, Rosner S: *Journal of Trauma* 2:494–501, 1962.
89. Pang L: *Laryngoscope* 81:1381–1387, 1971.
90. Rubin W: *Archives of Otolaryngology* 97:85–87, 1973.
91. Hohl M: *Clinical Orthopaedics and Related Research* 109:42–49, 1975.
92. Braakman R, Penning L: The hyperflexion sprain of the cervical spine. *Radiologica Clinics et Biologica* 37:309, 1968.
93. Howarth MB, Petrie JG: *Injuries of the Spine.* Baltimore, Williams & Wilkins, 1964.
94. Jeffreys E: *Disorders of the Cervical Spine.* London, Butterworths, 1980, pp 87–88.
95. Schaff RE et al: Lateral hyperflexion injuries of the cervical spine. *Skeletal Radiology* 3:73, 1978.
96. Bard G, Jones M: Cineradiographic recording of traction of the cervical spine. *Archives of Physical Medicine and Rehabilitation* August 1964.
97. Jeffreys E: *Disorders of the Cervical Spine.* London, Butterworths, 1980, pp 88–89.
98. Travell JG: Myofascial trigger points: Clinical view. In Bonica JJ, Albe-Fessard D (eds): *Advance in Pain Research and Therapy.* New York, Raven Press, 1976.
99. Schafer RC: *Chiropractic Management of Sports and Recreational Injuries.* Baltimore, Williams & Wilkins, 1982, p 246, 334–335.
100. Jaskoviak P, Schafer RC: *Applied Physiotherapy.* Arlington, Va, American Chiropractic Association. To be published in 1986.
101. Cailliet R: *Soft Tissue Pain and Disability.* Philadelphia, F.A. Davis, 1980, pp 128–130.
102. Moore KL: *Clinically Oriented Anatomy.* Baltimore, Williams & Wilkins, 1980, p 615.
103. Basmajian JV (ed): *Grant's Method of Anatomy,* ed 9. Baltimore, Williams & Wilkins, 1975, pp 533–541.
104. Hohl M, Baker HR: The atlantoaxial joint, roentgenographic and anatomical study of normal and abnormal motion. *Journal of Bone and Joint Surgery* 46A:1739, 1964.
105. Cailliet R: *Soft Tissue Pain and Disability.* Philadelphia, F.A. Davis, 1980, pp 107–119.
106. White AA, Panjabi MM: *Clinical Biomechanics of the Spine.* Philadelphia, J.B. Lippincott, 1978, pp 82–83.
107. Parke WW: Applied anatomy of the spine. In Rothman RH, Simeone FA (eds): *The Spine.* Phil-

adelphia, W.B. Saunders, 1975, vol 1, pp 24–26, 29–31, 43–45

108. Barham JN, Wooten EP: *Structural Kinesiology.* New York, Macmillan, 1973, pp 242–245.
109. Jeffreys E: *Disorders of the Cervical Spine.* London, Butterworths, 1980, pp 2–6.
110. Dove CI: The occipito-atlanto-axial complex. *Manuelle Medizin* 20:11–15, 1982.
111. Rude J: Morphology of the occipital condyles and movement of the atlanto-occipital joint. *Manuelle Medizin* 22:101–106, 1984.
112. Craton EF: Cranial vertebral junction autopsy. *Today's Chiropractic* September/October 1985, pp 29–30.
113. Kapandji IA: *Physiology of the Joints: The Trunk and Vertebral Column,* ed 2. New York, Churchill Livingstone, 1980, vol 3, pp 172, 180.
114. Fielding JW: Dynamic anatomy and cineradiography of the cervical spine. In Bailey RW (ed): *The Cervical Spine.* Philadelphia, Lea & Febiger, 1974.
115. Kapandji IA: *Physiology of the Joints: The Trunk and Vertebral Column,* ed 2. New York, Churchill Livingstone, 1980, vol 3, p 172.
116. Von Torklus D, Gehle W: *The Upper Cervical Spine.* New York, Grune & Stratton, 1972.
117. Johnson RM, Southwick WO: Surgical approaches to the spine. In Rothman RH, Simeone FA (eds): *The Spine.* Philadelphia, W.B. Saunders, 1975, vol 1, pp 83–85.
118. Kapandji IA: *Physiology of the Joints: The Trunk and Vertebral Column,* ed 2. New York, Churchill Livingstone, 1980, vol 3, pp 186–190.
119. Gehweiler JA Jr, Osborne RL Jr, Becker RF: *The Radiology of Vertebral Trauma.* Philadelphia, W.B. Saunders, 1980, pp 81–84.
120. Moore KL: *Clinically Oriented Anatomy.* Baltimore, Williams & Wilkins, 1980, pp 631–632.
121. Cailliet R: *Neck and Arm Pain.* Philadelphia, F.A. Davis, 1974, pp 17–20.
122. Dimnet J et al: Cervical spine motion in the sagittal plane: Kinematic and geometric parameters. *Journal of Biomechanics* 15:959–969, 1982.
123. Kapandji IA: *Physiology of the Joints: The Trunk and Vertebral Column,* ed 2, New York, Churchill Livingstone, 1980, vol 3, p 174.
124. Moore KL: *Clinically Oriented Anatomy.* Baltimore, Williams & Wilkins, 1980, pp 644–645.
125. Jeffreys E: *Disorders of the Cervical Spine.* London, Butterworths, 1980, pp 6–7.
126. Jeffreys E: *Disorders of the Cervical Spine.* London, Butterworths, 1980, pp 49–53.
127. White AA, Panjabi MM: *Clinical Biomechanics of the Spine.* Philadelphia, J.B. Lippincott, 1978, pp 65–70, 86.
128. Cailliet R: *Neck and Arm Pain.* Philadelphia. F.A. Davis, 1974, pp 11–15.
129. Fielding JW et al: Tears of the transverse ligament of the atlas: A clinical biomechanical study. *Journal of Bone and Joint Surgery* 56A:1683, 1974.
130. White AA, Panjabi MM: *Clinical Biomechanics of the Spine.* Philadelphia, J.B. Lippincott, 1978, pp 196–199, 201–202, 271.
131. Grice AS: A biomechanical approach to cervical and dorsal adjusting. In Haldeman S (ed): *Modern Developments in the Principles and Practice of Chiropractic.* New York, Appleton-Century-Crofts, 1980, pp 341–342.
132. Kapandji IA: *Physiology of the Joints: The Trunk and Vertebral Column,* ed 2. New York, Churchill Livingstone, 1980, vol 3, pp 176, 184, 228–232.
133. Jeffreys E: *Disorders of the Cervical Spine.* London, Butterworths, 1980, p 60, 62.
134. Bergmann T: Integrated Chiropractic Methods. Oklahoma seminar, April 23, 1983, Northwestern Chiropractic College, p 12.
135. Cailliet R: *Neck and Arm Pain.* Philadelphia. F.A. Davis, 1974, p 11.
136. Snijders CJ, Timmerman P: Motions and forces in the atlanto-occipital joint during flexion of the cervical spine. *Manuelle Medizin* 20:51–58, 1982.
137. Grice AS: A biomechanical approach to cervical and dorsal adjusting. In Haldeman S (ed): *Modern Developments in the Principles and Practice of Chiropractic.* New York, Appleton-Century-Crofts, 1980, p 345.
138. Kapandji IA: *Physiology of the Joints: The Trunk and Vertebral Column,* ed 2. New York, Churchill Livingstone, 1980, vol 3, pp 178, 182, 236.
139. Kapandji IA: *Physiology of the Joints: The Trunk and Vertebral Column,* ed 2. New York, Churchill Livingstone, 1980, vol 3, pp 184, 234.
140. Grice AS: A biomechanical approach to cervical and dorsal adjusting. In Haldeman S (ed): *Modern Developments in the Principles and Practice of Chiropractic.* New York, Appleton-Century-Crofts, 1980, pp 343–345.
141. Jirout J: Changes in the atlas-axis relations on lateral flexion of the head and neck. *Neuroradiology* 6:215, 1973.
142. White AA, Panjabi MM: *Clinical Biomechanics of the Spine.* Philadelphia, J.B. Lippincott, 1978, pp 65–68.
143. Kapandji IA: *Physiology of the Joints: The Trunk and Vertebral Column,* ed 2. New York, Churchill Livingstone, 1980, vol 3, pp 180–184, 228, 232.
144. Gillet H, Liekens M: *Belgian Chiropractic Research Notes.* Huntington Beach, Cal, Motion Palpation Institute, 1981, pp 40–42.
145. Gehweiler JA Jr, Osborne RL Jr, Becker RF: *The Radiology of Vertebral Trauma.* Philadelphia, W.B. Saunders, 1980, pp 78–81.
146. Kapandji IA: *Physiology of the Joints: The Trunk and Vertebral Column,* ed 2. New York, Churchill Livingstone, 1980, vol 3, pp 228–236, 240–244.
147. Miller MD et al: Significant new observations on cervical spine trauma. *American Journal of Roentgenology* 130:659, 1978.
148. Bohlman H: The pathology and current concepts of cervical spine injuries: A critical review of 300 cases. *Journal of Bone and Joint Surgery,* 54A:1363, 1972.
149. White AA, Panjabi MM: *Clinical Biomechanics of the Spine.* Philadelphia, J.B. Lippincott, 1978, pp 123–141, 183–184.
150. Barham JN, Wooten EP: *Structural Kinesiology.* New York, Macmillan, 1973, p 277.
151. Gehweiler JA Jr, Osborne RL Jr, Becker RF: *The Radiology of Vertebral Trauma.* Philadelphia, W.B. Saunders, 1980, pp 130–185.
152. Evans DC: Biomechanics of spinal injury. In Gonzna ER, Harrington IJ: *Biomechanics of Mus-*

culoskeletal Injury. Baltimore, Williams & Wilkins, 1982, pp 173–183.
153. Felding JW, Francis WR, Hawkins RJ: The upper cervical spine. In Feldman F (ed): *Radiology, Pathology, and Immunology of Bones and Joints: A Review of Current Concepts*, New York, Appleton-Century-Crofts, 1978, pp 303–312.
154. Yashon D: *Spinal Injury*. New York, Appleton-Century-Crofts, 1978, pp 104–125.
155. Abel M: *Occult Traumatic Lesions of the Cervical Vertebrae*. St. Louis, Green, 1971.
156. West HG: Vertebral artery considerations in cervical trauma. *ACA Journal of Chiropractic* December 1968, pp 18–19.
157. Cailliet R: *Soft Tissue Pain and Disability*. Philadelphia, F.A. Davis, 1980, pp 120–121.
158. Henderson DJ: Significance of vertebral dyskinesia in relation to the cervical syndrome. *Journal of Manipulative and Physiological Therapeutics* 2:1, 1979.
159. Brankman R, Penning L: *Injuries of the Cervical Spine*. London, Excerpta Medica, 1971.
160. Kattan JR (ed): *Trauma and No-trauma of the Cervical Spine*. Springfield, Ill, Charles C Thomas, 1978.
161. De Rusha JL: Upper cervical technic correlated with neurodiagnosis. *ACA Journal of Chiropractic* September 1961.
162. Nelson, WA: Personal communication 1980.
163. Gillet H: The anatomy and physiology of spinal fixation. *Journal of the National Chiropractic Association* December 1963.
164. Gillet H: Evolution of a chiropractor. *National Chiropractic Journal*, November 1945, January 1949, December 1949, January 1951.
165. Gillet H, Liekens M: *Belgian Chiropractic Research Notes*. Huntington Beach, Cal, Motion Palpation Institute, 1981.
166. Lombardi G: The occipital vertebra. *American Journal of Roentgenology* 86:260, 1961.
167. Janse J: *Principles and Practice of Chiropractic*. Lombard, Ill, National College of Chiropractic, 1976, pp 213–216.
168. Grove AB: *Chiropractic Technique—A Procedure of Adjusting*. Madison, Wis, Straus Printing & Publishing, 1979, pp 76–80.
169. Reinert OC: *Chiropractic Procedure and Practice*, ed 3. Florissant, Mo, Marian Press, 1972, pp 218–222.
170. Baltzell LG, Mackey RH (eds): *Firth's Technic Notes*. Publishing data not shown, 1967, pp 11, 13.
171. Craton EF: Condyle–paraglenoid ligament. *Today's Chiropractic* January/February 1985, p 46.
172. Craton EF: The actuality of occipital subluxation. *Today's Chiropractic* July/August 1985, pp 25–27.
173. Jackson H: Diagnosis of minimal atlanto-axial subluxations. *British Journal of Radiology* 23:672, 1950.
174. Coutts MB: Atlanto-epistropheal subluxations. *Archives of Surgery* 29:297, 1934.
175. Cattel HS, Filtzer DL: Pseudosubluxation and other normal variations in the cervical spine in children. *Journal of Bone and Joint Surgery* 47A:1295–1309, 1965.
176. Janse J: *Principles and Practice of Chiropractic*. Lombard, Ill, National College of Chiropractic, 1976, pp 216–219.
177. Grove AB: *Chiropractic Technique—A Procedure of Adjusting*. Madison, Wis, Straus Printing & Publishing, 1979, pp 66–76.
178. Baltzell LG, Mackey RH (eds): *Firth's Technic Notes*. Publishing data not shown, 1967, pp 13–17.
179. Kale M: The upper cervical specific. Parts 1 and 2. *Today's Chiropractic* July/August 1984, pp 28–29; September/October 1984, pp 27–30.
180. Janse J: *Principles and Practice of Chiropractic*. Lombard, Ill, National College of Chiropractic, 1976, pp 218–219.
181. Reinert OC: *Chiropractic Procedure and Practice*, ed 3. Florissant, Mo, Marian Press, 1972, pp 17, 204.
182. Janse J, Houser RH, Wells BF: *Chiropractic Principles and Technic*. Chicago, National College of Chiropractic, 1947, pp 283, 343, 399.
183. Sullivan AW: Subluxation of the atlanto-axial joint: Sequel to inflammatory process of the neck. *Journal of Pediatrics* 35:451, 1949.
184. Sweat RW: Scanning palpation: Cervical spine. *Today's Chiropractic* January/February 1985, pp 23–24.
185. Bolender N, Cromwell LD, Wendling AL: Fracture of the occipital condyle. *American Journal of Roentgenology* 131:729–731, 1978.
186. Woodring JH, Selke AC Jr, Duff DE: Traumatic atlanto-occipital dislocation with survival. *American Journal of Roentgenology* 137:21–24, 1981.
187. Finney HL, Roberts TS: Atlanto-occipital instability: Case report. *Journal of Neurosurgery* 48:636–638, 1978.
188. Norrell HA: Fractures and dislocations of the spine. In Rothman RH, Simeone FA (eds): *The Spine*. Philadelphia, W.B. Saunders, 1975, vol 2, pp 552–553.
189. White AA, Panjabi MM: *Clinical Biomechanics of the Spine*. Philadelphia, J.B. Lippincott, 1978, pp 203–208.
190. Powers B et al: Traumatic anterior atlanto-occipital dislocation. *Journal of Neurosurgery* 4:12, 1979.
191. Gehweiler JA et al: Fractures of the atlas vertebra. *Skeletal Radiology* 1:97, 1976.
192. Patzakis MJ et al: Posterior dislocation of the atlas on the axis. *Journal of Bone and Joint Surgery* 56A:1260, 1974.
193. Evarts CM: Traumatic occipito-atlanto dislocation: Report of a case with survival. *Journal of Bone and Joint Surgery* 52A:1653, 1970.
194. Sherk HH, Nicholson JT: Fractures of the atlas. *Journal of Bone and Joint Surgery* 52A:1017, 1970.
195. Jeffreys E: *Disorders of the Cervical Spine*. London, Butterworths, 1980, pp 66–67.
196. Arthur P: Emergency! Assessing the spinal cord injured athlete. *ICA International Review of Chiropractic* January/February 1984, pp 45–47.
197. Olson WH et al: *Practical Neurology for the Primary Care Physician*. Springfield, Ill, Charles C Thomas, 1981, p 356.
198. Maiman DJ, Cusick JF: Traumatic atlantoaxial

dislocation. *Surgical Neurology* 18:388–392, 1982.
199. Jefferson G: Fracture of the atlas vertebra: Report of four cases and a review of those previously recorded. *British Journal of Surgery* 7:407, 1920.
200. Iverson LD, Clawson DK: *Manual of Acute Orthopaedic Therapeutics*. Boston, Little, Brown, 1977, p 109.
201. Budin E, Sondheimer F: Lateral spread of the atlas without fracture. *Radiology* 87:1095, 1966.
202. Amyes EW, Anderson FM: Fractures of the odontoid process: Report of 63 cases. *Archives of Surgery* 72:377, 1956.
203. Greenberg AD: Atlantoaxial dislocations. *Brain* 91:655, 1968.
204. White AA, Panjabi MM: *Clinical Biomechanics of the Spine*. Philadelphia, J.B. Lippincott, 1978, pp 211–212.
205. Norrell HA: Fractures and dislocations of the spine. In Rothman RH, Simeone FA (eds): *The Spine*. Philadelphia, W.B. Saunders, 1975, vol 2, pp 553–557.
206. Brashear HR, Venters GC, Preston ET: Fractures of the neural arch of the axis: A report of 29 cases. *Journal of Bone and Joint Surgery* 57A:879, 1975.
207. Effendi B et al: Fractures of the ring of the axis: A classification based on the analysis of 131 cases. *Journal of Bone and Joint Surgery* 63:319–327, 1981.
208. Jeffreys E: *Disorders of the Cervical Spine*. London, Butterworths, 1980, pp 68–72.
209. Anderson LD, D'Alonzo RT: Fractures of the odontoid process of the axis. *Journal of Bone and Joint Surgery* 56A:1663, 1924.
210. Ryan MD, Taylor TFK: Odontoid fracture: a rational approach to treatment. *Journal of Bone and Joint Surgery* London 64B:416–421, 1982.
211. Sherk HH, Nicholson JT, Chung SMK: Fractures of the odontoid process in children. *Journal of Bone and Joint Surgery* 60A:921–924, 1978.
212. Fielding JW: Os odontoideum: An acquired lesion. *Journal of Bone and Joint Surgery* 56A:187, 1974.
213. Minderhound JM, Braakman R, Penning L: Os odontoideum: Clinical, radiological, and therapeutic aspects. *Journal of Neurological Sciences* 8:521, 1969.
214. Wollin DG: The os odontoideum: Separate odontoid process. *Journal of Bone and Joint Surgery* 45A:1459, 1963.
215. Johl M, Seerup KK: Os odontoideum. *Acta Orthopaedica Scandinavica* 54:113–118, 1983.
216. Seljeskog EL, Chou SN: Spectrum of the hangman's fracture. *Journal of Neurosurgery* 45:3, 1976.
217. Schneider RC et al: "Hangman's fracture" of the cervical spine. *Journal of Neurosurgery* 22:141, 1965.
218. Elliott JM et al: The hangman's fracture: Fractures of the neural arch of the axis. *Radiology* 104:303, 1972.
219. Wood-Jones F: The ideal lesion produced by judicial hanging. *Lancet* 1:53, 1913.
220. Parke WW: Applied anatomy of the spine. In Rothman RH, Simeone FA (eds): *The Spine*. Philadelphia, W.B. Saunders, 1975, vol 1, pp 20–24, 42–43.
221. Johnson RM, Southwick WO: Surgical approaches to the spine. In Rothman RH, Simeone FA (eds): *The Spine*: Philadelphia, W.B. Saunders, 1975, vol 1, pp 79–83.
222. Kapandji IA: *Physiology of the Joints: The Trunk and Vertebral Column*, ed 2. New York, Churchill Livingstone, 1980, vol 3, pp 172, 192,
223. White AA, Panjabi MM: *Clinical Biomechanics of the Spine*. Philadelphia, J.B. Lippincott, 1978, pp 83–84.
224. Fisk JW: *The Painful Neck and Back*. Springfield, Ill, Charles C Thomas, 1977, pp 28–32.
225. Bergmann T: Integrated Chiropractic Methods. Oklahoma seminar, April 23, 1983, Northwestern Chiropractic College, p 8.
226. Gehweiler JA Jr, Osborne RL Jr, Becker RF: *The Radiology of Vertebral Trauma*. Philadelphia, W.B. Saunders, 1980, p 74.
227. Fisk JW: *The Painful Neck and Back*. Springfield, Ill, Charles C Thomas, 1977, pp 35–37.
228. Kapandji IA: *Physiology of the Joints: The Trunk and Vertebral Column*, ed 2. New York, Churchill Livingstone, 1980, vol 3, p 154.
229. White AA, Panjabi MM: *Clinical Biomechanics of the Spine*. Philadelphia, J.B. Lippincott, 1978, pp 71–74, 86–87.
230. Kapandji IA: *Physiology of the Joints: The Trunk and Vertebral Column*, ed 2. New York, Churchill Livingstone, 1980, vol 3, pp 196–198, 216–228, 238–244.
231. Grice AS: A biomechanical approach to cervical and dorsal adjusting. In Haldeman S (ed): *Modern Developments in the Principles and Practice of Chiropractic*. New York, Appleton-Century-Crofts, 1980, pp 345–349.
232. Jeffreys E: *Disorders of the Cervical Spine*. London, Butterworths, 1980, pp 7–8.
233. Veleanu C: The cervical locking mechanism. *Morphology and Embryology* 21(1):3–7, 1975.
234. Cailliet R: *Neck and Arm Pain*. Philadelphia, F.A. Davis, 1974, pp 15–17.
235. White AA, Panjabi MM: *Clinical Biomechanics of the Spine*. Philadelphia, J.B. Lippincott, 1978, pp 211–218, 235.
236. Albright JP et al: Head and neck injuries in sports. In Scott WN, Nisonson B, Nicholas JA (eds): *Principles of Sports Medicine*. Baltimore, Williams & Wilkins, 1984, pp 40–85.
237. Kapandji IA: *Physiology of the Joints: The Trunk and Vertebral Column*, ed 2. New York, Churchill Livingstone, 1980, vol 3, p 200.
238. Jirout J: Patterns of changes in the cervical spine on lateroflexion. *Neuroradiology* 2:164, 1971.
239. Nash CL, Moe JH: A study of vertebral rotation. *Journal of Bone and Joint Surgery* 51:223, 1969.
240. Kapandji IA: *Physiology of the Joints: The Trunk and Vertebral Column*, ed 2. New York, Churchill Livingstone, 1980, vol 3, pp 202–213, 244.
241. White AA, Panjabi MM: *Clinical Biomechanics of the Spine*. Philadelphia, J.B. Lippincott, 1978, p 71.
242. Cailliet R: *Neck and Arm Pain*. Philadelphia, F.A. Davis, 1974, p 17.
243. Kapandji IA: *Physiology of the Joints: The Trunk*

and Vertebral Column, ed 2. New York, Churchill Livingstone, 1980, vol 3, p 214.
244. Bergmann T: Integrated Chiropractic Methods. Oklahoma seminar, April 23, 1983, Northwestern Chiropractic College, pp 12–14.
245. Pierce WV: The fifth cervical key. *The Digest of Chiropractic Economics* July/August 1982.
246. Bergmann T: Integrated chiropractic methods. Oklahoma seminar, April 23, 1983, Northwestern Chiropractic College, pp 9–11.
247. Pettibon Bio-Mechanics Institute: *Pettibon Spinal Bio-Mechanics: Theory and Implications*, ed 2. Vancouver, Wash, Pettibon BioMechanics, 1976, pp 44–46, 94–99.
248. Kapandji IA: *The Physiology of the Joints.* New York, Churchill Livingstone, 1974, vol 3, pp 20–21.
249. Sandoz R: A classification of luxation, subluxation and fixation of the cervical spine. *Annals of the Swiss Chiropractors Association* 6:219–276, 1976.
250. Schmorl G, Junghanns H: *The Human Spine in Health and Disease.* New York, Grune & Stratton, 1971.
251. Herbst RW: *Gonstead Chiropractic Science and Art.* City of publication unknown, Sci-Chi Publishers, (undated).
252. Ng, SY: The relationship between atlas deposition and cervical curvature. *ACA Journal of Chiropractic* 13:79–83, September 1979.
253. Rehberger LP: Reversal of the normal cervical curve. *Roentgenological Briefs*, Council on Roentgenology of the American Chiropractic Association, Des Moines, Ia, (undated).
254. Kapandji IA: *Physiology of the Joints: The Trunk and Vertebral Column*, ed 2. New York, Churchill Livingstone, 1980, vol 3, pp 196–197.
255. Barge FH: *Torticollis.* Davenport, Ia, Bawden Bros, 1979.
256. Whtie AA, Panjabi MM: *Clinical Biomechanics of the Spine.* Philadelphia, J.B. Lippincott, 1978, pp 141–166, 183–184, 294, 295–296.
257. Cailliet R: *Soft Tissue Pain and Disability.* Philadelphia, F.A. Davis, 1980, pp 121–124.
258. Mennell JMcM: *Back Pain.* Boston, Little, Brown, 1960, pp 205–214.
259. Baltzell LG, Mackey RH (eds): *Firth's Technic Notes.* Publishing data not shown, 1967, pp 17–19.
260. Grecco MA: *Chiropractic Technic Illustrated.* New York, Jarl Publishing, 1953.
261. Grove AB: *Chiropractic Technique—A Procedure of Adjusting.* Madison, Wis, Straus Printing & Publishing, 1979.
262. Janse J, Houser RH, Wells BF: *Chiropractic Principles and Technic.* Chicago, National College of Chiropractic, 1947, pp 17, 283, 311, 456.
263. Reinert OC: *Chiropractic Procedure and Practice*, ed 3. Florissant, Mo, Marian Press, 1972.
264. Reinert OC: Anatomical characteristics of subluxation—C2 through C7. *ACA Journal of Chiropractic* May 1984, pp 62–69.
265. Stoddard A: *Manual of Osteopathic Practice.* New York, Harper & Row, pp 120–123.
266. Nwuga, VC: *Manipulation of the Spine.* Baltimore, Williams & Wilkins, 1976, pp 39–40, 51–56.
267. Maitland GD: *Vertebral Manipulation*, ed 3. London, Butterworths, 1974.
268. Sprague RB: The acute cervical joint lock. *Physical Therapy* 63:1424–1428, 1983.
269. Brodin H: Cervical pain and mobilization. *Manuelle Medizin* 20:90–94, 1982.
270. Gehweiler JA Jr, Osborne RL Jr, Becker RF: *The Radiology of Vertebrae Trauma.* Philadelphia, W.B. Saunders, 1980, pp 187–258.
271. Norrell HA: Fractures and dislocations of the spine. In Rothman RH, Simeone FA (eds): *The Spine.* Philadelphia, W.B. Saunders, 1975, vol 2, pp 535–551.
272. Jeffreys E: *Disorders of the Cervical Spine.* London, Butterworths, 1980, pp 72–74.
273. Jackson R: *The Cervical Syndrome.* Springfield, Ill, Charles C Thomas, 1966.
274. Selecki BR, Williams HBL: *Injuries to the Cervical Spine and Cord in Man.* Australian Medical Association, 1970.
275. Woodring JH, Goldstein SJ: Fractures of the articular processes of the cervical spine. *American Journal of Roentgenology* 139:341–344, 1982.
276. Beatson TR: Fractures and dislocations of the cervical spine. *Journal of Bone and Joint Surgery* 45B:31, 1963.
277. Evans DC: Biomechanics of spinal injury. In Gonzna ER, Harrington, IJ: *Biomechanics of Musculoskeletal Injury.* Baltimore, Williams & Wilkins, 1982, pp 183–185.
278. Jeffreys E: *Disorders of the Cervical Spine.* London, Butterworths, 1980, p 60.
279. Clark WM, Gehweiler JA, Laib R: Significant signs of cervical spine trauma. *Skeletal Radiology* 3:201, 1979.
280. McKenzie JA: The dynamic behavior of the head and cervical spine during "whiplash." *Journal of Biomechanics* 4:477–490, 1971.
281. Evans DC: Biomechanics of spinal injury. In Gonzna ER, Harrington, IJ: *Biomechanics of Musculoskeletal Injury.* Baltimore, Williams & Wilkins, 1982, pp 185–192.
282. Schneider RC: The syndrome of acute anterior spinal cord injury. *Journal of Neurosurgery* 12:95, 1955.
283. Bauze RJ, Ardran GM: Experimental production of forward dislocation in the human cervical spine. *Journal of Bone and Joint Surgery* 60B:239–245, 1978.
284. Gehweiler JA et al: Hyperextension fracture-dislocations of the cervical spine. *Medical Imaging* 3:12, 1978.
285. Medical news: Will the real whiplash patient tip back his head? *Journal of the American Medical Association* 238:2341, 1977.
286. Evans DC: Biomechanics of spinal injury. In Gonzna ER, Harrington IJ: *Biomechanics of Musculoskeletal Injury.* Baltimore, Williams & Wilkins, 1982, pp 192–200.
287. States J, Dodd M, Masengil J: The enigma of whiplash injury. *New York State Journal of Medicine* December 15, 1970, p 2971.
288. Jahn WT: Acceleration-deceleration injury. *Journal of Manipulative and Physiological Therapeutics* 1(2):95–102, June 1979.
289. Sunderland S: Mechanisms of cervical nerve root

avulsion in injuries of neck and shoulder. *Journal of Neurosurgery* 41:705–714, 1974.
290. Braakman R, Vinkens PJ: Unilateral facet interlocking in the lower cervical spine. *Journal of Bone and Joint Surgery* 49B:249, 1967.
291. Gehweiler JA et al: Cervical trauma: the common combined conditions. *Radiology*, 130:77, 1979.

SUGGESTED READINGS

Fox TF: A review of cervical spine lines. Postgraduate orthopedic notes. St. Paul, Minn, Northwestern College of Chiropractic.

Frankel CJ: Medical-legal aspects of injuries to the neck. *Journal of the American Medical Association* 169(3):216, January 1959.

George AW: A method for more accurate study of injuries to the atlas and axis. *ACA Journal of Chiropractic* December 1983, pp 41–51.

Grotten N: Survey of 100 cases of whiplash injury after settlement of litigation. *Journal of the American Medical Association* 162:865, 1956.

Homewood AE: Cervical micro-manipulation. *The Digest of Chiropractic Economics* November/December 1985, pp 26, 28–29.

Kukurin GW: Normal characteristics of the cervical spinal curve. *The Digest of Chiropractic Economics* November/December 1985, p 12.

Mertz JA: Videofluoroscopy of the cervical and lumbar spine. *ACA Journal of Chiropractic* August 1981, pp 74–75.

Murphy C et al: Continuous recording of neck rotation: preliminary observations. *Spine* 9:657–658, 1984.

Panjabi MM et al: Stability of the cervical spine under torsion. *Journal of Biomechanics* 11:189–191, 1978.

Schafer RC: *Symptomatology and Differential Diagnosis.* Arlington, Va, American Chiropractic Association. To be published in 1986.

Teranel JA: *Chiropractic Orthopedics and Roentgenology.* Newark, NJ, Medusa Press, 1953.

Thompson GH, Hohl M: Healed untreated anterior cervical spine dislocation: a case report. *Spine* 3:113–115, 1978.

Van Dusen LG: *Chiropractic Relationship to Gravitational Force.* Sodus, NY, published by the author, 1968, pp 111–117, 121–127.

Wyke B: Clinical significance of articular receptor systems. *Annals of the Royal College of Surgeons of England* 60(2):137, 1978.

CHAPTER 9

Selected Clinical Problems of the Cervical Spine and Temporomandibular Joint

This chapter describes the underlying clinical factors involved in and the management of cervical subluxation syndromes, neurovascular deficit syndromes of the neck, traumatic brachial traction, flexion-extension injuries, cervical disc disorders, and torticollis. Chronic inflammatory diseases of the cervical spine are described, as are not infrequently seen deformities and anomalies of the cervical spine. The chapter concludes with a discussion of temporomandibular joint (TMJ) dysfunction, its relation to cervical function, and its holistic significance.

A classification of musculoskeletal disorders of the neck is given in Table 9.1.[1-3]

CERVICAL SUBLUXATION SYNDROMES[4-13]

Subluxations, regardless of region, are difficult to classify under normal categories of trauma because they can involve bone, joint, muscle, ligament, disc, nerve, cord, or lymphatic and vascular tissues.

Terminology

An osseous disrelationship or an abnormal degree of physiologic segmental motion is generally considered a finding, and associated soft-tissue aberrations are considered part of the syndrome. It may be either a contributing cause or an effect. Thus, in this context, describing a subluxation would not be a diagnosis. However, some may consider the spine as an organ; ie, a part of the body exercising a specific function,[14] and the spine readily meets this definition. In this context, it would be difficult not to consider a specifically defined primary subluxation complex as a diagnosis in that the description provides a determination of the nature of a disease (ie, a disorder of body function). A disease entity is characterized usually by at least two of the following criteria: (1) a recognized etiologic agent (or agents), (2) an identifiable group of signs and symptoms, or (3) consistent anatomical alterations.[15] Rarely does a subluxation-fixation entity have difficulty in meeting these criteria (Table 9.2).[3]

Pathoanatomical Considerations

Once a vertebra loses its ideal relationship with contiguous structures and becomes relatively fixed at some point within its normal scope of movement, it is no longer competent to fully participate in ideal coordinated spinal movement. The affected area becomes the target for unusual weight-bearing and traumatic stress. In addition to attending circulatory and static changes in the involved area, there is disturbed neural activity that may be exhibited as changes in superficial and deep reflexes, tremors and spasms, hyperkinesia, pupillary changes, and excessive lacrimation.[16]

Pertinent Functional Anatomy of the Cervical Plexus[17-19]

The dura mater of the spinal cord is firmly fixed to the margin of the foramen magnum and to the 2nd and 3rd cervical vertebrae. In other spinal areas, it is separated from the vertebral canal by the epidural space. Since both the C1 nerve and the vertebral artery pass through this membrane and both are beneath the superior articulation of the atlas and under the overhanging occiput, atlanto-occipital distortion may cause traction of the dura mater, producing irritation of the artery and nerve unilaterally and compressional occlusion contralaterally. De Rusha feels that this helps us understand

Table 9.1.
Classification of Musculoskeletal Disorders of the Neck

ADULT CERVICAL DISORDERS
- Trauma of the cervical spine and cord
  - Subluxation-fixation
  - Soft tissue or disc injury
    - Without neural deficit
    - With neural deficit
      - Root signs
      - Cord signs
  - Acute herniated disc
  - Fracture or dislocation
    - Without neural deficit
      - Stable
      - Unstable
    - With neural deficit
      - Complete quadriplegia
      - Incomplete quadriplegia
        - Anterior cord syndromes
        - Central cord syndromes
        - Brown-Séquard syndrome
      - Nerve root injury
- Degenerative disc disease
  - Traumatic
  - Geriatric
  - Spondylosis
- Congenital anomalies
  - Congenital stenosis
  - Cervical rib
- Systemic disease causing bone texture alterations
  - Anemia
  - Leukemia
  - Paget's disease
  - Osteoporosis
  - Hodgkin's disease
- Inflammatory diseases
  - Ankylosing spondylitis
  - Rheumatoid arthritis
  - Infections
- Tumors
  - Primary, of bone
  - Secondary, metastatic
    - Men: prostate, lung
    - Women: breast

CHILDHOOD CERVICAL DISORDERS
- Trauma
  - Soft tissue or disc injury
  - Cervical sprain
  - Cervical strain
  - Subluxation
  - Fracture or dislocation
- Acquired torticollis
- Congenital deformities
- Metabolic disease and bone dysplasias
  - Morquio's disease
  - Spondyloepiphyseal dysplasia
  - Diastrophic dwarfism
  - Central disc calcification
- Inflammatory disease
  - Juvenile rheumatoid arthritis
  - Ankylosing spondylitis
  - Vertebral/disc infections
- Tumors of the cervical spine
  - Primary (uncommon)
  - Secondary (rare)

INFANTILE CERVICAL DISORDERS
- Congenital disorders of cervical spine
  - Congenital torticollis
  - Atlanto-occipitalization
  - Basilar invagination
  - Odontoid process dysplasia
  - Vertebral fusion
  - Spinal dystrophia
- Birth injuries
  - Delivery-related subluxations
  - Cord injuries
  - Nerve injuries
  - Epidural hemorrhage
  - Bone injuries

those cases of suboccipital neuralgia in which a patient upon turning his head to one side increases the headache and vertigo that are relieved when the head is turned to the opposite side.[20]

There is also a synapse between the upper cervical nerves and the trigeminal nerve, which also supplies the dura mater. This may explain why irritation of C1 results in a neuralgia not only confined to the base of the skull but also referred to the forehead or eye via the supraorbital branch of the trigeminal nerve. The greater occipital (C2) nerve does not tend to do this. It exits between the posterior arch of the atlas and above the lamina of the axis (Fig. 9.1), referring pain to the atlanto-occipital area (Fig. 9.2) and often to the vertex of the head.

The superficial sensory cutaneous set of the cervical plexus (C1–C4) is frequently involved in subluxations of the upper four segments (refer to Table 8.4), particularly

Table 9.2.
Cervical Motion-Unit Dysfunction

Criteria	Nature of acute/chronic cervical subluxation-fixation complex: comon examples	
Etiologic agent	Abnormal structural support Contractures Inequal muscle balance Paralysis	Poor sleeping postures Somatic or visceral response Sprain Strain
Symptoms	Articular grating Headaches Neuralgia Numbness Pain (especially on motion) Possible remote somatic effects	Possible remote visceral effects Stiffness Tenderness Tension Upper extremity pain Weakness
Signs	Altered normal reflexes Boggy tissues (focal) Electromyographic signs Fibrosis Hyperemia Hypertonic/flaccid muscles Segmental atrophy	Skin electro-resistance alterations Skin temperature alterations Skin texture alterations Thermographic signs Trigger point development Visual postural imbalance
Anatomical alteration	Palpable malalignment Roentgenographic signs	Segmental motion alterations

when there are predisposing spondylitic degenerative changes. Janse[21] describes four resultant neuralgias: (1) *lesser occipital nerve neuralgia,* involving the posterior area of the occipitofrontalis muscle, mastoid process, and upper posterior aspect of the auricle; (2) *greater auricular nerve neuralgia,* extending in front of and behind the auricle, to the skin over the parotid gland, paralleling the distribution of the auriculotemporal branch of the trigeminus and easily misdiagnosed as chronic trifacial neuralgia; (3) *cervical cutaneous nerve neuralgia,* involving the area of the middle third of the platysma to the midline, possibly extending from the chin to the sternum; (4) *supraclavicular nerve neuralgia,* depending upon which rami are affected, the neuralgia may involve the suprasternal area, pectoral area, or deltoid area. Thus, sternoclavicular and acromioclavicular neuralgias may originate in the spinal levels of the supraclavicular nerve.

De Rusha[22] suggests that dysphagia and dysarthria may at times be due to upper cervical involvement rather than a central nervous system situation. The C1 joins the hypoglossal cranial nerve, which supplies the intrinsic muscles to the tongue. It then descends to join the descending cervical which is derived from C2 and C3. A loop of nerves, the ansi hypoglossi, which supplies muscles necessary for deglutition and speaking, is derived from C1–C3.

Irritative lesions involving the cervical articulations may in turn irritate the sympathetic nerve plexuses ascending into the head via the vertebral and carotid arteries. Some cases of visual and aural symptoms are related to upper cervical distortion in which the arch of the atlas snugly hugs the occiput, thus possibly irritating the sympathetic plexus near the vertebral artery as well as partially compressing the vessel. To appreciate this, note that the visual cortical area of the occipital lobe requires an ideal blood supply dependent on the sympathetics ascending the great vessels of the neck; this holds true for the inner ear as well. To test this syndrome, De Rusha[23] suggests having the supine patient read some printed matter while the examiner places gentle traction on the skull, separating the atlanto-occipital articulations. A positive sign is when the patient, often to his surprise, experiences momentarily enhanced visual acuity or a reduced tinnitus.

Cervical Nerve Root Insults[24–28]

Disturbances of nerve function associated with subluxation syndromes basically man-

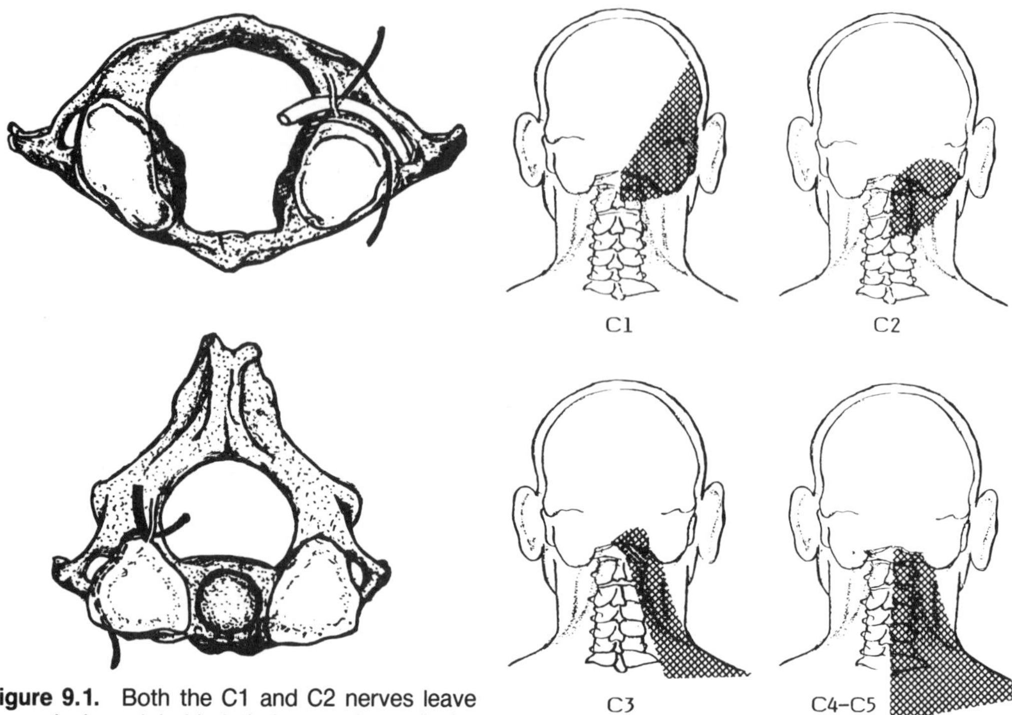

Figure 9.1. Both the C1 and C2 nerves leave the spinal cord behind their superior articular facets. *Top*, C1 follows a groove on the upper surface of the posterior arch of the atlas, posteroinferior to the atlanto-occipital capsule and beneath the vertebral artery as it crosses the atlas. *Bottom*, C2 transverses the arch of the axis behind the facet and in contact with the capsule. It exits the spinal canal through a small opening in the ligamentum flavum.

Figure 9.2. Areas of referred pain from C1–C5 nerve root irritation.

ifest as abnormalities in sensory interpretations and/or motor activities (Fig. 9.3). These disturbances may be through one of two primary mechanisms: direct nerve or nerve root disorders, or of a reflex nature.

Sensory Changes. When direct nerve root involvement occurs on the posterior root of a specific neuromere, it manifests as an increase or decrease in sensitivity over the dermatome. A typical example includes foraminal occlusion or irritating factors exhibited clinically as hyperesthesia, particularly on the dorsal and lateral aspects of the thumb and radial side of the hand, when involvement occurs between C5 and C6. Another example is on the dorsum of the hand, the index and middle fingers, and the ventroradial side of the forearm, thumb, index and middle fingers, when involvement occurs between C6 and C7. In other instances, this nerve root involvement may

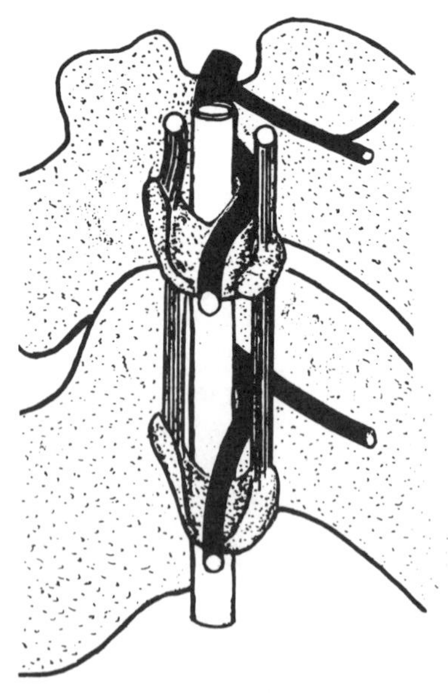

Figure 9.3. Schematic showing how a cervical nerve is forced against the medial aspect of the transverse process by the much larger vertebral artery. The vertebral vein is not shown.

cause hypertonicity and the sensation of deep pain in the musculature supplied by the neuromere. For example, in C6 involvement, there is deep pain in the biceps; or in C7 involvement, there is deep pain in the triceps and supinators of the forearm. Direct pressure near the nerve root or along its distribution may be particularly painful.

Motor Changes. Nerve root insults from subluxations may also be evident as disturbances in motor reflexes and/or muscle strength. Examples of these reflexes include the deep tendon reflexes, as seen in the reduced biceps reflex when involvement occurs between C5 and C6; or the reduced triceps reflex when involvement occurs between C6 and C7. These reflexes must also be compared bilaterally to judge whether hyporeflexia is unilateral. Unilateral hyperreflexia is pathognomonic of an upper motor neuron lesion. Prolonged and/or severe nerve root irritation may also cause evidence of trophic changes in the tissues supplied.

Underlying Factors. The common subluxation picture is rarely pure. It is often superimposed upon subclinical processes in the mature patient such as vertebral instability, osteochondrophytic ridges at the uncovertebral joints, apophyseal thickening and exostosis, or canal encroachment by a buckling ligamentum flavum, spinal stenosis, posterior vertebral body spurs, disc protrusions, dura and dentate thickening, arachnoid cysts, dura and arachnoid adhesions, and ossification of the posterior longitudinal ligament.

Loss of disc space, especially in the lower cervical area, may contribute as a source of chronic irritation to an already inflamed root by altering the angulation of the IVF tunnel. The sequence of inflammation, granulation, fibrosis, adhesion formation, and nerve root stricture may follow, along with a loss in root mobility and elasticity. These degenerative changes are not as pronounced during youth.

Subluxation-Induced Reflex Syndromes[24]

Certain spinosomatic and spinovisceral syndromes may result from cervical subluxation. For example, if the involvement is in the area of C1–C4, the cervical portion of the sympatheic gangliated chain or the 9th–12th cranial nerves as they exit from the base of the skull and pass into their compartments within the deep cervical fascia may be involved. The syndrome may include (1) suboccipital or postocular migraine; (2) greater occipital nerve extension neuralgia; (3) mandibular, cervical, auricular, pectoral, or precordial neuralgia; (4) paroxysmal torticollis; (5) congestion of the upper respiratory mucosa, paranasal sinuses, or eustachian tube with hearing loss; (6) cardiorespiratory attacks; (7) ocular muscle malfunction; (8) pathologic hiccups; (9) scalenus anticus syndrome; or (10) painful spasms in the suboccipital area.

Phillips[29,30] states that if a subluxation produces a stretching of the paravertebral musculature, there will be a continuous barrage of afferent impulses in the Group Ia fibers. "These afferent impulses monosynaptically bombard the alpha motor neurons causing the paravertebral musculature to go into tetany. There is a cessation of this afferent barrage when the stretch is released. The muscle stretching also initiates afferent impulses in the Group II afferents from flower spray endings which may reinforce the spastic muscle condition." He goes on to say that trauma to facet joints, disturbed articular relationships, spasms of closely related muscles, and overlying trigger points—all the result of a subluxation—set up a barrage of flexor-reflex afferent impulses via the Group II–IV fibers that converge upon the internuncial pool in lamina 7 of the spinal cord. "This abundant supply of flexor-reflex afferent impulses excites the alpha motor neurons through multisynaptic connections causing an excess of excitation of paravertebral muscles resulting in spasm."

Neurovascular Implications of Upper Cervical Subluxations[20,31]

Loss of mobility of any one or more segments of the spine correspondingly influences circulation. The resulting partial anoxia has a harmful influence upon nerve function. The artery and vein supplying a spinal nerve are situated in the foramen between the nerve and the fibrous tissue in the anterior portion of the foramen. It is unlikely that circulation to the nerve would be disrupted without first irritating or compressing the nerve because the arteries and veins are much smaller, the blood pressure within the lumen makes them resistant to compression, and nerve tissue is much more responsive to encroachment irritation.

The Vagus Nerve. As the vagus lies almost in immediate contact with the transverse process of the atlas, rotary subluxation of the atlas may cause pressure that produces a wide range of symptoms. The syndrome produced may exhibit as nasal and sinus congestion, swallowing and speech difficulties, cardiac arrythmias, functional coronary artery spasm, gastric and intestinal colic, and other symptoms of vagal disturbance.

The Medulla Oblongata. The medulla oblongata extends well into the lower reaches of the foramen magnum and the ligamentous ring that connects it with the atlas, thus any type of occipital or atlantal subluxation may produce abnormal pressure on this portion of the brain stem. Bilateral posterior shifting of the occiput or atlas may cause pressure upon the pyramids or adjacent olivary bodies producing a syndrome of upper motor neuron involvement characterized by a degree of spastic paralysis or ataxia. A lateral shifting of the occiput may cause pressure upon the tubercle of Rolando, producing pain in the area of trigeminal nerve distribution, headache, sinus discomforts, ocular neuralgias, and aches in the jaw.

The Vertebral Arteries. Janse relates that any cervical subluxation (particularly atlantal, axial, or occipital) producing muscle spasm may produce unilateral or bilateral constriction of the vertebral arteries resulting in circulatory impairment.[32] A large number of equilibrium, cardiac, respiratory, cranial nerve, extrapyramidal, vagal, visual, and auditory symptoms may follow. The vertebral nerve (sympathetic) runs along the vertebral artery within the arterial foramen of the cervical transverse processes. Irritation to this nerve is considered to occur from mechanical irritation to the vertebral artery anywhere along its course, producing symptoms of a vasomotor nature; eg, headache, vertigo, tinnitus, nasal disturbances, facial pain, facial flushing, and pharyngeal paresthesias. Cailliet[33] points out that although sympathetic fibers have not been found along the cervical roots, surgical decompression of an entrapped nerve root relieves symptoms attributed to the sympathetics. The mechanism for this effect is unclear.

The Vertebral Veins and Deep Cervical Veins. Spasm of the suboccipital muscles may cause a decided impediment of venous drainage from the suboccipital area via vertebral and deep cervical veins, resulting in a passive congestion with consequent pressure upon the sensory nerve endings in the area. This is perceived by the patient as unilateral or bilateral pain and a throbbing discomfort and may be palpated as knotty lumps within suboccipital muscles. The condition appears to be of a reflex nature more common among people under mental tension or those who work closely with their eyes over long periods.

Cerebrospinal Circulation. Any event that would cause constriction in the connecting area between the cerebral subarachnoid space and the vertebral canal limits the escape of cerebrospinal fluid into the inferior vertebral canal. This results in a degree of increased intracranial pressure. An atlanto-occipital subluxation may cause the dura mater of the cisterna cerebellaris to be pressed against the posterior medullary velum and to partially occlude the foramina of Luschka and Magendie and interfere with the flow from the 4th ventricle. The resulting increase of intraventricular fluid accumulation may create a large variety of symptoms such as deep-seated, stubborn, "internal pressure" headaches, nausea, a tendency toward projectile vomiting, bizzare and unusual visual disturbances, and protopathic ataxis.

Headaches of Cervical Origin[34–37]

It has been the experience of Markovich, the renowned neurologist, that the most common headache is the type caused by neuromuscular skeletal imbalance.[38] He points out that "the head in the human species has changed its position from the quadruped to the erect, thereby changing the basic relationship between the cervical spine and the head, with its important functional structures, and the rest of the body." For reference, he calls attention to the quite delicate interaction and highly sensitive biofeedback or servo-mechanisms that continually make adjustments in body balance, vision, pressure, and hearing with head and neck posture. "These regulatory, homeostatic mechanisms can be disturbed by a variety of conditions, originating at any level, including the inflammation and/or irritation of the cephalic projection of the upper cervical nerves (cervico-occipital neuralgias)."

In offering a neurologic appraisal of pain in the head, Kraus[39] states: "It has been my experience that the most common cause of headaches originates in the 'vicious circle' generated by the abnormal and painful contraction of the cervical-nuchal muscles, mainly the trapezius muscle. These contractions generate a type of 'ischemic irritation' that includes the entrapment of the second cervical nerves (greater occipital and lesser occipital) as they travel through the bulk of the muscle, ascending into the back of the head to innervate the posterior scalp region, the temporal areas, and the lobes of the ears, sending terminal branches into the angle of the jaw, the back of the eye, and the vertex of the head." This process can create a distinct clinical syndrome that is easily confused with atypical "vascular migraine" because of the unilaterality of the symptoms and the frequent complaints of pain in the back of the eye with or without visual disturbance.

Kraus[39] also states that the second most common entity is the TMJ pain dysfunction syndrome, which has been proven to be more common than many expect and has so many protean manifestations that it has become known as *The Great Imposter.* "The fact that a cervical nerve irritation can create a painful condition in the angle of the jaw or in the temple explains the possible common 'irritative' source of both syndromes."

Differentiation of various types of headaches is shown in Table 9.3, adapted from Markovich's data.[40] However, keep in mind that a patient may not exhibit such a clear-cut picture. For example, vascular migraine may be superimposed on occipitocervical neuralgia or episodes may be interposed, depending upon the causes involved.

Structural Fixations[41–49]

A vertebra may be fixed in a position it could normally occupy during any phase of physiologic movement; thus a fixated segment is hypomobile, enjoying a less than full range of movement but still occupying a position possible for a normal motion unit. In a typical vertebral fixation, nothing may be subluxated or "out of place." On the contrary, the involved segment is too much "in place"; ie, the full expression of movement is blocked. Such states are the most common form of chronic subluxation seen in chiropractic.

While fixations are not visible on static x-ray films, motion palpation reveals the subtleties of incomplete fixations as a loss of "joint play," an erratic jumpy motion at some point during the arc of movement, or as a paradoxical movement in which the involved segment moves in the opposite or divergent direction to the overall spinal movement.

Joint Play[50–52]

Every healthy articulation (spinal or extraspinal) can be moved through its planes of normal motion actively and passively without causing pain. In addition to this, there is an accessory movement called "joint play" that cannot be influenced except passively. Joint play can be defined as that degree of joint movement allowed passively that cannot be achieved through voluntary effort (Fig. 9.4).

Although joint play cannot be produced by phasic muscle contraction, voluntary action is greatly influenced by normal joint play. This is because the loss of joint play results in a painful joint that becomes involuntarily protected by secondary muscle spasm (splinting). Thus, motion palpation to detect restricted joint play is an important part of the biomechanical examination of any painful and spastic axial or appendicular joint.

When normal joint play is restored to a joint by correction manipulation, the pain caused by restricted joint play soon subsides and the associated muscle spasm relaxes. This manipulation usually requires a carefully directed dynamic thrust in the plane of restricted motion.

Motion Palpation of the Cervical Spine[4, 53–64]

The objectives of dynamic palpation are to note (1) normal and abnormal segmental

Table 9.3.
Differentiation of Common Types of Headaches

Symptom/Sign	Occipito-cervical neuralgia	Trigeminal neuralgia	Vascular migraine	Temporomandibular traction
Pain	Throbbing, paroxysmal, dull	Excruciating, paroxysmal	Severe, paroxysmal	Severe, dull
Quality	Muscle spasms	Stabbing	Throbbing	Dull ache
Location	Occipital	Facial	Unilateral	Facial
Aura	None	None	Visual	None
Duration	Days	Brief	Hours	Chronic
Associated symptoms and signs	Earache Eye pain Blurred vision Blepharospasm Hypersalivation Neck pain Paresthesias, scalp Anxiety Tinnitus Nausea/vomiting	Trigger zones in posterior neck, shoulder girdle	Vomiting Photophobia Scotomata Irritability	Bruxism Malocclusion Earache Joint clicks

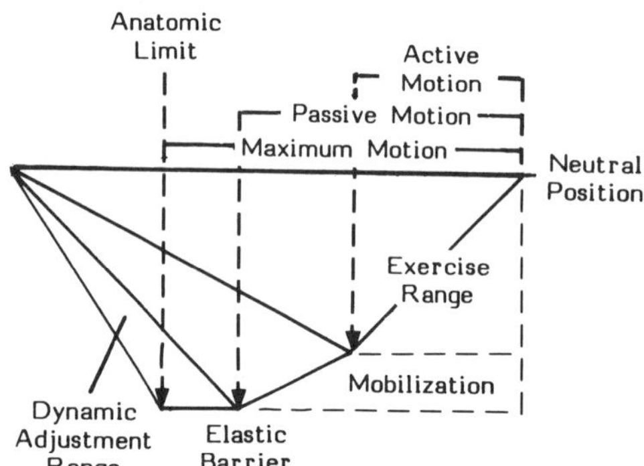

Figure 9.4. Comparative ranges of movement during exercise, mobilization, and dynamic adjustive techniques.

motion and (2) motion restrictions, "jumps," erratic gliding, and motion smoothness. Thus, quantity and quality of bilateral motion are concerns.

During motion palpation, each cervical vertebra is palpated during flexion, extension, rotation, and lateral flexion to assess segmental mobility. The amount of motion in any particular joint depends upon (1) the shape of the joint surface, (2) the laxity or tautness of supporting ligaments, and (3) the condition of the related musculature. Essentially, the extent of movement below the axis is dependent upon ligamentous and muscular laxity and the distortion and compressibility of the IVDs.

Atlanto-occipital Palpation. Spinal motion palpation usually starts with the articulation between the occiput and the atlas. Flexion, extension, rotation, and lateral flexion should be evaluated.

1. *Flexion-extension.* In cervical extension, the atlas projects forward as a unit; in flexion, the atlas rolls backward. The examiner's palpating finger is placed within the space between the tip of the transverse of the atlas and the ramus of the jaw, while the supporting hand on the patient's scalp forces the patient's head into extension so that the chin moves up and forward and then into flexion so that the chin moves down and inward. Note the change in space underneath the palpating fingertip. The space should normally open on extension and close on flexion. These movements, conducted several times, should be restricted as

much as possible to the upper cervical area and tested bilaterally.

2. *Rotation.* In rotating the atlas horizontally anteriorly without flexion or extension, there is normally a wider separation between the jaw and the transverse process. That is, the transverse-jaw space opens as the head is turned away from the palpating finger and closes as the head moves toward the palpating finger. This is a difficult motion to palpate because of the bulging of the sternocleidomastoideus.

3. *Lateral flexion.* The tip of the palpating finger is placed deep within the small space between the tip of the C1 transverse process and the mastoid process of the occiput. As the support hand rocks the patient's scalp laterally, the space change should be noted as the ipsilateral occipital condyle rolls laterally up and out on the atlas as the scalp moves away from the palpating finger, and down and in as the head is laterally flexed toward the palpating finger. On flexion to the right, the transverse-mastoid space should open on the left and close on the right.

Differentiating Atlanto-occipital Muscular and Ligamentous Fixations. The tip of the palpating finger is placed under the posterior occiput, midway between the occipital notch and the mastoid process. Some examiners prefer to cup the atlas in the web of the palpating hand so that the thumb palpates one side while the first finger palpates the other side. The supporting hand rocks the patient's head into flexion and extension. If a stubborn ligamentous fixation is present, the fibrous tissues will palpate as a hard mass that does not change texture during motion.

Posterior and Anterior Atlanto-occipital Fixations. During A-P examination, the ramus of the jaw may be felt to flip distinctly superiorly rather than rolling anteriorly. Gillet believes this hinge-type motion (rather than a rolling motion) is the result of hypertonicity of the rectus posterior minor muscle, either unilateral or bilateral, that produces restricted motion of the posterior atlas but free motion of the anterior atlas.[65] If this is the case, forced motion will produce a shear force. On the other hand, if the anterior muscles are hypertonic, the anterior aspect of the condyle(s) will be compressed against the anterior lateral mass(es) of the atlas, while the posterior aspect opens. This can be palpated on forced motion by placing the palpating finger in the posterior aspect of the transverse-mastoid space while the patient's head is forced into extension and flexion.

Atlantoaxial Palpation. The most important movements to evaluate here are rotation and lateral bending.

1. *Flexion-extension.* The palpating finger is placed in the space between the posterior tubercle of the atlas and the spinous of the axis. This space should open on flexion and close on extension, and the posterior tubercle should become more apparent on flexion and be lost to touch on extension.

2. *Rotation.* The tips of the first three fingers are placed horizontally in the suboccipital space so that the first finger firmly presses against the occipital notch and the third finger rests lightly on the tip of the C2 spinous process. The free hand is used to rotate the head. During rotation, several degrees of atlas rotation should take place before the axis begins to move. Normally, the third finger will slip upon the spinous process of the axis as the head is rotated because the head moves 1 cm or more prior to C2 motion. Bilateral atlantoaxial fixation is indicated if the axis immediately follows the movement of the head (essentially the atlas), noted by the third finger not gliding over the process of the axis. If unilateral (pivotal) fixation is present, this situation will occur during rotation to one side but not to the other, and the center of movement will be at the point of fixation rather than at the odontoid. If the axis is fixed unilaterally, rotary movement will also be felt on the free side during A-P motion.

3. *Lateral flexion.* It has been Gillet's experience that abnormal lateral flexion of the atlas on the axis is affected most by hypertonicity of the intertransversarii and/or the upper aspect of the longus coli.[66] Motion restricted can be determined by placing the tip of the palpating finger in the posterolateral space between the transverse processes of the atlas and axis. Space changes are checked during both lateral flexion and A-P motion. While intertransversarii hypertonicity restricts lateral bending, a small degree of lateral gliding of the atlas on the axis

is usually allowed. This does not appear to be true when hypertonus of the longus coli exists.

Illi's experiments showed that rotation of the occiput and atlas produced a 3–4-mm migration of the spinal root ganglia and spinal cord proper within the lower cervical and upper dorsal area. However, if the occiput and atlas were locked together and then rotated, the migration was 6 mm or more. This is evidence that spinal fixations, especially of the upper cervical area, produce an undue tension upon the cord, the dorsal root ganglia, and the meninges and their attachments.

Axis and Lower Cervical Palpation. Flexion, extension, rotation, and lateral bending motions should be evaluated for each segment when possible.

1. *Flexion-extension.* In flexion and extension, the interspinous spaces should be felt to open and close.

To check A-P joint play of any cervical vertebrae, place the thumb and middle finger on the articular pillars of the vertebra being examined. With the other hand (stabilizer), cup the patient's forehead in the palm. Place the patient's neck in full passive flexion and then extension, and check for additional joint play at the end of each passive motion by applying digital pressure with the contact hand.

2. *Rotation.* Areas of rotary fixation are quite easily determined except in the athlete with extremely heavy posterior neck muscles. The patient rotates the head as far as possible in one direction. Then the palpating fingers glide down the posterolateral aspect of the transverse processes. The contact is made by the tips of the palpating fingers pushing the belly of the sternocleidomastoideus anteriorly. A firm "bulge" will be evident over the restricted transverse, and this is usually attributed to a hypertonic multifidus or intertransversarii muscle.

To check rotational joint play of any cervical vertebrae, take the same contacts as above. Rotate the patient's head to one side and then to the other, checking for additional joint play at the end of maximum passive rotation.

3. *Lateral flexion.* The axis is palpated in lateral bending as moving away from the flexion. To evaluate lateral gliding of the axis, the examiner's thumb is firmly pressed against the posterolateral aspect of the C2 spinous process, while the supporting hand moves the patient's scalp in wide lateral flexion.

The third cervical may be palpated during lateral bending, flexion, and extension much like the axis, noting the separation and closure of the spinous process on A-P motion and rotation and lateral bending by palpating the posterolateral space between the transverse processes. Rotation reveals minimum motion and is difficult to palpate. The same procedure is applied to the rest of the cervical spine. However, palpation in the middle and lower cervical region is difficult because the palpating finger is usually against tender nerves. Some examiners prefer an interlaminae contact.

To check lateral flexion joint play of any cervical vertebra, make an index finger contact on the lateral aspect of the vertebra being examined. Laterally flex the patient's head over the contact finger, and check for additional joint play at the end of passive motion.

Common Types of Middle and Lower Cervical Fixation. The two most common types of fixation in this area are those of the interspinous and covertebral areas.

1. *Interspinous fixation.* Hypertonicity of one or more extensors tends to bind spinous processes together so that a local lordosis is formed. This condition, often found at the C3–C4 level, is palpable when the spinous processes refuse to open during forced flexion. It is also often evident on lateral flexion roentgenographs showing two or more vertebrae that do not follow the curve of the neck as a whole.

2. *Covertebral articular fixation.* Fixation is common at the lips of the joints of Luschka by longus colli hypertonicity, ligamentous shortening, and exostosis. Restricted motion can often be determined during A-P motion from the anterolateral by carefully pushing the esophagus laterally with two palpating fingers and evaluating the motion of the vertebral bodies. If, during passive extension, it is found that the patient's neck stops sharply at a point far short of normal extension, Gillet refers to this "brick wall" sign of strong restriction as an indication of cervical osteophytes.[67] This is

a classic sign of chronic degeneration found in the cervical joints of the elderly presenting a thin, "dry" cervical spine. These fixations usually produce a chronic brachialgia.

Upper Cervical Fixations from Hypertonicity[68, 69]

Because the cervical muscles are directly involved with the righting reflex, their stretch reflexes are normally relatively hyperactive. Chronic multimuscular contractions in the suboccipital area will often palpate as an area of tough ligamentous fixation, and, if this is the case, they should be considered as ligaments therapeutically.

Common Sites of Muscular Fixation. There are six major pairs of anterior and posterior muscles operating in the atlanto-occipital area to produce A-P rocking of the occiput on the atlas and atlas rotation. Any one or more of these muscles can be in a state of hypertonicity, thus maintaining the numerous types of upper cervical subluxation.

1. *Obliquus capitis superior.* This muscle joins the transverse process of the atlas to the occiput. Hypertonicity restricts contralateral extension and lateral flexion (Fig. 9.5).

2. *Obliquus capitis inferior.* This muscle spans between the spinous process of the axis and the transverse process of the atlas. Hypertonicity will tend to fixate the atlas-axis articulation, especially on rotation toward the opposite side. The spinous process of the axis will often be palpated as being distinctly pulled laterally.

3. *Rectus capitis posterior (minor and major).* The minor arises from the posterior tubercle of the atlas and the major from the spinous process of the axis. Both insert at the occiput and function in extension of the head upon the neck. Hypertonicity produces approximation of the C2 spinous process and the occiput, thus increasing upper cervical lordosis and restricting flexion mobility. Gillet feels this state is usually the manifestation of a lower fixation (eg, anterior thoracic).[70]

4. *Rectus capitis anterior and lateralis.* The anterior part originates on the lateral mass of the atlas and inserts in the basilar part of the occiput. The lateral aspect arises from the transverse process of the atlas and inserts at the jugular process of the occiput (Fig. 9.6). Both serve to flex and support the head. Hypertonicity restricts extension.

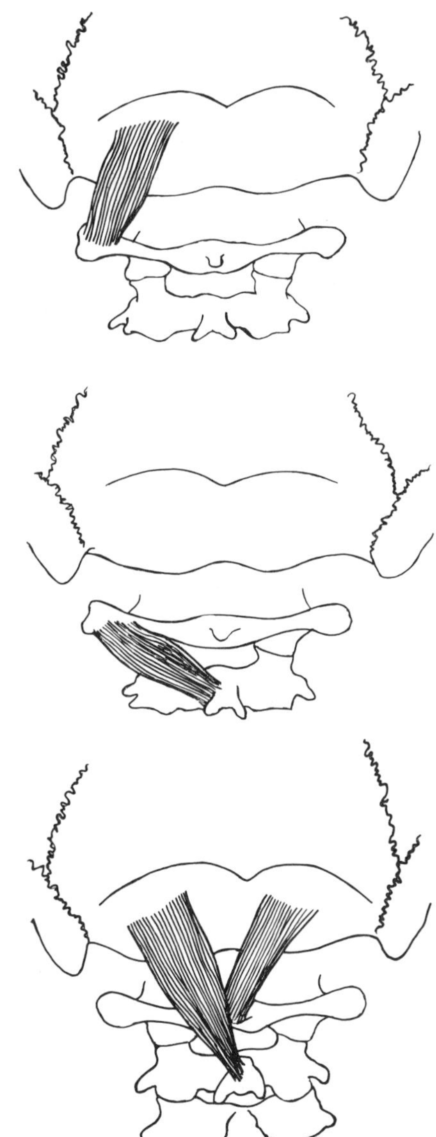

Figure 9.5. *Top*, left obliquus capitis superior muscle; *center*, left obliquus capitis inferior; *bottom*, left rectus capitis posterior major and right rectus capitis posterior minor.

5. *Longus colli.* Hypertonicity of the cervical branches of this muscle produces a greater fixed space between the C2 spinous process and the occiput. The picture is the converse of rectus capitis posterior shortening.

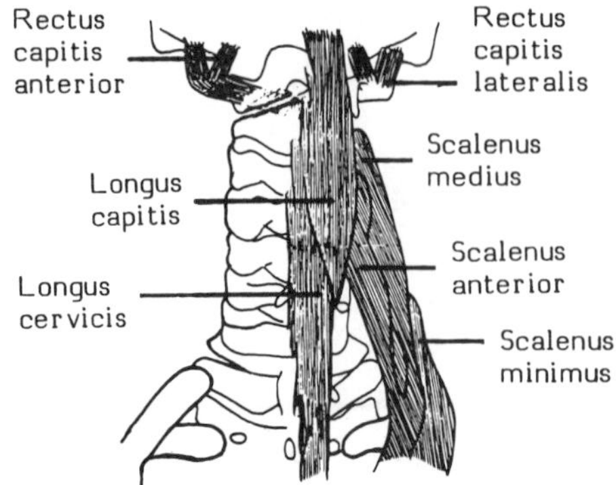

Figure 9.6. The major prevertebral muscles.

6. *Longus capitis.* This muscle arises from the transverse processes of the C3–C6 vertebrae and inserts at the basilar portion of the occiput. It functions in head flexion.

Occipitoaxial Locking. Although the occiput and axis are not contiguous, hypertonicity of the rectus capitis major posteriorly and/or longus colli anteriorly will tend to firmly bind these structures together. In the neutral position, a hypertonic rectus capitis major pulls the occiput against the spinous of C2, as seen in normal extension. This state remains palpable even in forced flexion by placing a palpating finger in the space behind the usually unpalpable posterior tubercle of the atlas. Conversely, a hypertonic longus colli tends to force the occipitoaxial space open, frequently allowing the posterior tubercle of the atlas to be palpated in the neutral position. This space does not appreciably close on forced extension, because the occiput and axis will move as a fixed unit if locked.

Secondary Fixations. Gillet feels that, although upper and lower cervical hypertonicities of the short muscles (eg, occipitoaxial locking) are quite common, they are often secondary effects from lower sites of fixation.[71, 72] Thus, they return quite quickly after correction unless the primary fixation is released.

Lower Cervical Fixations from Hypertonicity[73, 74]

The A-P Prime Movers. Hypertonicity of the sternocleidomastoideus (Fig. 9.7) and related flexors forces increased mobility upon the posterior arches, a decrease in height of the anterior anulus, and restricts

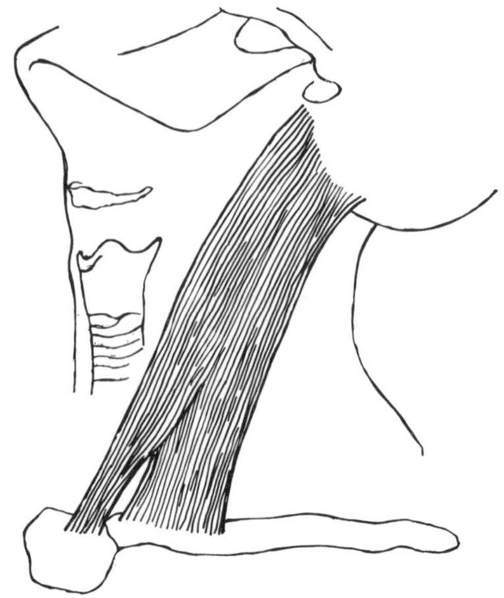

Figure 9.7. The left sternocleidomastoideus muscle.

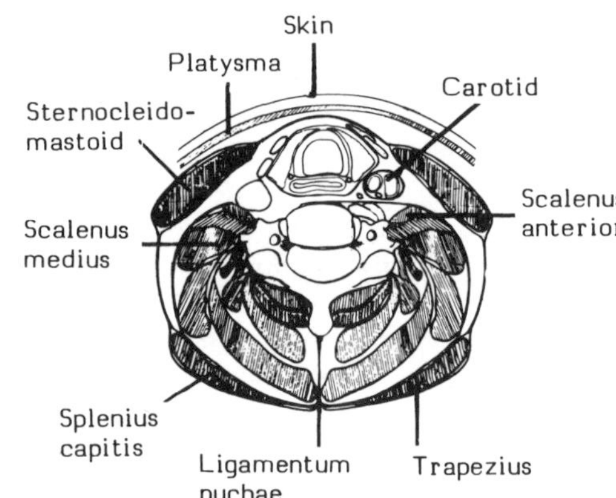

Figure 9.8. Diagram of transverse section at the midcervical area, showing the relative arrangement of the cervical musculature.

extension. The disorder may be either unilateral or bilateral. This is the converse of generalized posterior cervical muscle shortening that restricts flexion, decreases posterior IVD thickness, and forces increased mobility upon the anterior anular fibers. Either anterior or posterior hypertonicity tends to decrease the normal range of rotation but less so than hypertonicity of the rotatores (Fig. 9.8).

The Intertransverse Muscles. Because of the plane of the cervical facets, unilateral hypertonicity produces lateral flexion of the superior vertebra and a degree of rotation of the inferior vertebra. Bilateral hypertonicity exaggerates the cervical lordosis. If the curve has previously flattened, the kyphosis will be exaggerated.

The Interspinous Muscles. These muscles are often well developed in the cervical area. Bilateral hypertonicity produces a motion-unit lordosis that, more often than not, is asymptomatic except on deep palpation.

The Multifidi and Rotatores. The weak cervical multifidi are especially prone to fixation in the C4–C6 cervical area, while the rotatores are frequent sites at the C2–C3 levels.

Lower Cervical Fixations from Ligament Shortening[75]

The Anterior Longitudinal Ligament. This appears to be the only frequent site of adverse ligamentous fixation in the lower cervical region (Fig. 9.9).

The Intertransverse Ligaments. These ligaments are infrequent sites of pathologic fixation. They are usually palpable when the relaxed neck is laterally flexed.

Motion Measurements in Cervical Fixations[76]

Several investigators of cervical mobility have noticed that it is quite difficult to determine the effects of specific fixations on the overall mobility of the cervical region because each fixation is accompanied by an area of hypermobility. It appears on cineroentgenography that a degree of exaggerated mobility is capable of compensating for fixation restriction wherein the overall measurement appears normal.

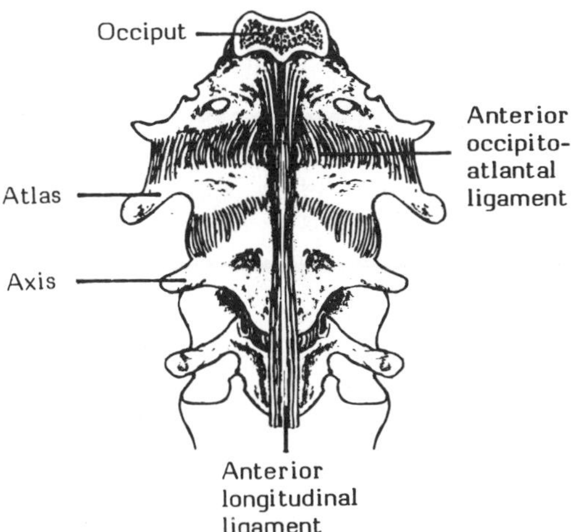

Figure 9.9. The major prevertebral upper cervical ligaments.

Gillet states that when the degree and number of fixations are such that there is no place for areas of consequent hypermobility, the overall ranges of movement are much more visibly restricted.[77] This is especially true when the fixations are bilateral; in which case, more gross methods can be used in assessment.

The degree of extension possible is calculated by Gillet by pulling the head and neck backward to a maximum degree short of pain and inspecting the patient in profile. An imaginary line is then made at the posterior edge of the ear, and a mark is made with a skin pencil at the point where this line cuts the shoulder. There will usually be a gain in mobility of a few centimeters after an adjustment. In nonosteophytic types of fixations of a principally muscular nature, the postadjustive change will be much greater.

The examiner measures the degree of anterior flexion by placing his chest against the patient's mid-dorsals to prevent thoracic movement and then directing the patient's head down and forward to a maximum short of pain. While the patient is in this position, the C7 spinous process is marked with a skin pencil. Then with a spirit level placed horizontally from that point to the ear, another mark is made where the horizontal line cuts the imaginary ear line. In a normally mobile neck, this point should meet the top of the auricle while the line in a stiff neck will cuts its base.

This offers the examiner two measures: one indicating restriction caused by fixation at the anterior aspect of the cervical spine and the other at the posterior aspect. One of these is usually greater than the other.

Gillet's research has shown that nearly all partial fixations found in the cervical region are secondary to more primary fixations in the remainder of the spine or in extraspinal joints (disappearing upon correction of the primary factors). The effects of these extracervical primary factors upon cervical rotation and lateral flexion mobility can also be measured. The examiner sits directly behind the patient and reaches forward, grasping the occiput of the patient in one hand and the chin in the other. The head of the patient is then rotated to an easy maximum with care taken not to force the patient's shoulders around at the same time. The examiner may hold the patient's shoulders back with his forearm. Then, holding the head in rotation with one hand, a point is drawn with a skin pencil on the patient's shoulder exactly under an arbitrary point to the ear. The head is then turned to the opposite side and a point is made on the other shoulder, exactly under the one made on the same point of the other ear. A third point is then marked on the C7 process, and the space between the two exterior points and the C7 will indicate the relative degree of mobility in rotation of the whole cervical spine. In a fairly supple neck, this distance should not be more than a centimeter; in a stiff neck, it may be up to 4 cm. These measurements can be used for all fixations in the cervical area; but because of the lesser degree of normal movement between the occiput and atlas, it will not be influenced as much by fixation there.

Some partial fixations hinder lateral flexion more than any other movement. This is especially true of the uncovertebral fixations, which are quite frequent in the C4–C6 region. To measure these fixations, the patient's head is flexed to the side to an easy maximum with one hand on the skull and the other on the ipsilateral shoulder to prevent it from following the movement. Again, an arbitrary point on the ear is selected and a mark is made on the shoulder directly under it while the patient's neck is in maximum lateral flexion. The same is done in lateral flexion of the opposite side, and, as in rotation, the space between the two shoulder points and the C7 process is measured. In a supple neck, the points should be quite close to the C7 spinous and may overlap it. In a stiff neck, this space may measure up to 3 cm on either side, but this is rare. Naturally, painful conditions of the neck influence the above measurements. In fact, they may be very difficult to measure in cases of acute torticollis.

Gillet found that most patients seemed to turn their heads less to the right than to the left, and no fixation could be found to be responsible for this anomaly in mobility.[78] It appears to be normal for right-handed people, and the opposite appears true for left-handed people.

Passive Cervical Sidebending

The importance of palpable asymmetry in response to passive cervical sidebending has been admirably brought out by Johnston and associates who concluded that it appears to be an early indicator of a measurable impairment of cervical function, even in the absence of pain or other complaints.[79] Thus, the role of segmental motion palpation in preventive health care is underscored.

Segmental motion studies should not be confused with gross motion studies. When a motion unit becomes dysfunctional, it exhibits asymmetrical behavior that is palpable. In addition, secondary (compensatory) effects spread to adjacent units, usually within three segments, which does not necessarily limit regional function.[80] Only in advanced stages in which multiple units are involved will overt regional motion be affected.

Visual Subluxation Patterns[81–86]

Clinical postural patterns reflect an individual's biomechanics that are responsive to underlying physiologic processes. This is readily appreciated clinically in many acute conditions such as the antalgic positions of sciatica, extremity dislocation, the opisthotonus of spinal meningitis, the orthopnea of asthma, the emprosthotonus of tetanus, the pleurothotonus of strychnine poisoning, the rigid abdominal spasm of peritonitis, and other postures that a patient might assume to gain relief.[87] However, the postures reflected in chornic subluxations are much more subtle and often assumed unconsciously through proprioceptive mechanisms.

The analysis of "body language" opens the way for much subjective interpretation, and there is a tendency to point to signs that confirm one's interpretation and ignore those that do not. Nevertheless, as shown in our previous discussion of gait, many specific neuromusculoskeletal disorders can be accurately judged by observing the body in stance and in action.[88, 89] The interpretation of spinal distortion patterns is likewise an art, and, as in any diagnostic art, its effectiveness is in knowing the normal from the abnormal and knowing where the normal or abnormal begins and ends.

Several chiropractic researchers feel that many postural distortions are essentially massive movement of structure held in fixation by impulse bombardment initiated by neural excitement. In this sense, a visual pattern is a clue that must be confirmed by other diagnostic methods such as static and dynamic palpation and roentgenography. Other researchers feel that it is most difficult to relate specific subluxations to gross postural patterns.

In this section and especially in the future chapters on the thoracic spine and the lumbar spine and pelvis, we will offer some of the basic premises of visual subluxation patterns with the hope that this will stimulate further research in spinal analysis.

Cervical Subluxation Patterns

In normal neutral posture, the ears (semicircular canals) and eyes will be held level and parallel to the shoulders for resting orientation.[90] Inspection is best made by using a double plumb line or a transparent grid and a foot-stabilizing device. De Jarnette feels that practically all subluxation patterns have some effect upon the occiput and upper cervical spine.[91,92] Any shifting of the cranial mass (eg, tilt) will have an effect upon the cervical muscles which, in turn, alter the stabilization of the position of the head upon the cervical spine. When the occiput, atlas, and axis are in good relationship, the ears will appear level and equally prominent, reflecting equal weight distribution bilaterally and good functioning of the righting mechanism (Fig. 9.10).

Occipital Subluxation Patterns[91, 93–95]

When viewed from the posterior, an occiput inferior on the right due to a compressed condyle, for example, will present a head tilt low on the right. The ears will be equally prominent. A purely rotational subluxation of the occiput on the atlas will exhibit a level skull with the ear on the side of relative posteriority more prominent (Fig. 9.11).

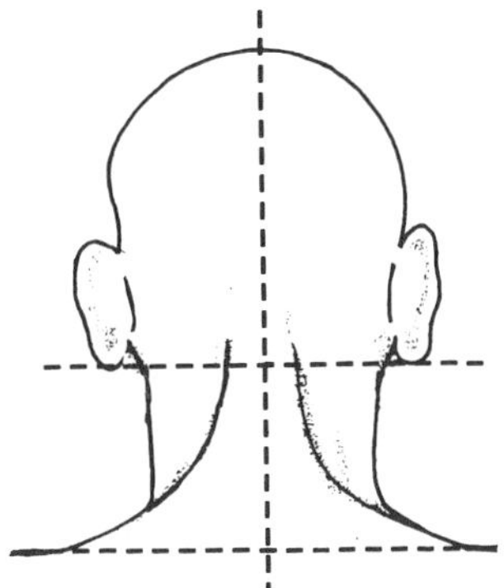

Figure 9.10. The normal cervical pattern.

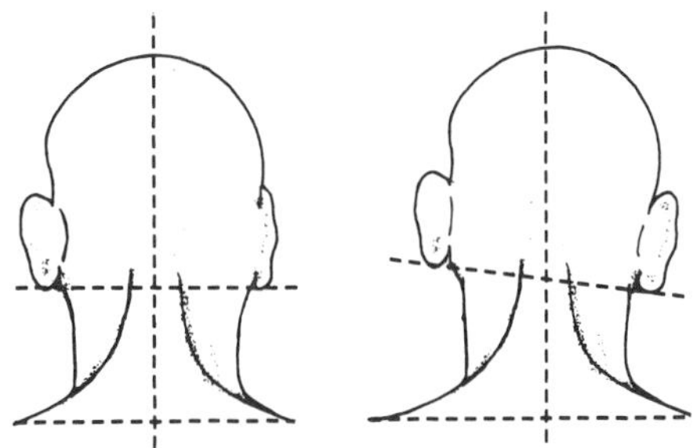

Figure 9.11. *Left*, occiput fixed in a left posterior rotation. The head is level but rotated as shown by the more prominent left ear. *Right*, visual pattern of a compressed condyle on the right or atlas lateral left. There is head tilt with equal prominence of the ears.

Atlas Subluxation Patterns[91, 93, 95–97]

It is theorized by many that every atlas subluxation changes the way that the skull adapts to body posture. When there is an occipital tilt and the ear is more prominent (rotated posteriorly) on the side of occipital superiority, an ipsilateral posterior or contralateral anterior atlas subluxation is suspected (Fig. 9.12).

When the atlas is fixed in a posterior rotation on the right or an anterior rotation on the left, the right ear and mandible will be more prominent (rotated posteriorly) than the left when viewed from the posterior. The prominence of the mandible is said to be due to the subluxation's effect upon the axis.

An atlas fixed in abnormal lateral flexion will present a tipped occiput shown by unlevel ears, but the ears will be equally prominent. This is the same picture as that of a contralateral sunken condyle. With such a

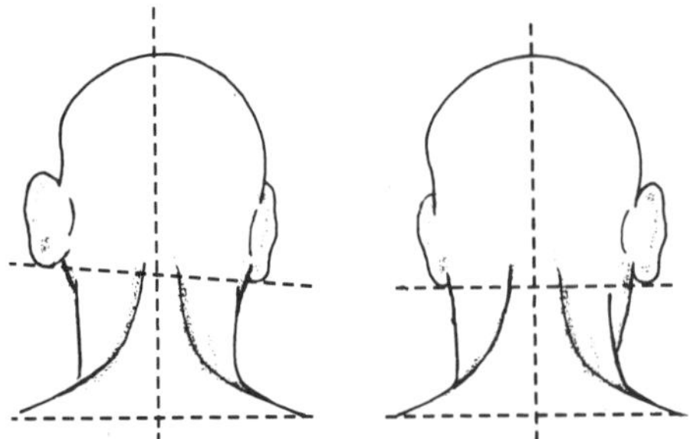

Figure 9.12. *Left*, cervical pattern of atlas rotated left posterior or right anterior with occipital tilt. *Right*, atlas rotated right posterior or left anterior without occipital tilt.

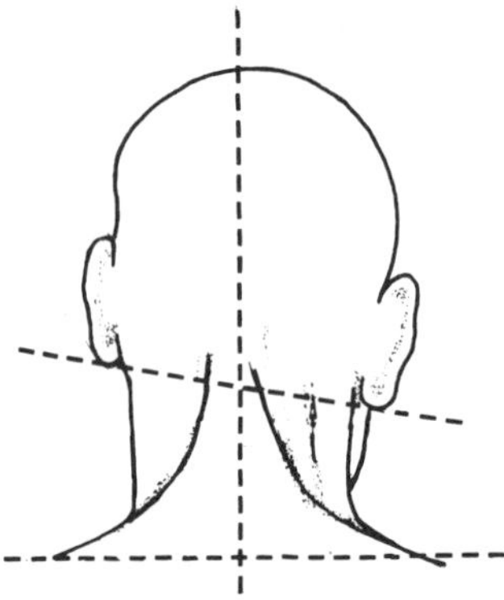

Figure 9.13. Cervical pattern of axis rotated posteroinferiorly on the right. The skull tips low on the right, and the right ear and mandible are more prominent. Distortion is exaggerated in the drawing.

subluxation, reports De Jarnette, the shoulders will be level or one will be slightly low on the side of atlas inferiority if shoulder problems are associated.[91] That is, the arm will be carried low on the side of atlas side slip.

Axis Subluxation Patterns[91, 93, 98, 99]

Rotary subluxations of the axis also appear to present a typical picture. An axis subluxation changes the way the skull balances upon the atlas. If the axis is fixed posterior and inferior on the right, for example, the right ear will be rotated posteriorly and be more prominent, and the skull will be tipped inferiorly on the right when viewed from behind (Fig. 9.13). A unilaterally prominent mandible is thought to be an effect only in axis subluxations or when the axis influences an atlas subluxation.

Cervical Subluxations with Sciatica Syndromes[100–102]

It is not unusual to see cervical complaints associated with a case of true sciatica. In right sciatica, for example, the patient's stance may exhibit very little distortion when viewed from the posterior. If the patient is asked to raise his left heel, however, a pronounced inferior tilt of the skull on the left may appear with the dorsolumbar spine forming a mild left scoliosis. When the patient is asked to lower his left heel and raise his right heel, the dorsolumbar curve increases, an acute right dorsocervical scoliosis develops, and the occipital tilt is increased (Fig. 9.14). The raising of the right heel invariably increases right sciatic pain, according to De Jarnette, and also produces cervical pain.[103] This manifestation is said to indicate a primary or secondary cervical subluxation, but other means will be necessary to isolate the exact segmental level of involvement.

Therapeutic Cervical Traction[104–107]

The term *traction* comes from the Latin *tractico,* which means to draw or pull.[108] In general, any procedure in which a longitudinal tensile force is applied to a part of the body in an effort to stretch soft tissues or open joint spaces can be called traction.

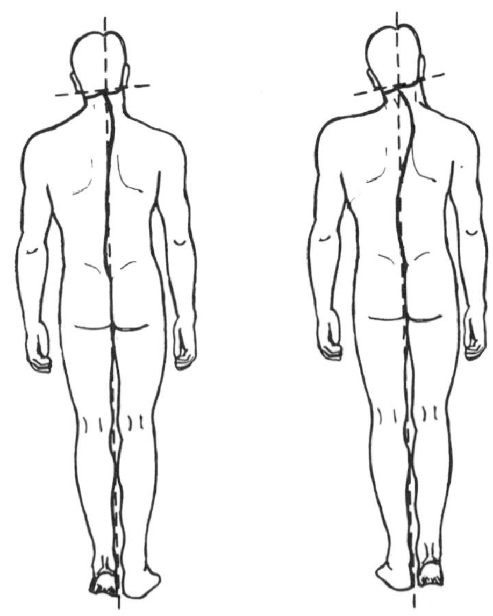

Figure 9.14. A typical thoracocervical subluxation pattern during heel lift with right sciatica.

Thus, traction is the opposite of joint approximation (compressed joint surfaces). Traction forces promote mobility, and compressive approximation of joints promotes stability. In either case, joint receptors are responsive to alterations in joint motion, tension, and position.[109]

Basically, traction encourages length, alignment, and functional stability. These goals become a priority in cases of mild structural compression that result in ischemia and pain sited either locally and/or distally, which in turn result in muscle spasm producing functional contraction. The associated nerve irritation, which may be sensory, motor, or both, may exhibit signs of pain, flaccidity, and diminished reflexes.[110]

Types of Traction and Their Objectives

Several types of traction are in common use today. The type selected depends partly on what objective(s) the practitioner wishes to achieve and partly on the patient's physical condition.

Continuous Traction. Continuous traction to the spine makes use of a constant pull that may be applied for periods of from several minutes up to several hours or days at a time. Its major effects are that it encourages plastic remodeling; immobilizes tissues; places muscles in a state of physiologic rest, which, in turn, relaxes muscle spasm; relieves the effects of compression on articular surfaces, effects that are due to muscle spasm or other compressive factors; and stimulates proprioceptive reflexes, thus relieving associated pain and tenderness. It also reduces the circumference of the IVD, thus aiding in restoring it to a position that allows for normal biomechanics (eg, by suction, molding, axial pull), and relieves compression effects of foraminal distortion and/or narrowing; ie, it increases the IVF's diameter. A by-product of these effects is the dissipation of congestion, stasis, edema, and dural-sleeve adhesions in associated tissues. In addition, it stretches perivertebral and intervertebral fibrotic tissues and adhesions (anticontracture factor), and relieves compression effects on articular tissues (eg, cartilage, discs) due to muscular spasm, gravity, or other compression forces (commonly seen in chronic subluxations) to restore connective tissue resiliency and contour.

Intermittent Traction. Intermittent traction is one of the more common types of traction applied today in general practice. With this type of traction, a mechanical unit applies a series of stretches interspaced with periods of relaxation. This method is used primarily to (1) reduce congestion in chronic musculoskeletal disorders and (2) provide increased mobility in patients with arthritic complaints. The pumping action created by alternating traction encourages soft-tissue elasticity and increases vascular flow and lymphatic drainage (suction aspiration effect), which tend to increase tissue flexibility and reduce stasis, edema, and coagulates in chronic congestion. The alternating pull and relaxation periods promote IVD hydration and nutrition by encouraging the expansion and contraction of disc tissues. The process tends to stretch and free periarticular and articular adhesions and fibrotic infiltrations, stimulate proprioceptive reflexes, and help tone muscles—all of which tend to reduce fatigue and restore elasticity and resiliency, thus serving as an efficient supplement to manual adjustments.

Positional Traction. Positional traction utilizes pillows, sandbags, rolls, or blocks, which are placed in such a way that a tensile force is placed on the involved perivertebral structures. The technique is usually performed to affect only one side of the spinal region being treated.

Miscellaneous Types. Other types of traction in use today include devices that the patient wears, special traction benches, roller tables, traction on split tables or inclined surfaces, and more recently, gravity inversion traction.

Application[111–119]

The primary indications for intersegmental spinal traction are IVD protrusion, degenerative disc disease, joint hypomobility, spinal nerve root impingement, muscle spasm, and compression fractures. A general rule, but one that must always be reconsidered in individual cases, holds that static traction should be used in acute conditions and intermittent traction in subacute and chronic disorders.

In order to achieve a beneficial traction

effect, the forces used must be of sufficient strength and duration and of appropriate direction and angle. The resistance offered by the patient to the traction forces depends on the weight of the patient plus such other factors as the size, contour, and texture of the two congruent surfaces (ie, the patient's skin and the table surface).

Force of Pull. As a general rule, continuous (sustained) cervical traction is started at 10 lb and increased gradually (eg, by 5-lb units) to patient tolerance. Do not exceed 30 lb. Intermittent (alternating) traction generally utilizes a force that is approximately 5–10% of the patient's total body weight. The usual range is from 15 to 30 lb maximum.

Duration of Pull. Experience has shown that (1) traction weight is relative to treatment duration; ie, less weight should be used for longer treatment times, and (2) heavier poundage can be used for shorter durations.[120] The time length of therapy depends on the specific condition being treated, the physical status of the patient, and patient tolerance. Intermittent traction is rarely applied for more than 30 minutes (15 minutes is average), while sustained traction of up to several hours may be appropriate. The duration of therapy must be adjusted to the circumstances. Undertreatment is better than excessive poundage or duration; these factors can always be increased after a trial period.

Direction of Pull. The patient should be placed in a position that will best affect the area of treatment. Pads, pillows, rolls, and other devices are helpful. It is usually best to have the patient in a horizontal or modified horizontal position. In this manner, longitudinal tensile forces can readily be effected to the cervical or lumbar regions. An adjustable table designed for this purpose is shown in Figure 9.15. With the patient in the sitting position, vertical traction forces can also be applied to the cervical region by using a harness, straps, weights, and a pulley system.

Angle of Pull. When applying the forces of traction to the cervical region, the head should be placed in 25–30° of flexion when the forces are applied to affect C3–C7, or in 0° of flexion when the forces are applied to affect the occiput, atlas, or axis. These examples refer to traction forces applied bilaterally. However, in some instances unilateral traction may be indicated, such as in unilateral joint hypomobility, spasticity, or spinal curvatures. When a protective (antalgic) scoliosis is present, traction is applied to the contralateral side of pain unless an unusual circumstance indicates otherwise.[121]

Precautions[122–124]

All apparatus should be kept in a sanitary condition. Have the patient remove dentures, ear-rings, glasses, or a wig before being harnessed. Secure attachment halters, straps, or other traction connections firmly but with ample padding to the skin, underlying soft tissues, and osseous structures. Care must be taken not to fasten halter straps too tightly. Ensure that the halter straps are not twisted, and carefully avoid jerking the rope when slack is removed from it.

Traction weight should be increased and/or decreased slowly to avoid abrupt reactions and adjusted to meet the conditions at hand. The amount of poundage utilized should be measured by a superimposed scale. Ensure that pressure points on the skin do not become irritated; eg, use facial tissue in the chain portion of the halter. Excessive traction will easily result in skin damage, thus one must carefully monitor proper padding, strapping, poundage, and angulation. Discontinue treatment immediately if adverse symptoms or signs appear; then seek and appraise the cause.

When the patient is placed in the horizontal position, the patient's feet should not be allowed to dangle in the air; ie, the legs should be well supported. During cervical traction in the seated position, the patient's arms should be placed on a lap pillow or cushion to relieve tension on the neck. Patients undergoing traction should not be allowed to read during treatment.

Postural Realignment[125, 126]

Because the center of gravity of the head lies anterior to the occipital condyles, definite force must be applied by the posterior muscles of the neck to hold the head erect. In addition, several groups of muscles are attached directly or indirectly to the anterior

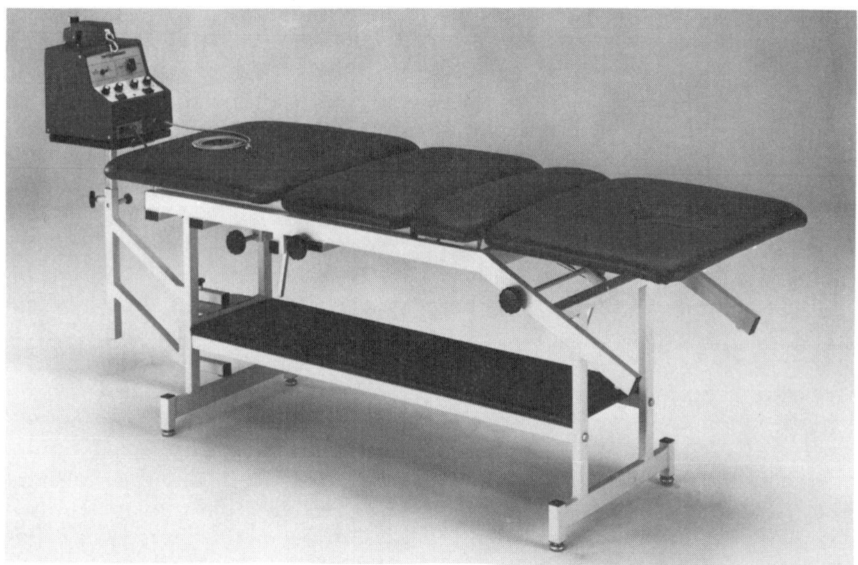

Figure 9.15. Adjustable traction table, Model TRF-24 (courtesy of the Chattanooga Corporation).

part of the head, and their function adds to the force of gravity to increase the load on the posterior cervical musculature. Gelb[127] feels that the most important anterior neck muscles are the masticatory and supra- and infrahyoid groups, which constitute a sort of chain with the hyoid bone and mandible to which they are attached. They join the head to the shoulder girdle anteriorly.

Deformity of cervical posture can be associated with or without neck pain. As discussed, the deformity may depict curvature exaggeration, flattening, occipital tilt, rotation, and areas of complete or partial segmental fixation. If pain is present, deviation may be toward or away from the site of pain, depending upon the primary site of irritation. Keep in mind that spinal stability is essentially under the control of neuromuscular mechanisms rather than the ligaments.

Although segmental spasm or instability may not be detectable by observation, it usually becomes evident by alert dynamic palpation. Careful localization of motion and muscle strength is necessary prior to prescribing any exercise program to assist postural realignment.

Proprioception[128–130]

In general, the abundant proprioceptors of the vertebral column enable the brain to know where each segment is and what it is doing at any given time without visual confirmation. More specifically, data about the degree of muscle tension and/or the length of muscles are relayed via the muscle spindles and Golgi tendon organs. Tension messages are moved through fast-conducting nerves from annulospiral endings and through higher threshold nerves from flower-spray receptors in the muscle spindle. The less complex Golgi tendon organs near the musculotendinous junctions discharge impulses initiated by either muscle contraction or stretch. Other receptors near the articular surfaces relay messages about joint speed and direction of motion.

In postural realignment, as Gelb[131] points out, restoring muscles to their physiologic resting length is a three-dimensional concept, which requires placing the origin and insertion of muscles in a correct three-dimensional relationship.

As mentioned previously, Lieb shows a number of full spine x-ray prints of severe spinal distortions greatly improved through improvement of dental occlusion.[132] If the temporomandibular joint has such a proprioceptive influence upon posture, it is no wonder that chiropractors who specialize in solely upper cervical or sacral correction exhibit a likewise abundance of such before- and-after exhibits—each spinal segment is richly endowed with equal or greater receptors than that of the jaw.

The Cervical Spinal Receptors[133]

The apophyseal joints of the cervical spine are richly innervated with mechanoreceptors and afferent fibers, endowed more than any other spinal region. Activity from the cervical articular receptors exerts significant facilitatory and inhibitory reflex effects on the muscles of the neck and both the upper and lower extremities.

Wyke[145] points out that the patterns of "normal cervical articular mechanoreceptor reflexes are profoundly distorted when cervical articular nociceptive afferent activity is added to that derived from the normally functioning cervical mechanoreceptors." To underscore this point, he states that (1) manipulation of the head on the neck can produce coordinated flexion and extension movements on the paralyzed arm and leg of a hemiplegic patient, (2) arm movement control in the absence of visual aid is considerably affected by rotation of the head, and (3) induced unilateral local anesthesia of the cervical joints in healthy subjects produces severe postural instability, dizziness, nystagmus, and muscular incoordination.[134] These signs and symptoms are similar to those experienced by some patients who suffer from cervical spondylosis, ankylosing spondylitis, and gross fixations, and some patients while wearing an orthopedic cervical collar.

Righting Mechanisms[135–137]

Several head extensors arise from the lower cervical and upper thoracic vertebrae that exert an oblique posteroinferior pull on the occiput. If the line of pull falls behind the atlanto-occipital joint, a rotary movement results that tilts the occiput posteriorly and lifts the face so that the neck is hyperextended. However, if this posterior rotation of the head is inhibited by the cervical flexors (which is normal), the oblique pull tends to have a posterior translatory component when the head is anterior to the midline. This serves to bring the head back toward the vertical gravity line and into better alignment.

In addition, the longus group exerts a bowstring action on the anterior cervicals that assists in axial extension of the neck. Thus, the extensors essentially serve to return the head to the midline following flexion, but axial extension is really completed by a straightening of the cervical lordosis produced by segmental *flexion*. If this segmental flexion did not occur during extension, the head would rest in the neutral position facing superiorly. Simultaneously, the thoracic extensors tend to straighten the dorsal curve so that the alignment of the entire cervicothoracic region is improved (Fig. 9.16).

Chronic flexion of the lower cervicals tends to produce elongation of the posterior upper thoracic soft tissues and adaptive shortening of the anterior elements (eg, anterior longitudinal ligament, anterior disc anulus, pectorals, intercostals). This is often seen in aging in which a contributing factor is degeneration of the normally fibroelastic ligamentum nuchae that helps to resist anterior deviation of the head. If this chronic flexion state occurs, cervical extension to the midline following flexion is fairly limited to increasing the cervical lordosis with little axial extension of the neck by segmental flexion. The neck angles forward, and the jaw juts out as the occiput rolls backward.

Weak Flexor Strength[138]

If weak neck flexion is evident (Fig. 9.17), emphasis should be on developing the sternocleidomastoideus, longus group, and rectus capitis anterior and lateralis. The longus groups and rectus capitis group are direct antagonists to the posterior cervical muscles.

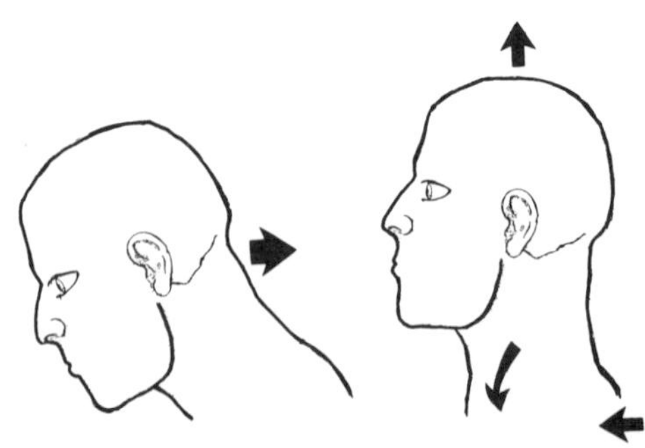

Figure 9.16. *Left*, in axial extension of the cervical spine, the cervical extensors return the neck to the midline. *Right*, the deep cervical flexors straighten the spine, and the thoracic extensors reduce the thoracic kyphosis.

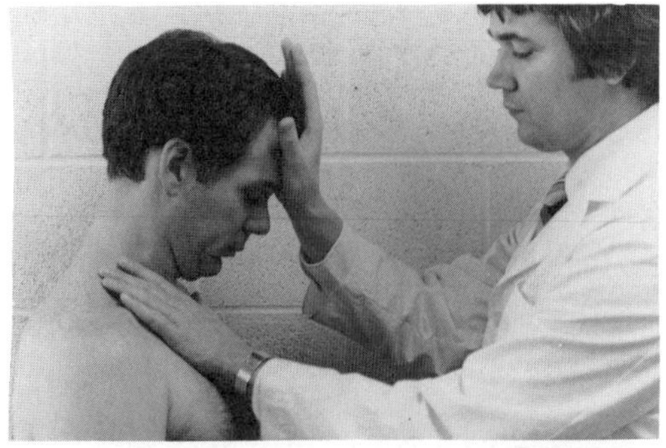

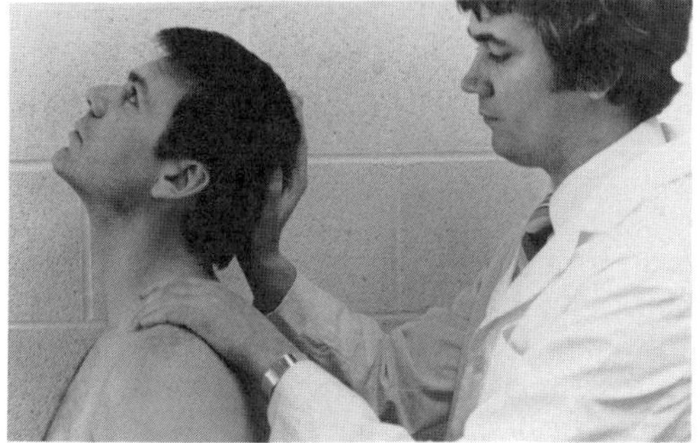

Figure 9.17. *Top*, testing flexion strength against resistance; *bottom*, testing extension strength.

They principally serve to right the neck after extension but have some activity in flexion from the neutral position. Hyperflexion, viewed as a flattened or kyphotic cervical curve, may be a manifestation of prevertebral hypertonicity, weak extensors, or a posteriorly displaced disc nucleus.

Weak Extensor Strength[139]

Clinical development of the trapezius, semispinalis capitis, splenius group, and erector spinae should be made if weak extension strength is evident. Only in the thoracic region do the erector spinae act solely as erectors. Their contraction in the cervical region produces hyperextension with a posterior rotation of the occiput so that the chin points upward. Hyperextension, viewed as hyperlordosis, may be a manifestation of extensor hypertonicity or weak prevertebral muscles.

With two exceptions, specific isotonic exercises will not be mentioned here—the literature abounds with many good regimens. However, the rationale behind isotonic exercises following trauma deserves attention.

The Cervicothoracic Interrelationship

The lateral gravity line of the body falls quite anterior to the midthoracic region. With fatigue, there is a tendency for thoracic kyphosis to increase. Thus when cervical alignment is poor, equal concern must be given to reduce an exaggerated thoracic kyphosis, for the positions of the cervical and thoracic regions are interrelated; ie, a thoracic kyphosis is usually accompanied by a compensatory cervical lordosis, and vice versa.

Exercises following Cervical Trauma[140,141]

Fisk points out that the reflex response to pain is an increase in isometric muscle activity by the small γ-fibers and a decrease in isotonic activity for the purpose of continuously resting (splinting) an irritated area.[142] This inactivity tends to reduce impulses from the large fibers of the muscle and joint proprioceptors so that the spinal cord's "gate" is kept open, according to the theory. As prolonged inactivity leads to muscle weakness and atrophy, shortening of related connective tissues, and deterioration of articular cartilage, restoring motion and strength of a stressed region is an important clinical and biomechanical objective.

Grieve states that post-traumatic soft-tissue changes that are secondary to joint derangement or irritability become progressively prominent with age: mild during youth, severe in the elderly.[143] The periarticular connective tissues adapt by shortening on one side of the joint and lengthening on the other side, resulting in a relatively permanent lateral flexion often accompanied by a degree of rotation. This makes chronic subluxations difficult to hold in a corrected position. However, prior to this chronic state is the state of prolonged isometric contraction mentioned above, which is readily amenable if comprehensive therapy is applied. Gillet and many others confirm this.

During the posttraumatic acute stage, when there is neural excitation from the inflamed area, temporary impulse activity over the large-fibered proprioception circuits can be encouraged by movement, pressure, stretching, heat, and cold stimuli. However, heat at this stage increases swelling and movement provokes spasms, and thus are contraindicated.[104] The logical alternative is to apply isometric exercises soon after the danger of recurrent hemorrhage has passed. This offers stretching without motion, which increases circulation without engorgement and activates the large-fiber circuits, allowing a more rapid recovery. Even in chronic disorders, vigorous active motion increases intradisc pressure and can aggravate inelastic degenerated soft tissues. This would not be true for isometric exercises.

Following are several isometric exercises recommended by Fisk for the cervical spine that can readily be modified to meet varying clnical situations.[144] They are designed to increase strength, but they also teach the patient the different perceptions of contraction and relaxation (helpful in controlling chronic tension, for example). As the head is held in the neutral position, these exercises are not contraindicated even in cases of uncomplicated hypermobility or arthritis if the patient is carefully instructed. Two or three exercise bouts daily are recommended.

Resisted Flexion. The patient sits erect with the head straight and is instructed to place clasped hands against the forehead, breathe normally, and attempt to push the head forward against the resisting hand contact (Fig. 9.18). This position should be held for about 7 seconds; then the patient relaxes for several seconds and repeats the exercise a few times.

In the alternative prone position, the patient lies face down with his forehead on a large folded towel to allow breathing in this position. The patient is instructed to tuck the chin in and firm the forehead against the towel while breathing normally. Pressure should be held for about 7 seconds; then the patient relaxes for several seconds and repeats the exercise twice.

Resisted Extension. The patient sits erect with the head straight and is instructed to clasp the hands behind the head above the cervical spine (Fig. 9.19). The patient is then asked to breathe normally, keep the head straight, and attempt to push the head back against the resisting hand contact. This position should be held for about 7 seconds; then the patient relaxes for several seconds and repeats the exercise a few more times.

This exercise can also be conducted in the supine position by having the patient lie face up on a firm surface. A small firm pillow or cushion should be placed under the neck to support the head. The patient is instructed to firm the head against the pillow and firmly tuck the chin in while breathing normally. This position should be held for about 7 seconds; then the patient relaxes for several seconds and repeats the exercise a few more times.

Resisted Lateral Flexion. The patient sits erect with the head straight and places

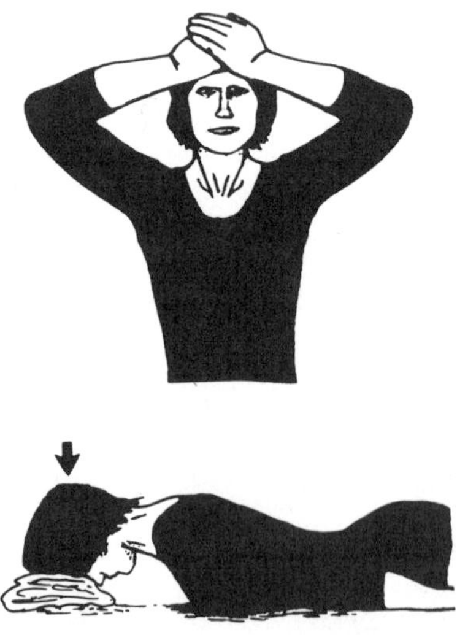

Figure 9.18. Isometric self-resisted cervical flexion: sitting and prone positions.

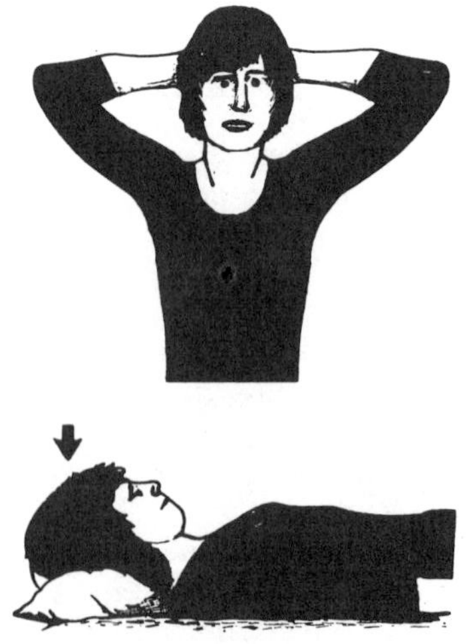

Figure 9.19. Isometric self-resisted cervical extension: sitting and supine.

the right hand over the right ear with the fingers extending over the scalp (Fig. 9.20). The patient is then asked to breathe normally and attempt to bend the neck toward the side of contact while resisting the effort with the contact hand. Again, this position should be held for about 7 seconds; then the patient relaxes for several seconds and repeats the exercise two or three times again. The hand positions are then interchanged, and the exercise is conducted for the other side.

This exercise can also be conducted in the lateral recumbent position. The patient lies on the side with the underside of the face against a firm pillow so that the spine is aligned in a straight line. The patient firms the head against the pillow while breathing normally. The position is held for about 7 seconds; then the patient relaxes for several seconds and repeats the exercise a few times. The patient is then instructed to lie on the other side and to repeat the exercise.

Resisted Rotation. The patient sits erect with the head straight. The patient is instructed to place the right hand on the right temple, and then asked to breathe normally and attempt to look over the right shoulder while resisting the movement with the hand contact (Fig. 9.21). This position is also held for about 7 seconds; then the patient relaxes for several seconds and repeats the exercise two or three more times. The left hand is then applied to the left temple and the exercise is conducted for the left side. This exercise can also be conducted in the supine position.

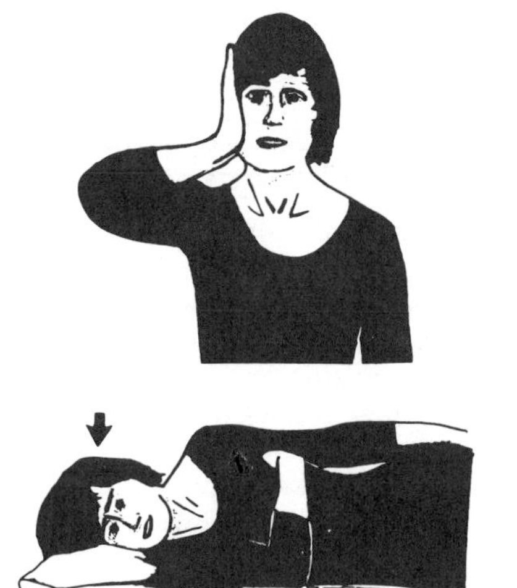

Figure 9.20. Isometric self-resisted lateral flexion: sitting and lateral recumbent.

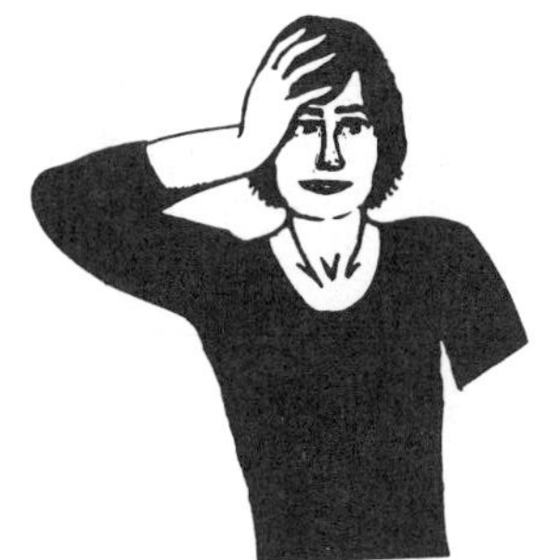

Figure 9.21. Isometric self-resisted rotation in the sitting position.

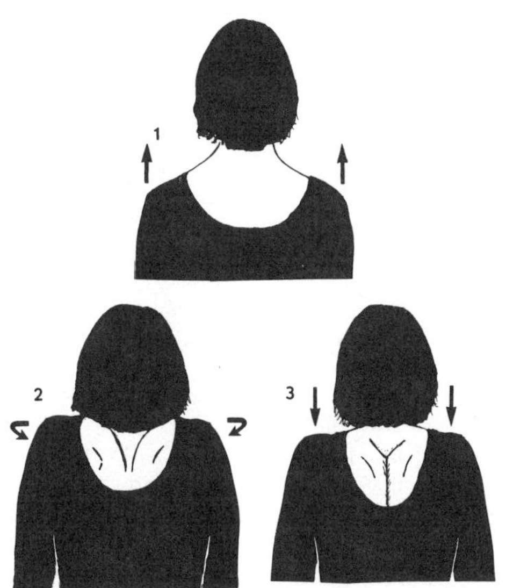

Figure 9.22. Shoulder shrugging exercise.

Two mild active isotonic exercises can be incorporated into the regimen when pain begins to diminish. These involve related shoulder and scapulae muscles that are often chronically tensed following cervical trauma.

Shoulder Shrugging. The patient stands or sits errect with the head straight, the neck aligned vertically, and the arms hanging loosely at the sides. The patient is instructed to breathe normally, elevate the shoulders as far as possible for several seconds, hold this position while the shoulders are retracted as far as possible for several seconds, and then to drop the shoulders in the retracted position and hold them there for several seconds (Fig. 9.22). The patient then relaxes for several seconds and repeats the exercise for several minutes until fatigued.

Arm Circling. Have the patient stand erect with the head straight, the arms hanging loosely at the sides, and the feet slightly apart to widen the base of support. The patient is instructed to breathe normally, flex forward at the waist, and then bring the arms back and up in an arc from the anterior to the posterior as far as can comfortably be managed (Fig. 9.23). This arm circling should be repeated without resting intervals for as many times as possible before fatigue occurs.

NEUROVASCULAR DEFICIT SYNDROMES

Several neurovascular deficit syndromes are related to the cervical spine. The two common general groups include the thoracic outlet/inlet syndromes and the vertebral artery syndromes.

Thoracic Outlet/Inlet Syndromes[145–152]

The cervicothoracic junction area is a unique spinal area that receives far less attention than it deserves in both medicine and chiropractic. It is a common site of developmental anomalies; it is a major site of arterial, lymphatic, and neurologic traffic; and it presents the juncture of the highly mobile cervical spine with the very limited thoracic spine. This latter point is biomechanically significant.

Background[80, 153–160]

There are several syndromes to consider under the classification of neurovascular compression syndromes (also termed thoracic outlet or inlet syndromes), each of which may produce the symptom complex of radiating pain over the shoulders and down the arms, atrophic disturbance, paresthesias, and vasomotor disturbances. These syndromes, however, do not necessarily indicate the specific cause of the problem.

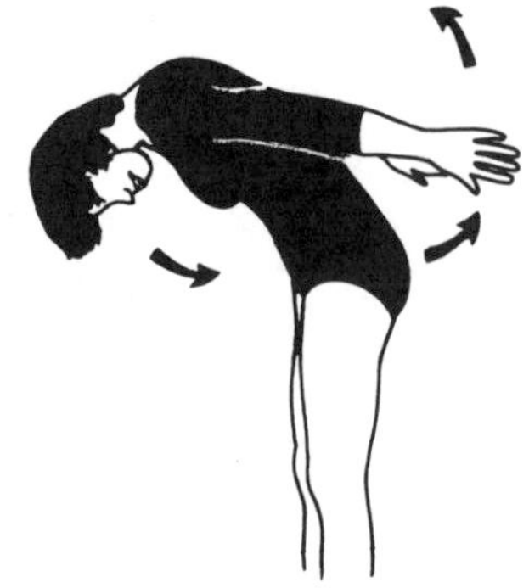

Figure 9.23. Arm circling exercise.

The Cervicothoracic Junction Area

The area of cervicothoracic transition is a complex of prevertebral and postvertebral fascia and ligaments subject to shortening. It offers a multitude of attaching and crossing muscles such as the longus colli, trapezius, scaleni, sternocleidomastoid, erector spinae, interspinous and intertransverse, multifidi and rotatores, splenius capitis, splenius cervicis, semispinalis capitis, semispinalis cervicis, longissimus capitis, longissimus cervicis, and the levator costarum and scapula—all of which are subject to spastic shortening and fibrotic changes that tether normal motion.

Incidence

The 4th and 5th decades mark the highest incidence of trouble in this area, probably because of regressive muscular changes. The incidence of disorders is more frequent in females by about 3:1. This is probably due to heavier upper-extremity work.

Etiology

Trauma to the head, neck, or shoulder girdle is a common factor. In some cases, poor posture, anomalies, or muscle contractures may be involved. Reduced tone in the muscles of the shoulder girdle, by itself, has been shown to allow depression of the clavicle that narrows the thoracic outlet and compresses the neurovascular bundle. In addition, subluxation syndromes (eg, retrolisthesis) may initiate these and other disturbances of the shoulder girdle and must be further evaluated. Cervical pathology such as spinal canal or IVD encroachment by a buckling ligamentum flavum, spinal stenosis, or spurs should be a consideration. During degeneration, the dura and dentates become thickened, dura and arachnoid adhesions become prevalent, and osteochondrophytes may develop from the borders of the canal or foramen—all of which tend to restrict the cord and/or nerve root during cervical motions. Osteochondrophytes near the foramen can readily compress the vertebral artery and root together.

Differential diagnosis must exclude a cervical rib etiology from infectious neuritis, banding adhesions, arthritis of the shoulder joint, clavicle fracture callus, bifid clavicle, cervical arthritis, subacromial bursitis, 1st rib subluxation and posttraumatic deformities, spinal or shoulder girdle malignancies, Pancoast's tumor of the lung apex, and cardiac disease. Aneurysms of the subclavian artery are rare.

Grieve[161] calls attention to "the poorly recognized part played by minor unilateral joint abnormalities of the upper three or four ribs, possibly often by tension of soft tissue attachments as a consequence of cervical joint irritability at higher segments, or due to the chronic sequelae of trauma. . . ."

Symptoms and Signs[162–169]

Symptoms usually do not occur until after the ribs have ossified. Two groups of symptoms are seen, those of scalenus anticus syndrome and those due to cervical rib pressure. The symptoms of cervical rib and scalenus syndrome are similar, but the scalenus anticus muscle is the primary factor in the production of neurocirculatory compression whether a cervical rib is present or not.

When symptoms are present, they usually result from compression of the lower cord of the brachial plexus and subclavian vessels and numbness and pain in the ulnar nerve distribution may occur. Pain is worse at night because of pressure from the recumbent position, and its intensity varies throughout the day. Tiredness and weakness of the arm, finger cramps, numbness, tingling, coldness of the hand, areas of hyperesthesia, muscle degeneration in the hand, a lump at the base of the neck, tremor, and discoloration of the fingers are characteristic. Work and exercise accentuate symptoms, while rest and elevation of the extremity relieve symptoms. Adson's and other similar compression signs will usually be positive.

Differentiation of Neural vs Circulatory Symptoms

Compression of nerve tissue results in numbness, pain, paralysis, and loss of function. Compression of vascular structures results in moderate pain and swelling. The obstruction of circulation can result in clotting within the vessels with possible consequent infarction in the tissues supplied. These unilateral phenomena are fairly limited to the cervicobrachial distribution.

Anatomical Considerations

Working above and behind to produce shoulder abduction and retraction (eg, painting a ceiling, repairing a ceiling fixture) will definitely cause temporary clavicle encroachment on the brachial plexus and press the subclavian artery against the scalenus medius. For many years, the cause was attributed to costoclavicular compression from shoulder depression. However, postmortem stress tests have shown the following:[170]

1. When the arm is depressed, the clavicle moves inferior and *anterior,* and this *widens* the space between the clavicle and 1st rib.
2. When the shoulder is depressed, the upper and middle trunks of the brachial plexus are stretched tightly over the tendinous edge of the scalenus medius and the lower trunks are pulled into the angle formed by the 1st rib and the scalenus medius tendon. Most symptoms found on shoulder depression will be the result of this traction. There is no compression of the subclavian artery against either scalenus.
3. When the shoulder is retracted, the clavicle does not impinge upon the subclavian vein but the tendon of the subclavius muscle compresses the vein against the 1st rib. The middle third of the clavicle pushes the neurovascular bundle against the anterior scalenus medius, and this could cause compression if a space-occupying lesion is also present (eg, cervical rib, extrafascial band).

Clinical Compression Tests[171–175]

X-ray films should always be taken before performing a cervical compression test, especially when the patient has experienced trauma or shows physical signs of advanced degeneration. It is important to rule out possible conditions that would be aggravated by any testing procedure.

Active Cervical Rotary Compression Test

The patient is seated and is observed while voluntarily laterally flexing his head toward the side being examined. With the neck flexed, the patient is then instructed to rotate his chin toward the same side, which narrows the IVF diameters on the side of concavity. Pain or reduplication of other symptoms probably indicates a physiologic narrowing of one or more IVFs.

Passive Cervical Compression Tests

Two tests are involved. First, the patient is seated and the examiner stands behind. The patient's head is laterally flexed and rotated slightly toward the side being examined. Interlocked fingers are placed on the patient's scalp and gently pressed caudally. If an IVF is physiologically narrowed, this maneuver will further insult the foramen by compressing the disc and narrowing the foramen, causing pain and reduplication of other symptoms. In the second test, the patient's neck is extended by the examiner who then places interlocked hands on the patient's scalp and gently presses caudally. If an IVF is physiologically narrowed, this maneuver mechanically compromises the foraminal diameters bilaterally and causes pain and reduplication of other symptoms.

Spurling's Test

This is a variation of the passive cervical compression test. The patient's head is turned to the maximum toward one side and then laterally flexed to the maximum. A fist is placed on the patient's scalp, and a moderate blow is delivered to it by the other fist. The patient's position produces reduced IVF spaces, and the blow causes a herniated disc to bulge further into the IVF space or an irritated nerve root to be aggravated, thus increasing the symptoms.

Shoulder Depression Test

The patient is seated and the examiner stands behind. The patient's head is laterally flexed away from the side being examined. The doctor stabilizes the patient's shoulder with one hand and applies pressure alongside the patient's head with the palm of the other hand, stretching the dural root sleeves and nerve roots or aggravating radicular pain if the nerve roots adhere to the foramina. Extravasations, edema, encroachments, and conversion of fibrinogen into fibrin may result in interfascicular, foraminal, and articular adhesions and inflammations that will restrict fascicular glide and the ingress and egress of the foraminal contents. Thus, pain and reduplication of other symptoms during the test suggest adhesions between the nerve's dura sleeve and other structures around the IVF.

Cervical Distraction Test

The patient is seated and the examiner stands to the side and places one hand under the patient's chin and the other hand under the base of the occiput (Fig. 9.24). Slowly and gradually the patient's head is lifted to remove weight from the cervical spine. This maneuver elongates the IVFs, decreases the pressure on the joint capsules around the facet joints, and stretches the paravertebral musculature. If the maneuver decreases pain and relieves other symptoms, it is a probable indication of narrowing of

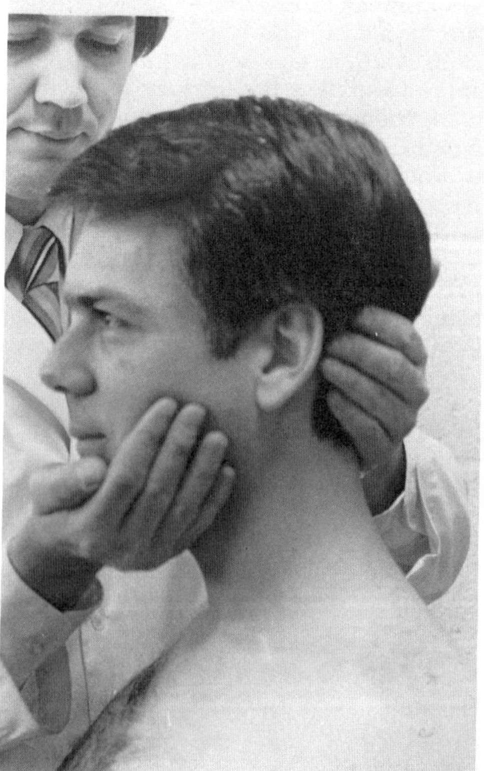

Figure 9.24. The cervical distraction test.

one or more IVFs, cervical facet syndrome, or spastic paravertebral muscles.

Adson's Test

With the patient seated, the examiner palpates the radial pulse and advises the patient to bend his head obliquely backward to the opposite side being examined, take a deep breath, and tighten the neck and chest muscles on the side tested. The maneuver decreases the interscalene space (anterior and middle scalene muscles) and increases any existing compression of the subclavian artery and lower components (C8 and T1) of the brachial plexus against the 1st rib. Marked weakening of the pulse or increased paresthesias indicate a positive sign of pressure on the neurovascular bundle, particularly of the subclavian artery as it passes between or through the scaleni musculature, thus indicating a probable cervical rib or scalenus anticus snydrome.

Eden's Test

With the patient seated, the examiner palpates the radial pulse and instructs the patient to pull the shoulders backward, throw the chest out in a "military posture," and hold a deep inspiration as the pulse is examined. The test is positive if weakening or loss of the pulse occurs, indicating pressure on the neurovascular bundle as it passes between the clavicle and the 1st rib, and thus a costoclavicular syndrome.

Wright's Test

With the patient seated, the radial pulse is palpated from the posterior in the downward position and as the arm is passively moved through an 180° arc. If the pulse diminishes or disappears in this arc or if neurologic symptoms develop, it may indicate pressure on the axillary artery and vein under the pectoralis minor tendon and coracoid process or compression in the retroclavicular spaces between the clavicle and 1st rib, and thus be a hyperabduction syndrome.

Vertebrobasilar System Patency

Cases of adverse effects (eg, paraplegia) from brain-stem ischemia due to mechanical compression of the vertebral artery, dislodgment of a plaque, or a reflex spasm following forced rotation and extension of the head are rare. One Swiss study reports that slight neurologic complications are observed in only 1 out of 400,000 manipulations.[176] However, such statistics are meaningless when you are personally involved.

Background[177–180]

The vertebral arteries are the major source of blood supply to the cervical spinal cord and brain stem, including the medulla oblongata, pons, and midbrain. They also supply the visual cortex of the cerebrum and cerebellum via the basilar artery.[181] For an unexplained reason, one artery is usually smaller than its mate.[182]

Any minor compromise (eg, compression, atherosclerosis, thrombosis, vasospasm, kinking, or longus colli and scalenus anticus spasm) producing an insufficiency of blood flow can lead to a singular symptom or a wide number of seemingly unrelated cranial manifestations. These manifestations include occipital headaches, memory lapses, dizziness, tinnitus, nausea and vomiting, lightheadedness or syncope, intermittent blurred vision, suboccipital tenderness, and, sometimes, retroocular pain (episodic), speech impairment, extremity paresthesia and weakness, drop attacks, and gait defects—all of which can be generally grouped under the title of *Barré-Lieau syndrome*, especially when cervical trauma and an underlying spondylosis are involved. These signs and symptoms, which sometimes fluctuate from side to side, can mimic a post-traumatic syndrome, multiple sclerosis, amyotrophic lateral sclerosis, or a tumor within the posterior fossa.

Severe interference (eg, thrombosis, osteophytic kinking, spondylotic foraminal impingement, extension effects of IVD degeneration) leads to involvement of the nucleus ambiguus of the vagus (dysphagia, ipsilateral palatal weakness), the descending root and nucleus of cranial V (ipsilateral facial hypoesthesia, especially around the lips), the descending sympathetic fibers (Horner's syndrome), the vestibular nuclei (rotary nystagmus), the midbrain and cerebellum (ipsilateral arm/leg malcoordination, intention tremor, ataxia), and the spinothalamic tract (contralateral hypoesthesia), and the effects from impaired venous drainage and cerebrospinal fluid (CSF) flow, often referred to as *Wallenberg's syndrome*.[183–188]

The vertebral arteries are unique in their course through several bony foramina, and in this intermittently channeled course from C6 upward, they must make four nearly right-angled turns (forming a half square) in just 20–30 mm between entering the C2 transverse and entering the foramen magnum. Added to this tortuous course are anomalous loops in about one in five people, and the C2 area is a common site for aneurysm—allowing additional vulnerability to compressive forces.[189,190]

The vertebral arteries also exhibit special features at particular sites of predilection for degeneration by the change of fixed and unfixed vessel parts, an increased vulnerability to bone and muscle movements, and the occlusion of peripheral arteries in their circulation area by difficult to diagnose pathologic changes of the vascular walls.[191] These factors mandate that advanced degenerative or inflammatory processes involving the vertebral arteries be ruled out prior to cervical manipulation or adjustments. Trauma to the vertebral artery has even been reported after emergency resuscitation procedures, when passive extension of the neck is usually necessary to insert an airtube.[192]

It can be readily projected that the many cranial-oriented symptoms that have been relieved by chiropractic adjustments to the cervical region can be attributed to normalization of vertebral artery blood flow. Here we have a clinical paradox: the same treatment may cause possible distress if unusual precautions are not taken with some patients.

Several clinical tests with only minor variations are portrayed in the literature. All include cervical rotation with extension. Five are described below.[193–195]

George's Test

The sitting patient closes the eyes, stretches the arms forward, and then is instructed to (1) rotate the head to a comfortable maximum, (2) extend the neck, and (3) hold this position for 30 seconds. Signs of swaying of the outstretched hands or symptoms of tinnitus, dizziness, nausea, or syncope suggest cerebral ischemia due to vertebral artery compromise. If no adverse signs appear, the test is repeated with contralateral cervical rotation-extension.

Maigne's Test

The examiner places the head of the seated patient in extension and rotation. This position is held for about 15–40 seconds on each side. A positive sign is indicated by nystagmus or symptoms of vertebrobasilar ischemia.

DeKleyn's Test

The patient is placed supine on an adjusting table, and the head rest is lowered. The examiner extends and rotates the patient's head, and this position is held for about 15–40 seconds on each side. A positive sign is the same as that in Maigne's test.

Hautant's Test

The examiner places the upper limbs of the seated patient so that they are abducted forward with the palms turned upward (supination). The patient is instructed to close his eyes, and the examiner extends and rotates the patient's head. This position is held for about 15–40 seconds on each side. A positive sign is for one or both arms to drop into a pronated position.

Underburger's Test

The patient is asked to stand with his upper limbs outstretched, his eyes closed, and then to march in place with his head extended and rotated. The examiner should stand close to the patient during the test because a positive sign is a loss of balance.

TRAUMATIC BRACHIAL PLEXUS TRACTION[196,197]

Trauma to the brachial plexus is often seen following severe cervical lateroflexion. The effects vary from mild to severe depending upon the extent of nerve contusion, crush, or laceration. Nerve "pinch" or "stretch" syndromes may be involved which respond well to conservative care, unless nerve severance or root avulsion has occurred.[198] The specific symptomatology, physical findings, roentgenography, and electromyography offer clues to the extent of damage, indicated therapy, and prognosis.

Background

In brachial plexus trauma, the entire plexus or any of its fibers may be injured (refer to Table 8.5). The lateral branches of the brachial plexus lie just anterior to the glenohumeral joint. The axillary nerve lies just below the joint.

As the roots of the plexus are fixed at their origin in the spinal cord, any sudden or severe traction of the upper extremity may avulse roots from the cord or stretch the plexus to the point of tearing. Stretching injuries are common; tearing injuries are rare. Such injuries may be divided into three general types: total arm palsies, upper arm palsies (most common), and lower arm palsies. The major sensory, motor, and reflex changes involved with the brachial radiculopathies are listed in Table 9.4.

Nerve Pinch or Stretch Syndromes[198]

Nerve "pinch" or "stretch" syndromes are common. They are often seen in the lower neck from overflexion, but the syndromes appear throughout the cranium, spine, pelvis, and extremities in many accidents. Hardly any peripheral nerve is exempt. Terms used synonymously include nerve compression, nerve contusion, nerve lesion, nerve pinch syndrome, nerve root syndrome, nerve stretch syndrome, radiculopathy, or traumatic neuritis.

A *nerve stretch syndrome* is commonly associated with sprains, excessive lateral cervical flexion with shoulder depression, or dislocations. Nerve fibers may be stretched, partially torn, or ruptured almost anywhere in the nervous system from the cord to peripheral nerve terminals.

A *nerve pinch syndrome* may be due to direct trauma (contusion), subluxation, a protruded disc that results in nerve compression, or fracture (callus formation and associated posttraumatic adhesions). Any telescoping, hyperflexion, hyperextension, or hyperrotational blow or force to the spine may result in a nerve "pinch" syndrome in which pain may be local or extending distally. Nerve pinch syndromes are less common than nerve stretch syndromes but are more serious.

Mild or Moderate Brachial Traction

After lateroflexion injuries of the neck (Fig. 9.25), a sharp burning pain may radiate along the course of one or more cervical nerves, the result of nerve contusion due to stretching. Scalenus anticus syndrome may be exhibited. This nerve stretch is often referred to as a "hot shot" by athletes. Recurring injury is common, especially in contact sports. It is not limited to sports, however, for any severe cervical lateral flexion can produce the syndrome.

Immediate pain may radiate to the back of the head, behind the ear, around the neck, or down toward the clavicle, shoulder,

Table 9.4.
Neurologic Signs in the Brachial Radiculopathies

Nerve root affected	Major sensory disorder (hypalgesia)	Major motor disorder (weakness)	Reflex impairment
C3	Shoulder region	Ventral diaphragm	No change
C4	Shoulder region	Dorsal diaphragm	No change
C5	Lateral arm	Biceps, supraspinatus, infraspinatus, deltoid	Biceps
C6	Lateral forearm and thumb	Brachioradialis	Brachioradialis
C7	Middle finger	Triceps	Triceps
C8	Little finger	Wrist and finger flexors	No change
T1	Medial forearm	Intrinsic hand muscles	Finger flexors

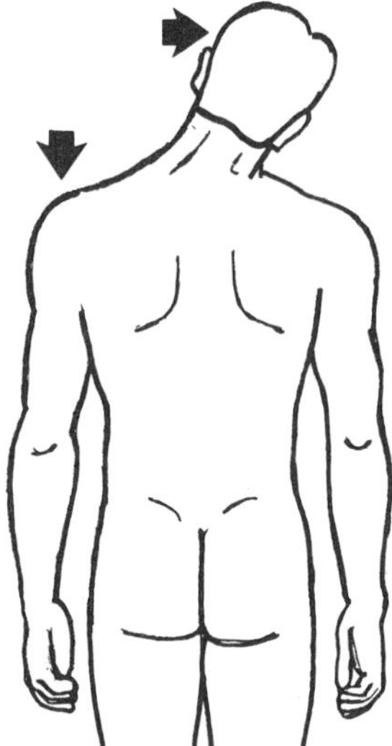

Figure 9.25. Typical forces involved in brachial plexus traction.

arm or hand. Frequently, there is arm paresthesia, severe arm weakness, diminished active motion, decreased biceps and triceps reflexes, forearm numbness, and cervical movement restriction. These signs and symptoms may disappear and reappear with greater severity.

Ipsilateral vs Contralateral Symptoms. If the symptoms appear on the opposite side of the forceful bending, undoubtedly a nerve has been "pinched" within the powerful muscles dorsal to the sternocleidomastoid. If this is the case, the symptoms usually subside in a few minutes with only slight residual tenderness and paresthesia, which disappear within a few hours. On the other hand, if symptoms appear on the same side as the direction of the forceful bending, deep skeletal injury such as severe rotary subluxation, fracture, dislocation, or nerve compression may be involved.

The Stinger Syndrome

The "stinger" syndrome is an apparently mild athletic brachial plexus injury that reflects a transient radiculopathy at the time of impact. Football "spearing" and head butting are common causes. Pressure against a misfitted shoulder pad and gymnastic accidents are other causes commonly reported. The injury usually occurs when the neck is forcibly hyperextended and laterally flexed, and symptoms can usually be precipitated in this position during examination.[201] The condition is initially felt as a painfully severe electrical shock–like dysesthesia that extends from the shoulder to the fingertips. This feeling passes within a few moments and is replaced by sensations of numbness and upper extremity weakness that may last from a few seconds to several minutes.

The most common site of injury is at the C5 or C6 root level; because of this, the most persistent sign will be weakness of the proximal shoulder muscles. An initial attack rarely leaves residual neurologic symptoms. Repetitive injuries of this nature, however, tend to have a cumulative effect that may lead to axonotmesis and chronic muscle weakness, which may take up to six months for full recovery. The most common lesion associated with the stinger syndrome is cervical sprain with traumatic compression neuritis. Infrequently, an acute cervical disc rupture or a spontaneously reduced hyperextension dislocation may be associated. These latter disorders are far more serious and may require hospitalization until the severity of the injury can be properly assessed.

Root Avulsion

A similar but more severe nerve injury is that to the brachial plexus or its roots which is usually caused by a fall on the shoulder, a blow to the side of the neck, forceful arm traction, or a combination of these mechanisms. The injury is essentially caused by acute shoulder depression that stretches the brachial plexus, especially in the supraclavicular area. The effect may be root tear near the vertebral foramen, spinal cord damage, dural cuff leaks of cerebrospinal fluid, and/or vertebral fracture or dislocation. During avulsion, the spinal cord itself is infrequently damaged and contralateral cord symptoms are found. Such severe manifestations are rarely seen in the well-conditioned patient in whom the picture is usually limited to pain radiating into the arm and/or hand.

Diagnosis and Management

Painstaking examination is required because multiple nerve injury, related tendon or other soft-tissue damage, and fractured bones may complicate the picture. The immediate site of injury should be first investigated, followed by the part's general appearance, voluntary motion, reflexes, and vasomotor changes. Trophic lesions of the joints, muscles (atrophy), skin, and nails are common in the late stage. They usually blend and are explained as the results of vasomotor changes. In addition to motor and sensory loss, the response to electrical stimulation should be evaluated.

Physical Findings

Damage to an individual peripheral nerve (eg, trauma) is characterized by (1) flaccid, atrophic paralysis of the muscles supplied by the involved nerve and (2) loss of all sensation, including proprioception, in the skin areas distal to the lesion. When partial destruction to various peripheral nerves occurs, the effects are usually more prominent in the distal extremities. The condition is characterized by muscular weakness and atrophy and poorly demarcated areas of sensory changes. Unless severe nerve injury has occurred to the nerve or its attachment at the cord, chiropractic care offers a conservative approach to case management.

In ulnar nerve damage, sensation is lost on the medial side of the hand, including the little finger and medial half of the ring finger. In median nerve damage, sensation of the remainder of the anterior surface of the hand is lost. However, motor involvement is the main feature because sensory loss is often obscured by overlapping innervation. As time goes by after severe nerve injury, the affected part assumes a posture and atrophy peculiar to the particular nerve involved; for example, "wrist drop" with the radial nerve, "claw hand" with the ulnar nerve, "flat hand" with the median nerve, and "ape hand" with the ulnar and median nerves.

Roentgenography

Films are often negative in mild to moderate cases. In severe cases, a unilaterally locked facet may be viewed as a positive sign of dislocation. This is caused by one facet displacing while the opposite side remains in position. It is easy to miss on physical examination because normal neck movements usually do not increase the dislocation.

On the standard A-P view, the spinous processes above the luxation will be out of alignment with the processes below the lesion. Displacement will be ipsilateral on the side of the locked facet.

On the lateral view, displacement is usually obvious even though it may not be pronounced. The facets inferior to the lesion are superimposed (often seen as one). Superior to the lesion, the facets are offset and viewed as being one in front of the other (bow-tie sign). In recurring cases, such as in football players, symptomatic or asymptomatic spur formation on cervical vertebrae is common.

Case Management

The effect of treatment depends largely upon early recognition of the nerve injury with removal of aggravating factors. Management consists of support to the affected part in the functional position and normal regimens for severe nerve contusion. As with most injuries, associated or concomitant subluxations or fixations must be adjusted to aid recovery, and sites of abnormal reflexes and stasis must be normalized.

Cold packs and/or especially ice massage are applicable in the acute stage to reduce adjacent swelling and bleeding. Vapocoolant sprays to isolated trigger points and meridian therapy often produce rapid spasm reduction of affected areas. After the acute stage subsides, massage, electric stimulation, progressive exercises, and reflex techniques may be utilized. Heat, massage, passive exercises, and nutritional control are also helpful during rehabilitation.

Prevention of aggravation requires correcting associated subluxations, strengthening cervical muscles, wearing a plastic roll within a stockinet as a cervical collar or applying a Thomas-type collar, and avoiding dangerous movements at work or play.

A reaction of nerve degeneration added to typical sensory and motor loss is indicative of complete anatomical or physiologic nerve damage usually requiring surgical intervention. If surgery is required, careful attention must be given to postoperative chiropractic care directed to maintaining, as much as possible, normal joint flexibility, fascia and ligamentous resiliency, muscle elasticity, and adequate nutrition to all tissues involved. Some postoperative improvement can be anticipated. Approximately one month before it can be detected clinically, an electromyogram will exhibit reinnervation.

Prognosis

If the lesion is due to stretching, contusion, or partial tearing, the prognosis is good and complete recovery may usually be anticipated. The prognosis is usually poor in avulsion from the cord. Fortunately, most injuries are neurapraxias, and full recovery can be anticipated in time.

When a peripheral nerve fiber is permanently destroyed by either trauma or disease, the portion distal to the nerve cell body completely degenerates, and the fiber loses its myelin sheath in the process. In time, the isolated fiber stump tries to sprout in random directions in an attempt to make a bridge with the severed portion of the nerve. Some of these sprouts may, apparently by chance, cross the gap and enter neurolemmal tubes leading to a peripheral motor or sensory terminal. Function may be restored if the connection is a suitable match. Fibers in the spinal cord and brain do not regenerate effectively; however, recent evidence discloses that some regeneration can occur.

MANAGEMENT OF CERVICAL STRAINS, SPRAINS, AND WHIPLASH[202–208]

The conservative management of cervical injuries is generally the same in Grades 1 and 2 sprains and strains, which are often associated with some degree of nerve contusion and osseous misalignment. The goals should be to restore bony alignment, relieve pain and spasm, reduce edema, and enhance healing by way of providing rest and support and assisting circulatory flow.

Treating Uncomplicated Cervical Strains and Sprains[209–212]

Cord injury, fracture, or dislocation, and severe root or vascular damage must be ruled out before conservative therapy is instigated.

Structural Alignment and Mobility

The benefits of structural adjustments when indicated are well known within the profession, thus there is no need to review the many techniques here. In most instances, spasticity should be relieved before mobilization techniques are applied.

Associated Spasm

To relieve muscle spasm, heat is helpful but cold packs and vapocoolant sprays have proved to be more effective in acute cases. Mild passive stretch is an excellent method of reducing spasm in the long muscles. Heavy passive stretch, however, destroys the beneficial reflexes. One techique is to place the patient prone on an adjusting table in which the head piece has been slightly lowered. Turn the patient's head toward the side of the spastic muscle. With head weight alone serving as the stretching force, the spasm should relax within 2–3 minutes. Thumb pressure, placed on a trigger area, is then directed toward the muscle's attachment and held for a few moments until relaxation is complete.

Other beneficial methods of relieving spasm include ice massage, ultrasound, and tetanizing galvanic or alternating currents. Keep in mind, however, that the purpose of spontaneous (antalgic) post-traumatic spasm is to splint the area to prevent injurious motion. Thus, if means are taken to remove this intrinsic splinting action, external support will likely be necessary.

Associated Trigger Points

The cervical and suprascapular areas of the trapezius frequently refer pain and deep tenderness to the lateral neck (especially the submastoid area), temple area, and angle of the jaw. The sternal division of the sternocleidomastoideus refers pain chiefly to the eyebrow, cheek, tongue, chin, pharynx, throat, and sternum. The clavicular division refers pain mainly to the forehead (bilaterally), back of and/or deep within the ear, and rarely to the teeth. Vapocoolant spraying during stretching of isolated sites often produces rapid spasm reduction of affected areas. Deep friction massage, high-volt current, and interferential currents have also proved to be effective.

Control of Persistent Pain

Peripheral inhibitory afferent impulses can be generated to partially close the presynaptic gate by acupressure, acu-aids, acupuncture, or other forms of transcutaneous nerve stimulation (eg, TENS). Many authorities believe that deep sustained manual pressure on trigger points is the best method, but a few others prefer sharp short-duration pressure (1–2 seconds). Deep pressure is contraindicated in any patient receiving anti-inflammatory drugs (eg, cortisone) because subcutaneous hemorrhage may result. The effects of cervical traction are often dramatic but sometimes short lived if a ruptured nucleus is involved. In uncomplicated chronic cases, relaxation training with biofeedback is helpful.

Nutrition and Metabolic Equilibrium

Vitamin C and Ligaplex supplementation tend to enhance connective tissue repair. An acid-base imbalance from muscle hypoxia and acidosis is sometimes the cause, and it may be prevented by Lindahl's alkalization mixture (potassium citrate, 33.5%; calcium lactate, 41%; sodium citrate, 12%; magnesium glyconate, 12%; lithium citrate, 1.5%).

Therapeutic Exercise

Isotonic exercises are useful in improving circulation and inducing the stretch reflex, especially in the cervical extensors. These exercises should be done in the supine position to reduce exteroceptive influences on the central nervous system. Specific remedial exercises for the cervical region have been described previously in this chapter.

Cervical Supports

Orthopedic Collars[104,213,214]

Torn muscle, ligament, capsule, and fascia fibers usually require immobilization during the initial stage of healing to prevent reinjury and offer the benefits of support and padding to weakened, sensitive tissues. A large variety of cervical collars and braces are available to meet different requirements. None affords complete immobilization, however, and the more flexible the appliance, the less effective it is (eg, a soft foam collar). Gross measuring guidelines for the more common supports are shown in Table 9.5.

Orthopedic Pillows[215–217]

Sleeping in awkward positions for long periods often leads to or aggravates cervical misalignment or motion-unit instability syndromes. These usually result from long-duration stretching (elongating) forces upon the passive resistance properties of the cervical and upper thoracic muscles, tendons, ligaments, and capsules—the end result of which is linear deformation.

The process of connective tissue elongation is governed by its properties of yield to biomechanical stress and strain—elasticity, plasticity, flexibility, viscosity, viscoelasticity, stiffness, and structural fatigue coefficients. These properties have been described in Chapter 3.

Background. Unlike ligaments, tendons, and capsules, muscles are not considered to be connective tissue straps. Nevertheless, studies have shown that most of the resistance imparted by muscles to passive stretch is derived from their connective tissue sheaths and intrinsic framework, and not from the myofibrils when a relaxed muscle is stretched.[218] Thus, regardless of the type of soft tissue involved, it is the connective tissue elements that provide resistance to passive stretch. This is also true of postinjury connective tissue products such as adhesions, scar tissue, or fibrotic contractures. This factor of connective tissue resistance to passive forces is important when considering the mobilization and holding aspects of chiropractic adjustments, postural realignment, and remedial exercises.

Elastic and Plastic Stretch Deformation. Elastic stretch (temporary) resembles that of a rubber band, in which the elongation deformation is released immediately when the tensile load is removed. Plastic stretch (relatively permanent) resembles that of putty, in which the deformation remains to a considerable degree after the load has been removed.[219] The effects of both elastic and plastic stretch are the products of force and time. Elastic deformation occurs to variable degrees when a substantial force is applied for a short duration (eg, acute strain/sprain, during a dynamic ad-

Table 9.5.
Common Cervical Supports

Type of support	Measuring guidelines
Firm cervical collar	Neck circumference and necessary height to position and support the cranium as desired.
Philadelphia collar	Neck circumference and necesasry height to position and support the cranium as desired.
Soft foam collar	Neck circumference and necessary height to position and support the cranium as desired.
Somi brace	Standard sizes of large, medium, and small, selected according to the dimensions of the patient.
Two- and four-poster	Standard sizes of large, medium, and small, selected according to the dimensions of the patient.

justment). Plastic deformation occurs when a low force (eg, gravity) is applied for a long duration (eg, unhealthy sleeping positions, stressful occupational postures, scoliosis, slow passive manipulation).

Associated Effects on Muscle Tissue. Elastic and plastic deformation forces stimulate muscle tissue receptors. Elastic stretch affects the muscle spindles because they monitor changes in muscle fiber length and rate of changes in length. Plastic stretch affects the Golgi tendon organs because they monitor tension produced from either contraction or stretch. The end result is reflected in a palpable tautness (hypertonicity). Thus, therapeutic elongation of muscle tissues that are in a state of plastic deformity would usually be counterproductive.

Advantages of Orthopedic Pillows. Cervical disorders that are caused or aggravated by improper sleeping positions contributing to plastic deformation will be benefited by a specially designed orthopedic pillow. The Pillo-Pedic line developed by Therapeutic Products to promote cervical flexion in acute conditions and cervical extension in chronic states is shown in Figure 9.26. A selection can be made between mild and moderate traction effects. A study of 400 patients with a flattened cervical curve concluded that 90% of the subjects showed distinct improvement after 90 days of use of this pillow.

Emergency Care in Suspected Cord Injury[221,222]

The immediate signs and symptoms of spinal cord injury parallel those of a fracture of the spinal column. In the on-site emergency-care situation, the patient with spinal cord injury must be treated as if the skull or spinal column were fractured, even when there is no external evidence. Shock must be prevented or reduced. If the patient is conscious, ask the location of pain. Ask if the patient can move arms and legs. Note pupil dilation bilaterally. Pinch the skin and check for pain perception. Check nose and ears for cerebrospinal fluid leakage. Clothing should be loosened, and everything removed from the pockets. Shoes and moist socks should be removed. Knee and ankle reflexes can be tested, but do not move the head or neck. The patient should be protected from temperature extremes, but heavy covers should not press against paralyzed parts during transportation.

CERVICAL DISC AND RELATED DISORDERS[223-227]

Grieve points out that the clinical picture of cervical disc disorders is typically a combination of "a hard osseocartilaginous spur, produced by the disc together with the adjacent margins of the vertebral bodies." Furthermore, "the mechanism by which pain and disability originate in the neck region,"

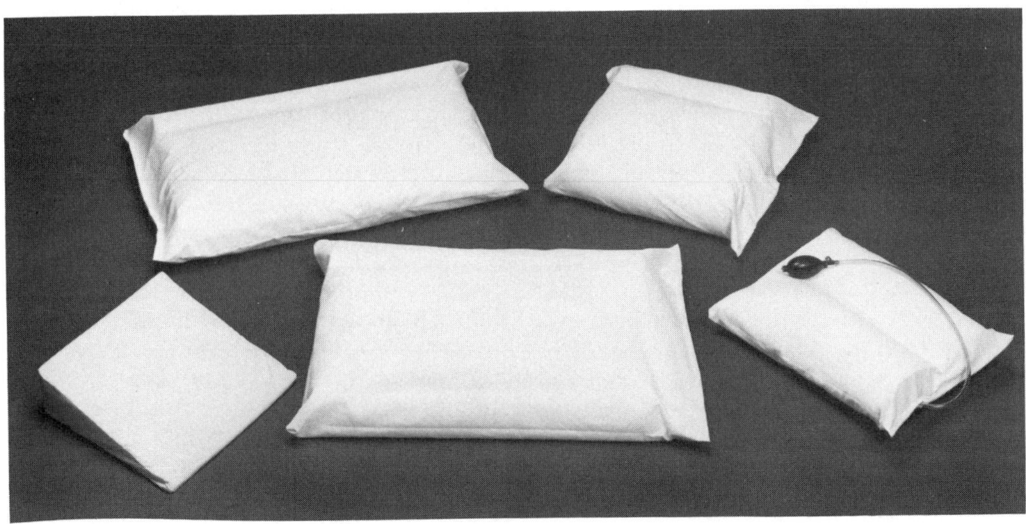

Figure 9.26. *Top left*, standard cervical traction pillow; *top right*, traction pillow for traveling; *bottom left*, wedge-shaped pregnancy pillow; *bottom middle*, cervical traction pillow for children and small-framed individuals; *bottom right*, adjustable (inflatable) cervical pillow that can also be used as a lumbar support (Courtesy of Foot Levelers, Inc).

contends Cailliet, "can be considered broadly to result from encroachment of space or faulty movement in the region of the neck through which the nerves or blood vessels pass."[228] This *encroachment of space* or *faulty movement* commonly comprises apophyseal subluxation with osteophyte formation, contributing to, or superimposed upon, disc degeneration and/or protrusion. This occurs most frequently in the C4–C6 area.

Disc Degeneration[229–234]

The cervical spine is readily subject to degenerative disc disease because of its great mobility and because it serves as a common site for various congenital defects. Bone changes are more common posteriorly in the upper cervicals and anteriorly in the lower cervicals. Cervical degenerative changes can be demonstrated in about half the population at 40 years of age and 70% of those at 65 years, many of which may be asymptomatic.

Various factors, individually or in combination, may be involved in initiating the process. These factors include trauma, postural and occupational stress, biochemical abnormalities (eg, hydration, mucopolysaccharide, collagen, or lipid changes), biologic changes (eg, aging), autoimmune responses, psychophysiologic effects (eg, the sodium retention of depression), and genetic predisposition (eg, identical development in twins).

Disc Encroachment[235–239]

Pure encroachment of a disc upon the spinal canal or IVF as seen in the lumbar region is not frequently seen in the cervical area. This is due to several reasons. First, the posterior longitudinal ligament completely covers the dorsal aspect of the disc and not just its central aspect as in the lumbar region. This ligament is also stronger and thicker (double-layered) in the cervical area. Second, the thickness of the cervical disc is so designed that it is wider anteriorly and narrower posteriorly, and horizontally wider and stronger in its posterior aspect. This tends to somewhat minimize posteriorly directed movement of the nucleus. Third, the dorsolateral disc herniation necessary for nerve root compression is minimized by the lips of the covertebral joints, which form a hard wall between the anulus and the exiting nerve.

Clinical Signs and Symptoms[240–246]

The discs below C3 exhibit a higher incidence and the greatest severity of herniation. The C5 disc is the most frequently involved, followed by the C6 disc. The C2 disc is the least frequently involved.

In acute disorders, interspace narrowing, straightening of the cervical curve, and instability may be the only roentgenographic signs present. Instability will be most evident as aberrant segmental movement in comparative lateral films made during full flexion and extension. If the protrusion is central, cord signs and symptoms present, such as lower extremity spasticity and hyperactive reflexes. Sensory changes are rarely evident. The gait may be ataxic. If the protrusion is posterolateral, the nerve root will be involved rather than the cord.

Several structural changes occur in chronic disorders. The vertebral bodies involved become elongated, the normal cervical lordosis flattens, the anterosuperior angle of the vertebral bodies becomes rounded, the involved body interspace narrows, the total height of the neck is reduced, and the inferior apophyseal facet above tends to subluxate posteriorly on the superior facet below and erode the lamina. Posterior osteophytes form at the disc attachment peripherally, often compromising the IVFs and vertebral canal. This may be noted by narrowing of the A-P dimension of the spinal canal in lateral films and foraminal encroachment on oblique films. These signs most frequently occur at the C6–C7 level. Anterior osteophytes are considered the result of abnormal ligamentous stress rather than part of the disc degeneration process. They occur most frequently below the C4 level, as do alterations of the covertebral joints.

Neurovascular Signs. The specific neurovascular manifestations of acute cervical disc herniation are:

- *C2 disc protrusion (C3 nerve root level)*: posterior neck numbness and pain radiating to the mastoid and ear. The reflexes test normal.
- *C3 disc protrusion (C4 nerve root level)*: posterior neck numbness and pain radiating along the levator scapulae muscle and sometimes to the pectorals. The reflexes are normal.
- *C4 disc protrusion (C5 nerve root level)*: lateral neck, shoulder, and arm pain and paresthesia, deltoid weakness and possible atrophy, hypesthesia of C5 root distribution over middle deltoid area (axillary nerve distribution). The reflexes test normal.
- *C5 disc protrusion (C6 nerve root level)*: pain radiating down the lateral arm and forearm into the thumb and index finger, hypesthesia of the lateral forearm and thumb, decreased biceps reflex, biceps and supinator weakness.
- *C6 disc protrusion (C7 nerve root level)*: pain radiating down the middle forearm to the middle fingers, hypesthesia of the middle fingers, decreased triceps and radial reflexes, triceps and grip weakness.
- *C7 disc protrusion (C8 nerve root level)*: possible pain radiating down the medial forearm and hand, ulnar hypesthesia, intrinsic muscle weakness of the hand. However, these symptoms are uncommon. The reflexes are normal.

The above symptoms will vary depending upon the direction of the disc bulge; eg, upon the nerve root, IVF vessels, spinal cord, or combinations of involvement. In some acute and many chronic cases, numbness may manifest without pain. In acute disorders, these cervical signs may be confused with those of shoulder or elbow bursitis, epicondylitis, or subluxation, especially when no local cervical symptoms exist.

Vertebral Artery Compression. Associated subluxation and osteophyte development may produce vertebral artery compression, especially if a degree of arteriosclerosis is present (Fig. 9.27). Symptoms of unsteadiness, dizziness, and fainting spells will occur, especially when the head is rotated to the opposite side.

Autonomic Involvement. Vague autonomic symptoms may be exhibited, such as dizziness, blurred vision, and hearing difficulties. These can usually be attributed to involvement of the plexus around the vertebral artery or intermittent disruption of the blood flow.

Lhermitte's Sign. With the patient seated, flexing of the patient's neck and hips simultaneously with the patient's knees in

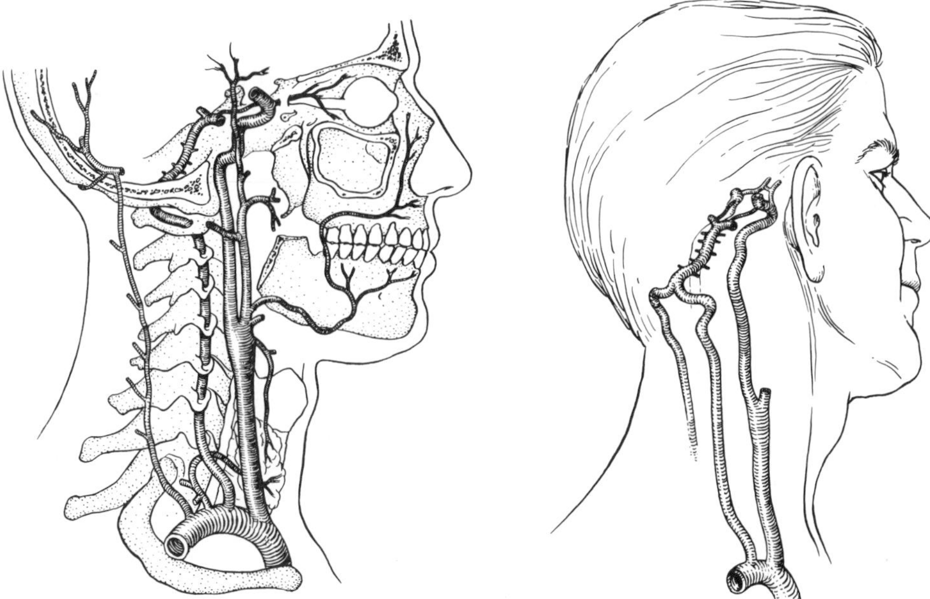

Figure 9.27. Course of the major arteries of the neck. Note the route of the vertebral artery through the cervical transverse foramina.

full extension may produce sharp pain radiating down the spine and into the upper or lower extremities. When pain is elicited, it is a sign suggesting irritation of the spinal dura matter either by a protruded cervical disc, tumor, fracture, or multiple sclerosis.

Therapeutic Considerations

Adjustive treatment consists of specific manipulation performed with manual or mechanical traction at the involved motion units to free impinged synovial fringes, reduce articular and disc displacements, and free areas of fixation. This should not be performed with the neck in extension, and extreme care must be taken to avoid joint, nerve, cord, or vascular insult.

Adjunctive therapy includes immobilization of the neck with a cervical collar; sleeping with the head between sand bags or in traction; heat (diathermy, ultrasound, infrared, moist hot packs) to reduce pain from muscle ischemia; trigger point therapy; and periodic bed rest with cervical traction by an orthopedic pillow. Gross vibrations (eg, long-distance automobile riding) and neck extension (eg, overhead work) must be avoided. Isometric exercises during rehabilitation to lengthen the cervical spine and strengthen the cervical muscles are extremely beneficial.

Referral for radical treatment is generally made if one of the following occurs: (1) conservative treatment fails to produce remission of symptoms; (2) attacks reappear after a short period; (3) severe nerve root compression with paralysis, indicated by muscle wasting and/or a persistent sensory deficit, has developed.

Cervical Spondylosis[247–250]

Three not infrequent diseases of the cervical spine with biomechanic implications are spondylosis, rheumatic spondylitis, and ankylosing spondylitis. In each of these conditions, severe subluxation is a cardinal manifestation.

Cervical spondylosis is a chronic condition in which there is progressive degeneration of the IVDs leading to secondary changes in the surrounding vertebral structures, including the posterior apophyseal joints. It is the result of direct trauma (ie, disc injury), occupational stress, or aging degeneration, or is found in association with and adjacent to subluxations and/or congenitally defective vertebrae.

Pathology

Spondylosis may produce compression of either the nerve root or spinal cord. During the degenerative process, intradisc pressure decreases, the anulus protrudes, and the endplates approximate because of reduction of disc thickness. As the disc protrudes, it loosens the attachment of the posterior longitudinal ligament and this allows the anulus to extrude into the cavity formed between the posterior vertebral body and the ligament. This portion of the anulus, in time, becomes fibrous and then calcifies (Fig. 9.28). It is because of this process that posterior osteophytes prevail in the cervical and lumbar regions, while anterior spurs are more common to the dorsal spine.

Incidence

Incidence is high in the second half of life with increasing severity in advancing years: 60% at 45 years, 85% at 65 years. The degenerative process, which may or may not progress, appears greatest in those segments below the maximum point of the lordosis because of the static and kinetic forces in the upright posture. It is most often seen at the C5 level, and next in frequency at the C6 level.

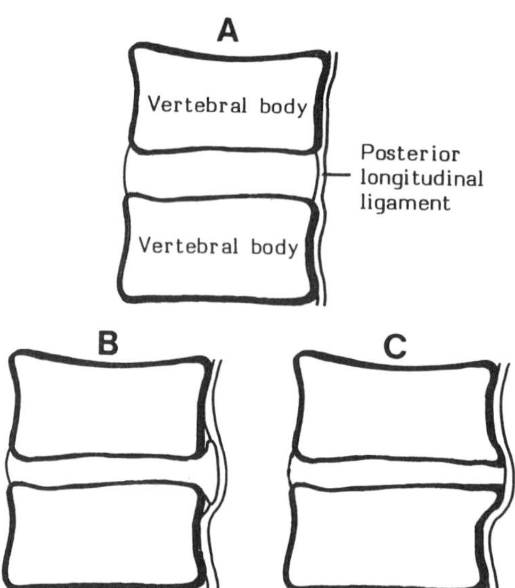

Figure 9.28. Mechanism of degenerative disc extrusion in spondylosis. *A*, normal vertebral motion unit. *B*, the first stage exhibits thinning of the degenerated disc and increased intradisc pressure separating the posterior longitudinal ligament from the vertebral bodies. *C*, the extruded disc later becomes fibrotic and then calcifies as part of the vertebral body, permanently narrowing the spinal canal.

Etiology

Pre-existing spinal stenosis, a thickened ligamentum flavum, a protruding disc, and spur formation not uncommonly complicate the picture of cervical spondylosis. There is almost no correlation between the degree of perceived pain in the neck and the degree of arthritic changes noted in x-ray films. The weight of the head in faulty posture (eg, exaggerated dorsal kyphosis and cervical lordosis) along with activity stress may contribute to chronic degenerative spondylosis often superimposed upon asymptomatic anomalies. Clinically, a vicious cycle is seen in which subluxation contributes to degenerative processes and these processes contribute to subluxation fixation.

Jeffreys points out that there appears to be a correlation of cervical spondylosis with carpal tunnel syndrome, lateral humeral epicondylitis, cervical stenosis, and low-back and/or lower extremity osteoarthritis.[251]

Signs and Symptoms

The onset is usually rapid and insidious but may be subjectively and objectively asymptomatic. The classic picture is one of a middle-aged person with greatly restricted cervical motion with marked muscle spasm, positive cervical compression test, insidious neck and arm pain and paresthesia aggravated by sneezing or coughing, acute radiculopathy from disc herniation, and usually some muscle weakness and fasciculations. Generally, central herniation produces local neck pain while lateral herniation produces upper extremity pain.

Whiting[252] lists the manifestations that develop in spondylosis to also include neck crepitus, subjective or objective; local neck tenderness; headaches; neck pain radiating to the scapulae, trapezius, upper extremities, occiput, or anterior thorax; extremity muscle weakness; paresthesia of the upper and/or lower extremities; dizziness and fainting; impaired vibration sense at the ankle; hyperactive patellar and Achilles reflexes; and positive Babinski responses.

Henderson and others also include many other local and remote effects such as:[253–258]

Ataxia	Memory faults
Atypical facial pains	Ménière's syndrome
Blurred vision	Mental confusion
Cold sweats	Nausea and vomiting
Deafness	Nystagmus
Diplopia	Pallor
Drop attacks	Paresis
Dysarthria	Poor concentration
Dysequilibrium	Precordial discomfort
Dysphagia	Pseudoangina
Dysphonia	Psychiatric disturbances
Epileptiform attacks	Retro-orbital pain
Fatigue	Tinnitus
Giddiness	Tonsillitis
Horner's syndrome	Upper extremity coldness
Indigestion	Vertigo
Irritability	
Lermoyez's syndrome	

Pathologic Mechanisms[259–263]

From the above, it is apparent that a subluxation complex leading to spondylosis can effect a wide variety of disturbances that may appear to be disrelated on the surface. Most of the remote effects can be grouped under the general classifications of nerve-root neuropathy, basilar venous congestion, cervical autonomic disturbances, CSF pressure and flow disturbances, irritation of the recurrent meningeal nerve, the Barré-Lieau syndrome, and/or the vertebral artery syndrome.

Roentgenographic Considerations

Because of the constant weight of the head, postural strains, occupational insults, degrees of congenital anomalies, and post-traumatic or postinfection effects with or without an associated disc involvement, the development of chronic degenerative spondylosis offers some distinct progressive characteristics: (1) flattening of the cervical spine from muscular spasm and adhesion development, (2) A-P fixation and restricted mobility, (3) thinning of the atlanto-occipital and atlantoaxial articular plates, resulting in motion restriction, (4) middle and lower cervical disc wearing and thinning which narrows the IVFs, (5) disc weakness encouraging nuclear shifting and herniation contributing to nerve encroachment, (6) osseous lipping and spurs with extensions into the IVFs, and (7) infiltration and ossification of paravertebral ligaments adding to inflexibility and pain upon movement.

The Davis series may suffice, but special views, tomography, myelography, or discography may be necessary for firm diagnosis.

Nelson[264] believes that head weight and postural strains are overemphasized; it has often been established clinically that "unless overt trauma can be shown, most neck problems are the result of reflex vasospasm where the reflex originates in the viscera below the diaphragm. Everyone would be affected if weight of the head and postural strains were common causes." Regardless of the merit of this controversial concept, it is important to avoid the pitfall of assuming that all the patient's symptoms involving the neck and upper extremities are caused by a cervical spondylosis when it is found radiographically. Cervical spondylosis is common, and symptoms may thus be associated with unrelated neurologic disease that may coexist with the spondylosis, making the diagnosis more difficult.

Case Management and Prognosis

Whiting brings out that it is fortunate that most people with cervical spondylosis are asymptomatic because there is no correction per se.[252] Treatment is aimed at reducing symptoms of neurologic and vasoneurologic involvement or treating the soft-tissue injury superimposed on the pre-existing spondylosis. A trial of conservative treatment is preferred in cases demonstrating signs of either cervical radiculopathy and/or myelopathy.

There is a natural tendency for a patient suffering with symptoms of radiculopathy related to cervical spondylosis to improve regardless of the treatment regimen. Unfortunately, the degenerative changes of the IVDs, vertebral bodies, and associated diarthrodial joints are permanent and, in most cases, progressive. Treatment is therefore aimed at reducing symptoms and future attacks by proper case management and prophylaxis. Exacerbation of symptoms is quite common, and months or years may elapse between attacks. With age and the gradual increase in degenerative changes, attacks are more closely spaced, and recovery from each attack is prolonged. Any trauma superimposed on silent cervical spondylosis can result in permanent partial disability of the cervical spine with symptoms far out of proportion to the severity of the injury.

In cervical myelopathy, there is a gradual increase in the neurologic signs and symptoms until a leveling off occurs and symptoms remain stationary, unless superimposed trauma ensues. Although conservative care does produce remission of subjective symptoms, especially in early diagnosed cases, objective signs are rarely changed and sensory symptoms often return and progress to a plateau. Thus, suggests Whiting, surgical intervention is probably the treatment of choice in myelopathy once symptoms return following a trial of conservative care, especially if there is evidence of paralysis.[252]

TORTICOLLIS[265–267]

Regardless of the cause of torticollis, the neck is rigid and tender, the head tilts laterally toward the side of spasticity, and the chin is usually rotated to the contralateral side. Care must be taken to determine the etiology and differentiate its many possible causes.

Background

Besides traumatic causes, torticollis may have an inflammatory, a congenital, or a neuropathic origin, or may result from various superimposed factors.

Severe Trauma

Traumatic dislocations of upper cervical vertebrae cause a distortion of the neck much like that of torticollis. A rotary fracture-dislocation of a cervical vertebra, especially of the atlas on the axis or the axis on C3, will produce neck rigidity and a fast pulse, but fever is absent. Local and remote trigger points are frequently involved. Even in mildly suspicious cases, the neck should always be x-rayed in two or more planes before it is physically examined.

Inflammation

"Wry neck" spasm (tonic, rarely clonic) of the sternocleidomastoideus and trapezius may be due to irritation of the spinal accessory nerve or other cervical nerves by swollen glands, abscess, acute upper respiratory infections, scar, or tumor. A spontaneous subluxation of the atlas may follow severe throat infection (eg, pharyngitis). Neck rigidity may also be the result of a sterile meningitis from blood in the cerebrospinal fluid. Thus, if a patient has slight fever, rapid pulse, and rigid neck muscles, subarachnoid hemorrhage should be suspected. Lateralizing signs are often indefinite.[268]

Congenital, Neuropathic, and Idiopathic Forms

The congenital form is commonly associated with Klippel-Feil syndrome, atlanto-occipital fusion, and pterygium colli. Focal neuropathic causes include ocular dysfunctions, syringomyelia, and tumors of the spinal cord or brain. Idiopathic forms are seen in acute calcification of a cervical disc, rheumatic arthritis, tuberculosis, or "nervous" individuals. Nelson feels that wry neck may also be the result of subdiaphragmatic or subclinical visceral irritation being mediated reflexly into the trapezius and cervical muscles.[264]

Subluxation

The most common direct cause is that from irritating cervical subluxation (eg, trauma, rotational overstress, unilateral chilling, unilateral lifting, instability). Subluxation may also be an asymptomatic complicating factor to those etiologic factors mentioned above.

Barge[269] states that the structural cause of torticollis is a rotary vertebral malposition and abnormal disc wedging, in which the nucleus of an involved disc has been forced to shift away from compressive forces. The patient's symptoms are often self-limiting with time and rest that allows the disc to expand in its non-weight-bearing (decompressed) state and the vertebral facets to be relieved of their jammed position. It can be theorized, however, that if the neck does not achieve this subluxation correction through disc imbibition, a rotary scoliosis is produced in adaptation so that the victim may at least have a straight eye level. But, as the now chronic subluxation has not been fully corrected, it can serve as a focus for morbid neurologic and degenerative processes, especially at the zygapophyses, covertebral joints, and IVFs.

The pain associated with acute torticollis is thought to be attributed essentially to zygapophyseal capsulitis and covertebral joint inflammation. This can generally be confirmed by palpation and should not be confused with the pain of stretching the rigid muscles on the side of the concavity.

Applied Anatomy

In the healthy cervical (or lumbar) spine that presents a moderate degree of lordosis, a good share of weight bearing is upon the zygapophyses because the line of cumulative loading of compressive forces is quite posterior to the center of the vertebral bodies. This produces a considerable degree of normal articular jamming as the result of loading that tends to restrict excessive rotation. That is, the rotary motion that occurs at the zygapophyses does so upon relatively compressed facets.

There is structural adaptation for this. For the normal adult spine, the cervical discs average 3 mm in thickness, there is a 2:5 disc/body ratio, a 4:7 nucleus/anulus ratio, and the nucleus sits in a position that is slightly posterior to the center of the disc. In addition, the surface area of the cervical facets is larger in proportion to the surface area of the vertebral body than at any other region of the spine. This contributes greatly to the overall segmental base of support in the neck. In fact, the area of weight-bearing surfaces of the two facets equal more than half (67%) that of the centrum. In addition, the superior facets below the axis face posterosuperiorly and medially to compensate for the normal anteroinferior tilt of the vertebral bodies.

The more the cervical curve becomes flattened, the more superimposed weight is shifted to the discs. With the shifting of the normal compressive forces at the posterior toward the anterior of the motion unit, the discs are forced to carry more weight and a greater responsibility in cervical stability. In time, this unusual compressive force on the nucleus can produce degenerative anular thinning, spurs, eburnation, and Schmorl's nodes. The posterior joints become relatively lax and predispose to retropositioning and posterior subluxations.

Clinical Classifications

Following is a classification, based on Barge's findings,[270] of three major types of torticollis that are the result of disc lesions.

Type I: Lateral Torticollis

The patient's neck is rigidly flexed laterally and locked, and this is usually accompanied by a degree of rotation of the chin away from the side of tilt. The spinous process of the involved vertebra will often palpate as being distinctly more lateral than its neighbor above and below.

From either traumatic or degenerative causes, the stiffness property of anular filaments may be so weakened as to allow considerable nuclear shifting within the disc. Barge feels that lateral shifting of the firm nucleus and consequent inferior tilting of the superimposed vertebra as it falls on a weakened anulus is the primary cause of lateral torticollis. Thus, a lateral nuclear shift to one side would be accompanied by disc compression on the other side, and the vertebral body above would tend to rotate away from the relatively higher side of the disc (nuclear site), following the plane of its base of support. It should be remembered that the nucleus serves as a ball-bearing–like fulcrum of movement of the superimposed vertebra.

The lateral tipping of the centrum causes the inferior apophyseal facet of the vertebra to ride down on the side of the thinned disc and up on the side to which the nucleus has shifted. This is usually within the range of physiologic movement. However, the added rotation of the centrum causes the inferior facet of the vertebra to separate (open) on the side of rotation, stretching the apophyseal capsule and covertebral synovial tissues beyond their normal limit, while the inferior facet on the other side merely rides up and serves as a pivot point for subluxation. This would encourage apophyseal capsulitis and covertebral inflammation, with profound reflex spasm to splint the affected area locked by the displaced nucleus.

Type II: Anterior Torticollis

The subject's cervical area is rigidly projected forward. In severe cases, all cervical motions are restricted. In mild cases, the complaint may be only a "stiff neck."

It should be kept in mind that the relatively small atlas must provide an upward push equal to the weight of the head. This is about a 14-lb static resistance force for a 200-lb individual. If the head is tilted so that its center of mass is not in line with both atlantal articulations, the cervical muscles opposite to the direction of tilt must contract to maintain equilibrium. If the muscles and ligaments at the base of the skull do not check the compressive and shear forces, failure can readily produce a degree of subluxation.

Using the same reasoning given for lateral torticollis, anterior torticollis is predisposed by a flattened area in the cervical spine that allows laxity of the zygapophyseal check ligaments, a posterior shifting of a nucleus, posterior disc bulge, and anteroinferior displacement of the superimposed vertebra (following the plane of its base of support) as its inferior facets ride up the superior facets of the subjacent vertebra. The spinous process can frequently be palpated as being distinctly superior.

As the inferior facets of the involved vertebra tip anteroinferiorly on the superior facets below, a pivot action occurs that overstretches the apophyseal capsules posteriorly. If severe, this will produce an apophyseal capsulitis and local tenderness will be acute. If the atlas has displaced anteriorly on the axis, a capsulitis may also occur at the atlantal-dens articulation and/or less frequently at the dens-cruciate junction.

Type III: Anterolateral Torticollis

This form of torticollis, the most frequently seen type, presents a combined lateral and anterior torticollis subluxation. The patient's neck is grossly projected forward and to one side, and the symptoms are usually intense. The disc mechanism involved is the same as that for lateral and anterior torticollis except that the involved nucleus is thought to shift obliquely in a posterolateral direction.

The types of torticollis described above are merely points of study. Within a clinical case, any type may occur singly or in combination and may involve one or more segements. If only one vertebra within an area is essentailly involved, a nuclear shift should be suspected after fracture and dislocation have been ruled out. Barge also explains contralateral attacks as being the result of a horizontal shifting of a nucleus from one side to the other.

In chronic cases, the patient may be asymptomatic if the sites of acute inflammation have become fibrotic. Most of the symptoms presented will usually be neurologic or vascular in nature, such as the paresthesias and referred pain of brachial plexus syndromes.

Selected Effects of Cervical Area Hypertonicity

Excessive hypertonicity of a muscle, confirmed by palpatory tone and soreness, will tend to subluxate its site of osseous attachment.[271] Below is a listing of common problem areas in the neck.

1. *Splenius capitis.* Increased tone tends to pull the C5–T3 spinous processes lateral, superior, and anterior, and to subluxate the occiput inferiorly, medially, and posteriorly.
2. *Scalenus anterior.* Increased tone tends to pull the C3–C6 transverse processes inferior, lateral, and anterior, and the 1st rib superior, and medial (see Fig. 9.28.).
3. *Scalenus medius.* Increased tone tends to pull the C1–C7 transverse processes inferior, lateral, and anterior, and the 1st rib superior and medial.
4. *Scalenus posterior.* Increased tone tends to pull the C4–C6 transverse processes inferior, lateral, and anterior, and the 2nd rib superior and medial.
5. *Obliquus capitis superior.* Increased tone tends to roll the occiput anterior and inferior and pull the atlas posterior and superior to produce lateral occiput tilt and condyle jamming.
6. *Obliquus capitis inferior.* Increased tone tends to produce a rotary torque of the atlas-axis motion unit.
7. *Rectus capitis posterior major.* Increased tone tends to pull the occiput posterior, inferior, and medial, and the spinous process of the axis superior, lateral, and anterior. Strong hypertonicity will lock the occiput

and axis together so that they appear to act as one unit even though they are not contiguous.

8. *Interspinales.* Increased tone tends to hyperextend the motion unit.

9. *Sternocleidomastoideus.* Increased tone tends to pull the sternum and clavicle posterior and superior, and the occiput inferior and anterior.

10. *Upper trapezius.* Increased tone tends to pull the occiput posteroinferior, the C5–C7 spinous processes lateral, and the shoulder girdle medial and superior.

The Troublesome Fifth Cervical Area

In the previous discussion on cervical fixation, it was pointed out that the multifidi are especially prone to fixation at the C4–C6 area. In the discussion on cervical disc disorders, it was stated that the encroachment of space, faulty movement, apophyseal subluxation, osteophyte formation, and disc degeneration and protrusion occur most frequently at the C4–C6 level. It was also stated that the highest incidence of cervical spondylosis is found at the C4–C6 level. This is also true for early osteoarthritis in the neck, IVD narrowing, apophyseal compression fracture, dislocation of pivot point, traumatic brachial traction, extension whiplash injury, lower cervical fixation, a dislodged disc nucleus, and ankylosing spondylitis. A common trigger point in "stiff neck" is found in the splenius cervicus, lateral to the C4–C6 spinous processes. These facts were derived from the work of a large number of separate researchers with various backgrounds (chiropractic, allopathic, osteopathic, bioengineering).

The clinical importance of the 5th cervical vertebra was brought out by pioneer chiropractor Clarence Reaver in the 1930s, and it has been emphasized recently by Pierce.[272] The biomechanical importance of the C5 vertebra becomes logical when we realize that the cervical curve often extends from C1 to D2, with its apex at C5. It is not functionally restricted to the C1–C7 vertebrae as depicted in most anatomy textbooks, in which the classic apex of the lordosis is located at C4.

Range of Motion

In a previous chapter, it was mentioned that normal spinal motion in the pure horizontal plane occurs only at the center of the curves (Fig. 6.6). While 50% of A-P motion of the cervical spine takes place between the occiput and the atlas, the remainder is distributed among the other cervical vertebrae, with C5 and C6 making the greatest contribution. This is also true in lateral bending and rotation below the axis. Thus, if C5 becomes fixed, compensatory effects (and symptoms) will be exhibited at the upper cervical and upper dorsal areas. This is readily confirmed empirically. In abnormal cervical kyphosis, it will be found that C5 is most frequently the center vertebra of the affected segmental region and symptomatic picture.

Neurology

We note in practice that upper extremity symptoms are far more frequently exhibited on the lateral (radial) aspect of the shoulder and arm than on the medial (ulnar) aspect. Abduction weakness of the shoulder is much more common than adduction weakness. A causative hypothesis is that this occurs because the C5 and C6 nerves comprise the upper aspect of the brachial plexus, supplying fibers to the musculocutaneous, axillary, radial, and median nerves—all but the ulnar. The deltoid muscle is innervated almost entirely by the C5 nerve. The biceps muscle receives dual innervation from the C5 and C6 nerves. Thus the strength of the deltoid and biceps are excellent sources to determine the motor integrity of midcervical innervation. It should also be noted that the C5 afferent pathway supplies sensation from the lateral arm, especially that over the deltoid—the site of the common "silver dollar sign" of hypesthesia.[273] Another important test is the biceps reflex, essentially determined by the C5 pathway with a lesser C6 component. Cervical compression tests usually stress the C5 segment more than any other area because of its horizontal plane.

CHRONIC INFLAMMATORY DISEASES OF THE CERVICAL SPINE

Rheumatoid Arthritis[274-276]

This common and highly deforming disorder is a generalized disease of connective tissue that initiates in joint synovium. Even when cervical symptoms are absent, periodic cervical roentgenographs should be taken to assess progress.

The initial target areas in the cervical spine are the apophyseal joints and the synovial tissues anterior and posterior to the dens where it articulates with the anterior arch of the atlas and the cruciate ligament. Other tissues affected include the IVDs, spinal ligaments, and extradural alveolar tissue. A genetic susceptibility factor has been shown to be involved in most cases.

The length of the cervical cord and cervical discs is greatest during flexion and least during extension in the normal spine. The opposite is true in the rheumatic spine because of loss of disc and vertebral body height from destruction and absorption.

Rheumatic Atlantoaxial Subluxation

Orthopedic subluxation is always a danger, proceeding from the synovitis, apophyseal erosion, and erosion of the vertebral bodies involved, which lead to instability from joint destruction and ligamentous laxity. As apophyseal erosion progresses, the dens migrates into the foramen magnum and the atlas becomes fixed to the axis to reduce the possibility of dislocation. These signs determine the severity and prognosis of the general disease.

The characteristic anterior subluxation of the atlas on the axis is generally considered to be an adaptation change to help increase the capacity of the spinal canal as rheumatoid tissue accumulates. If this is true, the decision for clinical reduction presents a dilemma. This anterior subluxation usually occurs only in flexion unless granulation tissue between the atlas and dens prevents reduction during extension. Thus, direct reduction of the orthopedic rheumatic subluxation by either manipulation or traction is usually contraindicated. Jeffrey states: "The incidence of neurological damage in subluxated (rheumatic) spines is very low," and "not infrequently the cord only becomes compromised when the subluxation is reduced."

Neurologic Damage

Nerve roots may become entrapped within one or more IVFs from a combination of subluxation, perivascular adhesions, dural adhesions, rheumatoid nodules, granulation tissue, and sequestrated disc tissue. Neck pain, with or without radiation to the arms, weakness, feelings of instability, ataxia, and paresthesias are common symptoms. However, these cervical symptoms are difficult to differentiate if the disease initiates in the peripheral joints where signs of peripheral entrapment, myositis, tenosynovitis, and subluxated joints from tendon rupture exist. Related giddiness and fainting spells suggest an associated vertebral artery ischemia that is usually associated with the upward migration of the dens, producing a kinking of the vertebral artery at the atlas level.

Differentiation from Spondylosis

In both degenerative and rheumatic spondylosis, involvement of the cervical cord first involves the anterolateral tracts and central gray matter of the cord. The effect is signs of an upper motor (pressure ischemia) lesion with a degree of tetraparesis produced by the reduced A-P dimension of the vertebral canal.

Degenerative spondylosis is differentiated from rheumatoid spondylosis in that the latter frequently involves the upper cervical area, and osteophyte formation and endplate sclerosis are usually absent, unless the two disorders are superimposed. The small peripheral joints are usually also involved in rhematoid arthritis.

Ankylosing Spondylitis of the Cervical Spine[277,278]

In ankylosing spondylitis, the tissues subjacent to articular cartilage are the first to be affected. Thus, the cartilage is invaded and erodes from below, in contrast to the surface erosion of rheumatoid arthritis.

Early diagnosis and management is important to reduce gross deformity. The first signs are not usually cervical but found in the dorsal spine (reduced chest expansion), lumbar spine (vertebral body "squaring"), and sacroiliac joints (erosion). The first cervical sign is usually that of reduced lateral flexion, followed by increasing gross neck flexion at rest and upper cervical subluxation. However, deformity is usually greatest at the lumbar spine and hips.

In addition to the disease process itself, a great danger in the ankylosing spine is the addition of trauma. Because the neck is unable to properly extend, any anteriorly directed force to the head can easily inflict a vertebral fracture. This usually occurs through a fused disc area, with or without residual displacement. Regardless, instability is great. Cord damage can result from impact if the shear forces produce posterior displacement.

CERVICAL DEFORMITIES AND ANOMALIES[279–281]

Congenital deformities of the cervical spine are extremely frequent but not frequently extreme. Those that have biomechanical significance vary in severity from minor to severe and occur multiply or singly. The cause is purely genetic transmission in about 35% of cases, and the remainder is due to environmental factors or a mixture of genetic and environmental factors.

Gross anomalies are rarely seen in chiropractic practice unless well adapted to the individual's life-style. However, subtle and asymptomatic anomalies in the cervical area frequently predispose subluxations from minor stress and underlie a pathologic process. Many anomalies do not become symptomatic unless the effects of trauma or degeneration are added. The primary concerns are whether the deformity will increase with growth and normal activity and how much the deformity contributes to the degree of cervical instability and neurologic deficit present.

Bony Anomalies of the Cervical Spine[282, 283]

Three general classifications can be made:

1. Cranio-occipital anomalies: basilar coarctation, occipital vertebrae, atlantoid assimilation, occipital dysplasia, and condylar hypoplasia.

2. Anomalies of the atlas and axis: atlas arch dysplasia and odontoid dysplasia.

3. Lower cervical anomalies (C3–C7): failure of segmentation (eg, Klippel-Feil syndrome); fusion failure (eg, spina bifida, spondylolisthesis); and cervical rib.

The above deformities are described in detail in standard radiologic atlases and do not require repetition here. However, a few points are worthy of review in this section.

Craniovertebral Malformations[284–288]

These many and varied anomalies arise from occipital malformations characterized by an abnormal shift upward of the atlas and axis with the odontoid protruding above Chamberlain's line (Fig. 9.29). Such anomalies are frequently associated with congenital neural malformations and with other osseous deformities (eg, Klippel-Feil syndrome). As these anomalies may remain asymptomatic unless precipitated by compressive forces following trauma or degeneration, a concern is that these anomalies may easily be confused with the root/cord signs and symptoms of lower cervical spondylosis. Headache, sensory loss, limb pain, and ataxia are often associated.

Congenital Basilar Coarctation and Platybasia

Basilar coarctation is the state in which the tip of the odontoid lies abnormally high above Chamberlain's or McGregor's line. The disorder should not be confused with platybasia, an anthropometric flattening of the base of the skull as seen in Down's syndrome. This is often associated with congenital atlantoaxial subluxation, which occurs in 20% of mongoloid children. Platy-

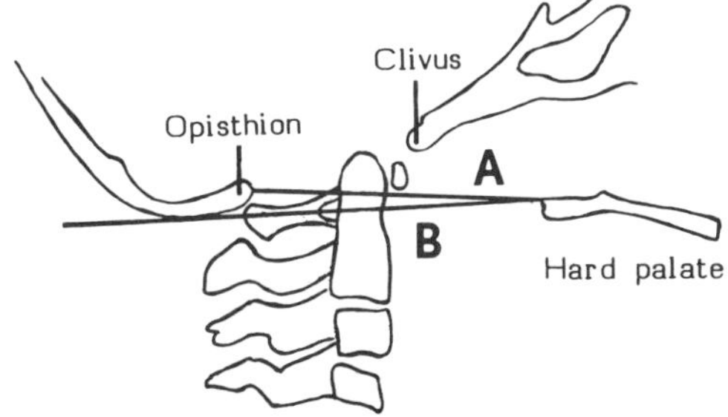

Figure 9.29. Diagnostic lateral atlanto-occipital roentgenographic lines. *A*, Chamberlain's line, extending from the posterior lip of the foramen magnum (opisthion) to the posterior margin of the hard palate. However, the opisthion is sometimes difficult to locate and a highly arched palate can distort this reference point. *B*, McGregor's line, drawn from the superior surface of the dorsal edge of the hard palate to the most caudal point of the curve of the posteroinferior occipital base. This line is usually used because the bony landmarks are commonly quite clear.

basia is measured by the angle extending from the clivus and the opisthion that is greater than 130°. Such developmental deformity must be differentiated from basilar impression.

Basilar Impression

This rare deformity is the result of a congenital or an acquired invagination of the odontoid process into the foramen magnum, measured by the height of the odontoid above Chamberlain's or McGregor's line on a lateral film. The diagnostic A-P line of Fischgold-Metzger is used to differentiate basilar impression from an abnormally long dens and/or high palate (Fig. 9.30). In basilar impression, the atlas appears to indent the base of the skull on an A-P film as the odontoid approaches the brain stem. During inspection, the ears will be closer to the shoulders even though the length of the cervical spine is normal. The congenital form is usually associated with other defects such as atlanto-occipital fusion, aplasia of the posterior arch of the atlas, and atlantoaxial dislocation. The acquired form is a sign seen in Paget's disease and osteomalacia or rickets. It is the result of head weight superimposed on softened structures at the base of the skull. Often, symptoms do not appear until later life and then can mimic a number of acquired neurologic disturbances.

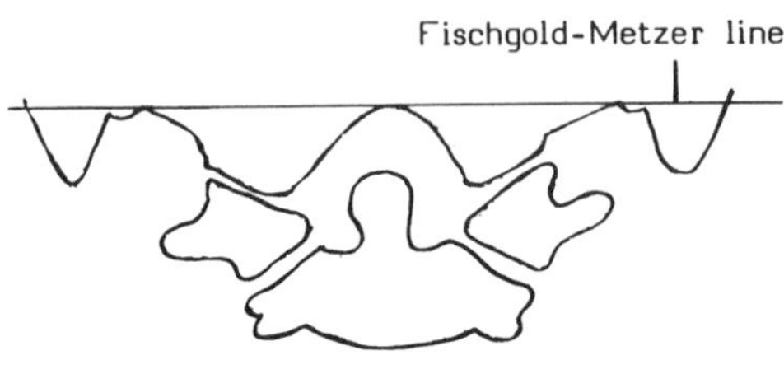

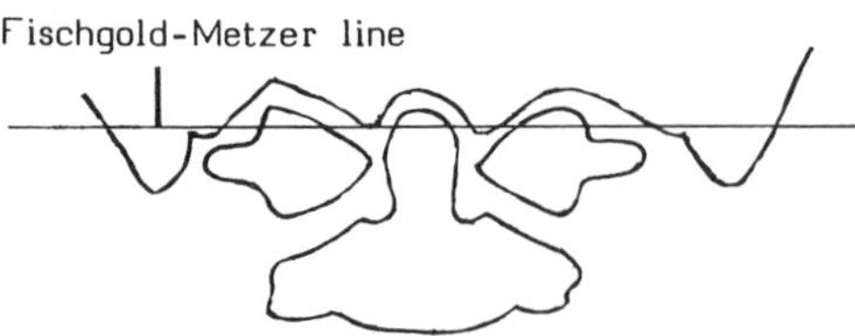

Figure 9.30. The line of Fischgold-Metzer is drawn on an A-P film through the digastric grooves located at the junction of the medial aspect of the mastoid process and the base of the occiput. This line should pass well above the tip of the dens unless basilar impression is present. *Top*, normal; *bottom*, basilar impression.

Occipitalization

Atlanto-occipital fusion (atlantal assimilation) is the most common anomaly of this joint, and C2–C3 fusion is associated in 70% of the cases. The gross features are those of Klippel-Feil syndrome.

Aplasia of the Arch of the Atlas

This rare deformity may vary from a slight opening to a complete loss of the anterior arch. Quite often the anomaly is asymptomatic unless precipitated by trauma.

Odontoid Anomalies

These rare deformities vary from an abnormally small size (hypoplasia) to a bifid odontoid, os odontoideum (suggesting congenital dysplasia or traumatic nonunion), or complete absence (agenesis). It is easy to confuse congenital absence with absorbed nonunion after fracture in early life.

Congenital Atlantoaxial Instability

Various precipitating factors may be involved in congenital predisposition to atlantoaxial instability. Most common are an abnormal odontoid, a loose cruciate ligament, and atlanto-occipital fusion—all of which can produce transient narrowing of the spinal canal and compression of its contents. The normal anterior atlas-dens interval is 3 mm in the adult and 4 mm in the child, particularly during flexion (Fig. 9.31). A distance greater than this indicates a ruptured or stretched transverse cruciate ligament following acute trauma. It should be noted that a hypermobile odontoid is also seen in mongoloids and rheumatoid arthritis. Of equal importance is the corresponding posterior dens-atlas interval that indicates the space available for the tissues within the spinal canal. It is rare to find an adult patient with less than 19 mm of posterior dens-atlas space who is asymptomatic, and cord compression is possible when the space is less than 17 mm.

Congenital Torticollis[289–291]

The clinical picture of this deformity is one of contracture of the sternocleidomas-

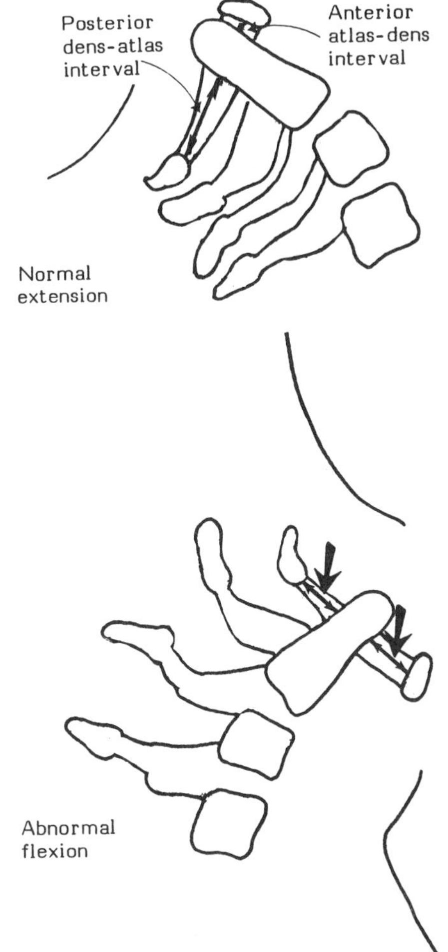

Figure 9.31. Drawings of atlantoaxial instability demonstrated during lateral flexion-extension stress films. *Top*, cervical extension with normal atlas-dens relationships; *bottom*, cervical flexion with abnormal anterior shifting of the atlas from the dens.

toideus; the head tilts toward the involved side and the chin rotates toward the contralateral side. A related facial deformity is often exhibited in later life.

Coventry and Harris[292] have reported that 90% of their infant patients respond to stretching exercises alone, yet undoubtedly a degree of subluxation exists (usually C1–C2) that should be corrected. The birth history will often portray a forceps delivery.

In skeletal torticollis, compensatory scoliosis below the defect may hide the physical picture or asymmetry of the occipital condyles that cause tilting of the atlanto-occipital and atlantoaxial joints. Differentiation must be made from acquired muscular torticollis.

Klippel-Feil Syndrome[293, 294]

This syndrome, which varies in degree of severity, classically consists of a short neck, a low hairline, and severe neck stiffness associated with fusion of the cervical (and possibly upper thoracic) vertebrae into bony blocks. It is sometimes referred to as congenital cervical synostosis. A case may be structurally severe yet asymptomatic of neurologic signs (eg, paresthesia, mirror movements of hands from an underlying neural defect) unless precipitated by trauma. Idiopathic deafness occurs in 30% of cases.

Associated deformities frequently include degrees of scoliosis and kyphosis; hemivertebrae; cervical rib; spina bifida; Sprengel's deformity, which is a small, elevated scapula often connected to the cervical spine; and Turner's syndrome, featuring webbing of the neck, gonadal hypoplasia, and cubitus valgus.

Acquired fusions are differentiated by the fact that (1) in acquired fusions, the margins of the vertebral body tend to be irregular, disc lines are wider than the adjacent vertebral bodies, the posterior arches are frequently subluxated, (2) congenital fusions are narrow, the disc remnants are no wider than the adjacent bodies, bony trabeculae tend to cross the disc line, and (3) associated deformities are not found.

Congenital Spinal Stenosis[295]

A degree of congenital narrowing of the cervical vertebral canal, for some reason seen only in males, will easily mimic cervical spondylosis in the young. Progressive thickening of the laminae is often initially diagnosed as multiple sclerosis because of the progressive tetraplegic spasticity produced.

Cervical Rib[166, 296–298]

Anomalous development of extra ribs in the region of the cervical vertebrae may be a single unilateral rib, bilateral, or multiple bilaterally. The condition is usually seen at C7, but may arise as high as C4, and the cause is a variation in the position of the limb buds. The anomaly may vary from a small nubbin to a fully developed rib. A small rudimentary rib may give rise to more symptoms than a well-developed rib because of a fibrous band attached between the cervical rib and sternum or 1st thoracic rib.

Significance

A cervical rib arising from C7 and ending free or attached to the T1 rib appears in the neck as an angular fullness which may pulsate owing to the presence of the subclavian artery above it. It rarely produces symptoms, and it is often first noticed when percussing the apex of the lung. The bone can be felt behind the artery by careful palpation in the supraclavicular fossa and demonstrated by roentgenography. Pain or wasting in the arm and occasionally thrombosis may occur from impaired circulation.

Grieve points out that some clinicians are far too anxious to blame upper limb paresthesia on the presence of a cervical rib just because it is there.[299] Many patients with a cervical rib have no complaints, many without a cervical rib have complaints, and many patients with complaints have symptoms on the contralateral side of a unilateral cervical rib. However, when any anomaly such as a cervical rib is seen roentgenographically, the examiner should be suspicious that other anomalies not as evident may be associated.

Differential Considerations

The etiologic theories of the cervicobrachial syndrome are compression of the nerve trunks, trauma to nerve trunks, injuries to the sympathetic and vasomotor nerves, trauma to the scalenus anterior muscle, embryologic defects, postural or functional defects, narrowing of the upper thoracic cap as a result of adjacent infections or anatomical defects, acute infection producing myositis, intermittent trauma to the subclavian artery, or a cervical rib.

Case Management

Palliative relief can be obtained in many cases by correction of posture and specific subluxations, gentle manipulation of the upper dorsal and lower cervical spine, cervical traction and other relaxing physiotherapy. Those cases treated conservatively usually show a recurrence of symptoms periodically, and those cases that do not respond to conservative treatment frequently require surgery.

TEMPOROMANDIBULAR JOINT DISORDERS[300–305]

During the last decade, recognition of the clinical importance of TMJ dysfunction to the cervical spine and body as a whole has greatly accelerated. During examination, remember that the TMJ is the most active joint of the body, moving up to 2000 times each day during talking, chewing, swallowing, yawning, and snoring.

Functional Anatomy

The TMJ hinges within the glenoid fossa, gliding forward to the eminentia during normal motion. The joint meniscus divides the joint cavity into two divisions. The lower part is used during gliding motion, and the upper part is used for hinge movements. This is accomplished by one head of the external pterygoid muscle pulling the meniscus forward while the second head opens the joint. Some assistance is provided by the mylohyoid, geniohyoid, and digastric muscles. Obviously, gravity is helpful in the upright position. Thus, the two heads of the pterygoid muscle, essentially, act asynchronously to open the TMJ. In closing the jaw (approximating the mandible and maxillae), the temporal, masseter, and internal pterygoid muscles are activated. All muscles that are active during TMJ function assist in maintaining the mandible in its resting position.

The head of the condyle and the glenoid fossa are covered with fibroid cartilage that serves as a shock absorber and wears quite thin when subjected to abnormal stress because it contains no direct blood supply. The articular space contains a small amount of viscous fluid for lubrication. The blood supply to the TMJ is from the superficial temporal branch of the external carotid artery; the disc itself, however, is avascular.

Etiology

TMJ dysfunction is four times more prevalent in women than in men. Numerous causative factors have been hypothesized. The more common general explanations include extrinsic trauma, intrinsic overstress, genetic disorders, nutritional factors, endocrine problems, and psychologic factors. The typical clinical picture includes several of these general factors, which express themselves mechanically in complete or partial dislocations of the articular disc.

It is hypothesized in several osteopathic papers that TMJ dysfunction is essentially imparted by stress factors that distort position of the temporal bone. For example, Magoun[306] states that the temporal bone usually rotates externally-internally on an axis that extends from the petrous apex to the jugular surface, depending on the stress pattern present. The temporomandibular fossa moves posteromedially during temporal external rotation (temporal protrusion) and anterolaterally during temporal internal rotation (temporal flattening), with the position of the mandible moving to correspond to the position of the temporomandibular fossae. Thus, the mandible will protrude if both temporals are in external rotation, and the mandible will retrude if both temporals are in internal rotation. Hruby[307] feels that it is more common to find that one temporal is in internal rotation and one is in external rotation, thus producing mandibular misalignment.

Mechanisms of Local Overstress

Joint sprain is usually the result of improper dentition, subluxation, or dislocation from trauma (eg, whiplash, eating an apple, traction). Relative muscle strain, capsule and ligament sprain, muscle spasm, and soft-tissue swelling may be involved, depending upon the extent of injury. Poor occlusion leads to a chronic sprain or strain as does bruxism (teeth grinding). Bruxism is commonly increased in anxiety states, thus TMJ dysfunction is often related to psychoneurosis. Overstretch results in pterygoid spasm and an asymmetrical lateral motion of the jaw. Restricted joint motion can be the result of muscle spasm, rheumatoid arthritis, osteoarthritis, joint ankylosis, scar tissue, trismus from spasm of the elevating muscles of mastication from hysteria, tetanus, congenital defect, or almost any type of local inflammation.

During examination, ask the patient to tap the teeth together and note the bite. The mandible normally moves backward during cervical extension and forward in cervical flexion, producing poor occlusion during flexion-extension. You can readily test this on yourself. Thus, a patient with a cervical spine in a chronic state of flexion or extension in the neutral position will exhibit a constant state of malocclusion, leading to TMJ dysfunction.

Articular Disrelationships

Mechanically, two major forms of joint malposition occur. They arise from either partial displacement or complete dislocation of the articular disc and occur in 10–12% of the population.[308]

In partial anterior displacements, condyle translation is not blocked; ie, when the patient moves the closed jaw forward and/or toward the contralateral side, the condyle will snap forward (opening click) into its normal position so that the mouth can be fully opened. However, when the jaw is retruded, the disc displaces with a snap (reciprocal click).[309]

In complete dislocation, the disc is usually dislodged anteriorly toward the front of the condyle so that its translation is restricted when the mouth is opened, increasing the joint space. Persistent condylar motion upon a dislocated disc encourages irregular adaptive remodeling and osteoarthritis to develop within the joint because the dislocated disc can no longer cushion the articular surfaces. Crepitus will be exhibited if bone-on-bone articulation occurs. In time, the collateral ligaments may perforate or tear and be drawn into the articular space and osteoarthritis will develop.

Neuromuscular Considerations

Within the immediate area of the TMJ are found the chorda tympani nerve, and branches of the superficial temporary artery, vein, and nerve; irritation in this area may cause reflex pain in other areas.

The external pterygoid muscle, the prime opener of the mouth, is supplied by the pterygoid branch of the mandibular division of the trigeminal nerve. Secondary force in opening is provided by the hyoid muscles and gravity when upright. The masseter and temporalis muscles, both supplied by the trigeminal nerve, are the primary closers of the jaw, with secondary effort provided by the internal pterygoid muscle. The capsule and structures of the TMJ are innervated by branches of the articular temporal nerve, filaments of the masseter nerve, and a sensory branch from the 7th cranial.

The TMJ nerves are not vulnerable to direct compression by the condyle, but the joint's proprioceptive bed is abundant with nerve endings. Thus, strain or subluxation, unilaterally or bilaterally, may not only cause symptoms within the joint and associated soft tissues but may also, by reflex action, mirror distorting effects within the musculature innervated by the gray cell motor columns of the C1–C4 neuromeres. A reflex aberrant stimulation transmitted downward via the tractus spinalis of the 5th cranial nerve, with attending atlanto-occipital jamming and atlantoaxial and/or C3 rotary subluxation, may result in suboccipital and cervical migraine (occipitofrontal neuralgia) caused by asymmetrical spasm of the suboccipital muscles and the upper extensions of the cervical multifidi.

Symptomatology[310–314]

The major symptoms of TMJ dysfunction are masticatory muscle fatigue and pain, which is usually described as a severe, unilateral (rarely bilateral), dull facial ache that is often fairly localized to an area just anterior to the tragus of the ear.

The onset of symptoms is gradual, progressively increasing over several days or months, and the pain is aggravated by chewing. It is often precipitated by eating an apple, a wide yawn, snorkeling, prolonged dental work, playing a wind instrument, prolonged chewing (eg, gum, a large quantity of popcorn), a blow to the mandible, sleeping in the prone position, or a cervical whiplash.

Joint clicking, popping, or grinding is often felt and/or heard (with or without auscultation). The mandible deviates to one side when opened, tenderness and muscle spasm are present, a nervous bruxism is usually present, and there is pain on opening and closing the mouth, or, sometimes, just by moving the head on the neck (Table 9.6). An associated referred earache is common, but note that an ear disorder can sometimes refer pain to the TMJ area.

The locations of associated muscle spasm in TMJ dysfunction, in order of incidence, are the external pterygoids, internal pterygoids, masseter, posterior cervical, temporalis, sternomastoid, trapezius, and mylohyoid. The rhomboids and scalene attachments to the first rib are also commonly tender and tight.

While pain is often referred from the TMJ to the scalp, supraorbital area, ear, or neck, it is rarely a site of referred pain except in cases of a tooth abscess in the mandible or an inflamed upper or lower wisdom tooth impaction. Nine of the 12 cranial nerves are in close relation to the temporal bones from which the mandible is suspended; thus, universal effects may be expressed. There is no doubt that TMJ dysfunction can have far-reaching effects, even to the point of involving peripheral circulation (eg, cold hands or feet, paresthesias). Smith, for example, reported a case in which major improvement in leg circulation directly corresponded to balancing a left TMJ compression by jaw repositioning.[304]

Inspection and Palpation

Inspect active joint motion by having the patient open and close his mouth and observe the movement of the mandible from the front and sides. Motion rhythm should be smooth, the arc should be continuous and unbroken, and the mandible should open and close in a straight line symmetrically, with the teeth easily separating and joining. Awkward arc, restricted range of motion, and lateral deviation during motion suggest an abnormality.

Palpation should include bony palpation and the soft-tissue palpation of the area, especially the external pterygoid muscle. During the initial palpation of the TMJs, the examiner sits in front of the patient and places the index finger of each hand in the patient's external auditory canals and applies pressure anteriorly while the patient opens and closes his mouth. Motion of the mandibular condyles will be felt on the fingertips. The motion felt should normally be smooth and equal on both sides.

Next, the lateral aspects of the joints are palpated by placing the first and second fingers just anterior to the tragi. Have the patient open and close the mouth, and note

Table 9.6.
Major Signs and Symptoms of TMJ Dysfunction

Local effects	Remote effects
Mandible deviates to one side when opened	Tenderness of posterior cervical muscles, usually unilateral
Joint click (palpable and/or audible) in displacement but not in dislocation	Pain radiates from TMJ area superiorly to temporoparietal region and/or inferiorly into the neck
Severe, unilateral, dull facial pain, aggravated by chewing and opening and closing the mouth.	Muscle spasm:
Crepitus of involved joint (sometimes)	Posterior cervicals
Tenderness at proximal mandible, usually unilateral	Sternocleidomastoid
Muscle spasm:	Trapezius
External pterygoids	Mylohyoid
Internal pterygoids	Scalenes
Masseter	Earache
Temporalis	Postural distortion (anywhere from the occiput to the feet)
Bruxism	Rib cage, spinal, and lower extremity sites of fixation and trigger points.
Malocclusion	Peripheral circulation disorders
Atypical facial neuralgia	Migraine

any abnormalities. A palpable crepitus suggests traumatic synovial swelling or meniscus damage, and a slight dislocation (painful) may be felt when the patient widely opens his mouth. If there is any doubt as to the presence of crepitus, auscult the joint for clicks or grating sounds (Fig. 9.32).

Palpate the middle fibers of the temporalis muscles between the eye and the upper ear. Palpate the body portion of the masseter muscles. Palpate the external pterygoid muscles by having the patient open his mouth. Point a gloved index finger posteriorly above the last molar, between the gum and the buccal mucosa, on the mandibular neck. The external pterygoid will normally be felt to tighten and relax as the patient opens and closes the mouth. The patient will report tenderness and pain upon palpation if the muscle has been strained or is in spasm. Palpate the internal pterygoid muscle intra- and extraorally simultaneously. Palpate the mylohyoid muscle beneath the tongue. The examiner may wish to test the jaw and Chvostek's reflexes at this time if they have not been checked previously, and then the posterior cervical, sternocleidomastoideus, and trapezius muscles for hypertonicity and tenderness.

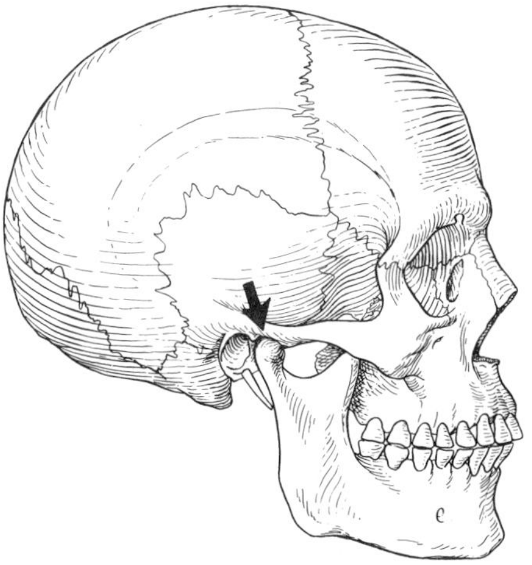

Figure 9.32. The temporomandibular joint.

Range of Motion and Muscle Strength

The adult range of motion is usually normal (1) if the examiner is able to insert three finger widths between the incisor teeth when the mouth is opened, and (2) if the patient is able to jut his jaw forward and place his lower teeth in front of his upper teeth. An accurate measurement of the interincisal opening can be made using a Boley gauge if necessary.

Test muscle strength by placing one hand on the patient's occiput to steady the patient and the other hand, palm up, under the patient's jaw. The patient opens his mouth while the examiner applies resistance with the palm. The patient should normally be able to open his mouth against the increasing resistance of the palm. When the patient is unable to close his mouth actively, the examiner checks to see if it can be closed passively.

If a patient with a subnormal range of mandibular motion can suddenly open the mouth wider after the TMJ area has been sprayed with a vapocoolant, muscle hypertonicity should be suspected as an important ingredient in the syndrome.

Craniospinal Mechanisms[315]

While the cranial sutures are immovable in cadavers and anatomical specimens, they are slightly movable in the living body, although it is often taught that they are not. The two uniting and five intervening layers between the edges of adjacent bones in the skull offer a strong bond of union but one which will permit definite though limited movement. This movement is thought to be necessary for tissue respiration of the brain and spinal cord. It is controlled by the following structures and motions: (1) the inherent motility of the brain and spinal cord, (2) the fluctuations of the cerebrospinal fluid, (3) the mobility of the intracranial and intraspinal membranes, (4) the articular mobility of the cranial bones, and (5) the involuntary mobility of the sacrum between the ilia.

Involuntary Cranial Motion

Every organ in the body exhibits a pulsation or inherent rhythmic action that features a slow, wormlike movement. The brain and spinal cord are no exception to this, manifesting a slow, rhythmic coiling and uncoiling of the hemispheres and a longitudinal movement of the spinal cord within the spinal dura. The combined motility of the central nervous system and movement of the cerebrospinal fluid manifest as a hydrodynamic "pump" and a bioelectric interchange. Upon very light palpation of the cranium, this pulsation can be felt to have a rate of about 10–14 cycles/minute. It is the result of the pull of the dural membranes, the fluctuating cerebrospinal fluid, and the inherent motility of the central nervous system.

The sphenobasilar symphysis appears to be the key cranial articulation. Prior to 25 years of age, it has a cartilaginous union; after this age, it has the resiliency of cancellous bone. Flexion of both the sphenoid and occiput increases the dorsal convexity and results in elevation of the sphenobasilar symphysis toward the vertex; extension does the reverse. In other words, flexion of the midline bones (occiput, sphenoid, ethmoid, and vomer) appears as a slight increase in convexity; extension as a slight decrease in convexity. The paired cranial bones move in synchronized internal and external rotation with the midline bones.

Associated Involuntary Sacral Motion

In addition to normal voluntary and postural motions of the sacrum between the ilia, the sacrum responds to the inherent motility of the central nervous system, fluctuation of the cerebrospinal fluid, and pull of the intracranial and intraspinal membranes in fashion similar to that of the cranial bones. Upon light palpation, this motion is felt as a slight rocking synchronized with cranial motion. Dysfunction of inherent craniospinal motion is also noted in every case of TMJ pain and dysfunction, thus the wide range of effects—from cranial nerve involvement to lower extremity disorders. Likewise, the spine, pelvis, and extremities also affect the head and TMJ via the temporals because there is a direct dura attachment of the sacrum to the cervical spine and occiput.

Diagnosis

Proper treatment of TMJ dysfunction must be based on a thorough case history, a complete physical workup, an evaluation of the cranial respiratory impulse and craniosacral mechanisms, and a detailed examination of the TMJ, cranium, and cervical spine. Unfortunately, radiographs to determine abnormal joint space are rarely successful unless over 30% of the bone has been destroyed.

Differentiation should first be made from angina or cardiac infarction, both of which often refer pain, aching, or throbbing to the angle and base of the mandible.[316] Sinusitis usually refers pain to the frontal area, but sometimes pain is referred to the jaw. Temporal arteritis and glaucoma can also refer pain to the jaw. Referred pain may also be due to dental pathology such as dental caries, pulpitis, impaction, occlusal trauma, periapical abscess, and cementitis. Referred pain from a lower molar is carried by the trigeminal, which also supplies the external pterygoid muscle.

As with most subluxation complexes, the TMJ entity may be a cause or an effect. If primary, its effects may express themselves through the whole functional-structural complex of the body. If secondary, its cause may be found at a source as the feet. Lay explains that the actions of muscles, ligaments, and fasciae throughout the body, from head to foot, coordinate the body as a functioning unit.[317] Thus, a functional or anatomical short leg, sacroiliac fixation, lumbar subluxation complex, rib-cage distortion (especially with scalene shortening), thoracic or cervical subluxations, or occipital malalignment may affect TMJ function.

Berkman points out that the jaw has been proven to influence the holding power of the atlas and axis, and, in turn, subluxations of the atlas and axis affect the stability of the TMJ.[318] The fascia colli binds the jaw and cervical spine into a unit; a fault of any one part affects the entire mechanism.

It has long been recognized in chiropractic that sacral imbalances will affect higher spinal segments, thus there is no need to elaborate this point here. Fairly new to the understanding of these remote biomechanical manifestations within the kinematic chain, however, is the influence of the cranium and TMJ and their part in contributing to the overall adverse neuromusculoskeletal synergisms involved.

Case Management[319-322]

The correction of structural disrelationships by chiropractic techniques and with the use of appropriate orthodontic and prosthodontic appliances (which are often necessary), provides the most practical approach to the treatment of TMJ dysfunction. The therapeutic approach must be structurally holistic inasmuch as TMJ dysfunction may affect any part or the whole of the axial skeleton, or vice versa. In other words, sites of fixation should be sought in the feet, ankles, knees, hips, pubes, sacroiliacs, spine, rib cage, and skull, and mobilized if found. If muscle groups are found to be weak, spastic, or shortened, appropriate therapy should be applied to restore their normal state.

Adjustive and Manipulative Approaches[317,323-327]

Invariably, motion palpation of the pubes and/or sacroiliac joints will reveal a fixation when TMJ dysfunction is present. When found, the fixation should be mobilized.

When TMJ joint compression is a factor, as it often is, physical correction can be aided by the doctor inserting gloved thumbs against the patient's lower molars, with the fingers wrapped around the jaw, and applying pressure to bring the mandible down and forward and then down and backward several times to open the joint space.

If a site of soft-tissue hypertension is found in one or both TMJs, gentle but firm passive pressure against the resistance until the tissues release is usually all that is necessary. This will be indicated when free mobility is restored. The same technique can be applied if abnormal tension is found in the sphenomandibular and stylomandibular soft tissues, as determined by exerting pressure on the angle of the mandible caudally and then cephally, and comparing the resistance found bilaterally.

Unilateral TMJ Anterior-Inferior Subluxation Adjustment. A fixated anterior-inferior misalignment of the TMJ may be found on one side while the other side is normal. The patient is placed in the sitting position facing forward, while the examiner stands behind the patient, cups the patient's chin within clasped fingers, and asks the patient to stabilize the occiput against his chest. The adjustment is made from the anterior-inferior to the posterior-superior. The thrust should be short, rapid, well-controlled, and in accord with normalizing the anatomical misalignment. In some cases, there will also be a degree of medial misalignment associated. If this is the case, the line of correction should be diagonal toward the patient's eye on the side of misalignment rather than directly posterior-superior (ie, posterior-superior-lateral). This will require the doctor to slightly rotate his shoulder anteriorly on the side contralateral to the lesion.

Unilateral TMJ Lateral Subluxation Ad-

justment. A TMJ joint may be found to be subluxated-fixated in an abnormal lateral position. This misalignment is usually accompanied by some superior jamming. The patient is placed in the sitting position facing forward while the examiner stands behind the patient, slightly to the side of the lesion. If the lesion is of the patient's right TMJ, the examiner's right palm is placed on the right side of the TMJ with the thenar eminence directly over the head of the affected condyle and above the angle of the mandible. The left stabilizing hand is placed in a similar position on the patient's left mandible. The examiner leans slightly forward so that his head is over the patient's head. In this position, the elbows will be bent and the wrists extended. The adjustment is from the superior-lateral to the inferior-medial against the stabilizing hand.

Unilateral TMJ Inferior Subluxation Adjustment. A TMJ may become subluxated (separated) and become fixed in a straight inferior position while the other side is normal. The patient is placed in the sitting position facing forward while the examiner stands behind the patient, slightly to the side of the lesion. If the lesion is of the patient's left TMJ, contact is made on the medial aspect of the mandible under the angle with the fingertips of the left hand. The right stabilizing hand should be cupped under the patient's right ramus. The patient is asked to stabilize the occiput against the examiner's chest. The adjustment is made by asking the patient to force his mouth open while the doctor applies pressure from the inferior to the superior.

Dislocation Reduction Technique. The most common example of mandibular dislocation is the anterior displacement of the mandibular condyle from its temporal articulation into the infratemporal fossa. The patient presents with the classic "mouth-agape," anxiety and helplessness, and aching and spastic temporal and masseter muscles. The mouth cannot be closed. It is often caused in a lax joint by a jaw blow or simply by a yawn, laughing, or eating an apple. During reduction of uncomplicated luxation confirmed by x-ray, take care to well pad the thumbs before placing them firmly on the molar and premolar surfaces. The patient should be supine. The thumbtips should be firm against the coronoid processes, and the eight fingers extended around the lower jaw. Apply an inferior-posterior thrust against the molars with the thumbs while the fingers tilt the mandible superiorly-anteriorly upward with a rotatory motion. Thumb padding is essential during leverage because reduction is usually immediately followed by an involuntary contraction of the masseter and temporal muscles in unison, causing the jaws to sharply snap shut. If only one side is involved, one contact thumb is used within the mouth, and the other hand is applied against the patient's forehead for counterpressure. After successful reduction, the chin should be mobilized for several seconds and then supported for 1–3 days.

Adjunctive Procedures[104, 328–330]

Just about any therapy with the objective of reducing pain and muscle hypertonicity is indicated. During the acute stage for example, cryotherapy, acupuncture, trigger-point therapy, and high-voltage or interferential currents are frequently recommended. After the acute stage, the common modalities utilized include moist heat over spastic areas, TENS, and ultrasound. Biofeedback has been reported to be effective in some stubborn cases. Nutritional muscle relaxants and anti-inflammatory agents are frequently recommended when pain and swelling is a major factor.

Trigger Points and Spasm. Several trigger points have been isolated that frequently refer pain and deep tenderness to the TMJ. The most common points are within the masseter, temporalis, and internal and external pterygoid muscles. Prior to correcting isolated subluxations, it is quite helpful to spray the peripherally located trigger areas with a vapocoolant. The patient's mouth should be comfortably propped open with a roll of gauze. The patient's eyes and nose are draped, and the patient's neck is laterally flexed away from the involved side. A few slow, even, interrupted sweeps of the spray in one direction only from jaw angle to temple should reduce any spasm and referred pain present. Do not frost the skin. Two or three applications, a few days apart, are usually sufficient. Application of high-voltage current over spastic masseter or temporal muscles for 15 minutes is an alternative approach.

Patient Education

Diet. During the acute stage, difficult to chew foods (eg, steak, nuts, raw vegetables) or those that require wide opening of the mouth (eg, sandwiches, apples) should be restricted in order to avoid masticatory overstretch.

Habits. The patient should be alerted to relax the jaw whenever muscle tension, jaw clenching, or teeth grinding are noticed. "Lips together, teeth apart" is the normal position of relaxation. Pipe smoking and sleeping in the prone position should be discontinued. Sleeping with an orthopedic pillow to maintain good cervical posture is often beneficial.

Remedial Exercises. Exercise against resistance is often helpful to relax cramped muscles and strengthen antagonists. The patient should be taught to slowly open the mouth as wide as possible without discomfort several times until the knuckles of the index and middle finger can be inserted between the front teeth. This should be followed by holding the chin between the index finger and thumb and resisting the opening and closing of the mouth. Next, resisted lateral movement of the jaw against the palm of the hand should be conducted, first on one side and then the other. Each exercise should be conducted about 10 times, with three to five bouts conducted each day.

REFERENCES

1. Maitland GD: *Vertebral Manipulation*, ed. 3. Boston, Butterworths, 1974, pp 2–8.
2. Bohlman HH: The neck. In D'Ambrosia RD (ed): *Musculoskeletal Disorders: Regional Examination and Differential Diagnosis*. Philadelphia, J.B. Lippincott, 1977, Chapter 6.
3. Schafer RC: *Symptomatology and Differential Diagnosis*. Arlington, Va, American Chiropractic Association. To be published in 1986.
4. Henderson DJ: Significance of vertebral dyskinesia in relation to the cervical syndrome. *Journal of Manipulative and Physiological Therapeutics* 2(1):3–13, March 1979.
5. Baltzell LG, Mackey RH (eds): *Firth's Technic Notes*. Publishing data not shown, 1967, pp 2–6, 12–23. Available from National College of Chiropractic.
6. Janse J: *Principles and Practice of Chiropractic*. Lombard, Ill, National College of Chiropractic, 1976, pp 43–44, 48–50, 205–221.
7. Reinert OC: *Chiropractic Procedure and Practice*, ed 3. Florissant, Mo, Marian Press, 1972, pp 51, 67–77.
8. Hadley LA: *Anatomico-Roentgenographic Studies of the Spine*. Springfield, Ill, Charles C Thomas, 1981, 128–132.
9. Kale M: The upper cervical specific. Parts 1 and 2. *Today's Chiropractic* July/August 1984, pp 28–29; September/October 1984, pp 27–30.
10. Jackson H: Diagnosis of minimal atlanto-axial subluxations. *British Journal of Radiology* 23:672, 1950.
11. Janse J, Houser RH, Wells BF: *Chiropractic Principles and Technic*. Chicago, National College of Chiropractic, 1947, pp 7–17, 201–205.
12. Mears DB Sr: *The Mears Technique*. St. Albans, Vt, published by the author, 1976, pp 56–59, 61–67.
13. Sullivan AW: Subluxation of the atlanto-axial joint: Sequel to inflammatory process of the neck. *Journal of Pediatrics* 35:451, 1949.
14. *Illustrated Stedman's Medical Dictionary*, ed 24. Baltimore, Williams & Wilkins, 1982, p 992.
15. *Illustrated Stedman's Medical Dictionary*, ed 24. Baltimore, Williams & Wilkins, 1982, p 403.
16. Schafer RC: *Chiropractic Management of Sports and Recreational Injuries*. Baltimore, Williams & Wilkins, 1982, p 343.
17. Bohlman HH: The neck. In D'Ambrosia RD (ed): *Musculoskeletal Disorders: Regional Examination and Differential Diagnosis*. Philadelphia, J.B. Lippincott, 1977, pp 178–186.
18. Chusid JG: *Correlative Neuroanatomy and Functional Neurology*, ed 19. Los Altos, Cal, Lange Medical, 1985, pp 137–138.
19. Reinert OC: *Chiropractic Procedure and Practice*, ed 3. Florissant, Mo, Marian Press, 1972, pp 15–19.
20. De Rusha JL: Upper cervical technic correlated with neurodiagnosis. *ACA Journal of Chiropractic* September 1961, pp 27–28, 54.
21. Janse J: *Principles and Practice of Chiropractic*. Lombard, Ill, National College of Chiropractic, 1976, p 210.
22. De Rusha JL: Upper cervical technic correlated with neurodiagnosis. *ACA Journal of Chiropractic* September 1961, pp 27–28.
23. De Rusha JL: Upper cervical technic correlated with neurodiagnosis. *ACA Journal of Chiropractic* September 1961, pp 28, 54.
24. Schafer RC: *Chiropractic Management of Sports and Recreational Injuries*. Baltimore, Williams & Wilkins, 1982, p 345.
25. Hadley LA: *Anatomico-Roentgenographic Studies of the Spine*. Springfield, Ill, Charles C Thomas, 1981, pp 431–443.
26. Mumenthaler M: *Neurology*, ed 2. Translated by EH Burrows. New York, Thieme-Stratton, 1983, pp 438–439.
27. Cleveland CS III: Spinal correction effects on motor and sensory function. In Mazzarelli JP (ed): *Chiropractic Interprofessional Research*. Torino, Italy, Edizioni Minerva Medica, 1983. Reprinted in

the United States by the International Chiropractors Association, Washington, DC, 1985.
28. Carrick FR: Cervical radiculopathy: The diagnosis and treatment of pathomechanics in the cervical spine. *Journal of Manipulative and Physiological Therapeutics* 6(3): 129–136, September 1983.
29. Phillips RB: The irritable reflex mechanism. *ACA Journal of Chiropractic* 8:S9–S12, January 1974.
30. Phillips RB: Upper cervical biomechanics. *ACA Journal of Chiropractic* 10: S127–S134, October 1976.
31. Janse J: *Principles and Practice of Chiropractic.* Lombard, Ill, National College of Chiropractic, 1976, pp 206–210.
32. Janse J: *Principles and Practice of Chiropractic.* Lombard, Ill, National College of Chiropractic, 1976, p 207.
33. Cailliet R: *Neck and Arm Pain.* Philadelphia, F.A. Davis, 1974, p 37.
34. Shu Yan NG: Upper cervical vertebrae and occipital headache. *Journal of Manipulative and Physiological Therapeutics* 3(3):137–141, September 1980.
35. Diamond S, Dalessio DJ: *The Practicing Physician's Approach to Headache,* ed 3. Baltimore, Williams & Wilkins, 1982.
36. Goodheart GL: *Collected Published Articles and Reprints.* Montpellier, O, Williams County Publishing, 1969, pp 15, 59–60, 65.
37. Cailliet R: *Soft Tissue Pain and Disability.* Philadelphia, F.A. Davis, 1980, pp 135–140.
38. Markovich SE: Painful neuro-muscular dysfunction syndromes in the head: A neurologist's view. Presented at the American Academy of Cranio-Mandibular Orthopedics Meeting, New Orleans, September 1976.
39. Kraus H: Muscular aspects of oral dysfunction. In Gelb H (ed): *Clinical Management of Head, Neck and TMJ Pain and Dysfunction.* Philadelphia, W.B. Saunders, 1977, pp 117–124.
40. Markovich SE: Pain in the head: A neurological appraisal. In Gelb H (ed): *Clinical Management of Head, Neck and TMJ Pain and Dysfunction.* Philadelphia, W.B. Saunders, 1977, pp 125–139.
41. Johnston WL: The role of static and motion palpation in structural diagnosis. In Goldstein M (ed): *The Research Status of Spinal Manipulative Therapy.* NINCDS Monograph, No. 15, DHEW Publication No. (NIH) 76-998, Stock No. 017-049-0-0060-7, Washington, DC, U.S. Government Printing Office, 1975, pp 249–252.
42. Stonebrink RD: Palpation for vertebral motoricity. *ACA Journal of Chiropractic* 3:S11–S14, February 1969.
43. Grove AB: *Chiropractic Technique—A Procedure of Adjusting.* Madison, Wis, Straus Printing & Publishing, 1979, p 40.
44. Northup, GW: Osteopathic lesions. *Journal of the American Osteopathic Association* 71:854–856, June 1972.
45. Beal MC: Motion sense. *Journal of the American Osteopathic Association* 53(3):151–153, 1953.
46. Stierwalt DD: *Fundamentals of Motion Palpation.* Davenport, Ia, published by the author, 1977.
47. Gillet H: A definition of the subluxation. *The Texas Chiropractor* February 1974.
48. Gates D: *Spinal Palpation.* Lakemont, Ga, published by the author, 1981, pp 44–59.
49. Taylor HH: Is a subluxation a lesion with a fixation causing joint dysfunction? *ACA Journal of Chiropractic* 15:S29–S30, March 1981.
50. Mennell JMcM: *Joint Pain.* Boston, Little, Brown, 1964, pp 3–5, 8–9, 15–16, 24, 28–31.
51. Stoddard A: *Manual of Osteopathic Practice.* New York, Harper & Row, 1969, p 75.
52. Nwuga VC: *Manipulation of the Spine.* Baltimore, Williams & Wilkins, 1976, p 8.
53. Gillet H, Liekens M: *Belgian Chiropractic Research Notes.* Huntington Beach, Cal, Motion Palpation Institute, 1981, pp 5–7, 38–43.
54. Johnson AC: *Palpation of Spine, Internal Organs, Muscles, Muscle Testing in Diagnosis.* Palm Springs, Cal, published by the author, 1980, p 3.
55. Bhalla K, Simmons EH: Normal range of intervertebral joint motion of the cervical spine. *Canadian Journal of Surgery* 12:181–187, 1969.
56. Conley RN: Stress evaluation of cervical spine mechanics. *Journal of Clinical Chiropractic* (special edition) 1(3), 1974.
57. Ferlic D: The range of motion of the "normal" cervical spine. *Bulletin of Johns Hopkins Hospital* 110:59, 1962.
58. Fielding JW: Cineroentgenography of the normal cervical spine. *Journal of Bone and Joint Surgery* 39A:1280, 1957.
59. Hahl M: Normal motions in the upper portion of the cervical spine. *Journal of Bone and Joint Surgery* 46:1777, 1964.
60. Gillet H: Occiput-atlas-axis fixations. *Journal of Clinical Chiropractic* 1:30–33, 1976.
61. Jirout J: Changes in the atlas-axis relations on lateral flexion of the head and Neck. *Neuroradiology* 6:215, 1973.
62. Jirout J: Patterns of changes in the cervical spine on lateroflexion. *Neuroradiology* 2:164, 1971.
63. Nash CL, Moe JH: A study of vertebral rotation. *Journal of Bone and Joint Surgery* 51:223, 1969.
64. Russell R: Diagnostic palpation of the spine: A review of procedures and assessment of their reliability. *Journal of Manipulative and Physiological Therapeutics* 6(4):181–183, December 1983.
65. Gillet H, Liekens M: *Belgian Chiropractic Research Notes.* Huntington Beach, Cal, Motion Palpation Institute, 1981, p 40.
66. Gillet H, Liekens M: *Belgian Chiropractic Research Notes.* Huntington Beach, Cal, Motion Palpation Institute, 1981, p 41.
67. Gillet H, Liekens M: *Belgian Chiropractic Research Notes.* Huntington Beach, Cal, Motion Palpation Institute, 1981, p 43.
68. Gillet H, Liekens M: *Belgian Chiropractic Research Notes.* Huntington Beach, Cal, Motion Palpation Institute, 1981, pp 11–13, 20, 69–71.
69. Van Dusen LG: *Chiropractic Relationship to Gravitational Force.* Sodus, NY, published by the author, 1968, pp 71, 121–127.
70. Gillet H, Liekens M: *Belgian Chiropractic Research Notes.* Huntington Beach, Cal, Motion Palpation Institute, 1981, pp 70–71.
71. Gillet H, Liekens M: *Belgian Chiropractic Research Notes.* Huntington Beach, Cal, Motion Palpation Institute, 1981, pp 70–71, 85–86.

72. Gillet H: Feet, hands, cranium, etc, *Bulletin of the European Chiropractors Union* (date unknown).
73. Van Dusen LG: *Chiropractic Relationship to Gravitational Force*. Sodus, NY, published by the author, 1968, pp 71, 93, 103–119
74. Gillet H, Liekens M: *Belgian Chiropractic Research Notes*. Huntington Beach, Cal, Motion Palpation Institute, 1981, pp 13–14, 16, 20, 42–43, 69–71.
75. Gillet H, Liekens M: *Belgian Chiropractic Research Notes*. Huntington Beach, Cal, Motion Palpation Institute, 1981, pp 14, 65–66.
76. Gillet H: Motion palpation—measurements. *Bulletin of the European Chiropractors Union* 23(2), 1974.
77. Gillet H, Liekens M: *Belgian Chiropractic Research Notes*. Huntington Beach, Cal, Motion Palpation Institute, 1981, pp 107–108.
78. Gillet H, Liekens M: *Belgian Chiropractic Research Notes*. Huntington Beach, Cal, Motion Palpation Institute, 1981, p 108.
79. Johnston WL, Vorro J, Hubbard RP: Clinical/biomechanic correlates for cervical function: Part I, a kinematic study. *Journal of the American Osteopathic Association* 85(7):429–436, July 1985.
80. Johnston WL, Hill JL: Spinal segmental dysfunction: Incidence in the cervicothoracic region. *Journal of the American Osteopathic Association* 81:67–76, September 1981.
81. Beatty HG: *Anatomical Adjustive Technic*, ed 2. Denver, published by the author, 1939, pp 71–91.
82. Grecco MA: *Chiropractic Technic Illustrated*. New York, Jarl, 1953, pp 25–28.
83. Logan VF: The value of inspection. *Chiropractic Palpation and Analysis*. Chesterfield, Mo, Logan College of Chiropractic (undated).
84. Levine M: *The Structural Approach to Chiropractic*. New York, Comet Press, 1964, pp 52–53, 67–68.
85. Gates D: *Spinal Palpation*. Lakemont, Ga, published by the author, 1981, pp 69–83.
86. Reinert OC: *Fundamentals of Chiropractic Techniques and Practice Procedures*. Chesterfield, Mo, Marian Press, 1983, pp 103–107, 120–122.
87. Firth JN: *A Textbook of Chiropractic Diagnosis*. Indianapolis, published by the author, 1948, pp 11–12.
88. Schafer RC: *The Magic of Self-Actualization*. Montezuma, Ia, Behavioral Research Foundation, 1977, pp 57–58, 67–68.
89. Cailliet R: *Neck and Arm Pain*. Philadelphia, F.A. Davis, 1974, p 10.
90. Johnson AC: *Postural Correction*. Los Angeles, Chiropractic Educational Extension Bureau, p 15 (undated).
91. De Jarnette MB: *Subluxation Patterns*. Nebraska City, published by the author, privately distributed, 1975, p 63.
92. De Jarnette MB: *Sacro Occipital Technic*. Nebraska City, published by the author, privately distributed, 1977, pp 163–169.
93. DeJarnette MB: *Sacro Occipital Technic*. Nebraska City, published by the author, privately distributed, 1977, pp 220–221.
94. Reinert OC: *Fundamentals of Chiropractic Techniques and Practice Procedures*. Chesterfield, Mo, Marian Press, 1983, pp 123–124.
95. Johnson AC: *Palpation of Spine, Internal Organs, Muscles, Muscle Testing in Diagnosis*. Palm Springs, Cal, published by the author, 1980, p 2.
96. Seemann DC: C1 Subluxations, short leg, and pelvic distortions. *International Review of Chiropractic* April/June 1979.
97. Reinert OC: *Fundamentals of Chiropractic Techniques and Practice Procedures*. Chesterfield, Mo, Marian Press, 1983, pp 124–126.
98. Reinert OC: *Fundamentals of Chiropractic Techniques and Practice Procedures*. Chesterfield, Mo, Marian Press, 1983, pp 126–127.
99. Johnson AC: *Palpation of Spine, Internal Organs, Muscles, Muscle Testing in Diagnosis*. Palm Springs, Cal, published by the author, 1980, p 3.
100. De Jarnette MB: *Sacro Occipital Technic*. Nebraska City, published by the author, privately distributed, 1977, p 218.
101. De Jarnette MB: *Subluxation Patterns*. Nebraska City, published by the author, privately distributed, 1975, pp 64–65.
102. Goodheart GJ: Applied kinesiology and muscle sound. *ACA Journal of Chiropractic* February 1967, pp S11–S13.
103. De Jarnette MB: *Subluxation Patterns*. Nebraska City, published by the author, privately distributed, 1975, pp 64–67.
104. Jaskoviak P, Schafer RC: *Applied Physiotherapy*. Arlington, Va, American Chiropractic Association. To be published in 1986.
105. ACA Council on Physiological Therapeutics: Physiotherapy guidelines for the chiropractic profession. *ACA Journal of Chiropractic* June 1975, p S68.
106. Cailliet R: *Neck and Arm Pain*. Philadelphia, F.A. Davis, 1964, pp 79–83.
107. Aston JN: *A Short Textbook of Orthopaedics and Traumatology*, ed 2. London, Hodder & Stoughton, 1976, p 178.
108. Saunders HD: *Orthopaedic Physical Therapy: Evaluation and Treatment of Musculoskeletal Disorders*. Minneapolis, published by the author, 1982, pp 143–146.
109. Voss DE et al: Traction and approximation. *Proprioceptive Neuromuscular Facilitation: Patterns and Techniques*, ed 3. Philadelphia, Harper & Row, 1985, p 294.
110. Schafer RC: *Chiropractic Management of Sports and Recreational Injuries*. Baltimore, Williams & Wilkins, 1982, p 203.
111. Rogoff JB (ed): *Manipulation, Traction, and Massage*, ed 2. Baltimore, Williams & Wilkins, 1980, p 191–198.
112. Lawson GA, Godfrey CM: A report on studies of spinal traction. *Journal of Medical Services* (Canada) 14:762–771, 1958.
113. Judovich BD: Herniated cervical disc: A new form of traction therapy. *American Journal of Surgery* 84:646–656, 1952.
114. McFarland JW, Krusen FH: Use of the Sayre head sling in osteoarthritis of cervical portion of spinal column. *Archives of Physical Therapy* 24:263–269, 1943.
115. Basmajian JV (ed): *Manipulation, Traction, and Massage*, ed 3. Baltimore, Williams & Wilkins, 1985, pp 184–187.

116. Zuidema GD et al: *The Management of Trauma*, ed 3. Philadelphia, W.B. Saunders, 1979, pp 241–244.
117. Yashon D: *Spinal Injury*. New York, Appleton-Century-Crofts, 1978, pp 134–144.
118. Fisk JW: *The Painful Neck and Back*. Springfield, Ill, Charles C Thomas, 1977, pp 134–135.
119. Hadler NM: *Medical Management of the Regional Musculoskeletal Diseases*. New York, Grune & Stratton, 1984, pp 97–98.
120. Hill LL: *Parameters of Physiotherapy Modalities*. Lombard, Ill, National Chiropractic College, class notes, pp 77–78 (undated).
121. Saunders HD: *Orthopaedic Physical Therapy: Evaluation and Treatment of Musculoskeletal Disorders*. Minneapolis, published by the author, 1982, pp 157–160.
122. Downer AH: *Physical Therapy Procedures: Selected Techniques*, ed 2. Springfield, Ill, Charles C Thomas, pp 155–164.
123. Rogoff JB (ed): *Manipulation, Traction, and Massage*, ed 2. Baltimore, Williams & Wilkins, 1980, p 199.
124. Hill LL: *Parameters of Physiotherapy Modalities*. Lombard, Ill, National Chiropractic College, class notes, pp 78–79 (undated).
125. Grieve GP: *Common Vertebral Joint Problems*. New York, Churchill Livingstone, 1981, p 199.
126. Johnson AC: *Postural Correction*. Los Angeles, Chiropractic Educational Extension Bureau, pp 5–9 (undated).
127. Gelb H: Patient evaluation. In Gelb H (ed): *Clinical Management of Head, Neck and TMJ Pain and Dysfunction*. Philadelphia, W.B. Saunders, 1977, p 79.
128. Gelb H: A review of the medical-dental relationship in craniomandibular syndromes. *New York Journal of Dentistry* 41:163, 1971.
129. Eversaul GA: Applied kinesiology and the treatment of TMJ dysfunction. In Gelb H (ed): *Clinical Management of Head, Neck and TMJ Pain and Dysfunction*. Philadelphia, W.B. Saunders, 1977, pp 480–505.
130. Todd M: *The Thinking Body*. New York, Dance Horizons, 1968.
131. Gelb H: Patient evaluation. In Gelb H (ed): *Clinical Management of Head, Neck and TMJ Pain and Dysfunction*. Philadelphia, W.B. Saunders, 1977, p 80.
132. Lieb MM: Oral orthopedics. In Gelb H (ed): *Clinical Management of Head, Neck and TMJ Pain and Dysfunction*. Philadelphia, W.B. Saunders, 1977, pp 58–71.
133. Fisk JW: *The Painful Neck and Back*. Springfield, Ill, Charles C Thomas, 1977, p 29.
134. Wyke BD: Articular neurology and manipulative therapy. In *Aspects of Manipulative Therapy*. Proceedings of Multidisciplinary International Conference on Manipulative Therapy, Melbourne, Lincoln Institute of Health Sciences, Carlton, Victoria, Australia, August 1979, pp 67–72.
135. Daniels L, Worthingham C: *Muscle Testing: Techniques of Manual Examination*, ed 4. Philadelphia, W.B. Saunders, 1980, p 49.
136. Kapandji IA: *Physiology of the Joints: The Trunk and Vertebral Column*, ed 2. New York, Churchill Livingstone, 1980, vol 3, pp 242–244.
137. White AA, Panjabi MM: *Clinical Biomechanics of the Spine*. Philadelphia, J.B. Lippincott, 1978, pp 71, 73.
138. Daniels L, Worthingham C: *Therapeutic Exercise for Body Alignment and Function*, ed 2. Philadelphia, W.B. Saunders, 1977, p 62, 64–65.
139. Daniels L, Worthingham C: *Therapeutic Exercise for Body Alignment and Function*, ed 2. Philadelphia, W.B. Saunders, 1977, p 63, 64–65.
140. Williams PC: *Low Back and Neck Pain*. Springfield, Ill, Charles C Thomas, 1982, pp 69–72.
141. Basmajian JV (ed): *Therapeutic Exercise*, ed 3. Baltimore, Williams & Wilkins, 1978, pp 358–359, 525–526.
142. Fisk JW: *The Painful Neck and Back*. Springfield, Ill, Charles C. Thomas, 1977, p 154.
143. Grieve GP: *Common Vertebral Joint Problems*. New York, Churchill Livingstone, 1981, pp 125–129.
144. Fisk JW: *The Painful Neck and Back*. Springfield, Ill, Charles C Thomas, 1977, pp 155–159.
145. McRae DL: The significance of abnormalities of the cervical spine. *American Journal of Roentgenology* 84:3, 1960.
146. Telford ED, Mottershead S: Pressure at the cervical brachial junction: An operative and anatomical study. *Journal of Bone and Joint Surgery* 30B:249–250, 1948.
147. Nelson JM: Conservative approaches to the management of thoracic outlet syndrome. In Coyle BA, Martinez DP (eds): *Proceedings of the Second Conference on Current Topics in Chiropractic: Reviews of the Literature*, May 4–5, 1985. Sunnyvale, Cal, Palmer College of Chiropractic—West, 1985, section B1.
148. Grieve GP: *Common Vertebral Joint Problems*. New York, Churchill Livingstone, 1981, pp 129–134.
149. Cailliet R: *Soft Tissue Pain and Disability*. Philadelphia, F.A. Davis, 1980, pp 142–148.
150. Hadler NM: *Medical Management of the Regional Musculoskeletal Diseases*. New York, Grune & Stratton, 1984, pp 123–126.
151. Bailey RW: *The Cervical Spine*. Philadelphia, Lea & Febiger, 1974.
152. Schafer RC: *Chiropractic Management of Sports and Recreational Injuries*. Baltimore, Williams & Wilkins, 1982, pp 331, 340–341, 357.
153. Bohlman HH: Cervical spine injuries: a critical review of 300 cards. *Journal of Bone and Joint Surgery* 54A:1353–1354, 1972.
154. Grieve GP: *Common Vertebral Joint Problems*. New York, Churchill Livingstone, 1981, pp 229–230.
155. MacBryde CM, Blacklow RS: *Signs and Symptoms*, ed 5. Philadelphia, J.B. Lippincott, 1970, pp 246–247.
156. Chusid JG: *Correlative Neuroanatomy and Functional Neurology*, ed 19. Los Altos, Cal, Lange Medical, 1985, p 337.
157. Salter RB: *Textbook of Disorders and Injuries of the Musculoskeletal System*. Baltimore, Williams & Wilkins, 1970, p 259.
158. D'Ambrosia RD: *Musculoskeletal Disorders: Regional Examination and Differential Diagnosis*. Philadelphia, J.B. Lippincott, 1977, pp 205–206
159. Friedman HH (ed): *Problem-Oriented Medical Di-*

agnosis, ed 2. Boston, Little, Brown, 1979, pp 34, 263, 339–3340.

160. Stanton PE et al: Thoracic outlet syndrome: A comprehensive evaluation. *Southern Medical Journal* 71:1070–1073, 1978.
161. Grieve GP: *Common Vertebral Joint Problems*. New York, Churchill Livingstone, 1981, p 130.
162. Schafer RC: *Chiropractic Physical and Spinal Diagnosis*. Oklahoma City, Associated Chiropractic Academic Press, 1980, pp V21–V22.
163. Jackson R: The positive findings in alleged neck injuries. *American Journal of Orthropaedics* 6:178–187, 1964.
164. Harvey AMcG, Bordley J III, Barondess JA: *Differential Diagnosis*, ed 3. Philadelphia, W.B. Saunders, 1979, p 106.
165. Hart FD (ed): *French's Index of Differential Diagnosis*, ed 12. Bristol, England, Wright, 1985, pp 629–630.
166. Mumenthaler M: *Neurology*, ed 2. Translated by EH Burrows. New York, Thieme-Stratton, 1983, pp 438–439.
167. Grieve GP: *Common Vertebral Joint Problems*. New York, Churchill Livingstone, 1981, pp 230–231.
168. Falconer MA, Li FW: Resection of first rib in costoclavicular compression of the brachial plexus. *Lancet* 1:59, 1962.
169. Lord JW, Rosati LM: *Thoracic-Outlet Syndromes*. Summit, NJ, Ciba Pharmaceutical, 1971.
170. Telford ED, Mottershead S: The costo-clavicular syndrome. *British Medical Journal* 15:4497, March 1947.
171. Schafer RC: *Chiropractic Management of Sports and Recreational Injuries*. Baltimore, Williams & Wilkins, 1982, pp 331–333.
172. Krupp MA et al: *Physician's Handbook*, ed 21. Los Altos, Cal, Lange Medical, 1985, p 62.
173. Jahn WT: Standardization of orthopaedic testing of the cervical and cervicobrachial regions. *Journal of Manipulative and Physiologic Therapeutics* 1(1):32–45, 1978.
174. White AA, Panjabi MM: *Clinical Biomechanics of the Spine*, Philadelphia, J.B. Lippincott, 1978, p 205.
175. Janse J: *Principles and Practice of Chiropractic*. Lombard, Ill, National College of Chiropractic, 1976, pp 222–223.
176. Dvorak J, Orelli FV: How dangerous is manipulation of the cervical spine? Case report and results of an inquiry. *Manuelle Medizin* 20:44–48, 1982.
177. Glerak RA: Vertebral artery compression and vascular insufficiency of the brain. *Archives of California Chiropractic Association* 2:28–39, 1972.
178. Keggi, Granger, Southwick: Vertebral artery insufficiency secondary to trauma and osteoarthritis of the cervical spine. *Yale Journal of Biology and Medicine* 38:471–478, 1966.
179. Mapstone T, Spetzler RF: Vertebrobasilar insufficiency secondary to vertebral artery occlusion. *Journal of Neurosurgery* 56:581–583, 1982.
180. Smith DM: Vertebral artery. *Roentgenological Briefs*. Council on Roentgenology of the American Chiropractic Association (undated).
181. Chusid JG: *Correlative Neuroanatomy and Functional Neurology*, ed 19. Los Altos, Cal, Lange Medical, pp 68, 297.
182. Sweat RW, Sievert T: Chiropractic and the vertebral arteries. Parts 1 and 2. *Today's Chiropractic* September/October 1984, pp 45–48; November/December 1984, pp 23–24.
183. Macnab I: Symptoms in cervical disc degeneration. In The Cervical Spine Research Society: *The Cervical Spine*. Philadelphia, J.B. Lippincott, 1983, pp 388–394.
184. Epstein BS: *The Spine: A Radiological Text and Atlas*. Philadelphia, Lea & Febiger, 1962, pp 268–269.
185. Toole J, Tucker SH: Influence of head position upon cerebral circulation. *Archives of Neurology* (AMA) :616–623, 1960.
186. Sheehan S, Bauer RB, Meyer JS: Vertebral artery compression in cervical spondylosis: Arteriographic demonstration during life of vertebral artery insufficiency due to rotation and extension of the neck. *Neurology* 10:968–986, 1960.
187. VonTorklus D: *The Upper Cervical Spine*. New York, Grune & Stratton, 1972, p 22.
188. Mumenthaler M: *Neurology*, ed 2. Translated by EH Burrows. New York, Thieme-Stratton, 1983, pp 157–158.
189. Hadley LA: *Anatomico-Roentgenographic Studies of the Spine*. Springfield, Ill, Charles C Thomas, 1981, p 162.
190. Duckworth JAW: Dissection seminar conducted at the Canadian Chiropractic College, Toronto, 1983.
191. Meyermann R: Possibilities of injury to the artery vertebralis. *Manuelle Medizin* 20:105–114, 1982.
192. Saternus KS, Fuchs V: Is the artery vertebralis endangered in resuscitation. *Manuelle Medizin* 20:101–104, 1982.
193. George PE: New techinques to identify the potential stroke victim. *International Review of Chiropractic* January/March 1981, p 23.
194. Bovee ML: *The Essentials of the Orthopedic and Neurological Examination*. City of publication not shown, published by the author, 1977, p 7.
195. Bergmann T: Integrated chiropractic methods. Oklahoma seminar notes, April 23, 1983. Northwestern College of Chiropractic, St. Paul, 1983.
196. Schafer RC: "Hot shots" and brachial plexus traction. *Journal of the American Chiropractic Association* September 1982.
197. Bryan EC: The traumatic cervical root syndrome. *ACA Journal of Chiropractic* April 1967, pp S25–S27.
198. Craig TT (ed): *Comments in Sports Medicine*. Chicago, American Medical Association, 1973, pp 22–23.
199. Duman S, Ginsburg SH: Selected neurogenic pain syndromes. In Friedman HH (ed): *Problem-Oriented Medical Diagnosis*, ed 2. Boston, Little, Brown, 1979, p 339.
200. Mumenthaler M: *Neurology*, ed 2. Translated by EH Burrows. New York, Thieme-Stratton, 1983, p 361.
201. Albright JP et al: Head and neck injuries in sports. In Scott WN, Nisonson B, Nicholas JA (eds): *Principles of Sports Medicine*. Baltimore, Williams & Wilkins, 1984, pp 41, 43, 68–70.

202. Wieland T: Cervical flexion and extension sprain/strain. In Hughes T: *Physical Therapy Class Notes*. Chesterfield, Mo, Logan College of Chiropractic, 1984, pp 595–597.
203. Aston JN: *A Short Textbook of Orthopaedics and Traumatology*, ed 2. London, Hodder & Stoughton, 1976, pp 49–51.
204. Kessler RM, Hertling D (eds): *Management of Common Musculoskeletal Disorders*. Philadelphia, Harper & Row, 1983.
205. Chusid JG: *Correlative Neuroanatomy and Functional Neurology*, ed 19. Los Altos, Cal, Lange Medical, 1985, p 378.
206. Schneider RC, Kennedy JC, Plant ML (eds): *Sports Injuries: Mechanisms, Prevention, and Treatment*. Baltimore, Williams & Wilkins, 1985, pp 676–687.
207. Dolan JP, Holladay LJ: *First-Aid Management*, ed 4. Danville, Ill, Interstate Printers & Publishers, 1974, p 298.
208. Dutro CL: Treatment of cervical flexion-extension injuries. In Coyle BA, Martinez DP (eds): *Proceedings of the Second Conference on Current Topics in Chiropractic: Reviews of the Literature*, May 4–5, 1985. Sunnyvale, Cal, Palmer College of Chiropractic—West, 1985, section B4.
209. Schafer RC: *Chiropractic Management of Sports and Recreational Injuries*. Baltimore, Williams & Wilkins, 1982, pp 334–335.
210. Johnson AC: *Chiropractic Physiological Therapeutics*. Palm Springs, Cal, published by the author, 1977, pp 61–64, 69–75.
211. Zuidema GD et al: *The Management of Trauma*, ed 3. Philadelphia, W.B. Saunders, 1979, pp 342–360.
212. Schaefer M: Acute cervical sprain/strain. In Hughes T: *Physical Therapy Class Notes*. Chesterfield, Mo, Logan College of Chiropractic, 1984, pp 591–594.
213. Hart DL et al: Review of cervical orthoses. *Physical Therapy* 58:857–860, 1978.
214. Fisher SV: Proper fitting of the cervical orthosis. *Archives of Physical Medicine and Rehabilitation* 59:505–507, 1978.
215. Therapeutic Products: Sleep and plastic deformation. *Research Bulletin No. 617*. Dubuque, Ia, Therapeutic Products (undated).
216. White AA, Panjabi MM: *Clinical Biomechanics of the Spine*. Philadelphia, J.B. Lippincott, 1978, pp 468, 470–472, 490, 498–500.
217. Root ML, Williams PO, Weed JH: *Normal and Abnormal Function of the Foot*. Los Angeles, Clinical Biomechanics Corporation, 1977, vol 2.
218. Banus MG, Zetlin AM: The relation of isometric tension to length in the skeletal muscle. *Journal of Cellular and Comparative Physiology* 12:403–420, 1938.
219. Johns RJ, Wright V: Relative importance of various tissues in joint stiffness. *Journal of Applied Physiology* 17:824–828, 1962.
220. Greenawalt MH: *Spinal Pelvic Stabilization*, ed 2. Dubuque, Ia, Foot Levelers, 1978.
221. Zuidema GD et al: *The Management of Trauma*, ed 3. Philadelphia, W.B. Saunders, 1979, pp 236–239.
222. Scott WN, Nisonson B, Nicholas JA (eds): *Principles of Sports Medicine*. Baltimore, Williams & Wilkins, 1984, pp 45, 65–71.
223. Grieve GP: *Common Vertebral Joint Problems*. New York, Churchill Livingstone, 1981, pp 90, 126–129.
224. Simeone FA, Rothman RH: Cervical disc disease. In Rothman RH, Simeone FA (eds): *The Spine*. Philadelphia, W.B. Saunders, 1975, vol 1, pp 387–415.
225. Bohlman HH: The neck. In D'Ambrosia RD (ed): *Musculoskeletal Disorders: Regional Examination and Differential Diagnosis*. Philadelphia, J.B. Lippincott, 1977, pp 213–217.
226. Yashon D: *Spinal Injury*. New York, Appleton-Century-Crofts, 1978, pp 147–161.
227. DePalma A, Rothman RH: *The Intervertebral Disc*. Philadelphia, W.B. Saunders, 1970.
228. Cailliet R: *Neck and Arm Pain*. Philadelphia, F.A. Davis, 1974, p 45.
229. Hadley LA: *Anatomico-Roentgenographic Studies of the Spine*. Springfield, Ill, Charles C Thomas, 1981, pp 230–240.
230. Fisk JW: *The Painful Neck and Back*. Springfield, Ill, Charles C Thomas, 1977, pp 25–27.
231. Rosse C, Clawson DK: *The Musculoskeletal System in Health and Disease*. New York, Harper & Row, 1980, pp 153–154.
232. Macnab I: *Backache*. Baltimore, Williams & Wilkins, 1977, pp 84–91, 158–159.
233. Salter RB: *Textbook of Disorders and Injuries of the Musculoskeletal System*. Baltimore, Williams & Wilkins, 1970, p 208.
234. Hadler NM: *Medical Management of the Regional Musculoskeletal Diseases*. New York, Grune & Stratton, 1984, pp 89–92.
235. White AA, Panjabi MM: *Clinical Biomechanics of the Spine*. Philadelphia, J.B. Lippincott, 1978, pp 162–163.
236. Macnab I: *Backache*. Baltimore, Williams & Wilkins, 1977, pp 91–97.
237. Hadley LA: *Anatomico-Roentgenographic Studies of the Spine*. Springfield, Ill, Charles C Thomas, 1981, pp 240–244.
238. Friedman HH (ed): *Problem-Oriented Medical Diagnosis*, ed 2. Boston, Little, Brown, 1979, p 339.
239. Wilson FC (ed): *The Musculoskeletal System: Basic Processes and Disorders*, ed 2. Philadelphia, J.B. Lippincott, 1983, p 78.
240. Fisk JW: *The Painful Neck and Back*. Springfield, Ill, Charles C Thomas, 1977, pp 8, 27.
241. Harvey AMcG, Bordley J III, Barondess JA: *Differential Diagnosis*, ed 3. Philadelphia, W.B. Saunders, 1979, p 105.
242. Mumenthaler M: *Neurology*, ed 2. Translated by EH Burrows. New York, Thieme-Stratton, 1983, pp 357, 360.
243. MacBryde CM, Blacklow RS: *Signs and Symptoms*, ed 5. Philadelphia, J.B. Lippincott, 1970, p 244.
244. Chusid JG: *Correlative Neuroanatomy and Functional Neurology*, ed 19. Los Altos, Cal, Lange Medical, 1985, p 376.
245. Rosse C, Clawson DK: *The Musculoskeletal System in Health and Disease*. New York, Harper & Row, 1980, pp 155–156.
246. Hart FD (ed): *French's Index of Differential Diag-*

nosis, ed 12. Bristol, England, Wright, 1985, pp 520, 624, 629.

247. Jeffreys E: *Disorders of the Cervical Spine*. London, Butterworths, 1980, pp 90–103.
248. Holt S, Yates PO: Cervical spondylosis and nerve root lesions. *Journal of Bone and Joint Surgery* 48B:407–423.
249. Hadley LA: *Anatomico-Roentgenographic Studies of the Spine*. Springfield, Ill, Charles C Thomas, 1981, p 264.
250. Pallis C, Jones AM, Spillane AD: Cervical spondylosis: Incidence, and implications. *Brain* 77:274–289.
251. Jeffreys E: *Disorders of the Cervical Spine*. London, Butterworths, 1980, p 90.
252. Whiting RJ: Cervical spondylosis. *Roentgenological Briefs*. Council on Roentgenology of the American Chiropractic Association (undated).
253. Henderson DJ: Significance of vertebral dyskinesia in relation to the cervical syndrome. *Journal of Manipulative and Physiological Therapeutics* 2(1):3–13, March 1979.
254. Blumenthal LS: Injury to the cervical spine as a cause of headache. *Postgraduate Medicine* 56:147–152, 1974.
255. Kovacs A: Subluxation and deformation of the cervical apophyseal joints. *Acta Radiologica* 43:1–16, 1955.
256. Ryan GMS, Cope S: Cervical vertigo. *The Lancet* December 1955, pp 1355–1358.
257. Gayral L, Neuwirth E: Oto-neuro-ophthalmologic manifestations of cervical origin. *New York State Journal of Medicine* 54:1920–1926, 1954.
258. Hanflig SS: Pain in the shoulder girdle, arm and precordium due to foraminal compression of nerve roots. *Archives of Surgery* 46:652–663, 1963.
259. Hargrave-Wilson W: The cervical syndrome. *Australian Journal of Physiotherapy* 18:144–147, 1972.
260. Giles LGF: Vertebral-basilar artery insufficiency. *Journal of the CCA* 21:112–117, 1977.
261. Burke GL: The etiology and pathogenesis of pain of spinal origin. *Applied Therapeutics* October 1966, pp 863–867.
262. Kunert W: Functional disorders of internal organs due to vertebral lesions. *Ciba Symposium* 13(3), 1966.
263. Gayral L, Neuwirth E: Clinical manifestations of the autonomic nervous system sequential to osteoarthritis of the cervical spine. *Lancet* May 1958, pp 197–198.
264. Nelson WA: Personal communication. San Francisco, 1980.
265. Barge FH: *Torticollis*. Davenport, Ia, Bawden Bros, 1979.
266. Bohlman HH: The neck. In D'Ambrosia RD (ed): *Musculoskeletal Disorders: Regional Examination and Differential Diagnosis*. Philadelphia, J.B. Lippincott, 1977, pp 193–194, 201–202.
267. Hadley LA: *Anatomico-Roentgenographic Studies of the Spine*. Springfield, Ill, Charles C Thomas, 1981, pp 130, 132, 431–438.
268. Visudhiphan P et al: Torticollis as the sign in cervical spine infection and tumor. *Clinical Pediatrics* 21:71–76, 1982.
269. Barge FH: *Torticollis*. Davenport, Ia, Bawden Bros, 1979, p v.
270. Barge FH: *Torticollis*. Davenport, Ia, Bawden Bros, 1979, pp vii, 17–19, 26, 32.
271. Van Dusen LG: *Chiropractic Relationship to Gravitational Force*. Sodus, NY, published by the author, 1968, pp 111–117, 121–127.
272. Pierce WV: The fifth cervical key. *The Digest of Chiropractic Economics* July/August 1982.
273. Hoppenfeld S: *Physical Examination of the Spine and Extremities*. New York, Appleton-Century-Crofts, 1976, p 31.
274. Jeffreys E: *Disorders of the Cervical Spine*. London, Butterworths, 1980, pp 106–113.
275. Bohlman HH: The neck. In D'Ambrosia RD (ed): *Musculoskeletal Disorders: Regional Examination and Differential Diagnosis*. Philadelphia, J.B. Lippincott, 1977, pp 208–212.
276. Cohen PL: Rheumatoid arthritis and other chronic inflammatory arthritides. In Wilson FC (ed): *The Musculoskeletal System: Basic Processes and Disorders*, ed 2. Philadelphia, J.B. Lippincott, 1983, pp 238–240.
277. Jeffreys E: *Disorders of the Cervical Spine*. London, Butterworths, 1980, pp 113–117.
278. Bohlman HH: The neck. In D'Ambrosia RD (ed): *Musculoskeletal Disorders: Regional Examination and Differential Diagnosis*. Philadelphia, J.B. Lippincott, 1977, p 208.
279. Bohlman HH: The neck. In D'Ambrosia RD (ed): *Musculoskeletal Disorders: Regional Examination and Differential Diagnosis*. Philadelphia, J.B. Lippincott, 1977, pp 192–193, 203–204.
280. Hadley LA: *Anatomico-Roentgenographic Studies of the Spine*. Springfield, Ill, Charles C Thomas, 1981, pp 69–113.
281. Inman OB (ed): *Chiropractic Manual of the Traumatized Cervical Spine*. Atlanta, Georgia Chiropractic Association, 1978, pp 36–37.
282. Jeffreys E: *Disorders of the Cervical Spine*. London, Butterworths, 1980, pp 32–33.
283. Kattan KR, Paris MJ: Some borderlands of the cervical spine: Part 1. *Skeletal Radiology* 8:1–6, 1982.
284. Hensinger RN, MacEwen GD: Congenital anomalies of the spine. In Rothman RH, Simeone FA (eds): *The Spine*. Philadelphia, W.B. Saunders, 1975, vol 1, pp 157–168.
285. Jeffreys E: *Disorders of the Cervical Spine*. London, Butterworths, 1980, pp 33–34.
286. Gehweiler J, Daffner R, Roberts L: Malformation of the atlas vertebra simulating the Jefferson fracture. *American Journal of Roentgenology* 140:1083–1086, 1983.
287. Wackenheim A: Occipitalization of the ventral part and vertebralization of the dorsal part of the atlas with insufficiency of the transverse ligament. *Neuroradiology* 24:45–47, 1982.
288. Schwartz AM et al: Posterior arch defects of the cervical spine. *Skeletal Radiology* 8:135–139, 1982.
289. Hensinger RN, MacEwen GD: Congenital anomalies of the spine. In Rothman RH, Simeone FA (eds): *The Spine*. Philadelphia, W.B. Saunders, 1975, vol 1, pp 195–199.
290. Hooker CW, Greene WB: Normal development of the musculoskeletal system. In Wilson FC (ed): *The Musculoskeletal System: Basic Processes and*

Disorders, ed 2. Philadelphia, J.B. Lippincott, 1983, p 16.
291. Chusid JG: *Correlative Neuroanatomy and Functional Neurology*, ed 19. Los Altos, Cal, Lange Medical, 1985, p 459.
292. Coventry MD, Harris LE: Congenital muscular torticollis in infancy: Some observations regarding treatment. *Journal of Bone and Joint Surgery* 41A:815–822, 1959.
293. Hensinger RN, MacEwen GD: Congenital anomalies of the spine. In Rothman RH, Simeone FA (eds): *The Spine*. Philadelphia, W.B. Saunders, 1975, vol 1, pp 179–194.
294. Jeffreys E: *Disorders of the Cervical Spine*. London, Butterworths, 1980, pp 37–42.
295. Bohlman HH: The neck. In D'Ambrosia RD (ed): *Musculoskeletal Disorders: Regional Examination and Differential Diagnosis*. Philadelphia, J.B. Lippincott, 1977, pp 204–205.
296. Grieve GP: *Common Vertebral Joint Problems*. New York, Churchill Livingstone, 1981, pp 131–134.
297. Jeffreys E: *Disorders of the Cervical Spine*. London, Butterworths, 1980, pp 31, 45.
298. Bohlman HH: The neck. In D'Ambrosia RD (ed): *Musculoskeletal Disorders: Regional Examination and Differential Diagnosis*. Philadelphia, J.B. Lippincott, 1977, pp 205–206.
299. Grieve GP: *Common Vertebral Joint Problems*. New York, Churchill Livingstone, 1981, pp 13, 131.
300. Hoppenfeld S: *Physical Examination of the Spine and Extremities*. New York, Appleton-Century-Crofts, 1976, pp 128–132.
301. Hruby RJ: The total body approach to the osteopathic management of temporomandibular joint dysfunction. *Journal of the American Osteopathic Association* 85(8):502–509.
302. "Doctor, my jaw hurts." *Patient Care* December 15, 1983, pp 108–136.
303. Common sense management for TMJ troubles. *Patient Care* January 15, 1984, pp 129–157.
304. Smith SD: Vascular analysis in temporomandibular orthopedics: Quantifying blood flow related to occlusal dynamics. *Osteopathic Medicine* October 1980, pp 29–32, 35–41, 71.
305. Gelb H (ed): *Clinical Management of Head, Neck and TMJ Pain and Dysfunction*. Philadelphia, W.B. Saunders, 1977.
306. Magoun HI Sr: *Osteopathy in the Cranial Field*. Kirksville, Mo, Journal Printing, 1966.
307. Hruby RJ: The total body approach to the osteopathic management of temporomandibular joint dysfunction. *Journal of the American Osteopathic Association* 85(8):506.
308. Farrar WB: Dysfunctional centric relation to the jaw associated with dislocation and displacement of the disc. *Compendium of the American Equilibrium Society* 13:63–67, 1973/1974.
309. Farrar WB, McCarty WL Jr: *A Clinical Outline of Temporomandibular Joint Diagnosis and Treatment*. Montgomery, Ala, Normandie Publications, 1982.
310. Guralnick W, Kaban LB, Merrill RG: Temporomandibular-joint afflictions. *New England Journal of Medicine* 299:123–129, 1978.
311. Mahan PE: Temporomandibular joint dysfunction: Physiological and clinical aspects. In Rowe NH (ed): *Occlusion: Research in Form and Function. Proceedings of Symposium*. East Lansing, University of Michigan, 1975, p 112.
312. Laskin DM: Etiology of the pain-dysfunction syndrome. *Journal of the American Dental Association* 79:147–153, 1969.
313. Bell WE: *Orofacial Pains: Differential Diagnosis*, ed 2. Chicago, Year Book Medical, 1979.
314. Marbach JJ, Lipton JA: Treatment of patients with temporomandibular joint and other facial pain by otolaryngologists. *Archives of Otolaryngology* 108:104, 1982.
315. Schafer RC: *Chiropractic Management of Sports and Recreational Injuries*. Baltimore, Williams & Wilkins, 1982, pp 309–310.
316. "Doctor, my jaw hurts." *Patient Care* December 15, 1983, p 115.
317. Lay EM: The osteopathic management of temporomandibular joint dysfunction. In Gelb H (ed): *Clinical Management of Head, Neck and TMJ Pain and Dysfunction*. Philadelphia, W.B. Saunders, 1977.
318. Berkman EH: The troublesome TMJ. *ACA Journal of Chiropractic* June 1971.
319. Smith SD: Head pain and stress from jaw-joint problems: Diagnosis and treatment in temporomandibular orthopedics. *Osteopathic Medicine* 5:35, February 1980.
320.. Shapiro BL: Changing views about temporomandibular pain-dysfunction. *Northwest Dentistry* 60:6, 1981.
321. Shore NA: *Occlusal Equilibration and Temporomandibular Joint Dysfunction*. Philadelphia, J.B. Lippincott, 1976.
322. Greene CS, Laskin DM: Long-term evaluation of conservative treatment for myofascial pain-dysfunction syndromes. *Journal of the American Dental Association* 89:1365–1368, 1974.
323. Schafer RC: *Chiropractic Management of Sports and Recreational Injuries*. Baltimore, Williams & Wilkins, 1982, pp 314–315.
324. Royder JO: Structural influences in temporomandibular joint pain and dysfunction. *Journal of the American Osteopathic Association* 80:460–467, March 1981.
325. Larsen NJ: Osteopathic manipulative contribution to treatment of TMJ syndrome. *Osteopathic Medicine* 3:15–27, August 1976.
326. Magoun HI Sr: Dental equilibrium and osteopathy. *Journal of the American Osteopathic Association* 75:981–991, June 1975.
327. Sutherland WG: Contributions of thought. Meridian, Ida, Sutherland Cranial Teaching Foundation, 1967.
328. Durbin K: TMJ dysfunction. In Hughes T: *Physical Therapy Class Notes*. Chesterfield, Mo, Logan College of Chiropractic, 1984, pp 616–619.
329. Travell JG, Simons DG: *Myofascial Pain and Dysfunction: The Trigger Point Manual*. Baltimore, Williams & Wilkins, 1983, pp 173–180, 240–271.
330. Hertling D: The temporomandibular joint. In Kessler RM, Hertling D (eds): *Management of Common Musculoskeletal Disorders*. Philadelphia, Harper & Row, 1983, pp 233–271.

SUGGESTED READINGS

Bogduk N: The clinical anatomy of the cervical dorsal rami. *Spine* 7:319–330, 1982.

Carver W: *Carver's Chiropractic Analysis,* ed 4. Oklahoma City, published by the author, 1921, vol one; 1922, vol two.

Gregory RR: Biomechanics of the upper cervical spine. *The Digest of Chiropractic Economics* September/October 1983.

Jones MD: Cineradiographic studies of the normal cervical spine. *California Medicine* 93:293, 1960.

Kotheimer WJ: *Applied Chiropractic in Distortion Analysis.* Ardmore, Pa, Dorrance & Company, 1977.

Robinson GK: Cinefluoroscopic motion studies of the post-traumatic cervical spine. *The Digest of Chiropractic Economics* November/December 1984.

Robinson GK: Videofluoroscopic joint motion studies of the cervical spine. *The Digest of Chiropractic Economics* March/April 1985.

Schafer RC: Procedures to save a life . . . avoid malpractice. *Journal of the Chiropractic Association of Oklahoma* March/April 1982.

Truscott LL, Frisbie GK: *Truscott System of Angular Analysis and Controlled Adjusting,* ed 2. San Jose, Cal, Rosicrucian Press, 1948.

Warfel JH: *The Head, Neck, and Trunk,* ed 5. Philadelphia, Lea & Febiger, 1985.

West HG: Vertebral artery considerations in cervical trauma. *ACA Journal of Chiropractic* December 1968, pp 18–19.

CHAPTER 10

The Thoracic Region and Related Clinical Problems

This chapter is concerned with the thoracic spine, the region of the primary spinal curvature. From a quantitative standpoint, it contains half of the spine segments and about three-fourths of the spinal cord. From a visceral standpoint, the sympathetic nervous system can be affected here more than in any other region of the spine.

To appreciate the normal thoracic biomechanics involved and how abnormal biomechanics can be corrected is the object of this chapter. This requires an understanding of thoracic kinesiology, the factors contributing to stability, and how to cope with the common biomechanical problems of this area.

BACKGROUND[1-3]

Severe biomechanical lesions of the thoracic spine are seen less frequently than those of the cervical or lumbar spine, but when they occur, they are often quite serious if related to a disc protrusion or facet position defect. Shoulder girdle, rib cage, spinal cord, cerebrospinal fluid flow, and autonomic visceral problems originating in the thoracic spine are far from being uncommon. The major biomechanical concern is the prevention of thoracic hyperkyphosis, flattening, or twisting; each of these can contribute to both local and distal and acute and chronic life-threatening manifestations, if not a life of poor quality.

Study of the thoracic spine in itself is often perplexing. Many thoracic problems have their origin in its base, the lumbar spine, while others are reflections of cervical disorders. By the same token, a thoracic lesion may manifest symptoms in either the cervical or lumbar spine. Foremost in our thoughts should be the recognition that the thoracic spine is the structural support and sympathetic source for the esophagus, heart, bronchi, lungs, diaphragm, stomach, liver, gallbladder, pancreas, spleen, kidneys, and much of the pelvic contents.

FUNCTIONAL ANATOMY OF THE THORACIC CAGE AND SPINE

The thoracic cage serves as a unique coupled system, composed of the sternal complex, 12 pairs of ribs, costal cartilages, and thoracic vertebrae. As a whole and individually, these structures are quite strong and elastic prior to the osteoporosis of old age. The thoracic cage of an infant can withstand compression loads of up to 200 lb without injury.[4] Young men can withstand up to 2800 lb.

Regional Characteristics

The most important structures to consider here that have significant biomechanical influences are the sternum, ribs, vertebrae, intervertebral discs (IVDs), and costal joints.

The Sternum[5, 6]

The sternum serves as a protective plate for the heart and aorta against anterior forces (Fig. 10.1). Anatomically, the sternum is divided into three main osseous parts: the manubrium, body, and xiphoid process.

The Manubrium. The thick manubrium at the superior part of the sternum articulates laterally with the medial clavicles and 1st ribs at its superolateral aspect and with part of the 2nd rib at its inferolateral aspect. The manubrium's superior aspect (jugular notch) is on a level with T2. Its inferior aspect, on a level with T4, joins the superior aspect of the body of the sternum in a synchondrosis. The symphysis here allows hinge-like movements during respiration.

The Body of the Sternum. The middle part of the body of the sternum is composed of four synchrondrotic segments that become fused in the young adult. Its lateral

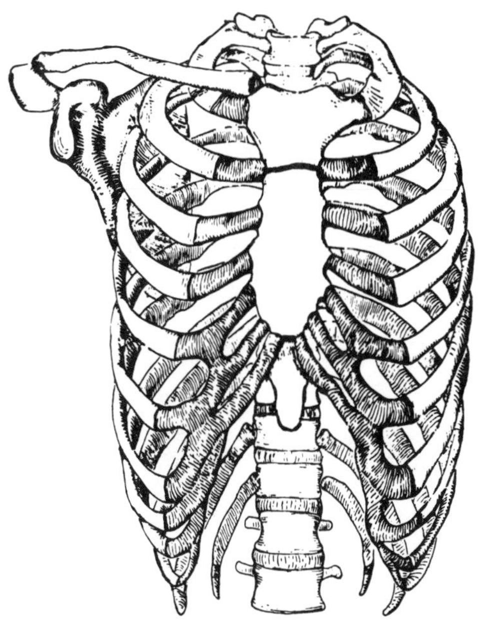

Figure 10.1. Schematic of the anterior aspect of an adult thoracic cage.

aspects offer a series of costal notches to accept the anterior aspects of the costal cartilages.

The Xiphoid Process. This coccyx-like process extends downward from the inferior aspect of the 4th segment of the sternal body and divides the superior aspect of the rectus abdominis. The joint between the body of the sternum and the xiphoid process, on a level with T8, is a synchondrosis that becomes a synostosis during middle age.

The Ribs[7–10]

With the exception of an anomaly, each of the 12 thoracic vertebrae normally has a corresponding pair of ribs. A typical rib is angled inferiorly from its vertebral attachment as it curves outward and serves as a curved lever. The lower the rib, the more acute the angle. At its anterior aspect, each rib curves medially and upward. Except for the short 1st rib, this means that the lateral aspect of a rib is lower than either its posterior or anterior attachment. The anterior attachment is lower than its posterior attachment.

This flattened, curved design of a rib, and the fact that a rib is under compression between the spine and the sternum, offers it special biomechanical advantages against anterior or posterior forces and rapid rebound when compressed linearly.[11, 12] Because a rib is preloaded through its long axis, it has a tendency to "spring open" if cut free from one of its fixed points. This tension is maintained essentially through the mechanical design and intercostal tonicity. Thus, an A-P force acting upon a rib must first overcome the expansion tendency of the rib before it can overcome the tensile strength of the bone.

Because inspiration increases tension on the thoracic elastic elements and elastic tension gives resistance to deformation or compression, an expanded thoracic cage is in a much better state to withstand a blow or support a load. It is for this reason that football players are taught to inspire just before making a block.

All rib cages increase with inspiration and decrease with expiration, and all rib lengths increase with inspiration and decrease with expiration.[13] This is called the "caliper," "ice tongs," or "pump handle" A-P effect. It occurs essentially at the costovertebral joints and is fairly restricted to the T2–T6 area.[14]

Also during respiration, the lateral aspect of a rib raises and lowers with inspiration and expiration. This lateral "bucket handle" effect is due to the relatively fixed points of articulation anteriorly and posteriorly and the lateral inferior-superior motion. The lateral aspects of the ribs are pulled away from the midline and the transverse diameter of the thoracic cage is increased.[15] This movement chiefly elevates and everts the lower borders of ribs T2–T10. The effect is most noticeable in the upper ribs.

The T1–T7 Area. These ribs, called "true" ribs, articulate with the sternum anteriorly. Their length progressively increases inferiorly. Because of strong attachments at the sternum and at the costovertebral and costotransverse joints, A-P distortion should be inhibited in this area. Yet, Grieve reports that it is not uncommon to find a flat midscapular area that is normal in all other respects.[16] This could indicate that acquired biomechanical forces have overcome inherent structural forces.

The T8–T10 Area. The ribs of this area, called "false" ribs, are joined anteriorly below the sternum by cartilage with no direct osseous support. Their length progressively decreases inferiorly.

The T11–T12 Area. These ribs, called "false floating" ribs, are relatively free anteriorly, lacking both osseous and cartilaginous support. They end within muscle tissue. They do not actually "float" because they articulate posteriorly with their numbered vertebrae (Fig. 10.2). Their length progressively decreases inferiorly. The 12th rib is attached to the tips of L1–L2 transverse processes by the lumbocostal ligament which runs anterior to the quadratus lumborum.

The Thoracic Vertebrae[17–19]

The Vertebral Body. The thoracic vertebral bodies from T1 to T3 diminish in size and then progressively enlarge to T12. The vertebral canal is small and circular. A forced index finger will completely fill the opening. Thus, any degree of buckling or stenosis of the canal ligaments or central protrusion of an IVD is likely to compromise the contents of the canal. (Figs. 10.3 and 10.4.)

Unlike the rectangular centrum of a cervical or lumbar vertebra when viewed laterally, the body of a thoracic vertebra is wedge shaped, with its posterior aspect 1–2

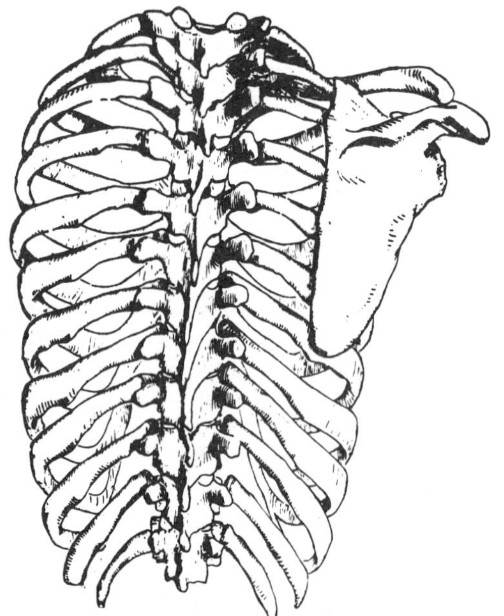

Figure 10.2. Drawing of the posterior aspect of an adult thoracic cage, spine, and right scapula.

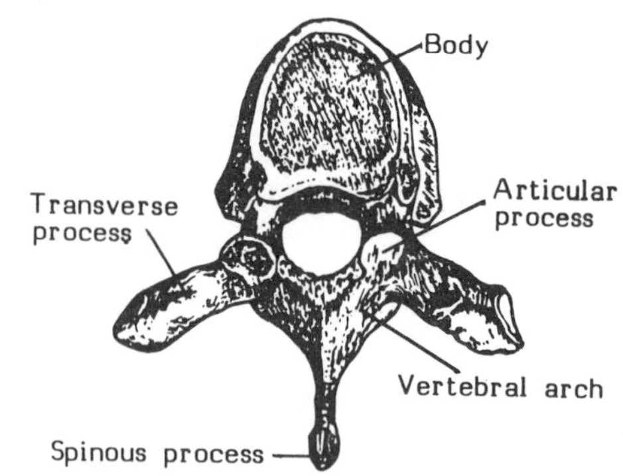

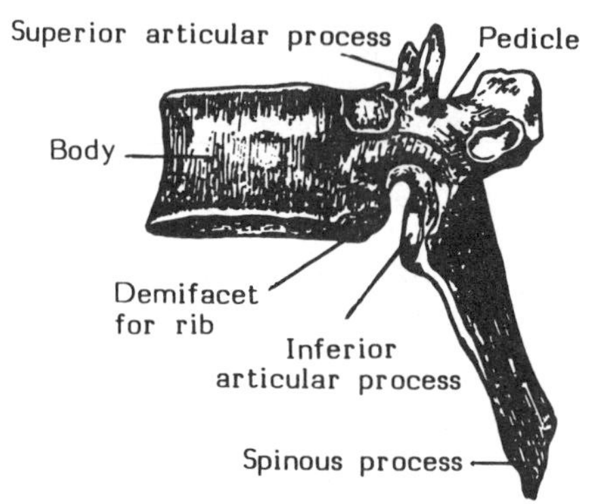

Figure 10.3. *Top*, view from the top of T6; *bottom*, view from the lateral.

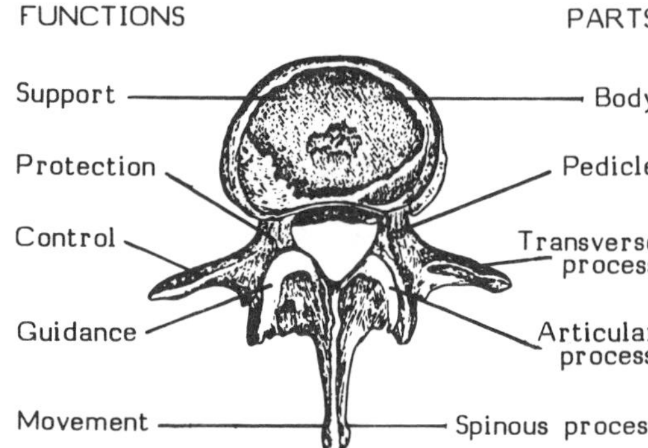

Figure 10.4. Major functional parts of a thoracic vertebra as seen from the superior.

mm higher than its anterior aspect. It is for this reason that lines drawn through the inferior vertebral body planes on a lateral roentgenograph will normally meet anteriorly. This osseous wedge produces the relatively stiff primary thoracic kyphosis and encourages acquired exaggeration after prolonged axial loading.

The Demifacets. The typical thoracic vertebra presents two demifacets (notches) to accept part of a rib head near the centrum's lateral posterosuperior and posteroinferior angle. The superior facet is usually much larger than the inferior facet.

The Spinous Processes. The midthoracic spinous processes project obliquely downward like a horse's tail or scales on a fish, with much less obliquity in the upper and lower segments. They are almost never bifid; but individuals will exhibit a wide degree of variation from the "norm," and this must be kept in mind during osseous palpation. Palpation between and around the spinous processes will disclose much more information than will the spinous processes themselves.

The Articular Facets. The flat, oval superior articular facets face posteriorly and superiorly at about a 60° angle, with a slightly lateral slant to match the inferior facets above (Fig. 10.5). From above, they appear as an arc of a circle whose axis is slightly anterior to the vertebral body.

The Transverse Processes. From T1–T8, the transverse processes are on a level with the superior border of their vertebral bodies. These processes are stouter and stronger in the thoracic region than any other region of the spine because they must buttress the ribs and serve as attachment points for strong muscles and ligaments. The anterosuperior aspect of the tip of most transverse processes presents a facet that articulates with a tubercle on the neck of a rib.

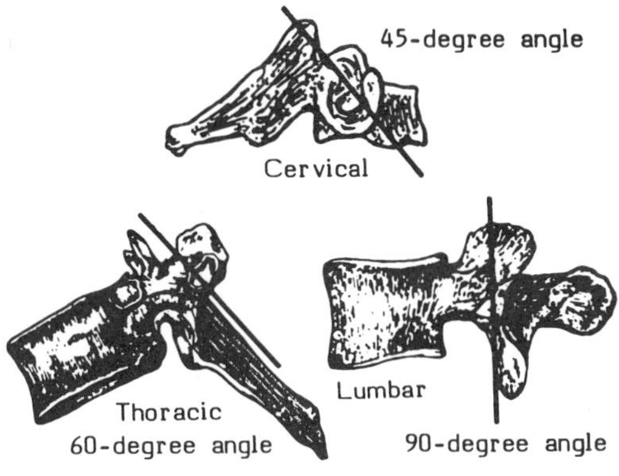

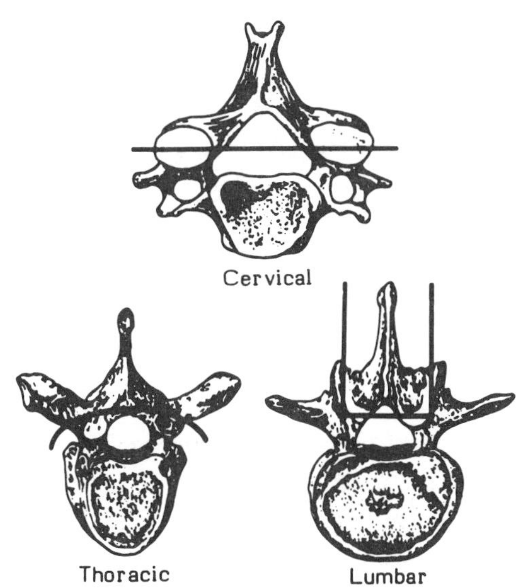

Figure 10.5. *Top group*, comparison of typical cervical, thoracic, and lumbar facet orientations; *bottom group*, views from above.

The Intervertebral Discs[20, 21]

Dorsal flexibility is minimal because disc height in comparison to vertebral body height is less in the thoracic spine than that of any spinal region. This is readily apparent by noting that there is little decrease in the thoracic curve on forward flexion or in the supine or sitting positions.

Unlike the cervical and lumbar regions, the disc spaces are fairly parallel rather than wedge shaped. Thus, the primary thoracic kyphosis is produced by bone while the secondary cervical and lumbar lordoses are produced by fibrocartilage. Also, the nucleus sits slightly more centrally within the anulus while it is more posterior to the midline in the cervical and lumbar regions. This means that the thoracic apophyses play less of a role in dispersing axial forces.[22]

The vertebral endplates show distinctive changes during growth, maturity, and old age. A gradual reduction in the width of the growth cartilage occurs up to 16–20 years of age. During adulthood and progressing into old age, the endplates consist of only articular cartilage, which undergoes calcification followed by resorption and replacement by bone.[23] During the degenerative process, an increasing number of collagen fibers arise from the endplates and course toward the center of the disc.

Cailliet and others contend that the adult IVD is devoid of nerve fibers.[24] In contrast, some think that the extreme posterior aspect of the anulus is impregnated with some pain-sensitive nerve fibers.[25] Adding to this controversy are the findings of recent studies of postmortem specimens of T10–L5 vertebrae showing that pain-sensitive fibers are present in the anterior anulus and probably also in vertebral bone.[26]

The Spinal Ligaments[27, 28]

In comparison to the cervical and lumbar regions, the elastic ligamentum flava and the anterior and posterior longitudinal ligaments are thicker and stronger. (Fig. 10.6.) On the other hand, the interspinous and capsular ligaments are thinner and looser in the neutral position. However, these latter ligaments receive support from ligaments radiating from the costovertebral and costotransverse joints.

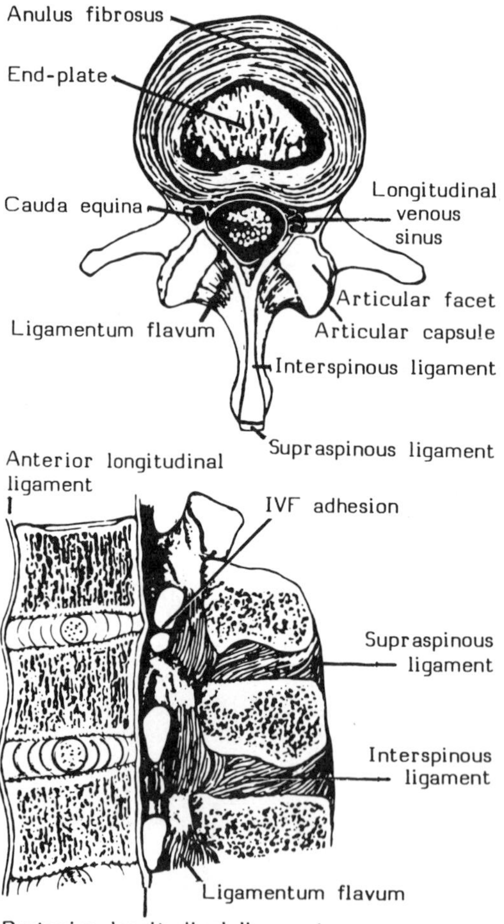

Figure 10.6. *Top*, the major spinal ligaments as viewed from above; *bottom*, lateral view of a midsagittal section.

The Costal Joints[29–32]

The Costovertebral Joints. Posteriorly, the convex head of a rib articulates (slides and pivots) upon two adjacent thoracic vertebral bodies at the concave demifacets, above and below disc level, in a single richly innervated synovial joint. Exceptions to this are the 1st rib and floating ribs whose heads articulate with only one vertebra. Typically, the capsule of a costovertebral joint is quite thin and weak by itself but stronger anteriorly than posteriorly. It is attached to the anulus by the intermediate intra-articular ligament that divides the cavity and attaches to the rib head between the facets. Interosseous fibers also extend from the rib head superiorly to the vertebral body above and inferiorly to the vertebral body below. These intermediate, superior, and inferior fibers greatly strengthen the inherently weak capsule proper. Posteriorly, capsule fibers merge with the lateral extensions of the posterior longitudinal ligament (Fig. 10.7). During inspiration, the rib heads undergo a slight rotary and gliding movement.

The Costotransverse Joints. As a rib is directed posteriorly from the attachment of

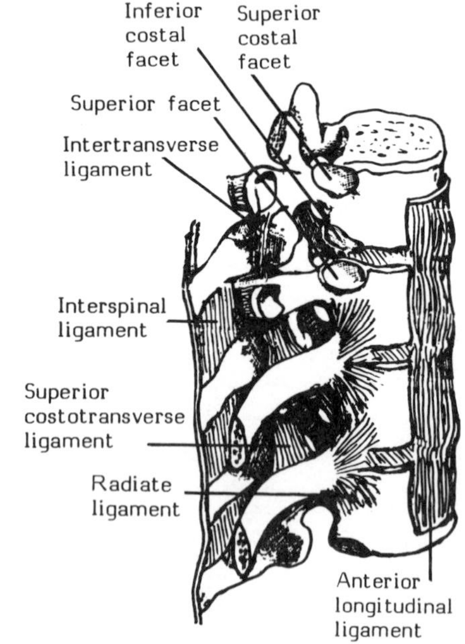

Figure 10.7. Highlights of the costovertebral joints and spinal ligaments of the midthoracic area as viewed laterally. Normal kyphosis is not depicted.

its head, a convex posterior tubercle on the rib articulates with a concave facet on the anterior tip of the transverse process of the same vertebra. This is also a richly innervated synovial joint that allows lubricated movement (Fig. 10.8). The T1–T7 joints are concave-convex to afford rotation, while the T8–T10 joints are flat to allow gliding. Strength is provided to the thin capsule by medial and lateral costotransverse ligaments. A strong superior costotransverse ligament connects an adjacent rib neck below to the transverse process above, but it offers only slight protection to the costotransverse capsule. During inspiration, the tubercles glide superiorly and posteriorly. The lower two or three ribs have neither articular tubercles nor costotransverse joints.

Costovertebral and Costotransverse Coupling. The costotransverse joint and the costovertebral joint serve as a mechanical couple that restricts normal movement to rotation about an axis that passes through the center of each of these joints.[13] These joints, along with the elasticity of the sternocostal articulations, produce pivot points from which the ribs elevate and depress laterally. Because the axis running through the costotransverse and costovertebral joints lies close to the frontal plane in the upper ribs and nearly parallel to the sagittal plane in the lower ribs, elevation of the ribs during inspiration appreciably increases only the A-P diameter of the upper thorax, increases both the A-P and transverse diameters in the midthorax, and increases only the transverse diameter of the lower thorax. All these

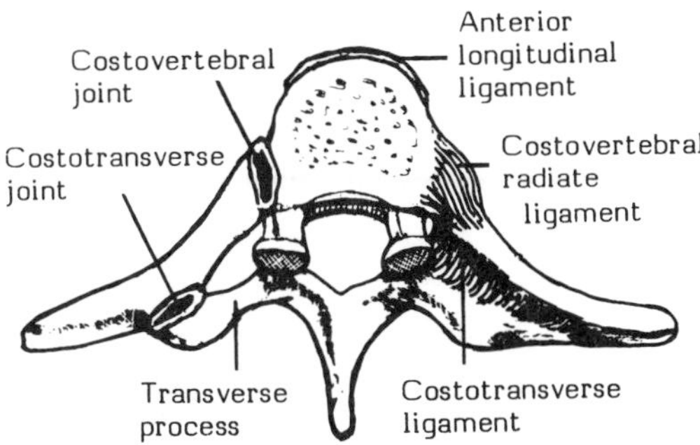

Figure 10.8. Highlights of the costovertebral and costotransverse joints of the midthoracic area as viewed from above.

changes in thoracic diameters can be accomplished by the diaphragm itself.

The Costochondral and Sternocostal Joints. The T1–T7 anteriorly cupped rib ends join their costal cartilages at synovial synchondrotic costochondral joints that are surrounded by periosteum. There is little motion at these joints. The anterior costal cartilages articulate with the sternum at synovial synchondrotic joints. The sternocostal joints are similar to the costovertebral joints; ie, synovial joints that are divided by an intra-articular ligament. The capsules are thin but strenghtened by anterior and posterior radiate ligaments.

During inspiration, the sternum moves anterior and superior when viewed from the side, the angle formed by the first rib and the manubrium closes when viewed from the side, and the costosternal angles open when viewed from above. The costal cartilages of the true ribs rotate upward and forward, and the false ribs slide upon each other at the interchondral joints. These mechanisms are reversed during expiration.

The Interchondral Joints. The T8–T11 ribs are held to the sternum by fused costal cartilage and anteriorly articulate (slide) superiorly and inferiorly within synovial-like joints that later become fibrous and then fuse in old age. The fibrous capsules are quite thin but strengthened by the interchondral ligaments. The articulation between T9 and T10 is usually united by a fibrous joint.

Kinesiology of the Thorax[33-35]

All movements in the thoracic spine are relatively limited compared to the cervical area, especially in the upper regions, because of the restrictions imposed by the costovertebral and costotransverse articulations, the direction and shape of the articular facets, the relatively thin discs, and the tension of the ligamentum flava. Movement of the thoracic spine cannot occur in any direction without the involved vertebrae somewhat carrying their attached ribs with them.[29]

Flexion and Extension

Thoracic flexion is provided essentially by the rectus abdominis with some assistance by the external and internal obliques (Table

10.1). At full flexion, all involved muscles relax except the iliocostalis dorsi. Extension power is dispersed among the erector spinae, semispinalis, spinalis, interspinalis, intercostals, longissimus dorsi, multifidus, and rotators (Figs. 10.9–10.11).

Rotation and Lateral Flexion

These movements are strongly coupled. Rotation is provided by (1) the unilateral internal oblique and erector spinae, and (2) the contralateral external oblique, semispinalis, and deep posterior intrinsics. The semispinalis is a prime mover of the thoracic spine, and the intrinsic muscles serve as synergists. Excessive tone of the synergists tends to produce abnormal coupled moments. Lateral flexion of the thoracic region is provided by the erector spinae, semispinalis, quadratus lumborum, deep posterior intrinsics, rectus abdominis, and the internal and external obliques.

Respiratory Movements[36, 37]

Quiet respiration is under the dominant control of the bellows-like diaphragm with some help from intercostal, levator costarum, and scalene activity. There is minimal movement in the thoracic joints. When the diaphragm contracts, its dome lowers so that the vertical length of the thoracic cavity is increased. This increase in vertical diameter is also contributed to by the raising of the upper ribs. When the diaphragm relaxes, the elastic rebound of the abdominal wall plus some contraction pushes the viscera and the diaphragm upward in expiration. The elastic recoil of the lungs and the subatmospheric pressure produced within the pleural cavity are also active during expiration.

During forced inspiration, the diaphragm, levator costarum, external intercostals, anterior internal intercostals, serratus posterior superior, and scalenes are the most active muscles. The thoracic spinal extensors, sternocleidomastoideus, scaleni group, pectoralis major and minor, trapezius, latissimus dorsi, serratus anterior and posterior inferior, subclavius, and levator scapulae are contributors. During respiratory activity, it is important that the quadratus lumborum fixates the 12th rib, or the diaphragm would not have a stable attachment from which to maintain its tension.

During forced expiration, the posterior internal intercostals, the abdominal group, and the serratus posterior inferior are the most active muscles. The latissimus dorsi, serratus posterior inferior, quadratus lum-

Table 10.1.
Major Muscles of the Trunk

Muscle	Major functions	Spinal segment
Diaphragm	Inspiration	C4
Erector spinae	Extension	T1–S3
External oblique	Rotation, flexion, forced respiration	T1–T11
Intercostals, external	Inspiration, extension	T1–T11
Intercostals, internal	Expiration, extension	T1–T11
Interspinalis	Extension, lateral flexion, rotation	T1–S3
Intertransversarii	Lateral flexion, rotation	T1–T8
Internal oblique	Rotation, flexion, forced respiration	T7–T11
Longissimus dorsi	Extension	T1–L5
Multifidus	Extension, lateral flexion, rotation	T1–S3
Quadratus lumborum	Extension	T12–L3
Rectus abdominis	Flexion, forced respiration	T7–T11
Rotatores	Extension, lateral flexion, rotation	T1–S3
Semispinalis	Extension, lateral flexion, rotation	T1–S3
Serratus posterior inferior	Expiration	T9–T11
Serratus posterior superior	Inspiration	T1–T4
Spinalis thoracis	Extension	T1–S3
Transverse abdominis	Forced respiration	T7–L1

Spinal innervation varies somewhat in different people. The spinal nerves listed here are averages and may differ in a particular patient; thus, an allowance of a segment above and below those listed in most text tables should be considered.

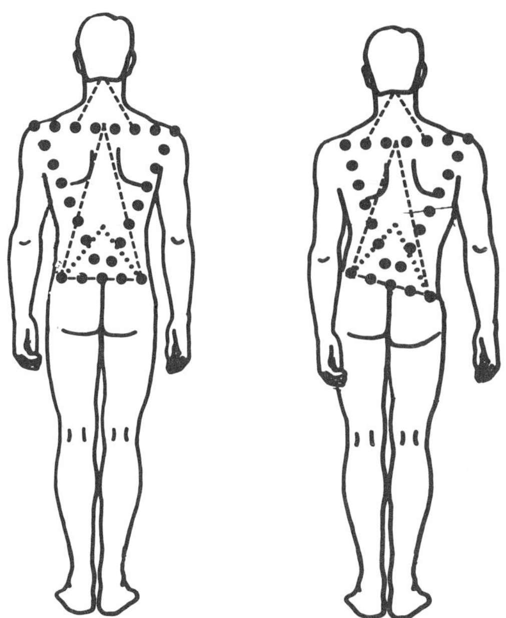

Figure 10.9. Diagrams of the triangular guy wire architecture of the large spinal muscles; *left*, in good posture; *right*, adaptation in a low right leg syndrome.

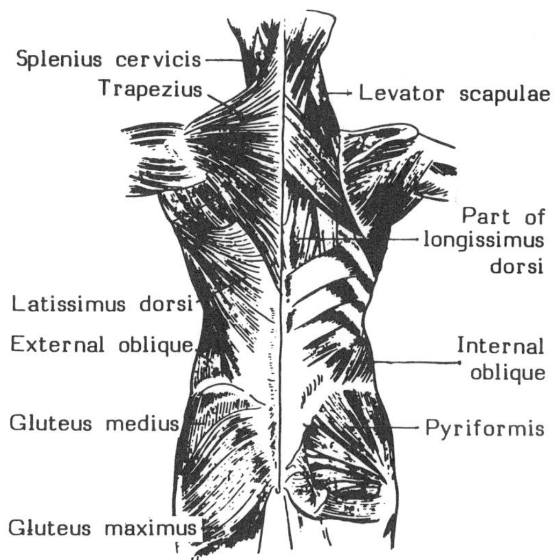

Figure 10.10. The large posterior muscles of the neck, back, and pelvis.

borum, and iliocostalis lumborum offer assistance. The muscles of the abdomen essentially serve as antagonists to the diaphragm during expiration.

Postural Effects. Gravity has a distinct effect upon the work of the diaphragm. In the upright position, the expiratory excursion of the diaphragm must overcome the gravitational pull upon the thoracic viscera. This is done by abdominal contraction that pushes the subdiaphragmatic viscera superiorly. Breathing is much easier when a patient is horizontal because the diaphragm is relieved of weight from above. Likewise, diaphragmatic excursion is much greater in the horizontal position than the vertical position. Excursion is inhibited more in sitting than in standing because the abdominals are relaxed in the sitting posture. When the abdominals are weakened by ptosis, hernia, or paralysis, respiration becomes purely thoracic. The reverse is true in pneumonia, pleurisy, and rib fracture.

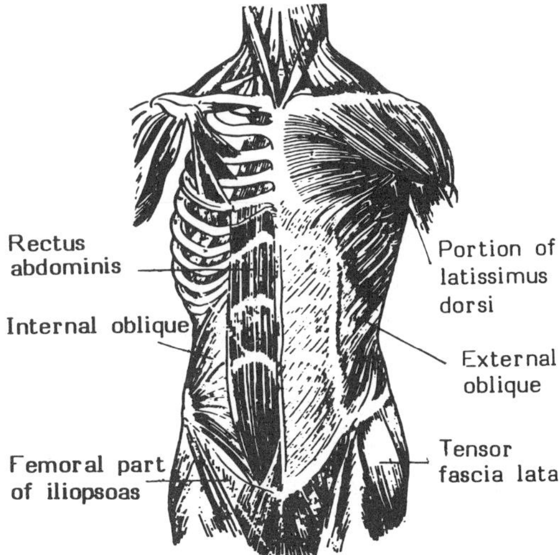

Figure 10.11. The large muscles of the anterior trunk.

Kinematics of the Thoracic Spine[38–45]

As in the lumbar spine, all thoracic movements are somewhat three-dimensional with rotation and lateral flexion being the most evident (Figs. 10.12 and 10.13).

Flexion and Extension

Flexion and extension of the thoracic spine are most limited (Fig. 10.14). An average of only 4° occurs in the upper discs, 6° in the middle discs, and about 12° in the lower discs. As in the other spinal areas, excessive A-P motion is restricted by the check ligaments, but the thoracic cage adds an additional mechanical barrier to flexion and intercostal straps to restrict extension.

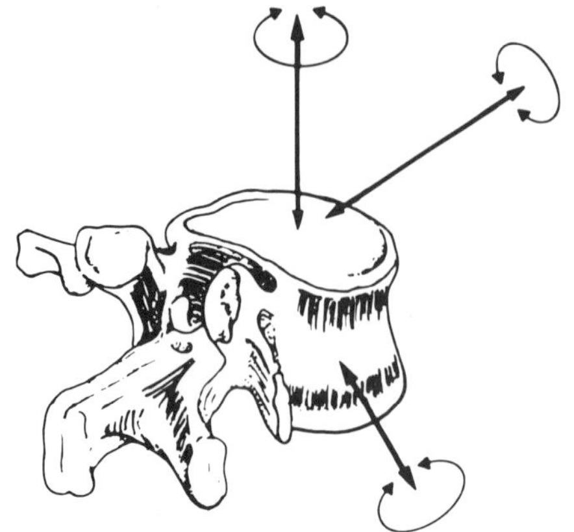

Figure 10.12. The six degrees of freedom involved in spinal kinematics.

Thoracic extension from full flexion takes place in two phases: (1) The articular surfaces glide posterior and inferior, the interspinous spaces appose, and the stretched posterior anulus of the disc returns to its normal shape as the individual achieves the erect position. There is no appreciable change in the anterior discs or nucleus. (2) It is not until the shingle-like facets, transverse processes, and spinous processes reach their limit as the spine is extended posterior to the midline that the anterior discs and anterior intercostal spaces begin to widen. On forced extension, the articular processes impact. The vertebrae then push between their ribs, and the rib heads and their angles are moved slightly aside by the transverse processes.[46]

Thoracic A-P mobility includes a good amount of facet gliding, but it is far less than that of the cervical region where the facets almost separate on forward flexion. In view of the rather limited normal movement of the thoracic spine, the gross idiopathic type of scolioses in this area are difficult to comprehend when little structural damage is present.

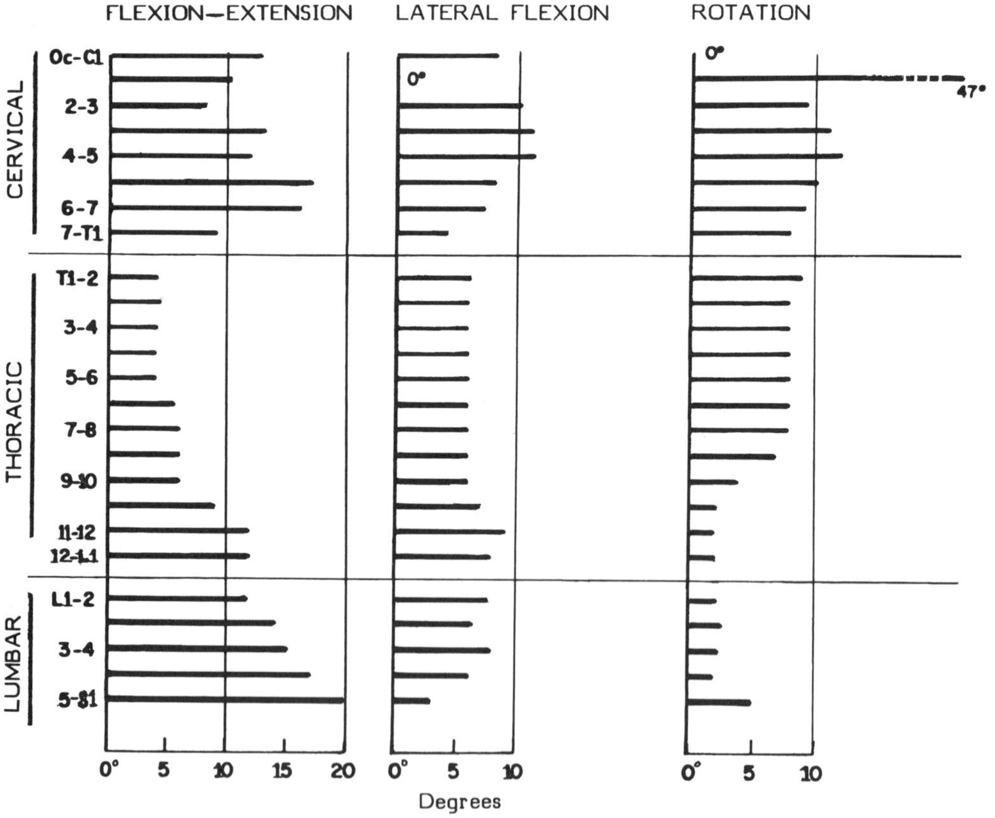

FLEXION—EXTENSION LATERAL FLEXION ROTATION

CERVICAL: Oc-C1, 2-3, 4-5, 6-7, 7-T1

THORACIC: T1-2, 3-4, 5-6, 7-8, 9-10, 11-12, 12-L1

LUMBAR: L1-2, 3-4, 5-S1

0° 0° 47°

0° 5 10 15 20 0° 5 10 0° 5 10

Degrees

Figure 10.13. Compared approximate values of flexion-extension, lateral flexion, and rotation, in degrees, for various spinal levels, as redrawn from data of White and Panjabi. Other authorities differ slightly from these figures.

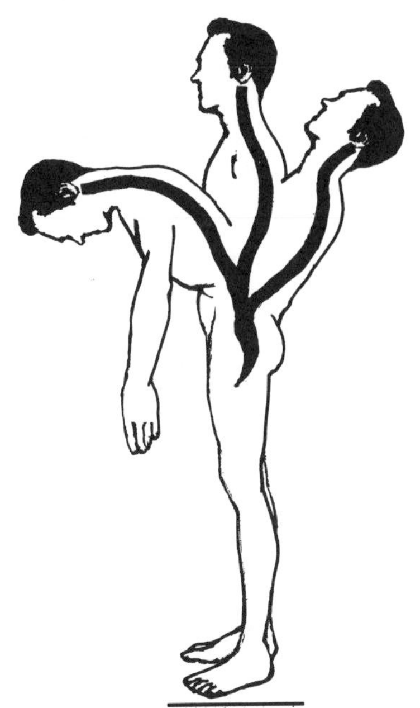

Figure 10.14. During spinal flexion-extension, note that the lumbar and cervical curves flatten considerably during flexion and increase slightly during extension. The thoracic curve exhibits little alteration in either flexion or extension.

As in other spinal areas, the anulus and its nucleus bulge in opposite directions during A-P and lateral bending moments to stabilize each other. During forced extension, the anulus thins and bulges posteriorly, and it stretches and contracts anteriorly. The nucleus bulges anteriorly without appreciable shifting. The anterior ligaments are put under tension while the posterior ligaments relax. At the end of forced extension, the inferior facets tend to pivot open at their anterior aspect as their posterior aspect jams on its neighbor below. These actions are quite minimal when the normal kyphosis is present, but it may be exaggerated in the flat "military" spine. During flexion, the mechanisms are essentially the opposite.

Rotation

Rotation of the thoracic spine, usually coupled with some vertebral body tilting, is somewhat greater than flexion and extension, which are approximately equal in range. Rotation up to about 10° occurs at the T1 segment but progressively diminishes inferiorly to a maximum of 2–3° at the T12 level. The total range of thoracic rotation is about 40°.

According to Grice, there are also a few degrees of coupled flexion during upper thoracic rotation and a few degrees of coupled extension during lower thoracic rotation.[47, 48] This becomes a significant point in analyzing scolioses.

Rib Changes. It can be readily noted during thoracic rotation that the spine does not rotate between the ribs but with the ribs, and this is accompanied by a degree of lateral gliding of the vertebrae involved. However, when rotation is forced beyond the limit of rib motion, there is a slight push by the transverse process against the rib head on the side moving anteriorly and a slight pull by the transverse process complex on the rib head on the side moving posteriorly. This motion is often revealed by palpation, rarely by roentgenography. It is recognized more easily in the upper thoracic region where rotation is greater and the ribs are firmly attached to the sternum than in the lower thoracic area where the floating ribs more readily follow vertebral movement. Because of its design, the thoracic spine would have a considerable range of rotary motion if it were not for the restricting thoracic cage. This is exhibited in scoliosis, in which every movement of the spine is registered by a corresponding movement in the attached ribs.[49, 50]

Some authors give more credit to the thoracic ligaments than they deserve because they study the thoracic spine separately from the rib cage. But it is not separate in vivo, and studying the spine by itself does not reveal the mechanics involved (eg, using a plastic model of the spine). A thoracic spine detached from the rib cage is fairly flexible in all directions except extension.

If the ligamentous attachments are supple (eg, those of a child), the ribs react to the movement of the transverse processes and enhance rotation. The rib spaces on the convex side will not open until the ribs on the concave side have reached their limit of approximation. In the adult thoracic spine, however, there is little rotation accompanying lateral bending except in the lower thoracic region where the ribs float. On forced lateral bending when the ribs approximate on the concave side and their limit is reached, the associated vertebrae are capable of slight additional lateral gliding.

Disc Changes. During axial rotation, the oblique anular fibers running in the direction of rotation become tensed, while those running in the opposite direction relax. This puts a twist on the anulus but there are no appreciable shear forces involved in the thoracic spine during pure axial rotation.

Lateral Flexion

Although lateral flexion is hampered by the rib cage, the average person should be able to touch the ipsilateral knee with the fingertips. In the average adult spine, less than 10° of motion occurs at the upper and middle discs, and a few more degrees of motion are attained by the lower discs. The total range of lateral flexion for the healthy thoracic spine is slightly greater than 50°.

Note that the position of a thoracic vertebra in lateral flexion is identical to that of the common subluxation in the neutral position in which one facet has slipped inferoposteriorly while its counterpart has glided superoanteriorly.

The subject of coupled rotation during thoracic lateral bending appears on the surface to be readily definable. This is not the case, however. Several authorities appear to disagree on what occurs, especially when flexion or extension is introduced. In regard to the cervical and upper thoracic spine, White and Panjabi[51] state that the direction of coupling of axial rotation with lateral bending is directed in such a manner "that axial rotation of the vertebral body causes its anterior aspect to point toward the concavity of the lateral bending curve. In other words, the spinous processes point more to the convexity of the physiologic curve." They also report that the same pattern occurs in the middle and lower thoracic spine, but to a lesser extent, is inconsistently present, and is possibly the reverse of the pattern occurring in the upper thoracic and cervical regions.

Grice[52] is in general agreement with this when he reports: "In the upper thoracic spine, rotation during lateral flexion is similar to that in the cervical spine; ie, the rotation of the spinous process is toward the convexity." He is more specific, however, when it comes to the lower thoracic spine during lateral flexion: " . . . the upper thoracic vertebrae behave similar to a cervical motion segment while the lower thoracic vertebrae behave similar to a lumbar segment."

On the other hand, in writing of the T3–T10 area, Grieve[53] states: "In neutral and extension, side-bending and rotation occur to opposite sides. In flexion, they occur to the same side, as in the cervical spine."

Shrader[54] appears at first to agree with White, Panjabi, and Grice: "When the spine is in a neutral position (easy normal) and side-bending is introduced, the bodies of the vertebrae will rotate toward the concavity." However, he goes on to report that "When the spine is either forward or backward bent and side-bending is introduced, the vertebrae will rotate toward the concavity."

In clinical application, however, the moot question of such "normal" movements may not be that important inasmuch as pathologic changes readily alter normal dynamics. Although Jirout[55] was referring to the cervical spine, his thoughts would be applicable here: "Any manipulation philosophy based on the supposed 'correctness' of this or that set movement 'logically' based on the plane of the facets may be fallacious." Grieve[56] underscores this point by stating that it may seem wise to " . . . allow the joints of individual patterns to speak for themselves, in the prime matter of the nature and direction of the most effective therapeutic movement" and " . . . clinical assessment of individual responses takes precedence over theories of biomechanics and theories of 'correct' techniques."

CLINICAL BIOMECHANICS OF THORACIC TRAUMA

The most common traumatic problems of the thorax are intervertebral, costovertebral, costotransverse, and sternocostal subluxations; fractures; joint separations, dislocations, and resulting fibrosis; contusions, strains, and resulting trigger points; and injuries to the internal organs.

Posttraumatic Assessment

Anterior chest and abdominal injuries can be life-threatening. Thus, the primary concern following trauma is to assure that there is normal breathing and circulation and that steps be taken to minimize shock. In regard to the thoracic spine, potential cord injury should be given priority consideration.

As in any musculoskeletal disorder after the possibility of fracture, dislocation, or bleeding have been eliminated, evaluation should include muscle strength grading, ranges of joint motion, sensory perception, appropriate tendon reflexes, and other pertinent clinical tests when indicated. A listing of various neurologic and orthopedic signs and tests relative to the thorax is shown in Table 10.2.

Pulmonary Contusion

Blunt chest injury commonly leads to pulmonary contusion, which is characterized by covert edema, reflex bronchorrhea, hemorrhage within the lung, and progressing atelectasis.[57] This is especially true in high-velocity accidents that produce a compression-decompression injury to the chest. Physical findings in from mild to moderate cases generally include a rapid respiratory and pulse rate, wet rales, and a copious cough that may be blood stained. In severe cases, hypoxia, respiratory acidosis, secondary pleurisy, and deteriorating respiratory insufficiency may lead to death in spite of heroic efforts.

Pitres' (Plumb Line) Chest Sign. The axis of the sternum is marked on the chest wall with a skin pencil, and a string is then stretched between the center of the sternal notch and the symphysis pubis. This line normally coincides with the line of the sternal axis. If this does not occur, as in cases of monolateral pleurisy, the angle that it forms with the sternal line indicates the degree of pleural effusion within the thorax.[58]

Biomechanical Instability[59–62]

As mentioned, it is fallacious to consider the thoracic spine biomechanically apart from the rib cage. The attached ribs, although individually quite flexible, offer increased stiffness and strength to the vertebral segments, and the thoracic spine's moment of inertia is increased by the rib cage which also increases the area's stiffness against torques and bending moments. The stiffness property of the thoracic spine is decreased by at least half in all loading directions once the ribs are removed.[44]

Unique Factors of the Thoracic Spine

Several unique factors have been considered in regard to stability of the thoracic spine. In review, the major points are that it: (1) is stiffer; (2) is less mobile; (3) has a smaller vertebral canal; (4) has a high incidence of cord damage associated with structural damage; (5) exhibits less vascularity for the cord; (6) has restricting costal articulations; (7) has an increased moment of inertia because of the added thoracic cage; (8) has an anatomical curvature directed posteriorly; (9) tends to be clinically unstable during flexion; (10) has relatively thin discs; (11) is a common site for bursting anterior centrum fractures (lower region only); (12) has the nuclei more centered within the anuli; (13) has thicker yellow ligaments; (14) has thinner and looser apophyseal capsules; (15) has thinner and weaker interspinous ligaments; (16) has a great resistance to extension; (17) possesses coupling variants from top to bottom; and (18) is the major source of supply of sympathetic fibers.

Table 10.2.
Neurologic and Orthopedic Maneuvers, Reflexes, Signs, or Tests Relative to Musculoskeletal Thoracic Syndromes

Adams' test	Lewin's supine test	Range of motion tests
Abdominal reflex	Light touch/pain tests	Schepelmann's sign
Barkman's reflex	Muscle strength grading	Soto-Hall's test
Beevor's sign	Obliquus reflex	Sternal compression test
Brudzinski's test	Naffziger's test	Spinal percussion test
Chest expansion test	Pectoralis flexibility test	Thomas's sign
Comolli's sign	Pitres' chest sign	Trousseau's line test
Forestier's bowstring sign		

Characteristics under Stress

During axial rotation, the thoracic cage is stressed so that the ribs are pushed posteriorly on the side of the movement and pulled anteriorly on the other side. This subjects the sternum to shear forces, and the sternum minutely tips obliquely toward the direction of rotation.

Motion is generally greater in the direction of loading in the thoracic spine than in other directions. The one exception is axial compression, which exhibits almost 50% more translation horizontally than axially.

The costovertebral joints exhibit their highest stiffness property in the lateral direction and their lowest stiffness against superior or inferior loading. The sternocostal joints are just the opposite: they exhibit higher resistance against vertical forces and lower resistance against A-P forces.

Sprains, Strains, and Subluxations[63-67]

The most common soft-tissue injuries of the thoracic region involve the costosternal, posterior musculature, thoracic spine, and tissues of the spinocostal joints.[68]

Costosternal Sprains and Separations

Rib cartilages may be ruptured at the costosternal junctions that are often impossible to view during roentgenography. Symptoms frequently mimic a gallbladder disorder or gastric ulcer. Management is the same as that for rib fracture, but pain is usually not as severe. A subtle shoulder dislocation may be associated. A rib belt often corrects pain in a few days, but healing may take several weeks because of the relative avascularity of cartilage. If conservative strapping and sprain therapy do not afford relief, surgery may be required to excise a cartilage fragment.

Rib Contusions

Impacts on the free ends of the floating ribs painfully involve related muscles. Pain and disability are severe and sometimes beyond the control of conservative measures. Both movement and breathing aggravate and prolong disability, even during bed rest. The possibility of concomitant kidney damage must be ruled out. Competitive activity should not be resumed until gradual exercises include vigorous running and twisting motions without discomfort.

Anterior Rib Pit Subluxation

This condition features a vague dull or sharp pain over the parasternal area at the costosternal junction. Some anterior intercostal neuralgia may be exhibited. One or more of the upper three ribs are most frequently involved.

Adjustment. The examiner stands almost perpendicular to the supine patient on the opposite side of the subluxation and with the cephalad hand, makes a pisiform contact over the anteriorly subluxated rib slightly lateral to the sternum. The caudal stabilizing hand is placed under the patient's scapula so that upward traction can be made during correction. At the end of patient exhalation, medial and slightly inferior traction is applied with the stabilizing hand while the contact hand makes a light pushing-type thrust, laterally and slightly superiorly to follow the curve of the rib. It frequently helps to have the patient internally rotate his ipsilateral humerous during the adjustment.

Alternative Adjustment Procedure. This is a slight adaptation of the adjustment for an anterior medial clavicular subluxation in which contact is made on the medial rib angle rather than on the medical clavicle.

Upper Thoracic Strain

The upper trapezius strain syndrome, often labeled cervical fibrositis is frequently found in patients who have a forward head and round upper thoracic hump. The compensatory head position is associated with a slumped and rounded upper spine, resulting in fixated hyperextension of the cervical spine.

Undue compression posteriorly on the facets of the vertebrae is characterized by a flattened area within the normal kyphosis. The clinical picture is one of posterior neck pain, weakness of anterior neck flexors, and tenderness of the upper dorsal transverse processes. Tension of the neck extensors, including the upper trapezius and cervical erectors, causes a constant fatigue and ache in the back of the neck. The patient frequently stretches the lower neck in an attempt to gain relief. A related impingement of the suboccipital nerves as they emerge through the fascial and muscular features at the base of the skull may account for the commonly associated occipital headaches.

Scapulocostal Syndrome

In this myofascial periostitis, a trigger area is often found at the site of the attachment of the levator scapula muscle to the upper medial angle of the scapula. The mechanism is postural with tension traction irritation of the attachment site.

Pain is located in the upper interscapular area and reported by the patient to be between the medial border of the blade and the underlying rib cage. The onset is often insidious. Discomfort may radiate (1) to the neck and occiput, (2) to the upper triceps and deltoid insertions, (3) around the chest to the anterior, or (4) to the medial forarm and/or the hands and fingers where numbness and tingling are sites of complaint. The course is frequently chronic and characterized by remissions and exacerbations.

Middle and Lower Thoracic Strain

A painful upper back disorder results from gradual and continuous tension on the middle and lower trapezius muscle (a stretch-weakness condition). The chief problem is one of excessive tension on the posterior muscles. There is also a problem of undue compression on the anterior surfaces of the bodies of the thoracic spine with a hyperkyphosis and a depression of the anterior rib cage.

Common causes are habitual posture position of forward (round) shoulders and rounded upper back, overdevelopment of the anterior shoulder girdle muscles with shortening, or heavy breasts that are not adequately supported. Nelson[69] points out that reflex vasoconstriction within the muscles may prevent normal adaptation to use.

This state of chronic muscle strain is rarely associated with an acute onset, but the symptoms may reach a point of severe pain after unusual physical activity. The clinical picture is characterized by soreness and fatigue, progressing to a burning sensation within the course of the middle and lower trapezius. Traction by the muscle on its bony attachments may cause complaints of an isolated sore spot. Palpation frequently elicits acute tenderness in the region of the dorsolumbar attachment of the lower trapezius.

Costovertebral and Costotransverse Subluxations

These subluxations feature misalignment of the costal processes in relation to the vertebral bodies and transverse processes independent of vertebral motion-unit subluxation (ie, primary), or misalignment of the costal processes in relation to the vertebral bodies and transverse processes as a result of vertebral motion-unit subluxation (ie, secondary). They present painful, difficult, and/or restricted respiratory movements of the ribs; shearing stress to the capsular ligaments and synovia; induction of a vertebral motion-unit subluxation; and/or are contributory to the chronicity of a subluxation, induction of spinal curvatures, and/or contribute to the chronicity of curvatures present, and irritation of the sympathetic ganglia and rami communicantes. Vague terms such as pleurodynia or intercostal fibrositis are often used in medical literature to describe the disorder.

Unilateral pain, which may be either stabbing or dull and usually episodic, may be expressed centrally and/or intercostally. The onset is usually rapid following a fall, push, misstep, stretch, sneeze, or cough. Transient but sharp neuralgia, angina, or dyspnea may be reported. Site tenderness, intercostal spasm, and tissue resistance are found at the rib angle and/or near the vertebral or sternal attachments. A midthoracic rib subluxation frequently presents pain radiating down the lateral arm, mimicking a scapulocostal syndrome. Symptoms are frequently aggravated during deep inspiration when the trunk is flexed.

Compressing the rib cage increases pain in fracture and sprain but not in intercostal strain. Springing the ribs from the posterior to the anterior in the prone and relaxed patient to create stress at the vertebral connections aggravates symptoms and causes an immediate apprehensive muscle-guarding response in sprain and subluxation. Overreaction should make the examiner suspicious of a hidden stress fracture.

Unilateral asymmetry point may be palpated inferior to the axilla by noting that one rib is unusually medial to the one above or below, indicating that some type of detraction mechanism is involved. In the nonscoliotic thoracic spine, detraction from the marginal line usually implies the existence of rotary alterations of the vertebral body to which the rib is attached (subluxation), flexion alteration of the same, or alteration of the costovertebral or costotransverse articulation.[70] Detraction would obviously involve numerous soft-tissue changes also.

To determine the exact site and direction of subluxation, Schoenholtz recommends that the patient be examined seated. The examiner should stand behind and ask the patient to laterally flex away from the painful side while lifting the ipsilateral arm over the head to open the ribs. As this is done, the examiner's fingertips are placed under the lower border of the suspected rib and pushed upward, then placed on the superior border and pushed downward. Pain will be increased in the direction of subluxation.[71]

Superior First Rib Head Subluxation. Of all rib head subluxations, those of the short, acutely curved 1st rib are the most common. The next in incidence are the 2nd, 5th, and 6th ribs, respectively, according to Schultz.[72] Palpation is aided if the patient's scapula is adducted. The 1st rib is frequently subluxated superiorly when lower cervical compression tests are positive (eg, scalenus anticus syndrome), in cervicobrachial neuralgias, and in various neurovascular shoulder-girdle, arm, and hand syndromes. Superior subluxation obviously narrows the costoclavicular space and places traction on the neurovascular bundle. It can also be the primary or a contributing factor in torticollis, herpes zoster, and vague anginal or breast aches. The 1st rib has no transverse articulation and only a small round articular facet with the body of T1. A superior 1st rib subluxation is frequently associated with quadratus lumborum muscle weakness and/or levator costarum and scaleni muscle spasm. The actual displacement mechanism is usually initiated by pushing with the elbows locked.

Adjustment of Superior First Rib Head Subluxation. With the patient supine, the examiner stands on the ipsilateral side of the involved rib, facing caudally and with the lateral hand, makes an open-web contact near the involved rib's crest that is high on the lateral index finger, with the thumb anterior and the fingers posterior to the patient's chest. The point of contact is about 4–5 inches lateral to the T1 spinous. The stabilizing palm is cupped over the patient's contralateral ear, with the fingers supporting the occiput. To relax the ipsilateral neck muscles, the examiner raises the patient's neck several inches with the stabilizing fingers, allowing the occiput to extend into the palm. The patient's head is rotated 20–30° away from the subluxation, and a moderate thrust is directed inferior and slightly posteromedial toward T4.

Some clinicians prefer the following alternative approach: With the patient prone, the examiner stands on the ipsilateral side of the involved rib facing the patient's contralateral shoulder and with the lateral hand makes an open-web contact on the rib's crest that is high on the lateral index finger, as described above. The examiner's lateral elbow will be flexed and pointing superiolaterally while leaning over the patient. A palm contact is made with the stabilizing hand on the patient's lateral occiput above the ear on the opposite side of involvement, and this hand is used to slightly extend the patient's head and rotate it away from the involved rib. Slight lateral flexion is applied to relax the ipsilateral muscles and, with the contact hand, a thrust is directed inferior and medial toward T4.

Inferior 2nd–7th Rib Head Subluxation. Palpation will reveal an increased intercostal space above and a decreased space below the rib that has subluxated inferiorly to its vertebra. Inferoextension displacements are infrequent in comparison to superoflexion subluxations, they take much greater force to correct, and they are more common at the lower ribs. The local pain often radiates to the abdomen with splinting lateral flexion on the contralateral side.

Adjustment of Inferior 2nd–7th Rib Head Subluxation. With the patient prone, the examiner stands on the ipsilateral side of the involved rib, facing cephally, and, with the lateral hand, makes a thumb-ball contact just below the inferior border of the subluxated rib between the rib's tubercle and angle. The contact-hand fingers will overlap the scapula. With the medial stabilizing hand, the examiner makes a soft pisiform contact over the contact thumb. Traction is applied superiorly to tighten the overlying tissues and to bring the contact thumb directly on the inferior border of the involved rib. The patient is asked to take a deep breath and to exhale deeply. At the end of exhalation, a short, moderate, anterior-superior recoil thrust is made by quickly extending the elbows.

Superior 2nd–7th Rib Head Subluxation. Palpation reveals an increased intercostal space below and a decreased space above the rib that has subluxated superiorly to its vertebra.

Adjustment of Superior 2nd–7th Rib Head Subluxation. This is essentially the opposite of the subluxation of a rib described as inferior. With the patient prone, the examiner stands above the ipsilateral side of the involved rib, facing caudally, and with the lateral hand, makes a thumb contact slightly above the superior border of the involved rib at the rib's angle. With the medial stabilizing hand, pisiform contact is made over the contact thumb. Traction is applied inferiorly to tighten the overlying tissues and to bring the contact thumb directly onto the rib's superior edge. At the end of patient exhalation, a short, moderate, recoil thrust is directed anterior and inferior.

"Bucket Handle" Complications

Costovertebral and costotransverse subluxations, and less frequently costosternal subluxations, are frequently complicated by reflex spasms in the thoracic cage. Hypertonicity of the scalene group, levator costarum, cervical longissimus, cervical and thoracic iliocostalis, and/or serratus posterior superior tends to raise and displace the upper ribs superiorly. On the other hand, hypertonicity of the thoracic longissimus, lumbar iliocostalis, and/or serratus posterior inferior tends to depress and displace the lower ribs inferiorly. Such attending hypertonicities or weakness of the antagonists should be corrected prior to structural adjustment, or the structural adjustment will not hold.[73]

Thoracic Spine Sprains

Acute traumatic spondylitis may follow contusions or wrenching of the spinal column. As in sprains of other joints, the symptoms are pain, tenderness, and reflex muscular rigidity that limits function. Symptoms may appear immediately after injury or not become apparent for a few hours or days. Diagnosis is based upon the history, physical findings, and x-ray to exclude fracture and destructive lesions.

Management. During the acute hyperemic stage, structural alignment, cold, strapping or bracing, positive galvanism, and rest are usually indicated. After 72 hours, passive congestion may be managed by light massage, gentle passive manipulation, sinusoidal stimulation, and ultrasound, and a mild range of motion exercise can be initiated. During the stage of consolidation, local moderate heat, moderate active exercise, motorized alternating traction, moderate range of motion manipulation, and ultrasound are beneficial. In the stage of fibroblastic activity, deep heat, deep massage, vigorous active exercise, motorized alternating traction, negative galvanism, ultrasound, and active joint manipulation tend to speed recovery and inhibit postinjury effects.

Vertebral Facet Subluxation Syndromes

Dorsal vertebral subluxations and/or fixations are attended in the same manner as in general practice. With the well-developed muscular person, however, subluxation is more commonly associated with acute symptoms of paravertebral strain and sprain. In such cases, leverage adjustive techniques on the medial transverse processes are preferred to pisiform recoil corrections with a spinous process contact. Because of the heavy musculature, heat prior to correction is necessary, as a rule, to relieve spasm unless acute symptoms (eg, swelling) contraindicate this.

Selected Effects of Thoracic Area Hypertonicity

A part of a muscle, a whole muscle, or a group of muscles may become chronically hypertonic as the result of noxious reflexes of a traumatic, visceral, postural, or psychomotor origin. This state of small fasciculation or gross splinting may predispose, initiate, or complicate a subluxation syndrome.

Excessive hypertonicity of a muscle, confirmed by palpatory tone and soreness, will tend to subluxate its site of osseous attachment. Such a state often exists unilaterally or bilaterally, within the whole muscle or part of a multi-innervated muscle.[74] Below is a listing of common problem areas in the thorax.

1. *Upper trapezius.* Increased tone tends to pull the head down and back, the spinal processes laterally, and the shoulder girdle medially.
2. *Lower trapezius.* Increased tone tends to pull the T6–T12 spinous processes lateral and the shoulder girdle medial and inferior.
3. *Latissimus dorsi.* Increased tone tends to pull the lower half of the spine and the pelvis anterior, lateral, and superior, and to internally rotate the arm.
4. *Rhomboid major.* Increased tone tends to pull the T2–T4 spinous processes lateral and inferior and the inferior vertebral border up and toward the midline.
5. *Iliocostalis dorsi.* Increased tone tends to lift the rib cage. If unilateral and chronic, a functional scoliosis will develop. Increased tone, especially if bilateral, also tends to flatten the normal thoracic kyphosis.
6. *Multifidus.* Increased tone tends to place a rotary torque on the vertebral motion unit.
7. *The quadratus lumborum.* Although this is considered a flank muscle, it has a most significant effect on the lower thoracic spine. Rarely is there a lower thoracic scoliosis that does not have a quadratus component. Increased tone tends to pull the lower spine inferior and lateral and the ilium superior and medial.

Fractures and Dislocations

Sternal injuries, rib fractures, "slipped" ribs, and vertebral body fractures are the most common effects of severe thoracic trauma seen in general practice.

Sternal Injuries[75–77]

Any injury strong enough to fracture the sternum is likely to produce severe damage to underlying parts (Fig. 10.15). The examiner should always seek signs of approaching cardiac tamponade and arrhythmias that will demand priority. A flail sternum may require ventilatory assistance and intubation. Developing tension pneumothorax is always a possibility. Sternum fractures are rare except in automobile injuries when the steering wheel is forced against the sternum.

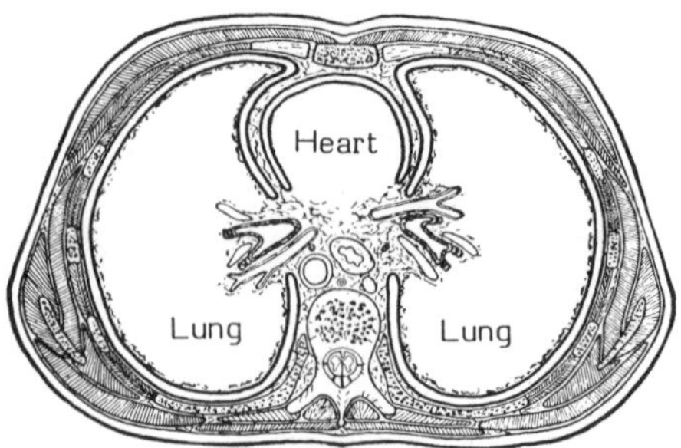

Figure 10.15. Diagram of a cross section of a normal thorax as viewed from above. Note that the heart and great vessels are located directly between the sternum and spine, and are thus readily subject to torsion forces of scoliosis.

Closed sternal fractures or those of the costal cartilages are most difficult to view on roentgenography except with elaborate techniques. The tenderness from a sternal bone bruise even without major damage lingers for an abnormally long time, frequently mimicking fracture.

Xiphisternal sprains are sometimes seen which are also persistently annoying and difficult to treat because of irritation from rectus activity. In rare instances, especially in somersaulting gymnastics, the manubrium may be ruptured from its attachments.

Rib Fractures[78–80]

Most rib fractures are extremely painful even if minor, because movements cause constant grating of highly innervated fracture endings. Both displaced fractures and fatigue cracks may be found. A compound fracture may communicate with the skin or the pleura and other thoracic contents. Cellular emphysema is a common complication but often disappears spontaneously.

The longest and most prominent ribs (5–9) are those most often fractured. The upper ribs are better protected; the lower ribs are more mobile and susceptible. The weakest site for compression injury is where the rib has its greatest change in curvature. This is just anterior to the costal angle.

Signs and Symptoms. Diagnosis must frequently be made without the classic signs of fracture. The history, pain, and point tenderness are the best clues. If present, pain is felt most sharply on inspiration or coughing. Localized tenderness is usually evident, the break can sometimes be felt with the fingers, and crepitus may be exhibited. However, crepitus is absent if the fracture is incomplete or if fragments override. Because ribs are highly mobile, preternatural mobility may have little value. Broken ribs cut like knives; if the lung is punctured, the patient may cough up bright red, frothy blood. Roentgenography may be obvious or nonconclusive. If a case presents no evidence on film, but pain, disability, and dyspnea persist for a few days and a localized periostitis is apparent, the disorder should be treated as a fracture even if evidence is lacking on film.

Roentgenographic Considerations. Rib fractures are usually obvious but may be missed with overlapping axial shadows. Fracture of a costal cartilage may be invisible unless partially calcified. Breaks run obliquely or irregularly where calcification has not yet occurred. In seeking signs of rib fracture, one should not overlook careful evaluation of the costospinal junctions (often associated with costovertebral subluxation) or the costosternal junction. Except for the very high or low ribs, costotransverse ligaments ruptured by a severe force may lead to superior subluxation of the ribs.

Golfer's Fractures. Some rib fractures are peculiar to certain sports. For example, novice golfers who complain of pain and discomfort in the upper back near the shoulder may present "golfer's fractures." This injury usually involves the posterior aspect of multiple middle ribs (4–7). Right-handed golfers exhibit left-sided fractures, and vice versa.[81]

Flail Chest. This traumatic distortion, often called a "staved-in" chest, is the result of several anterolateral segments being disrupted from the sternum so that they are freely movable because of fracture or dislocation. It is readily recognized by paradoxical breathing in which the chest wall sucks in with inspiration and pushes outward on expiration.[82, 83] It is a dangerous state that requires immediate respiratory assistance and surgical attention.

Management of Uncomplicated Rib Fractures

Uncomplicated rib fractures in which signs of displacement or hemothorax are absent can often be treated conservatively. Alert attention must be given to possible signs of a fat-embolism syndrome that can occur within three days after fracture, requiring immediate referral and hospitalization.

Because of respiratory and cardiac movements, fractured ribs are difficult and dangerous to immobilize. Strapping must be limited to one side and not cover the entire cage because encircling will restrict compensatory diaphragmatic and accessory muscle action. Shave the mature skin, cover the nipple with a gauze pad, and paint the area with benzoin. Each strap must be applied in an oblique fashion after forced exhalation (anchored high behind and low in front to follow the rib curve) for several inches above and below the fracture. The straps should be changed once a week for 3–4 weeks. Injuries to top ribs require a sling to rest and support the injured area. A rib belt with adjustable buckles and shoulder support has proved its merit. Sports activity can be resumed with padding in 3–4 weeks if there is no separation, but separated ends require termination of participation for the season as a safeguard against visceral puncture.

Rib Dislocations[84, 85]

The common "slipped rib" separation occurs at the junction of the osseous rib and its costal cartilage, and thus is easy to confuse upon palpation with a lateral rib fracture. The freed rib end springs open and invariably slips superiorly. It usually occurs at the 10th rib area in thin young women—often from a strong hug from a boyfriend or a lateral fall against blunt furniture.

Thoracic Vertebral Fractures[86–90]

Thoracic fractures most frequently occur at the T12 level, next in the midthoracic region. Most are compression fractures with collapse of a vertebral body.[91] Midthoracic fractures generally result from falls on the pelvis or when the head is severely forced between the knees.

Fractures of the thorax sometimes occur during convulsions or seizures. They usually occur in the T5–T7 region. The mechanism is strong abdominal contraction accompanied by paraspinal cervical and lumbar spasm. This places the midthoracic area under severe compression forces.

Bending moments and axial compressive forces produce compressive normal stresses that are cumulative at the anterior portion of the thoracic spine.[92] This fact helps to explain the high incidence of spinal fracture in the thoracic region.

Soto-Hall Test. This test is primarily employed when fracture of a vertebra is suspected. The patient is placed supine without pillows. One hand of the examiner is placed on the sternum of the patient, and a slight pressure is exerted to prevent flexion at either the lumbar or thoracic regions of the spine. The other hand of the examiner is placed under the patient's occiput, and the head is slowly flexed toward the chest. Flexion of the head and neck upon the chest progressively produces a pull on the posterior spinous ligaments from above, and when the spinous process of the injured vertebra is reached, an acute local pain is experienced by the patient.[93]

Roentgenographic Considerations. Fracture lines are rarely recognized within vertebral bodies unless the area is crushed. They are usually the result of considerable violence such as sudden extreme flexion, heavy crushing injury, or extreme muscular exertion. Abnormalities in outlines and relations with neighboring vertebrae are the usual findings, especially in the lateral view. There are two general types, compression fractures and comminuted fractures.

1. *Compression fractures* vary from a single slight irregularity in the anterior or lateral margins of the vertebral body similar to a long-bone torus fracture, to a complete collapse of a portion of the centrum. Milder forms are usually asymptomatic, but there may be persistent local tenderness. Chronic vertebral compression fractures such as in trampolining or horseback riding accidents are usually diagnosed without difficulty except in the active adolescent with endplate irregularities. Vertebral margin irregularities usually point to old trauma or infection.

2. *Comminuted fractures* are the result of greater trauma in which the vertebra is severely shattered either by direct violence or by another vertebra impacting it.

In comparison to vertebral body fractures, fractures of the neural arch including the articular processes are more disabling because of the neuroreceptor irritation increased by motion or distortion. Demonstration of a definite break is often difficult in the thoracic region, but callus formation offers indirect evidence. Unlike vertebral bodies, the posterior aspects readily form callus that becomes calcified in a few weeks. Severe acute traumatic subluxation may call attention to a subtle fracture.

Fractures of the transverse processes are usually multiple among adjacent vertebrae, but single processes may be broken by a blow from a sharp object. A slight callus can be expected, and fibrous union sometimes develops. The black lines formed by muscle shadows crossing transverse processes should not be confused with fracture. Muscle lines are smooth and straight, and extend beyond the bony margins.

Traumatic lesions are sometimes difficult to distinguish from infectious lesions. Traumatic lesions usually show a substantial portion of the intervening disc still present, while the disc commonly disappears or thins greatly in infection. The infectious process is frequently accompanied by or is an extension of a paravertebral abscess.

The Thoracolumbar Area. Computed tomography will often demonstrate fractures of the posterior elements that are not evident using conventional radiographic procedures.[94] Thoracolumbar fractures suffered as the result of vertical plunges (eg, jumping from a height) can generally be placed into two general categories: (1) compression or wedge fractures of the vertebral body not associated with permanent neurologic deficit, or (2) burst fractures with sagittal cleavage, usually associated with neurologic impairment.[95] Crush fractures at the thoracolumbar junction should be regarded as unstable with a risk of progressive flexion deformity, neurologic deterioration, and pain.[96]

Biomechanical Considerations. As hyperextension is strongly resisted in the thoracic region, which is normally in a state of structural flexion in the neutral position, fracture of the posterior element is rare. The biomechanical explanation is again offered by Gozna and Harrington:[97] "The distance between the flexion axis and the tip of the spinous process is three to four times greater than the distance between the axis and the anterior margin of the vertebral body. Therefore, when exposed to flexion stress, the anterior portion of the vertebral body experiences a compression load that is three or four times greater than the tensile load falling upon the spinous processes and supraspinous ligaments." Because of this, these researchers feel that hyperflexion forces will always produce an anterior wedge-shaped fracture of the vertebral body but never an avulsion or ligament rupture at the posterior element.

Fortunately, neurologic damage and severe disability are rare. Adequate management in uncomplicated cases can usually be provided by bed rest followed by extension exercises to stretch and strengthen the affected muscles. A light brace or corset should be worn by the patient when ambulated.

Common Mechanisms of Injury. Knowing the mechanism of injury focuses attention on the tissues most likely to be injured.

1. Anterior compression injuries commonly occur during flexion, because this position affords maximum protection to the face and vital organs. The normal thoracic kyphosis places the spine in flexion during the neutral position, thus even axial forces produce greater forces anteriorly than posteriorly. The most severe bending moment is at the apex of the kyphosis. When the thorax is flexed, compression forces distributed anteriorly are four times stronger than those distributed to the posterior elements. The nucleus serves as a fulcrum when forces are not centered.

2. The vertebral arch and posterior ligament complex are usually injured in severe hyperflexion that stretches the posterior elements or in vertical loading. This commonly occurs secondary to anterior injury. A degree of torsion is usually also involved. Roaf showed that it is almost impossible to tear the posterior ligament complex in pure flexion or the anterior longitudinal ligament in pure extension but quite easy to do either if torsion or horizontal shear are added.[98] The most severe forces occur at the thoracolumbar transition.

3. When a traumatic posterior lumbosacral shearing force is applied, a fracture dislocation of the thoracolumbar spine can occur in which the lower vertebra is displaced anteriorly under the upper vertebra by forward slipping of the posterior articular processes.[99]

4. Isolated fractures are sometimes seen in the posterior elements. Fractures of the upper thoracic spinous processes are usually the result of shoveling, severe cervical hyperextension, or a direct blow. They most frequently occur at the thoracocervical area. Fractures of the lower transverse processes are frequently associated with a direct blow from the posterior or to the flank in which a violent contraction of the quadratus lumborum occurs. An isolated fracture of an articular process is usually the result of severe lateral flexion with rotation about the long axis of the spine so that leverage is exerted against the jammed processes. Isolated fractures of the vertebral arch are extremely rare.

GROSS EVALUATION OF THE THORACIC REGION

Pain, both local and referred, and paravertebral thoracic spasm are common manifestations of local and/or visceral disorder. The possibility of myelopathy, nerve root irritation, and bone disease must always be weighed against the common complaints of a postural origin. Arthrosis, spondylosis, osteochondrosis, gout, and osteoporosis are common pathologies affecting the thoracic spine that may produce or contribute to biomechanical faults and spinal distortions affecting spinal design and equilibrium. Only a thorough physical, orthopedic, neurologic, and roentgenographic examination will help to differentiate the many possible syndromes that have their origin in the thoracic spine.

Background

Grieve points out that it is a rare thoracic spine that does not exhibit some areas of tenderness upon careful palpation.[100] There are probably more trigger points and reflex fasciculations located upon the thoracic walls than any other area of the body. Because trigger-point development has been shown to interfere with homeostasis, Hitchcock points out that a patient's condition can usually be improved by modifying or deleting an excessive reaction in the musculoskeletal system, especially when such a reaction is related to the same levels of the CNS that innervate the area of pathophysiologic disturbance.[101]

Probably much more than any other region, the thoracic region can be considered a most critical zone, even though the predominance of current literature emphasizes the importance of its neighboring regions. It can be said that the thoracic spine suffers the "middle child syndrome" from an orthopedic viewpoint. It is just as important as its structural brother and sister, yet fails to receive the same attention.

May we remember that chiropractic pioneers took their greatest steps forward when "Meric analysis" was in vogue—long before our preoccupation was placed upon the atlas and sacrum. These were the days when the profession was accused of being undereducated and overmotivated. But these were the days when "miracles" were taken for granted.

Postural Evaluation

A comprehensive postural evaluation should include a comparative analysis of the physical signs found in the standing, sitting, Adams, prone, and supine positions, both with and without use of a plumb line or grid (Figs. 10.16 and 10.17). An overview of this evaluation will be discussed in the next chapter.

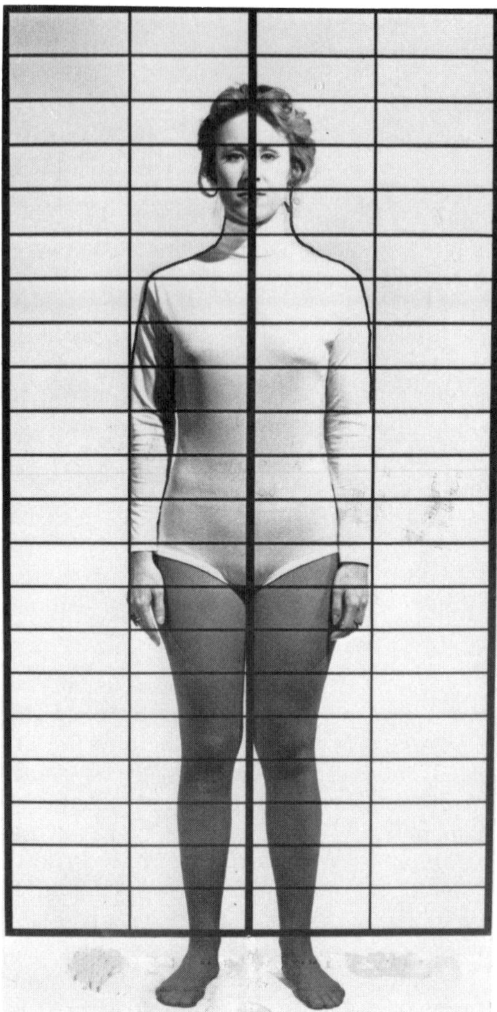

Figure 10.16. A postural grid. (With the permission of Reedco Research, Auburn, N.Y.)

To maintain an erect posture with whatever postural abnormality may be present, the righting reflexes (if intact) attempt to distribute the weight of the body over the area occupied by the feet. To some extent, this accommodation process is limited by the gravitational forces involved, which in turn direct the postural variations that are possible. The components that are distinguishable in the majority of postural defects when viewing the body from the lateral plane are (1) an increase or decrease in the angle of the sacral base, (2) the presence or absence of a fixed thoracolumbar tendency toward kyphosis, (3) the presence or absence of a midthoracic hyperkyphosis, (4) the presence or absence of a flattening of the thoracic spine (Pottenger's saucering), and/or (5) an increase or decrease in the A-P cervical curve.[102] Some of these distortions will be readily apparent on visual analysis, especially when a grid or plumbline is used. However, the determination of the cause(s) of the distortion must be based on detailed physical and roentgenographic analyses.

Goniometry of the Thoracolumbar Spine

Thoracic and lumbar motion are measured as a whole, and the following proce-

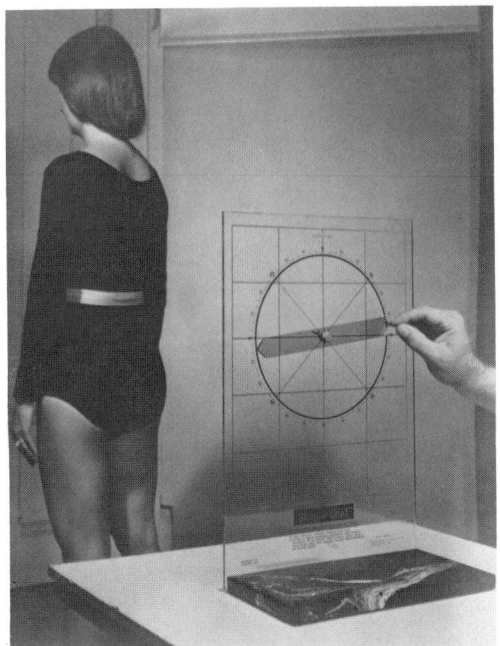

Figure 10.17. The Skan-a-Graf postural permagrid. (With the permission of Reedco Research, Auburn, N.Y.)

dures are used for measuring restricted motion.[103] In ankylosis, the goniometer is placed as if measuring the neutral position and the deviation from the neutral position is recorded. The number and position of ankylosed vertebrae are determined by roentgenography.

Thoracolumbar Flexion-Extension

The standing patient is placed in the neutral position. The goniometer is centered by the examiner along the patient's midaxillary line at the lowest rib level and the neutral reading is recorded by the examiner. The patient flexes as far forward as possible, while the examiner keeps the goniometer base in line with the patient's femur. The end of motion is recorded by the examiner. When the examiner measures extension, the patient should start from the neutral and bend as far backward as possible. The end of motion is recorded by the examiner.

Thoracolumbar Lateral Flexion

The patient is placed in the neutral position with the goniometer so centered that its base is over the posterior iliac spines and its arm is extended along the midline of the spine. The neutral reading is recorded. The patient bends as far as possible to the left and to the right, and readings at the end of each motion are recorded by the examiner.

Thoracolumbar Rotation

The patient is placed in the neutral position, and the examiner steadies the patient's hips. The goniometer is not used. The patient twists to the right and to the left. Each motion is recorded separately as the examiner estimates the arc described by the frontal plane of the patient's body as it turns.

STRUCTURAL FIXATIONS AND MOTION PALPATION[104–107]

The entire thoracic region is prone to a number of types of muscular, ligamentous, and costovertebral fixations. In addition, Gillet believes that primary thoracic fixations tend to produce secondary areas of fixation in the cervical spine.

The lower thoracic region (T9–T12) is probably more prone to fixation development than any other area of the spine (Figs. 10.18 and 10.19). This is probably due to the abrupt change in facet planes between the superior and inferior processes of the transitional vertebra, the altered stiffness between thoracic and lumbar vertebrae, the lack of strong supporting muscles enjoyed by the lumbar region, the lack of firm anterior support of the floating ribs, and the large compressive forces concentrated at this area. A sudden change in the stiffness properties of a structure at a given point will subject the structure to stress concentration at that point. This can lead to eventual mechanical failure.

Etiologic Factors

Muscle Hypertonicity[108]

Most fixations seen in the thoracic area are muscular in type. This is fortunate because difficult to manage fibrous ankylosis can readily develop in the thoracic spine. While fibrous ankylosis does not contraindicate manipulation, the tissues adapt slowly and correction takes frequent care utilizing a wide scope of therapy over many months, if not year, to obtain an appreciable

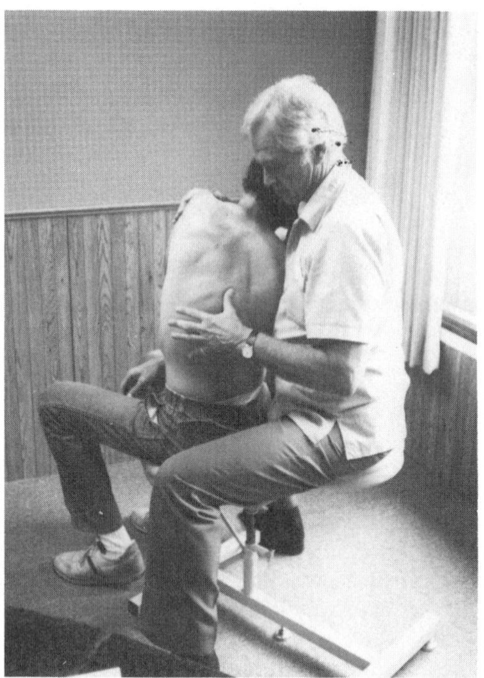

Figure 10.18. Dynamic palpation during lateral flexion to the right of a left lower thoracic costotransverse joint (courtesy of Dynamic Palpation Institute).

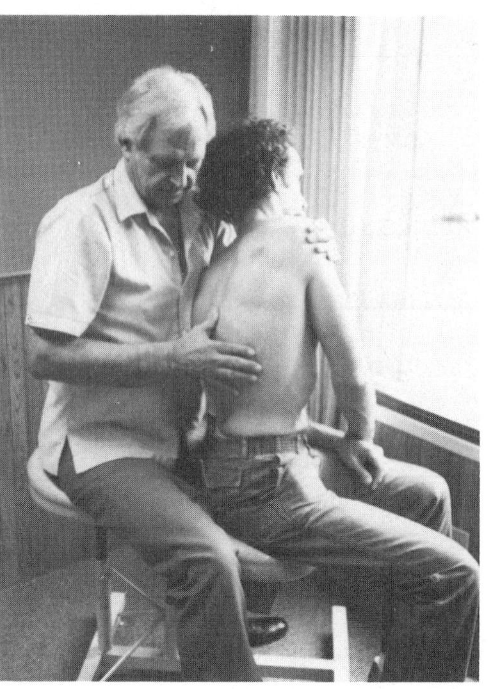

Figure 10.19. Dynamic palpation during body rotation to the left of a lower thoracic vertebra (courtesy of Dynamic Palpation Institute).

change because of the poor vascularity of the tissues involved.

The Interspinous and Intertransverse Muscles. Bilateral interspinous and/or intertransverse muscle hypertonicity produces extension fixation. In unilateral intertransverse hypertonicity, the transverse processes approximate, the disc thins ipsilaterally and the height of the intervertebral foramen is reduced. The superior articulation is pulled into a stressed position away from the inferior process (facet syndrome).[109] The articular space exhibits an abnormal "V"-shaped appearance. The IVD space increases at the anterior and decreases at the posterior. The acute stage is due to muscular spasm, but in prolonged conditions, the ipsilateral muscles become fibrotic and the paravertebral ligaments shorten. Stretching occurs on the contralateral side.

The Rotatores. A unilateral hypertonic rotatores, which courses in the groove between the spinous and transverse processes, will pull the corresponding spinous process into rotation and the transverse process below into counterrotation, similar in effect to that of intertransverse hypertonicity.[110] This unilateral state, usually acute, commonly extends over several thoracic segments.

Bilateral rotatores hypertonicity, often a generalized reflex condition in the thoracic spine, tends to initiate the interspinous syndrome. Rotation is restricted and lateral bending is inhibited to slightly less a degree. The condition is more readily palpable in the upper dorsal area and usually accompanied by bulging levator costarum muscles. Gillet feels that this disorder is frequently secondary to a primary fixation in one or both feet.

The Rhomboids. The rhomboideus major arises from the spinous processes of T2–T5 and inserts at the vertebral margin of the scapula. The rhomboideus minor connects the spinous processes of C7–T1 and the lower part of the nuchal ligament to the vertebral margin of the scapula at the root of the scapular spine. As their function is to retract and fix the scapula, hypertonicity of these muscles produces this normal function in a fixed state. In unilateral involvement, the scapula is pulled medially and upward so that the ipsilateral shoulder is higher than the other.[111] This state, often secondary, is infrequently symptomatic even though a postural distortion may be quite evident.

Pectoralis Flexibility Test. The patient lies supine with the hands clasped behind the head, and the elbows are allowed to slowly lower laterally toward the table. If the elbows do not approximate the tabletop, shortening (eg, spasm, inflexibility, contracture) of the pectoralis group is indicated.

Ligament Shortening

The Anterior Longitudinal Ligament. Shortening of the anterior longitudinal ligament is a common site of fixation in the thoracic spine, but it is rare in the lumbar region. It is manifested by an increased kyphosis and a decreased anterior disc space on a lateral roentgenograph and may be confused with anulus degeneration which may or may not be present. The normal IVF space will appear elongated. Gillet feels that this traction appears to have considerable effect on the sympathetic nerves (visceral symptoms), to be a source of noxious reflex activity, but to have little or no effect on the somatic nerves.[112]

The Posterior Longitudinal Ligament. For some unexplained reason, shortening of this ligament is rarely seen. This could possibly be explained by the greater flexion exercise required in normal activity, keeping in mind that P-A thoracic motion is minimal at best. While this may explain the thoracic state, one would think that these ligaments would be shortened in chronic cervical or lumbar lordosis, but this is rarely demonstrated.

When it occurs, ossification of the posterior longitudinal ligament in the cervical region is often associated with signs of radiculomyelopathy. However, when this ligament ossifies in the thoracic spine, it is typically, but not always, asymptomatic.[113–115] For an unknown reason, the disorder occurs predominantly in females when the thoracic region is involved and almost always in Japanese males when the cervical region is affected.

Fixations

Sternal Fixations

Articular fixations at the costosternal articulations can produce hypermobility in the related thoracic vertebrae. This is usually manifested as an increased spread of the spinous processes on full flexion. However, if a costosternal area is in a state of fixation and the corresponding anterior longitudinal ligament is in a state of shortening, the local area will be forced into an exaggerated state of kyphosis even in the erect position.

Anterior Rib Pit Fixations. Anterior rib fixations resulting in decreased chest excursion can be determined by motion palpation of the thoracic cage during deep inspiration with the patient either standing or supine. First, the examiner should traction the skin of the patient's lateral thorax toward the midline with broad bilateral palmar contacts. The examiner's thumbs are placed near the patient's sternum on the rib being examined. As the patient inhales deeply, the examiner should note whether both of his or her thumbs move equally. Thumb motion restricted unilaterally suggests the side of fixation.[116]

The Manubrium-Sternum Joint. The hinge joint between the manubrium and the body of the sternum is normally active in forced breathing and extreme A-P movements. Fixation at this joint will restrict these motions. Such fixations are frequently mobilized spontaneously during an upper thoracic adjustment directed anterosuperiorly of a prone patient.[117]

Intercostal Fixations

If the intercostal muscles are in a state of hypertonicity, the ribs will abnormally appose and the thoracic cage will exhibit an area of lateral flattening that restricts mobility on contralateral bending. The patient will assume a somewhat "hunched" posture in the neutral position, depending upon the extent of fixation.

Intercostal fixations are best determined laterally near the rib angles. Palpation should reveal opening posteriorly during flexion, anteriorly during extension, on the convex side during lateral bending, and on the side opposite to the direction of vertebral body rotation.

Costovertebral Fixations

The articulation between the rib head and vertebral body or between the rib tubercle and the transverse is a common site of fixation, commonly due to serratus and/or levator costarum hypertonicity. Gillet believes this type of fixation is contributed to by capsular shortening that allows enough torsion for unrestricted breathing during nondemanding activities. Associated adhesion-type bands could very easily irritate an entrapped sympathetic ganglia during normal motion. Costovertebral fixations are rarely complete. They usually tend to restrict mobility in one or more directions but not in all directions.

Posterior Rib Head Fixations. Posterior rib fixations resulting in decreased chest excursion can be determined by motion palpation of the thoracic cage during deep inspiration with the patient either standing or prone. First, the examiner should traction the skin of the patient's lateral thorax toward the spine with broad bilateral palmar contacts. The examiner's thumbs are placed near the patient's dorsal midline on the rib being examined. As the patient inhales deeply, the examiner should note whether both of his or her thumbs move equally. If the rib rises and the interspace opens, it is considered normal; if it remains down or down to some extent in relation to the opposite side, it is considered "locked." Thumb motion restricted unilaterally suggests the side of fixation.[118]

Once identified, a general rib mobilization technique with and without traction on the ipsilateral iliac crest or shoulder can then be applied on the angles of the ribs involved to loosen restrictions. This is usually best followed by a regimen of heat and graduated stretching exercises.

Dynamic Palpation of the Thoracic Spine and Ribs[70,71,104,106,119,120]

Motion palpation in the thoracic spine must of necessity encompass the apophyseal joints, the costovertebral joints, and the sternocostal joints. Areas of total fixation are found most commonly at the upper and middle thoracic segments and invariably involve the posterior facets before the costal joints. Joint play is extremely difficult to appraise.

Lateral Flexion

The thoracic spine is usually first palpated during gross lateral flexion of the head and neck. It can be demonstrated that lateral flexion of the head of only 30° will yield palpable motion in the lumbar spine. With the patient seated, palpation for vertebral motion is accomplished with the thumbtips over the inferolateral aspect of the spinous process of the segment being examined and the fingers extending over the paravertebral musculature. The inside of the thumb may be placed over the corresponding zygopophysis for further kinesthetic awareness. Some examiners prefer to use one hand for the contact with the index finger placed on the tip of the spinous process and the thumb and middle finger placed over the transverse processes of the vertebra below the segment being examined. Thus, comparative movement of the superior segment upon its base may be appraised. The other arm of the examiner may be placed anteriorly around the patient's shoulders to guide him through the various spinal movements.[121]

During lateral bending, the movements felt will be (1) vertebral lateral gliding, (2) vertebral lateral tipping, and (3) rib tipping as the vertebra carries the rib with it. You will find that rotational coupling during lateral flexion is much stronger in children than adults. This is normal because of the more supple spine in youth.

Gillet feels that a lateral fixation at C7–T2 is a secondary manifestation that is commonly linked to shortening of the pelvic sacrotuberous ligament. He reports that stretching the ligament in the knee-chest position immediately corrects this secondary fixation. This effect, however, has not been widely confirmed.

Flexion-Extension

The patient is then asked to slowly and completely flex and extend his spine while the examiner evaluates the corresponding segmental kyphotic and lordotic motions. Failure of or incomplete symmetrical motion, ankylosis, fixation, or excessive motion (hyperkinesia) is easily noted, the latter being particularly evident because of the usually associated palpable instability of the supraspinal ligament.[122]

When the thoracic spine is normally extended from a flexion position, there is first an inferior gliding of the inferior facets upon the superior facets below, and the interspinous spaces close. This can be determined by placing a palpating finger or thumb within the interspinous space being examined. During forward flexion, the spinous process will open unless there is an interspinous fixation.

According to Gillet, the first partial fixation to occur is usually that which resists forced extension. The involved segment will be kyphotic. When hyperextension is forced, the spinous process will normally be felt to move slightly anterior as the inferior facets of the vertebra above pivot (open anteriorly) on the superior facets of the vertebra below. This anterior shift is a normal action that can be restricted by shortening at the anterior motion unit (eg, anterior longitudinal ligament).

Asymmetrical movement that is due to underlying subluxation may also be evaluated: (1) Extension subluxations show a lesser degree of kypthotic movement on flexion and much greater degree of hyperextension motion. (2) In the case of flexion subluxations, the motion is opposite; ie, flexion of the segment shows a greater tendency for segmental kyphotic movement and hyperextension of the spine causes less segmental lordosis.

Rotation

Next, the patient is asked to rotate to the right and left. A rotary subluxation, by being further accentuated, may be confirmed by palpating just lateral to the spinous process. Assisted lateral flexion to the right or left helps to confirm the analysis of a fixated form of subluxation. Further confirmation of ankylosis, fixation, or segmental hyperkinesia may also be made during these range of motion studies.

Normal vertebral rotation can be greatly impaired by a rib fixation because the ribs must move with the rotating transverse processes. Similarly, hypertonicity of the rotatores, multifidi, and levator costorum will restrict rotation. These conditions are often found in the upper thoracic area. The intertransverse muscles may be a cause of fixation extending from the middle to the lower thoracic area and can be best determined by intertransverse palpation during lateral flexion.

Screening Tests for Ankylosis

Chest Expansion Test

With the patient standing, chest measurements are taken around the circumference of the thorax near the nipple level: first after the patient inhales and then after the patient exhales completely. A 2-inch difference (possibly less in females) is a negative sign. A positive sign is indicated by no or very little difference in measurements and encourages suspicions of osteoarthritic ankylosis or ankylosing spondylitis.[123–127] Roentgenography should offer confirmatory evidence.

Forestier's Test

The patient in the upright position is asked to bend laterally, first to one side and then to the other. Normally, the contralateral paravertebral muscles will bulge because of the normal coupling rotation of the lumbar spine (exhibited by the spinous processes pointing to the ipsilateral side of lateral flexion). However, in ankylosing spondylitis (Marie-Strumpell's disease) or a state of extensive spinal fixation, the musculature will appear to bulge more prominently on the side of the curve's concavity (Forestier's bowstring sign).[124]

Lewin's Supine Test

This test is identical to Chapman's test, except that Lewin believes that a positive sign is indicative of an ankylosing dorsolumbar lesion. The patient is placed supine, and the examiner fixes the patient's extended knees firmly against the table top. The patient is then instructed to attempt to sit up without utilizing the hands; inability to do so is said to constitute a positive sign.[128–130]

BASIC THERAPEUTIC CONSIDERATIONS

Almost any therapy that is applicable elsewhere in the body can be used to treat neuromusculoskeletal disorders of the thoracic region, with the obvious exception that electric currents should not penetrate the heart. Thoracic traction is described in Chapter 13.

Commonly Used Modalities

Cryotherapy, heat, high-voltage currents, hydrotherapy, interferential currents, low-voltage currents, massage, mechanical vibration/percussion, meridian therapy, traction, etc, can be used effectively in treating many neuromusculoskeletal disorders of the thoracic region. The reader should refer to a general text on physiologic therapeutics in chiropractic practice for specific indications and contraindications.[131–134]

Manual Methods

Tissue Goading and Pressure[135–137]

Deep tissue goading has been applied in the profession for many decades as a means to arouse driving impulses, break up areas of stasis, and stretch contractures and adhesions.

An area of localized stasis producing muscle fasciculation, approximately the size and shape of a small pea or coin, is often the site of noxious reflexes and referred pain. Quite frequently, such areas are found in the deep tissues of the iliac crest and associated with sciatic-like referred pain that persists in spite of vertebral and disc correction. Such foci may by found almost anywhere in the musculoskeletal system.

A thumbtip, pad of a finger, or small, blunt instrument is used to deeply massage, up to patient tolerance, a localized tender spot within subcutaneous tissues. During goading, with strokes about 1 inch in length, the skin should not be moved. The therapy is quite uncomfortable but often brings dramatic relief in a few hours when more conservative measures have failed.

Hanes feels that many disorders are the result of a post-traumatic neuritis, produced intrinsically or extrinsically, and has isolated several specific points of major irritation. The sites are palpated as excessively tender local spasms. He recommends a firm, constant pressure with no thumb motion which is easily bearable for the patient. The typical pressure duration is 10–30 seconds.[138]

Neurotherapy and Spondylotherapy[139]

Neurotherapy refers to the inhibition of overly active nerve function or the activation of sluggish function. Spondylotherapy is the treatment by physical methods applied to the spinal region. A nerve fiber may be stimulated artifically (eg, mechanically, thermally, chemically, electrically) anywhere along its course.

Certain nerve fibers function specifically for certain sensory and motor acts and may be stimulated at either their central or receptor ends; ie, efferent nerves are stimulated centrally and afferent nerves peripherally. The ability of sensory nerve stimulation to produce a motor or granular response is readily demonstrated in eliciting any tendon reflex in which superficial percussion produces the characteristic jerk, in the muscle spasm reflex resulting from skin exposure to a cool wind or proprioceptive excitement from strain or sprain, or in the salivary response from seeing a person eat a lemon.

Neuroinhibition. Abnormal reflexes appear to be inhibited more by pressure, polar traction, and cold than by any other method. For example, a painfully splinting erector-muscle spasm can be relaxed by placing the muscle in a position of functional rest and then applying mild continuous stretching or pressure. Cold is an excellent neuroinhibitor, especially with nerves that are located superficially. Functional inhibition can be gained by stimulating a nerve whose chief function is inhibitory (eg, a parasympathetic).

Pressure may be applied digitally or with a pressor instrument at or near the paravertebral spaces. Steady pressure on the surface of the body, usually applied digitally, over the course of a nerve tends to be a restraining influence. There also appears to be specific reflex influences upon vessels, lymphatics, and glandular secretions. Certain skin areas (eg, suboccipital, paraspinal, parasacral, perianal, peripheral-meridian) are highly responsive to specific pressure from which reflexes of vasodilation, muscle relaxation, and pain-impulse blocking can be initiated.

Neurostimulation. Deep and rapid short-duration percussion, applied either by hand or by a percussion-type vibrator, upon spinous processes at a rate of 1–2 impulses per second for about 20 seconds with 30-second rest intervals can be used to stimulate a spinal center. Prolonged stimulation such as periods of 3 minutes or longer fatigue excitability and produce an inhibitory effect. When a medium-strength electric current passes through a position of nerve, an impulse is created at the instant the current is initiated and broken, as evidenced by muscle contraction. Experience has shown that sinusoidal current is an excellent method to contract involuntary muscle without irritation, but pulsating ultrasound is also effective in stimulating spinal centers. Therapeutic heat in almost any form increases nerve conductivity.

Acupuncture has proved itself to be an acceptable procedure for balancing visceral and somatic systems. However, the system is far too complicated to be even briefly mentioned here.

Effects of Spinal Center Stimulation[140–142]

Certain spinal segments have been mapped out empirically to produce the highest degree of physiologic response. These appear to include:

C1–C2: to initiate vagal responses of increased gastric secretion and peristalsis; to increase nasal, buccal, and pulmonary mucosal secretions.

C3: to initiate phrenic influence to increase depth of diaphragmatic excursions. Note that C3 inhibition is helpful in chronic cough, hiccups.

C4–C5: to initiate lung reflex contraction (eg, used in expiratory dyspnea, emphysema) and pulmonary vascular vasoconstriction.

C6–C7: the reflex center for increasing generalized vasoconstriction and myocardial tone.

T1–T3: to initiate lung reflex dilation (eg, inspiratory dyspnea), relax the stomach body, and contract the pylorus; to inhibit heart action (ie, antitachycardia reflex) and gastric hypermotility.

T4: to initiate cardiac and aortic dilation and inhibit viscerospasms.

T5: to initiate pyloric and duodenal dilation when applied to the right side.

T6: to initiate gallbladder contraction when applied to the right side.

T7: to initiate slight visceromotor renal dilation when applied bilaterally and stimulate hepatic function.

T8–T9: to initiate gall duct dilation.

T10–T11: to initiate slight visceromotor renal contraction, enhance pancreatic secretion, relax intestines and colon, and stimulate adrenals when applied bilaterally; to initiate splenic contraction (and circulatory red blood cells) when applied on the left.

T12: to initiate prostate contraction and tone of cecum and bladder sphincter.

L1–L3: to initiate uterine body; round ligament, and bladder contraction; pelvic vasoconstriction; vesicular sphincter relaxation.

L4–L5: to initiate sigmoidal and rectal contraction; increase tone of lower bowel.

Vagal Tone[143]

Johnson states that the tone of the parasympathetics may be increased through several methods such as (1) applying sinusoidal stimulation to the area C7, (2) moderate percussion of the C7 spinous process, (3) extending the neck to raise the hyoid, (4) mild percussion of the upper cervical area, (5) pressure in an intercostal space, and (6) rectal dilation.[144]

It has been Johnson's experience when sinusoidal current is used that stimulation should not exceed 30 seconds, with current alternated 5 seconds on and 5 seconds off, at 6–8 cycles, otherwise the reflex becomes exhausted. Others have found that vagal inhibitory action can also be aroused through such methods as (1) pinching the sternocleidomastoideus between the thumb and the forefinger and working deeply under the muscle's medial margin, (2) bilateral submastoid pressure, (3) concussion over the T2–T4 spinous processes, and (4) paravertebral pressure near T4.

Postural Realignment

In postural alignment of the thoracic spine and shoulder girdle, the primary muscles requiring strengthening are (1) the quadratus lumborum on the side of concavity, (2) the upper and lower trapezius and the major and minor rhomboids to improve scapular adduction and rotation, and (3) the infraspinatus and teres minor to improve lateral rotation of the shoulder.

It is also unusual in thoracic distortions for certain muscles not to need stretching such as (1) the quadratus lumborum on the side of lower thoracic convexity, (2) the latissimus dorsi, teres major, and subscapularis to improve shoulder adduction and medial rotation, and (3) the pectoral group to improve shoulder adduction and medial rotation. Invariably, stretching of the intercostals on the side of thoracic concavity is necessary.[145]

McGall and associates have shown that long-term immobilization in plaster casts for scoliosis, including the duration of the adolescent growth spurts, leads to an increase in height of the vertebral bodies and a decrease of their height-to-width ratio.[146] These changes appear to be at the expense of the disc, which is *reduced* in thickness. It is thought that this stimulating effect on vertebral body is due to the alteration of mechanical forces.

PATHOLOGY

The disease processes that are commonly involved with thoracic biomechanical defects are chronic pulmonary disorders, disc protrusions and diseases, infections, epiphyseal disorders, tumors, and adverse metabolic manifestations. Thoracic chordomata presenting as posterior-superior mediastinal tumors occur infrequently, but they may be highly malignant lesions.[147]

Pulmonary Impairment

Maximum breathing capacity is considered to be reduced in proportion to the degree of thoracic scoliosis present. According to Gucker's studies, gross rotary deformity appears to affect cardiopulmonary function to a greater extent than gross lateral deformity.[148] Pulmonary impairment is not usually a priority concern unless the deformed rigid thoracic cage reaches a point that restricts the pulmonary volume and vital capacity adequate for the demand. This is not to say that restriction far below this threshold will not predispose the patient to numerous cardiorespiratory disorders even though there are no signs of obstructive pulmonary disease. As the spinal deformity increases, the heart is pushed inferior and traction is placed on its superior nerves and vessels.

Arterial restriction in the lung fields leads to right ventricular hypertrophy. While the effects may be perceived by cardiac auscultation, its cause is almost impossible to detect on roentgenography. Cardiorespiratory failure is so slow in these cases that the distortion and its neuromuscular and neurovascular causes are rarely given the credit they deserve.

The reduced vital capacity in spinal deformity may not be due solely to mechanical restriction inasmuch as weakened thoracic and possibly abdominal muscles, costal fixations, thoracic venous and lymph flow restrictions, and portal pooling are invariably involved in scoliosis. Most of these nonmechanical influences can be attributed to subtle secondary sympathicotonia.

Thoracic Disc Herniation[149–151]

Not infrequent thoracic cord signs are probably due to the fact that there is less vertebral canal space here for the spinal cord than in the other regions of the supine. Thus, a slight posterior disc protrusion may manifest cord and cerebrospinal flow symptoms and referred neurovascular signs and symptoms in the thoracic region that would never manifest in the cervical or lumbar spine. Added to this fact is the relatively poor vascularity of the thoracic cord compared to the cervical cord or even the cauda equina. Although the thoracic cord is relatively small, its free space is extremely limited.

Fortunately, overt disc herniation is less common in the thorax than in any other spinal region. Only about 1 in every 1000 disc operations involves a thoracic disc. The costovertebral joints serve to inhibit the development of a posterolateral disc protursion in the same manner as the covertebral joints in the cervical region.

When disc protrusion does occur, it occurs predominantly in males over 50 years of age and most likely in the transitional T11–L1 area. Almost all cases involve forward flexion injuries with locked extensors in which the nucleus is forced forward. Thus, cord or nerve-root compression is rare except in "bursting" fractures. Bowel and bladder incontinence and impotence are rarely associated. If disc protrusion interferes with spinal fluid flow, symptoms may mimic multiple sclerosis, arteriosclerotic myelopathy, etc.

In less severe cases, the clinical picture is one of relative pain, usually unilateral in chronic cases or bilateral in acute cases, with girdle-like distribution (Fig. 10.20). Spastic paraparesis with sensory complaints may be involved. Motion restriction and tenderness on percussion may be the only local physical signs. Hyperactive tendon reflexes in the lower extremity and a positive Babinski reflex are sometimes seen. Differentiation must be made from intercostal neuralgia, ankylosing spondylitis, metastatic or intramedullary spinal cord tumors, neurofibroma, disc space infection, or viscerosomatic reflexes.

The position of the protrusion determines the clinical picture. A midline protrusion usually produces intermittent pain, sensory impairment, pyramidal signs, and possibly bowel and bladder symptoms. Protrusion laterally causes more pain, is radicular in distribution, and is associated with fewer cord signs.[152]

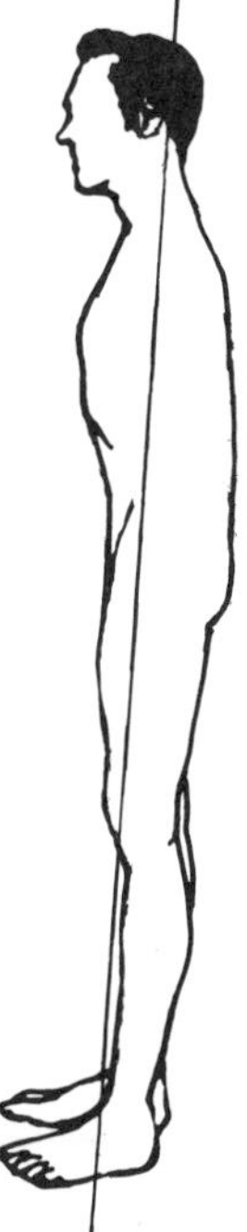

Figure 10.20. A typical lateral view of a patient with a posterior disc protrusion in the lower thoracic area. The upper body is flexed forward to the midline and the lower pelvis is posterior to the midline to place more weight on the anterior aspect of the motion unit. The erectors, and often the abdominals, are splinted to minimize motion. The involved superior vertebra is invariably locked in a position of extension.

The Upper Thoracic Spine

The pain radiates anteriorly along the affected intercostal nerve. If the T1 root is involved, pain usually radiates down the medial aspect of the arm to the little finger. Sensory loss may be found on the medial side of the forearm, hand, little finger, and half of the ring finger. Weakness is typically exhibited in the intrinsic muscles of the hand. If the T2 root is involved, pain will be referred to the axilla and the medial aspect of the arm.

The Midthoracic Spine

Pain and sensory impairment are typically intercostal (dermatomal) in nature.

The Lower Thoracic Spine

The pain is referred anteriorly to the abdomen, pelvic organs, or groin, depending on the level of involvement. Segmental sensory impairment will help to isolate the lesion.

Thoracic Disc Disease

The common concerns are calcification, adjacent exostoses, infection, arthritis, spondylitis, and associated paravertebral fibrositis. Calcification, usually the consistency of toothpaste, can occur either peripherally or at the endplates. Infection results from a contaminated inoculation, from venous extension of pelvic or genital disease, or an aseptic irritation (eg, avulsion). Arthritis is predisposed by subluxation, trauma, disc degeneration, occupational stress, and congenital or acquired structural deformities. Rare is the middle-aged spine that does not show some signs of osteoarthritis.[153]

It should also be noted that vertebral lipping can be a sign of covert visceral pathology. A high incidence of osteophytic lipping in the thoracic region has been described in patients with gastrointestinal disorders, diabetes mellitus, and coronary heart disease.[154] Bergfeldt and associates have shown a strong correlation between asymptomatic ankylosing spondylitis and sacroiliitis with disturbances of the cardiac conduction system.[155]

Spontaneous Vertebral Collapse and Fracture

Care must be taken to differentiate pure traumatic injury from trauma superimposed upon a pathologic process. Turek lists the most common causes of spontaneous vertebral collapse in their order of frequency as osteoporosis, malignant bone disease, rheumatoid arthritis treated by corticosteroids, and osteomalacia.

Spinal Tuberculosis

Both tubercular spondylitis or osteomyelitis commonly occur in the vertebral bodies and progresses to marked osteoporotic and sclerotic changes, collapse, wedging, and gibbus deformity.[156] Roentgenographic obliteration of adjacent endplates points toward infection rather than neoplasm in cases of vertebral collapse. In Pott's disease, in which there are caries of the bodies of the vertebrae, there often is a sharp curvature of the spine in the dorsal or the lumbar region as a result of the weight upon the weakened vertebral bodies. These are usually present as an abrupt and permanent area of kyphosis.[157]

Scheuermann's Kyphosis

In children and adolescents of either sex, moderate anterior wedging of one or more hyperkyphotic vertebrae, usually extending from the middle to the lower thoracic spine; IVD space narrowing; Schmorl's nodes; endplate cupping; and sclerosis are the cardinal signs of vertebral epiphysitis. Disc substance becomes replaced by fibrous tissue. A history of trauma is invariably associated, thus the disease is easily confused with compression fractures.[158] Differentiation must also be made from infectious spondylitis, tumors, and the osteochondrodystrophies. Mild cases are usually asymptomatic, and the only outward sign is a rounded "tractor back."[159]

Helfet and Lee[160] jointly point out that postural exercises are just as important in the management of serious Scheuermann's osteochondritis as they are in nonpathologic postural weakness.

Vertebra Plana

Calvé's disease of the spine is characterized by rapid collapse and flattening of a single vertebral body associated with an aseptic necrosis. It is seen in children with an insidious onset of localized pain and muscle spasm that is followed by hyperkyphosis or scoliosis.[161]

Spondylitis

The ankylosed osteoporotic spines of patients with chronic spondylitis are prone to fracture from what may appear to be trivial forces.[162] These injuries, which have a higher incidence in the cervical region than the thoracic region, can easily be overlooked when neurologic signs are absent.

SELECTED DEFORMITIES AND ANOMALIES[163–165]

Almost any congenital anomaly may present itself in the thoracic spine. Asymptomatic odd-shaped spinous and transverse processes, hemivertebrae, closed-clefted vertebrae, and supernumerary vertebrae are sometimes seen on films taken for other reasons. As in the cervical region, those anomalies that have biomechanical significance vary in severity from minor to severe and occur multiply or singly. Congenital torticollis, Klippel-Feil syndrome, cervical rib, Sprengel's deformity, and spinal stenosis frequently involve both the cervical and upper thoracic area.

In cases of congenital coarctation of the aorta or neurofibromatosis, sometimes notching of the ribs is the only obvious clinical sign. Enlarged intercostal arteries or nerve tumors tend to erode the inferrior borders of the involved ribs.

Absent floating ribs, lumbar ribs, and bifid ribs are not uncommon, but they rarely are the initial cause of biomechanical faults. Wedged segments, hemivertebrae, and unsegmented bars are the most common conditions that have severe biochemical implications.

Lumbar, Bifid, and Fused Ribs

Lumbar ribs are more common than cervical ribs.[166] They are usually shorter than the 12th rib and articulate with L1, either at a costovertebral joint, costotransverse joint, or both.

Bifid (forked) ribs are usually unilateral and invariably split on the anterior aspect of the rib. They usually confuse palpation in the T1–T8 rib area at the costosternal junction. Fused ribs are rare unless associated with other gross genetic defects.[167]

Wedged Segments and Hemivertebrae[164, 168]

These common anomalies are frequent causes of asymmetrical growth and spinal distortion. If the hemivertebra is incarcerated in good alignment, it has less tendency to produce an exaggerated curve. As the direction of growth is most difficult to predict, careful monitoring should be made during maturation.

Unsegmented Bar[169, 170]

This congenital defect in vertebral segmentation and asymmetrical growth requires early detection and surgical correction to prevent severe spinal distortion, especially if it is unilateral. Fusion may occur at almost any point on the vertebra, but it usually involves the centrum. The most common point is on the posterolateral aspect of the vertebral body. It is fairly limited to the thoracic spine, and ribs tend to fuse on the side of the bony bar. As normal growth continues unilaterally, severe spinal distortion occurs. This becomes evident either at birth or before 3 years of age.

REFERENCES

1. Benson DR: The back: Thoracic and lumbar spine. In D'Ambrosia RD: *Musculoskeletal Disorders: Regional Examination and Differential Diagnosis*. Philadelphia, J.B. Lippincott, 1977, pp 247–253.
2. White AA, Panjabi MM: *Clinical Biomechanics of the Spine*. Philadelphia, J.B. Lippincott, 1978, pp 236–239.
3. Jones L: *The Postural Complex: Observations as to Cause, Diagnosis, and Treatment*. Springfield, Ill, Charles C Thomas, 1955.
4. Morehouse LE, Cooper JM: *Kinesiology*. St. Louis, C.V. Mosby, 1950, p 44.
5. Basmajian JV (ed): *Grant's Method of Anatomy*, ed 9. Baltimore, Williams & Wilkins, 1975, pp 392–394.
6. Moore KL: *Clinically Oriented Anatomy*. Baltimore, Williams & Wilkins, 1980, pp 15–16.
7. Barham JN, Wooten EP: *Structural Kinesiology*. New York, Macmillan, 1973, p 246.
8. Basmajian JV (ed): *Grant's Method of Anatomy*, ed 9. Baltimore, Williams & Wilkins, 1975, pp 394-398.
9. Edwards LF, Gaughram GRL: *Concise Anatomy*. New York, McGraw-Hill, 1971.
10. Moore KL: *Clinically Oriented Anatomy*. Baltimore, Williams & Wilkins, 1980, pp 4–7.
11. Agostoni E et al: Forces deforming the rib cage. *Respiratory Physiology* 2:105, 1966.
12. Nahum AM et al: Deflections of human thorax under sternal impact. Presented at the International Automobile Safety Conference, Detroit, 1970.
13. Kapandji IA: *The Physiology of the Joints: The Trunk and the Vertebral Column*, ed 2. New York, Churchill Livingstone, 1974, vol 3, p 138.
14. Grice AS, Fligg DB: Class notes. Department of Biomechanics/Kinesiology, BK202. Toronto, Canadian Memorial Chiropractic College, pp 81–82 (undated).
15. Daniels L, Worthingham C: *Therapeutic Exercise for Body Alignment and Function*, ed 2. Philadelphia, W.B. Saunders, 1977, p 73.
16. Grieve GP: *Common Vertebral Joint Problems*. New York, Churchill-Livingstone, 1981, pp 33, 235.
17. White AA, Panjabi MM: *Clinical Biomechanics of the Spine*. Philadelphia, J.B. Lippincott, 1978, p 236.
18. Gates D: *Correlative Spinal Anatomy*. Lakemont, Ga, published by the author, 1977, pp 67–71.
19. Moore KL: *Clinically Oriented Anatomy*. Baltimore, Williams & Wilkins, 1980, pp 1, 4.
20. Hollinshead WH, Jenkins DB: *Functional Anatomy of the Limbs and Back*, ed 5. Philadelphia, W.B. Saunders, 1981, pp 203–205.
21. Reinert OC: *Fundamentals of Chiropractic Techniques and Practice Procedures*. Chesterfield, Mo, Marian Press, 1983, pp 84–87.
22. Ponsetti IV et al: Biomechanical analysis of intervertebral discs in idiopathic scoliosis. *Journal of Bone and Joint Surgery* 54:1993, 1972; 56A, 1973.
23. Bernick S, Cailliet R: Vertebral end-plate changes with aging of human vertebrae. *Spine* 7:97–102, 1982.
24. Cailliet R: *Low Back Pain Syndrome*, ed 2, Philadelphia, F.A. Davis, 1968, p 25.
25. Grieve GP: *Common Vertebral Joint Problems*. New York, Churchill Livingstone, 1981, p 10.
26. Hilton RC, Bail J: A systematic pathological study of the dorsolumbar spine. *Journal of Rheumatology* 9:95–96, 1983.
27. Gehweiler JA Jr, Osborne RL Jr, Becker RF: *The Radiology of Vertebral Trauma*. Philadelphia, W.B. Saunders, 1980, pp 76–78.
28. Rosse C, Clawson DK: *The Musculoskeletal System in Health and Disease*. New York, Harper & Row, 1980, pp 122–124.
29. Barham JN, Wooten EP: *Structural Kinesiology*. New York, Macmillan, 1973, p 247.
30. Gates D: *Correlative Spinal Anatomy*. Lakemont, Ga, published by author, 1977, pp 97–99.
31. Rosse C, Clawson DK: *The Musculoskeletal System in Health and Disease*. New York, Harper & Row, 1980, p 129.
32. Miller MA, Leavell LC: *Kimber-Gray-Stackpole's Anatomy and Physiology*, ed 16. New York, Macmillan, 1972.
33. Warfel JH: *The Head, Neck, and Trunk*, ed 5. Philadelphia, Lea & Febiger, 1985, pp 65–72.

34. Cooper JM, Glassow RB: *Kinesiology*, ed 3. St. Louis, C.V. Mosby, 1972.
35. Logan AL, McKinney WC: *Kinesiology*. Dubuque, Ia, W.C. Brown, 1970.
36. Moore KL: *Clinically Oriented Anatomy*. Baltimore, Williams & Wilkins, 1980, pp 18–28.
37. Kapandji IA: *The Physiology of the Joints: The Trunk and the Vertebral Column*, ed 2. New York, Churchill Livingstone, 1974, vol 3, pp 146–150.
38. White AA, Panjabi MM: *Clinical Biomechanics of the Spine*. Philadelphia, J.B. Lippincott, 1978, pp 74–78.
39. Andriacchi T et al: A model for studies of mechanical interactions between the human spine and rib cage. *Journal of Biomechanics* 7:497–507, 1974.
40. Haller JS, Gurewitsch AO: An approach to dynamic posture based on primitive motion patterns. *Archives of Physical Medicine* 31:632–640, 1950.
41. White AA, Panjabi MM: Spinal kinematics. In Goldstein M (ed): *The Research Status of Spinal Manipulative Therapy*. NINCDS Monograph, No. 15, DHEW Publication No. (NIH) 76-998, Stock No. 017-049-00060-7, Washington, DC, U.S. Government Printing Office, 1975.
42. Morris JM: Biomechanics of the spine. *Archives of Surgery* 107:418–423, 1973.
43. Panjabi MM et al: Mechanical properties of the human thoracic spine. *Journal of Bone and Joint Surgery* 58A:642–651, 1976.
44. Panjabi MM et al: Three dimensional flexibility and stiffness properties of the human thoracic spine. *Journal of Biomechanics* 9:185–192, 1976.
45. Weis EB Jr: Spinal geometry: Normal and abnormal. In Goldstein M (ed): *The Research Status of Spinal Manipulative Therapy*. NINCDS Monograph, No. 15, DHEW Publication No. (NIH) 76-998, Stock No. 017-049-00060-7, Washington, DC, U.S. Government Printing Office, 1975.
46. White AA, Panjabi MM: Basic kinematics of the human spine. *Spine* 3:1, March 1978.
47. Grice AS: A biomechanical approach to cervical and dorsal adjusting. In Haldeman, S (ed): *Modern Developments in the Principles and Practice of Chiropractic*. New York, Appleton-Century-Crofts, 1980, pp 339–340, 351–352.
48. Grice AS: Radiographic biomechanical and clinical factors in lumbar lateral flexion: part I. *Journal of Manipulative and Physiological Therapeutics* 2(1):26–34, March 1979.
49. Roaf R: Rotation movements of the spine with special reference to scoliosis. *Journal of Bone and Joint Surgery* 40B:312–332, 1958.
50. Gregerson GG, Lucas DB: An in vivo study of axial rotation of the human thoracic-lumbar spine. *Journal of Bone and Joint Surgery* 49A:247, 1967.
51. White AA, Panjabi MM: *Clinical Biomechanics of the Spine*. Philadelphia, J.B. Lippincott, 1978, p 93.
52. Grice AS: A biomechanical approach to cervical and dorsal adjusting. In Haldeman, S (ed): *Modern Developments in the Principles and Practice of Chiropractic*. New York, Appleton-Century-Crofts, 1980, pp 351–352.
53. Grieve GP: *Common Vertebral Joint Problems*. New York, Churchill-Livingstone, 1981, p 48.
54. Shrader TL: Council on technic (column). *ACA Journal of Chiropractic* December 1985, p 90.
55. Jirout J: Pattern of changes in the cervical spine in lateroflexion. *Neuroradiology* 2:164, 1971.
56. Grieve GP: *Common Vertebral Joint Problems*. New York, Churchill-Livingstone, 1981, p 47.
57. Orringer MB: Chest injuries in the athlete. In Schneider RC, Kennedy JC, Plant ML (eds): *Sports Injuries: Mechanisms, Prevention, and Treatment*. Baltimore, Williams & Wilkins, 1985, pp 826–827.
58. Robertson WE, Robertson HF: *Diagnostic Signs, Reflexes, and Syndromes*, ed 3. Philadelphia, F.A. Davis, 1947, p 261.
59. White AA, Panjabi MM: *Clinical Biomechanics of the Spine*. Philadelphia, J.B. Lippincott, 1978, pp 237–240, 250–251.
60. Branton P: Behavior, body mechanics, and discomfort. *Ergonomics* 12:316–327, 1969.
61. Craig AS: Elements of kinesiology for the clinician. *Physical Therapy* 44:470–473, 1964.
62. Frankel VH, Burstein AH: *Orthopedic Biomechanics*. Philadelphia, Lea & Febiger, 1970.
63. Bowerman JW: *Radiology and Injury in Sport*. New York, Appleton-Century-Crofts, 1977, pp 87–94.
64. Moore KL: *Clinically Oriented Anatomy*. Baltimore, Williams & Wilkins, 1980, pp 7–12.
65. Zuidema GD et al: *The Management of Trauma*, ed 3. Philadelphia, W.B. Saunders, 1979, 379–383.
66. Williams JGP, Sperryn PN (eds): *Sports Medicine*, ed 2. Baltimore, Williams & Wilkins, 1976, p 369.
67. Hirata I Jr: *The Doctor and the Athlete*, ed 2. Philadelphia, J.B. Lippincott, 1974, pp 177–180.
68. Schafer RC: *Chiropractic Management of Sports and Recreational Injuries*. Baltimore, Williams & Wilkins, 1982, pp 422–425.
69. Nelson WA: Personal communication, 1980.
70. Maurer EL: The thoraco-costal facet syndrome with introduction of the marginal line and the rib sign. *ACA Journal of Chiropractic* 10:S158–S159, December 1976.
71. Schoenholtz F: Conservative management of costovertebral subluxation. *ACA Journal of Chiropractic* 14:S77–S78, July 1980.
72. Schultz AI: *The Shoulder, Arm and Hand Syndrome*. Mitchell, S Dak, published by the author, 1969, p 165.
73. Daniels L, Worthingham C: *Therapeutic Exercise for Body Alignment and Function*, ed 2. Philadelphia, W.B. Saunders, 1977, pp 73–74.
74. Van Dusen LG: *Chiropractic Relationship to Gravitational Force*. Sodus, NY, published by the author, 1968, p 71.
75. Schafer RC: *Chiropractic Management of Sports and Recreational Injuries*. Baltimore, Williams & Wilkins, 1982, p 421.
76. Bowerman JW: *Radiology and Injury in Sport*. New York, Appleton-Century-Crofts, 1977, p 189.
77. Zuidema GD, et al: *The Manaqement of Trauma*,

ed 3. Philadelplhia, W.B. Saunders, 1979, pp 12–13, 383–384.
78. Hirata I Jr: *The Doctor and the Athlete*, ed 2. Philadelphia, J.B. Lippincott, 1974, pp 175–176.
79. Krupp MA et al: *Physician's Handbook*, ed 21. Los Altos, Cal, Lange Medical, 1985, pp 16–17.
80. Bowerman JW: *Radiology and Injury in Sport*. New York, Appleton-Century-Crofts, 1977, pp 87–92.
81. Curwen IHM: Golf. In Armstrong JR, Tucker WE (eds): *Injury in Sport*. London, Staples, 1964, pp 200–204.
82. Moore KL: *Clinically Oriented Anatomy*. Baltimore, Williams & Wilkins, 1980, p 9.
83. Zuidema GD et al: *The Management of Trauma*, ed 3. Philadelphia, W.B. Saunders, p 384.
84. Moore KL: *Clinically Oriented Anatomy*. Baltimore, Williams & Wilkins, 1980, p 12.
85. Mills KLG: *Guide to Orthopaedics*. New York, Churchill-Livingstone, 1981.
86. Gehweiler JA Jr, Osborne RL Jr, Becker RF: *The Radiology of Vertebral Trauma*. Philadelphia, W.B. Saunders, 1980, pp 259–373.
87. White AA, Panjabi MM: *Clinical Biomechanics of the Spine*. Philadelphia, J.B. Lippincott, 1978, pp 166–179, 240–244.
88. Zuidema GD et al: *The Management of Trauma*, ed 3. Philadelphia, W.B. Saunders, 1979, pp 610–616.
89. Salter RB: *Textbook of Disorders and Injuries of the Musculoskeletal System*. Baltimore, Williams & Wilkins, 1981, pp 489, 496–498.
90. Howorth MB, Petrie VG: *Injuries of the Spine*. Baltimore, Williams & Wilkins, 1964.
91. Howe JW: Frequently missed fractures. *Roentgenography Briefs*, American Council on Roentgenography of the ACA (undated).
92. Orne D, Liu YK: A mathematical model of spinal response to impact. *Journal of Biomechanics* 4:49–71, 1971.
93. Schafer RC: *Basic Chiropractic Procedural Manual*, ed 3. Des Moines, Ia, American Chiropractic Association, p III-26.
94. McAfee PC, Yuan HA, Lasda NA: The unstable burst fracture. *Spine* 7:365–373, 1982.
95. Kilcoyne RF et al: Thoracolumbar spine injuries associated with vertical plunges: Reappraisal with computed tomography. *Radiology* 146:137–140, 1983.
96. Willen J et al: The thoracolumbar crush fracture. An experimental study on instant axial dynamic loading: The resulting fracture type and its stability. *Spine* 9:624–631, 1984.
97. Gonza ER, Harrington IJ: *Biomechanics of Musculoskeletal Injury*. Baltimore, Williams & Wilkins, 1982, p 202.
98. Roaf R: A study of the mechanics of spinal injuries. *Journal of Bone and Joint Surgery* 42B:810–823, 1960.
99. De Oliveira JC: A new type of fracture-dislocation of the thoracolumbar spine. *Journal of Bone and Joint Surgery*, 60A:481–488, 1978.
100. Grieve GP: *Common Vertebral Joint Problems*. New York, Churchill Livingstone, 1981, p 134.
101. Hitchcock ME: Myofascial considerations in the thoracic area. *Osteopathic Medicine* 85, December 1978.
102. Sweere JJ: Type II round back deformity. *Orthopedic Brief*. ACA Council on Chiropractic Orthopedics, August 1985.
103. Schafer RC: *Chiropractic Physical and Spinal Diagnosis*. Oklahoma City, Associated Chiropractic Academic Press, 1980, p X-27.
104. Stonebrink RD: Palpation for vertebral motoricity. *ACA Journal of the Chiropractic* 3:S11–S14, February 1969.
105. Johnston WL: The role of static and motion palpation in structural diagnosis. In Goldstein M (ed): *The Research Status of Spinal Manipulative Therapy*. NINCDS Monograph, No. 15, DHEW Publication No. (NIH) 76-998, Stock No. 017-049-00060-7, Washington, DC, U.S. Government Printing Office, 1975, pp 249–252.
106. Stierwalt DD: *Fundamentals of Motion Palpation*. City of publication not shown, published by the author, 1977, pp 18–24.
107. Gillet H, Liekens M: *Belgian Chiropractic Research Notes*. Huntington Beach, Cal, Motion Palpation Institute, 1981, pp 43, 69, 106.
108. McAndrews JF: Spinal motion examination. *ACA Journal of Chiropractic* 3:S38–S39, May 1969.
109. Van Dusen LG: *Chiropractic Relationship to Gravitational Force*. Sodus, NY, published by the author, 1968, p 93.
110. Gillet H, Liekens M: *Belgian Chiropractic Research Notes*. Huntington Beach, Cal, Motion Palpation Institute, 1981, p 18.
111. Van Dusen LG: *Chiropractic Relationship to Gravitational Force*. Sodus, NY, published by the author, 1968, pp 105, 107.
112. Gillet H, Liekens M: *Belgian Chiropractic Research Notes*. Huntington Beach, Cal, Motion Palpation Institute, 1981, pp 27–28.
113. Ono M et al: Ossification of the thoracic posterior longitudinal ligament in a fixed population. *Radiology* 143:469–474, 1982.
114. Miyasaka K, Kaneda K, Ito T: Ossification of spinal ligaments causing thoracic radiculomyelopathy. *Radiology* 143:463–468, 1982.
115. Chin WS, Oon CL: Ossification of the posterior longitudinal ligament of the spine. *British Journal of Radiology* 52:865–869, 1979.
116. Schafer RC: *Chiropractic Management of Sports and Recreational Injuries*. Baltimore, Williams & Wilkins, 1982, p 420.
117. Gillet H, Liekens M: *Belgian Chiropractic Research Notes*. Huntington Beach, Cal, Motion Palpation Institute, 1981, p 92.
118. Schafer RC: *Chiropractic Management of Sports and Recreational Injuries*. Baltimore, Williams & Wilkins, 1982, p 425.
119. Gillet H, Liekens M: *Belgian Chiropractic Research Notes*. Huntington Beach, Cal, Motion Palpation Institute, 1981, pp 7–8.
120. Schafer RC: *Chiropractic Physical and Spinal Diagnosis*. Oklahoma City, Associated Chiropractic Academic Press, 1980, p X-26.
121. Weitz EM: The lateral bending sign. *Spine* 6:4, July/August, 1981.
122. Walters RL, Morris JM: An in vitro study of

normal and scoliotic interspinous ligaments. *Journal of Biomechanics* 6:343, 1973.

123. Schafer RC (ed): *Basic Chiropractic Procedural Manual*, ed 4. Des Moines, Ia, American Chiropractic Association, 1984, p 85.
124. Mazion JM: *Illustrated Manual of Neurological Reflexes/Signs/Tests, Orthopedic Signs/Tests/Maneuvers*, ed 2. Arizona City, published by the author, 1980, p 246.
125. Schafer RC: *Chiropractic Physical and Spinal Diagnosis*. Oklahoma City, American Chiropractic Academic Press, 1980, p X-29.
126. Schafer RC: *Chiropractic Management of Sports and Recreational Injuries*. Baltimore, Williams & Wilkins, 1982, p 427.
127. Cipriano JJ: *Photographic Manual of Regional Orthopaedic Tests*. Baltimore, Williams & Wilkins, 1985, p 43.
128. Schafer RC (ed): *Basic Chiropractic Procedural Manual*, ed 4. Des Moines, Ia, American Chiropractic Association, 1984, pp 92–93.
129. Schafer RC: *Chiropractic Physical and Spinal Diagnosis*. Oklahoma City, American Chiropractic Academic Press, 1980, p XIII-25.
130. Mazion JM: *Illustrated Manual of Neurological Reflexes/Signs/Tests, Orthopedic Signs/Tests/Maneuvers*, ed 2. Arizona City, published by the author, 1980, p 312.
131. Jaskoviak P, Schafer RC: *Applied Physiotherapy*. Arlington, Va, American Chiropractic Association. To be published in 1986.
132. Betge G: *Physical Therapy in Chiropractic Practice*. Via Tesserete, Switzerland, published by the author, 1975.
133. Johnson AC: *Chiropractic Physiological Therapeutics*. Palm Springs, Cal, published by the author, 1977.
134. Langilotti FT: *Adjunctive Therapy for the Chiropractor*. Publisher not shown (undated).
135. Baltzell LG, Mackey RH (eds): *Firth's Technic Notes (Revised)*. City of publication not shown, 1967, pp 45–48.
136. Janse J: *Principles and Practice of Chiropractic*. Lombard, Ill, National College of Chiropractic, 1976, p 99.
137. Johnson AC: *Chiropractic Physiological Therapeutics*. Palm Springs, Cal, published by the author, 1977, pp 46–47.
138. Hains G: *Post-Traumatic Neuritis*. Trois-Rivieres, Quebec, published by the author, 1978, p 10.
139. Schafer RC: *Chiropractic Management of Sports and Recreational Injuries*. Baltimore, Williams & Wilkins, 1982, p 271.
140. Johnson AC: *Chiropractic Physiological Therapeutics*. Palm Springs, Cal, published by the author, 1977, pp 44–45.
141. Janse J: *Principles and Practice of Chiropractic*. Lombard, Ill, National College of Chiropractic, 1976, pp 105–109
142. Janse J, Houser RH, Wells BF: *Chiropractic Principles and Technic*, ed 2. Chicago, National College of Chiropractic, 1947, pp 256–267, 512–518.
143. Schafer RC: *Chiropractic Management of Sports and Recreational Injuries*. Baltimore, Williams & Wilkins, 1982, p 272.
144. Johnson AC: *Chiropractic Physiological Therapeutics*. Palm Springs, Cal, published by the author, 1977, pp 37–38.
145. Daniels L, Worthingham C: *Therapeutic Exercise for Body Alignment and Function*, ed 2. Philadelphia, W.B. Saunders, 1977, pp 66–71.
146. McGall IW et al: Alterations in vertebral growth following prolonged plaster immobilisation. *Acta Orthopaedica Scandinavica*, 52:327–330, 1981.
147. Cotler HB et al: Intrathoracic chordoma presenting as a posterior superior mediastinal tumor. *Spine* 8:781–786, 1983.
148. Gucker T: Changes in vital capacity in scoliosis: preliminary report on the effects of treatment. *Journal of Bone and Joint Surgery* 44:469, 1962.
149. Turek SL: *Orthopaedics: Principles and Their Application*, ed 3. Philadelphia, J.B. Lippincott, 1977, pp 1358–1359.
150. Evans DC: Biomechanics of spinal injury. In Gonza ER, Harrington IJ: *Biomechanics of Musculoskeletal Injury*. Baltimore, Williams & Wilkins, 1982, pp 200–204.
151. Albrand OW, Corkill G: Thoracic disc herniation: Treatment and prognosis. *Spine* 4:41–46, 1979.
152. Blits J: Thoracic disk herniation. *Ortho Briefs*. ACA Council on Chiropractic Orthopedics, Spring 1982, pp 8–9.
153. Winsberg F: Roentgenographic aspects of aging. In Rossman, I (ed): *Clinical Geriatrics*. Philadelphia, J.B. Lippincott, 1971, p 267.
154. Cox J, Gideon D, Rogers F: Incidence of osteophytic lipping of the thoracic spine in coronary heart disease: Results of a pilot study. *Journal of the American Osteopathic Association* 82:837–838, 1983.
155. Bergfeldt L et al: Ankylosing spondylitis: An important cause of severe disturbances of the cardiac conduction system. *American Journal of Medicine* 73:187–191, 1982.
156. Wilkins RW, Levinsky NG (eds): *Medicine: Essentials of Clinical Practice*. Boston, Little, Brown, 1978, p 154.
157. Teranel JA: *Chiropractic Orthopedics and Roentgenology*. Newark, NJ, Medusa Press, 1953, pp 107–108.
158. Salter RB: *Textbook of Disorders and Injuries of the Musculoskeletal System*. Baltimore, Williams & Wilkins, 1970, pp 279–281.
159. Turek SL: *Orthopaedics: Principles and Their Application*, ed 3. Philadelphia, J.B. Lippincott, 1977, pp 1380–1381.
160. Helfet AJ, Gruebel Lee DM: *Disorders of the Lumbar Spine*. Philadelphia, J.B. Lippincott 1978, pp 3–4.
161. Holmes GW, Robbins LL: *Roentgen Interpretation*. Philadelphia, Lew & Febiger, 1947, pp 111, 170.
162. Hunter T, Dubo H: Spinal fractures complicating ankylosing spondylitis. *Annals of Internal Medicine* 88:546–549, 1978.
163. Salter RB: *Textbook of Disorders and Injuries of the Musculoskeletal System*. Baltimore, Williams & Wilkins, 1981, pp 117, 119–123.
164. Benson DR: The back: Thoracic and lumbar spine. In D'Ambrosia RD: *Musculoskeletal Dis-*

orders: Regional Examination and Differential Diagnosis. Philadelphia, J.B. Lippincott, 1977, pp 308–309.

165. Gehweiler JA Jr, Osborne RL Jr, Becker RF: *The Radiology of Vertebral Trauma*. Philadelphia, W.B. Saunders, 1980, p 361.
166. Moore KL: *Clinically Oriented Anatomy*. Baltimore, Williams & Wilkins, 1980, pp 9–10.
167. Moore KL: *Clinically Oriented Anatomy*. Baltimore, Williams & Wilkins, 1980, p 10.
168. Hadley LA: *Anatomico-Roentgenographic Studies of the Spine*. Springfield, Ill, Charles C Thomas, ed 5, 1981, p 44.
169. Hadley LA: *Anatomico-Roentgenographic Studies of the Spine*, ed 5. Springfield, Ill, Charles C Thomas, 1981, pp 36–37, 42–45.
170. Barge FH: *Scoliosis*. Davenport, Ia, published by the author, 1981, vol 3, pp 147–149.

SUGGESTED READINGS

Carver FJ: Postural adjusting. *Journal of the National Chiropractic Association* April 1940.

Goldthwait JE et al: *Essentials of Body Mechanics*. Philadelphia, J.B. Lippincott, 1952.

Kelley DL: *Kinesiology: Fundamentals of Motion Descriptions*. Englewood Cliffs, NJ, Prentice-Hall, Inc, 1971.

Kendall HO et al: *Posture and Pain*. Baltimore, Williams & Wilkins, 1952.

Kendall HO et al: *Muscles: Testing and Function*, ed 2. Baltimore, Williams & Wilkins, 1971.

Logan HB: *Textbook of Logan Basic Methods*. St. Louis, Logan Chiropractic College, 1950.

Nelson RC, Morehouse CA (eds): *Biomechanics IV*. Baltimore, University Park Press, 1974.

Petersen AP: *Segmental Neuropathy*. Toronto, Canadian Chiropractic College, 1970.

Schmorl G, Junghanns H: *The Human Spine in Health and Disease*, ed 2. New York, Grune & Stratton, 1971.

Steindler A: *Kinesiology of the Human Body Under Normal and Pathological Conditions*, ed 3. Springfield, Ill, Charles C Thomas, 1970.

Wells KF: *Kinesiology*, ed 5. Philadelphia, W.B. Saunders, 1971.

CHAPTER 11

The Lumbar Spine and Pelvis

Deranged patterns of action of the lumbar spine and pelvis have been noted since primitive civilizations. This chapter investigates this complex area with emphasis upon the biomechanical influences in back pain and postural faults. Although the lumbar spine, sacrum, pelvis, and hips operate as a closed kinematic chain, the abdomen, lumbar spine, and pelvic components are discussed separately with concern for their functional interrelationships. Within each major topic, the highlights of pertinent anatomy, kinesiology, and kinematics are offered.

PREVERTEBRAL FUNCTION OF THE ABDOMINAL AREA

Studies in spinal loading expose the vulnerability of the spine to the mechanical stresses placed upon it, especially in people with poor muscle tone. When the spine is loaded during the act of lifting, the lumbosacral area is subjected to forces from both the upper body plus the weight being lifted. It is also being subjected to the bending torque caused by these forces because they are some distance from the trunk's center of mass.

The load on the lumbosacral disc is therefore the sum of the upper body, any weight held, and the spinal muscle forces and their respective lever arms to the disc. This load must be dissipated to prevent collapse of the vertebra. It is dissipated through the paraspinal muscles and, importantly, by the abdominal cavity which acts as a hydraulic chamber to absorb and thus diminish the load applied.

Functional Anatomy of the Abdominal Muscles[1–6]

The major muscles of the lower trunk include the rectus abdominis, external and internal obliques, and transversus abdominis anteriorly, and the quadratus lumborum posteriorly (Fig. 11.1).

The *rectus abdominis* spans between the pubic crest and the costal cartilages of the 5th–7th ribs and is attached medially in the linea alba. Laterally, it blends with the three layers of flank muscle. It is separated at different levels by transverse-oblique fibrous bands. Unilateral action produces lateral flexion of the trunk, and bilateral action flexes the thoracic and lumbar regions of the spine.

The *external oblique* attaches superiorly on the external surfaces of the lower 8 ribs by tendinous fibers that intertwine with those of the serratus anterior. It attaches inferiorly at the anterior half of the iliac crest and medially in the linea alba. Unilateral action produces spinal lateral flexion and rotation to the opposite side, and bilateral action flexes the thoracic and lumbar regions of the spine.

The *internal oblique* lies under the external oblique. It attaches superiorly on the inferior borders of the last three ribs, medially in the linea alba and pubic crest, inferiorly on the thoracolumbar fascia and iliac crest, and laterally at the lateral aspect of the inguinal ligaments. Unilateral action produces lateral flexion and rotation of the spine to the same side, and bilateral action flexes the thoracic and lumbar regions of the spine.

The unpalpable *transversus abdominis* lies under the internal oblique. Its transverse fibers attach medially in the linea alba and pubic crest and laterally at the cartilages of the lower six ribs, inguinal ligament, iliac crest, and thoracolumbar fascia. This is essentially a respiratory muscle and its action produces depression of the lower ribs and compression of the abdomen.

The *quadratus lumborum* spans up the lateral aspect of the lumbar spine. It attaches superiorly at the transverse processes of L1–L4 and inferiorly on the iliac crest and iliolumbar ligament. Its sole but important role is in lateral flexion of the lumbar spine.

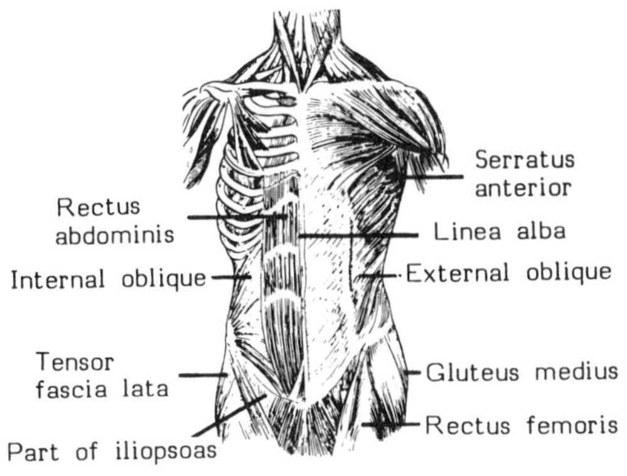

Figure 11.1. The major anterior abdominal muscles.

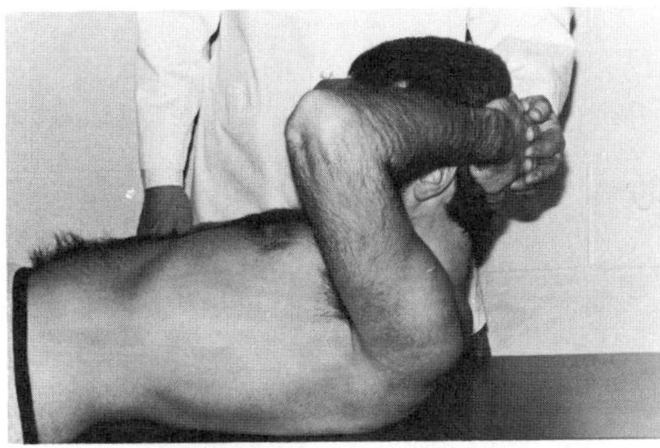

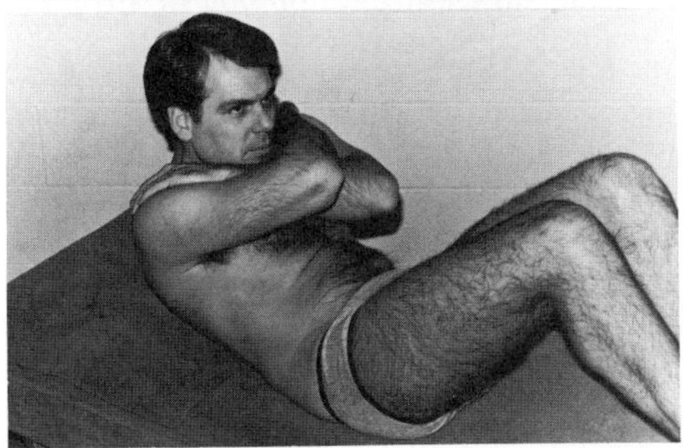

Figure 11.2. Screening active trunk flexion strength.

Trunk Movements[7-12]

Flexion and Extension

Any muscle with vertical or oblique fibers that connects the thorax with the pelvis assists in flexion of the trunk. The major actions involved are bilateral activity of the rectus abdominis, external and internal oblique, and psoas major (Fig. 11.2).

Extension is the product of bilateral action of the thoracic and lumbar erector spinae and the semispinalis, with some assistance provided by the deep posterior spinal muscles (Fig. 11.3).

Lateral Flexion and Rotation

All trunk flexors and extensors can produce lateral flexion when acting unilaterally. The major muscles involved are the rectus abdominis, external and internal obliques, erector spinae, semispinalis thoracis, latissimus dorsi, deep posterior spinal muscles, quadratus lumborum, and psoas.

Thoracolumbar rotation to the opposite side is produced essentially by unilateral action of the external oblique, semispinalis, and the deep posterior spinal muscles. Rotation to the same side is produced by the internal oblique and erector spinae.

THE LUMBAR SPINE: ANATOMICAL AND KINEMATIC CONSIDERATIONS

Body weight is carried in the lower back essentially by the L5 disc and dissipated to the sacral base, sacroiliac joints, and acetabulae. This weight on the L5 disc is forced slightly anteriorly on the load surfaces. The lateral line of gravity cuts a point just antero-inferior to S2.

Functional Anatomy[13-17]

The lumbar vertebrae, along with their articulations and intervertebral foramina (IVFs), offer distinct characteristics that have significant biomechanical influences (Fig. 11.4).

The Lumbar Vertebrae[18-23]

Weight distribution in the lumbar region is governed chiefly by the inclination of

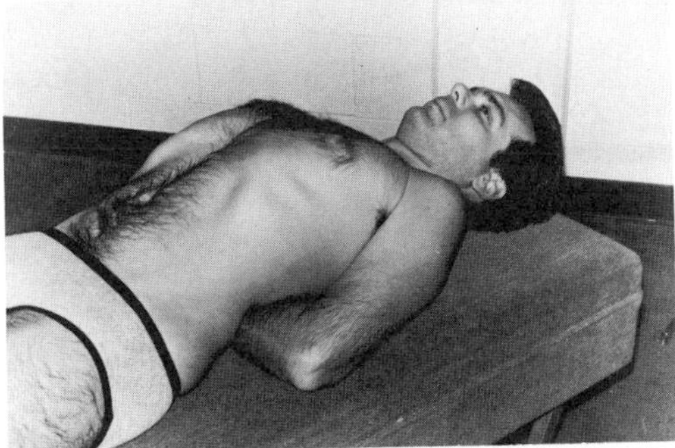

Figure 11.3. Screening active trunk extension strength with the patient supine.

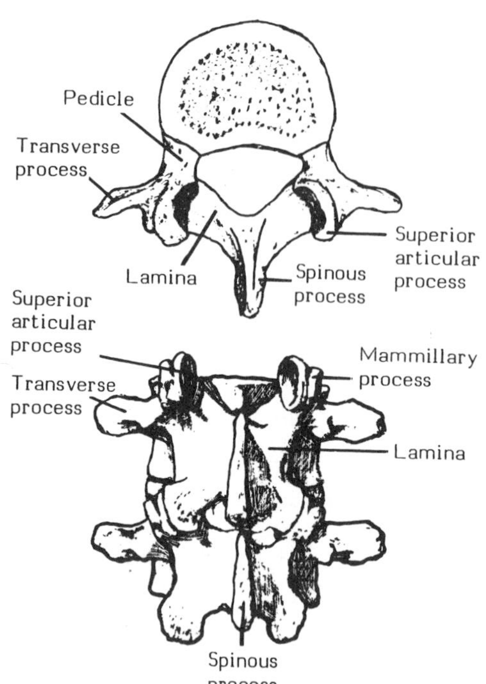

Figure 11.4. A middle lumbar vertebra as viewed from above and behind.

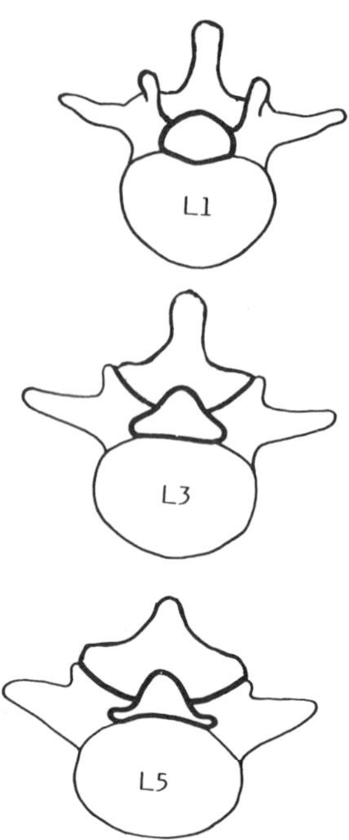

Figure 11.5. Schematic of the changing articular planes and shape of the lumbar vertebral canal as viewed from above.

each vertebral body articulation. The lateral center line of gravity falls upon the spinal points because of gradual changes in the angles of the inclined planes of the various articular surfaces. This tends to force each lumbar vertebra more inferior, medial, and anterior or posterior until gravity brings the apex of the curve back toward the balancing point.

Planes of Articulation The lumbar facets are moderately sloped surfaces rather than a single-plane angle as seen in the cervical and thoracic area, and they are fairly parallel to the vertical plane at L1 and L2. The laterally convex inferior facets mate with the concave superior facets. From L1 to L5, the planes of the articular facets change from mediolateral to anteroposterior and lie, for the most part, in the sagittal plane. There are considerable differences between the plane of articulation and the shape of the vertebral canal that progress from L1 to L5 (Fig. 11.5). Rotation and lateral flexion is anatomically inhibited by the articular planes in the L1–L2 segments but not in the L4–L5 segments.

Facet Angle Variations. Interspinal posture is directed by the facet facing of each posterior intervertebral joint, with altered facings most commonly occurring in the lumbar and lower cervical regions. Articular facings are altered more frequently between L4 and L5 than at any other level in the vertebral column. Normal symmetrical facets glide with little friction produced. However, if the facets deviate in their direction of movement, the unparallel articulating surfaces "scrub" upon one another. Over a period of time, even in the absence of overt injury at the level of abnormality, articular variations will present marginal sclerosis. This hardening is usually followed by hypertrophy or exostosis. Coexistent with this finding, the interarticular spaces gradually become narrowed, hazy, obscured, and even obliterated on x-ray films.

Facet Strength. In genearl, the facets normally carry about 18% of a vertebra's total axial load but can contribute up to 33% of its compression strength, depending upon posture. The lower facets of the lordotic curve (L3–L5) carry more weight than those of other areas. The posterior processes and their capsular ligaments provide up to 45% of torsional strength of a vertebral motion unit, in contrast to 45% by the disc and longitudinal ligaments and 10% by the interspinous ligaments. These percentages, however, will vary with different postures. In torsion during flexion, for example, the lumbar joints are quite susceptible to rotational stress.

The Lumbar Intervertebral Foramina[24–27]

All vertebrae move in the planes of their articulations, and it is the posterior intervertebral articulations that most subluxations occur and influence the IVFs. Changes in the diameter of normal IVFs result in an abnormal joint formation which predisposes further subluxation and begins altering the curves of the particular region of the spine where this structural defect is found.

Size and Shape. Lumbar IVFs are shaped laterally like inverted teardrops or kidney beans, with the diameter of the vertical axes about double the anteroposterior (A-P) dimensions (Fig. 11.6). There is normally adequate space for changes in vertical dimension during normal movements without injury to the IVF contents, as long as there is adequate fat and fluid present and stenosis and adhesions are absent. However, reduction of the already short transverse diameter can produce a number of noxious effects. For this reason, disc collapse anteriorly is often asymptomatic, while a slight posterolateral herniation may protrude upon the IVF and produce severe symptoms.

IVF Contents. Each foramen widens and expands with spinal motion. From one-third to one-half of the foraminal opening is occupied by the spinal nerve root and its sheath, with the remaining portion filled essentially by fat, connective tissue, and various vessels. The IVF contains the anterior nerve root, the posterior nerve root, a part of the dorsal nerve root ganglion, a bilaminar sleeve of dura and arachnoid membrane to the ganglion, a short continuation of the subarachnoid space with cerebrospinal fluid which ends just after the ganglion, the recurrent meningeal nerve, the spinal ramus artery, the intervertebral vein, and lymphatic vessles.

IVF Diameter Changes Common factors altering the diameters of the IVFs are the disrelation of facet subluxation; the changes in the normal static curves of the spine; the presence of induced abnormal curves of the spine; degenerative thinning, bulging, or extrusion of the related intervertebral disc (IVD); the swelling and sclerosing of the capsular ligaments and the interbody articulation; and marginal proliferations of the vertebral bodies and articulations.

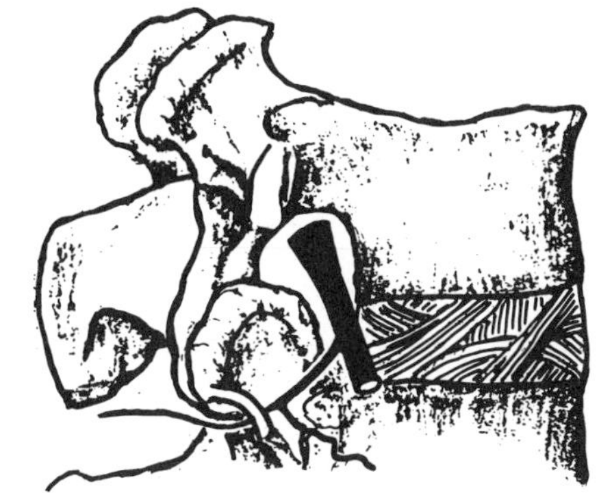

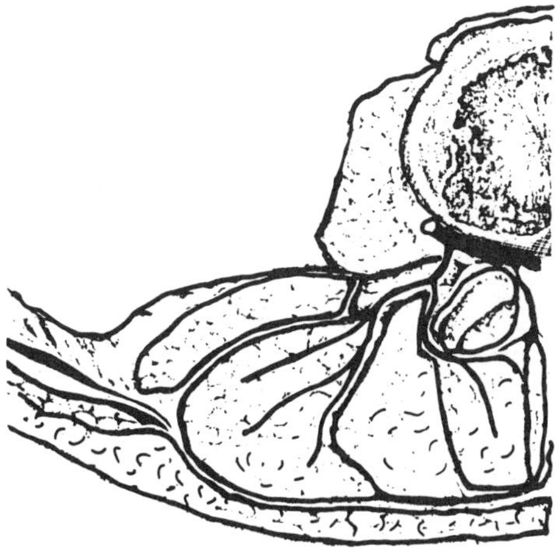

Figure 11.6. *Top*, the lumbar nerve root descends obliquely through the upper IVF, posterior to the vertebral body. The dorsal ramus runs laterally across the superior articular process and through a ligamentous tunnel. Only a small portion of this ligamentous channel is shown in the diagram. *Bottom*, the posterior division of the nerve root as viewed from above. Only the main branches are shown.

These factors affecting the IVF diameter insult the viable contents of the IVF. The result is nerve-root pressure, traction, or torque; constriction of the spinal blood vessels; intraforaminal and paraforaminal edema; induration and sclerosing of the periarticular ligaments with trauma to the receptors; forcing of the foraminal contents into protracted constriction and altered position; and such other consequences. Acute phenomena are usually the result of friction, severe or repeated trauma, and encroachment from degenerative thickening or exostosis, rather than of neurologic origin.

Lumbar Nerve Roots[28–30]

Several authorities state that the nerve roots are not normally fixed to the margins of the IVFs. Wyke and others report that they are. We can suspect that fibrotic changes following the granulation tissue of irritation, especially in the lumbosacral region, frequently fix the sleeve at one or more points, which contributes to traction on the sheath and its contents during movements such as exhibited in a straight-leg-raising test (Fig. 11.7). These abnormal attachments increase in strength with repetitive trauma, aging, and other degenerative changes.

Impingement Factors. In the lumbar spine, the nerve root runs anterior and superior to the facets. The nerve root is often compressed in the IVF by a subluxated articular facet and less often by a herniated disc or a spur from the posterior aspect of the vertebral body. These disorders can be worsened by a state of spinal stenosis which narrows the vertebral canal and the tunnel in which the nerve roots exit the IVFs.

Sensory Mechanisms. There are about twice as many sensory fibers as motor fibers in the lumbar roots. When the anterior root is irritated, pain is felt in the muscles supplied and often becomes self-perpetuating from the focal spasm produced. In posterior root irritation, pain can be felt in its dermatome, myotome, sclerotome, and possibly the viscerotome.

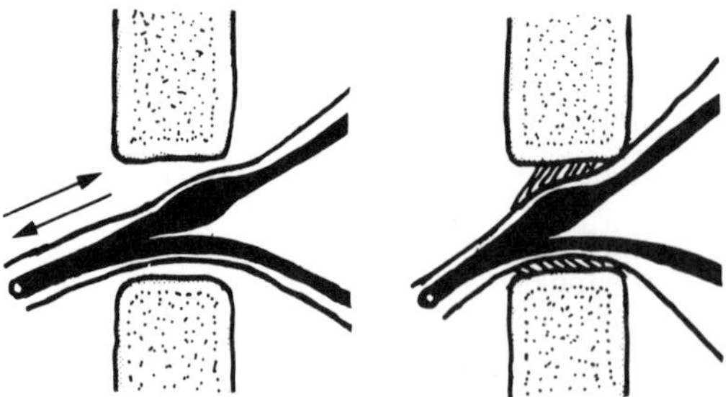

Figure 11.7. *Left*, a normal nerve root within the IVF is quite free to shift in and out of the foramen. *Right*, intraforaminal dural adhesions place considerable traction on the root complex during normal movements that stretch the sensitive tissues of the complex.

Developmental Defects[31–33]

Genetic factors frequently leave the lumbar spine in defect and instability, and the gross and subtle implications of anteroposterior balance, lateral balance, and rotational balance are manifold. The incidence of low-back disorders of a protracted and recurring nature is much higher in those patients whose spines show evidence of developmental defects and anomalies. This is especially true in the young.

Bipedism greatly augments the mechanical and neurologic complications of the lumbosacral complex. Such lumbosacral defects and complications as asymmetrical facet facing, imbrication, sacralization (especially the pseudo type), lumbarization, pars defect, discopathy, iliotransverse ligament sclerosing, retrolisthesis, and L5–S1 reverse rotation are important concerns.

Body weight during development wedges the sacrum between the innominates because of their peculiar laterally inclined planes. This allows the sacrum to move inferior, anterior, and medial, coupled with the anteroinferior angulation of the sacral base. Many of the abnormal orientations found in the lower spine are because the lumbar facet joints are not determined until the secondary curves are developed in the erect position. Forces imposed during maturation contribute greatly to the high incidence of asymmetry.

Nerve Distribution[34–38]

The segmental innervation of the lumbosacral spine to the major musculature supplied and the related skin and tendon reflexes are shown in Table 11.1. The major nerves of the lumbosacral plexus and their functions are given in Table 11.2. The main dorsal rami branches from a nerve root extend between the mutifidus muscle medially and the longissimus muscle laterally (see Fig. 11.6).

Kinesiology[8,39–43]

The trunk is held erect by the flexors and extensors of the spine and the extensors of the hip. The muscles and ligaments that hold the trunk erect are much stronger as a

Table 11.1.
Segmental Innervation of the Lumbosacral Spine

Segment	Major muscles supplied
L1–2	Cremaster
L1–5	Iliopsoas
L2–3	Sartorius, pectineus, abductor longus
L2–4	Quadriceps, gracilis, adductor brevis
L3–4	Obturator externus, adductor magnus and minimus
L4–5	Tibialis anticus
L4–S1	Semimembranosus, semitendinosus, extensor hallucis longus, popliteus, plantaris, extensor digitorum longus, extensor hallucis brevis, gluteus medius and minimus, quadratus
L5–S1	Peroneus longus and brevis, tibialis posticus, flexor digiti brevis, abductor hallucis
L5–S2	Gluteus maximus, obturator internus, biceps femoris, soleus, gastrocnemius, flexor hallucis longus
S1–2	Lumbricales, piriformis, abductor digiti, flexor digiti, opponens, quadratus plantae, interossei
S2–4	Levator ani, bulbocavernosus, ischiocavernosus
S4–5	Sphincter vesicae
S5–Cx1	Sphincter ani, coccygeus
Skin reflexes	
L1–2	Cremasteric
L4–S1	Gluteal
S1–2	Plantar
S5–Cx1	Anal
Tendon reflexes	
L2–4	Patellar
L5–S2	Achilles

whole than those of the pelvis. After a long illness, for example, a patient can sit erect long before he can stand.

Testing Muscle Weakness

Extension. Because A-P trunk motions are the most common movements used in daily living and because flexion is assisted by gravity, the spinal extensors are the most important muscles of the trunk from a biomechanical viewpoint (Fig. 11.8). It is also for this reason that back muscles are rarely weak unless paralysis is present. Kendall places the incidence of weak spinal erectors at less than 1% in the nonparalytic.[44] When signs of extension weakness are evident (Fig. 11.9), differentiation must be made between weak spinal extensors and weak hip extensors. A screening test can easily be done with the patient prone (Fig. 11.10).

Lateral Flexion. Trunk raising from the lateral recumbent position exhibits the strength of trunk lateral flexors and hip abductors. A simple screening test to differentiate weakness in these groups is shown in Figure 11.11.

Flexion. Leg raising from the supine position is a two-phase combination between strong abdominals and strong hip flexors. A screen test to differentiate weakness of the two groups is shown in Figure 11.12.

Testing Muscle Shortening

The postural patterns exhibited in forward flexion from the supine position can offer distinct clues to shortening of specific muscles and muscle combinations. Six typical patterns are shown in Figures 11.13 and 11.14.

Kinematics[45–52]

If lumbar active motions are normal, there is no need to test passively. A patient may be observed, however, who replaces normal lumbar motion by exaggerated hip motion, or vice versa. In such a situation, the range of motion of the restricted lumbar or hip joints should be passively tested. Any disorder of the hip joint itself (eg, fracture,

Table 11.2.
Nerve Function of the Lumbosacral Plexus

Nerve	Function
Iliohypogastric	Sensory to skin over hypogastric and lateral gluteal areas
Ilioinguineal	Sensory to skin over genitalia and upper medial thigh area
Genitofemoral	Sensory to skin over scrotum, upper anterior thigh area; motor to cremaster
Lateral femoral cutaneous	Sensory to skin over lateral thigh
Obturator	Motor to adductor longus, brevis, magnus; obturator externis; gracilis
Muscular branches	Motor to major and minor psoas, quadratus femoris, gemellus inferior and superior, piriformis, obturator internus
Femoral	Sensory to skin over anterior and medial thigh, knee, leg, dorsum of foot to base of 1st metatarsal
	Motor to iliacus, pectineus, sartorius, quadriceps femoris
Superior gluteal	Motor to gluteus minimus and medius, tensor fascia lata
Inferior gluteal	Motor to gluteus maximus
Posterior femoral cutaneous	Sensory to skin over inferior buttock, posterior thigh, popliteal space, perineum, external genitalia
Sciatic	Sensory to skin over posterolateral aspect of leg and lateral foot; heel; over upper third of lateral aspect of leg below knee; over anterolateral aspect of leg and dorsum of foot and toes; medial aspect of sole, great toe, 2nd to 4th toes; lateral aspect of sole, 4th and 5th toes; on dorsum of foot between great toe and 2nd toe
	Motor to hamstrings, adductor magnus; gastrocnemius; plantaris; soleus; popliteus; tibialis anterior and posterior; flexor and extensor digitorum longus and brevis; peroneus longus, brevis, and tertius; abductor and adductor hallucis; flexor hallucis brevis; extensor hallucis longus; quadratus plantae; abductor digiti quinti brevis; all interossei; 1st through 4th lumbricals
Pudendal	Sensory to skin of genitalia, anus, scrotum, labium majorus, penis, clitoris
	Motor to levator ani, coccygeus, sphincter ani externus, transversus perinei superficialis, profundus, bulbocavernosus, ischiocavernosus, sphincter urethrae membranaceae

tuberculosis, osteoarthritis) or of the hip flexor, adductor, abductor, or extensor muscles may result in limited hip motion.

The range of lumbar motion is determined by the disc's resistance to distortion, its thickness, and the angle and size of the articular surfaces. As in the thoracic spine, the movements of the lumbar spine are flexion, extension, lateral bending, and rotation. While lumbar motion is potentially greater than that of the thoracic spine because of the lack of rib restriction, facet facing and heavy ligaments check the range of rotary motion.

Joint Function

The lumbosacral facet planes are slightly more horizontal than those above them, allowing greater A-P and lateral motion but less joint locking than in the vertebrae above. This horizontal and anterior inclination of L5, spreading out toward the coronal plane, becomes progressively more vertical upward from L4 to L1. The upper joints are J-shaped when viewed from the lateral, thus the anterior aspect of the articulations resists forward displacement.

When the spine is in good alignment, facet articulation offers minimal friction. In

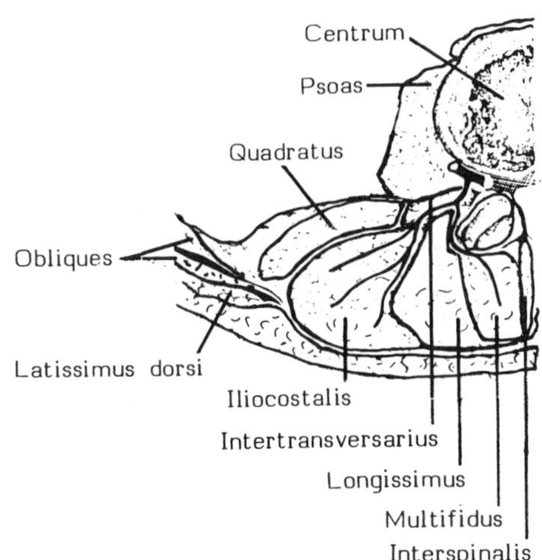

Figure 11.8. A cross section showing the major paraspinal muscles of the lower left back.

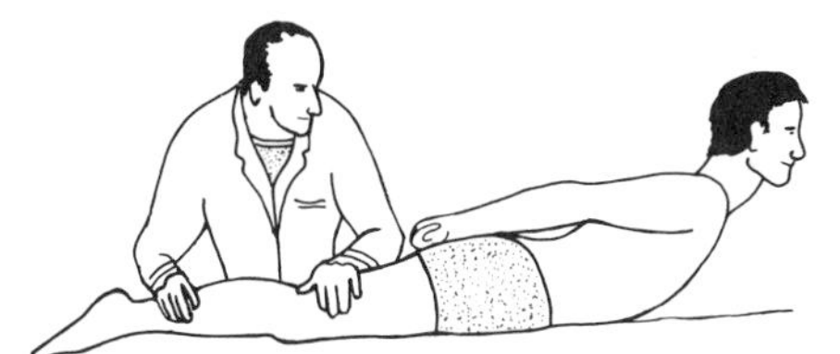

Figure 11.9. Screening active trunk extension strength with the patient prone.

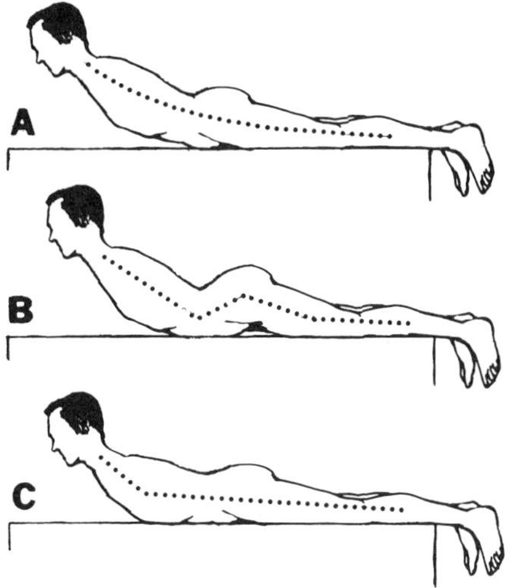

Figure 11.10. *A*, if both the back extensors and the hip extensors are strong, the patient will smoothly coordinate hip extension with spinal extension. *B*, if the spinal extensors are strong but the hip extensors are weak, the patient will hyperextend the trunk but the pelvis will fail to rotate posteriorly. *C*, if the spinal extensors are weak but the hip extensors are strong, the trunk will fail to arch but the pelvis will rotate posteriorly.

scoliosis, the articular surfaces are no longer parallel and the result is articular friction leading to impingement, erosion, and arthritis. This is the result of normally reciprocal articulating surfaces operating in an oblique position.

Motion of the Thoracolumbar Transitional Area

Because of the restriction of normal movements in the thoracic spine and the relatively mobile lumbar spine below, the intervening thoracolumbar area must achieve a degree of hypermobility in all three body planes. Because of this, as is true to some extent in all spinal transitional areas, the thoracolumbar junction is more prone to stress from both above and below because of its unusual design.

The superior facets of the transitional vertebra resemble thoracic facets and are designed for rotation and lateral flexion, even though these motions are restricted somewhat by the free ribs. While the stiff thoracic spine tends to move as a whole, most rotation takes place in the lower segments that are not restricted by the rib cage. The inferior facets of the transitional vertebra are of the lumbar type and are designed for flexion and extension. Although we readily observe great curves in the lumbar area, most of the apparent rotation seen is from distortion of the lumbar spine's base, tipping, and the lumbar lordosis viewed out of its normal plane.

Lateral Flexion

In the lumbar spine as a whole, lateral flexion is relatively free, followed in order of mobility by extension, flexion, and minimal rotation. Most significant to movements in the lumbar spine is the fact that all movements ae to some degree three-dimensional; ie, when the lumbar spine bends laterally, it tends to also rotate posteriorly on the side of convexity and assume a hyperlordotic tendency.

In evaluating lateral flexion of the lumbar spine, the standing or seated patient's right iliac crest should be stabilized as he leans to the left as far as possible. Then the same

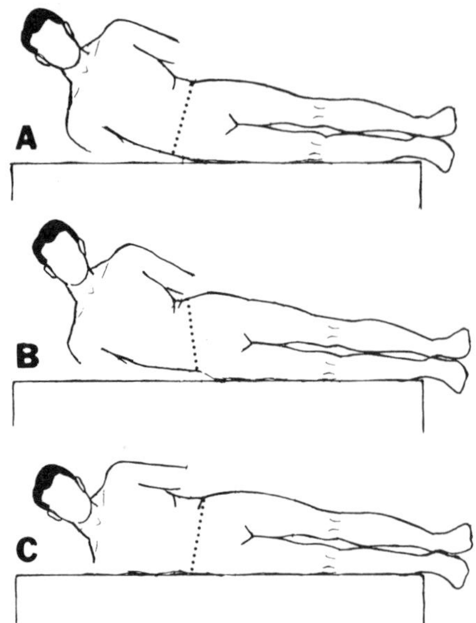

Figure 11.11. *A*, if both the flank muscles and the hip abductors are strong, the patient will smoothly coordinate trunk and hip lateral flexion, *B*, if the flank muscles are strong but the hip abductors are weak, the upper shoulder will flex and the upper pelvis not fixed by body weight will tend to move cephalad, reducing the rib-ilium distance. *C*, if the flank muscles are weak but the hip abductors are strong, the upper shoulder will fail to move much but the pelvis will tend to move caudad, increasing the rib-ilium distance.

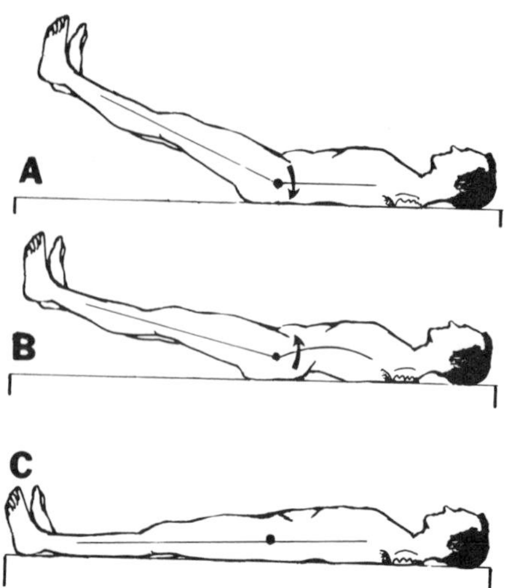

Figure 11.12. Slow leg raising and lowering in the supine position evaluates the strength of the abdominals and hip flexors. *A*, if the abdominals and hip flexors are both strong, leg raising and lowering can be accomplished by the patient consciously rotating the pelvis backward so that the lumbar spine is kept flat on the table. *B*, if the abdominals are weak but the hip flexors are strong, the lumbar spine will arch acutely into hyperlordosis at the higher degrees, the pelvis will rotate anterior, and the abdominals will stretch, increasing the sternal-pubic distance. *C*, if the abdominals are strong but the hip flexors are weak, the patient will be unable to lift the extremities from the table but there will be strong abdominal contraction that tends to decrease the sternal-pubic distance.

maneuver is repeated for the other side, and the degree of lateral flexion is noted.

During lateral bending in the erect position, considerable rotation accompanies the abduction motion if there is a significant degree of lordosis. However, if the lumbar spine is relatively flat or if the lateral bending is performed in the sitting position the amount of associated rotation is minimal. The intertransverse spaces of the normal spine open on the convex side and approximate on the concave side. In distinct lordosis, however, the facets are relatively locked and lateral flexion is so restricted that the vertebrae must severely rotate to allow lateral bending.

Flexion

During lower back flexion or extension, there is far less vertebral gliding than seen in other areas of the spine during A-P motion. Opening of the anterior disc space on extension or of the posterior disc space on flexion does not occur until movement nears its full range of motion. Even then, it is much less than that seen in other areas of the spine. The anterior longitudinal ligaments relax during flexion, and the supraspinal and interspinal ligaments stretch.

To measure flexion, the standing patient flexes forward and attempts to touch the floor with his fingertips. Measure the floor-fingertip distance. Such flexion in the adult will not normally result in a kyphosis of the lumbar area as flexion does in the cervical area. While a number of disorders result in decreased flexion, paraspinal muscle spasm is the prime suspect.

Extension

To test lumbar extension, the standing patient bends backward as far as possible. The patient is given support by the examiner

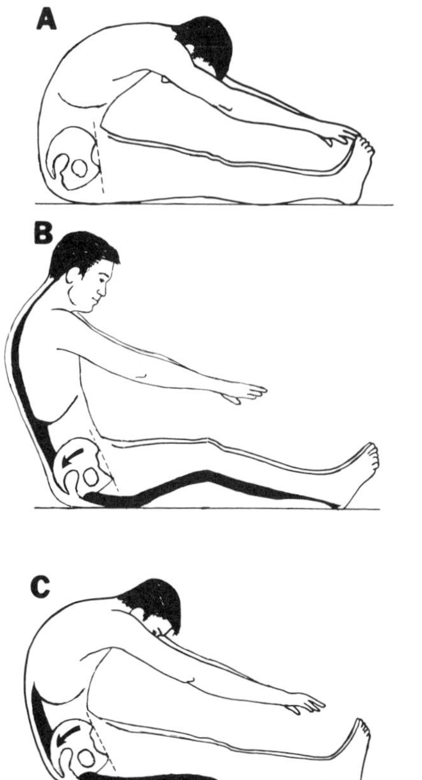

Figure 11.13. Testing length of some posterior muscle combinations. *A*, if the posterior spinal, thigh, and calf muscles have not shortened, forward flexion from the sitting position will produce a smoothly curved spine with little if any movement of the pelvis or knees. *B*, if the posterior muscles of the spine, thigh, and calf muscles have all shortened, forward flexion will be extremely limited, the pelvis will rotate posteriorly, and the knees will flex. *C*, if the lower back and hamstrings are moderately tight but the upper spinal and the calf muscles are not shortened, flexion will be restricted with the upper thoracic region arching smoothly, the lumbar region flattening, and the pelvis rotating posteriorly, but the knees will remain flat on the table.

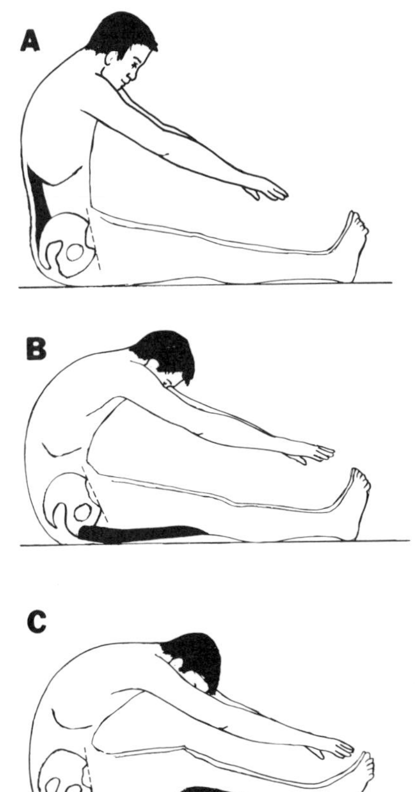

Figure 11.14. More tests for posterior muscle shortening combinations. *A*, if the posterior lower back muscles are severely shortened but the upper thoracic, hamstrings, and calf muscles are flexible, flexion will be restricted with the lumbar region holding some lordosis but the pelvis and knees remaining stable. *B*, if the hamstrings are shortened but the spinal and calf muscles are flexible, flexion will be restricted with the pelvis rotating posteriorly. The spine will curve smoothly and the knees will remain extended. *C*, if the calf muscles have shortened but the spinal and posterior thigh muscles are flexible, the spine will curve smoothly, the pelvis will remain stable, but the knees will flex.

placing one hand firmly on the patient's sacrum and the other hand on the patient's anterior chest.

The degree of extension is controlled by stretching of the anterior longitudinal ligament and rectus abdominis, relaxation of the posterior ligaments, and contraction of the spinal extensor muscles (Fig. 11.15). If posterior disc protrusion, facet inflammation, or spondylolisthesis exist, pain will be increased during extension.

Loss of lumbar extension is usually the result of poor sitting posture and/or inadequate extension mobilization following injury in which shortened scar tissue prevents a full range of extension. Reduced extension (1) causes chronic stress on the soft tissues of the posterior motion unit and an increased intradisc pressure during sitting; (2) restricts a fully upright posture during relaxed standing, leading to a stooped appearance in stance and gait; and (3) pro-

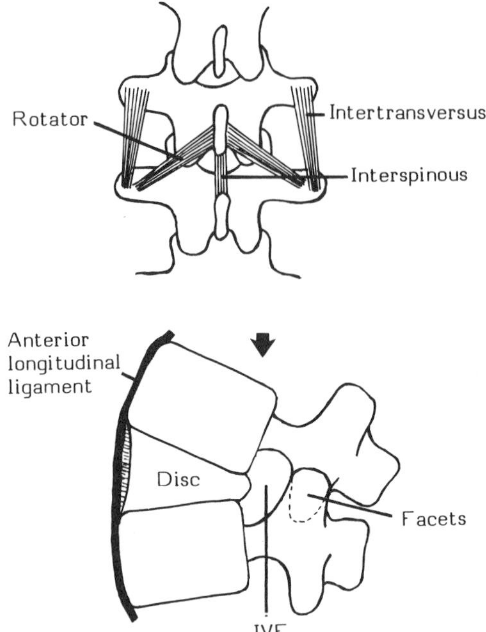

Figure 11.15. *Top*, the deep spinal extensor muscles. *Bottom*, a motion unit in extension. Note the movement required at the anterior longitudinal ligament, disc, and posterior facets. As the disc contracts anteriorly during extension, the fibers of the anterior longitudinal ligament that connect to the IVD become stressed.

duces a *premature* fully stretched lumbar posture when arising from a forward flexed posture.

It should be remembered that the fibers of the posterior anulus are the weakest. The anterior and lateral aspects of the anulus are almost twice as thick as the posterior aspect. The anular fibers at the posterior aspect of the disc are less numerous, narrower, and more parallel to each other than at any other portion of a disc.

If a person must work habitually in a prolonged forward flexed position, periodic lumbar extension will relieve the stress of the posterior anulus and tend to shift a loose nucleus pulposus anteriorly; ie, away from the spinal cord and IVF. Many manual workers do this maneuver automatically.

Rotation

If the axis of rotation of lumbar vertebrae were at the tips of the spinous processes, as sometimes is taught, the spinous process of L1 would be directly in line with the process of L5 during rotation while the vertebral bodies rotate to a greater degree toward the direction of movement. But because the center of rotation of T12 is distinctly anterior, it must pull L1 with it during rotation. This forces the lumbar region into rotation and flexion that jams the facets on the side moving posteriorly and opens the facets on the side moving anteriorly. This lumbar effect is continued to the sacrum, which also flexes and rotates with the lumbars.

Only a slight degree of rotational fixation is necessary to affect A-P and lateral bending motions. Because the facial planes are no longer reciprocal, normal motion becomes restricted. To grossly screen trunk rotation, the standing or sitting patient's pelvis is stabilized, and he is asked to turn his shoulders as far as possible to the left and then to the right.

Kinetic Tests in Distortion Patterns

A feature of any spinal and pelvic distortion is the fact that the segment or segments can be carried into the deviation of the distortion pattern much more readily than out of the gravitational pattern of the deviation. Two examples relative to the lumbar spine illustrate this: (1) If there is a right structural scoliotic deviation of the lumbar area, the patient sitting to fix the pelvis will find it easier to rotate the torso to the right than to the left. (2) If there is a left wedging of L5, L4, or L3, lateral flexion to the left is noticeably easier than lateral flexion to the right.

Biomechanical Instability[53–56]

Primary instability of the lumbar spine is considered to be a common cause of low-back pain. This refers to a loss of soft-tissue integrity leading to diminished intersegmental control, weakness, and liability to yield under normal stress and produce abnormal articular sliding (subluxation). The cause is frequently traumatic and most often seen in middle-aged males. The most common level involved is at the L4–L5 interfaces (90%).

Instability may be the result of rotation with or without much tilting, flexion with or without much rotation, lateral displacement (rare without fracture), lateral tilt and wedging, or extension overstress with or without spinous process impingement.

Segmental Stability

It is obvious that each spinal segment rests upon the one beneath it and that the interposed joint surfaces serve as the support base of the separate segments. The force of gravity acting upon each segment must be individually neutralized if the body as a whole is to be in complete gravitational balance. Thus, joint stability is partially dependent on (1) the size of the joint surfaces, (2) the height of the segmental centers of gravity above the joint surface, and (3) the horizontal distance of the common gravity line to the joint's center.

In the adult lumbar spine, the interspinous and supraspinous ligaments play a minimal role in segmental stability. White and Panjabi[57] report that these ligaments are frequently absent, degenerated, or ruptured.

Instability Characteristics

Painful attacks with severe splinting, often with brief episodes of paresis and paresthesia, are sudden in onset and frequently bilateral as opposed to the unilateral pain of a posterolateral disc protrusion. The paravertebral ligaments are extremely tender, and pain is increased by rotation. Neurologic signs and Lasegue's test are usually negative. In most cases, the acute attacks of instability are quickly relieved by rest and support.

The Role of Ligaments in Static Balance

When we stand in static equilibrium, we rest on our axial joints and ligaments. There is only light and intermittent muscular activity. As ligamentous support does not consume much energy, it does not contribute to fatigue. Chronic ligament tension, however, must be intermittently relieved by muscle activity and position changes to avoid chronic sprain.

The important ligaments involved in static balance are the lumbar anterior longitudinal ligament, which restricts lumbar "sinking"; the iliofemoral "Y" ligaments at the anterior hip, which guard hip hyperextension; the tensor fasciae latae, which assist the "Y" ligaments, restrict lateral sway, and help the knees to lock; and the posterior knee ligaments, which lock the knees in extension (Fig. 11.16). The ankles cannot be locked, thus they require slight intermittent contraction of the leg muscles.

The pelvic angle is the key to ligament stability. Lateral pelvic tilting from a unilateral short leg, for example, is accompanied by load shifting to the lower hip and pelvic rotation that unlocks the weight-bearing joints of the lower extremities. The lumbar spine will not bend laterally without some rotation. This change in equilibrium forces imposes increased muscular effort to maintain balance, and this leads to general fatigue.

GENERAL FULL SPINE POSTURAL EXAMINATION CONSIDERATIONS[58–64]

A comprehensive postural evaluation should include a comparative analysis of the physical signs found in the standing, sitting, Adams, prone, and supine positions,

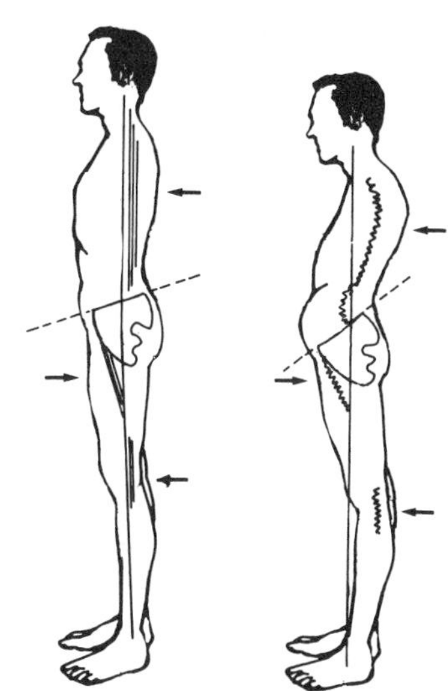

Figure 11.16. *Left*, the major ligaments involved in maintaining static balance are the anterior longitudinal ligament of the spine, the anterior iliofemoral ligaments of the pelvis, and the posterior ligaments of the knees. *Right*, typical posture of severe ligament laxity. Note loss of height, flattened chest and thoracic kyphosis, pot belly and lumbar hyperlordosis, anterior rotation of pelvis, and genu recurvatum. This posture exhibits biomechanical failure (sinking) from the pull of gravity.

both with and without use of a plumb line or grid.

In the horizontal positions, the lumbar spine is in extension when a person is supine on a firm mattress or prone on either a firm or soft mattress. The lumbar spine is in flexion when a person is supine on a hammock or an extremely soft mattress. In the relaxed lateral recumbent position, the lumbar region glides laterally (with some coupled rotation) toward the floor—especially if the mattress is soft.

The Standing Position

The patient stands with the heels together and hands hanging normally at his sides. He should be encouraged to stand normally and not try to assume "good posture" or the "military stance." Then the following are noted:

1. Abnormal rotation or tilt of the patient's head. The cervical and suboccipital muscles are digitally explored. Asymmetrical fullness of the suboccipital musculature usually indicates upper cervical rotation.

2. Overall curvatures of the spine. They are evaluated as normal, lordotic, kyphotic, or scoliotic.

3. The comparative height of the scapulae. The cervicobrachial spine is always scoliotic toward the side of the high shoulder. Winged scapulae or scapulae failing to lie smoothly upon the chest wall are sought. The midthoracic spine is always scoliotic toward the side on which the vertebral margin of the scapula is more prominent and flaring. If the shoulder is high on the right and the scapula flares on the right, the entire cervicobrachial and thoracic spine is scoliotic toward the right. If the shoulder is high on the right yet the left scapula flares, it indicates that the cervicobrachial spine is scoliotic to the right and the midthoracic spine is scoliotic to the left. The contours of the area muscles are digitally explored to seeks signs of abnormal tightness or tenderness.

4. The angles of the ribs. In pelvic mechanical pathologies on the side of involvement, there is a reduction in the height and depth of the body angle as observed from the A-P. A difference in the height of the scapula and the iliac crests usually indicates a scoliosis. The transverse processes of the lumbar vertebrae are palpated. Lateral positions of the spinous processes and anterior or posterior positions of the transverse processes together with an elevation of the angles of the ribs would indicate a rotation of vertebrae. The possibility of a spinous process being asymmetrical, deviated to the right or left, without the body of the vertebra being involved should be kept in mind.

5. The comparative height of the iliac crests. A low and less prominent iliac crest will be best observed from the front. If chronic sciatic neuralgia is on the high iliac crest side, degenerative disc weakening with posterolateral protrusion should be suspected. If occurring on the side of the low iliac crest, the possibility of a sacroiliac slip and lumbosacral torsion should first be considered as a causative factor.

6. Seated behind the patient, the examiner reaches around the crests and places a finger of each hand upon the ASISs. As the patient leans slightly forward, it is noted whether there is abnormal pressure on the finger on one iliac spine as compared with the other.

7. The position of the gluteal cleft. A line passed through the crease of the buttocks should demonstrate its lower end equally between the feet and its upper end over the C7 spinous process and the occipital protuberance. Tension of the gluteals and the comparative height and depth of the sacral dimples are noted.

Elderly patients may lose considerable height compared to their height in early maturity due to the thickening of the ligaments, weakening of the musculature, and thinning of the IVDs. The range of motion of the spine is, of course, considerably less.

Although the lumbar spine falls into full flexion during relaxed or prolonged sitting, prolonged standing in a relaxed posture places the lower lumbar spine into full extension. Thus, if symptoms are aggravated by prolonged standing, it is evident that sustained lumbosacral extension is causing a mechanical deformation. If symptoms are relieved by prolonged standing, therapy should be directed to obtaining sustained extension. Forward bending puts the lumbar spine in hyperflexion, and overhead work puts the lumbar spine into hyperextension.

The most common standing postural fault associated with low-back pain is not hyperlordosis; it is an abnormal flattening of the lumbar area. Frequently associated is a lateral shift (scoliosis) away from the midline.

Plumb Line Analysis[65]

Lateral. From each side, the line should cut through the ear lobe, slightly posterior to the mastoid process, through the odontoid, through the tip of the shoulder, the anterior edges of T2 and T12, through the centrum of L3, just anterior to S2, just posterior to the axis of the hip, posterior to the patella, anterior to the lateral malleolus of the ankle, through the cuboid-calcaneal junction, and through the 5th metatarsal of the foot.

Posterior. From the back, the line should cut through the occipital protuberance, through the spinous processes, through the gluteal crease, through the coccyx, and bisect the knees and ankles. The horizontal level of the ears, shoulders, scapulae, rib angles, iliac crests, greater trochanters, knee joints, and malleoli should be noted.

Anterior. From the front, the line should cut between the eyes, through the nose and neck, through the sternum, xiphoid process, navel, pubic symphysis, and bisect the knees and ankles. The horizontal level of the ears, shoulders, nipples, rib angles, iliac crests, hips, patellae, and malleoli should be noted.

An alternative to the simple plumb line that offers multiplane postural measurements is the Stan-a-Graf (Fig. 11.17). This instrument provides a means to record postural distortion in degrees.

The Sitting Position[66]

The patient sits on an examining stool, thus immobilizing the pelvis. He rotates his body first to the right and then to the left. Then he laterally bends first to the right and then to the left. Finally, he flexes and then extends the spine, and the integrity of the column during these movements is observed. Any abnormal motion should be noted.

A spinal segment always rotates or deviates into a distortion pattern with greater ease than out of the distortion pattern. We previously discussed that, if the atlas shows a left lateral shift, right lateral flexion of the head is greater than the same effort to the left. If the upper cervical segments indicate vertebral body rotation to the right, the head and neck actively and passively rotate to the right with greater ease than to the left. If there is a right cervicoscoliosis, the patient can laterally flex his head to the left much more readily than to the right. The same principles apply in the thoracic and lumbar regions. If there is a right structural scoliotic deviation of the lumbar area, the patient sitting, with pelvis fixed, will find it easier to rotate the torso to the right than to the left. Later flexion will be further on the side of concavity than the side of convexity.

McKenzie's experiences[67] indicate that "almost all low-back pain is aggravated and perpetuated, if not caused, by poor sitting postures in both sedentary and manual workers." Watching a relaxed patient's posture during the history and examination will tell the alert examiner almost as much as the history of low-back pain itself.

The typical sitting posutre leading to low-back pain is characterized by the common decrease or the less common increase of the normal lumbar curve to the extent that the involved ligaments are placed under maximum stretch for a prolonged period. This eventually leads to pain. As few chairs contain a lumbar roll to maintain the normal lordosis, the longer a person sits in a relaxed position, the more the muscles relax and weight-bearing stress must be absorbed by the ligaments. Thus, if poor sitting posture (eg, lumbar flexion) is within the patient's history of low-back pain, continued poor sitting posture will perpetuate the problem and often enhance the symptoms while seated or when arising from a seated position. Likewise, if symptoms are aggravated by prolonged sitting, it is evident that sustained flexion is causing a mechanical deformation and therapy should emphasize lumbar extension. If symptoms are relieved by prolonged sitting, therapy should be directed to obtaining sustained flexion.

People who habitually sit with the lumbar area stretched (flexed) constantly place abnormal tension upon the weak posterior aspect of the anuli and the soft tissues and facets of the posterior motion units. In addition, habitual sitting in lumbar flexion leads to a loss in the range of motion of

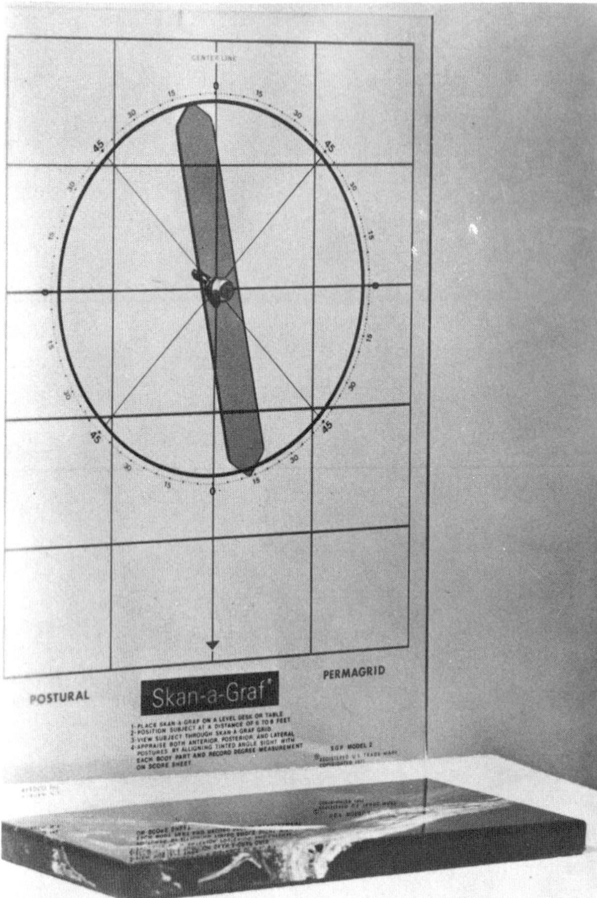

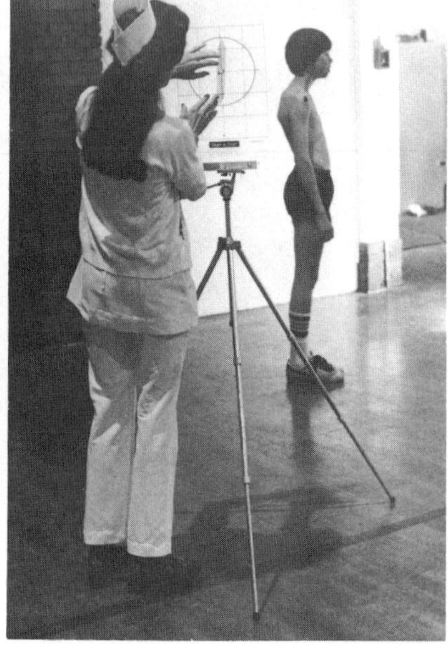

Figure 11.17. The Stan-a-Graf posture analyzer. Objective postural analysis that offers numerical data is best made by an instrument that does not touch the subject's skin. Even slight cutaneous stimulation will produce reflex muscle actions that may give erroneous findings. (With the permission of Reedco Research, Auburn, N.Y.)

lumbar extension, which influences segmental motions in sitting, standing, and gait.

The Adams Position

The patient assumes the Adams position by standing erect, with his heels together, then bending forward with his fingers as near the floor as possible without straining. For an indication of gross spinal flexibility, the distance between the fingertips and the floor should be measured or at least observed. In bending, the knees should not flex. As a patient advances in age and the spine settles, there will of course be less flexibility. Stiffness would also occur with hypertonic or spastic paravertebral muscles.

While the patient goes in and out of the flexed Adams position, the following points are noted: (1) Is flexion unrestricted? (2) Is flexion straight forward or deviated laterally? (3) Do the spinous processes line up straight during forward flexion and extension from flexion? This is more easily determined by dotting the spinous processes with a skin pencil when in the standing position. (4) Are there abnormal prominences or movements of the angles of the ribs during A-P motion? Is the pelvis level? The two most common clinical signs that appear are (1) restriction of end motion (motion block, with or without pain) in which the patient's fingers stop far above the floor, and/or (2) scoliotic rotation of the spine in which the vertebral bodies follow the plane of least resistance (structural or antalgic).

Repetitive Loading

As previously discussed in earlier chapters, repetitive loading has beneficial effects on shortened tissues and adverse effects on the disc or an area of inflammation (eg, sciatic neuritis). To test the effects of repetitive lumbar flexion loading, the standing patient is asked to flex forward to the *maximum* and return to normal stance ten times in succession. If the patient's pain increases, a disc involvement or area of inflammation is probably the factor involved. If the patient's pain reduces, shortened tissues are most likely the origin of the patient's pain.

Common Causes of Idiopathic Scoliosis

There are several biomechanical influences expressed in idiopathic scoliosis when viewed in the Adams position. They can be best appreciated by test movements that place normal stress on normal or abnormal tissues. The most common factors involved are: (1) A rotatioal subluxation, causing the superior segment to follow the plane of its base. (2) An area of acute or subacute inflammation (eg, myositis, strain, sprain), causing deviation away from the site of pain. (3) An anatomical or functional short leg, causing the lumbar spine to follow the tipped base of the sacrum. (4) The presence of scar tissue from repeated attacks of disc or facet injury, causing restricted forward flexion and a slight swing toward the side of abnormal stiffness. (5) A laterally displaced nucleus pulposus, causing flexion away from the painful side. (6) The presence of a fixed nerve root (mechanically entrapped or locked by adhesions), causing lateral deviation during forward flexion toward the side of binding. Forward flexion in the standing position places considerable stretch on the sciatic nerve. (7) Bilateral or unilateral fixation of a posterior motion unit, causing restricted forward flexion. (8) Asymmetrical facets or facets facing in an unusual plane.

Lumbosacropelvic Rhythm

The Adams maneuver is possibly the best to detect unusual vertebral rotation and ascertain the integrity of lumbosacropelvic rhythm. This latter point is an excellent method of gathering accurate clues of biomechanical faults, and it may be well to briefly review the mechanisms involved. Forward flexion takes place in two phases. During the first 60° of flexion, the pelvis is locked by the posterior pelvic muscles. About 70% of this motion occurs at the lumbosacral joint, 20% between L5 and L4, and 10% between the L1 and L3 vertebrae. The motion is smoothed by the counterforce of the spinal extensors. During the second phase, from 60° to 85°, the hip releases and the pelvis rotates bilaterally forward around the transverse axis of the hip joints. Near the end of spinal flexion, the sacral base slightly follows L5 anteroinferiorly as the sacral apex pivots posterosuperiorly. Perfect synchronization of these lumbar-sacral-pelvic motions must be achieved to obtain minimal biomechanical stress. Abnormalities in these mechanisms will quickly point out and help differentiate sites of lumbar, sacral, or hip restrictions or instability (Fig. 11.18).[68]

Flexion from Neutral

During the first stage of flexion, the normal lumbar lordosis gradually flattens and then gradually develops a smooth curved kyphosis. In many people, the degree of lumbar flexion is up to and only slightly over the flattening of the normal lordosis, thus total possible flexion must be achieved by hip rotation. In fact, some people can bend forward to touch the floor with little

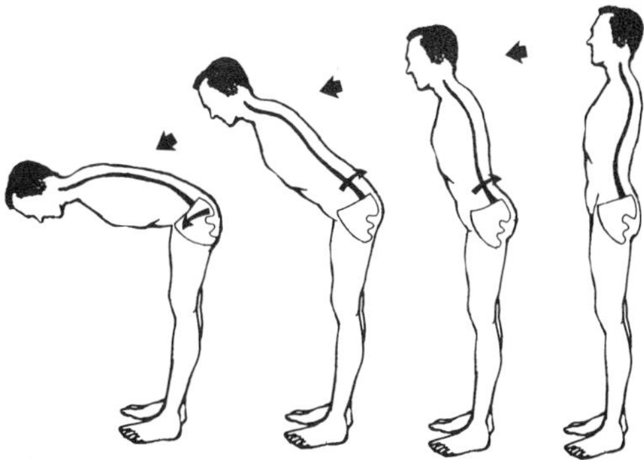

Figure 11.18. In normal lumbosacropelvic rhythm, the lumbar lordosis flattens and is smoothly coordinated with anterior pelvic rotation during flexion. Lumbar motion is dominant during the first 60° of flexion, then pelvic motion about the femurs becomes dominant.

change in the spinal curves. This is often due to hypermobile ilia and hips adapting to lumbar fixation.

If the lumbar curve fails to flatten during trunk flexion, the first suspicions should be restriction of the posterior elements from muscular hypertonicity, ligamentous shortening, or abnormal articular planes. Unilateral facet asymmetries will often be revealed by a distinct scoliosis exhibited in the Adams position that is not apparent at all in the erect position. If pelvic rotation fails to occur, the first suspicions should be sciatic irritation, hip restriction, or tight hamstrings. If a hamstring fails to elongate unilaterally, distinct contralateral lumbar rotation will be seen during flexion as L5 follows the low sacrum.

Segmental Faults

As the patient goes into and out of the Adams position, the vertebral column should be examined for individual segments that flatten or arch at the wrong time or do not move evenly with their neighbors. Palpation should be done with the fingerpads upon the interspinous spaces. With motion by the patient, the various segments of the spine can be felt to glide closer together or further apart. Should an area be found that remains rather immobile or without the normal gliding action, further tests and x-ray studies should be made of this section of the spine.

When one or more spinous processes are out of alignment, spinal lesions, subluxations, or an abnormality of the spinous process are indicated. Frequently, two or more spinous processes that are out of alignment will indicate multiple subluxations in portions of the vertebral column, perhaps with the exception of the middle thoracic column, but even these may sometimes be involved.

Rotation during Flexion

Where the spine does not bend straight forward, but deviates to one side, even slightly, a search should be instituted for contractured, thickened, or shortened muscles, tendons, and/or ligaments of the column existing on one side and not on the other. If the spine shows rotation to the right, the patient in a forward bent position can swing his torso into right rotation much more readily than to the left.

In common pelvic mechanical pathologies on the side of involvement, there is an observable slanting and anteriority of the pelvis in the forward bending position. There will be a noticeable lumbar scoliosis to the side of involvement.

Elevation or prominence of the ribs on either side denotes a rotation of the vertebrae upon their axes. Shortening of the ligaments with contracture of the musculature of the spine will be exhibited by abnormal stiffness or hardness of the muscles on the side of the spine that suffers from contractures. Compare the position of the dots over the spinous processes with their appearance when the patient was in the anatomical position.

Extension from Flexion

Return extension occurs in reverse order of these two phases, and just as much information can be gathered as the patient returns to the neutral position as during flexion. If a load is being lifted, the vast majority of the force is upon the posterior lumbar ligaments until about 60° when the back muscles become active and the abdominals serve to smooth the action. The main function of the longitudinal ligaments is to restrict abnormal motion. If there is segmental restriction, excessive motion is forced upon the adjacent segments and the hips. Hip restriction forces excessive motion upon the lumbar spine and sacrum. If there is excessive joint laxity, subluxation with or without sprain or strain may occur. The most common fault recognized in extension from full flexion is premature return of lumbar lordosis (Fig. 11.19). If this occurs, the first suspicion should be weak hamstrings and/or other pelvic extensors. Associated weak abdominals will contribute to faulty pelvic stabilization.

Standing Hyperextension

The standing patient is asked to place his palms in the small of his back, bend backward, and then move his hands distally down his buttocks and the back of his thighs as far as possible. The examiner's fingertips should be placed in the lumbar interspinous spaces to note segmental motion. Extension

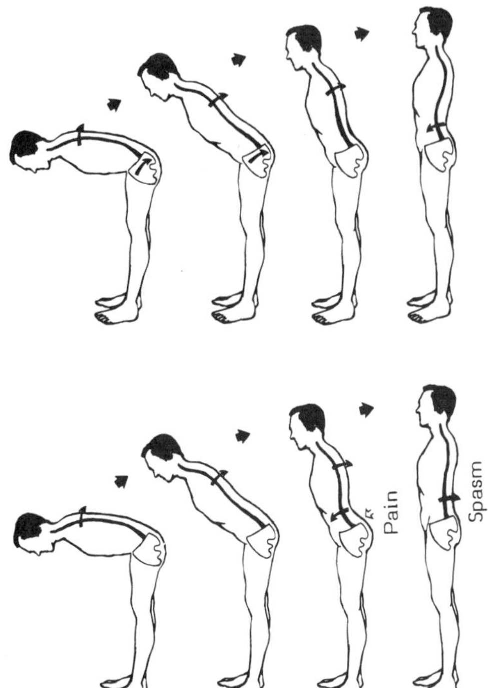

Figure 11.19. *Top*, normal extension from flexion. First phase of return is primarily pelvic, with lumbar lordosis returning only near the neutral position. *Bottom*, if the pelvis fails to rotate posteriorly during extension because of weak hip extensors (rarely painful) or hyperactive lumbar extensors (often painful), the lumbar spine will develop a hyperlordosis near 60° that places severe stress upon the lumbosacral joint. In approaching the neutral position, this stress is often reacted to by a flattening (spasm) of the lumbar curve, exhibiting an antalgic stiff spine.

occurs from above downward. The maximum range of motion, and the production, increase, or reduction of pain and its distribution should also be evaluated. Before concluding this part of the examination, the examiner should test the effects of repetitive loading.

Restricted extension is usually the result of fixation at the posterior motion unit that prevents facet gliding. Increased pain during hyperextension suggests a rotational subluxation. When a fixed posterolateral herniation is present, the patient will have restricted extension with deviation away from the side of pain.

Standing Lateral Bending

The standing patient is asked to flex sideward and move his hand on the side of bending distally down the side of his thigh as far as possible. This point should be recorded. Lateral flexion should occur from above downward. The examiner's fingertips should be placed in the lumbar interspinous spaces to evaluate segmental motion. The maximum range of motion and the production, increase, or reduction of pain and its distribution should also be evaluated. It is not unusual to find that one side is unrestricted and the other side is blocked. This suggests a degree of scoliosis, with restricted movement on the side of convexity. A laterally displaced nucleus pulposus would have the same effect. Before concluding this part of the examination, the examiner should test the effects of repetitive loading.

The Prone Position

This is the typical position in which many chiropractic examiners palpate the spine. It is important that the patient lie on a flat surface rather than on a table with built-in convolutions that may confuse findings.

As the patient lies prone, the dots over the spinous processes are again observed. They may be quite altered and decidedly changed from their appearance in either the anatomical or Adams position. Patients in poor health and/or with chronic disease tend to have an increased distortion of the spinal column when in the prone position. However, this distortion may diminish or disappear when the patient assumes a supine position.

A stiff distortion of the spinal column may suggest spondylitis deformans. In this condition, the movements of the spine are diminished or may perhaps eventually be lost. It is important to note in spondylitis that the curvatures of the spine are not influenced by movements or by changes in the examining position of the patient. In fact, many spinal curvatures and disorders might be missed if the spine is examined with the patient only in the prone position.

A scoliosis will sometimes present a lordosis and a somewhat anterior curvature of the spine between the scapulae. When this condition exists, there is generally a flattening of the anterior curvature of the lumbar vertebrae. In conditions in which the paravertebral musculature is weakened, we may see a lateral curvature of the spinal column with no appreciable rotation of the vertebra. This lateral deviation will disappear when the patient assumes different positions. The paravertebral muscles can be weakened by long illness, chronic degenerative conditions, malnutrition, or by chronic hysteria or emotional stress.

In common pelvic mechanical problems on the side of involvement, (1) the posterior superior iliac spine (PSIS) palpates as being prominent and inferior in comparison with that of the opposite side due to the posterior innominate rotation; (2) the ischial tuberosity palpates as being less prominent and anterior; and (3) the spinous process of S1 approximates the PSIS on the side of involvement due to the anteroinferior shifting of the sacrum which carries its centrum toward the posterior innominate.

With the patient in the prone position, a re-examination by palpation of the spinous processes, transverse processes, and the paravertebral musculature should be made.

Recumbent Hyperextension

A patient's spine is automatically placed in extension when the prone position is assumed. The prone patient is asked to lift his trunk upward by extending his elbows, yet keeping his lower pelvis firm against the examining table. This is similar to a push-up in which the pelvis is not raised. A much greater degree of lumbosacral hyperextension can be achieved in the prone position than in the standing position. As in the other tests, the examiner's fingertips should be placed in the lumbar interspinous spaces to note segmental motion; the maximum range of motion and the production, increase, or reduction of pain and its distribution should be evaluated. Before concluding this part of the examination, the examiner should test the effects of repetitive loading.

A small disc protrusion would be reduced by segmental extension, thus extension should relieve pain. However, an entrapped fragment or protrusion would not be benefited and might be aggravated.

The Supine Position

This position is often neglected by practitioners in performing their spinal examination, diagnosis, and/or analysis. This is unfortunate because it is an excellent position for accurately palpating cervical and upper thoracic vertebrae and related soft tissues.

With the patient lying in the dorsal recumbent position, the examiner, while standing at the patient's head, holds the patient's head between his two hands with the tips of the index and middle fingers palpating and easily determining the alignment of the spinous processes of the upper dorsals and of the entire cervical column. If the head is sufficiently flexed, the forward curve of the cervical spine will be reduced and so changed that the spinous processes of the cervical vertebrae will be separated, enabling their positions to be more easily palpated. In this position, the comparative size of the interspaces of the spinous processes of each consecutive vertebra should be examined.

The advantage of this position in the palpation of the spinous processes is that the extensor muscles of the neck are at rest while the head is being slightly raised; consequently, they are nonresistant to the palpating fingertips. It is only the flexor muscles of the cervical region that may be put into action by the patient, providing he tries to assist the palpator to raise or hold his head in the elevated position. This assistance should be discouraged.

In common pelvic mechanical problems on the side of involvement, (1) the ASIS palpates as being superior, (2) there is increased tenderness over the lateral portion of the inguinal ligament, and (3) there is increased tenderness over the origin of the sartorius muscle.

Upon fully extending the legs in pelvic mechanical pathologies, the leg on the side of involvement will be retracted ¼–½ inch shorter than the opposite leg because the posterior innominate rotation causes the acetabulum to be carried superior and anterior—the superior position producing the retraction of the limb. However, upon bringing the extremities upward to an extended position at right angles to the body, the short leg now measures the longest. It is the anterior position of the acetabulum that now produces the added length.

This multiposition visual and palpatory examination is one of the first steps in physical spinal analysis. In no way should it preclude the use of necessary instrumentation, laboratory procedures, or thorough roentgenography.

Recumbent Hyperflexion

The supine patient is asked to grasp his flexed knees, pull them toward his abdomen, and flex his neck forward in an attempt to touch his forehead between his knees. In this position, flexion should occur from below upward and a greater stretch is placed on the lumbosacral area than can be achieved in the standing position. The examiner's fingertips should be placed in the lumbar interspinous spaces to evaluate segmental motion. At the same time, the examiner should note the maximum range of motion and the production, increase, or reduction of pain and its distribution. Before concluding this part of the examination, the examiner should test the effects of repetitive loading.

In contrast to forward flexion in the standing position, flexion in the supine position places little tension on the sciatic nerve. Thus, sciatica that is aggravated by both standing and supine flexion suggests a disc involvement. Sciatica that is aggravated in the standing but not the supine position suggests a nerve root involvement.

Gait Analysis

The most stressful action in gait on a painful lumbar spine appears to be that point at which lordosis is increased by the propelling hind leg in extension. Thus, if symptoms are aggravated by prolonged walking, it is evident that repetitive lumbosacral extension is causing a mechanical deformation. If symptoms are relieved by prolonged walking, therapy should be directed to obtaining sustained lumbosacral extension.

The degree and timing of body oscillation, pelvic coronal tilt, axial rotation, horizontal displacement, knee and ankle flexion, out-of-phase vertebral motion, stride width, and walking speed should be carefully noted. Signs of an antalgic posture during gait should be sought, and if present, an immediate attempt to isolate the cause should be made. These points have been discussed in Chapter 4.

THE PELVIS AND SACRUM: ANATOMICAL AND KINEMATIC CONSIDERATIONS

The pelvis (basin) is the anatomical link between the axial skeleton and the lower extremities. Each half of the pelvic girdle consists of the ilium, ischium, and pubic bones, which are three separate bones during early life that retain their separate identity in adulthood, even though they become completely fused. Although the hip joint is anatomically considered part of the lower extremity, it is so closely linked biomechanically to the sacrum and lumbar spine that it must be considered in any discussion of the pelvis.

Functional Anatomy[69–77]

Pelvis design differs greatly between the sexes (Fig. 11.20). In addition, there are wide individual variations, and asymmetry is more the rule than the exception. Thus, static palpation alone can lead to many erroneous conclusions.

The common pelvic landmarks are the anterior superior iliac spine (ASIS), posterior superior iliac spine (PSIS), and anterior inferior iliac spine (AIIS). The summit of the iliac crest is normally on a level with the L4 spinous process, and the PSIS is on a level with the S2 spinous and near the midline of the lower third of the sacroiliac articulation.

The Ilia[78,79]

The ilia serve as the superior elements of the pelvis. They articulate anteriorly via the symphysis pubis and posteriorly at the sacrum. The superior flared wings of the ilia (false or major pelvis) support the lower abdomen. The lower half of the pelvis forms the true or minor pelvis which is surrounded by the pubes, lower iliac, ischia, and sacrum. The inferior aspect of the lateral ilium forms the superior aspect of the acetabulum.

The Iliac Facet. Anterolateral to the PSIS and the PIIS of the ilium is the convex facet that articulates with the sacrum. As it resembles a rough, bony ear facing backward, it is called the auricular surface. Some refer to it as being boot-shaped, with the toe pointing backward (Fig. 11.21). Regardless, it is slightly wider than its mate on the sacrum, but the surface area of the sacral facet is

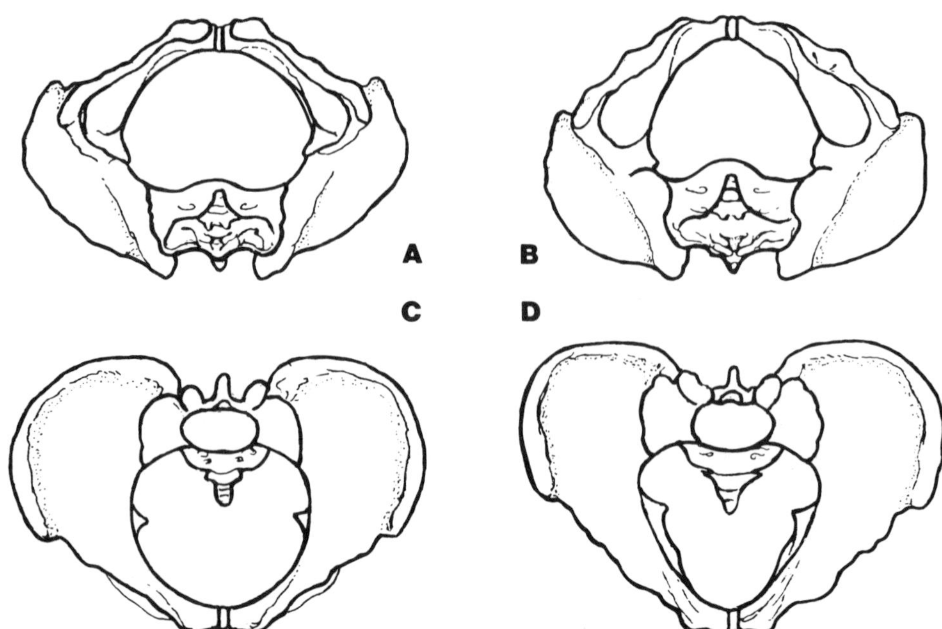

Figure 11.20. Schematic comparison of the architecture of the female pelvis from below (*A*) with that of the male pelvis from below (*B*), and the female pelvis from above (*C*) with the male pelvis from above (*D*).

slightly longer than that of the ilium. The anterior-superior aspect of the iliac facet, which articulates with the superiolateral aspect of S1 at the foot of the boot, contains a much deeper pit than that of its inferior-posterior aspect. This pit and the reciprocal sacral tubercle enlarge with age.

Boorsma[80] reports that this boot-shaped articular design is relatively deep, oblique, mobile, and especially related to a hyperlordotic spine. When associated with a flattened lumbar spine, the sacroiliac articulation is more bean-shaped, vertical, shallow, and less mobile.

This short arm or foot of the articulation allows a sliding motion anteroinferior or posteroinferior and a rotating action about the pit. The foot of the boot articulates with the S2–S3 segments. This design has a distinct influence on traumatic iliosacral motion. The upper pit also serves to offer osseous relief to the relatively weak superoanterior ligaments. An important role of this design is to prevent sacral displacement during loaded movements. Superior and posterior to the articular surface is a larger area of rough bone that serves for the attachment of strong sacroiliac ligaments.

During aging degeneration, calcium infiltration of the joint appears within the fibrocartilage of the ilium long before changes occur in the hyaline coated sacral facet. This is most likely because the sacral cartilage is three times thicker than the iliac cartilage.

The Sacrum and Coccyx[81–83]

The adult sacrum is composed of five fused segments. As a whole, it resembles the keystone of an arch. Some authors such as Boorsma take exception to this analogy, and from a gross aspect they are correct inasmuch as the sacral base is tipped anteriorly and inferiorly.[80] The keystone image cannot be appreciated unless one visualizes all sacral bone chipped away except that between the sacroiliac joints.

The sacrum also resembles an inverted pyramid from the front, back and sides (Fig. 11.22). Its dorsal surface is convex while its anterior surface is concave. To meet with the flared ilia, the S1–S3 segments are wider anteriorly than posteriorly. The concave sacral articulation with the ilia is congruently boot-shaped, and its numerous bumps and depressions offer stability and limit motion. These ridges and furrows,

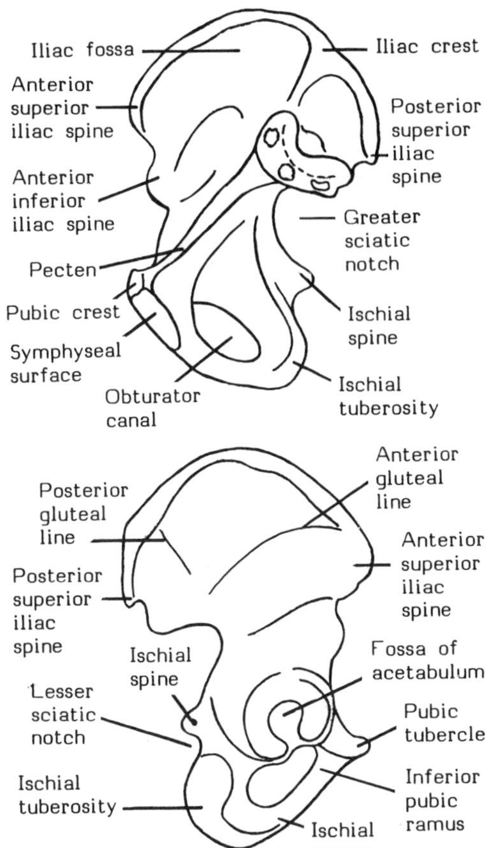

Figure 11.21. Major features of the medial aspect of the pelvis (*top*) and the lateral aspect (*bottom*).

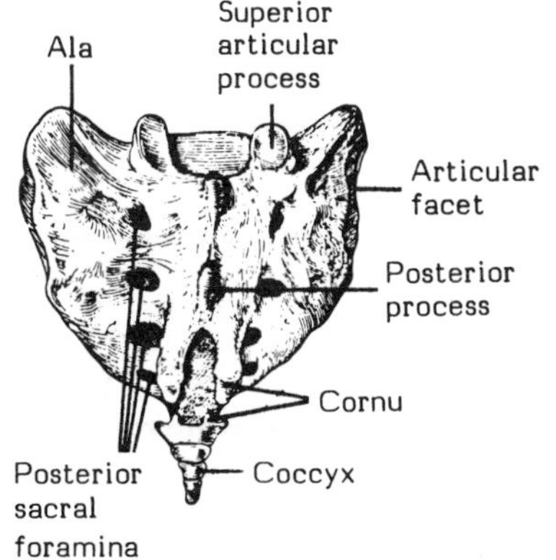

Figure 11.22. Schematic of the sacrum, as viewed from the posterior.

however, are not always ideally reciprocal with those of the ilium, nor are the bilateral planes of articulation commonly symmetrical.

The much smaller coccyx is formed from three or four segments that fuse in later life. It is also pyramidal in shape and is convex posteriorly and concave anteriorly.

The Ischia and Pubic Bones[84]

The body of the inferior ischium serves as the posterior half of the lower two-thirds of the acetabulum. The ischial ramus forms the posterior wall of the lower pelvis and the inferior wall of the obturator (closed) foramen. This foramen, although seen as a large opening in the dried skeleton, is completely closed in vivo by a tough membrane that serves to attach several strong muscles to the circumference of the opening.

The pubis serves as the anterior extension of the ilium and ischium. Posteriorly, its superior ramus forms the anterior aspect of the lower two-thirds of the acetabulum while its inferior ramus curves down and back to join the ischial ramus to form the superior wall of the obturator foramen.

The Sacroiliac Joints[85–89]

The slightly sliding, gliding, pivoting, and rotating sacroiliac joints serve as the sole point where the axial skeleton is attached to the pelvis (Fig. 11.23), thus the necessity of this joint's being bilaterally strong.

Uniquely, the sacroiliac joints are both diarthrotic and amphiarthotic.[90] Gehweiler[91] is one of several authorities who state that the sacral facet is covered by hyaline cartilage and that the iliac facet is covered

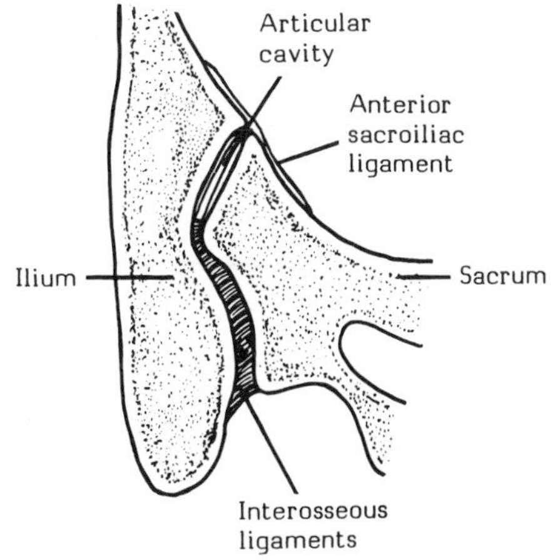

Figure 11.23. The left sacroiliac joint, as viewed from above.

by fibrocartilage, but others report a variety of different findings. The inferior two-thirds of the joint is considered a true synovial articulation, while the superior third is a fibrocartilaginous amphiarthrosis supported by the short but strong sacroiliac ligaments. Thus, a true polysynovitis will involve only the caudad aspect of the joint. The synovial membrane covers the whole joint cavity except at its posterior aspect where large ligaments attach to the articular cartilage.

Grieve states that one of three patients will exhibit accessory sacroiliac joints formed between the PSIS area and either S2 or S1.[92] These articulations, lined with fibrous cartilage or sometimes synovial membrane, are common sites of early osteoarthritic changes.

Denton has classified five different types of sacroiliac design.[93] Each type appears to have different motion and instability characteristics.

Major Ligaments. Excessive motion is strapped posteriorly by the interosseous ligaments, the short posterior sacroiliac ligament on the superolateral aspect of the sacrum, the long posterior sacroiliac ligament, and the sacrotuberous ligament on the inferolateral aspect of the sacrum (Fig. 11.24).

White and Panjabi state that the interosseous sacroiliac ligaments that support the thin fibrous capsule posteriorly and inferiorly are the strongest of the body.[71] These ligaments, considered the chief bond between the sacrum and ilia, are so thick that they fill the roughened space between the sacral and iliac tuberosities behind the sacroiliac joint. There is an upper part that spans between S1 and S2 and the anterior medial iliac crest. Immediately below is the lower part of the ligament that arises from S3 and inserts into the iliac crest. The strength of these ligaments helps prevent displacement of the sacrum even during forceful jumping.

The major straps anteriorly are the thinner anterior sacroiliac ligaments on the superolateral aspect of the sacrum and the stronger sacrospinous ligament that extends from the inferolateral aspect of the sacrum and coccyx to the ischial spine. The superolateral ligaments appear to be little more than extensions from the anterior capsule.

Macnab states that 30% of the population

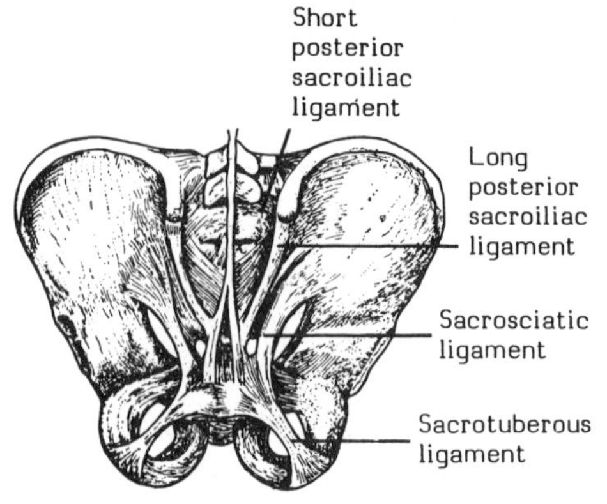

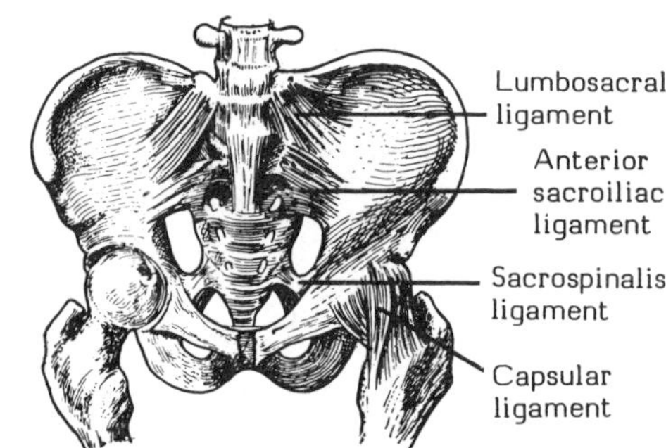

Figure 11.24. Ligaments of the pelvis, as viewed from the posterior and anterior.

over the age of 45 years has an anterior sacroiliac capsule that is ossified.[94] Several other authorities report quite free movement during advanced age even in the presence of gross changes noted on roentgenography. A variety of interarticular adhesions appear within the joint with age, but they are not reported to restrict motion. Illi has found an interarticular ligament at the toe of the boot that he feels has a considerable influence on sacral motion.[95]

Associated Muscles.[96,97] Strong muscles surround the joint, but there are no intrinsic muscles as seen in the spine. Muscle action is indirect via ilia, ischia, hip, and lumbar attachments. Nevertheless, several muscles have close connections with sacral ligaments. For example, (1) fibers of the lower quadratus lumborum mix with the iliolumbar ligament; (2) fibers of the iliopsoas mingle with the anterior sacroiliac ligament; (3) fibers of the multifidi and sacrospinalis mix with the long posterior sacroiliac ligament; (4) fibers of the gluteus maximus and hamstring fibers intertwine with the sacrotuberous ligament; and (5) fibers of the piriformis also mix with the sacrotuberous ligament and some enter directly into the sacroiliac capsule.

It is important to appreciate in studying sacroiliac motion that although there are no intrinsic muscles of the sacroiliac joints, the intermingling of muscle fibers within the ligamentous tissue allows the ligaments to serve almost as tendons. Thus, all sacroiliac motion need not be considered purely passive as is so commonly taught. This point is underscored by the discovery of mechanoreceptors, as reported by Denton, throughout the sacroiliac ligamentous complex that are similar to Golgi tendon organs.[93]

Innervation. The posterior aspect of the joint is innervated by the posterior rami from L5–S2. An irritation at the posterior joint usually refers pain to the buttocks and back of the thigh, following the dermatomes. The anterior aspect of the joint is supplied by both posterior branches from the L3–S2 roots and the superior gluteal nerve (L5–S2). Anterior joint irritation commonly refers pain to the groin and anterior thigh. If the sciatic nerves pierces the piriformis rather than exiting the pelvis over or under the muscle, sacroiliac distortion or inflammation may involve any of the numerous sciatic fibers.

Load Carriage Effects. By puberty, in adaptation to walking and other stresses, all articulating bony surfaces develop a variety of incongruities and small projections where dynamic stress would be concentrated if not for the smoothing effect of articular cartilage. In comparison to most other articulations, the sacroiliac joint contains a larger array of reciprocal bony hills and valleys. This joint surface roughness, more prominent in males, is generally considered the result of its segmental heritage; ie, the fused lateral tips of the transverse processes and the intertransverse spaces.

The articular surfaces of both the sacrum and ilium are quite smooth during childhood and do not exhibit their rough ridges and furrows until after puberty. Like fingerprints, their exact design is unique to the individual. In the child, stability is essentially ligamentous.

There are three articular areas of primary concern in adult sacroiliac dysfunction: an iliac elevation and sacral depression in the upper third of the joint, an iliac depression and sacral elevation in the middle third of the joint, and an iliac elevation and sacral depression in the lower third of the joint (Fig. 11.25).

The characteristic of a roughened articular surface allows deformation during loading to increase the contact area and significant recovery during the unloaded stage. Load carriage is particularly enhanced by the ability of the cartilage's hydrophilic proteoglycans to retain matrix water and of its collagen to resist matrix tensile forces.

Sacroiliac stability is so great that experimental overloading of S1 results in fracture of the lateral sacrum, pubis, or hip while the sacroiliac joints remain intact. Thus, complete fractures or greatly advanced destructive processes are the sole causes of clinical instability of the sacrum.

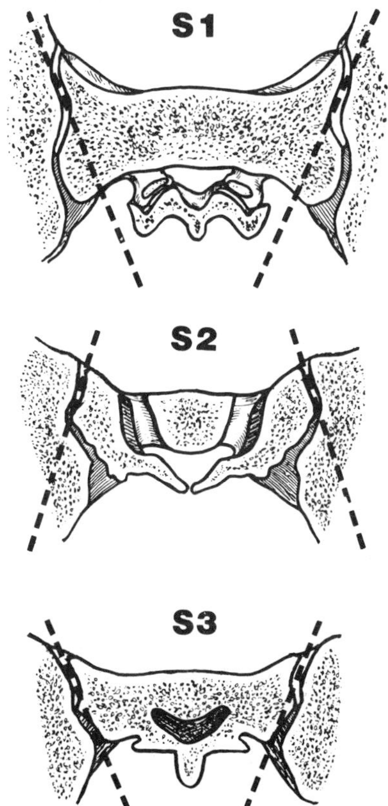

Figure 11.25. Coronal sections through S1, S2, and S3 showing the various planes of sacroiliac articulation.

The Sacrococcygeal Joint

The atypical joint between the sacrum and coccyx, usually considered a symphysis, is formed by the last sacral segment and the first coccygeal segment. It is united by a rudimentary IVD and tough ligamentous bands around its circumference. Slight posterior motion is normally exhibited during defecation, gait, and more so during parturition.

The Symphysis Pubis[98]

The anterior aspects of the hyaline-coated pubes join at the fibrocartilaginous pad (a nuclear disc) of the pubic symphysis. Slight but important movement takes place at this joint by yielding of the interpubic fibrocartilage. Iliac motion imposes reciprocal compression, tensile, and torsional forces on the pubis. Excessive movement is strapped by the superior and inferior pubic ligaments, and fusion is rare even in old age. Pubic innervation is from L1–S4 fibers; thus referred pain is often diffuse or unpredictably specific.

Kinematics[99–105]

The pelvis and its associated articulations are located fairly central to the kinematic chain extending from the cranium to the feet. Thus, any alteration in normal dynamics such as a unilateral fixation must manifest biomechanical effects both above and below. Fixation at a link or links of any kinematic chain forces hypermobility on the nearest possible segments.

Within the lumbar spine, Illi locates the axis of rotation posterior to the articular facets.[106] This permits a wide range of vertebral body rotation (Fig. 11.26), restricted essentially by the facial planes and the paravertebral ligaments. The inclination of the sacral base directs the lumbar curve. However, the axis of movement of the thoracic spine lies far anterior to the facets, near the nucleus of the IVD. Thus thoracic rotation is characterized by deviation of the spinous processes in a wider arc than the vertebral bodies.

The thicker anterior aspect and thinner posterior aspect of the lumbar discs provide the lumbar spine with its unique rotation, lateral bending, or combined phenomena.

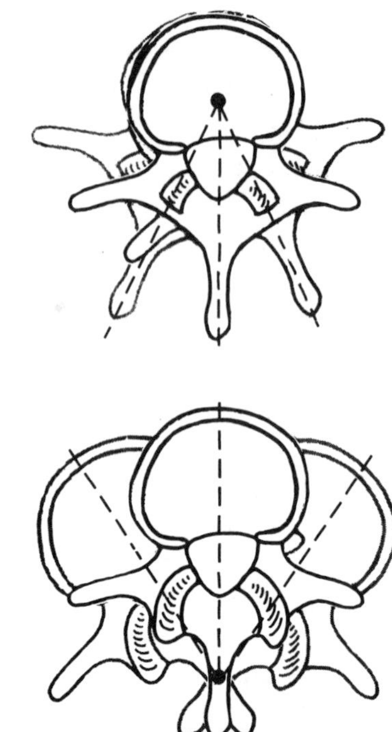

Figure 11.26. White/Panjabi and Farfan place the axes for transverse rotation near the nucleus pulposus for the cervical, thoracic, and lumbar regions. Illi's studies also place the axis for thoracic rotation (*top*) near the nucleus, but that of lumbar rotation posterior to the articular facets (*bottom*). This would simplify the explanation of the different coupling mechanisms in thoracic and lumbar scolioses.

The coupled lateral bending and rotation of the lumbar spine during forward flexion (1) protects the axial length of the lumbar spine and its contents from excessive tension; and (2) causes the peripheral fibers of the anulus to draw inward, thus securing the nucleus more firmly as a protection against displacement. This helps to further explain why fixation inhibiting rotation during flexion invites IVD protrusion. If rotation is not freely allowed during flexion, the segment tends to slide laterally and produce excessive shear forces upon the subjacent IVD and posterior facets. These basic characteristics of the lumbar spine coupled with the mechanics of the ilia are the factors that govern sacral dynamics.

Motion of the Transitional Lumbosacral Area

The junction of L5–S1 constitutes a rather unique "universal joint." For example, when the sacrum rotates anteroinferior on one side within the ilia, L5 tends to rotate in the opposite direction because of the restraint of the iliolumbar ligament. The effect is a mechanical accommodation of the lumbar spine above assuming a posterior rotation on the side of the unilateral sacral antero-inferiority. It also tends to assume an anteroflexed position, thus producing the three-dimensional movements of the lumbar spine. In view of the intricacy of the lumbosacral junction, anomalies such as asymmetrical facets have a strong influence on predictable movements in this area.

The iliolumbar ligaments connect the transverse processes of L5 to the crests of the ilia and sacral base. Aside from the articular facets, the iliolumbar ligaments are the most important structures limiting axial rotation of L5 on the sacrum and preventing forward gliding of L5 on the sacrum.

Because of its deep position below the iliac crests and the strong strapping by the iliolumbar ligaments and spinal extensors, L5 is only as movable as the sacral base will allow. Thus when lipping of or spurs at the inferior L5 body are seen, a history of instability can be presumed.

The Resolution of Pelvic Static Forces

When erect, body weight and any extrinsic loading of the upper body are transmitted from L5 to the sacral base, the sacroiliac joints, ilia, and ischia. Impact forces from below arise from the foot through the tibia and femur. These axial forces meet at the acetabulum and are essentially dissipated transversely to be absorbed by the cartilages and ligaments of the hip joints, sacroiliac joints, symphysis pubis, and the spongiosa of pelvic bone (Fig. 11.27). The gross effect is locking of the involved joints by opposing forces traveling around each side of the pelvis anteriorly and posteriorly from the acetabulum.

If these counterdirected axial forces are not equalized, the pelvis cannot be in a state of equilibrium according to Newtonian principles. When the force from below is greater, the head of the femur tends to jam within the acetabulum. If the force from above is greater, the L5 and S1 endplates or sacroiliac joints tend to displace.

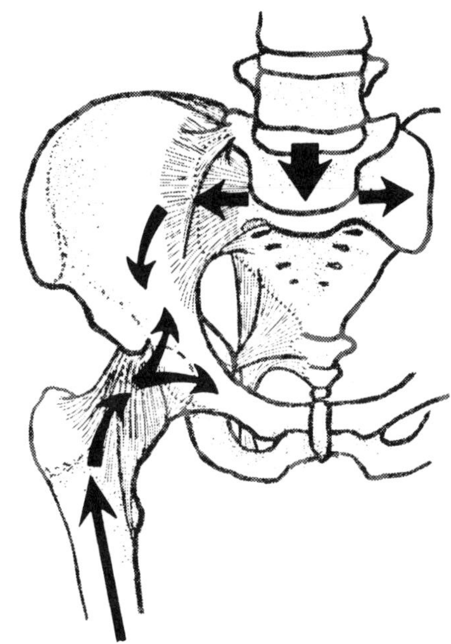

Figure 11.27. The forces developed in the pelvis from body weight and reactive ground forces.

The Pelvic Three-Joint Complex

The three-joint complex of a vertebral motion unit has been previously discussed. This complex consists of the disc anteriorly and the apophyseal facets posteriorly. A similar three-joint complex is seen in the pelvis. This complex consists of the symphysis pubis anteriorly and the sacroiliac facets posteriorly (Fig. 11.28). Thus, the pelvis as a unit has six degrees of freedom just as a vertebral motion unit.

Pelvic Tilt and Horizontal Rotation[107–110]

In the neutral position, the ASISs normally lie in the same transverse plane and in the same vertical plane as the symphysis pubis (Fig. 11.29).

The movements of the pelvis as a whole are forward and backward tilt around the transverse interfemoral axis, lateral tilt (associated with lumbar scoliosis), and rotation in the horizontal plane. None of these motions is produced by intrinsic pelvic muscles; rather, they are made by muscles of the trunk and/or hip that attach to the pelvis or sacrum. These motions occur at and affect the lumbosacral junction, the heads of the femurs, and the sacroiliacs (to a far lesser extent).

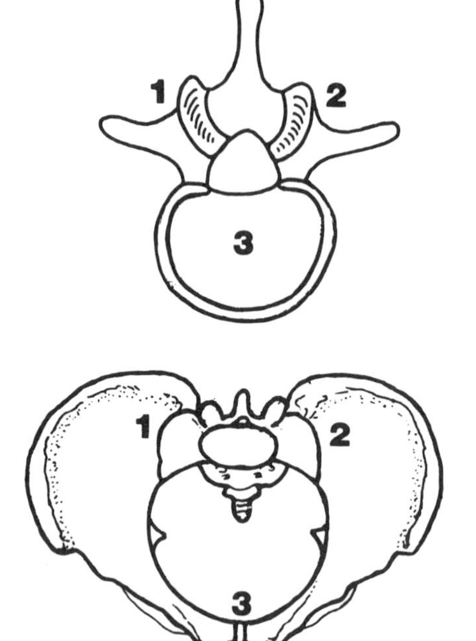

Figure 11.28. The three-joint complex in a vertebral segment and the pelvis.

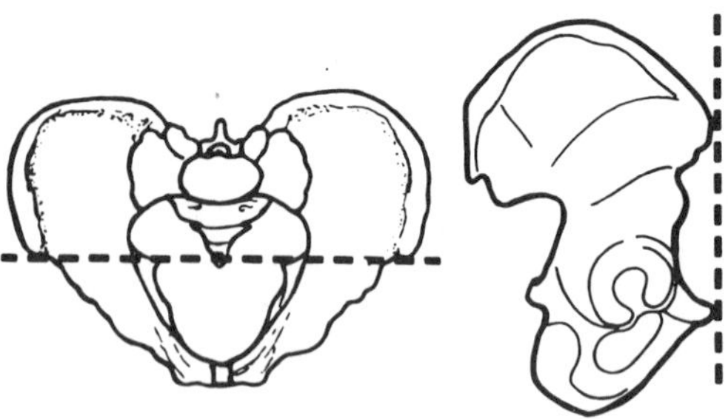

Figure 11.29. The normal analytical planes of the anterior pelvis.

Forward and backward pelvic tilts describe an arc that appears to follow the arcuate (bow-shaped) ridge and groove of the sacroiliac facets. Forward tilt is related to lumbar hyperlordosis and hip flexion. The anterior thigh muscles are also a strong component in this motion, and thus the frequent involvement of these muscles in pelvic distortions. Backward tilt is associated with lumbar flattening and hip extension. The major actions come from the posterior pull of the hamstrings and the anterior pull of the rectus abdominis with help from the obliques.

When a person shifts most of his weight to one leg, passive lateral pelvic tilt becomes evident. The pelvis on the unsupported side is restricted actively by the gluteus medius and minimus and passively by the iliotibial tract of the fascia lata. When weight is distributed bilaterally, lateral tilting of the pelvis is associated with lumboscoliosis, sacroiliac distortion, or a unilateral short leg.

Axial or lateral rotation of the pelvis about a fixed femoral head is produced by actions of the muscles of the thigh, loin, and the abdominal obliques. This is exhibited in walking.

Normal Motion of the Sacroiliac Articulations[111–114]

For many years, it was the allopathic opinion that there was no normal sacroiliac or pubic motion in the absence of disease and that the sacrum and ilia moved as a whole. This opinion has long been disputed empirically by chiropractic and osteopathic physicians and in recent years been proved a fallacy through cineroentgenographic studies. Only since the 1970s has sacral motion been widely recognized in allopathic literature.

Illi believes that a human being is the only vertebrate with a movable sacroiliac articulation.[115] At birth, the joint is only slightly movable. Because of bipedism, sacroiliac function is produced. However, because the sacroiliac and pubic articulations are readily subject to fixation, normal movement is not always exhibited in the adult within modern society where physical activity is minimal. Yet, several autopsy studies report freely movable joints in individuals over the age of 80.

Slight but smooth movement is permitted upward, downward, forward, and backward, and axial rotation occurs around a transverse axis to allow pelvic tilting. Because the sacrum does not have distinct articular planes but moves within the pelvic ring, its motion is multidirectional for 1–3 mm rather than in restricted directions. This multidirectional movement of the sacrum is probably the result of the wider iliac facet, the longer sacral facet, and the thick articular cartilage of the sacrum. This multidirectional motion is especially passive in the non-weight-bearing positions and affected above from lumbar forces and/or laterally and below from iliac-ischial forces.

Theories Regarding Sacral Motion[80,116–119]

While back pain has been a concern since early civilization, it was not until just before the turn of the century that the studies of Farabeuf and Bonnaire and their differing conclusions brought attention to the complexity of sacroiliac motion. A hundred years later, there is still more controversy concerning sacral motion than any other joint motion in the body.

1. *Farabeuf* contributed the classic theory that places the axis of rotation at the level of short strong axial interosseous ligament fibers within the deep layer of the sacroiliac ligaments. These fibers are attached laterally to the lateral aspect of the posterior PSIS and medially to the anterior foramina of S1 and S2. Farabeuf felt that angular displacement took place along the arc of a circle whose center was located posterior to the articular facet at the interosseous ligament (Fig. 11.30). De Jarnette[93] concurs with this finding, as far as weight bearing is concerned.

2. *Bonnaire* stated that the axis of rotation is at the lateral sacral tubercle (and iliac depression) located within the articular facet just posterior to the heel of the boot. Cassidy's findings concur. Fisk and several others place the axis for rotation at the ankle of the boot-shaped joint where the tubercle is located. This axle site would appear to be especially logical in the 5th decade when this tubercle becomes quite prominent.

3. *Weisl* placed the axis of rotation just anteroinferior to the sacrum and the axis of translation along the caudal aspect of the articular surface (Fig. 11.31).

4. *Illi* has conducted extensive studies that appear to tie the above three theories together. He discusses rotational pivoting during weight bearing around the S2 tubercle (Bonnaire). He has also found that two components arise during the figure 8 motion of gait. One component arcs around a center posterior to the sacrum (Farabeuf), and a second component is centered around a point about 10 cm anterior and inferior to the sacral promontory (Weisl).

5. *Shrader* has developed dry models that indicate that the axes for innominate rotation rest in common planes that extend from the torsional center of the symphysis pubis through the center of each femoral head (Fig. 11.32).[120] This concept would appear

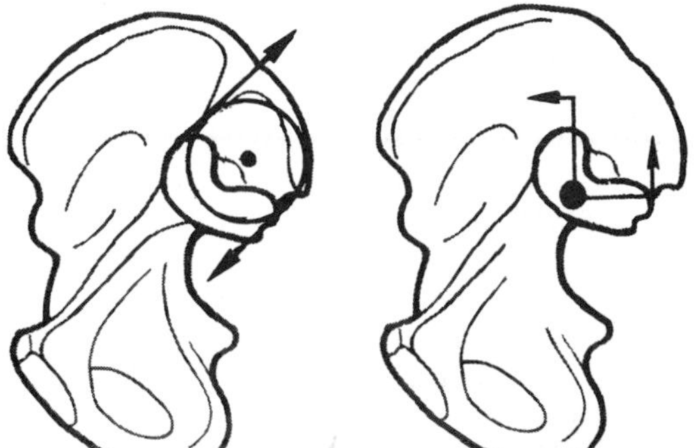

Figure 11.30. *Left*, Farabeuf's axis of sacral rotation; *right*, Bonnaire's axis of sacral rotation.

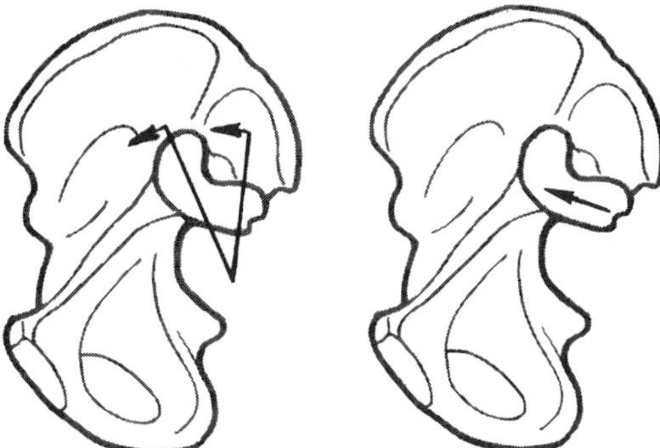

Figure 11.31. *Left*, Weisl's axis of sacral rotation; *right*, Weisl's plane of translation.

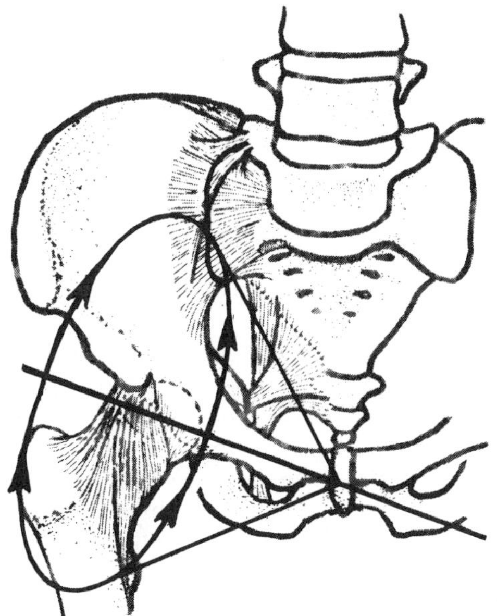

Figure 11.32. Shrader's axis of innominate rotation.

to conflict with the sites found by others and certainly deserves further investigation with fresh cadavers and in vivo.

Sacroiliac Movements[121–124]

For the sake of study, specific motions will be described. In vivo, these motions are always coupled. There is no one normal movement of the sacrum upon the ilia.

Intrapelvic mobilities are classified by Gillet[125] into three categories: (1) the A-P rotations of the ilia in relation to the sacrum, and to each other at the pubis; (2) the various movements of the sacrum itself in relation to the ilia; and (3) the sitting-standing changes in the relationship of the ilia to the sacrum and to each other. Another mobility is that motion of the sacrum at the lumbosacral joint in which it moves passively with the ilia, as seen in lateral flexion of the pelvis during gait. Weisl, Gonstad, and others also give an inferior or superior gliding motion along the caudal aspect of the sacroiliac facet.

Sacral Changes from Recumbent to Standing Positions. The sacrum approaches its nearest state of static equilibrium in the prone position when inferior and superior forces are removed. This is probably why sacral and para-anal reflex techniques achieve their effect in this position. Several studies have shown that there is distinct sacral motion in changing position from the recumbent, to the sitting, to the standing postures. These changes will be discussed later.

General Sacroiliac Motion during Pelvic Tipping. During forward flexion of the trunk in either the standing or sitting position, the sacral base pivots further anterior and inferior while the sacral apex moves posterior and superior. Simultaneously, the PSISs moves posterior, inferior, and obliquely medial so that the space between the spines is reduced. The ischia concurrently move obliquely anterior and superior and fan laterally. During extension, these pelvic actions are reversed.

Standing A-P Sacroiliac Motion. During erect weight bearing, the sacral base tends to rotate (pivot) anterior and inferior about the lateral S2 tubercles. When the standing patient lifts his right knee to a maximum, for example, as in taking a high step, the right ilium tends to follow the femur in its motion, rotating in the A-P plane with the approximate center of movement being at the femoral head. At the same time, the right arm of the pubis moves upward in relation to its opposite, and this is palpable. The iliac portion of the sacroiliac articulation glides posterior and inferior relative to its contact with the sacrum. Thereafter, the sacrum must arc posterior and inferior with the left ilium. If both the pubic and sacroiliac articulations reach their limits of mobility and the knee is lifted still further, the pubis starts serving as the center of rotation and, at the posterior pelvis, the ilium will start pulling the sacrum down in its course, forcing it to articulate with the opposite ilium. As this latter movement does not follow the sacroiliac facet plane, a certain degree of joint separation must take place. If the knee lifting test is carried still further, the normal limit of the other articulation (the left in this example) will be reached, and then the whole pelvis will rotate backward.

In the above standing position, motions of the sacrum in relation to the ilia are sometimes difficult to detect because of coupled acetabular changes; thus it may be necessary to seat the patient to restrict these movements. Sitting fixes the pelvic base, alters its shape, and permits a totally different type of motion than that of the standing position.

Sitting Sacroiliac Rotational Motion. In the sitting position, the sacrum readily flexes and turns between the two ilia. To produce this movement, the stabilizing arm of the examiner grasps the opposite shoulder of the patient across his chest and rotates the patient to a maximum while the examiner's palpating fingers follow the sacral spinous processes in their movement. The lumbar region will also rotate and flex in order to follow the line of the dorsal vertebrae which move laterally in a wide arc. The placement of the sacrum can also be roughly judged by the direction of the buttocks line.

There is a fundamental difference between A-P standing mobility of the ilia on the sacrum, which does not carry the sacrum with it until the limit of movement is reached, and the rotation and flexion of the sacrum in the sitting position, which will carry the ilia along with it to a degree. This partial iliac mobility in the sitting position can be palpated by putting the thumb on the crest or on the PSIS and following it forward and downward as the thorax rotates in that direction. Most authorities agree that any degree of sacral rotation has a related translatory component.

Sacroiliac Motion during Lateral Flexion. In lateral flexion, a similar movement of the sacrum takes place with a maximum of flexion and a minimum of rotation. To feel this, the shoulders of the patient must be put into a complete lateral bending posture and an attempt must be made to concentrate the movement in the area being palpated. Again, the ilia make an effort to follow this movement into lateral flexion, with the distal ilium flaring away.

Sacroiliac Motion during Gait.[126,127] Sacroiliac motion allows for reciprocal movement of the innominates and a gyroscopic motion of the sacrum during gait (Fig. 11.33). These motions tend to dampen the axially directed forces of heelstrike. Illi has shown that as the heel strikes, the ilium rotates posteriorly and inferiorly, the sacral base rotates anteriorly and inferiorly, and the ipsilateral transverse of L5 is pulled backward.[128] This vertebral action of functional lumbar scoliosis diminishes cephally. At midstance, the pelvis moves over the femoral head in a neutral position. As the contralateral extremity is abducted forward, the sacrum is positioned posteriorly and superiorly on that side. This reciprocal motion between the sacrum and ilium describes a horizontal figure 8 between the ilia when viewed during gait. One side of the sacral base arcs down and forward, and rotates toward the ipsilateral side, while the other side swings upward and backward, and the sacral apex rotates toward the contralateral side. The path of this arc appears to be the product of sacral translation and torque having various components, depending on the planes of the bilateral facets, the force vectors, and the bilateral integrity of the involved restraining ligaments.[129]

Sacral Motion during Respiration. The majority of references to this mechanism

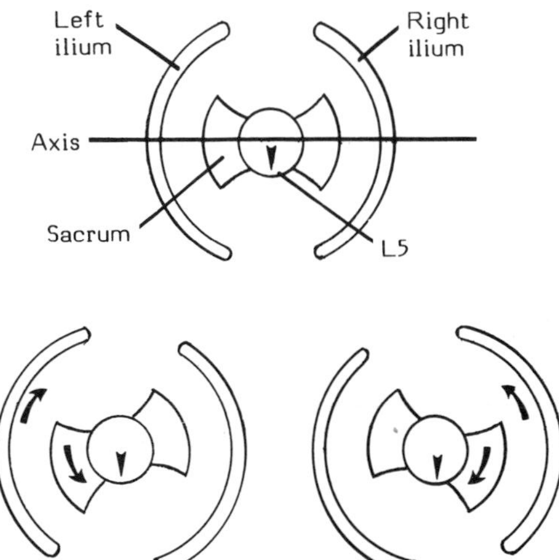

Figure 11.33. The gyroscopic motion of the sacrum during gait. *Top*, neutral position; *bottom left*, left swing phase; *bottom right*, right swing phase. Note that L5 maintains a relatively stable state.

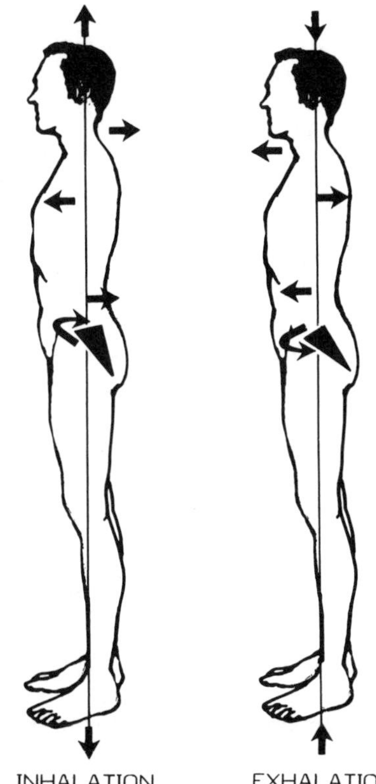

Figure 11.34. The sacrorespiratory mechanism. During inhalation, the sacral base pivots posteriorly; the lumbar, thoracic, and cervical curves reduce; and height is increased. During exhalation, the sacral base pivots anteriorly, the lumbar lordosis increases, the thoracic kyphosis increases, the cervical lordosis increases, and height is decreased.

have been published by De Jarnette, Goodheart, and a number of osteopaths researching cranial manipulation and reflexes.[130] They have found that there is also slight sacral A-P motion during respiration and Valsalva maneuvers (Fig. 11.34). The sacral base tends to pivot posteriorly during inspiration (or increased intra-abdominal pressure) and anteriorly during expiration of 1–7 mm. The rate is about 14 excursions per minute. This sacral mechanism, synchronized with a reciprocal cranial action, appears to manifest a pumping action on cerebrospinal fluid circulation. This is made possible by the continuous dural sheath that descends from the cranial vault, attaches at the foramen magnum, connects to the posterior ring of the atlas and odontoid and then descends through the spinal canal to insert near S2. This helps to explain why sacral and upper cervical dysfunctions are so frequently associated.

Pelvic Changes during Sitting and Standing[131–133]

In the sitting posture when weight is borne essentially by the ischial prominences, the body tries to widen its base of support by slightly separating the ischia, which in turn slightly close the iliac crests. As the inferior sacral space opens, the apex of the sacrum juts backward to remain in contact with it. That is, because of the oblique slant of the sacral facets, the sacral base moves anteriorly and the apex moves posteriorly. The axis of this motion is commonly a horizontal plane approximately at the S2 level. Articulation for this motion takes place at the pubic and sacroiliac articulations.

A different mechanism is seen in the standing posture. Upon arising, the ischia are passively brought together to permit body weight to lie directly on the heads of the femurs. It is then that the iliac crests open laterally (flare out). This closes the inferior sacral angle, opening the space that holds the base of the sacrum. In adaptation, the sacral base moves slightly posterior and the apex rotates to the anterior.

In considering A-P nodding of the sacrum, remember that the position of the ilia are not rigid and that the slant of the articulations force the ilia to adapt themselves to flexion by lateral flexion of their own. Thus, we rotate each hip backward and forward each time we walk. Each time we sit and arise, we cause our ilia to flare out and in. Each time we bend or turn in a seated position, we cause the sacrum to move within the interiliac space.

REFERENCES

1. Finneson BE: *Low Back Pain.* Philadelphia, J.B. Lippincott, 1973, pp 19–23.
2. Barham JN, Wooten EP: *Structural Kinesiology.* New York, Macmillan, 1973, pp 248–250, 259–262.
3. Hollingshead WH, Jenkins DB: *Functional Anatomy of the Limbs and Back.* Philadelphia, W.B. Saunders, 1981, pp 372–375.
4. Basmajian JV (ed): *Grant's Method of Anatomy,* ed 9. Baltimore, Williams & Wilkins, 1975, pp 175–183, 246.
5. Moore KL: *Clinically Oriented Anatomy.* Baltimore, Williams & Wilkins, 1980, pp 127–137.
6. Kapandji IA: *Physiology of the Joints: Lower Limb,* ed 2. New York, Churchill Livingstone, 1981, vol 3, pp 88–106.
7. Esch D, Lepley M: *Musculoskeletal Function: An Anatomy and Kinesiology Laboratory Manual.* Minneapolis, University of Minnesota Press, 1974, pp 49–53.
8. Morehouse LE, Cooper JM: *Kinesiology.* St. Louis, C.V. Mosby, 1950, pp 73–76.
9. Grieve GP: *Common Vertebral Joint Problems.* New York, Churchill Livingstone, 1981, pp 48–52.
10. Kendall HO, Kendall FP, Wadsworth GE: *Muscles: Testing and Function,* ed 2. Baltimore, Williams & Wilkins, 1971, pp 201–240.
11. Van Dusen LG: *Chiropractic Relationship to Gravitational Force.* Sodus, NY, published by the author, 1968, pp 87, 91, 93, 97, 103.
12. Barham JN, Wooten EP: *Structural Kinesiology.* New York, Macmillan, 1973, pp 266–269.
13. White AA, Panjabi MM: *Clinical Biomechanics of the Spine.* Philadelphia, J.B. Lippincott, 1978, pp 251–254.
14. Cailliet R: *Soft Tissue Pain and Disability.* Philadelphia, F.A. Davis, 1980, pp 41–54.
15. Grieve GP: *Common Vertebral Joint Problems.* New York, Churchill Livingstone, 1981, pp 17–29, 34, 53–55, 60–62.
16. Kapandji IA: *Physiology of the Joints: Lower Limb,* ed 2. New York, Churchill Livingstone, 1981, vol 3, pp 74–78, 86.
17. Reinert OC: *Fundamentals of Chiropractic Techniques and Practice Procedures.* Chesterfield, Mo, Marian Press, 1983, pp 13–14.

18. Helfet AJ, Gruebel Lee DM: *Disorders of the Lumbar Spine.* Philadelphia, J.B. Lippincott, 1978, pp 27–30.
19. Cailliet R: *Low Back Pain Syndrome,* ed 3. Philadelphia, F.A. Davis, 1981, pp 1–21, 49–51.
20. Hollingshead WH, Jenkins DB: *Functional Anatomy of the Limbs and Back.* Philadelphia, W.B. Saunders, 1981, p 200.
21. Moore KL: *Clinically Oriented Anatomy.* Baltimore, Williams & Wilkins, 1980, pp 617–618.
22. Parke WW: Applied anatomy of the spine. In Rothman RH, Simeone FA (eds): *The Spine.* Philadelphia, W.B. Saunders, 1975, vol 1, p 27.
23. Finneson BE: *Low Back Pain.* Philadelphia, J.B. Lippincott, 1973, pp 7–9.
24. Kapandji IA: *Physiology of the Joints: Lower Limb,* ed 2. New York, Churchill Livingstone, 1981, vol 3, p 120.
25. Helfet AJ, Gruebel Lee DM: *Disorders of the Lumbar Spine.* Philadelphia, J.B. Lippincott, 1978, p 27.
26. Dvorak J: Neurological and biomechanical aspects of back pain. In Buerger AA, Greenman PE (eds): *Empirical Approaches to the Validation of Spinal Manipulation.* Springfield, Mo, Charles C Thomas, 1985, pp 241–262.
27. Schafer RC: *Chiropractic Management of Sports and Recreational Injuries.* Baltimore, Williams & Wilkins, 1982, pp 283–286.
28. White AA, Panjabi MM: *Clinical Biomechanics of the Spine.* Philadelphia, J.B. Lippincott, 1978, p 295.
29. Hollingshead WH, Jenkins DB: *Functional Anatomy of the Limbs and Back.* Philadelphia, W.B. Saunders, 1981, pp 222–224, 229, 248–250.
30. Helfet AJ, Gruebel Lee DM: *Disorders of the Lumbar Spine.* Philadelphia, J.B. Lippincott, 1978, pp 45–48.
31. Evans DP: *Backache: Its Evolution and Conservative Treatment.* Baltimore, University Park Press, 1982, pp 21–30, 40–43, 48, 55–63, 161–165.
32. Hadley LA: *Anatomico-Roentgenographic Studies of the Spine.* Springfield, Ill, Charles C Thomas, 1981, pp 399, 401, 404.
33. Janse J: *Principles and Practice of Chiropractic.* Lombard, Ill, National College of Chiropractic, 1976, pp 45–46.
34. Chusid JG: *Correlative Neuroanatomy and Functional Neurology,* ed 19. Los Altos, Cal, Lange Medical, 1985, pp 150–161.
35. Wilson FC: *The Musculoskeletal System: Basic Processes and Disorders,* ed 2. Philadelphia, J.B. Lippincott, 1983, pp 67–69.
36. Mumenthaler M: *Neurology,* ed 2. Translated by EH Burrows. New York, Thieme-Stratton, 1983, pp 361–363.
37. Schafer RC: *Chiropractic Physical and Spinal Diagnosis,* Oklahoma City, American Chiropractic Academic Press, 1980, pp XIII-15–XIII-16.
38. Hoppenfeld S: *Orthopaedic Neurology,* Philadelphia, J.B. Lippincott, 1977.
39. Fosse M: A Clinical Study of Lumbar Spine Movement Using an External Method of Measurement. Thesis, Anglo-European College of Chiropractic. Brussels, Prestoprint, 1972.
40. Goodheart GJ: *Applied Kinesiology.* City of publication not shown, published by the author, privately distributed, 1964, pp 33–37.
41. Goodheart GL: *Collected Published Articles and Reprints.* Montpellier, O, Williams County Publishing, 1969, pp 44–46, 64–67.
42. Daniels L, Worthingham C: *Muscle Testing: Techniques of Manual Examination,* ed 4. Philadelphia, W.B. Saunders, 1980, pp 22–29, 34–35.
43. Warfel JH: *The Head, Neck, and Trunk,* ed 5. Philadelphia, Lea & Febiger, 1985, pp 51–60, 73–79.
44. Kendall HO, Kendall FP, Wadsworth GE: *Muscles: Testing and Function,* ed 2. Baltimore, Williams & Wilkins, 1971, p 208.
45. White AA, Panjabi MM: *Clinical Biomechanics of the Spine.* Philadelphia, J.B. Lippincott, 1978, pp 78–81.
46. Cailliet R: *Low Back Pain Syndrome,* ed 3. Philadelphia, F.A. Davis, 1981, pp 53–67.
47. Kapandji IA: *Physiology of the Joints: Lower Limb,* ed 2. New York, Churchill Livingstone, 1981, vol 3, pp 80–82, 114–118.
48. Helfet AJ, Gruebel Lee DM: *Disorders of the Lumbar Spine.* Philadelphia, J.B. Lippincott, 1978, p 220.
49. Grice AS, Fligg DB: Class Notes: Spinal Dynamics. Department of Biomechanics/Kinesiology, BK202. Toronto, Canadian Memorial Chiropractic College, pp 36–41 (undated).
50. Finneson BE: *Low Back Pain.* Philadelphia, J.B. Lippincott, 1973, pp 24–34.
51. Evans DC: Biomechanics of spinal injury. In Gonzna ER, Harrington IJ: *Biomechanics of Musculoskeletal Injury.* Baltimore, Williams & Wilkins, 1982, pp 204–212.
52. Gates D: *Correlative Spinal Anatomy.* Lakemont, Ga, published by the author, 1977, pp 129–132.
53. White AA, Panjabi MM: *Clinical Biomechanics of the Spine.* Philadelphia, J.B. Lippincott, 1978, pp 254–264, 272.
54. Helfet AJ, Gruebel Lee DM: *Disorders of the Lumbar Spine.* Philadelphia, J.B. Lippincott, 1978, pp 42–44, 219–220.
55. Helfet AJ, Gruebel Lee DM: *Disorders of the Lumbar Spine.* Philadelphia, J.B. Lippincott, 1978, pp 69–82.
56. Finneson BE: *Low Back Pain.* Philadelphia, J.B. Lippincott, 1973, pp 10–13.
57. White AA, Panjabi MM: *Clinical Biomechanics of the Spine.* Philadelphia, J.B. Lippincott, 1978, p 212.
58. LACC Technic Department: Multiposition spinal examination. *The Chirogram* April 1976.
59. White AA, Panjabi MM: *Clinical Biomechanics of the Spine.* Philadelphia, J.B. Lippincott, 1978, pp 297–302.
60. Cailliet R: *Low Back Pain Syndrome,* ed 3. Philadelphia, F.A. Davis, 1981, pp 69–78.
61. Fisk JW: *The Painful Neck and Back.* Springfield,

Ill, Charles C Thomas, 1977, pp 54–76.
62. McRae R: *Clinical Orthopaedic Examination*, ed 2. New York, Churchill Livingstone, 1983, pp 71–96.
63. Hoppenfeld S: *Physical Examination of the Spine and Extremities*, New York, Appleton-Century-Crofts, 1976.
64. Schafer RC: *Chiropractic Physical and Spinal Diagnosis*, Oklahoma City, American Chiropractic Academic Press, 1980, pp XIII-1–XIII-8, XIII-16–XIII-19.
65. Johnson AC: *Postural Correction*, Los Angeles, Chiropractic Educational Extension Bureau, pp 15–16 (undated).
66. McKenzie RA: *The Lumbar Spine: Mechanical Diagnosis and Therapy.* Waikane, New Zealand, Spinal Publications, 1981, pp 4–5, 87–90.
67. McKenzie RA: *The Lumbar Spine: Mechanical Diagnosis and Therapy.* Waikane, New Zealand, Spinal Publications, 1981, pp 1–2.
68. Cailliet R: *Low Back Pain Syndrome*, ed 3. Philadelphia, F.A. Davis, 1981, pp 44–49.
69. Kapandji IA: *Physiology of the Joints: Lower Limb*, ed 2. New York, Churchill Livingstone, 1981, vol 3, pp 54–57, 68.
70. Grieve GP: *Common Vertebral Joint Problems.* New York, Churchill Livingstone, 1981, pp 29–31, 34–35.
71. White AA, Panjabi MM: *Clinical Biomechanics of the Spine.* Philadelphia, J.B. Lippincott, 1978, p 264.
72. Esch D, Lepley M: *Musculoskeletal Function: An Anatomy and Kinesiology Laboratory Manual.* Minneapolis, University of Minnesota Press, 1974, pp 11–12.
73. Rosse C: The hip region and the lumbosacral plexus. In Rosse C, Clawson DK (eds): *The Musculoskeletal System in Health and Disease.* Hagerstown, Md, Harper & Row, 1980, pp 253–254, 256–257, 268–272.
74. Basmajian JV (ed): *Grant's Method of Anatomy*, ed 9. Baltimore, Williams & Wilkins, 1975, pp 271–278, 290–292, 298–301.
75. Grice AS, Fligg DB: Class Notes: Spinal Dynamics. Department of Biomechanics/Kinesiology, BK202. Toronto, Canadian Memorial Chiropractic College, pp 15–17 (undated).
76. Finneson BE: *Low Back Pain.* Philadelphia, J.B. Lippincott, 1973, pp 15–17.
77. Reinert OC: *Fundamentals of Chiropractic Techniques and Practice Procedures.* Chesterfield, Mo, Marian Press, 1983, pp 9–12.
78. Barham JN, Wooten EP: *Structural Kinesiology.* New York, Macmillan, 1973, pp 197–199.
79. Hollingshead WH, Jenkins DB: *Functional Anatomy of the Limbs and Back.* Philadelphia, W.B. Saunders, 1981, pp 231–232.
80. Boorsma JD: Architecture of the sacro-iliac joint. In *Biomechanics of the Pelvis.* Council on Technic of the American Chiropractic Association, Denver Conference, June 17–20, 1980, pp 5–7.
81. Moore KL: *Clinically Oriented Anatomy.* Baltimore, Williams & Wilkins, 1980, pp 618–620.
82. Parke WW: Applied anatomy of the spine. In Rothman RH, Simeone FA (eds): *The Spine.* Philadelphia, W.B. Saunders, 1975, vol 1, pp 27–28.
83. Finneson BE: *Low Back Pain.* Philadelphia, J.B. Lippincott, 1973, p 9.
84. Hollingshead WH, Jenkins DB: *Functional Anatomy of the Limbs and Back.* Philadelphia, W.B. Saunders, 1981, pp 232–233, 235.
85. Gehweiler JA Jr, Osborne RL Jr, Becker RF: *The Radiology of Vertebral Trauma.* Philadelphia, W.B. Saunders, 1980, pp 85–88.
86. Barham JN, Wooten EP: *Structural Kinesiology.* New York, Macmillan, 1973, pp 202–203.
87. Hollingshead WH, Jenkins DB: *Functional Anatomy of the Limbs and Back.* Philadelphia, W.B. Saunders, 1981, pp 235–236.
88. Kapandji IA: *Physiology of the Joints: Lower Limb*, ed 2. New York, Churchill Livingstone, 1981, vol 3, pp 58–63.
89. Fisk JW: *The Painful Neck and Back.* Springfield, Ill, Charles C Thomas, 1977, pp 46–47.
90. Helfet AJ, Gruebel Lee DM: *Disorders of the Lumbar Spine.* Philadelphia, J.B. Lippincott, 1978, p 219.
91. Gehweiler JA Jr, Osborne RL Jr, Becker RF: *The Radiology of Vertebral Trauma.* Philadelphia, W.B. Saunders, 1980, p 85.
92. Grieve GP: *Common Vertebral Joint Problems.* New York, Churchill Livingstone, 1981, pp 29–31.
93. Denton DG: Sacro-occipital technique biomechanics of the pelvis. In *Biomechanics of the Pelvis.* Council on Technic of the American Chiropractic Association, Denver Conference, June 17–20, 1980, pp 24–42.
94. Macnab I: *Backache.* Baltimore, Williams & Wilkins, 1977, p 64.
95. Illi FW: *The Vertebral Column: Life-Line of the Body.* Chicago, National College of Chiropractic, 1951, pp 13–14.
96. Goodheart GJ: *Applied Kinesiology.* City of publication not shown, published by the author, privately distributed, 1964, pp 11–12, 23–24, 38–43.
97. Goodheart GL: *Collected Published Articles and Reprints.* Montpellier, O, Williams County Publishing, 1969, pp 80–81.
98. Barham JN, Wooten EP: *Structural Kinesiology.* New York, Macmillan, 1973, p 202.
99. White AA, Panjabi MM: *Clinical Biomechanics of the Spine.* Philadelphia, J.B. Lippincott, 1978, pp 264–270, 272.
100. Weisl H: Ligaments of the sacro-iliac joint examined with particular reference to their function. *Acta Anatomica (Basel)* 20:201–213, 1954.
101. Barham JN, Wooten EP: *Structural Kinesiology.* New York, Macmillan, 1973, pp 270–271.
102. Barge FH: *Scoliosis.* Davenport, Ia, Bawden Bros, 1982, pp 10–49.
103. Hollingshead WH, Jenkins DB: *Functional Anatomy of the Limbs and Back.* Philadelphia, W.B. Saunders, 1981, pp 269–270.
104. Grice AS, Fligg DB: Class Notes: Spinal Dynamics. Department of Biomechanics/Kinesiology, BK202. Toronto, Canadian

Memorial Chiropractic College, pp 17–23 (undated).
105. Janse J: The concepts and research of Dr. Fred W. Illi. In *Notes on Correlative Techniques*. Chicago, National College of Chiropractic (undated).
106. Illi FW: *The Vertebral Column: Life-Line of the Body*. Chicago, National College of Chiropractic, 1951, pp 61–73.
107. Kendall HO, Kendall FP, Wadsworth GE: *Muscles: Testing and Function*, ed 2. Baltimore, Williams & Wilkins, 1971, p 22.
108. Gatterman B: Motion palpation of the sacroiliac joints. In *Biomechanics of the Pelvis*. Council on Technic of the American Chiropractic Association, Denver Conference, June 17–20, 1980, pp 76–80.
109. Mawhiney RB: *Scoliosis Manual*. Waukesha, Wis, published by the author, 1982, pp 9–61.
110. Barge FH: *Scoliosis*. Davenport, Ia, Bawden Bros, 1982, pp 51–118, 155–176.
111. Hemauer JD: Sacroiliac anatomy, movement, and subluxation. In *Biomechanics of the Pelvis*. Council on Technic of the American Chiropractic Association, Denver Conference, June 17–20, 1980, pp 112–119.
112. Janse J: Investigations and observations on the sacroiliac. In *Biomechanics of the Pelvis*. Council on Technic of the American Chiropractic Association, Denver Conference, June 17–20, 1980, pp 121–128.
113. Colachis SC Jr et al: Movement of the sacroiliac joint in the adult: a preliminary report. *Archives of Physical Medicine and Rehabilitation* 490–498, September 1963.
114. Wood J: Motion of the sacroiliac joint. *PCC Research Forum* 1(3):95–101, Spring 1985.
115. Illi FW: *The Vertebral Column: Life-Line of the Body*. Chicago, National College of Chiropractic, 1951, p 11.
116. Cassidy JD: Anatomy and biomechanics of the sacroiliac joint. In *Biomechanics of the Pelvis*. Council on Technic of the American Chiropractic Association, Denver Conference, June 17–20, 1980, pp 20–22.
117. Faucret BH: Introduction to pelvic biomechanics. In *Biomechanics of the Pelvis*. Council on Technic of the American Chiropractic Association, Denver Conference, June 17–20, 1980, pp 51–58.
118. Kapandji IA: *Physiology of the Joints: Lower Limb*, ed 2. New York, Churchill Livingstone, 1981, vol 3, pp 64–67.
119. Grice AS, Fligg DB: Class Notes: Spinal Dynamics. Department of Biomechanics/ Kinesiology, BK202. Toronto, Canadian Memorial Chiropractic College, pp 12–15 (undated).
120. Shrader TL: A model for simulation of pelvic biomechanics. In *Biomechanics of the Pelvis*. Council on Technic of the American Chiropractic Association, Denver Conference, June 17–20, 1980, pp 143–151.
121. Kapandji IA: *Physiology of the Joints: Lower Limb*, ed 2. New York, Churchill Livingstone, 1981, vol 3, p 70.
122. Weisl H: Movements of the sacro-iliac joint. *Acta Anatomica (Basel)* 23:80–91, 1955.
123. Weisl H: The articular surfaces of the sacro-iliac joint and their relation to movements of the sacrum. *Acta Anatomica (Basel)* 22:1–14, 1954.
124. Campbell JR: Gonstead analysis of pelvic biomechanics. In *Biomechanics of the Pelvis*. Council on Technic of the American Chiropractic Association, Denver Conference, June 17–20, 1980, pp 9–18.
125. Gillet H, Liekens M: *Belgian Chiropractic Research Notes*, ed 11. Huntington Beach, Cal, Motion Palpation Institute, 1981, pp 100–106.
126. Grice AS, Fligg DB: Class Notes: Introductory Concepts to Clinical Analysis of Joint Movement and Muscle Testing. Department of Biomechanics/Kinesiology, BK101. Toronto, Canadian Memorial Chiropractic College, pp 100–102 (undated).
127. Banks SD: Sacro-iliac biomechanics and its effects on gait. *Journal of the ACA Council on Sports Injuries* 1(3):9–14, April 1983.
128. Illi FW: *The Vertebral Column: Life-Line of the Body*. Chicago, National College of Chiropractic, 1951, p 19.
129. Gatterman MI: Sacroiliac motion and pelvic tilt. In *Biomechanics of the Pelvis*. Council on Technic of the American Chiropractic Association, Denver Conference, June 17–20, 1980, pp 81–92.
130. Upledger JE, Vredevoogd JD: *Craniosacral Therapy*. Seattle, Eastland Press, 1983, pp 46–52.
131. Grice AS: Clinical analysis of the sacroiliac joint. In *Biomechanics of the Pelvis*. Council on Technic of the American Chiropractic Association, Denver Conference, June 17–20, 1980, pp 96–109.
132. SantoMauro A: Bio-statics of the pelvis. In *Biomechanics of the Pelvis*. Council on Technic of the American Chiropractic Association, Denver Conference, June 17–20, 1980, pp 139–141.
133. Kapandji IA: *Physiology of the Joints: Lower Limb*, ed 2. New York, Churchill Livingstone, 1981, vol 3, p 112.

SUGGESTED READINGS

Albright JA, Brand RA: *The Scientific Basis of Orthopaedics*. New York, Appleton-Century-Crofts, 1979.

Barge FH: *Tortipelvis*. Davenport, Ia, Bawden Bros, 1980.

Cox JM: *Low Back Pain: Mechanism, Diagnosis and Treatment*, ed 4. Baltimore, Williams & Wilkins, 1985.

Coyle BA, Martinez DP (eds): *Proceedings of the Second Conference on Current Topics in Chiropractic: Reviews of the Literature*, May 4–5, 1985. Sunnyvale, Cal, Palmer College of Chiropractic—West, 1985.

D'Ambrosia RD: *Musculoskeletal Disorders*. Philadelphia, J.B. Lippincott, 1977.

Goldstein M (ed): *The Research Status of Spinal Manipulative Therapy* Monograph No. 15, U.S. Department of Health, Education, and Welfare, Public Health Service, DHEW Publication No. (NIH) 76-998. Bethesda, Md, National Institutes of Health, 1975.

Kirkaldy-Willis WH (ed): *Managing Low Back Pain.* New York, Churchill Livingstone, 1983.
Mennell JMcM: *Back Pain.* Boston, Little, Brown, 1960.
Salter RB: *Textbook of Disorders and Injuries of the Musculoskeletal System.* Baltimore, Williams & Wilkins, 1970.
Spengler DM: *Low Back Pain: Assessment and Management.* New York, Grune & Stratton, 1982.
Williams PC: *Low Back and Neck Pain.* Springfield, Ill, Charles C Thomas, 1982.
Yashon D: *Spinal Injury.* New York, Appleton-Century-Crofts, 1978.

CHAPTER 12

Selected Disorders of the Lumbar Spine and Pelvis

This chapter portrays a large number of clinical problems involving the lumbar motion units and pelvic articulations that are often encountered in private practice. Emphasis has been placed on the biomechanical and pathophysiologic mechanisms involved and the direction of their clinical management. The major topics include regional muscle weakness and hypertonicity syndromes, postural realignment, structural fixations and their dynamic palpation, the etiology of lumbopelvic pain, traumatic disorders, and degenerative and entrapment syndromes. Several pathologies that affect this region, which may cause or contribute to low-back pain syndromes, are described.

CLINICAL PROBLEMS OF THE ABDOMINAL MUSCLES

The abdominal muscles offer considerable protection to the viscera when active, but when they are relaxed, they are easily damaged by intrinsic or extrinsic forces. This is especially true of the rectus abdominis. Muscle contractures, stitches, strains, ruptures, and direct blows are the most common somatic causes of pain in the abdominal wall.

Intrinsic Muscle Problems

Effects of Muscle Weakness and Shortening[1-3]

Rectus Abdominis Weakness. This is portrayed by a loss in trunk flexion and posterior pelvic rotation strength. In the upright posture, a lengthening of the sternal-pubic distance, lumbar hyperlordosis, and anterior pelvic tilt will be evident. The rectus is rarely shortened by itself.

Oblique Weakness. This is exhibited by decreased respiratory efficiency and loss in abdominal support. Trunk flexion and posterior pelvic tilting strength are diminished in bilateral weakness. This is overtly suggested by anterior pelvic tilt and lumbar hyperlordosis or an exaggerated "S" curve laterally (Fig. 12.1). Ipsilateral weakness of the external oblique with contralateral weakness of the internal oblique encourages lumbar scoliosis with rotation and tilting, while unilateral weakness of these two muscles promotes a "C" curve toward the side of weakness.

Oblique Shortening. Bilateral shortening anteriorly reduces the sternal-pubic distance. This tends to produce a flat chest and a long thoracic hyperkyphosis. Unilateral lateral shortening of both obliques reduces the rib-ilium space and produces a "C" curve with a contralateral convexity. Ipsilateral shortening of the external oblique with contralateral internal oblique shortening produces an "S" scoliosis. Bilateral shortening of the internal oblique and lateral stretching of the external oblique produces the anterior rotation of the pelvis and thoracic hyperkyphosis so often seen in a "slumped" posture.

Transversus Abdominis Weakness. This is exhibited best by the lateral bulging of the flanks during arching of the back in the prone position.

Relationship to Low-Back Pain

In studying abdominal (spinal flexors) and back extensor muscle function (strength and endurance) and the relation to chronic low-back pain, Smidt and associates[4] found that, in those with chronic low-back dysfunction, the abdominals were more susceptible to fatigue than the back extensors and women demonstrated more endurance than men. Similar findings are reported by Suzuki and Endo.[5]

Abdominal Wall Injuries[6-10]

Solar Plexus Impaction[11,12]

The large plexus of nerves located in the peritoneal cavity near the level of L1 con-

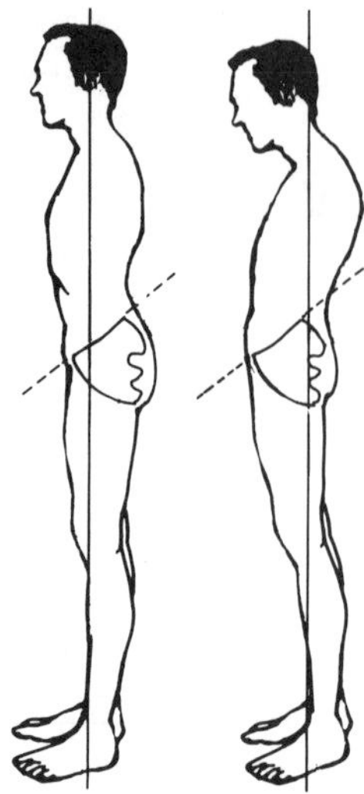

Figure 12.1. Evaluating oblique weakness from the lateral. *Left*, weaknes resulting in anterior pelvic tilt that is well compensated; *right*, weakness resulting in anterior pelvic tilt with forward pelvic displacement and poorly compensated thoracic hyperkyphosis and cervical projection.

tains two large ganglionic masses and a dense network of nerve fibers. It supplies nerves to the abdominal viscera and is indirectly associated with the respiratory mechanism. Thus, a strong blow to the abdominal area can inhibit breathing (winding) and result in unconsciousness. An abdominal blow overstimulates the fibers of the plexus and causes delayed venous return to the inferior vena cava.

The clinical picture is one of neurologic shock: faintness, prostration, dyspnea, clammy skin, and pallor. The air hunger often leads to panic. Fortunately, symptoms subside spontaneously in 2–3 minutes. Then, deep abdominal injury should be ruled out. A far more serious condition that should be considered is an associated splenic or hepatic rupture producing hemorrhage within the abdominal cavity.

Strains[13]

Unless a muscle is weakened by prior injury, it usually takes severe force to rupture an abdominal muscle. Symptoms of stress are pain, localized swelling, tenderness at the point of torn muscle or tendinous fibers, and ecchymosis occurring later. Motion increases pain. If a rupture has occurred, there is usually depression and hematoma at the site.

Local support by strapping in a position of relaxation and cold packs for 24–72 hours are advised.[14] This should be followed by heat, massage, and other appropriate physiotherapeutic and support measures. Stretching exercises are important during rehabilitation. If proper care is not administered, contractures may result that lead to spinal distortions.

Rectus Abdominis Rupture[15]

Although tearing of the abdominis muscle is rare, diagnosis must be rapid to avoid secondary lesions from hematoma. The common site is at the right inferior aspect. Because of its sheath of strong transverse bands, bleeding easily pools; and because of its extension from the lower ribs to the pubis, difficult breathing (thoracic) and coughing spells are usually exhibited. These signs are followed by severe "stomach ache," rigidity, and inability to forward flex the trunk when supine.

A torn inferior epigastric artery may be involved, characterized by shock and a large tender hematoma. When bleeding is suspected, apply ice packs to the area and refer immediately for surgical attention.

Avulsion from the anterior superior iliac spine (ASIS) may be involved. This is most common in adolescents.[16] Traction stress exhibits localized tenderness at the pubic attachment; later, roentgenography will show osseous sclerosis.

POSTURAL REALIGNMENT OF THE LUMBAR SPINE[17-20]

Low-back pain has been the second most frequent health complaint in the United States for many years, second only to headaches. More lost working hours are attributed to this affliction than any other factor, and the vast majority of these complaints find their cause in biomechanical failures. These failures are often complex, often accumulative, and often subtly hidden by the body's marvelous adaptive mechanisms—a diagnostic problem when pain is soley referred.

In general, faults in weight bearing can be attributed to the anterior portion of the vertebral motion unit, while faults in the direction of distortions can be blamed on the posterior aspect of the motion unit.

Body Balance and Equilibrium[21–28]

Posture is most efficient in the standing position when the vertical line of gravity falls through an aligned column of supporting bones. If the segments are aligned so that the gravity line passes directly through the center of each joint, the least stress is placed upon the adjacent ligaments and muscles. This ideal situation is impossible in the human body because the centers of segmental links and the movement centers between them cannot be brought to accurately meet with a common line of gravity.

Thoracolumbar Balance. When gravitational forces on a vertebral segment are in a balanced position, the pull is equal on all sides about the center of gravity; ie, its center of gravity is directly above its base of support and the segment is quite stable. The amount of body mass outside this base does not affect the equilibrium unless the center of gravity of the mass is altered. If mass is laterally shifted to one side without a compensatory shift of another part of equal weight, the center of gravity is displaced sideward.

Action Lines. Accumulative body weight on a lumbar segment offers resistance to movement because gravity is acting on the part only in a downward direction with the part's mass acting as if it were at its center of mass. The effectiveness of this weight for rotating a part can be changed by shifting its position in relation to the fulcrum (nucleus pulposus): the farther the gravity line falling through the center of mass is from the axis of motion, the longer will be the moment arm and the greater will be the moment. Keep in mind that the gravitational action line of any part can be moved nearer to or farther from the axis of a joint simply by changing the part's position.

Common Torques. In each given segment during lumbopelvic motion, the partial center of gravity or its axes of motion do not coincide with the common line of gravity. In fact, most partial centers are quite distant from the common line. This produces active rotary torques in many joints during static and dynamic postures because gravity forces must be neutralized by antigravity muscles. A weight-bearing joint is considered to be in equilibrium if the gravity line of the supported structure is equal to the joint's axis of rotation. If the gravity line is posterior to the joint's axis of rotation, the superior segment tends to rotate posteriorly in compensation; if it is anterior to the axis, the superior segment tends to rotate anteriorly.

Common Mechanical Causes of Nondisc Functional Pain[29–33]

Because more research has been done on the IVD than any other structure, there is an orthopedic tendency to attribute almost any type of backache to some type of disc disorder. This leads to tunnel vision because many disorders, both spinal and extraspinal, may simulate disc disease. The most common causes of nondisc functional pain are postural fatigue, spinal strains (acute and chronic), and IVF syndromes. Certain pelvic disorders may also be involved such as chronic adominal collapse, sacroiliac sprain, and coccygeal stress.

Postural Fatigue. After exercise, the unconditioned individual will experience aching, stiffness, and soreness in overexerted muscles (Fig. 12.2). This is common in the lower back muscles. In most cases of

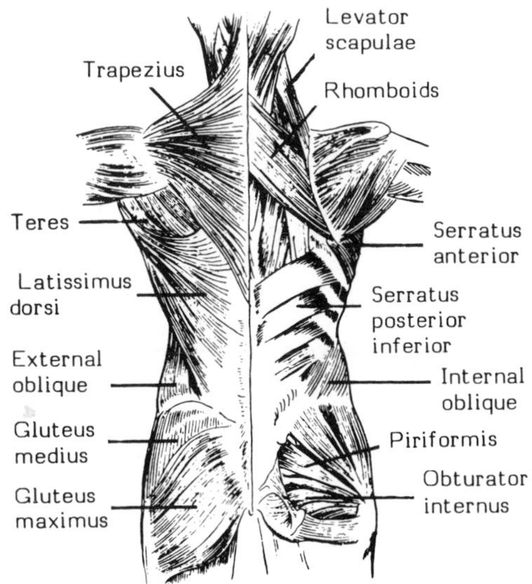

Figure 12.2. Some major muscles of the back. Superficial muscles are shown on the *left*, deeper muscles on the *right*.

such overstress, warmth and rest offer immediate relief and symptoms disappear with progressive conditioning. However, if at least stretching exercises are not offered, chronic strain can lead to the typical posture of spinal "sag," exhibiting drooping shoulders, a rounded thoracic region, inhibited rib and diaphragm motion, shallow breathing, lumbar hyperlordosis, anterior longitudinal ligament stretching, anterior pelvic rotation, chronic apophyseal synovitis, backache, disc collapse, bulging abdomen, visceroptosis, digestive disturbances, flatulence, and chronic tiredness.

While specific spinal adjustments are necessary to correct immediate symptoms, a most carefully supervised regimen of progressive corrective exercise (eg, isometric, isotonic, deep breathing) interspersed with adequate rest is a must if more than palliative care is to be offered. Care must be taken to avoid overexertion that would contribute to the chronic stress on weakened muscles and stiffened joints. In women, the initial cause can often be traced to poor postpartum management during which the stressed abdominal and pelvic muscles were not properly reconditioned.

Sitting Postures. In the erect sitting posture, body weight should be supported upon the ischial tuberosities and the adjacent soft tissues. The center of gravity is forward of the ischia, the lumbar lordosis is but slightly flattened, and about 25% of body weight is transmitted to the floor through the lower extremities. In the slouched sitting position, however, the center of gravity is posterior to the ischia, the lumbar lordosis is reversed, and far less body weight is transferred to the floor via the lower extremities.

The degree of the lumbar curve during the sitting posture depends upon sacral angulation, which is governed by pelvic posture and the degree of mobility of the involved segments. Lumbar IVD pressure is *higher* during sitting than in the standing posture because intradisc pressure increases with the tendency toward lumbar kyphosis.

Problems during Aging

Common Problems in Youth[34–36]

Intrinsic backache is not frequent in the preadolescent. When it occurs, it is painfully acute and has its highest incidence in the thoracic or thoracolumbar spine. The typical clinical picture exhibits severe antalgic spasm, thoracolumbar hyperkyphosis, muscular tenderness, no bony tenderness, positive Lasègue's sign, tight hamstrings, and negative roentgenographs. These signs suggest instability that is rarely confirmed by physical examination. Initial differentiation must be made from forgotten trauma and early Scheuermann's disease. Relief usually comes spontaneously after rest, but idiopathic episodes may occur and then disappear with further maturation.

Common Problems in Adulthood[37,38]

A loss of tissue elasticity and other signs of repeated trauma or degeneration are common during middle age. Quite frequently, psychologic stress superimposed on a biomechanical fault precipitates episodes of backache. The overt symptoms are increased by activity and relieved by rest. These must first be differentiated from the claudication-type backache and buttock pain associated with aortic block, aneurysm, and spinal stenosis.

Helfet and Lee describe the vertebral degenerative process after severe trauma as follows: compression injury fractures the end-plates which leads to disc and posterior joint changes. In following years, new bone forms markedly on the posterior articular processes and this leads to spinal stenosis at the level of injury. Fixation at this level produces added stress above and below, leading to extension of the degenerative arthritis and spinal stenosis.

Common Problems in Later Years[39–41]

In treating the fragile elderly, the cardinal concerns in both diagnosis and therapy are arteriosclerosis, demineralization, and diminished collagen. These disorders are said to affect 25% of females and 18% of males over 70 years of age.

Symptoms first arise in those joints under the greatest chronic stress such as the hip joint and the T11–L1 area. The loss of systemic collagen will be most noticeable on the dorsal aspect of the hands, where the skin will appear atrophic, thin, marbled and capillary fragility will usually be apparent. Unless the metabolic defect can be corrected, progressive thoracic kyphosis, pulmonary symptoms, disc degeneration and failure, vertebral collapse, and wedge fractures can be expected.

Muscle Conditioning[42,43]

The rectus abdominis, obliques, gluteus maximus, psoas major, iliacus, and hamstrings are the common muscles that need strengthening in lumbopelvic postural faults. Inasmuch as trunk or leg flexion in the supine position strongly activates the iliopsoas, such exercises must be avoided in cases of psoas hypertonicity. Some strengthening exercises are shown in Figure 12.3.

The erector spinae and quadratus lumborum are the muscles that usually need stretching in poor lumbopelvic posture. In most cases, pelvic tilting stretching to correct anterior or posterior fixation and weak muscles must be included in the regimen. Some stretching exercises are shown in Figures 12.4 and 12.5.

TRAUMATIC DISORDERS OF THE LUMBAR SPINE[44–48]

The lumbar spine, sacrum, ilia, pubic bone, and hips work as a functional unit. Any disorder of one part immediately affects the function of the other parts. A wide assortment of muscle, tendon, ligament, bone, nerve, and vascular injuries in this area are witnessed in general practice.

The Mechanics of Lifting[49–56]

During forward flexion, the trunk moves anteriorly and the spinal erectors contract to equalize the force of gravity in proportion to the degree of flexion. However, no erector action is present at full flexion and the load must be borne solely by the ligaments. Even though the muscles are strong and the bony segments are in good alignment, it takes a degree of mechanical ingenuity to lift without creating an overstress.

In the forward lifting position, the lumbosacral joint serves as a fulcrum with the extensors serving as a long arm of a lever (Fig. 12.6). An anterior rotational torque is placed on the spine by the weight of the body above the L5 disc and the load lifted. An analysis of the dynamics involved shows that the more the trunk is displaced from the neutral midline during flexion, the more the spinal and pelvic extensors are stressed. This is the result of (1) the increased distance from the fulcrum and (2) the more acute angle of pull of the spinal extensors, both of which contribute to greatly increased compression forces.

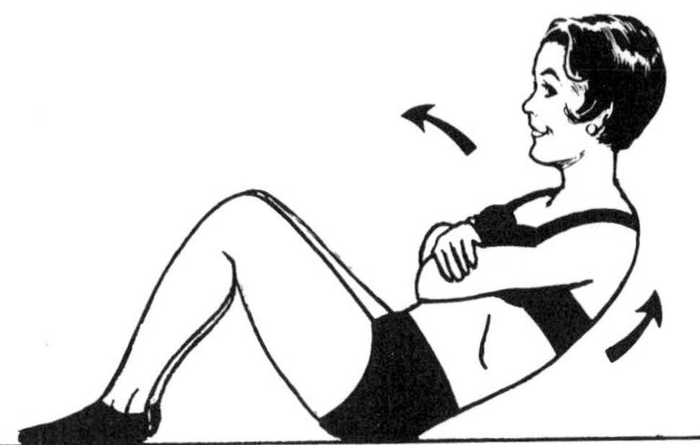

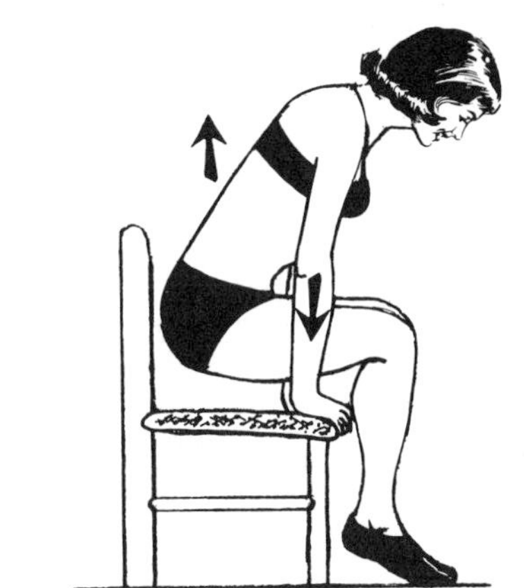

Figure 12.3. *Top*, abdominal strengthening exercise from the supine position. During flexion, instruct the patient to bring her nose to a site several inches lateral to the knee, alternating sides during an exercise bout of about 6 times, two or three times daily. *Bottom*, abdominal and spinal extensor strengthening exercise in the sitting position. As the patient flexes slightly forward, the front corners of the chair should be firmly grasped. The patient is instructed to lift the thighs and buttocks off the chair against body weight, hold this position for a few seconds, and then relax. This should be repeated at least 3–5 times, two or three times daily.

Body weight at the lumbosacral joint is resolved into two major components: one perpendicular to the sacral base offering a compressive force, and one parallel to the sacral base producing a shearing force. A 200-lb person with a normal sacral angle standing in the erect position carries a 75.5-

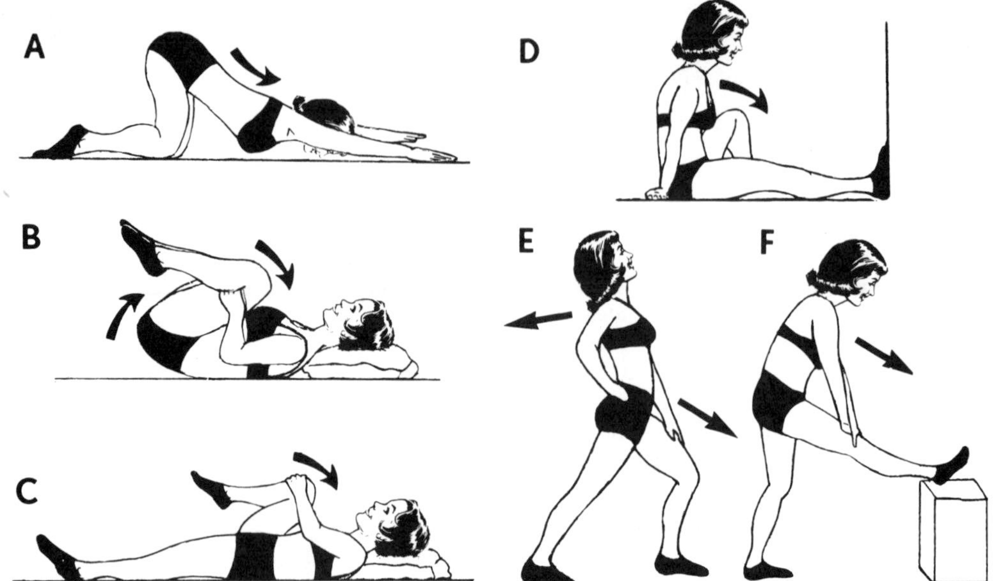

Figure 12.4. Stretching exercises. *A*, prone thoracolumbar stretch; *B*, supine thoracolumbar stretch; *C*, supine iliopsoas stretch; *D*, sitting hamstring stretch; *E*, standing iliopsoas stretch; *F*, standing hamstring stretch. Each exercise should be done at least 3–5 times, two or three times daily.

lb compressive force and a 65.6-lb shearing force on the lumbosacral joint. If a degree of lordosis exists so that the sacral angle is 60°, the individual would carry a 50-lb compression force and a 86.6-lb shearing force. Any sacral angle over 52° subjects the joint to severe stress, even in the erect position. If the lumbar area has flattened so that the sacral angle is only 30°, the forces reverse so that the compression force would be 86.6 lb and the shearing force would be 50 lb.

It is in such a mechanism that many back injuries occur. Overstress can be minimized by (1) keeping the load as close to the body as possible, (2) maintaining a comfortably wide stance to broaden the base of support, (3) keeping the trunk as erect as possible, (4) seeking mechanical aids if possible, and (5) only partially flexing the knees when lifting an object from the floor. Full knee flexion reduces quadriceps efficiency, thus placing an additional burden on the back. The strong plantar flexors should be utilized in gaining momentum.

Intradisc pressure within the lumbar IVDs increases as the lumbar spine flattens (flexes) and decreases as it curves forward (extends). It is for this reason that a professional weight lifter is taught to maintain a lumbar lordosis when his spine is loaded. Thus, if low-back pain is increased by lumbar flexion and decreased by extension, a disc problem is either responsible or a contributing factor in the syndrome.

Low-Back Strains[57–61]

Low-back disability has an extremely high incidence, and acute strains are frequently superimposed on chronic strains. The associated pain may be immediate or not occur for several hours after the tissues warmed by exercise begin to cool. Because of the increased lever arm operating on the lumbar segments, the incidence of injury is two times higher in taller individuals than shorter people.

The mechanism of injury is usually intrinsic rather than extrinsic. The precipitating cause is often through overbending, a steady lift, or a sudden release—all of which primarily involve the musculature. The most damaging forces are compression with torsion. When a weight is lifted, the arms and trunk can be considered as a long anterior lever that is counteracted by the extremely short lever extending from the disc nucleus (fulcrum) to the spinous process. This has

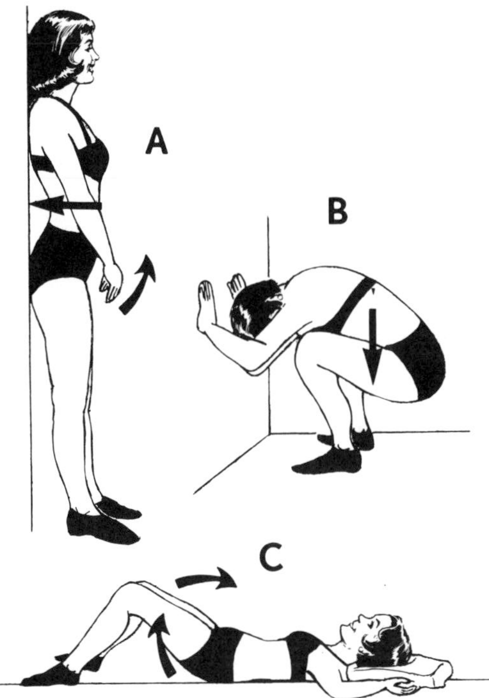

Figure 12.5. Pelvic tilt exercises to improve hyperlordosis. *A*, standing pelvic tilt exercise. With the patient's feet several inches from the wall and the knees slightly flexed, the thoracic and lumbar spine are flattened against the wall. Once the patient is able to do this with minimal strain, the heels should be progressively brought closer to the wall and the knee flexion reduced. *B*, squatting exercise with wall support to stretch the posterior calf and Achilles tendon. Ideally, this exercise should be done barefooted and the heels must be kept on the floor throughout the exercise. The feet should be placed about 5 inches apart and far enough from a wall so that a knee will not touch the wall during the exercise. Progressive shoe heel lowering and uphill walking (eg, treadmill) are recommended. *C*, prone pelvic tilt exercise. This is accomplished in two phases. First, the pelvis is rotated posteriorly so that the pubis moves toward the sternum and the lower back is flattened. Second, a push is made by the feet and the pelvis is raised toward the ceiling while the back is pushed against the floor. Each exercise is repeated at least 3–5 times, two or three times daily.

been estimated as a 15:1 ratio; thus, holding a 20-lb weight in front with the arms held horizontal must be counteracted by at least a 300-lb contraction of the spinal extensors to maintain equilibrium.

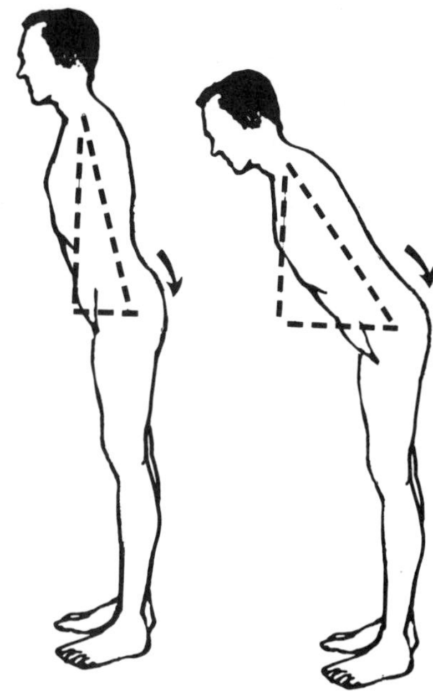

Figure 12.6. The further the trunk is flexed during a lift, the greater the torque on the lumbosacral joint.

Low-Back Sprains[62–65]

In the well-conditioned individual, IVD conditions are more often, but not exclusively, attributed to extrinsic blows and wrenches. An accurate and complete history is vital to arrive at an accurate diagnosis and offer the best management and counsel.

Horizontal shear forces appear to be the most damaging forces for disrupting the ligamentous strapping between vertebrae. Because of the lax capsules, a minor sprain can produce a severe synovitis at the posterior joints. If the synovium is torn on the side of tension, irritating hemarthrosis results and fragments of fractured articular cartilage and periosteum may form loose bodies in the joint. The distorted articular surface may produce chronic instability from erosion and degeneration, leading to reactionary osteophytoses which in turn are subject to fracture. Repeated episodes of minor trauma and tissue changes predispose progressive degenerative arthritis.

Chronic Strain and Sprain

Chronic strain results in fine fibrous intramuscular adhesions that interfere with normal motion. The features are a history of trauma, palpable swelling within the involved muscles, and trigger point tenderness. Helfet and Lee feel that this occurs most frequently at the junction of tissues of differing elasticity (eg, attachments).[66] Overstress disrupts muscle fibers, and this produces bleeding, swelling, and exudate organization leading to further adhesions. These adhesions respond well to manipulative therapy, but they will recur unless the joint is exercised a few minutes a day to its maximum range of motion.

In general, the process can be described in two phases. (1) Stress is applied to weakened muscles, which produces stretching and inflammation. Initially, the stretched soft tissues will be lax and the joint will exhibit a degree of instability once spasm subsides. (2) Later, protective and fibrotic soft-tissue shortening develops as soft tissue readily adapts to activity needs. If articular subluxation is also involved, the result is shortening on one side of the joint and stretching on the other side that tend to hold the joint in chronic subluxation. In time, articular "gluing" and periarticular bony overgrowth will develop to fix the joint in the misaligned state.

Subluxations, Fractures, and Dislocations[67–69]

Subluxations are discussed throughout this chapter, but a few general points are well to make here. The apices of curvatures and rotations are logical points for spinal listings since they are frequently the location of maximum vertebral stress. Subluxations may occur at other points in curves and rotations, particularly at the beginning point of a primary defect in balance such as in the lower lumbar and upper cervical sections. Subluxations also frequently occur at the point where a primary curve merges into its compensatory curve. A posterior subluxation of L3 is rare when the apex of the lumbar curve is too high or too low, but common at L4, L5, or the sacral base. When the apex of the lumbar curve is too low, a posterior subluxation will most likely be found in the upper lumbar area.[70]

Rotational Subluxations. Rotational malpositions of the lower lumbar vertebrae are frequently seen and invariably associated with changes in the related disc and posterior joints. It is usually impossible to tell what is primary and what is secondary because each can cause the other. In addition, rotation is coupled with tilting and vice versa. Periodic recurrence after correction can usually be attributed to congenital asymmetry of the facet planes or acquired asymmetry from the repeated deformation forces of trauma.

Roentgenographic Considerations. As in other areas of the body, x-ray views of the spine must be chosen according to the part being examined and the injury situation. And as with the cervical spine, careful evaluation must be made of the vertebral structures, the IVDs, and the paraspinal soft tissues. The L5–S1 and sacroiliac joints, the pelvis, and its contents deserve careful scrutiny. Acute injuries to the supporting soft tissues about a vertebra are not clearly demonstrable, but their presence is suggested when the normal relations of bony structures are disturbed. When ligamentous lesions heal, hypertrophic spurs and sometimes bridges may develop locally on the margins of the bones affected.

Avulsions. The lower back and pelvis are the most common sites for avulsion-type injuries. Severe, sudden muscle contraction, especially during rotation in flexion, can produce fragmented osseous tears near sites of soft-tissue origin and insertion. Avulsions in the lumbar area often occur with transverse process fragmentation at the site of psoas insertion. Helfet and Lee feel that this is the most common avulsion fracture of the body.[66]

Transverse Process Fractures. Although the transverse processes of the lumbar spine are quite sturdy, multiple fractures are seen after severe accidents. Such fractures are sometimes not evident or are poorly visualized in roentgenography, unless they are markedly displaced or angled, due to overlying gas and/or soft-tissue shadows that obscure detail. Howe[71] suggests a cleansing enema or other means of clearing overlying soft-tissue shadows whenever all bony processes are not well visualized. Transverse process fractures are frequently asymptomatic or nearly so and often lack the symptoms to encourage the careful examination necessary.

Spinal Cord Injuries[72]

Any trace or sensory abnormality, objective or subjective, should immediately raise suspicion of injury to the spinal cord or cauda equina. White and Panjabi mention studies showing that during severe spinal trauma, relaxed muscles appear to be associated with less cord injury than when the muscles are strongly tensed.

Injuries to the lumbar cord or its tail occur from vertebral fractures, dislocations, or penetrating wounds in severe accidents. In other rare instances, the cord may be damaged from violent falls with trunk flexion. The T12–L1 and L5–S1 areas are the common sites of injury, especially those of crushing fractures with cord compression. Neurologic symptoms develop rapidly, but the lower the injury, the fewer roots will be involved. More common than these rare occurrences are cord tractions, concussions, and, less frequently, contusions.

Pathologic Traction of the Spinal Cord. A lumbar scoliotic deviation must always be attended by a commensurate vertebral body rotation to the convex side. If this does not occur, it is atypical and most likely pain-producing. If the vertebral bodies were not subject to the law of rotation during bending, the spine would have to lengthen during bending and its contents (ie, cord, cauda equina, and their coverings) would be subjected to considerable stretch. Thus, in a case of scoliotic deviation in the lumbar area without body rotation toward the convex side, signs indicating undue tension within the vertebral canal should be sought. It should also be noted that atlanto-occipital, atlantoaxial, and coccygeal disrelation with partial fixation places a degree of traction upon the cord, dura, and dural sleeves in flexion-extension and lateral bending efforts.

Concussion of the Spinal Cord. Immediate signs are usually not manifested in mild or moderate injuries; but weeks later, lower extremity weakness and stiffness may be experienced. It takes time for nerve fibers to degenerate. Deep reflexes become exaggerated and originally mild sensory, bladder, and rectal disturbances progress. The picture is cloudy, often mimicking a number of cord diseases (eg, sclerosis, atrophy, syringomyelia). Life is rarely threatened, but full recovery is doubtful.

Contusions of the Spinal Cord. Cord concussion usually complicates cord contusion. If laceration occurs, shock is rapid. Deep reflexes, sensation, and sphincter control are lost. The paralysis is flaccid. Obviously, a prognosis cannot be made until the shock is survived.

Kernig's Neck Test. Biomechanically, this test is the cephalad representation of Lasègue's straight-leg-raising test. The supine patient is asked to place both hands behind his head and forcibly flex his head toward his chest. Pain in the neck or lower back, or down the lower extremities indicates meningeal irritation, nerve root involvement, or irritation of the dural coverings of the nerve root. That is, something is being aggravated by the tensile forces.

Kernig's Leg Test. The examiner flexes the thigh at a right angle with the torso and holds it there with one hand. With the other hand, the ankle is grasped and an attempt is made to extend the leg at the knee. If pain or resistance is encountered as the leg extends, the sign is positive, provided there is no hip or knee stiffness or sacroiliac disorder.

Milgram's Test. The supine patient is asked to keep his knees straight and lift both legs off the table about 2 inches and to hold this position for as long as possible. The test stretches the anterior abdominal and iliopsoas muscles and increases intrathecal pressure (Fig. 12.7). Intrathecal pressure can be ruled out in the typical adult if the patient can hold this position for 20 seconds without pain. If this position cannot be held or if pain is experienced early during

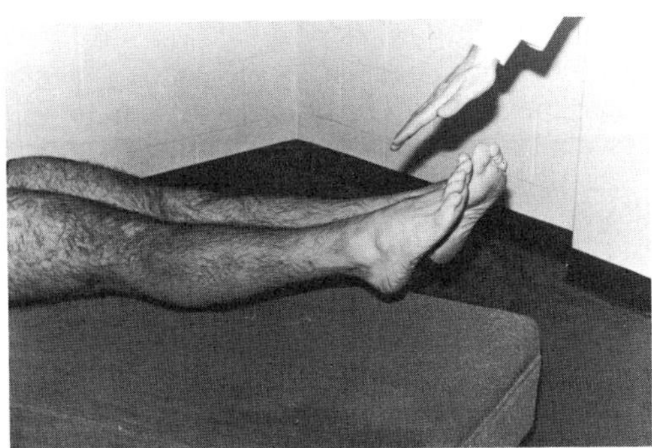

Figure 12.7. Milgram's test.

the test, a positive sign is offered that indicates, for example, intrathecal pathology, herniated disc, or pressure upon the cord from some source.

LUMBAR PAIN AND SPASM

Once the difference between normal and abnormal is well understood, changes in posture, muscle tone, and movement offer fundamental clinical clues to diagnosis and therapy. And once the biomechanical mechanisms involved are appreciated, painful effects can often be reproduced or relieved at will. Knowing exactly *where, when,* and *how* motion increases or decreases pain are the major clues that lead the examiner to find and correct the biomechanical fault, whether it be functional or structural.

Low-Back Pain[31,73–81]

The major predisposing factors to low-back pain appear to be a poor sitting posture, a loss of motion within the normal range of lumbar extension, and/or excessive hyperflexion activities. The primary precipitating factors usually involved are a sudden stress at an unguarded moment of lifting with inadequate mechanical advantage.

Incidence

A survey of questionnaire of 1221 males between the ages of 18 and 55 years seen in family practice was conducted by Frymoyer and associates[82] to determine the prevalence of a history of low-back pain and associated risk factors. The results are shown in Table 12.1.

The Lumbar Nociceptive Receptor System[62,83,84]

Static postural support of the lumbar spine in the prolonged relaxed erect or seated postures is provided essentially by the passive elastic tension of the involved ligaments and fascia rather than the spinal muscles, whose role can be considered insignificant during a state of relaxation. This shifting of support from the muscles to the ligaments, however, occurs slowly over a period of several minutes before significant EMG activity can be considered absent.

The lumbar ligaments and fascia are richly innervated by nociceptive receptors. When the lumbar spine is in a relaxed neutral position, its nociceptive receptor system is relatively inactive. However, any mechanical force that will stress or deform receptors, with or without overt damage, or any irritating chemical of sufficient concentration will depolarize unmyelinated fibers and enhance afferent activity.

Mechanical and Chemical Factors of Traumatic Low-Back Pain[85–88]

Pain experienced after trauma can be the result of mechanical factors, chemical factors, or both.

Characteristics of Mechanical Pain. Normal mechanical force applied to normal tissue does not produce pain. However, abnormal mechanical deformation occurs whenever (1) abnormal stress is applied to normal tissues (eg, postural pain), (2) abnormal stress is applied to abnormal tissues, or (3) normal stress is applied to abnormal tissues (eg, soft-tissue shortening). Pain from mechanical causes is sharp, acute, and occurs immediately. If mechanical pain does not occur until several minutes or hours after an activity, it is most likely that the position assumed following the activity is the cause of the pain rather than the activity itself.

Mechanical pain may be intermittent, appearing and disappearing, or vary in intensity according to aggravating and beneficial circumstances. It is usually intermittent be-

Table 12.1.
Risk Factors in Low-Back Pain

History of low-back pain	Percentage of survey	Risk factors
No history	30.1	No specific identifiable factors
Moderate pain	46.3	Jogging, cross-country skiing
Severe pain, with more lower extremity complaints	23.6	Heavy lifting, using jackhammers, operating motor vehicles, cigarette smoking

cause of increased and decreased mechanical deformation forces. *In cases of pain of mechanical origin, the examiner should always be able to reproduce the patient's symptoms by test movements.* Constant pain from constant mechanical deformation (eg, irreducible disc protrusion) is always possible but not common. The rule to remember is that *pain of mechanical origin is always affected by movement,* for better or worse.

Characteristics of Chemical Pain. Chemical irritants accumulate in damaged tissue soon after injury. As soon as the nociceptive receptor activity is enhanced, pain will be experienced. Chemical irritation an be the result of any inflammatory, infectious, or traumatic process of sufficient degree. It can also be the result of any abnormal metabolic by-product, especially that of ischemia, of sufficient concentration to irritate free nerve endings in involved tissues.

In contrast to pain of mechanical origin, pain from chemical causes is constant, dull, and aggravated by normal movements as long as the chemical irritants are present in sufficient concentration. It may not occur until several minutes or hours after an injurious event has taken place. Chemical pain subsides during the natural healing process as scar tissue forms. Rarely does chemical pain from trauma extend past 20 days after the accident.

Considerations in Adjustive Therapy. The motion that eases pain the most (reduces mechanical deformation) usually determines the plane of adjustive therapy. An exception to this would be the pain produced by motion that stretches shortened tissues. This type of pain subsides immediately when passive stress is removed and the joint returns to its neutral position.

In either subluxation or displaced IVD substance (ie, end-plate, anulus, nucleus pulposus), a dynamic adjustment should be given in the direction that *decreases* mechanical deformation and pain. When shortened tissues are involved, slow rhythmic manipulation increasing in force should be given in the direction that stretches the contracted tissues and temporarily *increases* pain. In some instances, a dynamic adjustment will be necessary to free adhesions and locked facets. Obviously, this requires careful differentiation prior to therapy.

Oriental Concepts. Spinal manipulative techniques have been a part of Chinese traditional medicine for over 1000 years. It is interesting to note than in modern China, in contrast to the many chiropractic and osteopathic techniques suggested in this country, only six steps of maneuver in three positions are generally practiced. (1) *In the supine position:* traction on the spine, hip rotation with leg flexed, straight-leg raising with gentle flexion and extension of the knee, flexion of the lower back in the knee-chest position, and correction of the spinal listing. (2) *In the lateral recumbent position:* waist rotation and hyperextension of the waist and hip by pulling the lower limb backward. (3) *In the prone position:* waist vibration by manual or automatic manipulation. Kuo and Tang[89] followed up 850 cases in which these procedures were utilized and found that excellent to good results were rated in 81.9%, with a recurrence rate of 35.9%.

Prognostic Clues

While prognosis in a case of acute low-back pain must be founded upon specific findings, the patient's age and occupation, and a multitude of other factors, Murphy and Cornish[90] arrived at a profile that appears to offer some guidance as to whether or not the disorder would become chronic. Their study of 48 patients concluded that patients whose disorders became chronic complained in the acute stage of pain over a wider area of the body, pain that was deeper and more central, higher anxiety, and lower activity levels.

Posture

Watching the body move offers the best clues to muscle trouble. If a posterior disc protrusion or an irritated nerve root is involved, the patient will invariably assume the antalgic position shown in Figure 12.8. The posteriorly rotated pelvis, the flattened lumbar area, and the slight flexion of the knees and hips, bilateral or unilateral, is an unconscious attempt to lessen the tension of the involved sciatic nerve and/or to reduce intradisc pressure. The greater the pain, the greater will be this "semi-squatting" posture in the upright position. Golfers will recognize this position of balance.

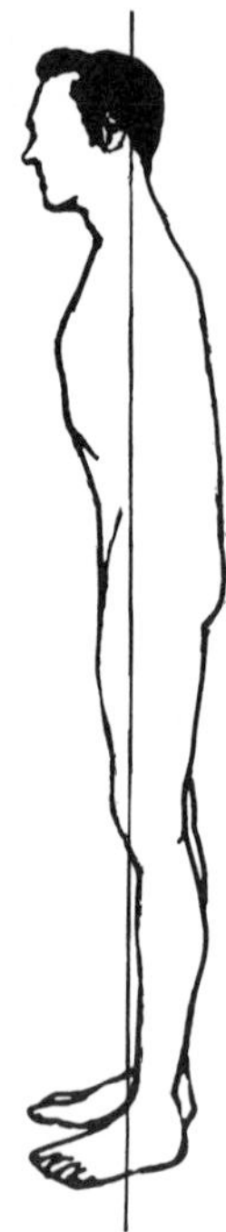

Figure 12.8. A patient with an IVD protrusion in the upper lumbar area. The thorax is flexed slightly forward of the midline and the pelvis is posterior to the midline to place more weight on the anterior aspect of the involved motion unit. The erectors, and often the abdominals, are splinted to minimize spinal motion. The vertebra superior to the involved segment is invariably locked in a position of extension.

Muscle Considerations

Spasm[91–93]

General spasm of the spinal muscles guarding motion in the vertebral joints can be tested by watching the body attitude (eg, stiff, military carriage) and by efforts to bend the spine forward, backward, and to the sides. If we are familiar with the average range of mobility in each direction and at the different ages, this test is usually easy and rapid. Care should be taken to differentiate phasic spasm (usually antalgic) from frequently exhibited reflex hypertonicity.

It is one thing to find muscle spasm present and another to determine whether it is protective, compensatory, hysterical, or a causative factor. Careful analysis of gait is an important method of gaining differential clues. Limitations of motion due to muscular spasm are seen with special frequency in joint pathology and subluxation-fixations, but they may occur in almost any form of joint trouble, particularly in the larger joints.

Muscle Enlargement

Hypertrophy and spasm must be differentiated from the muscular enlargement following exercise. The increase in muscle bulk following exercise is caused by two factors: (1) there is an opening of capillaries during activity that are closed during rest, and (2) prolonged activity appears to increase the size of individual muscle fibers, which is thought to result from an increase in sarcoplasm. A few authorities believe that even the number of myofibrils may increase during increased exercise over several weeks. If this is true, it rescinds the old "law" that the quantity of myofibrils does not increase after birth.

Muscular Pain from Lymph Dysfunction

Low-back pain of muscular origin is often a complex problem. Although skeletal muscle tissue lacks an intrinsic lymph supply, a muscle's connective tissue sheath and tendons are richly endowed with lymphatic vessels. During the normal physiologic exchange of fluids through capillary walls, the quantity of fluid leaving the capillary is usually greater than that entering the venule. The related lymphatic network takes up this excess and eventually delivers it to the venous system. It is this process that allows a continuous exchange of tissue fluids and maintains a constant pressure of interstitial fluid.

The flow of lymph is increased during activity as is capillary circulation, but this flow can be restricted by excessive pressure exerted by a constantly hypertonic or phasic contracted muscle. De Sterno[94] shows that inhibited lymph drainage contributes to muscular pain during prolonged activity by (1) causing a buildup of interstitial fluids that increase hydrostatic pressure, and (2) encouraging the accumulation of metabolic waste products that would normally be drained by the lymphatics and venules.

Selected Effects of Hypertonicity in the Lower Trunk

As the spine is never completely static, even during sleep, proprioceptive activity and its neuromuscular responses are continuous throughout life. If structural disrelationship exists, neural firing is magnified by increased muscle stretch, hypertonicity, ligament tension, and abnormal joint position to the point of unconscious central bombardment. The result is fatigue, muscle soreness, myofibrosis, and possible osteoarthritis.

Excessive hypertonicity of a muscle, confirmed by palpatory tone and soreness, will tend to subluxate its site of osseous attachment. Below is a listing of common problem areas in the lumbar area.[95]

1. *Latissimus dorsi.* Increased tone tends to pull the lower half of the spine and the pelvis anterior, lateral, and superior.
2. *Quadratus lumborum.* Increased tone tends to subluxate the ilium superiorly and pull the 12th rib and lumbar transverse processes posteroinferior.
3. *Iliocostalis lumborum.* Increased tone tends to pull the pelvis superior and posterior and the rib cage and lower thoracic transverse processes inferior and anterior.
4. *Psoas group.* Increased tone tends to pull the lumbar spine into anterior and inferior flexion.
5. *Erector spinae.* This muscle group arises from the iliac crests, sacrum, and spines of the L5–T11 segments, then splits and inserts as iliocostal, longissimus, and spinal muscles. Hypertonicity puts the lumbar area into hyperlordosis.
6. *Interspinales.* Increased tone tends to hyperextend the segments affected.
7. *Multifidus.* Increased tone tends to rotate the lumbar spine by pulling the involved spinous processes anterior and lateral.
8. *Rectus abdominis.* Increased tone tends to roll the pubis superior and posterior and pull the medial thorax inferior.

Muscular Pain

Many acute spinal pains with a history of overexertion are muscular in origin. This overexertion may be from (1) continuous contractions of long duration in a normal physiologic state, (2) vigorous jerky movements of short duration, or (3) a combination of stretch reflex and relaxation reactions if fibers have been stretched to a pathologic length. It has been shown that repeated stress can produce more soreness if a short rest interval is allowed between movements (eg, shoveling) because a great workload is demanded.

Types of Postexertion Pain of Muscular Origin. There are two types. They may be found most anywhere in the body but are more common to the lumbar area.

1. *Immediate pain,* which can persist for hours. This is largely attributed to diffusible metabolic end-products (eg, potassium and lactic acid) acting upon pain receptors within the involved muscles.

De Sterno[94] states that "an isometric contraction of only 60% of maximum strength results in almost complete occlusion of the blood vessels that supply muscle tissue. This results when the pressure of the contracted muscle exceeds systolic arterial pressure." Such contraction and vascular compression reduces oxygen supply, reduces the removal of metabolic ash, lowers muscle pH, increases receptor-irritating lactic acid, and increases the osmotic pressure within the muscle—all of which contribute to fatigue, pain, decreased contractility, and a breakdown in homeostasis.

2. *Delayed pain,* characterized by localized spasm and soreness that does not appear for 24–48 hours (often called myositis). While the same mechanisms involved in immediate pain can explain some of the etiology of delayed pain, two other explanations can be put forth. One involves fatigue, the other tonicity.

The Fatigue Theory. Repeated contractions with short rest intervals (1–2 seconds) produce a decrease in contraction amplitude accompanied by fatigue. This results in an inability to achieve complete relaxation and leads to spasm.

The Spasm Theory. Exercise to the level at which capillaries are occluded by muscle contraction produces intrinsic ischemia and potassium leakage into extracellular tissue which, in turn, elevates osmotic pressure. This increased pressure irritates pain receptors that initiate a reflex tonic contraction which, in turn, enhances the ischemia. Thus a pathologic cycle is created (Fig. 12.9).

The Stretch Reflex. Antalgic muscle spasm is common to acute lumbar dysfunction. Keep in mind that the myotatic stretch reflex uses a single sensory neuron and is

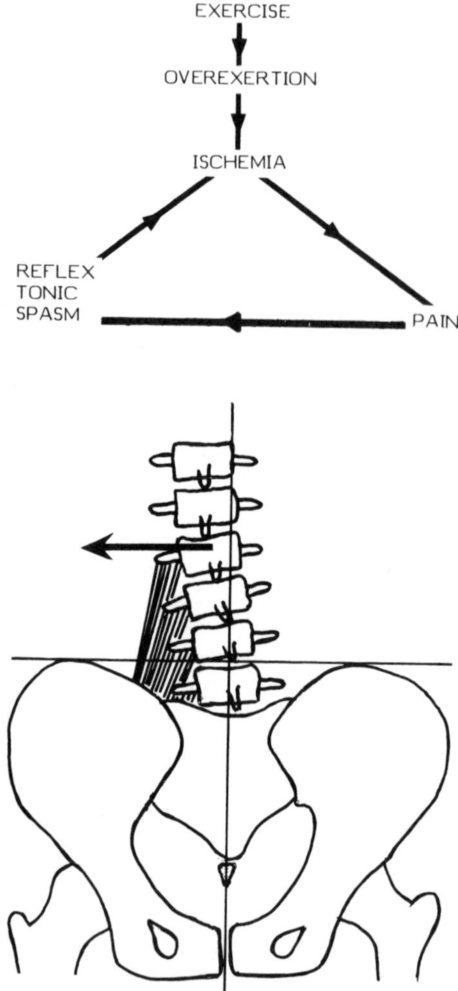

Figure 12.9. *Top*, the pathologic cycle as commonly seen in acute lumbago following overexertion. *Bottom*, schematic of erector spinae reflex spasm following irritation of a nerve root at an IVF. *Arrow* indicates direction of scoliosis.

initiated by elongation of muscle spindle's annulospiral receptors. The effect is a protective contraction designed to protect against further stretch so that the muscle may maintain a constant length. This reflex action is many times more severe if initiated by a sudden stretch than by a slow stretch. In addition, inhibitory impulses are transmitted to the motor neurons of the antagonists (reciprocal inhibition) and facilitating impulses are transmitted to the synergists—both of which enhance the response. The stretch reflex is not normally initiated by voluntary contraction. If there is spasm present after trauma, the irritating focus can usually be attributed to irritating ischemia initially and blood debris later.

Thoracolumbar Trigger Points[96–100]

The most common trigger points of the thoracic region are the scalene, pectoralis minor, and serratus anterior (Fig. 12.10). These points are often sites of secondary reaction to lumbar dysfunction.

The most common trigger points for the lumbar area are located (1) alongside the T12–L1 spinous processes and (2) alongside the L5–S1 spinous processes. The T12–L1 trigger, often associated with a T12 spinous process tipped posterosuperiorly, frequently refers pain to the iliac crest with secondary nodules found deep along the posterosuperior crest (Fig. 12.11). The L5–S1 trigger is usually within the multifidi. Trigger points may also be found in the erector spinae, when the patient is prone, about 1 inch lateral to the spinous processes. Specific trigger points for the multifidus and iliocostalis and their areas of referred pain are shown in Figure 12.12.

Management

Rest and warmth (to increase oxygen supply) are the best therapy in immediate pain following muscle overexertion. Delayed spasms are best treated by stretching to activate the Golgi tendon organs and the myotatic stretch reflex. Stretching reduces

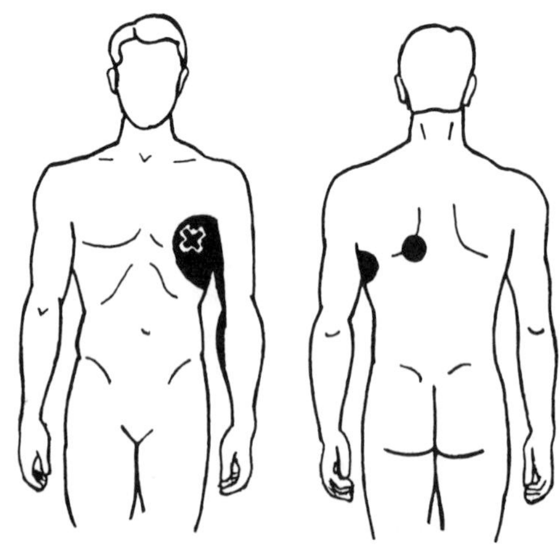

Figure 12.10. Serratus anterior trigger point; *X*, common site. *Blackened areas* indicate typical sites of referred pain.

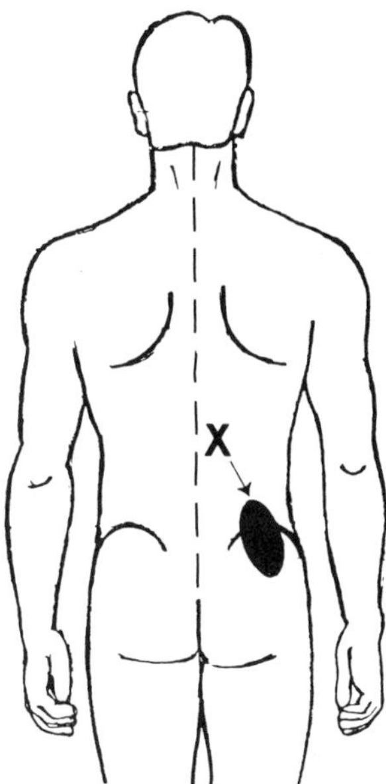

Figure 12.11. The thoracolumbar transitional trigger point on the right; *X*, common site. *Blackened area* indicates typical site of referred pain and often referred tenderness.

electromyographic activity but is contraindicated during the acute stage if fresh muscle tears are present.

STRUCTURAL FIXATION AND MOTION PALPATION OF THE LUMBAR SPINE[101–113]

While 15% of asymptomatic patients indicate hypomobility of the lumbar region, a recent study has shown that as many as 43% of patients with low back pain have decreased movement of the lumbar spine.

Muscle and Ligament Fixations

Whenever a segment is in a state of prolonged distortion, the involved connective tissues histologically adapt to their biomechanical requirements. Fibers on the side of the concavity shorten and fibers on the side of the convexity lengthen. This process occurs in all connective tissues but becomes more overt in muscular and ligamentous tissues because motion is no longer symmetrical. Unless corrective action is taken, this state becomes progressively degenerative as the result of the abnormal weight distribution during static and dynamic activity.

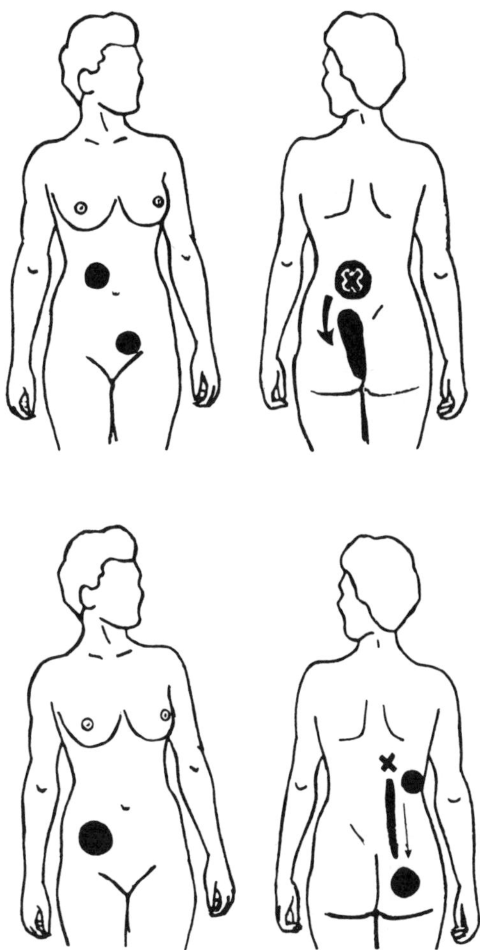

Figure 12.12. *Top*, multifidus trigger point; *X*, common site. *Blackened areas* indicate typical sites of referred pain. *Bottom*, iliocostalis trigger point; *X*, common site. *Blackened areas* indicate typical sites of referred pain.

The Interspinous Muscles. Chronic hypertonicity of the lumbar interspinous muscles leading to fibrotic changes is probably the most common finding associated with the fixed lordosis related to chronic low-back pain. Such a lordosis does not fully flatten in the supine position. The focal superior articulation is pulled into a stressed position away from the inferior process (facet syndrome). On a lateral roentgenograph, the involved articular space exhibits an abnormal V-shaped appearance and the disc space will appear increased at the anterior and decreased at the posterior. In the more acute stage, it is due strictly to muscular spasm. In the chronic stage, the muscles become fibrotic and the paravertebral ligaments shorten, often to an area extended quite lateral from the midline.

The Quadratus Lumborum. This quadrate muscle, which acts as one large muscle on each side of loin, connects the iliac crest and thoracolumbar fascia to the 12th rib and transverse processes of the lumbar vertebrae. Its primary role is that of lumbar lateral flexion and rotation during lateral flexion of the trunk. When active bilaterally, it stabilizes the lumbar spine. If involved in either local or reflex hypertonicity, the posterior lumbar articulations on the side of fixation are forced open in an abnormal arc. If severe, this can force the inferior process into the IVF and produce direct impingement of the IVF contents. The typical result is sciatica on the *convex* side of the lumbar scoliosis.

The Intertransverse Muscles. Chronic hypertonicity of the intertransverse muscles is another common cause of low-back pain. The transverse processes approximate, the disc thins ipsilaterally, and the height of the IVF is reduced. In contrast to quadratus lumborum fixation, hypomobility of this muscle causes sciatica on the *concave* side of the lumbar scoliosis.

The Erector Spinae. When these muscles become fibrotic, gentle and progressive stretching is required, often for many months because these muscles are largely fascia to begin with. Because of their placement bilaterally, the most helpful exercise is lateral bending in the standing position; A-P motions may overexert the lower lumbar area.

The Iliolumbar Ligaments. Functionally, L5 acts as part of the pelvis. This is probably due to the usually strong iliolumbar ligaments that connect the L5 transverse processes to the iliac crests.

When lumbar and pelvic muscles become fibrotic, a search should be made for other areas within the lower extremity, such as the hip flexors and the gastrocnemius (eg, the "high heel" syndrome).

Dynamic Lumbar Palpation

The lumbar spine can be palpated in the same manner as the cervicals and dorsals, except that rotation is normally quite limited in the upper lumbar segments. Most examiners prefer that the patient be seated during dynamic palpation of the lumbar spine. Segmental flexion and extension motions are difficult to feel and are useful only in classic retrolisthesis and anterolisthesis.

Flexion-Extension. The palpating fingers are placed within the interspinous spaces of the units being examined. Two or three motion units may be examined simultaneously by separate fingers. An interspinous space normally opens during flexion and closes during extension, and the spinous processes tend to move posteriorly during flexion and anteriorly during extension. Erratic motions are noted and interspinous spaces are compared during movement.

Rotation. Motion is felt best when the spine is slightly flexed during rotation. First, the palpating fingers are placed in the interspinous spaces being examined and evenness of movement is noted. Normally, the spinous processess will fan slightly anterior and lateral opposite the side of posterior rotation. Any segmental restriction or hypermobility is noted. Next, a thumb is placed on each transverse process of the unit being examined and the patient is asked to make the same movements actively.

Lateral Flexion. The palpating fingers are placed on the spinous processes being examined. When the trunk is laterally flexed, the spinous processes normally fan slightly apart and move toward the concavity. Erratic motions, restrictions, and excessive movements are noted. The L4–L5 joint is best palpated in lateral flexion with the thumbs lateral to the interspinous space. If the PSIS opposite lateral flexion of L5 moves inferior, this is normal motion. Any other motion indicates a fixation of the L4–L5 joints.

LUMBOSACRAL ANGLE SYNDROMES[114-117]

In the erect position, the line of gravity typically falls through the posterior edge of the lumbosacral joint. The average sacral angle during stance is about 40°. The normal range appears to be between 35° and 55°, depending upon the reference used (Fig. 12.13). Thus, function, alignment, and

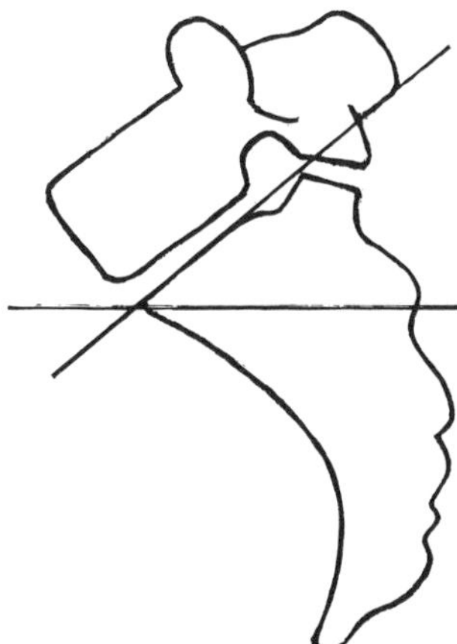

Figure 12.13. The lumbosacral angle is formed by a horizontal line and a line drawn through the superior surface of the sacral base. The greater the angle, the greater the "step off" of the lumbar lordosis.

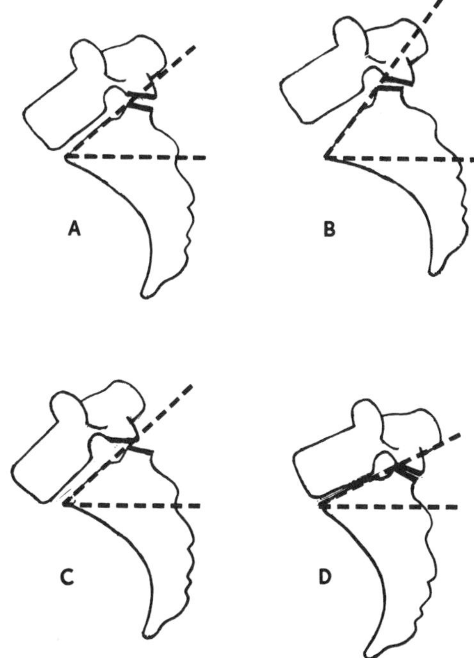

Figure 12.14. Common lumbosacral articular relationships. *A*, normal lumbosacral relationship, about 40°. *B*, increased angulation with posterior subluxation of L5 or, more likely, an anterior subluxation of the sacral base. *C*, spondylolisthesis with normal angulation and anterior subluxation of L5 or posterior subluxation of the sacral base. *D*, disc degeneration syndrome exhibiting decreased angulation and narrowing of the IVF without subluxation but with apophyseal jamming.

dynamic signs and symptoms are better criteria than exact angulation requirements.

In the erect position, the abdominal and spinal erectors should be relaxed, and the lumbosacral joint is loaded only by the weight of the body above. Flexion is the most pronounced spinal motion. About 75% of all spinal flexion below the neck occurs in the lumbar spine, and about 70% of all lumbar flexion occurs at the lumbosacral joint.

Lumbosacral Instability[118–120]

Lumbosacral instability is a mechanical aberration of the spine that renders it more susceptible to fatigue and/or subsequent trauma by reason of the variance from the optimal structural weight-bearing capabilities. Harriman states that between 50% and 80% of the general population exhibit some degree of the factors that predispose to lumbosacral instability, whether by reason of anomalous development of articular relationships or altered relationships due to trauma or disease consequences.[121] It is the most common finding of lumbosacral roentgenography and often brought to light after an acute strain (Fig. 12.14).

Disturbance of the physiologic response of the spinal segment is the primary finding, with the sequela of "stress response syndrome" which may take the form of any degree ranging from sclerosis of a tendon to and including an ankylosing hypertrophic osteophytosis or arthrosis. Frequent trauma to the articular structures as a result of excessive joint mobility results in repetitive microtrauma. The scope of involvement and the tissue response is determined by the type of severity of the instability.

Signs and Symptoms. Unusual early fatigue is a constant symptom, and this leads to strain, sprain, and subsequent disc pathologies. Symptom susceptibility increases with the age of the individual. Postural evaluation is especially important during the physical diagnosis of the sequelae as well as to an extraspinal causation (eg, short leg syndrome).

Roentgenographic Considerations. Roentgenographic diagnosis is the best manner of delineating the type and severity of the underlying productive agent of the condition of instability. However, there is no characteristic finding except the recognition of the various anomalies and pathologies present. Care should be taken to include the entire pelvis in this determination because, for instance, a sacroiliac arthrosis may lead to instability.

Acute Lumbosacral Stress[122, 123]

Any movement or distortion of the lumbar spine affects the pelvis, and any movement or distortion of the pelvis affects the lumbar spine. Thus, postural distortions of the lumbar area with a muscular etiology should never be considered apart from the pelvis. However, occasionally a case will be seen that exhibits a major lumbar distortion with normal pelvic function.

Finneson states that the diagnosis of lumbosacral spasm is probably given more frequently than any other diagnosis related to back dysfunction.[124] He also feels it is a "wastebasket" diagnosis into which any low-back dysfunction that is not readily identified is erroneously placed.

Lumbosacral Sprain. Acute lumbosacral sprains have a high incidence. They occur most commonly in the 25–50 year age group, and sedentary workers are involved just as frequently as workers doing heavy labor. Heavy loads or severe blows, especially at an unguarded moment, may rupture some associated ligaments and/or subluxate the joint. Pain may be local or referred. Overt symptoms are usually relieved by rest and aggravated by activity and high heels, but fatigue is chronic regardless of adequate rest. Care must be taken to differentiate these sprains from a sacroiliac, hip, rectal, or pelvic lesion. Localized tenderness and the standard clinical tests are helpful in differentiation.

In almost every case of acute lumbosacral stress, the local multifidi will be stiff or possibly mildly splinted. Cailliet states that when this happens, the motion unit will be kyphotic. This cannot be true because the multifidi are hyperextenders in the erect position that can only produce locking in lordosis. Shortened abdominals and possibly the psoas major would be the logical muscles in the lumbar area responsible for kyphotic fixation. Anterior disc will collapse or a fixed facet separation would be a more logical cause if a segmental kyphosis is present. An associated lumbar scoliosis with pain on the side of the concavity is evidence of psoas major involvement.

The Lumbosacral Triangle. When viewed from the posterior, a clinical triangle can be drawn between the high points of the iliac crest and the sacral apex. This area includes the vast majority of structures that are most commonly involved in low-back pain syndrome. Here we find the L4–L5, lumbosacral, sacroiliac, and sacrococcygeal joints; the psoas, quadratus lumborum, iliocostal, longissimus, multifidi, interspinal and intertransverse muscles; the iliolumbar and transverse ligaments; and the extensive lumbosacral fascia (Fig. 12.15).

Degenerative Changes. Cartilage is found between all articular surfaces, and undue stress during weight bearing on the lumbosacral facets can cause injury to the cartilage which will progress with degenerative changes. The degeneration may cause L5 to skip forward (degenerative disc disease), portray decreased disc space (discogenic disease), or exhibit decreased space with eburnation (discopathy). Sacralization is the only condition in which it is normal to have a decreased disc space, unless the disc is underdeveloped (hypoplasia).

Associated Facet Syndrome. In lumbosacral stress, the acute angulation of L5 on S1 is twofold.[125] (1) There is bursal involvement due to an overriding of the facets

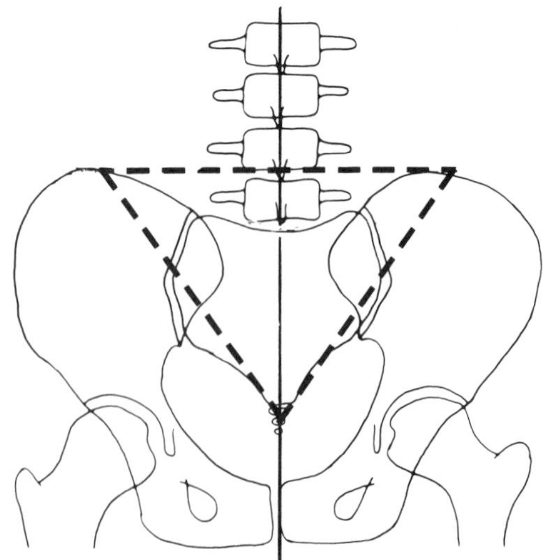

Figure 12.15. The lumbosacral clinical triangle.

which stretches the bursa. (2) There is a narrowing of the IVF causing a telescoping from the superior to the inferior of the facet joints. Radiographically, the type of bursitis cannot be defined, but orthopedically the problem can be described as a facet pain syndrome. This facet syndrome can occur with (1) an anterior-base sacrum with a normal lordosis, (2) an anterior-base sacrum with an accentuated lordosis, (3) an anterior-base sacrum with a "sway back," or (4) a normal sacral base angle and the "swayback" type individual with shortened "Y" ligaments. Thus, along with the facet syndrome, there may also be an increased lordosis of the entire lumbar spine.

Roentgenography. Evaluation is made by drawing a line through the superior border of the sacral base and through the inferior border of L5. If these lines cross within the IVF or anterior to it, this indicates a facet syndrome. Olsen[125] recommends the use of *Ferguson's angle*: the body of L3 is X'ed and a line is dropped perpendicularly from the center of the vertebral body (Fig. 12.16). This line normally falls over the anterior edge of the sacrum and reveals normal lumbosacral weight bearing (Ferguson's line of gravity). The L5 disc spacing is seen normally as symmetrical with the one above, and the actual weight bearing is on the nucleus pulposus.

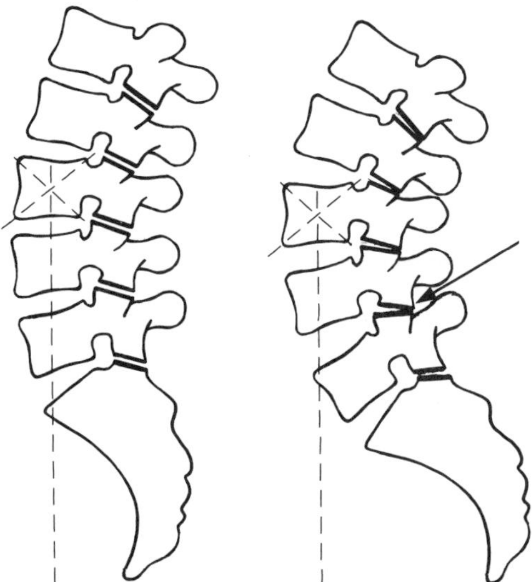

Figure 12.16. *Left*, normal alignment of Ferguson's line. *Right*, anterior displacement of Ferguson's line in hyperlordosis. Note jamming of posterior facets.

A persistent notochord may be seen where the disc is normal but embedded in the body of one or both adjacent vertebrae. This is seen in a postural facet syndrome in which the anterior disc space is wide at the expense of narrowed disc space posteriorly. It is not pathologic. The disc is healthy, but the symmetry of the disc interspace is broken.

Roentgenography during lateral bending has been a common procedure used as one noninvasive method to determine lumbosacral instability.[113] However, Vernon's study of lumbar static and dynamic roentgenography appears to indicate that the lumbar spine does not seem to demonstrate isolated segmental pathomechanical behavior during stress films. That is, the complex nature of the highly variable situations appears to discount a reliable degree of predictability of the exact level involved prior to surgical intervention.[126]

Management. Acute cases are rarely a problem in chiropractic, but chronic cases can be frustrating. This is due to the stubborn soft-tissue changes that resist normalization. In such cases, rest on a firm mattress, heat, progressive sole lifts if necessary, and carefully supervised progressive hamstring and paraspinal stretching and abdominal strengthening exercises should be an important part of the regimen. A lumbosacral support for several weeks may be necessary during acute episodes. Finneson warns that care must be taken not to encourage a low-back neurosis.[127]

Type II Round-Back Deformity

This infrequently seen distortion of unknown cause is usually asymptomatic until the 2nd or 3rd decade of life. The symptomatology usually includes chronic low-back pain, general fatigue, femoral bursitis or tendinitis, menstrual distress, and bowel and bladder disturbances. Common remote complaints may include chronic recurrent headaches, neck pain, thoracodynia, upper-dorsal stiffness, knee pains, and leg aches. If the disorder is discovered after full bone maturity, it is a stubborn condition to correct.

The following roentgenographic criteria

were established by Wiles, according to a paper by Sweere:[128]

1. Ferguson's perpendicular line is *posterior* to the sacral base and the shadows of the head of the femur.

2. The sacral base angle is *decreased* (35° or less) from the norm.

3. A fixed (structural) thoracolumbar kyphosis is present that begins at the L4–L5 level. It is visible in the standing, sitting, or prone positions.

4. A measurable posterior-inferior (extension) subluxation is present at either L5 or L4, which is often sufficiently severe to produce facet imbrication at the posterior intersecting lines of the superior and inferior vertebral body end-plates.

5. The upper lumbar or lower thoracic vertebral bodies *may* be wedge-shaped, with the posterior aspect of the centrum of the involved segments increased in their vertical height compared to the anterior aspect. It is not clear whether this wedge-deformity is the result of the gross distortion or a part of its cause.

Chronic Hyperlordosis

Strong abdominals and posterior thigh muscles are necessary to prevent thoracic hyperkyphosis, lumbar hyperlordosis, and visceroptosis. Weakness leads to visceroptosis which in turn tends to produce lumbopelvic sagging and compensatory thoracic hyperflexion. Strong abdominals and hamstrings keep the pubic arch horizontal so that most visceral weight is in the basin. This inhibits pelvic tilt and hyperlordosis.

In the upright position, the greater the lordosis, the greater the compressive forces upon the posterior elements of the vertebral segments and the greater the shearing forces on the discs. The greater the lordosis, the more (1) the IVFs are narrowed, (2) the posterior discs are compressed and bulged, and (3) the higher the intradisc pressure.

An increase or decrease in the sacral angle determines the direction of the lumbar spine. These A-P changes must be made within the lumbar spine because of the different facet angles and degree of stiffness of the thoracic spine. Cailliet[129] feels that 75% of all postural low-back pain can be attributed to hyperlordosis, while Barge[130] attributes most low-back pain to lumbar kyphosis. Unfortunately, such figures are useless when dealing with an individual patient.

Regardless of the degree of lordosis, L3 is usually fairly horizontal, thus it is subjected to minimal shear forces. It is for this reason that L3 in hyperlordosis is usually asymptomatic unless the forces on its posterior elements produce symptoms, such as in "kissing" spines.

Screening Reflexes, Signs, and Tests in Lumbosacral Syndromes

Giegel's (Inguinal) Reflex. With the patient supine, the skin of the upper thigh is stimulated from the midline toward the groin. A normal response is an abdominal contraction at the upper edge of Poupart's ligament. This reflex (L1–L2) is essentially the female counterpart of the cremasteric reflex in the male.

Adductor Reflex. With the patient supine and the thigh moderately abducted, a normal response is seen when the tendon of the adductor magnus is tapped and a contraction of the adductor muscles occurs. This reflex reaction tests the integrity of the obturator nerve and L2–L4 segments of the spinal cord, as does the patellar reflex.

Double-Leg-Raise Test. This is a two-phase test. (1) The patient is placed supine, and a straight-leg-raising (SLR) test is performed on each limb, first on one side, and then on the other. (2) The SLR test is then performed on both limbs simultaneously; ie, a bilateral SLR test. If pain occurs at a lower angle when both legs are raised together than when performing the monolateral SLR maneuver, the test is considered positive for a lumbosacral-area lesion.

O'Connell's Test. This test is conducted similarly to the double-leg-raise test except that both limbs are flexed on the trunk to an angle just below the patient's pain threshold. The limb on the opposite side of involvement is then lowered. If this exacerbates the pain, the test is positive for sciatic neuritis.

Nachlas' Test. The patient is placed in the prone position. The examiner flexes the knee on the thigh to a right angle, then, with pressure against the anterior surface of the ankle, the heel is slowly directed straight toward the homolateral buttock. The contralateral ilium should be stabilized by the examiner's other hand. If a sharp pain is elicited in the ipsilateral buttock or sacral area, a sacroiliac disorder should be suspected. If the pain occurs in the lower back area or is of a sciatic-like nature, a lower-lumbar disorder (especially L3–L4) is indicated. If pain occurs in the upper lumbar area, groin, or anterior thigh, quadriceps spasticity/contracture or a femoral nerve lesion should be suspected.

Hyperextension Tests. These two tests help in localizing the origin of low-back pain. (1) The patient is placed prone. With one hand the doctor stabilizes the contralateral ilium, and the other hand is used to extend the patient's thigh on the hip with the knee slightly flexed. If pain radiates down the front of the thigh during this extension, inflamed L3–L4 nerve roots should be suspected, if acute spasm of the quadriceps or hip pathology have been ruled out. (2) With the patient remaining in the relaxed prone position, the examiner stabilizes the patient's lower legs and instructs the patient to attempt to extend the spine by lifting the head and shoulders as high as possible from the table by extending the elbows bilaterally. If localized pain occurs, the patient is then asked to place a finger on the focal point.

Hamstring Reflex. The patient is placed supine with the knees flexed and the thighs moderately abducted. The tendons of the semitendinosus and semimembranosus are hooked by the examiner's index finger and the finger is percussed. Normally, a palpable contraction of the hamstrings occurs. An exaggerated response indicates an upper motor neuron lesion above L4, and it may be associated with a reflex flexion of the knee (Stookey response). An absent response signifies a lower motor neuron lesion affecting the L4–S1 segments, as do absent Achilles and plantar reflexes.

Heel Walk Test. A patient should normally be able to walk several steps on the heels with the forefoot dorsiflexed. In the absence of a localized heel disorder (eg, calcaneal spur) or contracted calf muscles, an inability to do this because of low-back pain or weakness can suggest an L5 lesion.

Toe Walk Test. Walking for several steps on the base of the toes with the heels raised will normally produce no discomfort to the patient. In the absence of a localized forefoot disorder (eg, plantar wart, neuroma) or an anterior-leg syndrome (eg, shin splints), an inability to do this because of low-back pain or weakness can suggest an S1–S2 lesion.

Gower's Maneuver. The patient uses the hands on the thighs in progressive short steps upward to extend the trunk to the erect position when arising from a sitting or forward flexed position. This sign is positive in cases of severe muscular degeneration (eg, muscular dystrophy) of the lumbopelvic extensors or a bilateral low-back disorder (eg, spondylolisthesis).

Facet Syndrome[131–135]

It has been the popular belief among allopathic orthopedists that damage to the facet joint is always secondary to disc failure. However, Farfan, Grieve, and others state that autopsy evidence clearly shows that varying degrees of facet damage can and frequently do occur that are not secondary to disc failure. Helfet and Lee affirm that lesions of the posterior joints always have an effect on the disc, and disc lesions always have an effect on the posterior joints.

The subluxation of lumbar facet structures is a part of all lumbar dyskinesias and must be present if a motion unit is deranged.[71] In a three-point articular arrangement, such as that present at each vertebral segment, no disrelationship can exist that does not derange two of the three articulations. Thus, determination of the integrity of or subluxation of the facets in any given motion unit is important in assessing that unit's status.

The common cause of facet syndrome is not a weak back but a weak abdomen. When the healthy spine extends from flexion, the lumbar spine does not create its lordosis until near the upright position when body weight becomes centered on the discs. This is because the pelvis accommodates by rotating posteriorly. However, if the abdominals and/or hamstrings are weak, the lordosis begins to occur at about 45° to compensate for the abnormally increased sacral angle. This produces excessive stress at the lower lumbar facets, and the "catch" comes at this angle (Fig. 12.17).

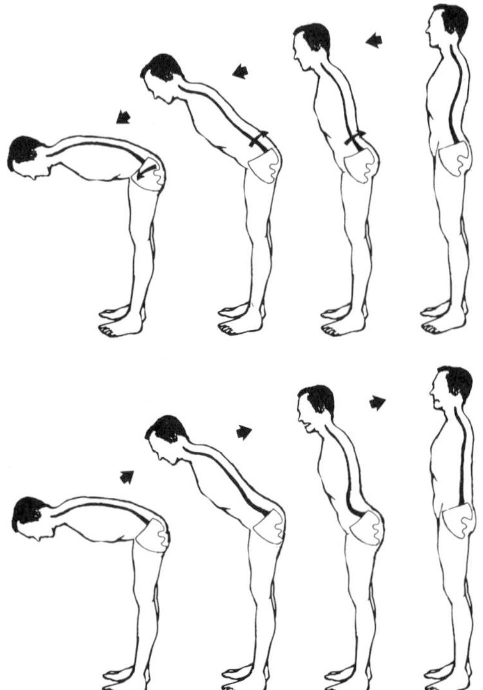

Figure 12.17. Facet impingement extension syndrome. *Top*, normal (usually painless) flexion from the upright in facet syndrome. *Bottom*, premature development of the lumbar lordosis causing a painful "catch" in extension from the flexed position, resulting in acute temporary erector splinting that flattens the lumbar region until the pain subsides.

After observing 1063 cases, Peters[136] reports that an increase in the sacral base angle, posteriority of the gravity line, an increase in the lumbosacral disc angle, and a decrease in lumbar mensuration tend to increase the incidence of facet syndrome.

Loading Factors

The articular facets have been shown to be load-bearing structures that are a common site for low-back pain. A study by Yang and King[137] revealed that normal lumbar facets carry only 3–25% of the load. However, if the facet joint was arthritic, the load could be as high as 47%. When loaded to failure in compression, the inferior lumbar facets rotated posteriorly relative to the superior facets of the vertebra below and caused the capsule to rupture at about 6 kilonewtons without bony fracture. The transmission of compressive facet load occurs through contact of the tip of the inferior facet with the pars of the vertebra below. The data also showed that an overloaded facet will cause posterior rotation of the inferior facet, resulting in the stretching of the joint capsule. These researchers also developed a model of a lumbar motion segment to simulate the transmission of facet load and to study the effects of disc degeneration on facet loads. This model predicted an increase in facet load due to a decrease in disc height. From these experiments, it was projected that excessive facet loads stretch the joint capsule and can be a definite cause of low-back pain.

Roentgenographic Considerations

Any method of spinographic interpretation that utilizes strict millimetric measurements from any set of preselected points is most likely to be faulty because structural asymmetry and minor anomaly is universal in all vertebrae. However, the estimation of the integrity of facet joints is a reliable method of assessing the presence of intervertebral subluxation. An evaluation of the alignment of the articular processes comprising a facet joint may be difficult from the A-P view alone when the plane of the facet facing is other than sagittal or semisagittal. In this case, oblique views of the lumbosacral area are of great value in determining facet alignment, since the joint plane and articular surfaces can nearly always be visualized.

When disrelationships of the facet articular structures cannot be visually identified, Howe[71] suggests use of Hadley's S curve. This is made by tracing a line along the undersurface of the transverse process at the superior and bringing it down the inferior articular surface. This line is joined by a line drawn upward from the base of the superior articular process of the inferior vertebra at the lower edge of its articular surface. These lines should join to form a smooth S (Fig. 12.18). If the S is broken, subluxation is indicated. This A-P procedure can also be used on an oblique view.

Differentiation

To help differentiate the low-back and sciatic neuralgia of a facet syndrome from that of a protruding disc, several physical clues are available.

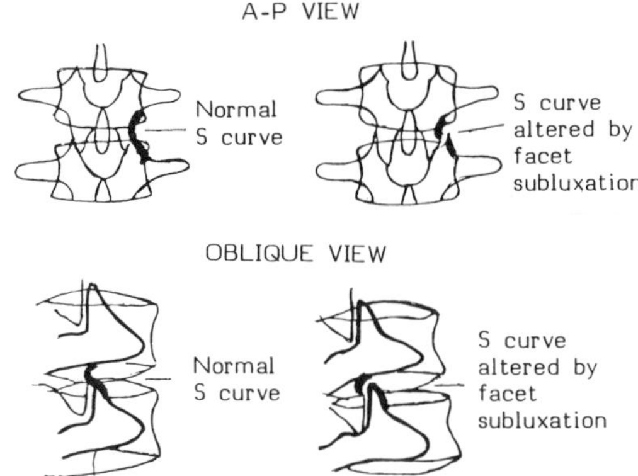

Figure 12.18. Determination of lumbosacral facet subluxations by "S" curve analysis.

The patient stands with feet moderately apart, and the doctor from behind the patient firmly wraps his arms around the patient's pelvis and firms his lateral thigh against the back of the patients' pelvis. The patient is asked to bend forward. If it is a facet involvement, the patient will feel relief. If it is a disc that is stressed, symptoms will be aggravated.

In facet involvement, the patient seeks to find relief by sitting with feet elevated and resting upon a stool, chair, or desk. In disc involvement, the patient keeps knees flexed and sits sideways in his chair and moves first to one side and then to the other for relief. If lumbosacral and sacroiliac pain migrates from one to the other side, it is suspected to be associated with arthritic changes.

Management

The associated pain, accentuated by hyperextension of the trunk, results when an inferior apophyseal facet becomes displaced upward so that it impinges on the IVF contents of the inferior vertebral notch (eg, nerve root) of the superior vertebra. Cryotherapy and other forms of pain control are advisable during the acute stage for 48 hours. Considerable relief will be achieved by placing the patient prone with a roll under the lower abdomen to flex the lumbar spine while applying manual traction techniques. This should be followed by corrective adjustments to relieve associated fixations and abnormal biomechanics, traction, and other physiotherapy modalities. A regimen of therapeutic exercises and shoe inserts designed to improve postural balance and lessen gait shock is helpful during recuperation.

PATHOLOGIC DISPLACEMENTS AND IMPINGEMENTS[138–140]

The primary concerns that involve pathologic displacements and impingements with overt biomechanical implications are spondylolisthesis, spondylolysis, spinal stenosis, IVD syndromes, nerve root insults, and disc degeneration.

Center of Gravity Adaptation in Pathology

In health, it takes little conscious effort to balance the center of gravity over the feet. However, in trunk or lower limb paralysis and muscular dystrophies, body balance becomes a major problem if a fall is to be avoided. Here, the delicate position interplay between pelvis, shoulders, and head must be consciously controlled. Whenever one part is moved in one direction, another part must be alertly moved in an opposite manner.

In lower paralysis or weakness in which there is control of the shoulders and head, movement of the upper mass helps to place the pelvis during locomotion. When the trunk muscles are weakened by disease (eg, muscular dystrophy), the individual must arch the spine in an exaggerated lordosis to delicately balance in the upright position. Locomotion is extremely slow because this delicate balance must be repositioned over each supporting foot as it is swung forward.

Spondylolisthesis[141–147]

The anterior or posterior sliding of one vertebral body on another (spondylolisthesis or retrolisthesis) usually results from either traumatic pars defects or degenerative disease of the facets (Fig. 12.19). Congenital, acquired, or pathologic factors may also be involved or superimposed.[148,149] There is a separation or elongation of the posterior motion unit from the anterior motion unit, which allows the vertebral body to slip forward on the segment below, carrying with it a portion of the neural arch and severely altering weight distribution.

Incidence. Davis[150] points out that many

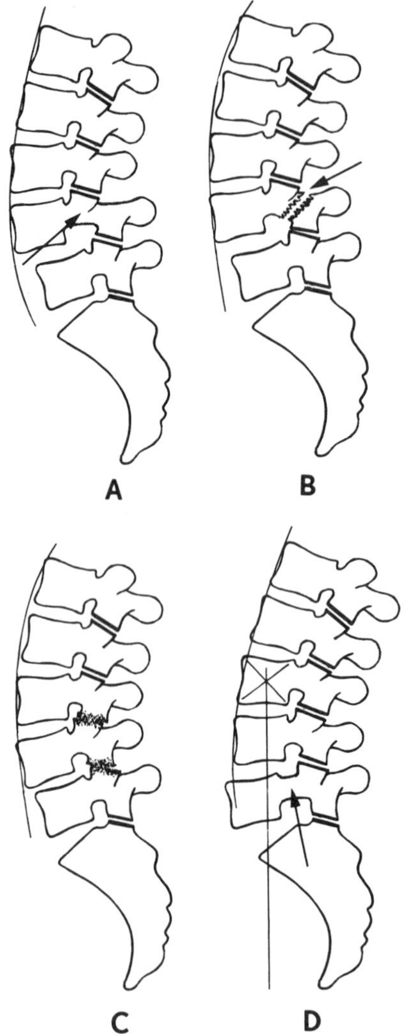

Figure 12.19. Various types of spondylolisthesis. *A*, forward displacement of vertebral body of L4 due to elongation of the pars interarticularis. *B*, bilateral separation of neural arch of L4. *C*, subluxated facets of L4 leading to apophyseal degeneration that allows forward displacement of L4 on L5. *D*, pedicle elongation producing a spondylolisthesis of L5 on S1.

authorities consider the condition congenital, while others are of the opinion that trauma in early childhood is more often responsible. Regardless, when witnessed in an adult, the lesion dates from childhood rather than from some recent injury. Rehberger states that it occurs in 4–6% of the population, but it is present in about 25% of people complaining of chronic backache.[151]

An increase in the S1 sagittal diameter in spondylolisthesis occurs during teenage maturation. Displacement tends to increase before the age of 30 years, but this trend sharply decreases thereafter, unless there is an unusual cause such as chronic fatigue coupled with a prolonged unusual posture. Predisposing spinal instability is frequently related to a degenerated disc at the spondylolisthetic level.

Fredrickson and associates[152] studied the natural history of spondylolisthesis and spondylolysis in 500 cases and came to the conclusion that the incidence of spondylolysis at the age of 6 years was 4.4%, and increased to 6% in adulthood. The degree of spondylolisthesis was as much as 28%, and progression was unusual. The data supported the hypothesis that the spondylolytic defect is the result of a defect in the cartilaginous anlage of a vertebra. There is a hereditary predisposition to the defect and a strong association with spina bifida occulta. The study showed that progression of the slip was unlikely after adolescence, and the slip was never symptomatic in the random population studied.

Physical Signs and Symptoms. Quite often the lesion is asymptomatic during the first two decades of life. Dimpling of the skin above the level of the spondylolisthesis may be observed or extra skin folds may be seen because of the altered spinal alignment. A distinct "step off" or depression is usually palpable. Hamstring tightness of a varying pattern, flattened heart-shaped buttocks when viewed from the posterior, and flared ilia are commonly associated during youth, but nerve root irritation is rare until adulthood. Lasègue's test is resisted and accommodated by early posterior rotation of the pelvis. Restricted hip flexion is often obvious in gait.

When the condition becomes symptomatic, the pain is usually recurrent and increases in severity with subsequent episodes. Low-back pain often develops after insignificant injury or strain, with recurrent pain gradually increasing in intensity. A functional scoliosis is invariably associated that reduces as pain subsides. Weakness, fatigue, stiffness, unilateral or bilateral sciatic pain, and extreme tenderness in the area of the spinous process of L5 are associated. Pain usually subsides in the supine position.

Roentgenographic Considerations. Disc tone is best analyzed through neutral, flexion, and extension views. As with spondylolysis, the most common site of spondylolisthesis is in the lower spine, but it has been reported in all areas of the lumbar spine and the cervical area. The typical situation is slippage of L5 on the sacral base (75%–80%) or of L4 on L5.

Spondylolisthesis is graded by dividing the superior surface of the base segment into four equal parts when viewed in the lateral film: the *Meyerding method*[153] (Fig. 12.20). The part occupied by the posterior-inferior tip of the vertebra above indicates the degree of forward slip. In suspected cases in which no obvious gross slippage has occurred, the *Meschan method* is used on the lateral projection. A line is drawn across the posterosuperior and posteroinferior tips of the L5 vertebral body. A second line is drawn from the posterosuperior tip of the sacrum to the posteroinferior tip of L4. Normally, these two lines should overlap or nearly so. If they are parallel or form an angular wedge at the superior, it indicates an anterior movement of L5. If the lines are separated more than 3 mm, a spondylolisthesis is present (Fig. 12.21).

To determine the degree of instability, flexion and extension studies in the lateral projection are utilized. The degree of angulation formed in flexion is subtracted from the degree of angulation formed in extension, because the maximum degree of slippage is seen during extension. The result of these two measurements offers an appraisal of the degree of instability present.

Oblique views show a defect in the isthmus or pars interarticularis, where the neural arch is visualized as a picture of a terrier's head. The pedicle and transverse process form the head of the dog, the ears are formed by the superior articular process, the neck by the pars interarticularis, the body by the lamina, and the front legs by the inferior articular process. When the defect appears as a collar on the dog, a spondylolysis is present (Fig. 12.22). If the terrier is decapitated, a spondylolisthesis is present. In some cases, spondylolisthesis develops without spondylolysis by osseous elongation of the pars interarticularis and pedicles. This is usually attributed to bone softening or a congenital alteration from the norm.

Other roentgenographic findings include an unusual lumbar lordosis with increased lumbosacral angle and overriding of facets adjacent to the defect, which is usually vis-

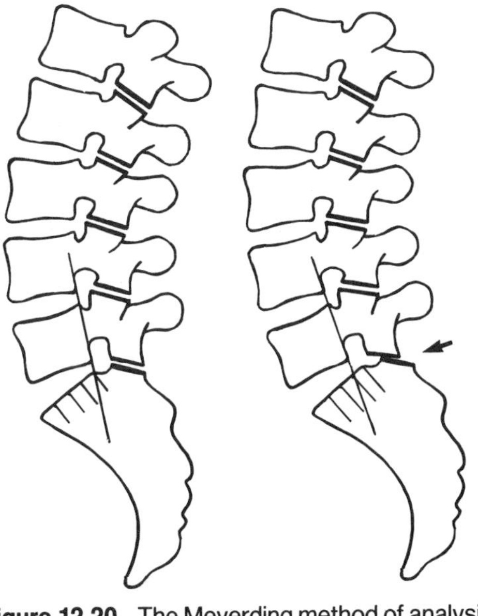

Figure 12.20. The Meyerding method of analysis of L5. *Left*, normal alignment; *right*, first degree spondylolisthesis.

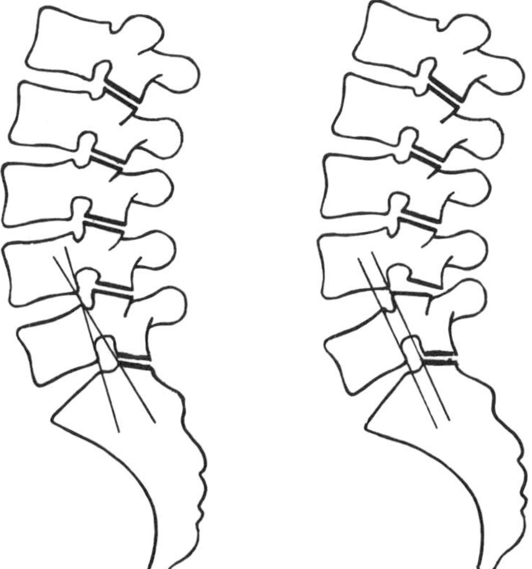

Figure 12.21. The Meschan method of analysis. *Left*, normal alignment; *right*, L5 spondylolisthesis.

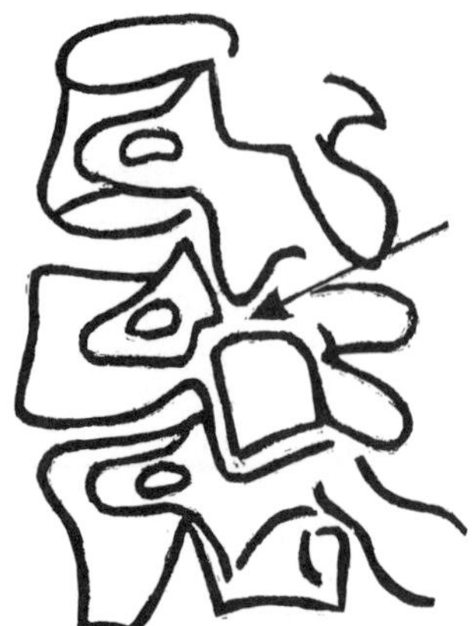

Figure 12.22. Isthmus defect as seen on an oblique roentgenographic view.

ible on the A-P view. In time, the overriding apophyseal joints show osteoarthritic changes. The amphiarthrodial joint between the vertebral bodies frequently shows narrowing, spurring, and associated osteoarthritic changes. A functional lumbar kyphosis is sometimes associated, indicating the possibility of a herniated disc.

Boxall and associates[154] have found that the angle of slipping (measurement of the kyphotic relationship of L5 to S1) was as important a measurement as the percentage of slipping in measuring instability and progression of slipping. They also found that hamstring tightness did not correlate with the neural deficit present.

Management. Symptoms progress from mild stiffness and low-back spasm after working or lifting in the forward flexion position to a sharp pain upon mild hyperextension of the trunk. Pain elicited by spinal percussion exhibits late, but depression of the spinous process is an early physical sign. Cryotherapy and other forms of pain control are advisable during the acute stage (eg, 48 hours). Considerable relief will be achieved by placing the patient prone with a small roll under the lower abdomen to flex the lumbar spine while applying manual traction techniques. This should be followed by corrective adjustments to release attending fixations, improve abnormal biomechanics, and help reduce the separation.[155] Traction and other physiotherapy modalities are helpful adjuncts. A regimen of mild stretching exercises, with emphasis on flexion, is extremely helpful during recuperation. Sole lifts or lowered heels may be necessary if the sacral angle is abnormally wide. Lifting should be prohibited until the patient has been unsymptomatic for several weeks, and then initiated only with caution.

Intermittent Lumbar Flexion-Distraction. Cox's technique[156, 157] of intermittent lumbar flexion-distraction has shown good results in the conservative treatment of uncomplicated spondylolisthesis. Robertson[158] conducted a trial with 20 patients and found that only 20% reported a poor response. Moist heat and ultrasound were administered prior to therapy, then distraction was conducted for 3–5 minutes. A nonrigid lumbosacral support was then applied, and the patient was instructed to wear the appliance during waking hours.

Reverse Spondylolisthesis

Retrolisthesis is often the result of some infectious or degenerative disc process according to Finneson,[159] but Gehweiler[160] feels that such changes may be absent. It is common at the L2 and L1 segments. It is occasionally seen at the L5–S1 joint and associated with a traumatic herniated disc. Some authorities feel that the cause can be attributed to a decreased sacral angle that flattens the lumbar lordosis and forces the upper lumbar segments into kyphosis.

Regardless of the initial cause, the disc space narrows and the posterior facets compress and "telescope" as the superior segment tends to slide posteriorly upon the inferior segment of the motion unit (Fig. 12.23). This tears or at least stretches the posterior aspect of the capsules. This process establishes a chronic inflammatory process within the apophyseal joints that is easily aggravated by stretching of the involved posterior elements (eg, flexion, hyperextension). The result is pain and spasm of the erectors.

Spondylolysis and Spondylosis[161–167]

The term spondylolysis literally refers to the destruction of vertebral structure and spondylosis refers to vertebral ankylosis. Thus, they can be considered the first and second stages of the same degenerative process. Spondylolysis is similar to spondylolisthesis in that there is also a defect in

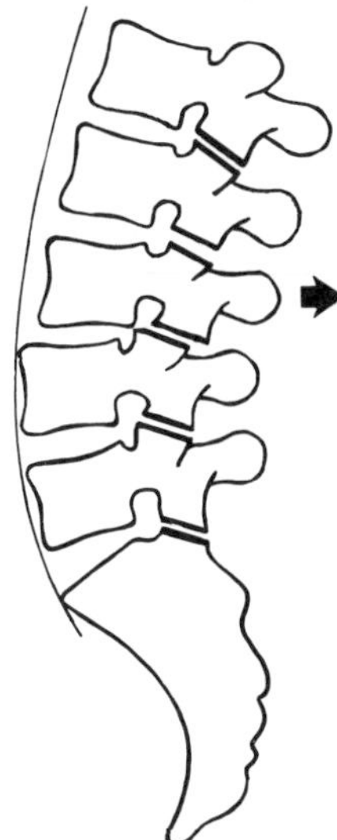

Figure 12.23. Reverse spondylolisthesis of L3, producing bilateral posterior-inferior subluxation of the segment.

the pars interarticularis, but there is no anterior slipping of the vertebral body. Disc narrowing and facet sclerosis are usually associated. In time, a picture of degenerative arthritis, ankylosis, and IVF narrowing is produced.

Incidence. Spondylolysis is a degenerative condition generally associated with early middle life, is more common to males, and is often associated with athletic or occupational overstress. The most common site of spondylolysis is the lower spine. There is a high incidence of trauma and strenuous physical activity in the history of spondylolysis, such as fatigue fractures from falling on the buttocks. Spondylolysis is more common in the obese, robust, endomorphic individual.[168] A large percentage of cases show a degree of associated spondylolisthesis, usually with normal neurologic signs. Because of chronic lumbar overstress, heavy lifting is commonly associated with an increased incidence in spondylolysis and disc herniation at the lower lumbar area. Infrequently, vertebral body fracture is associated.

Eisentein considers it possible that the defects in bilateral cases represent established nonunion of fractures of the pars interarticularis resulting from excessive mobility, and are not due to dysplasia of bone.[169] This study notes, for the first time, that the superior facets of affected vertebrae are abnormally enlarged, and that the inferior facets of the separate neural arch are characteristically elliptical.

Pathology. The disc narrowing is the result of anular tears that decrease intradisc pressure and allow the vertebral bodies to approximate and the IVFs to narrow. As the process continues, the involved disc becomes dehydrated and thinning increases. Elastic anular fibers become replaced by fibrous tissue. The ligamentum flavum may buckle (Fig. 12.24) and/or the anulus may exude between the ligament and the vertebral body (Fig. 12.25) and form a hard mass (ie, canal stenosis). Helfet and Lee feel that the ligamentum flavum rarely thickens in itself and that the appearance of thickening is due to underlying laminal growth and a

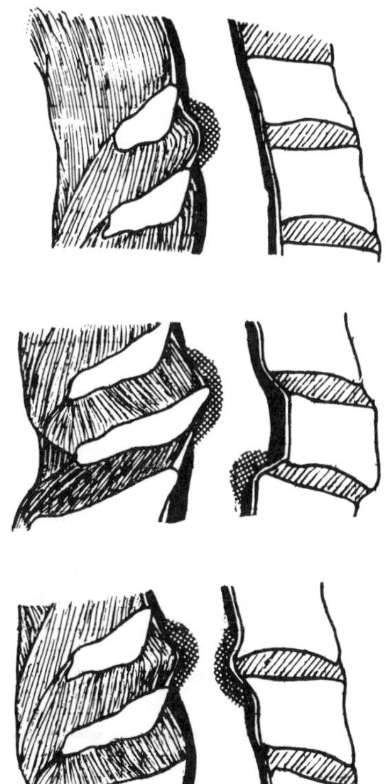

Figure 12.24. *Top*, spinal cord encroachment by thickening of the yellow ligament. *Center*, "pincher phenomenon" produced by the posterior arch of the middle vertebra that has slipped anteriorly and the superior edge of the body of the subjacent vertebra. *Bottom*, pincher encroachment posteriorly by ligament hypertrophy and anteriorly by a protruded disc and a spur on the superior lip of the subjacent vertebra.

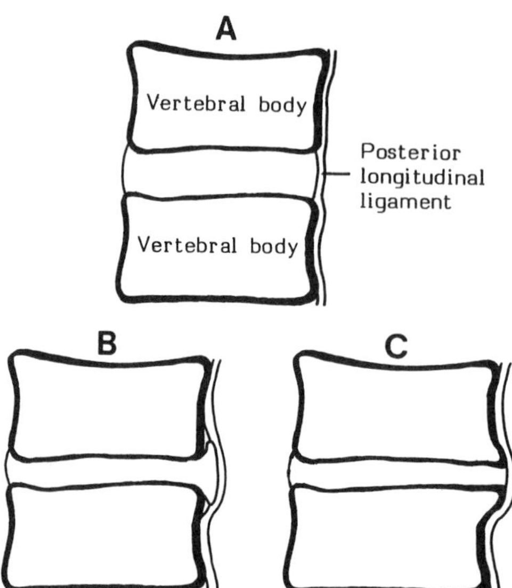

Figure 12.25. Mechanism of degenerative disc extrusion in spondylosis. *A*, normal vertebral motion unit. *B*, the initial stage exhibits thinning of the degenerated disc and increased intradisc pressure which separates the posterior longitudinal ligament from the vertebral bodies. *C*, the extruded disc later becomes fibrotic and finally calcifies as part of the vertebral body, permanently narrowing the spinal canal.

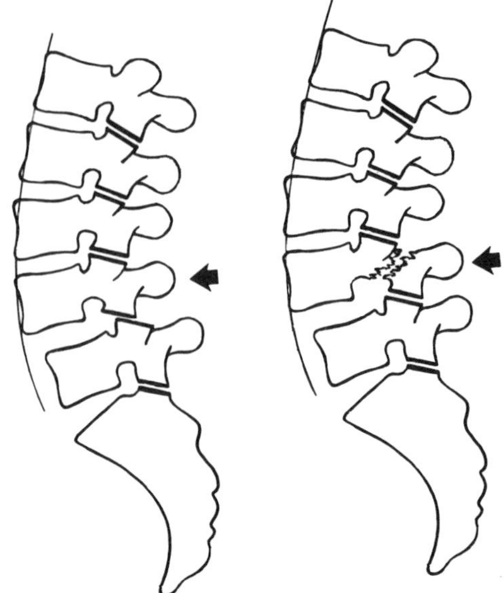

Figure 12.26. Comparison of L4 nonspondylolytic spondylolisthesis with intact vertebral arch (*left*) and L4 spondylolytic spondylolisthesis with arch defect, anterior centrum displacement, but aligned spinous process (*right*).

layer of superimposed fibrous tissue.[170] The anterior longitudinal ligament may also weaken and lead to spur formation. This process of disc and associated tissue destruction places excess weight on the apophyseal facets. The capsules weaken and allow increased shear, and this produces joint synovitis, articular degenerative changes, capsular thickening, adhesions, osteochondral fractures, loose bodies in the joint, and possible nerve root entrapment. Figure 12.26 compares nonspondylolytic with spondylolytic spondylolisthesis.

In describing spondylolysis, Davis[150] states that the term "pre-spondylolisthesis" as used by Finneson and others is a misnomer because it indicates that spondylolisthesis will occur. This term is also inaccurate to describe an exaggeration of the sacral base angle. It is true that spondylolysis will contribute to spinal instability in much the same way as an exaggerated sacral base angle, but it is *not true that spondylolisthesis must progress* in either condition. Degenerative arthropathy of the apophyseal joints will most likely result from the stress and strain placed upon the facets. This defective arrangement will also predispose the individual to spinal fatigue. The condition is also referred to as hypertrophic osteoarthritis, and this is also a misnomer because there is no inflammatory involvement present. The appropriate nomenclature is discogenic spondylosis.

Roentgenographic Considerations. Turner describes the findings as primary changes in the IVD with progressive loss of turgor and elasticity contributing to softening and weakening of the disc margin.[171] Marginal spurring, lipping, and the consequence of osteophytic formation ensues. The sacroiliac areas are not usually involved. Narrowing of one or more IVD spaces may develop when the disc space together with changes in the curvature of the spine appear narrowed. The clinical picture, often associated with spondylosis deformans, is usually referred to the area of structural deformity that results in compromise of contour and diameter of the related IVF.

Spinal Stenosis[172–179]

A large variety of congenital or acquired factors may be responsible for narrowing of the vertebral canal or IVF. Movements that would never produce symptoms in the normal spine will often cause difficulty in the spine whose vertebral canals are narrowed. The common factors are congenital narrowing, degenerative hypertrophic stenosis of the anterior or posterior elements, posterior or posterolateral disc herniation, spondylolisthesis, post-traumatic stenosis, or post-surgical stenosis, pathologic stenotic enlargement (eg, Paget's disease), ligament thickening or buckling, or a combination of these factors. In unusual cases, tumors, cysts, and inflammatory swelling may be responsible.

Figure 12.27 exhibits a number of possibilities. In most cases, regardless of the initial cause, the process progresses from IVD degeneration to apophyseal arthritis, segmental instability, and various attempts at repair that result in fibrotic or new bone encroachment on the cord, nerve root, arteries, veins, or a combination of factors. The most common sites are at the L3–L4 or L4–L5 levels. When spondylosis is accompanied by spinal stenosis, cauda equina claudication is likely (Fig. 12.28).

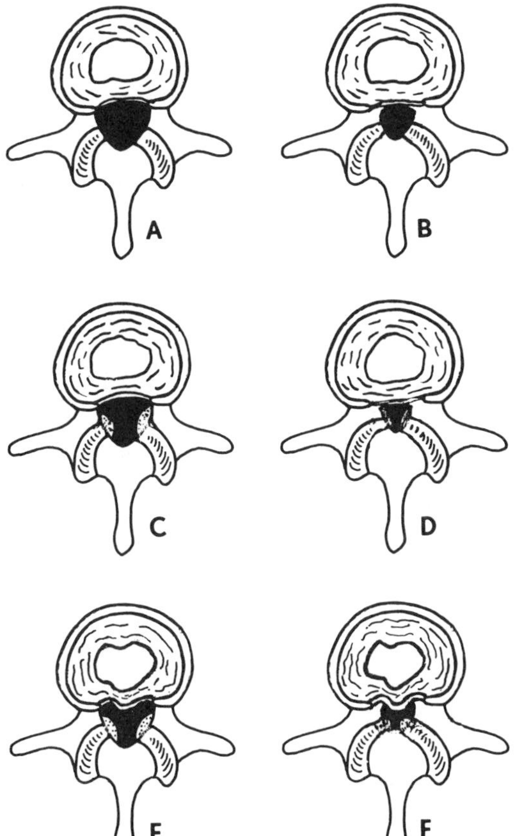

Figure 12.27. Various types of central spinal stenosis as viewed from above. *A*, normal canal (*black*); *B*, congenitally small canal; *C*, degenerated canal; *D*, combined congenitally small and degenerated canal; *E*, combined degenerated canal with disc protrusion; *F*, combined congenitally small and degenerated canal with disc protrusion.

Intermittent neurogenic claudication is a common manifestation secondary to lumbar spinal stenosis. The syndrome features low-back pain and sciatica, which are usually aggravated when the spine is hyperextended or when walking. Gait, bowel, bladder, and sexual dysfunction are commonly associated. Dejerine triad is negative, and the femoral, popliteal, and pedal pulses are normal.[180]

Narrowing of the IVD space with sclerosis of the adjacent vertebral bodies may occur as a consequence of infection, neoplasm, trauma, or rheumatic disease.[181,182] When lumbar disc degeneration reaches the point of rotary and lateral instability, posterolateral bulging of the anulus fibrosus into the root canal occurs when weight is taken on the ipsilateral lower limb. Symptoms of the spinal stenosis syndrome do not arise until the development of this instability.[183,184]

When a case becomes symptomatic, constant or intermittent pain may be local or referred to the lower extremities, especially the posterior thighs and calves. Muscle weakness, sensory deficits, and reduced circulation of the lower extremities that differ bilaterally are usually associated. Exercise usually aggravates the symptoms, but walking often relieves night pain if there is circulatory impairment.

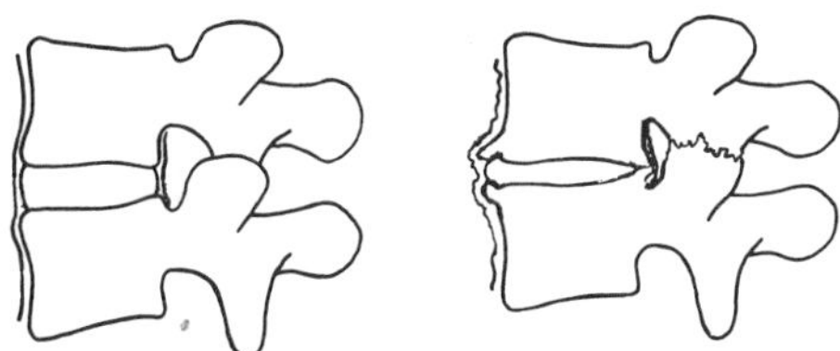

Figure 12.28. *Left*, normal relationships of vertebrae. *Right*, the main products of degenerative spondylosis, including disc degeneration, slackening of the anterior and posterior longitudinal ligaments, osteophyte formation, facet degeneration, and apophyseal stenosis, all of which contribute to IVF narrowing.

The spinal canal is relatively wide in children, reaches a maximum diameter in the late teens, and reduces slightly by late adult life.[185] The size of the canal is particularly significant in patients who have neurogenic claudication and disc symptoms, but size is less significant in root entrapment syndromes.

If the ratio of the sagittal diameter of the neural canal to the sagittal diameter of the adult vertebral body is 1:4.5 or greater, stenosis should be suspected. The average sagittal diameter of the neural canal is 20–25 mm at L1 and gradually decreases to 16–20 mm at L5. Any measurement less than 15 mm at any level suggests stenosis, and a measurement less than 10 mm indicates stenosis.[180] If the stenotic condition extends through the lumbar spine, it is usually congenital in origin. If acquired, L5 is the most vulnerable segment.

Intervertebral Disc Syndromes[186–190]

It is generally agreed that a true diagnosis of disc herniation with or without fragmentation of the nucleus pulposus can only be made on surgical intervention. Thus the term *intervertebral disc syndrome* is generally used when conservative diagnostic means are used exclusively. Unfortunately, there is considerable dogmatism associated with both diagnosis and management.

The IVD syndrome usually has a traumatic origin and occurs more commonly between the ages of 20 and 60 years. There may be a history of low-back complaints with evidence of organic or structural disease. Most protrusions seen occur at the L4–L5 or L5–S1 level, involving the L4, L5, or S1 roots. A unilateral sciatic pain following a specific dermatome segmentation and not remissive except by a possible position of relief is often presented. There is usually a "C" scoliosis away from the side of pain, splinting, and a flattening of the lumbar spine. Lasègue's, Kemp's, and Naffziger's tests are positive. There may be diminished tendon reflexes of the involved segment and possible weakness and/or atrophy of the musculature innervated.

The Typical Herniation Process. A lifestyle with frequent flexion activities will cause the nucleus to migrate posteriorly, and the ability of the motion unit to fully extend will become restricted. The result is chronic stress on the posterior anulus and anterior disc thinning, leading to anular tears, posterior herniation, and anterior lipping. Once the posterior anulus becomes weakened by radial fissures, the disc will bulge both anteriorly and *posteriorly* during flexion. This causes extension to be further restricted to avoid stress upon the posterior extrusion of the anulus.

Anular and endplate tears lead to fragmentation, displacement, and the development of scar tissue. As the scar tissue contracts, the involved area of the disc becomes less elastic and the motion unit becomes less mobile. On repeated injury, the stiffened area fragments and the cycle repeats itself to an even more advanced state. Whenever a patient presents a history of recurring attacks with greater severity, adaptive changes can be assumed to have occurred. While episodes of low-back pain may be self-limiting within 4–6 weeks, they tend to recur and each successive attack tends to become progressively more severe.

The Progression of Disc-Related Low Back Pain. Wyke believes that a disc protrusion initially impinges on the recurrent meningeal nerve in or just medial to the IVF.[191] At this stage, he feels, the centralized pain produced (without sciatica) is the result of pressure interrupting afferent mechanoreceptor activity and irritating the afferent nociceptive fibers. As the protrusion increases, impingement begins to involve the dorsal nerve roots and their dura sleeves, leading to increased pain extending more peripherally and the development of paresthesias within the distribution of the sciatic nerve. The initially central pain in the midline spreads across the lumbosacral area, into the buttocks and thigh, and possibly as distal as the calf and heel as the lesion becomes worse.

It has been the experience of several investigators that this process will reverse itself under corrective care; ie, progressively subsiding distally (retracing). This is believed to be an indication that reduction of the derangement is taking place, even when the pain appears to increase proximally as it subsides distally.

The phenomenon of pain progressing from a central to a peripheral area as a patient's lesion worsens or retraces itself during correction seems to be limited to a disc derangement syndrome. It does not appear to be associated with a postural or a fixation syndrome.

Clinical Classes. The terms protrusion, rupture, and herniation are often used interchangeably to describe the pathologic grade of an IVD lesion. However, to establish a practical guideline in the management of such lesions, many physicians refer to a Grade I, II, or III disc syndrome based primarily on symptomatology. These grades are explained in Table 12.2.

Supine Lasègue's Straight-Leg-Raising Test. The patient lies supine with legs extended (Fig. 12.29). The examiner places one hand under the heel of the affected side and the other hand is placed on the knee to prevent the knee from bending. With the limb extended, the examiner most cautiously flexes the thigh on the pelvis to the point of pain, keeping the knee straight. The patient will normally be able to have the limb extended to almost 90° without pain. If this maneuver is markedly limited by pain, the test is positive and suggests sciatica from a disc lesion, lumbosacral or sacroiliac lesion, subluxation syndrome, tight hamstring, spondylolisthetic adhesion, IVF occlusion, or a similar disorder.

Some examiners feel that pain below 30° indicates sacroiliac involvement because there is no traction of roots at the foraminal level in this range. Pain above 30° begins traction on the L5 root, and the more the leg is raised the greater the tension applied to the more cephalad roots. However, an extremely sensitive lumbar irritation will show signs quite early (eg, 30°). Thus, all that can be determined in this and similar tests is that pain is elicited at a certain point.

Many reports confirm that when Lasègue's sign is positive, the pupils will dilate, blood pressure will rise, and the pulse will become more rapid. However, these signs are not unique to low-back pain. They are only helpful in that these phenomena are not present in the malingerer or psychoneurotic individual.

Lasègue's Rebound Test. At the conclusion of a positive sign during Lasègue's supine straight-leg-raising test, the examiner may permit the leg to drop to a pillow without warning. If this rebound test causes a marked increase in pain and muscle spasm, then a disc involvement is said to be suspect. However, it would appear that any site of irritation in the lower back and pelvis would be aggravated by such a maneuver.

Standing Lasègue's Test. Another method described by Lasègue is to have the patient attempt to touch the floor with the fingers while the knees are held in extension during the standing position. Under these conditions, the knee of the affected side will flex, the heel will slightly elevate, and the body will elevate more or less to the painful side. This would also be true with shortened posterior thigh and calf muscles.

Kemp's Test. While in a sitting position, the patient is supported by the examiner who reaches around the patient's shoulders and upper chest from behind. The patient is directed to lean forward to one side and then around to eventually bend obliquely

Table 12.2.
Classes of Intervertebral Disc Syndromes

Grade	Description
Grade I	The patient has intermittent pain and spasm with local tenderness. There is very little or no root compression. Paresthesia and/or radiculitis may extend to the ischial area.
Grade II	Some nerve root compression exists along with pain, sensory disturbance, and occasionally some atrophy. Paresthesia and/or radiculitis may extend to the knee.
Grade III	Marked demonstrable muscle weakness, pronounced atrophy, and intractable radicular pain. Paresthesia and/or radiculitis may extend to the ankle or foot.
Frank herniation	Complete extrusion of the nucleus through the anulus into the canal or IVF. All above symptoms are found in herniation, and, in addition, pain is worse at night and not generally relieved by most conservative therapies.

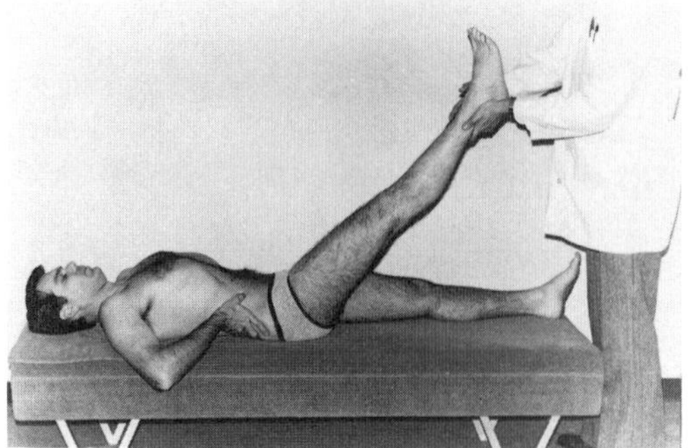

Figure 12.29. Lasègue's supine straight-leg-raising test.

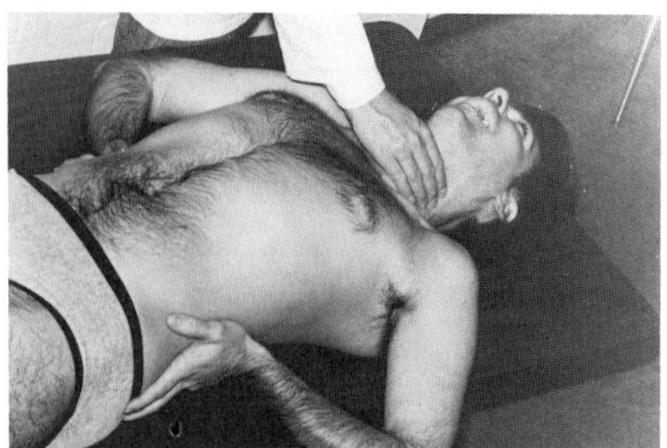

Figure 12.30. Naffziger's test.

backward by placing his palm on his buttock and sliding it down the back of his thigh and leg as far as possible. The maneuver is similar to that used in oblique cervical compression tests. If this compression causes or aggravates a pattern of radicular pain in the thigh and leg, the sign is positive and suggests nerve root compression. It may also indicate a strain or sprain and thus be present when the patient leans obliquely forward or at any point in motion. Not to be dismissed lightly would be the possibility of shortened contralateral paraspinal ligaments and tendons that would force erratic motion on the side of lateral flexion.

Since the elderly individual is less prone to an actual herniation of a disc because of lessened elasticity involved in the aging process, other reasons for nerve root compression are usually the cause. Degenerative joint disease, exostoses, inflammatory or fibrotic residues, narrowing from disc regeneration, tumors—all must be evaluated.

Naffziger's Test. This test essentially offers a suspicion of an abnormal space-occupying mass such as a spinal tumor or disc protrusion. It is performed by having the patient sit or recline while the examiner holds digital pressure over the jugular veins for 30–45 seconds (Fig. 12.30). The patient is then instructed to cough deeply. Pain following the distribution of a nerve may indicate nerve root compression. Though more commonly used for low-back involvements, thoracic and cervical root compression may also be aggravated. Local pain in the spine does not positively indicate nerve compression; it may indicate the site of a strain, sprain, or another lesion. The sign is almost always positive in the presence of cord tumors, particularly spinal meningiomas. The resulting increased spinal fluid pressure above the tumor or disc protrusion causes the mass to compress or pull upon sensory structures to produce radicular pain. The test is contraindicated in geriatrics, and extreme care should be taken with anyone suspected of having atherosclerosis. In all cases, the patient should be alerted that jugular pressure may result in vertigo.

Bechterew's Test. The patient in the seated position is asked to extend first one knee with the leg straight forward (parallel to the floor). If this is performed, the patient is asked to extend the other knee likewise. If this can be performed, the patient is asked to extend both limbs simultaneously. If the patient is unable to perform any of these tests because of sciatic pain or is able to do so only by leaning far backward to relieve the tension on the sciatic nerve, a lumbar disc disorder or acute lumbosacral sprain should be suspected.

Dejerine's Sign. If sneezing, coughing, and straining at the stool (Dejerine's triad) or some other Valsalva maneuver produces or increases a severe low-back or radiating sciatic pain, a positive Dejerine's sign is present. This is indicative of some disorder that is aggravated by increased intrathecal pressure (eg, IVD lesion, cord tumor, etc).

Astrom's Suspension Test. This is a confirmatory test for sciatic neuritis and/or lumbar traction therapy. The patient is asked to step on a low stool, grasp a horizontal bar, and hang suspended for several seconds. In most cases, the traction effect produced will be sufficient enough to retract a protruding disc, separate the articular facets, open the IVFs, and, thus, relieve the patient's discomfort. A variation of this test is for the examiner to conduct a spinal percussion test while the patient is suspended.

Intradisc Shifting[192–195]

There is considerable controversy about nuclear shifting. This is because some authors describe nuclear action under loading in a healthy disc while others study the loading responses of a degenerated disc. Because anular protrusion and abnormal nuclear shifting are more common in the lumbar region, a review of the biomechanical mechanisms involved should help clarify the processes.

It is well to appreciate that the nucleus and the anulus are antagonists. Without any extrinsic loading involved, a major role of the anulus and yellow ligament is to pull adjacent vertebrae together. A major role of the nucleus is to push adjacent vertebrae apart. The pressure within a disc is considerable—about 30 psi. Jessen has pointed out that this is about equal to the air pressure in an automobile tire.[196] Thus, it is not an insignificant force.

In the healthy disc, the nucleus is not a pliable pearl that slips around within the anulus. It is quite fixed within its position transversely by a firm honeycomb of strong crisscrossed fibers. Vertical fibers also connect the nucleus with the endplates. Some of these fibers even pierce the endplates and enter the spongiosa. In the lumbar spine, disc thickness is one-third that of the vertebral body, and 40% of the disc is the nucleus. As the disc is mostly liquid, there is little compressibility. Segmental motion is only a product of total disc deformation.

Nuclear Actions in the Healthy Disc. During loading, the anulus thins and bulges only slightly on the side of compression and widens and contracts on the side of tension. In opposition, the nucleus pulposus bends toward the side of convexity, contracts on the side of concavity, and shifts minutely toward the side of convexity during unilateral loading (eg, in lateral bending). This nuclear bulging and shifting is negligible, and for all general purposes the healthy nucleus can be considered to retain its shape and position under loading.

In moving from full extension to flexion or from full flexion to extension, there is normally a slight but significant posterior or anterior movement, respectively, of the nucleus within the anulus. It can thus be appreciated that the normal nucleus tends to move away from the site of compression forces whether a force is applied P-A, A-P, or ipsilaterally in side bending.

To understand why the nucleus makes this slight shift to the side of convexity is to appreciate that (1) the healthy disc is honeycombed with oblique fibers running in opposite directions, and these preloaded fibers are firmly attached to the endplates above and below; (2) a disc widens much more contralaterally to the force than it compresses ipsilaterally as the result of strong tensile forces during asymmetrical loading and the fact that most discs are not square to the axial line; (3) the greatest tendency under heavy compression loads is for the nucleus to bulge the very thin endplates axially into adjacent spongiosa rather than to shift peripherally. It is this endplate bending that produces what is generally referred to initially as disc "thinning."

Traumatic malalignment of vertebral bodies commonly displaces the superior endplate of the inferior vertebra either anteriorly or laterally with little nuclear displacement. Sharp nuclear shifting in a healthy disc requires violent shearing forces applied at the end of a range of motion. Under severe compressive loading, the vertebral body will crush while the nucleus will remain unharmed.

Nuclear Actions in a Degenerated Disc. The anulus and nucleus function the same in a degenerated disc as in a healthy disc with a few important exceptions. The nucleus tends to shift sharply toward the convexity for several reasons. (1) With fiber degeneration, the disc loses its honeycombed design and takes on more of the appearance of a gelatinous sac. Weakened and broken fibers fail to offer preloaded straps between the end-plates. (2) There is relatively greater ipsilateral thinning than contralateral stretching because of diminished disc stiffness and reduced paravertebral elasticity. (3) These combined conditions place greater transverse and shearing forces upon the nucleus when heavy compression loads are applied. (4) When a nucleus shifts laterally, it serves *somewhat* as a fulcrum for a lever with a short and a long arm with the longer arm travelling a longer distance. However, Farfan[197] has shown that there is no evidence to support the assumption that the superior vertebra see-saws or teeters on the subjacent nucleus, which occupies almost half the disc area, as claimed by Barge.[198]

Relatively few spinal operations on patients with a history of severe chronic back pain show overt indications of disc degeneration or nuclear displacement unless there is a distinct rupture. Most protrusions are anular in nature and are associated with a weakened posterior longitudinal ligament. Most degenerated discs in the adult are found in patients who have advanced degenerative processes elsewhere. However, disc degeneration in middle life is not rare.

Peripheral anular tears are more common in hyperlordosis when the discs are severely wedged. Unlike a degenerated anulus, the nucleus does not shrivel during the degeneration process. Rather, it is prone to swelling (ie, increased tension). Finneson states that a degenerated nucleus is unable to adequately distribute its load radially but fails to explain why. Broken anular fibers would be one answer.

Slipped Endplates. As explained, the likelihood of endplate shifting is much greater than that of nuclear shifting per se (Fig. 12.31). Helfet and Lee point out that end-plate fractures occur most frequently

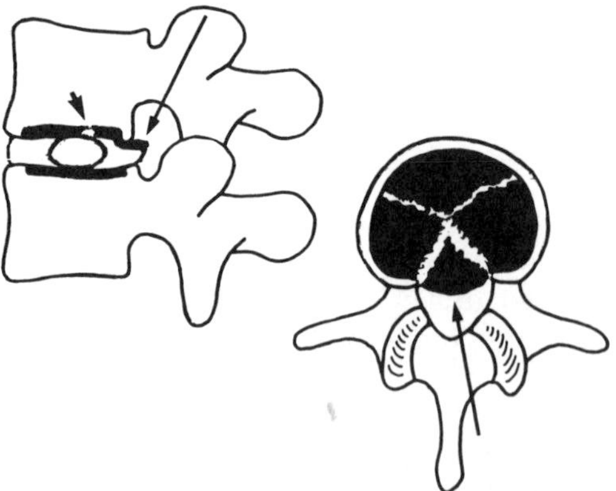

Figure 12.31. Slipped endplate (in *black*) mimicking nuclear protrusion, as viewed from the lateral and superior. *Arrows* point to IVF encroachment.

when the lumbar curve has flattened.[199] Statistically, for what that is worth in examining a specific individual, displaced buckled endplate fragments are frequently associated with trauma of the tall, lean, well-conditioned subject with long, smooth spinal curves.

Roentgenographic Considerations in Disc Disorders[200–202]

As a major adaptive change to the carrying of weight, there is normally a flattening of the lumbar lordosis and a mild rotation of the sacrum into a more vertical position. The maximum adaptation occurs at the lumbosacral junction with only minor adjustments at the higher levels. The L5 disc assumes a more nearly horizontal position with widening posteriorly and compression anteriorly, which results in a decrease in the downward sliding force (shear) applied at the S1 level. These comments by Olsen[125] go on to state that the usual manifestation of disordered function of any part of the motion unit is weakness. He quotes De Jarnette's 1967 notes that "the position of the sacral base is often compensatory to keep severe situations from becoming worse through weight bearing."

When an IVD leaves its normal anatomical position, routine radiographic examination without contrast medium may present diagnostic characteristics such as narrowing of the intervertebral space (most typical), retrolisthesis of the vertebral body superior to the herniated disc, posterior osteophytes on the side of the direction of the herniated disc or apophyseal arthrosis, and sclerosis of the vertebral plates as a result of stress on denuded bone (frequent). Such malformations as asymmetrical transitional lumbosacral vertebra and spina bifida are seen more frequently with herniated disc than in cases in which these anomalies do not exist. Torsion is more common in the L4–L5 disc than in the L5–S1 disc.

Points to especially evaluate are asymmetry and unilateral elevation of disc spaces, limited and impaired mobility on the affected side, blocked mobility contralaterally one segment above the L5–S1 level, and slight rotation of the L4 or L5 vertebral body toward the side of collapse. Abnormal findings suggesting a fixed prolapse in these functional views include flattening of the lumbar curve, posterior shifting of one or more lumbar vertebral bodies, impaired mobility on forward flexion so that the disc space does not change compared to the findings in the neutral position, and impaired mobility on dorsiflexion.

Management

The cause of pain may vary from a mild bulge to a severe protrusion to frank prolapse and rupture of the IVD into the vertebral canal. While physical signs are helpful, but not conclusive, in determining the extent of damage, subjective symptoms are often misleading.

Cryotherapy and other forms of pain control are advisable during the acute stage for 48 hours or more. Some relief will be achieved by placing the patient prone with a small roll under the lower abdomen to flex the lumbar spine while applying manual traction techniques. This should be followed by adjustments to correct attending fixations and abnormal biomechanics and by traction and other physiotherapy modalities to control the pain and spasm and improve the biomechanical fault. A regimen of therapeutic exercises to improve torso strength, a temporary lumbopelvic support, and shoe inserts designed to improve postural balance and lessen gait shock are extremely helpful during recuperation.

Nerve Root Insults[203–210]

Disturbances of nerve function associated with subluxation syndromes manifest as abnormalities in sensory interpretations and/or motor activities. These disturbances may be through one of two primary mechanisms: from direct nerve or nerve root disorders, or of a reflex nature.[211,212] The major neurologic signs found in lumbosacral radiculopathies are listed in Table 12.3, and points in differentiating nerve lesions from root or cord lesions are presented in Table 12.4.

Lumbar Nerve Root Entrapment. Entrapment of lumbar nerves may occur (1) at the lateral aspect of the central canal, (2) at the lateral aspect of the IVF, (3) at the posterior aspect of the IVD, (4) at the posterior aspect of the zygapophyseal joints, or (5) in the cauda equina.[213] A wide variety of degenerative changes can occur in both the posterior joints and the disc area, which can produce central stenosis, IVD herniation, lateral entrapment, and/or ligamentous instability. Kirkaldy-Willis feels that pain from an IVD lesion or canal stenosis may come from irritation and inflammation of the dura. He also states that the motor loss in these lesions may be due to reflex inhibition and vascular insufficiency rather than nerve compression. In the vast majority of cases, astute chiropractic management will prove to be highly beneficial. If an adequate trial of conservative management fails, referral for surgical decompression, fusion, or other techniques should be considered.

Pain from Disc Protrusion. If the protrusion is lateral to the nerve root, the patient will lean laterally away from the side of the lesion and the sciatic pain (Fig. 12.32). If the protrusion is medial to the nerve root, the list of the trunk will be toward the side of the lesion and the sciatica.[214]

Referred Pain. Root pain usually has a dermatomal distribution that is aggravated by a Valsalva maneuver. In contrast, abnormal stimuli arising from the lumbar paravertebral soft tissues often refer a dull, diffuse, sclerotomal ache to the sacroiliac joints, buttocks, or posterior thighs.

The term *sclerotome* refers to tissues with the same embryonic origin. Sclerotomal pain may be the sole cause of pain or it may be superimposed on dermatomal radicular pain and greatly confuse the clinical picture. Sclerotomal pain may originate from numerous sources. Poole[215] lists the subcutaneous tissues overlying the motion unit, the posterior aspect of the disc, the dura mater and epidural adipose tissue, the adventitial sheaths of the epidural and paravertebral veins, the walls of the vertebral arteries and arterioles, the articular capsules, the longitudinal ligaments, the ligamentum flavum, the interspinous ligaments, the paravertebral muscles and their tendons, and the periosteum.

Root Traction. Whereas peripheral nerves have considerable tensile strength against stretch, nerve roots do not. Thus, excessive traction forces can create considerable stress, dural leaks, etc. Traction (tension) on the root can pull the IVF contents outward, subjecting the thicker intracanal

Table 12.3.
Major Neurologic Signs in the Lumbosacral Radiculopathies

Feature	L3 Root	L4 Root	L5 Root	S1 Root
IVD space	L2–L3	L3–L4	L4–L5	L5–S1
Back pain radiates to	Buttocks, dorsal thigh, anterior knee	Buttocks, dorsal thigh, medial calf	Buttocks, lateral calf, dorsal foot, great toe	Buttocks, midcalf, plantar foot, heel
Lasègue's sign	Usually negative	+ at 80° or more	+ at 50–60° or more	+ at 30–40° or more
Patellar reflex	Normal	Diminished	Normal	Normal
Ankle reflex	Normal	Normal	Normal	Diminished
Sensory sign	Knee numbness	Lower medial leg numbness	Numbness at cleft between 1st and 2nd toe dorsal, foot	Numbness inferoposterior to lateral malleolus, heel, lateral foot, dorsal calf
Muscle weakness	Quadriceps femoris group	Quadriceps, iliopsoas	Gluteus medius, tibialis anterior, hallucis exterior	Gluteus maximus, hamstrings, gastrocnemius, soleus

portion of the root complex to adverse pressure and irritation.

Sensory Changes. In the lumbar spine, the sensory posterior nerve root is twice the thickness of the anterior motor root. When direct nerve root involvement occurs on the posterior root of a specific neuromere, it manifests as an increase or decrease in awareness over the dermatome; ie, the superficial skin area supplied by this segment. Typical examples might include foraminal occlusion or irritating factors exhibited clinically as hyperesthesia, particularly on the (1) anterolateral aspects of the leg, medial foot, and great toe, when involvement occurs between L4 and L5; and (2) posterolateral aspects of the lower leg and lateral foot and toes when involvement occurs between L5 and S1. In other instances, this nerve root involvement may cause hypertonicity and deep pain in the musculature supplied by the neuromere; for example, L4 and L5 involvement, with deep pain or cramping sensations in the buttock, posterior thigh and calf, or anterior tibial musculature. In addition, direct pressure over the nerve root or distribution may be particularly painful.

Reflexes. Nerve root insults from subluxations may also be evident as disturbances in motor reflexes and/or infrequently as loss of muscular strength. Examples of these reflexes include the deep tendon reflexes, such as seen in reduced patella and Achilles tendon reflexes when involvement occurs at L2–L4 or L5–S2, respectively. These reflexes should be compared bilaterally to judge whether the hyporeflexia is unilateral. Unilateral hyper-reflexia is highly indicative of an upper motor neuron lesion.

Atrophy. Prolonged and/or severe nerve root irritation may also cause evidence of trophic changes in the tissues supplied. This may be characterized by obvious atrophy. Such a sign is particularly objective when the circumference of an involved limb is measured at the greatest girth in the initial stage and this value is compared to measurements taken in later stages.

Chronic L5 root compression exhibits weak dorsiflexion of the foot, characterized by a slapping foot drop during gait. In contrast, chronic L4 root compression manifests weak quadriceps associated with knee pain and buckling during stance. Many knee operations have been unsuccessful because the focal irritation was of the L4 root rather than in the knee.

Sciatic Irritation.[216–218] Although it is the largest nerve of the body and supplies through its branches all the muscles below the knee, the sciatic nerve is rarely injured by sudden trauma. It is often affected, however, by sciatic neuritis (sciatica) which is frequently due to intermittent intrinsic trauma.[219] Sciatic neuralgia or neuritis is

Table 12.4.
Differentiation of Nerve, Root, and Cord Lesions

Nerve lesions	Caudal-root lesions	Lumbosacral cord lesions
Usually unilateral	Usually bilateral, but not symmetrical	Usually bilateral and symmetrical
Pain on pressure over nerve trunks common	Not present; superficial hyperalgesia or anesthesia dolorosa	Not present
Symptoms present in nerve distribution	Symptoms in segmental distribution	Symptoms in segmental distribution
Pain often aggravated by movement, but spontaneous pain not severe	Spontaneous pain is often severe; movement of limbs not painful; coughing, sneezing are painful	Pain absent unless nerve roots are implicated
Sensory loss involves pain, touch, temperture	Same	Sensory dissociation may be present with unilateral lesions in upper lumbar segments
Reflexes lost in areas affected; others are not increased	Same	Achilles reflex may be absent and patellar increased or vice versa, or all reflexes may be lost
Seldom involve dorsal divisions of peripheral nerves	Involve both dorsal and ventral distributions	Involve both dorsal and ventral distributions
Muscle atrophy and reaction of degeneration may be present	Same	Same
Fibrillation in muscles absent or slight	Same	Fibrillation of muscles active
Trophic sores absent	Trophic sores unusual or mild	Trophic sores common and severe
Sphincters not affected	Sphincters may be affected	Sphincters usually affected
No loss of sexual power	Often some loss of sexual power	Sexual power lost or dissociated
X-ray negative	X-ray may show pathology below L1 (fracture, dislocation, caries)	X-rays may show some pathology in T11, T12, or L1

characterized by pain of variable intensity to a maximum that is almost unbearable. The pain radiates from the lumbosacral or sacroiliac area down the posterior thigh and even to the sole of the foot. In time, muscular atrophy and the characteristic limp are usually present.

Sciatic neuropathy must be differentiated from a lumbar impingement radiculopathy, and this is often challenging. The latter can be considered a nerve compression syndrome. As disc herniation rarely involves several segments, neuropathy is first suspected when multiple segments are involved.

When Lasègue's straight-leg-raising test is made just short of pain, internal rotation of the femur increases pain and external rotation decreases pain in sciatic neuropathy but has little effect upon lumbar radiculopathies. During Lasègue's supine test, sciatic pain is almost always increased by forced dorsiflexion of the foot and relieved by flexion of the knee. As the point of pain is reached, active flexion of the patient's neck will increase pain in radicular involvement because of the increased tension in the dura. This test is considered a positive Lasègue confirmation, but it does not pinpoint the exact site of the lesion.

Lumbar Dorsal Ramus Syndrome.[220] This syndrome features low-back pain that is referred to the lower extremity. Spasm of the lower back, gluteal area, and hamstring muscles are associated. Careful differentiation must be made to exclude an IVD lesion or nerve root irritation, because only the lumbar dorsal ramus is affected. Recogni-

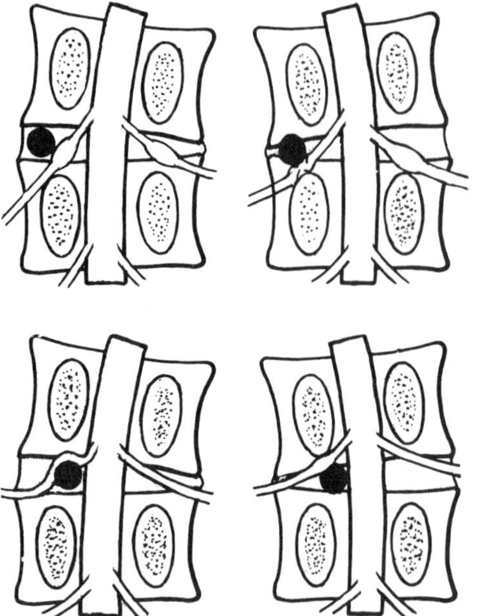

Figure 12.32. Spinal movements in the presence of disc herniation (shown in *black*) may offer distinct diagnostic clues. *Top*, when protrusion exists lateral to the nerve root, the patient obtains relief by bending *away* from the lesion and pain (*top left*). Pain is increased by bending toward the lesion, when the root is caught between the hernia and the inferior pedicle (*top right*). *Bottom*, on the other hand, when a left protrusion exists medial to the nerve root, pain is increased by bending away from the side of pain because the hernia places an irritative traction on the nerve root (*bottom left*). The patient obtains relief by bending *toward* the side of pain (*bottom right*), which relaxes the tension on the nerve root.

tion of this syndrome will eliminate the need for unnecessary surgical referral.

Clinical Signs. Note the comparative height of the iliac crests. If chronic sciatic neuralgia is on the high iliac crest side, degenerative disc weakening with posterolateral protrusion should be suspected; if occurring on the side of the low iliac crest, one should first consider the possibility of a sacroiliac slip and lumbosacral torsion as the causative factor. There is a lessening or lack of the patellar tendon reflex in sciatica (*Babinski's sciatica sign*). When the patient's great toe on the affected side is flexed, pain will often be experienced in the gluteal region (*Turney's sign*). Also in sciatica, the pelvis tends to maintain a horizontal position despite any induced degree of scoliosis (*Vanzetti's sign*), unlike other conditions in which scoliosis occurs in which the pelvis is tilted.

Lasègue's, Kemp's, and Naffziger's tests have been previously described in this chapter, but several other orthopedic and neurologic tests will be summarized as aids in differentiation. It should be kept in mind that the originators of these tests make specific claims, but they are rarely so. Wyke has shown that because the nociceptive receptor system of the lumbar spine has such an extensive distribution, testing procedures designed to selectively stress individual components and segments by orthopedic stress tests are extremely difficult if not impossible to perform.[191] Only by visualizing the structures being affected and the biomechanical forces being applied will such tests be meaningful to the examiner.

Bragard's Test. If Lasègue's test is positive at a given point, the leg is lowered below this point and dorsiflexion of the foot is induced (Fig. 12.33). The sign is negative if pain is not increased. A positive sign is a finding in sciatic neuritis, spinal cord tumors, IVD lesions, and spinal nerve irritations but is certainly not limited to these disorders. Tight calf muscles and hamstrings would also resist dorsiflexion. Several authorities state that Bragard's test helps to differentiate the pain of sciatic involvement from that of sacroiliac involvement: the sacroiliac articulation is not stressed by the Bragard maneuver, nor is the lumbosacral joint. However, the sacroiliac joint would be stressed if the calf muscles and hamstrings have shortened because the ilium would be pulled posterior if the limb were raised to any significant degree.

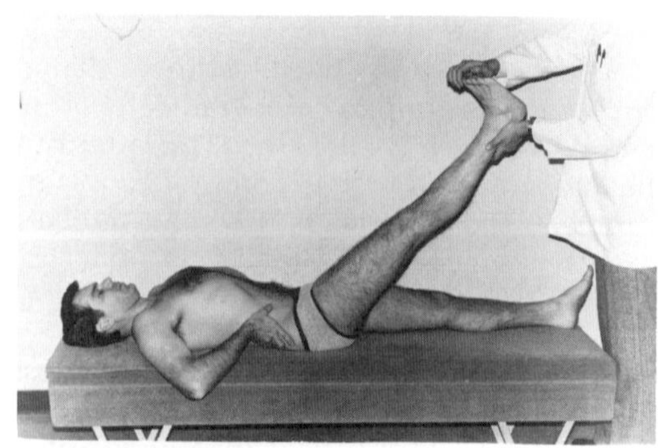

Figure 12.33. Bragard's test.

Fajersztajn's Test. When straight leg raising and dorsiflexion of the foot are performed on the asymptomatic side of a sciatic patient and this causes pain on the symptomatic side, there is a positive Fajersztajn's sign, which is said to be particularly indicative of a sciatic nerve root involvement such as a disc syndrome, dural root sleeve adhesions, or some other space-occupying lesion. This is sometimes called the well or crossleg straight-leg-raising test. From a biomechanical viewpoint, this test would be suggestive and not indicative.

Demianoff's Test. This is a variant of Lasègue's test used by many in lumbago and IVF funiculitis with the intent of differentiating between lumbago and sciatica. When the affected limb is first extended and then flexed at the hip, the corresponding half of the body becomes lowered and with it the muscle fibers fixed to the lumbosacral segment. This act, which stretches the muscles, can induce sharp lumbar pain. Lasègue's sign is thus negative because the pain is caused by stretching the affected muscles at the posterior portion of the pelvis rather than stretching the sciatic nerve. To accomplish this test with the patient supine, the pelvis is fixed by the examiner's hand firmly placed on the ASIS, and the other hand elevates the leg on the same side. No pain results when the leg is raised to an 80° angle. When lumbago and sciatica are coexistent, Demianoff's sign is negative on the affected side but positive on the opposite side unless the pelvis is fixed. The sign is also negative in bilateral sciatica with lumbago. The fixation of the pelvis prevents stretching the sciatic nerve, and any undue pain experienced is usually associated with ischiotrochanteric groove adhesions or soft-tissue shortening.

Deyelle-May Test. This test may be helpful in differentiating the various etiologies of sciatic pain and is particularly designed to differentiate between pain from pressure on the nerve or its roots and pain due to other mechanisms in the lower back. Compression or tractional pressure on muscles, ligaments, tendons, or bursae may cause reflex pain that often mimics actual direct nerve irritation. Reflex pain does not usually follow the pattern of a specific nerve root, is more vague, does not cause sensory disturbances in the skin, comes and goes, but may be a very intense ache. The procedure in the sitting position is to instruct the patient to sit very still and brace himself in a chair with his hands. The painful leg is passively extended until it causes pain, then lowered just below this point. The leg is then held by the examiner's knees and deep palpation is applied to the sciatic nerve high in the popliteal space, which has been made taut (bow string) by the maneuver. Severe pain on palpation indicates definite sciatic irritation or a root compression syndrome as opposed to other causes of back and leg pain such as the stretching of strained muscles and tendons or the movements of sprained articulations.

The Bent-Knee Pull Test. This is a relatively new maneuver described by Jabre and Bryan[221] to elicit the pain pattern in patients with an upper lumbar root lesion. The examiner pulls the half-prone patient's bent knee backward while putting forward pressure on the ipsilateral buttock. This test may prove positive even if the straight-leg-raising (SLR) test is negative.

Minor's Sign. A patient with sciatica will arise from the seated position in a particular supporting position. If the chair has arms, both will be grasped and the trunk will be flexed forward. When arising, the elbows extend to push the trunk forward and upward, the hand on the uninvolved side will then be placed on the thigh, the other hand will be placed on the hip of the involved side, and the knee on the involved side will remain flexed to relieve the tension on the sciatic nerve. The knee on the uninvolved side is then extended to support the majority of body weight.

Buckling Sign. With the patient supine, the examiner slowly raises the involved lower limb (flexes it on the trunk) with the unsupported knee extended. A patient with radiculitis will automatically flex the knee to relieve the tension from the sciatic nerve.

Lindner's Sign. The patient is placed supine. A positive sign is found when conducting Brudzinski's test (progressive occiput, cervical, and upper thoracic flexion) if the patient's ipsilateral sciatic pain is reproduced or aggravated. It is indicative of lower lumbar radiculitis and is in contrast to the sharp but diffuse pain experienced in meningitis.

Sicard's Sign. A patient with sciatica-like symptoms is placed in the supine position. The limb on the involved side is raised with the knee extended to the point of pain; it is then lowered about 5°, and the examiner firmly dorsiflexes the large toe. Because this will increase tension forces on the sciatic nerve, pain will be reproduced in the posterior leg and/or thigh in cases of sciatic neuritis.

Lewin's Punch Test. This test, which should be reserved for the young and muscular, is conducted with the patient in the relaxed standing position. If local pathology has been ruled out, a positive sign of lower lumbar radiculitis is seen when a sharp blow to the ipsilateral buttock over the area of the belly of the piriformis elicits a sharp pain, but a similar blow to the contralateral buttock does not elicit pain.

Bonnet's Sign. A patient with sciatica is placed supine. The examiner lifts the involved limb slightly, adducts and internally rotates the thigh while maintaining the knee extended, and then continues to flex the thigh on the trunk to patient tolerance, as in a SLR test. If this maneuver exaggerates the patient's pain or the pain response is sooner than that seen in Lasègue's SLR test, sciatic neuritis, psoas irritation, or a hip lesion is indicated.

Lasègue's Differential Sign. This test is used to rule out hip disease. A patient with sciatic symptoms is placed supine. If pain is elicited on flexing the thigh on the trunk with the knee extended, but is not produced when the thigh is flexed on the trunk with the knee relaxed (flexed), coxa pathology can be ruled out.

McKenzie's Low-Back Pain Syndromes

R. A. McKenzie of New Zealand has developed a different approach to the classification of low-back pain syndromes. He describes postural, dysfunction, and derangement syndromes, and explains his clinical approach for each. Following is a brief summary of his findings.[31]

The Postural Syndrome

The postural syndrome is characterized by mild to moderate soft-tissue strain with no or very minor pathology or gross structural distortion involved. It is the effect of mechanical deformation of soft tissues of the motion unit as the result of acute overactivity or prolonged postural stress that leads to pain.

Physical Effect. There is no loss of passive motion.

Pain. The pain, intermittent in character, is increased on active motions but not on passive manipulation. The syndrome is initiated by certain postures and positions that induce a dull ache that later progresses into acute pain minutes or hours after the aggravating activity. Conversely, this pain subsides with a corrective change in position or posture.

Cardinal Signs. Intermittent pain is relieved by a position change.

Position of Relief. Any position of rest of the involved soft tissues eases the discomfort.

Home Therapy. Warmth and massage progressing to stretching exercises are indicated.

The Dysfunction Syndrome

The dysfunction syndrome features pathologically involved muscles, ligaments, fascia, apophyseal joints, and the IVD. The major factor is adaptive soft-tissue shortening (fixation) of the motion unit causing chronic mechanical deformation and loss of joint play prior to ligamentous restraint. The precipitating cause is usually a by-product of trauma, spondylosis, or poor posture. If end motion in a certain plane causes pain or discomfort, the patient will avoid such movement and the tissues will shorten to accommodate the more limited range of motion.

Physical Effect. There is partial restriction of passive movement in one or more planes. Subjective stiffness is greater after rest (eg, in the morning) and less after exercise.

Pain. In the restricted plane of motion, pain will be produced by passive manipulation prior to the end of the normal range of motion; ie, when the fibers of the shortened tissues reach their functional limit. Conversely, this pain subsides within minutes when the overstress is discontinued.

Cardinal Signs. Intermittent pain and

partial loss of motion are typical. A loss in extension motion is commonly associated with a flattened lumbar region; a loss in flexion motion is commonly related to hyperlordosis.

Position of Relief. Pain is eased in the supine position (lumbar spine in flexion) when extension loss is present and in the prone position (lumbar spine in extension) when flexion loss is present. Although these positions afford temporary relief, they also contribute to chronic structural deformation.

Adjustive Therapy. Preadjustment passive stretching will indicate which position relieves the patient's pain and mechanical deformation the most. In a case presenting extension loss, for example, gentle, rhythmic pressure can be applied P-A over the involved segment of the prone patient, slowly increasing the force to the patient's tolerance. The object is to increase extension mobility of the involved segments and "remodel" the soft tissues of the involved joint. If symptoms do not begin to subside within two weeks, a dynamic adjustment can be made to free locked facets, IVF adhesions, or other types of fixations. The patient's complete clinical picture will indicate whether the adjustment should be conducted in the prone or lateral recumbent position. Rarely is it necessary to make a forceful dynamic adjustment twice on the same patient for the same condition if proper home therapy is conducted. In a case presenting flexion loss, the standard adjustive procedures for spondylolisthesis should be used.

Caution. The doctor must use care in avoiding overstretch that would produce microtrauma and another cycle of post-traumatic shortening. While some "strain" pain must be obtained if elongation is to be achieved, "sprain" pain must be avoided. Overstretching contracted tissues can be the result of too forceful a technique or too frequent therapy. Overstretching will be indicated by an ache persisting more than 20 minutes following therapy, suggesting pain of chemical origin. At least a one-week interval should be allowed between treatments to allow for tissue accommodation between structural treatments.

Home Therapy. When extension loss is present, pain is eased initially by extension stretches while standing. Exercises in the prone position should not be conducted until standing exercises are advanced, progressing to sustained and repetitive lumbar extension. When flexion loss is present, the static supine position should be used, progressing to sustained and active lumbar flexion stretching. When recumbent exercises are advanced, standing flexion exercises may be incorporated in the patient's routine. Home therapy is essential to maintain the corrective influences of professional therapy.

Symptoms do not subside rapidly in dysfunction syndromes because the involved soft tissues take several weeks to adapt to corrective procedures. Symptoms will not subside until shortened tissues have been elongated to the length necessary for pain-free function.

The Derangement Syndrome

The derangement syndrome features internal derangement of the IVD, causing mechanical deformation of soft tissues (eg, end-plate, anular, or nuclear alterations) that results in an abnormal position of function of the involved spinal segments. It should be noted, however, that fixations producing dysfunction are far more common than IVD derangements.

Physical Effect. There is partial restriction of passive movement in one or more planes.

Pain. Discomfort is usually intermittent, but sometimes episodes of pain extending over many hours are experienced.

Cardinal Signs. Intermittent pain and partial or complete loss of extension motion are typical.

Position of Relief. Relief is usually found in the prone position (lumbar spine in extension) in typical posterolateral or posterior herniation. It may require 10–20 minutes of complete relaxation in this position for the protruded anulus to recede. This position may be initially uncomfortable to the patient, but the pain should subside distally when complete relaxation is attained. Only rarely does the nucleus migrate anteriorly, making the prone position contraindicated.

Adjustive Therapy. Preadjustment passive stretching will indicate which position relieves the patient's pain and mechanical deformation the most. Gentle, rhythmic pressure can then be applied P-A over the involved segment of the prone patient, slowly increasing the force to the patient's tolerance. The object is to encourage anterior migration of the posteriorly displaced IVD substance (ie, end-plate, anulus, or nucleus). Once acute symptoms subside, a dynamic adjustment can be made to reduce a posterior subluxation if indicated.

Home Therapy. The initial stage should incorporate standing extension stretches and resting in the static prone position. Later, progression to sustained and active lumbar extension stretching in the prone position can be used. Standing or sitting flexion exercises should not be used until late in the program. Home therapy is essential to maintain the corrective influences achieved at the doctor's office.

Disc Degeneration Syndromes[222–229]

Pathologic disc processes are rarely a specific entity. They invariably represent several superimposed processes, and atypical cases are numerous. Episodic back pain is probably the only consistent symptom, and even this may not be present until the late stage.

The relationship between disc degeneration and low-back pain is not always clear. Many patients with chronic or recurring low-back pain exhibit no evidence of a degenerative process, and many patients that display obvious signs of a degenerative process have no low-back pain.

Bipedism and Disc Degeneration

The effects of bipedism have clinical significance. Anthropologists suggest that erect biped posture began about 12,000,000 years ago during the early Pliocene Era, and adaptation to this upright position has not been ideal. This is witnessed in such afflictions as degenerated IVDs, scoliosis, hemorrhoids, varicose veins, and hernia.

To show that these biomechanical effects of maladaptation are not unique to mankind. Yamada[230] amputated the forelegs and tails of rats during the first week after birth. The rats that survived soon assumed an upright bipedal posture. In time, histologic examination of their IVDs showed the same degenerated changes that are typically found in humans.

Voloshin and Wosk[231] found that low-back pain complaints correlate with the reduced capacity of the human musculoskeletal system between the femoral condyle and the forehead to attenuate incoming shock waves. Results of their investigation supported the idea that the repetitive loading resulting from gait generates intermittent waves that propagate through the entire human musculoskeletal system from the heel up to the head. These waves are gradually attenuated along this course by the natural shock absorbers (bones and soft tissues).

History and Physical Examination[232,233]

A thorough case history, comprehensive physical examination, and appropriate roentgenographic and laboratory tests are always necessary to differentiate a sinister and sometimes subtle disease process from a mimicking biomechanical lesion. Static and dynamic inspection, palpation, percussion, sensory and reflex integrity, joint motion tests, motor evaluation, and peripheral vascular function tests must be meticulously conducted.

During early disc degeneration, it is impossible to differentiate disc failure from other causes of backache such as instability or postural overstress. Sciatica is frequently absent during the early stage, but it may be elicited by a strong Valsalva maneuver.

Differential Diagnosis[234–236]

The first disease processes to be ruled out should be referred pelvic disease, primary or secondary neoplasm, metabolic diseases, and local infection. Spinal neoplasms usually have their peak pain during sleeping hours. Infection invariably presents local bone tenderness as opposed to the soft-tissue tenderness of strain and sprain. The major clues are visceral signs and symptoms and paravertebral spasm in all directions.

After fracture, the first gross structural processes to be ruled out should be disc involvement, apophyseal involvement, ligament instability, spinal stenosis, spondylolisthesis, ankylosing arthritis, spinal osteoporosis, and hip pathology. Postural analysis, orthopedic evaluations, and neurologic tests are vital for accurate differentiation.

Spinal strain sprain, and IVD herniation often resemble each other. In each, the onset of pain is usually sudden, activity is aggravating, mobility is diminished in the area involved, the normal lordosis is reduced, there are no signs of systemic disease, and x-ray and laboratory findings are usually negative. The typical clinical points of spinal sprain, strain, and disc protrusion are shown in Table 12.5.

Disc pain is usually intermittent and mechanically aggravated by standing, lifting, coughing, prolonged flexion (eg, while shaving or stooping), or a slight misstep. Rothman and Simeone point out that for some unknown reasons these episodes often occur early in the day when nuclear turgor is at its maximum.[237]

Most radicular involvement associated with a protruded disc occurs at the lower lumbar level. The L1–L4 roots leave the cord below the disc level, and the L5 root usually cuts across both the L4 and L5 disc as it descends and the S1 root crosses the L5 disc.

Pathology[238–242]

The reason why discs degenerate has not been solved. Degenerated discs have been found in some postadolescents and not found in some senior citizens. It is strange that neither gender, body type, nor even occupation appear to have a great influence on incidence. This fact would tend to point to a hereditary predisposition, but this theory drawn from gross statistics is hard to accept by most clinicians who treat laborers who constantly lift, shovel, or drive tractors.

During compression with torque, the peripheral fibers receive the greatest stress because they are farthest from the axis of rotation, and those near the nucleus receive the least stress. When the nucleus begins to fail, further stress is placed upon the peripheral anulus. Concentric interanular tears first appear, and with repeated trauma they enlarge and coalesce to form radial tears (Fig. 12.34). They occur most frequently in the compact but weak posterolateral part of the disc.[243] When a radial tear splits the peripheral anulus, extrusion of disc substance occurs. Even in the absence of frank herniation, an attempt at healing is made by granulation tissue that is richly endowed with unmyelinated nerve endings. When this occurs, there can be discogenic pain without overt disc protrusion.

Discs whose posterior aspect tends to be convex (eg, L5) have a high incidence of central herniations, while discs whose posterior aspect tends to be concave (eg, L2–L4) have a high incidence of posterolateral herniation. This correlates with the site of maximum stress and instability (Fig. 12.35).

Table 12.5.
Typical Signs of Spinal Strain, Sprain, and Disc Protrusion

Feature	Strain	Sprain	Disc protrusion
Initial feeling	Tearing	Snap	Lock
Onset of pain	During lifting	Unprepared joint	Minor trauma
Area of pain	Over muscle	Convex side of curve	Concave side of pain
Location of pain	Involved muscle	Lumbosacral or sacroiliac area	Segment
Most painful action	Flexion	Hyperextension	Hyperextension with torsion
Major cause of pain	Myositis	Synovitis	Root/cord irritation
Deep pressure pain	Usually bilateral, large area, in muscle	Unilateral pain, localized, often one joint	Often bilateral, localized, usually one joint
Percussion	Little increased discomfort	Sharp local pain	Sharp pain that radiates
Position of rest	Moves frequently	Still position	Still position
Effect of rest	Stiffens area	Relieves pain	Relieves pain
Curve pattern	Antalgic, if any	Segmental distortion	Segmental distortion
Iliac position	High on pain side	High on pain side	Low on pain side

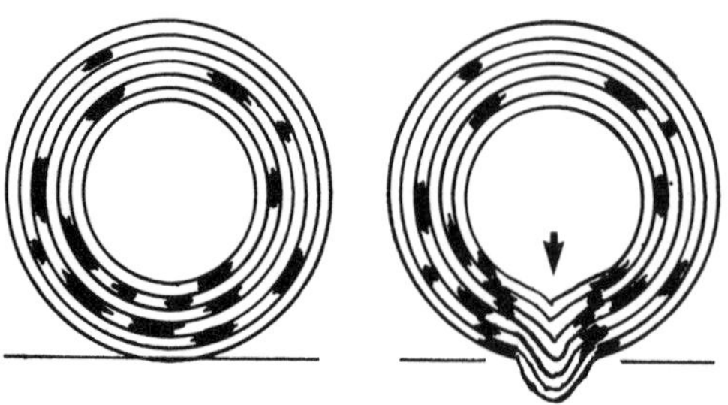

Figure 12.34. *Left*, concentric anular tears within a degenerating disc; *right*, later progression to anular protrusion.

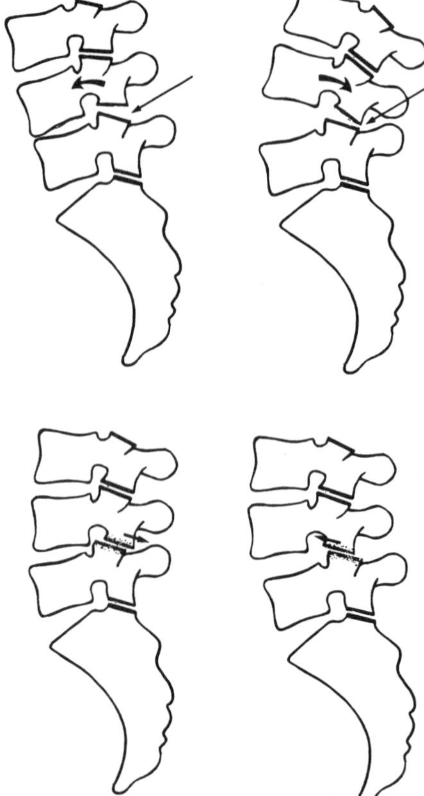

Figure 12.35. *Top*, mechanical A-P instability of L4, allowing facet rocking rather than gliding. *Bottom*, late stage of instability of L4, exhibiting facet degeneration and either posterior (*left*) or anterior (*right*) subluxation.

The L5 disc is affected 75% of the time and is usually the first disc to be involved. This is the site of greatest disc angulation and of greatest A-P motion of the trunk.

In addition to disc protrusion, disc ballooning, Schmorl's nodes, disc thinning, foraminal encroachment, pedicle migration, and osteophyte formation are commonly associated with the disc pathology. Ballooning of the IVD into the endplates is commonly associated with the early stage of weakening bone structure (eg, osteoporosis). Nuclear herniation into centrum spongiosa is the result of an endplate defect (eg, fracture). This often occurs at a site of a nutrient blood vessel channel that failed to close during maturation.

Disc thinning without anular rupture first suggests nuclear degeneration with evasion of granulation tissue into the anulus or an IVD dehydration process. As the disc thins, there must be an accompanying posterior subluxation of the inferior facets down onto the superior facets, which may impinge the nerve root to some degree (Fig. 12.36). Also

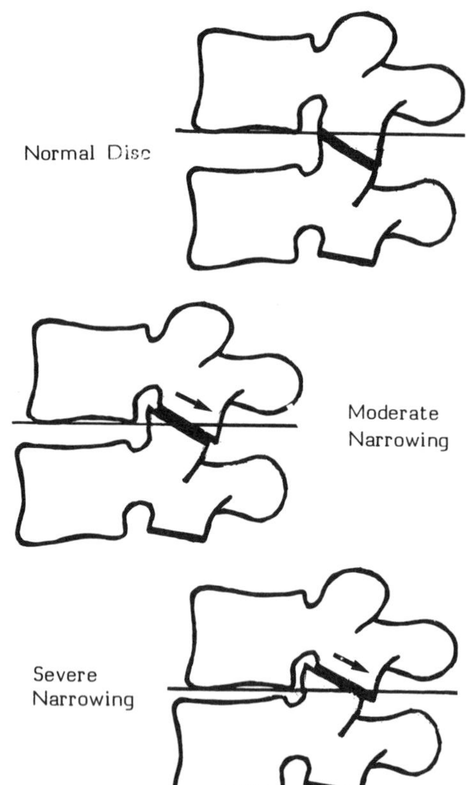

Figure 12.36. Degrees of facet subluxation associated with IVD thinning. A horizontal line drawn across the inferior surface of the vertebral body should just touch the tip of the superior facet of the subjacent vertebra. As the IVD thins and/or the vertebra subluxates inferoposterior, this line will cut a greater portion of the superior process below.

with disc thinning, Macnab shows that the pedicles will migrate caudad to the nerve root and tether the root as it descends.[244] If this occurs, unrelenting radiculitis and possible neurologic failure from compression will develop (Fig. 12.37). Horizontally directed osteophytes associated with disc degeneration usually signify new bone formation resulting from pathologic stimulation (eg, hypermobility from instability) at the attachments of the anterior longitudinal ligament.

Relationship of Facet Plates to Disc Disease

Studies by Farfan and Sullivan[245] have shown a distinct correlation between the asymmetry of the facet planes and the level of disc pathology, as well as a correlation between the side of the more oblique facet and the side of sciatica. They show that the orientation of the lumbar articulation contributes to greater shear forces on the IVDs during axial rotation. These forces are especially increased at the L4 and L5 discs because of their angle from the horizontal plane. Such continued torsional loading readily predisposes to failure of the anular fibers leading to disc disease.

Roentgenography

The common indirect x-ray signs of disc degeneration are disc space narrowing, retrolisthesis, posterior subluxation, traction spurs, and facet degeneration (Fig. 12.38).

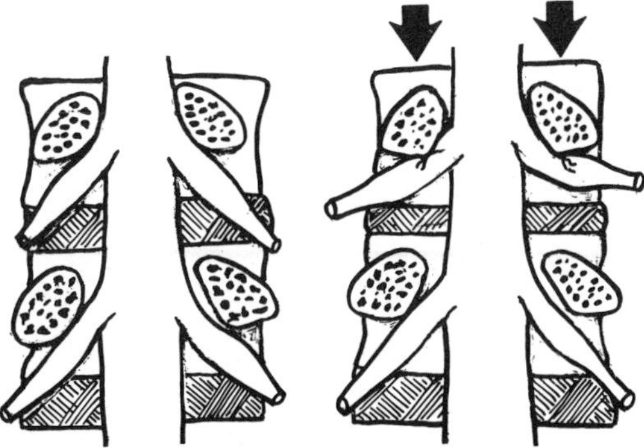

Figure 12.37. *Left*, normal relationship of the pedicle and nerve root. *Right*, caudad migration of the pedicles of the upper segment of the motion unit during IVD thinning, producing nerve root compression.

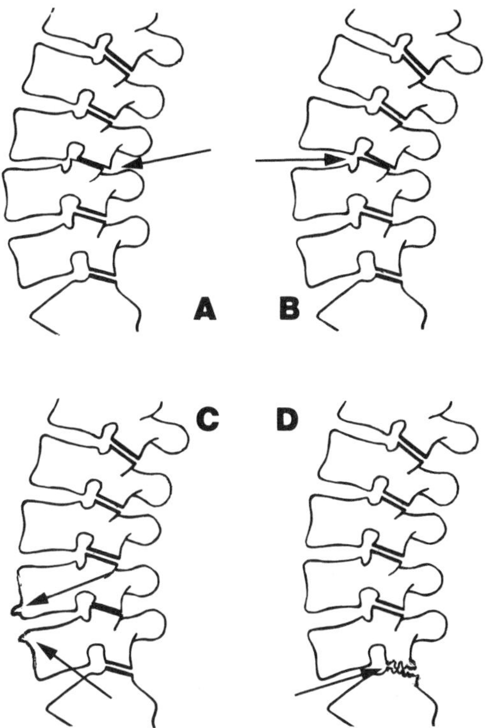

Figure 12.38. Common roentgenographic changes seen in advanced disc degeneration. *A*, L3 disc thinning and retrolisthesis. *B*, encroachment of the IVF by the superior articular process of L4 (posterior subluxation of L3). *C*, development of anterior traction spurs at the L4–L5 attachment of the anterior longitudinal ligament. *D*, gross irregularity of the L5 posterior joints indicating advanced degenerative changes.

Entrapment Syndromes

In addition to the common nerve compression syndrome in the IVF by impingement (eg, subluxation complex), other types of entrapment may occur.

After studying the interrelation between lumbosacral nerves and their surrounding tissue, Hasue and associates[246] found several mechanisms leading to sciatica and lower-extremity intermittent claudication. Typical mechanisms were the course of nerve roots altered by congenital anomalies or acquired lesions (eg, facet compression) and root compression by ossified ligaments. They also found that the space around the nervous tissue, both in the spinal canal and in the IVF, is narrower in males than in females.

Wiltse and associates[247] describe entrapment of L5 by the alar transverse process. They refer to it as the *far-out syndrome*. It appears to be linked with elderly individuals with degenerative scoliosis or younger adults with isthmic spondylolisthesis with at least a 20% slip. Classical symptoms of nerve compression arise, usually at the L5–S1 level. Surgical decompression is usually required.

General Aspects of Conservative Management[248–259]

As with nerve root insults, therapy is directed to (1) relieve pain by normalizing biologic imbalances, (2) correct biomechanical dysfunctions, and (3) rehabilitate to improve balance and stability to reduce the possibility of recurrence. Conservative treatment is primarily based upon articular normalization, rest on a firm surface in appropriate postures, postural balancing, support during the acute stage, and appropriate stretching and strengthening exercises.

Of all nerves in the body, the sciatic is one of the slowest to regenerate. Corrective osseous adjustments, disc manipulation, muscle techniques, and reflex techniques should be applied where indicated. The application of cold during the acute stage to reduce swelling followed by local heat to speed the removal of metabolic wastes and corrective muscle rehabilitation to stretch contractures and strengthen exhibited weakness speed recovery when applied in the appropriate stages.

Any irritated tissue initially needs the cause of the irritation removed, rest to speed healing, and good support to avoid further irritation. The techniques to achieve these goals must be adapted to the situation at hand (eg, severity, age, tissue integrity, complications).

Painful and Antalgic Maneuvers[260–262]

In both nerve root irritations and IVD protrusions, pain is increased by any Valsalva maneuver. Sneezing, coughing, or abdominal straining are mechanically related. Each increases subarachnoid pressure, and the subarachnoid space extends well into the IVF. Existing inflammation, swelling, stasis, or engorgement near the cord or within the IVF makes this area highly irritable and susceptible to even a slight increase in subarachnoid pressure or nerve root stretch. It is for this reason that the patient will find most relief when resting on a firm mattress with the knees and hips flexed at right angles (ie, the spine "Z" position). This position reduces tension on the sciatic nerve, eases pressure within the lumbar discs, and tends to reduce a posterior disc protrusion if the lumbar spine is extended by a small pillow or roll.

Adjustive Techniques[263–267]

As direct external trauma to a lumbar nerve is so rare, careful evaluation of lumbar, sacral, and sacroiliac subluxations and fixations must be made, as well as lower back, pelvic, and hip musculature and trigger points. The feet, upper, cervical area, thoracolumbar junction, and overall posture should be evaluated for signs of predisposing defects in biomechanics. The first concern should be the reduction of irritation (eg, impingement); second, the increase in mobility and the support of instability.

The transition points of the spinal curvatures (ie, the atlanto-occipital cervicobrachial, thoracolumbar, and lumbosacral points) serve as mobile differentials about which flexion, extension, circumflexion, circumduction, and compensatory scoliotic deviations should occur. *If these areas are kept mobile, the adaptive, compensatory, and ordinary motor functions of the spine are enhanced.*

Rest, Limited Activity, and Exercise[43, 268–270]

When pain is moderate to severe, rest and limited activity become automatic and thorough counsel is usually necessary. The American Chiropractic Association has detailed patient instructions along this line prepared by this author a few years ago. These padded sheets (Form E-10), titled "41 Hints for Care of Low-Back Disorders," will reduce explanation time and avoid the possibility of forgetting an important instruction.

Corrective exercises for low-back disorders are also available (Form E-8). In the vast majority of cases, the major muscular problems will be anterior weakness (eg, abdominals, quadriceps) and posterior contraction and shortening (eg, psoas, piriformis, hamstrings, gastrocnemius).

Because repetitive stimulation of joint receptors tends to block the central transmission of nociceptive impulses, Wyke suggests in cases of low-back pain or lower extremity pain the frequent use of a rocking chair.[191] The continual and rhythmic oscillation of the lower spine, pelvis, hips, knees, and ankles during rocking (along with the stretching of muscle spindles) provides a simple yet effective means to produce blockage of nociceptive impulses.

Bell and Rothman[271] report that the mainstay of rational conservative medical treatment of sciatica involves bed rest (eg, 2 weeks) followed by gradual mobilization for 7–10 days and anti-inflammatory/analgesic therapy (10–15 grains of buffered aspirin every 4 hours), with counsel given to low-back hygiene and aerobic exercises. They feel that, in the absence of absolute indications for surgery such as cauda equina syndrome or marked progressive muscle weakness, 3 months of conservative therapy should be given before recommending surgery.

Traction[14,272–275]

If traction is to be successful, conservative treatment mandates a total management program, thorough patient education, and a gradual/cautious return to normal activity.[276] The primary indications for intersegmental spinal traction are IVD protrusion, degenerative disc disease, joint hypomobility, spinal nerve root impingement, muscle spasm, and compression fractures. A general rule, but one that must always be reconsidered in individual cases, holds that static traction is used in acute conditions and intermittent traction is applicable to subacute and chronic disorders.

Basically, traction encourages length, alignment, and functional stability. These goals become a priority in cases of mild structural compression that result in ischemia and pain sited either locally and/or distally, leading to muscle spasm that produces functional contraction. The associated nerve irritation, which may be sensory, motor, or both, may exhibit signs of pain, flaccidity, and diminished reflexes.[277]

Continuous moderate traction tends to immobilize and "splint" strained musculoskeletal tissue, to relieve spasms by placing them in physiologic rest, and to stimulate proprioceptive reflexes, thus relieving associated pain and tenderness. It stretches fibrotic tissues and adhesions (anticontracture factor), and relieves compression effects on articular tissues (eg, cartilage, discs) due to muscular spasm, gravity, or other compression forces (commonly seen in chronic subluxations) to restore connective tissue resiliency and contour. Traction can reduce edema in an extremity if the traction unit elevates the affected part above the heart.

Intermittent traction effects include increased vascular and lymphatic flow (suction aspiration effect), which tends to reduce stasis, edema, and coagulates in chronic congestions. It tends to stretch and free periarticular and articular adhesions and fibrotic infiltrations, is an efficient supplement to manual adjustments, stimulates proprioceptive reflexes, and helps to tone muscles and thus reduce fatigue and restore elasticity and resiliency. In the spine, intermittent traction encourages the expansion and contraction of disc tissues, thus improving their nutrition.

Extreme care must be taken in post-traumatic cases to eliminate the possibility of instability prior to traction. For example, the use of traction following traumatic spondylolisthesis in which the anterior longitudinal ligament has been separated can produce severe displacement with catastrophic effects.

Many of the adverse disc effects from traction can be avoided with knowledge of IVD pressures during traction. Anderson and associates[278] have shown that during active traction, an increase in pressure was always recorded in their in vivo studies in the L3 disc, with greater increases corresponding to larger traction forces. During passive traction, the pressure remained near (slightly above or below) that of resting pressure. It was concluded that when traction is applied so that the back muscles contract, disc pressures will increase.

If traction is used on a lordotic spine in which the sacral angle is increased, care must be taken that the angle of pull is correct. Traction applied to the legs is a most inadequate method when compared to the effectiveness of pelvic traction. Direct horizontal pull on the legs tends to rotate the pelvis forward and increase the sacral angle and lordosis. To correct this, the pelvic pull must be inferoanterior from the posterior with the hips and knees flexed so that body weight will tend to flatten the lumbar curve and the pelvis will curl into slight extension (Fig. 12.39).

Joint Hypomobility and Muscle Spasm. Almost any case of hypomobility may respond favorably to traction. Traction in chronic arthritis, for example, often encourages a greater range of motion.[279] Muscle spasm and antalgic guarding frequently respond to traction.

Disc Herniation with Protrusion. There is strong evidence that an intervertebral disc protrusion can be reduced and spinal nerve root symptoms relieved to some extent when spinal traction is applied. For example, Mathews recommends sustained traction of 120 lbs for 20 minutes,[280] and several others suggest using 60–80 lbs every three or four hours until acute symptoms subside. Spinal traction tends to reduce the circumference of intervertebral discs, thus helping to restore normal positioning (eg, from suction, molding, axial pull), and relieves compression effects of foraminal distortion and/or narrowing; ie, it increases the intervertebral foramen's diameter. A byproduct of these effects is the dissipation of congestion, stasis, edema, and dural-sleeve adhesions in associated tissues. However, the effects of traction are often dramatic but sometimes short lived if a herniated disc is involved.

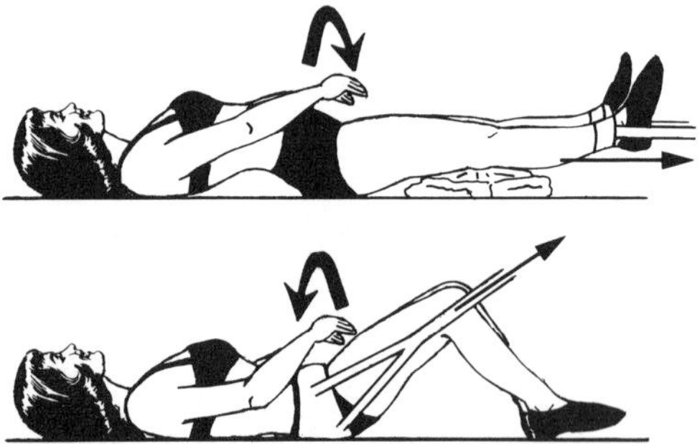

Figure 12.39. *Top*, improper horizontal leg traction tends to anteriorly rotate the pelvis clockwise and produce a hyperlordosis. Excessive stress is also placed on the knees and hips. *Bottom*, diagonal pelvic traction directed counterclockwise on the pelvis produces posterior rotation, and the lumbar curve flattens. For simplicity, counterforce harnesses are not shown in the drawings.

Root Impingement. Spinal nerve root impingement caused by spondylolisthesis, spinal nerve root swelling, osteophyte encroachment, narrowing of the intervertebral disc, ligamentous encroachment, hyperlordosis, or herniated disc may respond favorably to traction.

Degenerative Disc Disease. Many cases of degenerative disc disease show periods of relieved symptomatology for months or years following a series of treatments with traction. Other patients, for reasons unknown, do not respond, and a small percentage of patients with spondylosis report an aggravation of symptoms.

Support

The objectives and indications of spinal supports have been discussed in the previous chapter. If a brace or more restrictive corset is advisable during the acute stage, several objectives must be obtained in fitting: (1) the support should contain a firm anterior abdominal lift to raise and keep the viscera well within the pelvic basin and minimize the lumbar lordosis; (2) the support should contain several flat steel stays to replace the need for splinted muscles and to restrict motion to the hips; (3) the support must be long enough to extend from the sacrum to the midthoracic area posteriorly and from just below the pubis to the upper abdomen anteriorly; (4) bony prominences should be well padded. Short-waisted elastic supports that compress tissues but do not restrict motion or support weakened muscles or ligaments have little more than a psychologic benefit.

Any fitting of a support should be made with a time goal in mind. Contractures and atrophy from immobilization develop quickly in the lumbar area. Simultaneous isometric exercises, passive stretching, and postural training will help reduce the development of myofascial contractures, disuse atrophy, and psychologic dependence. All regimens must be well adapted to the patient's age and the degree of structural changes involved.

Surgical Indications[281–283]

If a patient does not respond to a reasonable session of conservative care (eg, 4–6 weeks), the first thing to seek is an error in diagnosis. Once this possibility is eliminated, certain signs may point to the necessity of referral for surgical or chemonucleolytic attention. These signs include increasing pain on motion, increasing pain on coughing, unrelenting pain, diminishing time intervals between episodes, articular signs changing to dural and neural signs, signs of associated bladder or bowel dysfunction, diminishing straight-leg-raising tests, and progressing motor or sensory deficits. Although disc herniation with or without disc degeneration is usually amenable to chiropractic care, frank protrusion in which the anulus has extruded deep into the canal usually requires referral for surgical correction.

Once disc degeneration has become advanced, forward lumbar flexion widely opens the posterior aspect of the motion unit. The posterior ligaments and the posterior aspect of the anulus become taut, and the anulus usually bulges posterolateral toward an IVF, either unilaterally or bilaterally. If this occurs, symptoms become aggravated. When the spine is extended, the posterior ligaments and posterior aspect of the anulus relax, the nucleus moves anteriorly, and the symptoms ease. In frank rupture, however, the extruded disc becomes locked and is not reduced by active or passive lumbar extension. The patient will be in a state of constant pain regardless of position.

In frank IVD hernia, the typical patient cannot tolerate the prone position. The antalgic lumbar kyphosis may temporarily be relieved by arching the prone patient over several pillows or lifting the chest piece and pelvic piece of an adjusting table upward so that the lumbar spine is arched (kyphotic). In a few cases, some reduction of the protrusion may be gained from this positioning alone if the patient is able to relax.

Management of Surgical Failures

Orthopedic data indicate that only about 50% of disc operations are successful in freeing the patient completely from pain. While manipulative care directly over an area of fusion is contraindicated, many postoperative patients can be helped with conservative care.

If an operation has failed to offer much relief, a misdiagnosis should be suspected. Remote sites should be sought of referred pain or a focus at a distant region (eg, upper cervical or pelvic muscle lesion). Often the simple use of a heel or sole lift to balance the patient's posture will bring relief in a few hours. Reflex techniques, trigger-point therapy, high-voltage therapy, acupuncture techniques, and carefully supervised muscle therapy often bring dramatic results (Fig. 12.40) even after several unsuccessful operations.

Poor surgical technique or psychoneurosis should always be considered, but they are not frequently involved. Only an impartial surgeon or psychiatrist should make a qualitative determination of the work of another colleague.

POSTURAL REALIGNMENT PROBLEMS OF THE PELVIS AND SACRUM

Any patient presenting pelvic complaints should be given a thorough physical examination. This would include a rectal examination for the male and a vaginal examination for the adult female to exclude pathology.

Basic Considerations[284-293]

Any movement or distortion of the lumbar spine affects the pelvis, and any movement or distortion of the pelvis affects the lumbar spine. Thus, postural distortions of the pelvis with a muscular etiology should

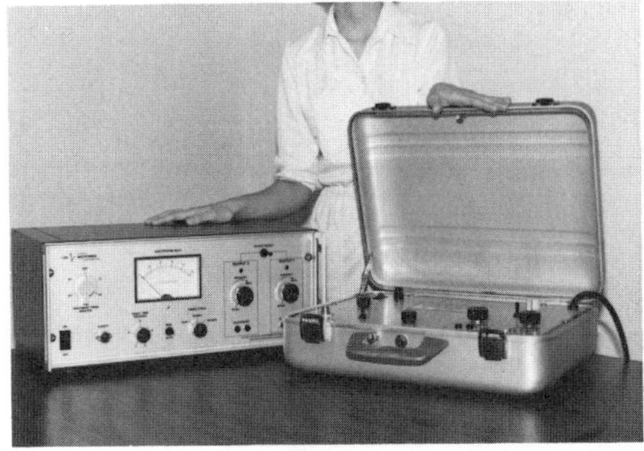

Figure 12.40. Muscle stimulation can be applied to relieve pain, build muscle strength and size, re-educate function, increase arterial and venous circulation, loosen adhesions, and improve contraction velocity. The portable model shown is an Electrostim 180. (With the permission of Nu-Med Surgical/Dental Supply, Inc., Joliet, Ill.)

never be considered apart from the lumbar spine. However, occasionally a case will be seen that exhibits a major pelvic distortion with almost normal lumbar function.

Therapeutic Goals

Postural alignment is not a conscious activity. Temporary modifications can obviously be made, but permanent correction is a product of postural reflexes. Some authorities feel that therapy directed solely at increasing muscle size and power alone will have little long-term benefit. Here the emphasis is upon the development of postural "habits" and muscle re-education to influence the righting and myotatic reflexes. However, any therapy that is directed to improve biomechanical influences and relieve stress, including the normalization of noxious reflexes, will soon become habitual simply because it will be more comfortable.

Regardless of the emphasis, optimal postural therapy is usually best offered in three stages: (1) restoring sufficient mobility, (2) gaining voluntary control, and (3) establishing permanent reflex control. The first two stages essentially involve soft-tissue stretching and muscle strengthening.

Be alert that pelvic-acting and lumbar muscles are easily irritated by strong passive stretching, thus provoking an adverse reflex contraction. If this occurs, strong contraction of the antagonist against resistance will afford the necessary relaxation of the agonist without patient discomfort. The results of this simple procedure are often spectacular in offering a patient relief.

In this context of postural realignment, Bosshard feels that isometric contractions of the major postural muscles involved, along with chiropractic mobilization of restricted joints, is far superior to that of prolonged isotonic exercise.[294] Isometric and stretching bouts of 5 minutes each should be conducted from three to five times each day.

To know what to advise is one thing. To have the patient do it is another. Thus, motivation must be an important part of the regimen if it is to be successful.

Anterior and Posterior Pelvic Tilt[295]

Forward tilt of the ilium is essentially the product of weak abdominals, hamstrings, or both, hypertonicity of the lumboextensors or hip flexors, and contractures of the rectus femoris. This distortion is by far the most common postural fault of muscular origin. Strengthening the inferior pull of the hamstrings posteriorly and the rectus abdominis superiorly comprise an in-line force couple to correct anterior pelvic tilt. The erector spinae, quadratus lumborum, and iliopsoas usually need stretching. Conversely, posterior tilt of the ilium is typically the result of hypertonic abdominals, shortened hamstrings, or weakened lumboflexors or hip extensors. In either case, biomechanical correction must incorporate (1) mobilization of fixated facets, (2) strengthening of weak musculature, (3) stretching of contractures, and (4) relaxation of hypertonicity.

Lateral Pelvic Inclination

A pelvic sag when viewed from the front or behind can be caused by several abnormalities. The most common causes are muscular shortening or weakness, a unilateral lower extremity deficiency, sacroiliac dysfunction, and hip or lower extremity alignment problems. Muscular fixation from lack of stretch is the second most common cause, second only to the common leg-length deficiency.

After studying 200 patients with a presenting complaint of low-back pain, Greenman found that 64% exhibited lateral pelvic tilt (sacral base inferiority).[296] This lateral tilt was exhibited in several types (Fig. 12.41).

It can be appreciated in the biomechanical sense that pelvic inclination directs the lumbar curvature and that pelvic inclination is essentially determined by posture of the hips. Thus, the muscles of the hips are strategically involved in controlling pelvic inclination and the lumbar curve. In the upright position, the thighs are fixed points from which these muscles act. For example, shortening of the pelvic extensors (eg, glutei, hamstrings) reduces the A-P dimension of the lumbar curve and rotates the pelvis posteriorly. Shortening of the pelvic flexors (eg, iliopsoas, rectus femoris) increases the lumbar lordosis and tips the pelvic basin forward. Likewise, weakness of the antagonists would have the same effect. Thus, rehabilitation should be directed to relax and stretch muscles shortening by spasm or contracture and strengthen counterparts weak-

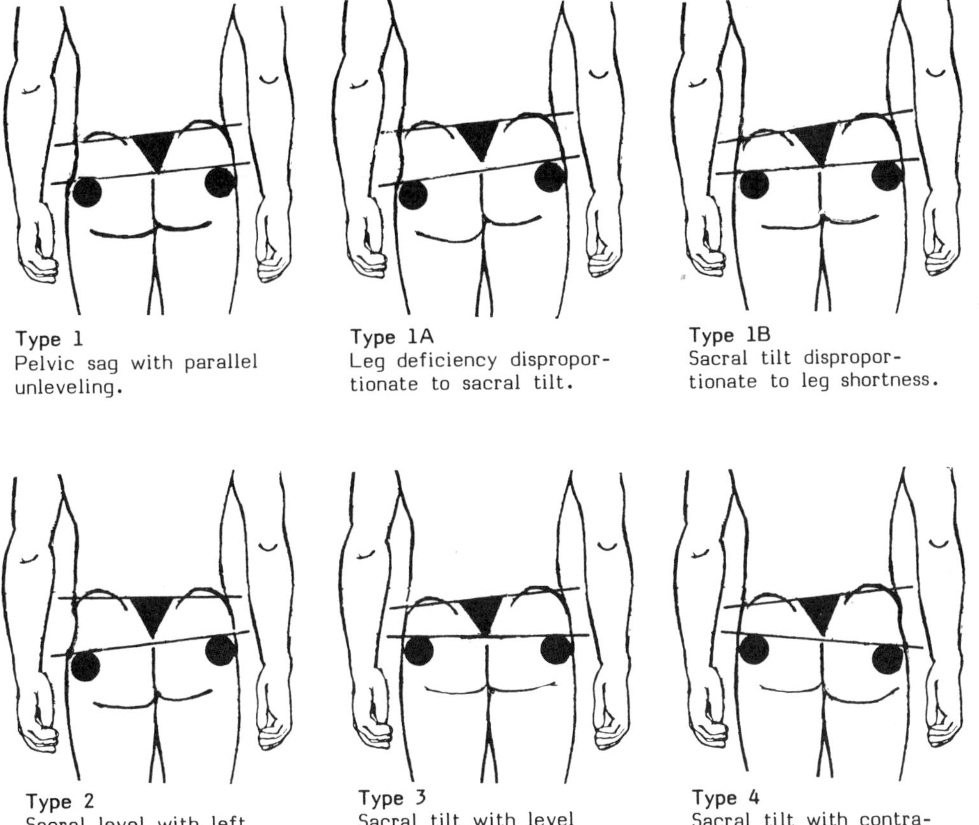

Figure 12.41. Greenman's classes of lateral pelvic tilt.

ened by inactivity or constitutional factors. This need not be a dual activity because a muscle relaxes as its antagonist contracts against resistance.

Several kinesiologists state that, in bilateral muscle checking during posture analysis, the overwhelming majority of patients presenting postural defects have muscle weakness rather than primary spasm. It appears to be this weakness that causes the contralateral muscles to contract into an apparent spasm. Thus, the weakness is said to be primary and the spasm to be secondary. The spasm is thought to be the result of the prime-mover/antagonist reciprocal relationship. For example, an elevated iliac crest on the right relative to the left may be due to weakness on the right of the psoas, gluteals, and tensor fascia lata or weakness on the left of the adductors, quadratus lumborum, rectus or transverse abdominis, or the sacrospinalis. In the same regard, an elevated shoulder on the right relative to the left may be due to weakness on the right of the latissimus dorsi, lower trapezius, anterior serratus, pectoralis major and minor, subscapularis, teres minor, infraspinatus, and levator scapulae or weakness on the left of the upper trapezius. However, these viewpoints, originated by Goodheart[297] have not been accepted by several authorities.

Pelvic Height

Anthropometric analyses by Merriam and associates;[298] have confirmed previous reports that people prone to back pain have a greater standing height than individuals of lower stature. In calculating suprapelvic height, pelvic height, and subischial height (which when added equal the standing height), they found that the relatively large standing height of the subject prone to back pain was due to the pelvic component.

Muscle Weakness[299–301]

Posterior rotation of the innominates in the erect position is essentially produced by contraction of the hamstrings, gluteus maximus, and fascia lata. Anterior innominate rotation is produced by the iliopsoas and anterior muscles of the thigh. Abduction is the product of the gluteus medius and minimus and the muscle fibers of the fascia lata, and adduction is made by the adductor group of the medial thigh. Lateral flexion is essentially the product of unilateral and reciprocal action of the pelvic extensors, flexors, and rotators.

The Gluteus Maximus

This large quadrangular muscle is the most superficial muscle of the buttocks (Fig. 12.42). It arises from the posterior sacral ligaments, the PSIS, the coccyx, and the sacrotuberous ligament. It inserts superiorly into the fascia lata and divides inferiorly to insert into the iliotibial band and at the ischial tuberosity. Gross weakness is evaluated by testing thigh abduction and external rotation against resistance.

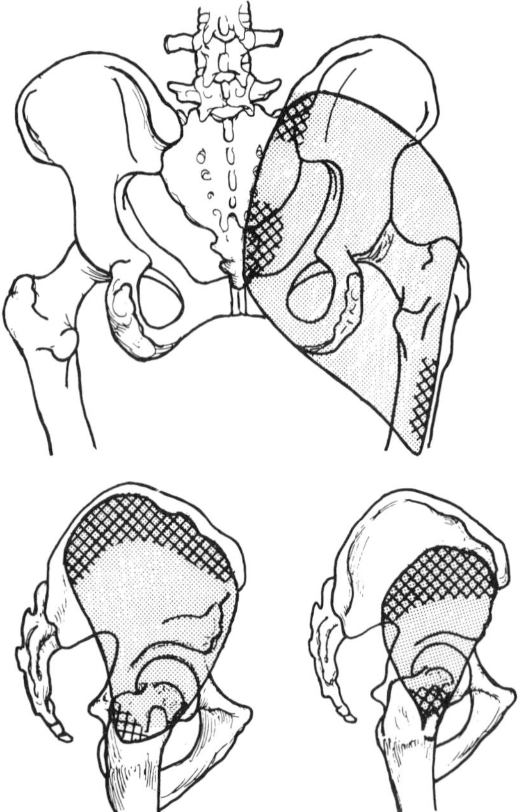

Figure 12.42. *Top*, the gluteus maximus muscle. *Hatchmarks* indicate sites of origin and insertion. *Bottom left*, the gluteus medius; *bottom right*, the gluteus minimus.

Several studies have shown that the gluteus maximus is the *most atonic muscle of the body* in the nonathlete, with the rectus abdominis a close second. This fact of gluteal weakness is often hidden by the overlying fat of the buttocks or a lumbar hyperlordosis and anterior pelvic tilt that projects the buttocks posterosuperior so that the glutei appear firm and well developed. Possibly that is why so many ladies prefer high heels.

A S1 lesion may be exhibited indirectly by unilateral weakness of the gluteus maximus (Fig. 12.43). The view from the posterior will show a unilateral sag of the buttock crease, which can be confused at first with a short-leg syndrome (Fig. 12.44).

The Gluteus Medius and Minimus

The gluteus medius and minimus act within the pelvis as the deltoid does in the shoulder. During gait, they rotate the pelvis over the femur on the side of stance. The gluteus medius lies under the maximus. It arises from the upper lateral periosteum of the iliac wing and fascia and inserts at the greater trochanter of the femur. The accessory gluteus minimus muscle lies under the belly of the gluteus medius. It arises from the dorsal aspect of the ilium between the anterior and posterior gluteal lines and also inserts at the greater trochanter. Gross weakness of these two muscles is evaluated by testing high abduction and medial rotation against resistance (Fig. 12.45).

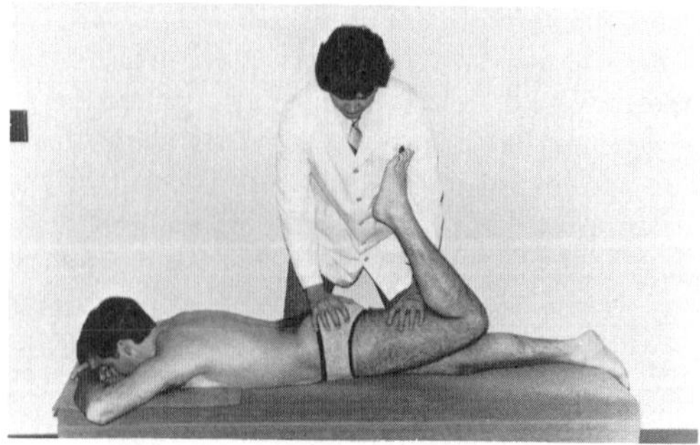

Figure 12.43. Testing the strength of the hip extensors against resistance.

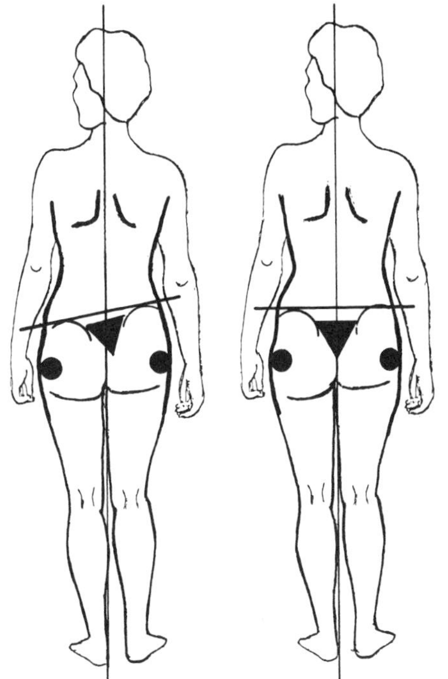

Figure 12.44. Typical "short-leg" left pelvic sag (*left*) compared to gluteal maximus atrophy from S1 root compression (*right*). While both syndromes exhibit a low buttock on the left, the sacrum and iliac crests are relatively level in the right diagram. In gluteal medius weakness, however, there would be a pelvic tilt and related scoliosis away from the weak side.

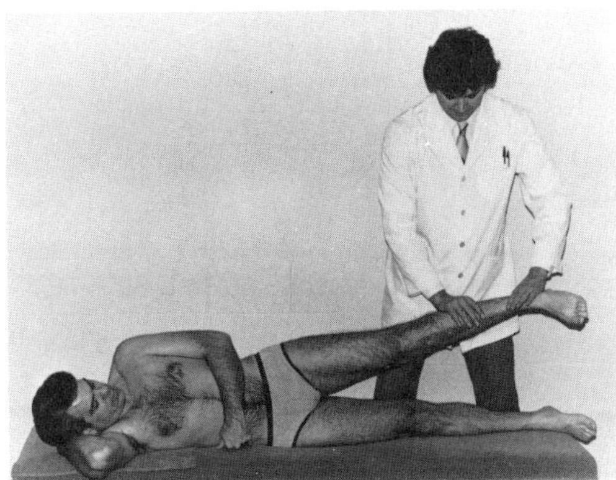

Figure 12.45. The position for testing hip abduction or adduction strength against resistance.

The Tensor Fascia Lata

The tensor muscle of fascia lata arises from the iliac crest and inserts into the iliotibial tract. Gross weakness is evaluated by testing thigh flexion and medial rotation against resistance.

The Piriformis[302]

This pear-shaped muscle spans between the ilium and S2–S4 sacral segments and the greater trochanter. It functions in rotating the thigh externally, abducting the thigh when the hip is flexed, and holding the head of the femur within the acetabulum.

To determine piriformis strength, the patient is placed supine, the hip is fully flexed, and the knee is flexed to a right angle. The foot on the side being tested is brought across the patient's opposite leg by the examiner, the patient's knee is stabilized with the other hand of the examiner, and adduction pressure is applied to the ankle by the examiner against patient resistance (thigh abduction).

The Iliopsoas[303, 304]

The psoas muscles as a whole (major and minor) arise from the sides and transverse processes of the lumbar vertebrae and often the T12 and insert at the lesser trochanter and arcuate line of the hip bone. According to Goodheart,[305] psoas hypertonicity is rare, weakness is common, and hypertonicity is usually the contralateral response to an ipsilateral weakness, but not all authorities agree with this hypothesis. The psoas minor has a short weak belly and a long tendon. It assists the psoas major but has an insignificant role in humans. It is absent in 40% of the population, and there is little clinical need for specific testing.

A large triangular sheet of iliacus muscle lies on the lateral side of the lower psoas. It originates from the upper iliac fossa and psoas tendon and inserts into the lesser trochanter of the femur. The psoas group and iliacus are collectively called the iliopsoas, which is the most powerful flexor of the thigh.

To test iliopsoas strength, the seated patient is asked to raise each knee by hip flexion against resistance of the examiner's hand placed on the distal anterior thigh (Fig. 12.46). Then test in the supine position. The ability to flex the thigh in the supine position but not in the seated position indicates an iliopsoas lesion. To further test with the patient in the supine position, raise the leg

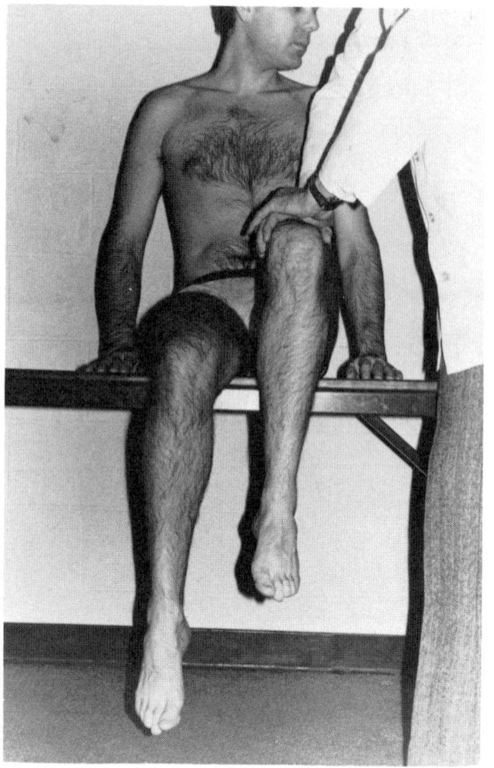

Figure 12.46. The position for testing iliopsoas strength against resistance in the sitting position.

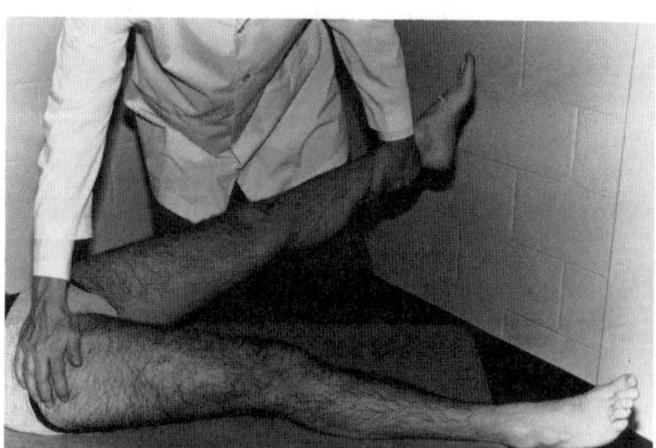

Figure 12.47. The position for testing iliopsoas strength against resistance in the supine position.

to be tested to about 45°, keeping the knee extended. The patient is asked to resist a downward and slightly lateral force when the examiner exerts pressure against the lower anteromedial leg (Fig. 12.47). A quick method is offered by Goodheart, who states that simple internal rotation of the femurs of a relaxed supine patient will offer quick evaluation. The side of greatest rotation medially is said to designate the weaker psoas.[305]

Bilateral iliopsoas weakness tends to flatten the lumbar curve or displace the pelvis forward to the lateral midline (Fig. 12.48). Unilateral weakness produces a "C" curve away from the weakness with a compensatory ipsilateral high hip when viewed from the posterior (Fig. 12.49).

The Hamstrings[306, 307]

The semimembranosus arises from the ischial tuberosity and inserts at the lateral condyle of the femur and the medial condyle and border of the tibia. The semitendinosus arises from the ischial tuberosity and inserts on the upper part of the medial surface of the tibia. The long head of the biceps femoris arises from the ischial tuberosity and the short head from the linea aspera of the femur. Both insert via a common tendon at the head of the fibula and lateral condyle of the femur. Gross weakness is evaluated by testing simultaneous extension of the thigh and flexion of the knee against resistance.

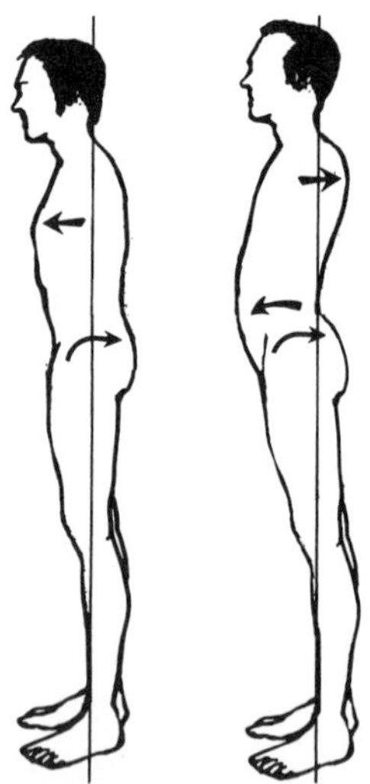

Figure 12.48. *Left*, bilateral iliopsoas weakness exhibiting posterior pelvic rotation, lumbar flattening, and forward lean of the upper body. *Right*, a later picture of bilateral iliopsoas weakness in which the pelvis is shifted far forward of the midline and the upper body is arched back from the midline. It is important to note how the forward shift of the pelvis masks the lumbar flattening and posterior pelvic rotation so that the posture falsely resembles a lumbar lordosis.

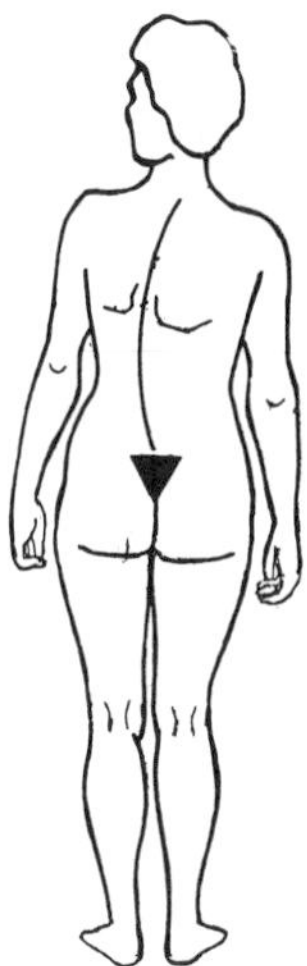

Figure 12.49. Unilateral psoas weakness frequently exhibits a "C" scoliosis away from the side of weakness in spite of good strength in the other hip flexors. Such a scoliosis is often related to a relatively level pelvis, in contrast to the pelvic tilt associated with gluteus medius weakness.

The Quadratus Femoris

This small muscle spans transversely between the ischial tuberosity and the posterior surface of the femur at the intertrochanter crest between the greater and lesser trochanters. Gross weakness is evaluated by testing adduction and external rotation of the thigh against resistance.

The Obturator Internus and Externus

The thick fan-shaped obturator internus muscle arises from the anterolateral pelvic surface of the ilium, obturator membrane, and margin of the foramen. It inserts at the medial surface of the greater trochanter. The externus arises from the pubis, ischium, and external surface of the obturator foramen and inserts at the trochanteric fossa of the femur. Gross weakness is evaluated by testing external rotation of the thigh against resistance when the hip is flexed.

The Superior and Inferior Gemelli

The superior gemelli muscle spans between the ischial spine and the internal obturator tendon. Its inferior partner arises from the ischial tuberosity and inserts at the internal obturator tendon, which runs below the piriformis. Gross weakness is evaluated by testing external rotation of the thigh against resistance (Fig. 12.50).

Muscle Spasm

Muscle spasms in the pelvis generally reflect themselves in the trunk, thigh, or both. Fixation of most major muscles acting on the pelvis has a restrictive influence upon the mobility of the femur and an effect upon an individual's stance. When evaluating relative muscle function, note that mild unilateral hypertonicity is most difficult to differentiate from contralateral hypotonicity. In differentiation, palpation may reveal more than kinetic tests.

Piriformis Spasm[302, 308, 309]

If the patient has deep gluteal pain, sciatic neuralgia, and walks with the foot noticeably everted on the side of involvement, involvement of the piriformis should be suspected. Increased piriformis tone tends to subluxate the sacrum anteriorly and externally rotate the thigh.

The sciatic nerve should pass under the piriformis and follow the "wisdom" of the textbooks. In many cases, however, the nerve takes a different course and is found on surgery to be stretched over or even to pass through the muscle in 15–20% of the population (ie, about one of every 5–7 patients).

To test for piriformis spasm, the patient is placed supine on a firm flat table. His heels are grasped and firmly inverted and abducted, and his feet are externally rotated. If one foot resists this effort and the act is

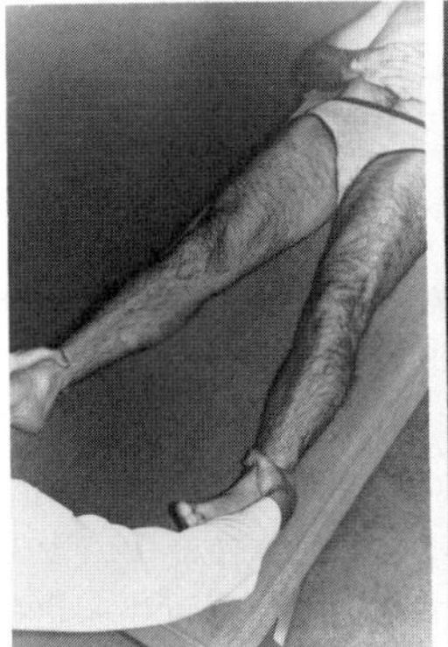

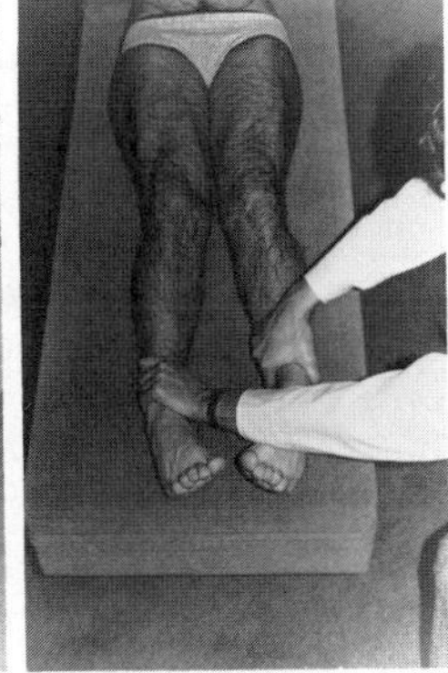

Figure 12.50. *Left*, testing hip abduction strength against resistance. *Right*, testing adductor strength.

attended by pain in the gluteal area, the piriformis should be suspected. Differentiation of piriformis spasm from other causes can often be elicited by reproducing the pain on internal rotation of the femur when it is at a lower level than the original point of pain.

To test for piriformis myofascitis, the patient is seated on a table with his hips and knees flexed. Resistance is applied by the examiner as the patient attempts to separate the knees. In piriformis myofascitis, pain and weakness will be noted on resisted abduction and external rotation of the thigh. Inflammation will be confirmed by rectal examination exhibiting acute tenderness over the lateral pelvic wall proximal to the ischial spine.

Iliopsoas Spasm[310, 311]

In the normal erect posture, only about 12% of the weight of the abdominal organs is borne by the suspensory ligaments. The majority of weight is supported by the inclined psoas and held there by the abdominal wall.

Increased tone tends to pull the lumbar spine into anterior and inferior flexion and to externally rotate and flex the thigh. The psoas minor, which runs between the T12 and L1 to the arcuate line of the hip bone, assists its "big brother."

In psoas spasm, the thigh is usually somewhat flexed on the trunk, although this is usually concealed by forward bending of the trunk. Iliopsoas hypertonicity can be confirmed by tension and pain during deep palpation of the abdomen below the umbilicus, lateral to the linea alba, medial to and slightly inferior to the ASIS. It will feel as a taut longitudinal bundle. It is also palpable in the upper sulcus of the pubic arch.

Effects of Iliopsoas Shortening. Bilateral iliopsoas shortening results in lumbar rigidity, anterior pelvic tilt, and hip flexion. When associated with acute back pain, the patient tends to flex the knees and the hip to help decrease the degree of pelvic tilt and lordosis (Fig. 12.51). When the hip flexors are short, the lumbar region does not flatten in the supine position unless the knees and hips are flexed.

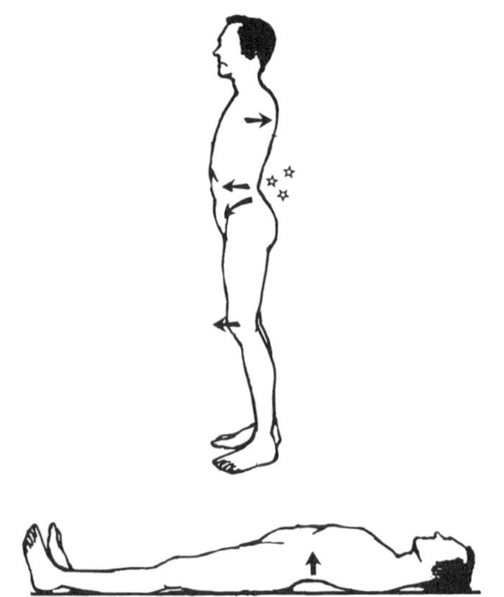

Figure 12.51. *Top*, typical posture of bilateral iliopsoas shortening with back pain. Note knee flexion, anterior pelvic tilt, increased lumbar curve, and compensatory high thoracic hyperkyphosis. *Bottom*, failure of the lumbar spine to flatten in the supine position because of bilateral iliopsoas shortening.

Nachemson's electromyographic studies indicate that the iliopsoas is just as important a lumbar stabilizer against gravitational forces in standing as it is a hip flexor during gait.[312] Some authorities feel that the iliopsoas is the key to postural correction. Michelle, who asserts that 30% of the population has an iliopsoas imbalance, makes the bold charge that any and all defects of the spine and hip structures should be evaluated in terms of iliopsoas dysfunction.[313] His theory presents some evidence that practically all conditions working against the "straight child" are attributable to the failure of the iliopsoas to elongate during bipedal maturation. "When the abnormal force of the nonelongated iliopsoatic musculature is presented bilaterally, the directional force is symmetrical, with the formation of an exaggerated dorsal kyphosis," he claims.

Pelvic Irritation. If the kidney-bladder complex, colon, appendix, pancreas, or lumbar lymph nodes or nerves are diseased, the sheath of the psoas is likely to be secondarily inflamed and painful. As the muscle also crosses the sacroiliac joint, inflammation is likely to lead to a protective reflex to fix the joint from irritating motion.

Thomas' Test. This is another test to determine excessive iliopsoas tension. The supine patient holds one flexed knee against his abdomen with his hands while the other limb is allowed to fully extend (Fig. 12.52). The patient's lumbar spine should normally flatten. If the extended limb does not extend fully (ie, the knee flexes from the table) or if the patient rocks his chest forward or arches his back, a fixed flexion contracture of the hip is indicated, as from a shortened iliopsoas muscle. Michele uses the degree of pain elicited on forceful extension of the flexed knee as his criterion of iliopsoas tension.[313] This should always be tested bilaterally.

Ely's Test. To support iliopsoas spasm suspicions, the patient is placed prone with his toes hanging over the edge of the table, legs relaxed. One or the other heel is approximated to the opposite buttock. After flexion of the knee, pain in the hip will make it impossible to carry out the test if there is any irritation to carry out the test if there is an irritation of the psoas muscle or its sheath. The buttock will tend to rise on the involved side. However, a positive Ely's sign can also be an indication of a lumbar lesion, a contracture of the tensor fascia lata, or an osseous hip lesion.

Differentiating General Hip Spasm. In the hip joint, two forms of spasm are common: (1) that which is due to irritation of the psoas alone, and (2) that in which all the muscles moving the joint are more or less contracted. The normal range of hip flexion is 120°. In isolated psoas spasm, motions of the hip (rotation, adduction, abduction, and flexion) are not impeded. General spasm of the hip muscles is tested with the patient supine upon a table or bed and the leg flexed at a right angle, both at the knee and at the hip. A child may be tested on its parent's lap. Using the sound leg as a standard of comparison, the examiner then draws the knee away from the midline (abduction), and toward the patient's chest (flexion). Rotation is tested by holding the knee still and moving the foot away from the median line of the body or toward and across it.

Selected Effects of Other Types of Pelvic Hypertonicity[95]

Excessive hypertonicity of any strong muscle, confirmed by palpatory tone and soreness, will tend to subluxate its site of osseous attachment. Below is a list of common problem areas in the pelvis other than piriformis or psoas spasm.

Gluteus Maximus. Increased tone tends to pull the pelvis posterior, inferior, and lateral, and rotate the thigh laterally. Trigger points in this area, especially along the crest, are a common cause of low-back pain.[314, 315]

Gluteus Medius. Increased tone tends to pull the ilium posterior, inferior, and lateral, and internally rotate the thigh.

Tensor Fascia Lata. Increased tone tends to pull the ilium down, sway the

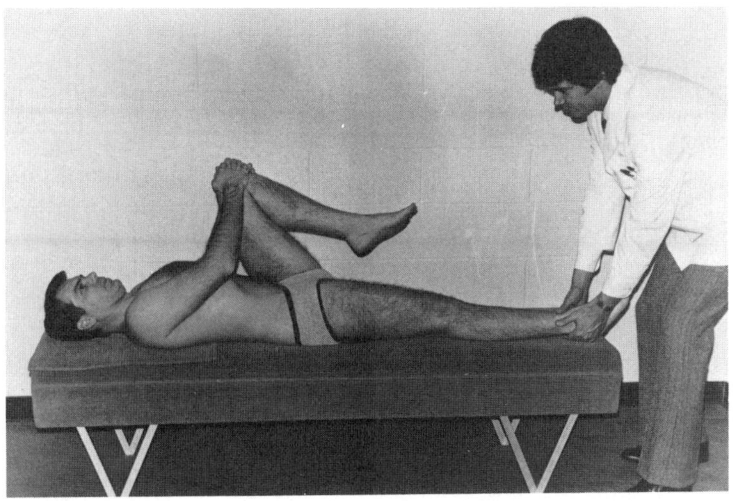

Figure 12.52. Thomas' test.

pelvis to the lateral, and subluxate the femur superiorly.

Common Pelvic Distortions from Muscular Dysfunction

During lateral flexion in the standing position, a plumb line will move from its sacral position and cut the buttock on the side of lateral flexion. This represents normal pelvic shifting and rotation about the ipsilateral head of the weight-bearing femur.

If the plumb line remains central during lateral bending, Grice feels that the first suspicion should be contraction of the contralateral gluteus medius.[316] The pelvis will remain relatively level. If the spine laterally flexes sharply at the lower thoracic area, splinting of the spinal erectors or contralateral iliopsoas contraction are most likely involved. If the lumbar concavity is exaggerated unilaterally and reduced on opposite lateral flexion, suspect hypertonicity of the quadratus lumborum on the exaggerated side.

Muscular dysfunction in the lower extremities frequently exhibits in pelvic distortions, often mimicking higher lesions. For example, shortening of the hip flexors rotates the pelvis anteriorly and overworks the hamstrings in maintaining balance (Fig. 12.53). Shortened calf muscles produce knee flexion and ankle dorsiflexion that incline the body forward from the midline and overwork the spinal extensors and stabilizers. In contrast, weak calf muscles produce hyperextension at the knees that must be compensated by a forward projection of the pelvis that which also overworks the spinal extensors and stabilizers.

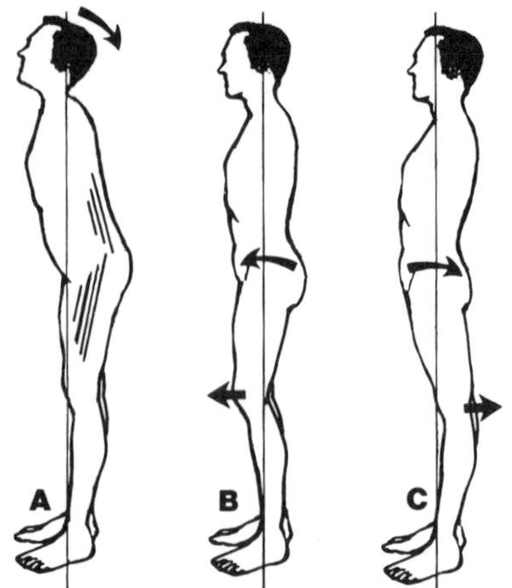

Figure 12.53. *A*, chronic postural hip flexion. In this syndrome, shortening of the hip flexors and spinal extensors, adapting to chronic hypertonicity of poor posture, causes the trunk to rotate over the femur heads. Note posterior deviation of the pelvis, anterior tilt of the trunk, and compensatory cervical hyperlordosis. *B*, this semi-squat posture is the result of soleus weakness producing chronic knee flexion and compensatory anterior iliac rotation to maintain balance. *C*, weakness of the gastrocnemius produces genu recurvatum and compensatory posterior rotation of the ilia to maintain balance. In time, a sharp lumbar hyperlordosis and long thoracic hyperkyphosis will develop.

Reflexes[317]

Trigger Points[96, 97, 318]

Trigger points of the pelvis are commonly located (1) over the greater sciatic notch through the gluteal muscles, (2) over the crest of the ilium, (3) over the belly of the tensor fascia lata, (4) in the ischiorectal fossa apex, and (5) at the sciatic outlet onto the back of the thigh from under the gluteus maximus. Specific trigger points for the gluteus medius and minimus, longissimus dorsi, and abductor longus are shown in Figure 12.54.

Viscerosomatic Reflexes[319, 320]

The sacral parasympathetics as well as the thoracolumbar sympathetics innervating the viscera are accompanied by a meager but sufficient quantity of viscerosensory fibers. These afferent fibers have extensions into the dorsal horns of the cord at the same level and from three to four segments above and below. Any visceral disturbance will therefore register itself upon the synaptic fields of the dorsal horns and in turn provide impulse bombardment via internuncial neurons to the ventral horns. This results in a reflex contraction of the muscles supplied. In this context, Janse feels that the muscles most directly affected by this noxious reflex from an irritated viscus are the multifidi, rotatores, intertransverse, and psoas major muscles.[321]

The local contraction of these muscles usually unilateral, may prevent one or more vertebra from participating in normal scoliotic compensations or the segment(s) may

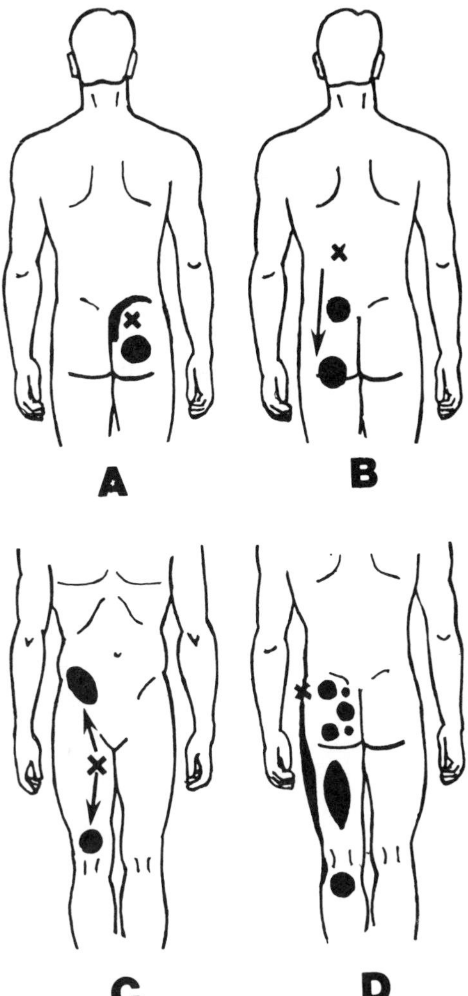

Figure 12.54. Trigger points of the gluteus medius (*A*), longissimus dorsi (*B*), abductor longus (*C*), and gluteus minimus (*D*); common site of trigger point indicated by *X*. Areas of referred pain shown by the *blackened areas*.

be pulled into an exaggerated displacement (subluxation), depending on which side of a scoliotic curve the unilateral contraction occurs. Thus, once a site of incompatible deviation (Lovett negative) or fixation is found, it is a great aid in the diagnosis of segmentally related visceral complaints and identifies a specific site of primary spinal therapy.

Craniosacral Respiratory Reflexes

Denton reports that anything disturbing the craniosacral respiratory mechanism such as altered body balance secondary to a functional pelvic distortion or dysfunction of a weight-bearing sacroiliac mechanism will result in palpatory swelling of the supine patient somewhere on the posterolateral aspect of the upper cervical transverse processes or mastoid process.[322] He also reports that a sacral base lesion will produce an indicator of increased nuchal tension and tenderness between the occiput and C5.

Heel Checks

At the risk of incurring the wrath of many eminent colleagues, it should be stated that pre- and postadjustment leg checks of the levelness of the heels when the patient is supine or prone offer highly erroneous conclusions. According to Logan's 1-2-4 ratio, it only takes a ⅛-inch intrinsic shift of the lower trunk to change the heel level ½ inch. Several factors can be involved singularly or in combination that will produce such a minute change in posture. (1) It is unnatural for a patient to remain in a completely static posture without some type of conscious or unconscious movement. (2) Any examination or manual procedure that requires touch sets up cutaneous reflexes that must manifest within the musculoskeletal system. (3) If the doctor-patient relationship is in good rapport, suggestion alone will produce the change anticipated. This response has been repeatedly shown even at the nonverbal level within clinical suggestion-hypnosis experiments.

TRAUMATIC DISORDERS OF THE PELVIS[323–329]

In evaluating pelvic trauma and distortions, inspection, palpation, muscle strength and length, and joint movement tests offer the most significant physical signs.

Sacroiliac Sprain[330–333]

Sacroiliac sprains with overt rupturing are of infrequent occurrence. Overloading and severe blows are the typical allopathic explanations, but these causes are considered infrequent by chiropractors and osteopaths unless severe ligament rupture and acute subluxation are associated. Careful differentiation is important because the intrinsic strength of the posterior ligaments makes severe sprain unlikely and because the joint is the common site of diffuse referred pain and tenderness.

Because the sacroiliac joint is so often the site of referred pain and tenderness (eg, lumbar disc, upper cervical fixation), it is unrealistic to automatically attribute these signs to the joint itself. However, we should also avoid the tendency to generalize that all such symptoms and signs are referred.

Etiology and Direction of Therapy. Straightening up or lifting from a stooped position can cause a traumatic unilateral or bilateral displacement of the sacrum within the ilia (Fig. 12.55), thus spraining the sacroiliac and iliolumbar ligaments. In this position, body weight (plus loading) pulls the sacrum anterior, while taut pelvic extensors pull the ilia posterior.

Most sacroiliac sprains, however, are not the result of severe overloading or drastic trauma. They are more frequently the result of a misstep, an awkward twist during flexion, or torsional overexertion (eg, shoveling). These common occurrences could hardly be classified as traumatic enough to tear the strongest ligaments of the body. The question arises: what makes this normally strong and slightly movable joint displace? The explanation is the same as that previously given for the cause of many vertebral subluxations.

Inhibited motion at some point within the normal range of sacroiliac movement is compensated by hypermobility at adjacent segments such as the lumbosacral, pubic, and proximal femur articulations. Likewise, a degree of lumbosacral or hip fixation leads to adaptive sacroiliac and pubic loosening and instability that predisposes sprain by normal activity forces. It is for this reason that the direct cause of a sacroiliac sprain-subluxation may not be within the joint itself and recurrence can only be avoided if the coupled joints, ligaments, and muscles are kept elastic. Once the coupled restrictions are normalized, the unstable joints will slowly tighten to meet their natural requirements.

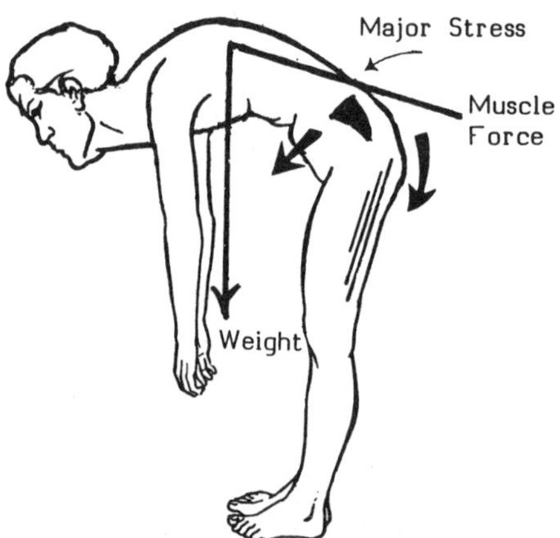

Figure 12.55. Lifting stresses placed on the sacroiliac joint when trunk load pulls the sacral base anteriorly while contraction of the hamstrings and gluteus maximus rotate the ilia to the posterior.

Pregnancy is another cause of adaptive loosening of the sacroiliac and pubic joints, but the cause is hormonal rather than adjacent fixation. Grieve's studies showed that the normal symphysis pubis width of 4 mm increases to 9 mm, and some separations have been recorded up to 2 cm.[334] Obvious changes can be recognized as early as the fourth month of pregnancy, and normalization does not return until 6–12 weeks after delivery.

Some chiropractors have considered bowling very stressful to the sacroiliac joints because of the unilateral weight activity. Biomechanical principles, however, do not support this hypothesis. Most sacroiliac injuries that occur during bowling do not occur during the locomotion phase. During delivery with "good form," the unilateral loading is compensated by a shift in body mass and the momentum of the ball. The greatest force is made when the body is balanced on *one* extremity. Translational and torsional forces are automatically relieved by the body sliding and turning on the ball of the foot with minimal friction. When injuries do occur, they result from poor technique and especially when the ball is lifted from the return rack in flexion when body weight is balanced on *both* extremities, thus fixing the base of support. Rather than the body responding as a whole, the weight-bearing joints must adapt or fail.

Symptoms. Jarring the spine causes a sharp localized pain in the affected joint. The pain usually radiates over the ipsilateral hip and down the anterior thigh. These symptoms are usually relieved by rest and aggravated by activity. When the gluteus medius shortens to abduct the hip when the patient is laterally recumbent, the contraction tends to separate the ilium from sacrum. If the sacroiliac joint is inflamed from trauma or disease, abduction of the thigh against resistance is acutely painful.

Signs. Stress upon the joint should increase pain such as in lateral compression or torsion of the iliac crests. A variety of clinical stress tests have been developed. Tenderness will be found inferomedial to the PSIS and often at the pubic symphysis, contralateral anterior acetabulum, and fascia lata. Care must be taken not to confuse sacral base tenderness from local ligamentous stress with that of tender sacrospinalis muscle fiber insertions. Lasègue's test is unpredictable. If the sprain is "hot," Lasègue's test will definitely be positive between 30° and 60°.

Visual Analysis. The patient assumes the characteristic standing posture with a flatened lumbar area and weight placed on the unaffected side. The trunk is inclined away from the painful lesion. There is a guarded gait and limited spinal motion, especially spinal flexion due to hamstring tension. Trunk rotation is rarely inhibited because this takes place primarily in the thoracic spine. Because of gluteal inhibition, a definite Trendelenburg lurch may be exhibited during gait. In most cases, restricted mobility will be found in thigh flexion or hyperextension.

Differentiation. Care must be taken to differentiate the symptoms of sacroiliac sprain from a sacral base lesion, lumbar subluxation, or pelvic pathology. Special roentgenographic and laboratory analyses are necessary if symptoms do not respond as anticipated. Localized point tenderness and the standard kinesiologic and orthopedic tests are helpful in differentiating mimicking musculoskeletal disorders.

It should be apparent that a sacroiliac or lumbar adjustment may release an adjacent lumbar, hip, or pubic fixation and lead to erroneous cause-effect conclusions. This is an example of why empiric results often lead to the various misleading theories often expounded at seminars.

Gaenslen's Test. In this test, the patient is placed supine with knees, thighs, and legs acutely flexed by the patient who clasps his knees with both hands and pulls them toward his abdomen. This brings the lumbar spine firmly in contact with the table and fixes both the pelvis and lumbar spine. With the examiner standing at right angles to the patient, the patient is brought well to the side of the table. The examiner slowly hyperextends the opposite thigh by gradually increasing force by pressure of one hand on top of the knee while the examiner's other hand is on the flexed knee for support in fixing the lumbar spine and pelvis (Fig. 12.56). Some examiners allow the hyperextended limb to fall from the table edge. The hyperextension of the hip exerts a rotating force on the corresponding half of the pelvis. The pull is made on the ilium through the "Y" ligament and the muscles attached to the anterior iliac spines. The test is positive if the thigh is hyperextended and pain is felt in the sacroiliac area or referred down the thigh, providing that the opposite sacroiliac joint is normal and the sacrum moves as a unit with the side of the pelvis opposite to that being tested. It should be tested bilaterally. A positive sign may be elicited

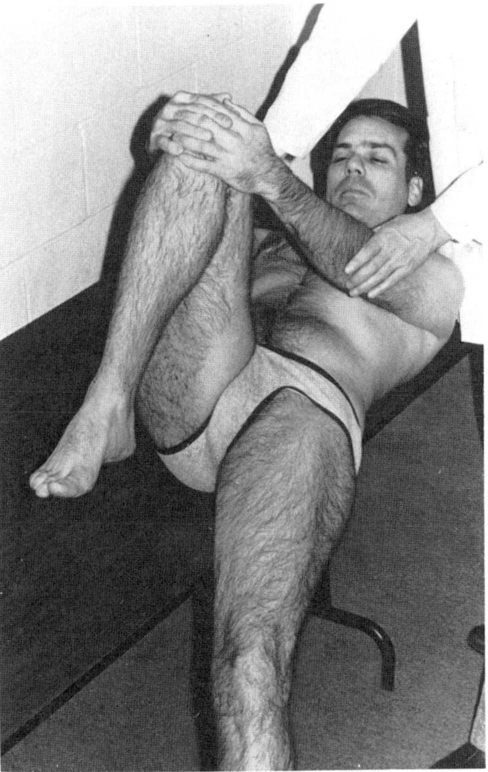

Figure 12.56. Gaenslen's test.

in a sacroiliac, hip, or lower lumbar nerve root lesion. If the L4 is involved, pain is usually referred anteriorly to the groin or upper thigh. If the sign is negative, a lumbosacral lesion should be first suspected. This test is usually contraindicated in the elderly.

Erichsen's Pelvic Rock Test. With the patient supine, the examiner places his hands on the iliac crests with his thumbs on the ASISs and forcibly compresses the pelvis toward the midline (Fig. 12.57). This tends to separate the sacroiliac joints. If conducted carefully, this test can be quite specific. Pain experienced in the sacroiliac joint suggests a joint lesion that may be postural, traumatic, or infectious in origin.

Iliac Compression Test. The patient is placed on his side with the affected side up. The examiner places his forearm over the iliac crest and exerts pressure downward for about 30 seconds. This tends to compress the sacroiliac and pubic joints. A positive sign of joint inflammation or sprain is seen with an increase in pain; however, absence of pain does not necessarily rule out sacroiliac involvement. This test is usually contraindicated in geriatrics and pediatrics or with any sign of a hip lesion or osseous pelvic pathology.

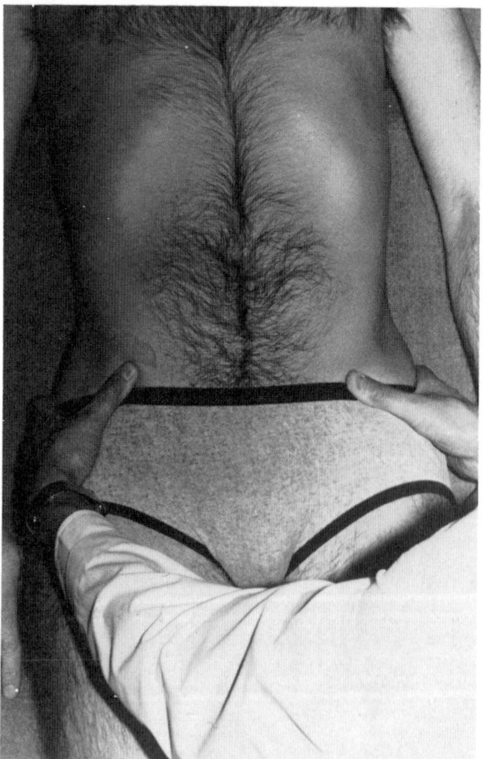

Figure 12.57. Erichsen's pelvic rock test.

Hibb's Test. With the patient supine, the examiner extends the patient's thigh on the affected side and rotates the hip joint internally by rotating the leg at the knee. An increase in pain is a positive indication of a sacroiliac lesion if the possibility of a hip lesion has been eliminated.

Mennel's Test. The patient is placed prone, and one hand is used to stabilize the contralateral pelvis. With the palpating hand, the examiner places a thumb over the patient's PSIS and exerts pressure, then slides his thumb outward and then inward. The sign is positive if tenderness is increased. When sliding outward, trigger deposits in structures on the gluteal aspect of the PSIS may be noted. If when sliding inward tenderness is increased, it is indicative of sprain of the superior sacroiliac ligaments. Confirmation is positive when tenderness is increased when the examiner pulls the ASIS posteriorly while standing behind the patient or when the examiner pulls the PSIS forward while standing in front of the supine patient. These tests are helpful in determining that tenderness is due to overstressed superior sacroiliac ligaments.

Yeoman's Test. The patient is placed prone. With one hand, firm pressure is applied by the examiner over the suspected sacroiliac joint, fixing the patient's anterior pelvis to the table. With the other hand, the patient's leg is flexed on the affected side to the limit, and the thigh is hyperextended by the examiner by lifting the knee off the examining table. If pain is increased in the sacroiliac area, it is significant of a ventral sacroiliac or hip lesion because of the stress on the anterior sacroiliac ligaments. Normally, no pain should be felt on this maneuver.

Goldthwait's Test. The patient is placed supine. The examiner places one hand under the lumbar spine with each fingerpad pressed firmly against the interspinous spaces. The other hand of the examiner is used to slowly conduct an SLR test. If pain occurs or is aggravated before the lumbar processes open (0–30°), a sacroiliac lesion should be suspected. Goldthwait felt that if pain occurred while the processes were opening at 30–60°, a lumbosacral lesion was suggested; at 60–90°, an L1–L4 disc lesion was suggested.

Smith-Peterson's Test. If it is possible during Goldthwait's test to raise the limb on the unaffected side to a greater level without pain than on the involved side, a positive Smith-Peterson's sign is found, which confirms a sacroiliac lesion; ie, pain usually occurs at the same level for either leg when a lumbosacral lesion is present.

Sacroiliac Stretch Test. The patient is placed supine. The examiner, standing to face the patient, crosses his arms and places one hand on the contralateral anterior-superior iliac spine and the other hand on the ipsilateral anterior-superior iliac spine. Oblique (posterolateral) pressure is then applied to spread the anterior aspects of the ilia laterally. A positive sign of sacroiliac sprain is a deep-seated pelvic pain that may radiate into the buttock or groin. While the iliac compression test is designed to stretch the posterior sacroiliac ligaments, this test stretches the ligaments on the anterior aspect of the joints.

Gillis' Test. With the patient prone and the examiner standing on the side of involvement, the examiner reaches over and stabilizes the uninvolved sacroiliac joint while the thigh on the involved side is extended at the hip. Pain initiated in the sacroiliac area of the involved side by this maneuver is a positive sign of an acute sacroiliac sprain/subluxation or sacroiliac disease.

Management. Management of acute sacroiliac sprain with or without subluxation rarely presents a clinical problem. Standard sprain therapy will relieve the acute pain. A trochanteric belt is helpful in the acute stage, but if ligamentous rupture is extensive a larger support will be necessary. Mobilization of fixations, correction of subluxations, activity and lifting counsel, and muscle therapy incorporating strengthening and stretching where indicated are the best procedures to avoid recurrence. A back support while sitting may be helpful (Fig. 12.58).

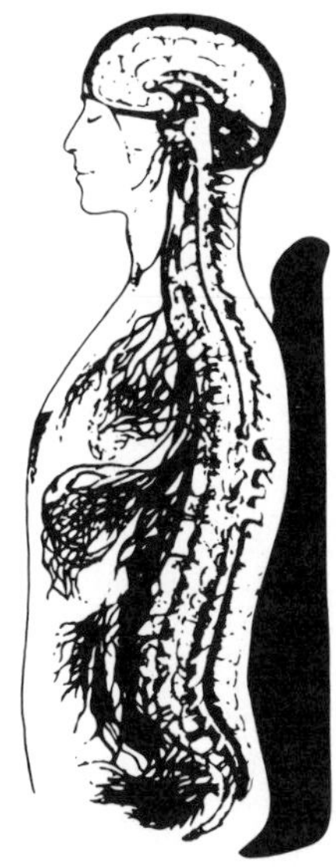

Figure 12.58. Sitting postural support. (With the permission of Posture Support Mfg., Inc., Solon, Ohio.)

Sacroiliac Subluxation[335–340]

Sacroiliac subluxations produce (1) irritative microtrauma to the interarticular structures, (2) induction of a vertebral motion unit subluxation and/or are contributions to chronicity of subluxations, (3) induction of spinal curvatures and/or are contributions to the chronicity of curvatures present, and (4) biomechanical impropriety of the pelvis in static postural accommodation and in locomotion.

Local pain and acute tenderness are rarely seen in chronic cases unless the fixated site is irritated by trauma. Old lesions appear to enjoy confusing the examiner by referring signs and symptoms far above or below. Roentgenography is quite helpful, but rarely is it an end in itself. Thus, immobility, stress tests, and spinal balance are the most reliable clues.

Piedallu's Sign.[341] When a sacral base is unilaterally subluxated anteroinferiorly and laterally so that the adjacent ilium is subluxated posteroinferiorly and medially, the ipsilateral PSIS on the side of inferiority will be low in the standing and sitting positions. If this PSIS becomes higher than the contralateral PSIS during forward flexion, the phenomenon is called a positive Piedallu's sign. Such a sign signifies either ipsilateral sacroiliac locking in which the sacrum and ilium move as a whole or muscular contraction that prevents motion of the sacrum on the ilium. Regardless, it shows that sacral dysfunction is probably present.

Sacroiliac vs Lumbosacral Differentiation. To differentiate these two common disorders, the patient is placed supine on a firm flat table. A folded towel is placed transversely under the small of the patient's back. The doctor stabilizes the patient's pelvis by cupping his hands over the ASISs and exerting moderate pressure. The patient is instructed to raise both extremities simultaneously with legs straight. If the patient senses discomfort or an increase of discomfort in the low back or an increase of discomfort in the low back or over the sacrum and gluteal area at about 25–50° leg raise and before the small of the back wedges against the towel, sacroiliac involvement is suspected. If, on the other hand, discomfort is experienced or augmented only after the legs have been raised beyond 50° and the small of the back wedges firmly against the towel, lumbosacral involvement should be the first suspicion.

Belt Test. The standing male patient flexes forward with the examiner holding the patient's belt at the back. If bending over without support is more painful than with support, it suggests a sacroiliac lesion. Conversely, if bending over with support is more painful than without support, it suggests a lumbosacral or lumbar involvement.

Beery's Sign. If backache is relieved when the patient goes from a standing to sitting position, such relief is said to be indicative of a pelvic lesion rather than a lumbar condition. This relief, a positive Beery's sign, comes from hamstring relaxation.

Structural Listings[342–352]

The sacrum and ilium move upon each other in a reciprocal manner (Fig. 12.59). When a unilateral anterior sacral base is listed, a unilateral posterior sacral apex, unilateral posterior ilium, or unilateral anterior ischium listing could be substituted. As the PSIS can be considered to be a point at the end of a long lever from the axis of rotation, it moves a greater distance than points closer to the axis. A rotational displacement of the sacrum cannot occur without opposite effects upon the ilium even though one mechanism of injury is usually involved. Similarly, in rotational displacements a listing is made for one side. It is understood that a reciprocal state exists on the contralateral side unless it is fixated. It is the doctor's choice whether to use a sacral base, sacral apex, iliac, or ischial listing. There is little standardization, unfortunately, even among our colleges.

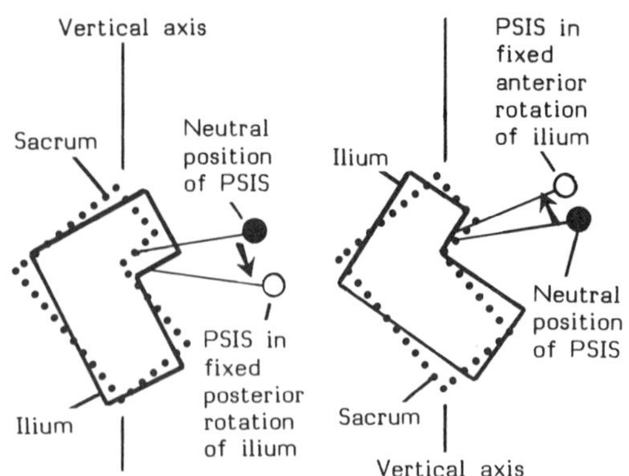

Figure 12.59. Reciprocal rotational motion leading to subluxation between the sacrum and ilium, and the position changes of the posterior superior iliac spine.

Anterior and posterior listings refer to displacements around a horizontal lateral axis. Superior and inferior iliac listings refer to displacements that are obliquely vertical across the joint. Superior and inferior sacral listings refer to displacements around an A-P transverse axis. Medical and lateral iliac listings refer to displacements around a vertical axis.

Because of the slant of the articular surfaces, forward displacement of the sacrum must be in an oblique anterior, inferior, and lateral direction. It is common practice to shorten such a listing to a simple *base anterior* (right or left), but this is not meant to ignore the accompanying inferiority and laterality. Other common abbreviations include:

• Sacral base posterior: posterior, superior, medial rotational misalignment.

• Posterior ilium: posterior, inferior, medial rotational misalignment, in which the posteriority is the more prominent motion fixated.

• Anterior ilium: anterior, superior, lateral rotational misalignment, in which the anteriority is the more prominent motion fixated.

• Superior ilium: superior, anterior, lateral translational misalignment, in which the superiority is the more prominent motion fixated.

• Inferior ilium: inferior, posterior, medial translational misalignment, in which the inferiority is the more prominent motion fixated.

• Medial ilium: posterior transverse rotation of the ilium on the sacrum, in which medial translation is the more prominent motion fixated.

• Lateral ilium: anterior transverse rotation of the ilium on the sacrum, in which lateral translation is the more prominent motion fixated.

Not understanding this abbreviated form, some have unfairly criticized chiropactors for such "anatomically ignorant" terminology in allopathic literature. As medical literature abounds with such shortened forms with implied omissions, no apology is necessary.

Any of these misalignments may be unilateral or bilateral. While there are many exceptions to any clinical rule, it is generally held that unilateral subluxations will usually have a history of trauma while bilateral lesions are usually related to postural origins.

Rarely is the sacral apex or ischium used as a listing, but the same process of abbreviation described would apply. The most common listings are anterior and posterior sacral base and iliac listings. These are the typical mechanical distortions found. However, it is not unusual to see sacroiliac distortions that have not completely followed the plane of articulation (eccentric lesions). In these circumstances, we may infrequently find, for example, a sacral base that appears anterior and superior or an ilium that is posterior and superior. Such combinations are almost endless because of the multidirectional movement capabilities of this important joint.

Anterior Sacrum Listings. According to Logan,[353] Illi,[354] and several other investigators, the primary sacroiliac subluxation features sacral fixation in the anterior position (Fig. 12.60). As the sacrum slips anterior and the ilium moves posterior, the iliolumbar ligament pulls the ipsilateral transverse process of L5 posterior. This produces a torque at the lumbosacral junction. In addition, there is always a secondary torsion at the pubes, but this is usually automatically corrected when the sacroiliac joint is normalized.

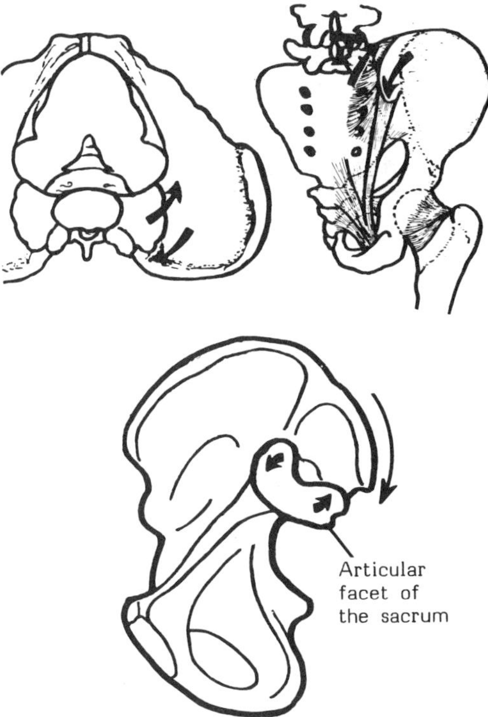

Figure 12.60. Direction of original sacral and iliac motion when the sacral base is fixed in an anterior position. Such forces create a severe rotational torque within the joint.

When the sacral base slips unilaterally anterior and the ilium posterior, the standing patient will flex his hip so that his thigh is carried upward against his abdomen (thus rotating the innominate further posterior) much more readily than he can extend his thigh backward and thus rotate the innominate anterior. With the patient supine and the pelvis fixed by the examiner, the patient will find it somewhat more difficult to abduct the leg upward on the side of sacroiliac subluxation. These are purely mechanical signs.

Bilateral sacral base anteriority is commonly associated with lumbar hyperlordosis. Traumatic causes usually result from jumping when the trunk is flexed: the sacrum is caught between body weight directed inferiorly and impact forces from the ground traveling toward the superior that meet at the anteroinferiorly tilted sacral base where much of the force must be resolved.

Posterior Sacrum Listings. Posterior base subluxations are unusual but not rare (Fig. 12.61). They are never due to a postural weight-bearing fault because of the natural anteroinferior tilt. When they occur, they are associated with the concavity of a lumbar scoliosis, a fall on or blow to the sacral apex that stretches the strong posterior ligaments, or a contralateral anterioinferior sacral fixation that has caused adaptive joint instability on the ipsilateral side.

Bilateral sacral base posteriority is usually associated with the stiff "military spine" with severe lumbar flattening or trauma against the sacral apex.

Posterior Ilium Listings. These subluxations are the converse of anterior sacral base listings. When an ilium is subluxated posterior, medial, and inferior on the sacrum, the ischium is relatively rotated anterior, lateral, and superior. This will produce the classic functional short leg on the side of the lesion because the acetabular level is raised in the standing weight-bearing position. The ipsilateral pubis will also be raised and sometimes tender. The pelvis as a whole rotates horizontally anterior on the side of the short leg. Associated contralateral tenderness at the hip joint is usually related.

Anterior Ilium Listings. These are the converse of posterior sacral base listings.

Inferior or Superior Ilium Listings. These subluxations result from a blow directed from the inferior or superior through the sacroiliac joint (Fig. 12.62). They are rare except from an injury similar to a football block. In most cases, the force from the inferior results from a fall directly on the inferior ischium or landing from a jump on the heels while the femoral heads hold. In cases of rickets, the sacrum can slide inferior within the softening sacroiliac joints—thus resembling bilateral iliac superiority without rotation.

Inferior or superior listings must not be confused with the "short leg" or "long leg" phenomena related to A-P ilial-ischial rotation. In inferior and superior listings, the ilium has translated up or down obliquely on the sacrum or the sacrum has translated on the ilium with little rotation involved. In rotational subluxations, the unilateral vertical height of the ilium increases on the side of the short leg and decreases on the side of the long leg (Fig. 12.63). Correction of a posterior ilium will improve a functional short leg, and correction of an anterior ilium will improve a functional long leg.

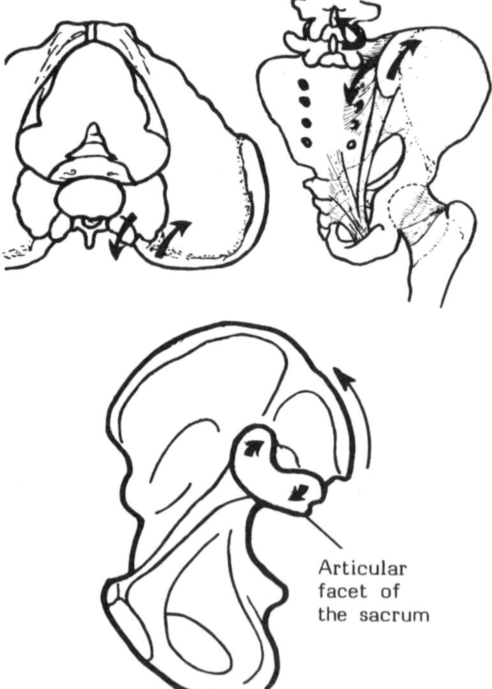

Figure 12.61. Direction of original sacral and iliac motion when the sacral base is fixed in a posterior position. Such forces create a severe rotational torque within the joint.

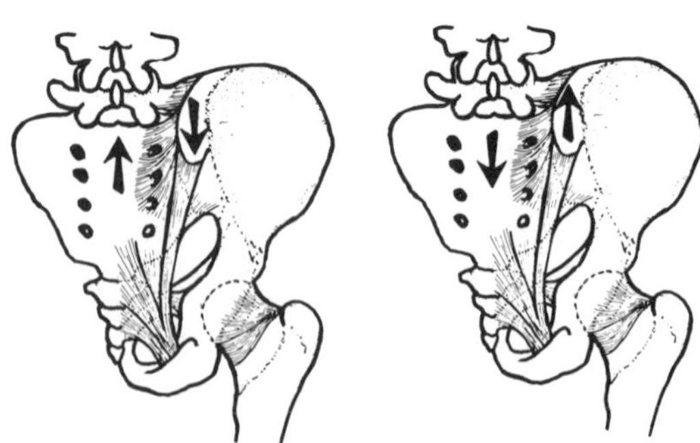

Figure 12.62. Direction of original sacral and iliac motion when the ilium is fixed in an inferior position (*left*) or a superior position (*right*). Such forces create severe shear stress within the joint.

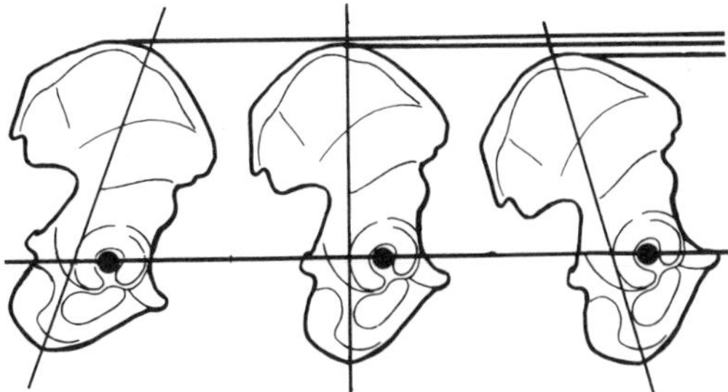

Figure 12.63. Changes of apparent iliac crest vertical height due to normal rotation. *Left*, anterior iliac rotation; *center*, neutral position; *right*, posterior iliac rotation. The pivot point around the femoral head is represented by the *black dot.*

In cases of a structurally deficient extremity, the body usually makes the corrective rotation of the ilium spontaneously. This biomechanical adaptive mechanism should not be treated unless it becomes symptomatic or produces adversee effects elsewhere.

Medial or Lateral Ilium. It has been explained that during forward flexion, the sacral base tends to bulge toward the posterior at the upper third of the joint and further separate the PSISs. During hyperextension, the sacral base tends to sink at the level of the upper joint and the distance between the PSISs reduces. Similar motions occur when changing from the recumbent to the standing positions, or visa versa. If the joint becomes fixed in one of these extreme ranges of normal motion with minimal rotation involved, the involved ilium can be listed as medial or lateral (Fig. 12.64). Some authorities use the terms interior (medial) or exterior (lateral) ilia for the subluxation-fixations.

Analytical Cautions

The most common errors of analysis stem from misleading visual signs, subjective responses to testing procedures, structural symmetry, and subjective descriptions of pain.

Visual Signs in Acute Cases. Any severe sprain or strain will produce reflex muscle splinting as a protective mechanism. This spasm around any joint will not release until the neuron excitation subsides. A basic clue of an antalgic posture associated with lumbar or pelvic dysfunction is the head far

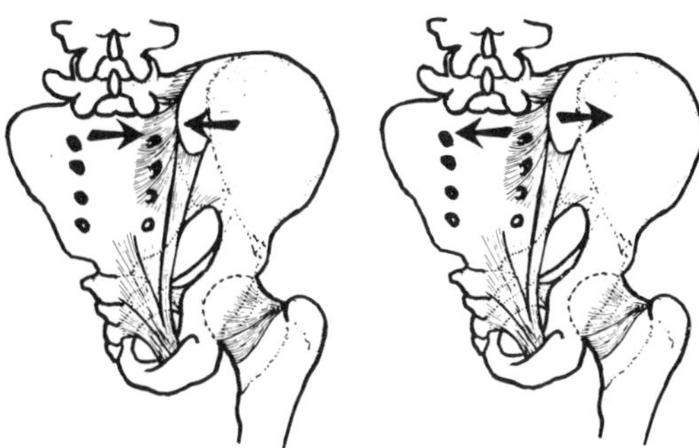

Figure 12.64. Direction of original sacral and iliac motion when the ilium is fixed in a medial (*left*) or lateral (*right*) position. Such forces create severe compressive and tensile forces, respectively, within the posterior aspect of the joint and an opposite effect at the anterior sacroiliac joint and pubic symphysis.

removed from the midline when viewed from the A-P—much farther lateral than that seen in uncompensated or decompensated scolioses. The pelvis will often be severely tilted and twisted with the spine torqued in several opposite directions above (corkscrew reaction). The trunk will usually be flexed in the basic protective position. Thus, pain and splinting produce temporary antalgic postures that invariably mask and sometimes reverse basic distortions, rendering visual analysis of basic balance patterns useless at the time. While antalgic postures have a predictable pattern with each individual, they vary widely from patient to patient because of uniquely acquired conditioned reflexes, different pain thresholds, and the stage of related inflammation.

Subjective Responses to Testing Procedures. A description of many standard tests are offered within this book. Most kinetic tests are highly subjective in response and unspecific. To differentiate physical restriction from psychologic restriction is a laborious process, and it is almost impossible to stress the tissues of one joint without stressing the tissues of adjacent joints. Thus, the conclusions from several tests must be compared. And there is always the human tendency to find that which prejudgment would like to find.

Structural Asymmetry. Grieve points out that the most common error in many structural methods of analysis is the assumption of bilateral symmetry.[355] Optimal manipulative therapy for a specific patient must be based on the *individual* patient's response to a variety of testing procedures and not on theoretical notions based on structural averages. Cineroentgenographic studies of the sacroiliac joint have shown that sacroiliac movement is highly variable and patterns of movement difficulties differ widely from patient to patient. They are often attributed to differences in lateral sacral or iliac dimensions, articular variances, calcified ligaments, unusual pelvic designs, and oddities at the lumbosacral articulation.

Clinical Judgment. Most authorities state that sacroiliac pain will always be on the side of hypermobility, while others of equal credentials place the pain on the side of fixation. Some state that the side of fixation is always the major, while others say that the side of hypermobility is always the major because the joint is normally hypomobile. This confuses everybody except the mentors' disciples. It is my opinion that the typical pain of sacroiliac stress is diffuse across the sacroiliac area and most difficult for the patient to isolate. It is not uncommon for referred pain to detour from textbook descriptions (eg, gallbladder distress does not always refer to the right scapula, anginal pain does not always refer to the left arm). Even palpable tenderness may be referred. The most reliable clues are the site of consistently increased pain on biomechanical stress tests and, conversely, opposite maneuvers that relieve pain, tenderness, and structural imbalance. When dealing with individual patients, each of which is unique, *the doctor is best directed by what he or she finds to be true in the situation at hand and not by the theories of others based upon their patients.*

Strains and Inflammations[356–358]

Gluteal Contusions

The gluteus maximus receives an independent nerve (inferior gluteal) from the sacral plexus that leaves the pelvis below the piriformis muscle close to the lateral edge of the sacrotuberous ligament. This nerve and accompanying inferior gluteal artery and vein pierce the gluteal fascia and then spread between the fascia and the muscle. The gluteus medius is supplied by the superior gluteal nerve and vessels that exit the pelvis above the piriformis muscle.

This large muscle is firmly enclosed in strong fascia, especially its deep surface. Because of this, it is often involved in a compartment syndrome that is misdiagnosed as sciatica when a kick to or a fall upon the buttocks is in the history. Because its fascia is continuous with that of the fascia lata, differentiation must be made from "hip pointer" and proximal femur lesions.

Contusions, especially to the ischial tuberosity and the well-developed buttocks, are sometimes seen. Just walking may be aggravating, but pain is usually not severe. Swelling and bleeding may be extensive, but it is reduced quickly if cold is applied immediately. Recurrent bleeding is always a problem, but its likelihood is reduced if cold is continued for 3–4 days. Full healing will usually take place within a month if reinjury does not occur.

Gluteal Strains

In many cases of what is first thought of as being sacroiliac sprain, palpable tenderness will be most acute just lateral or superolateral to the PSIS rather than medial over the joint. This first suggests gluteal strain (eg, hip overstress), sacrospinalis or latissimus dorsi attachment strain, or hypertonicity emitted from L5 irritation.

Strain may be seen in the muscles that rotate the thigh and stabilize the hip such as the glutei, piriformis, gemelli, and quadratus femoris. Awkward slips are the typical injury mechanism, and the dysfunction is extremely debilitating. Strains of the origin of the hamstring muscles, associated with lower-buttock pain on exercise and ischial tenderness on forward flexion, are common. An unimpeded forceful, full swing of an object (eg, golf club) may cause an avulsion of the ischial apophysis. Sciatica tests will be negative. Heat in the postacute stage, gentle passive stretching, and graduated active exercises should be incorporated into the standard strain management program.

When the gluteus maximus is injured, it will manifest increased pain on hip extension from a flexed position, walking up stairs, external hip rotation against resistance, thigh adduction against resistance when the limb is extended, and thigh abduction against resistance when the hip is flexed. Injury of the gluteus medius and minimus will exhibit increased pain on resisted thigh abduction and medial rotation of the femur.

Adductor Strains

An adductor strain referring pain to the pelvis is frequently suffered by athletes. The complaint will be one of stiffness, tenderness, and pain during abduction that is high in the groin. In addition to regular strain therapy, treatment should include applying progressive adductor tendon stretch up to patient tolerance.

A severe "scissors" kick frequently leads to instability of the sacroiliac and symphysis pubis joints. Groin pain is aggravated during running, jumping, and in the stretching motion of kicking with power. A periosteal reaction may be noted at the origin of the adductor muscles (gracilis syndrome).

Pelvic Bursitis

A bursa is formed between the lateral capsule of the proximal femur and the gluteus maximus muscle's tendon as it passes over the greater trochanter to insert into the iliotibial tract. Inflammation from an external blow is not unusual.

Another bursa is formed at the internal obturator tendon and the superior and inferior gemelli. It runs below the piriformis and passes posteriorly to round the sciatic notch, largely filling the lesser sciatic foramen. Inflammation is evaluated by testing external rotation of the thigh against resistance and signs of tenderness upon deep palpation.

Pubic Sprain and Subluxation

This frequently occurring condition is often mistaken for sacroiliac slip, although sacroiliac displacement may have occurred and been spontaneously reduced.[359] (The disorder is also associated with lateral hip subluxations. In pure pubic subluxation, the predominant evidence will be found at the pubic symphysis. The sacroiliac area will not be excessively tender, but acute tenderness will be found over the painful pubis. After severe trauma, pubic and sacroiliac displacement may coexist.

It should be kept in mind that there is a good degree of bone elasticity between the extreme A-P points of the pelvis except in the very elderly or osteoporotic pelvis. Healthy bone is not brittle. Normal iliac movements are bilaterally reciprocal. This places a torsion on the pubic fibrocartilage that can be likened to slowly wringing a damp cloth by hand (Fig. 12.65). Thus, it is no wonder that the symphysis often becomes fibrotic.

When pain in the area of the symphysis pubis is the complaint, x-ray views should be taken in the weight-bearing position, first with full weight on one limb and then the other to seek signs of instability. Oval or semicircular lucency and avulsion sites may be exhibited at the pubis near the symphysis at the origin of the gracilis muscle and the adductors longus and brevis. In addition, symphysis widening, instability, ragged corners, fluffy margins, pubic osteoporosis, and muscle attachment periosteal reactions may be seen. Stress sclerosis of the iliac aspect of the sacroiliac joints are often associated in these conditions.

Osteitis Pubis

This is a rare disability that is becoming more common with the increase of poorly conditioned joggers. It is frequently chronic and episodic. The picture is one of severe groin pain sometimes radiating to the hips,

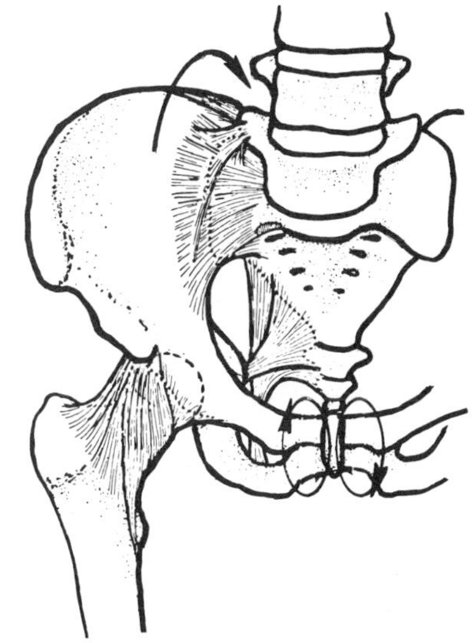

Figure 12.65. Direction of motion in a subluxated posterior right ilium and the torque forces at the symphysis pubis.

groin, or abdomen that is aggravated by hip rotation, abdominal flexion, and sometimes by iliac compression. Swelling and tenderness will be noted over the symphysis pubis. A slight epiphyseal slip may be a predisposing factor during youth. Roentgenography may reveal an eroded symphysis with joint widening, tending to calcification in later stages. Fever, dysuria, leukocytosis, and an increased sedimentation rate are inconsistent associations. Differentiation must be made from ankylosing spondylitis, adductor-origin strain, and perineal disease.

Coccyx Sprain and Subluxation[360-363]

An irritating coccygeal displacement referring pain to the sacroiliac area is sometimes overlooked. It is more common among women than men. The typical coccyx lies in the same curved plane as the sacrum when viewed during inspection, and slight displacements are never obvious on x-ray films. The direction of displacement is usually anterior, but it is infrequently posterior. The cause is usually a fall in the sitting position. Ligamentous tears may be associated with subluxation and/or fracture. If a gluteus maximus is unilaterally weak, the coccyx will deviate contralaterally.

Coccygodynia may be from mild to severe, and urogenital, rectal, and sciatic-like complaints and general nervousness may be related. The associated pain is usually far greater than the degree of displacement would indicate. In traumatic situations, pain and local levator ani spasm may be pronounced and often episodic. Local tenderness is consistently present, and pain is aggravated by pressure in the direction of displacement.

Keep in mind that the terminal of the spinal cord is attached to the cornua of the coccyx. As the segment moves anteriorly, the apex of the sacrum acts as a fulcrum. As the cornua moves backward and downward, traction is applied to the spinal cord. Thus, symptoms from the resulting cord tension need not be confined to the pelvic region alone (eg, occipital headaches, torticollis).

The coccyx enjoys confusing smug examiners. Ossification of the sacrococcygeal disc, for example, is easily mistaken for a fracture. A congenital lateral deviation of the coccyx from the midline can be mistaken for a dislocation by those who use roentgenography exclusively to confirm their diagnosis.

Pelvic Avulsions and Fractures[364-369]

After pelvic injury, all related structures should be carefully evaluated. Direct buttock falls upon a hard surface (eg, ice or roller skating, skateboarding) often result in vertical or sometimes oblique sacral fractures associated with other unilateral pelvic fractures, dislocation of the coccyx, and lumbar subluxation. After pelvic or leg injury, hip dislocation or gross instability is sometimes missed.

Note pelvic symmetry, deformity, and carefully palpate for bony crepitus about the ischium, rami, and hip areas. Rolling injuries are usually at fault in pelvic ring fractures such as seen in horseback riding accidents, falls against a hard surface, and vehicular accidents. Vascular, bladder, and perineal injuries are often associated. Even when the ilium and/or sacrum is fractured, the strong sacroiliac joint remains intact.

Pelvic Avulsions. Fatigue and avulsion fractures are far from uncommon, but the most typical injuries are associated with muscle, tendon, fascia, and cartilage injuries of the lower extremity. The most common sites of avulsion fractures in one 2-year study occurred at the ischial tuberosity at the hamstring origin, the ASIS at the sartorius origin, and the AIIS at the origin of the rectus femoris muscle. In running strains, sudden severe pain in the area of the hip or buttock may be traced to an avulsion of the hamstring attachments at the ischial tuberosity. Roentgenography may indicate large crescent-shaped bone masses near the injured ischium.

Pelvic Fractures.[370] While pelvic fractures are not common, they should never be taken lightly because they are reported to be the second most common cause of traumatic death—second only to head injuries. They are usually due to violent injuries, are frequently multiple, and result in severe deformity. The most common area involved is that about the sacroiliac joints and the symphysis pubis. A fracture or dislocation of a pubis is frequently associated with separation of a sacroiliac joint or fracture of the adjacent sacrum, ilium, or pubis.

Pelvic fractures often cause severe internal bleeding difficult to halt even on surgery. Shock is present in 40% of the cases. The patient will be unable to stand or walk, complains of pain in the pelvic region or back and, if the bladder or kidney is injured, passes blood in the urine. A pelvic girth injury is suggested by severe low-back pain (especially in retroperitoneal bleeding), severe pain with compression of the iliac crests, or acute pubic tenderness.

In roentgenography, fractures of the ilium are visible as sharply defined lines of diminished density that are possibly stellate. Sacral fractures are most difficult to visualize unless there is some displacement. Colon or rectal gas may mimic or obscure a pelvic fracture, but these shadows are not constant and can be ruled out on future examination. Other sources of error are the blood-vessel grooves in the ilium, but their branching character and bilaterality help in identification. In examining the young, keep in mind that the pelvic epiphyses are among the last to unite. They are open until 20–25 years of age.

Pubic Fatigue Fractures. On rare occasions, the adductor muscle attachment area at the inferior pubic ramus may be the site of a stress factor.[359,371] This usually occurs from a fall or a sudden stop while delivering a bowling ball or throwing a heavy package in an unbalanced position. Avulsion of the inferior pubic ramus and rupture of the adductor longus' origin may be associated, as well as laceration to scrotal vessels.

Sacral Fractures.[372,373] Isolated sacral fractures are invariably related to a direct blow from the posterior or the inferior. The mechanism of injury is sometimes associated with *shear* when a blow to the sitting erect knee (eg, dashboard injury) drives the femur posteriorly, superiorly, and medially; *rotation* when the hip is severely hyperextended; and/or *leverage* when the A-P dimension of the pelvis is flattened. The fracture line is usually through the sacral foramina which weakens the bone at these points.

Referred Trauma. Howe points out that after falls or trauma to the back, particularly when the blow is applied to the bottom of the pelvis with the force traveling up the spinal column, compression fractures of vertebral bodies frequently result.[71] The most often missed of these occur at the T12–L1 junction, but they may possibly extend as high as T10 or T11. The reason they are often missed is that the pain is usually referred to the lumbosacral area, and there may be no spasm or even tenderness in the fracture area. If the x-ray beam is centered at the location of pain, the coned view may not extend high enough to include the lower thoracic area. A compression fracture is frequently not evident until several days later when deformity becomes more pronounced.

STRUCTURAL FIXATIONS AND MOTION PALPATION OF THE PELVIS[101,374–384]

Many references state that the sacrum and pelvis can be considered a biomechanical unit in which rocking of the pelvis is accompanied solely by a change in the sacral angle. Cineroentgenography shows that this is true *only* when the sacroiliac and pubic articulations are completely fixated in all directions of movement.

Illi[354] has shown that sacroiliac fixation of any degree inhibits the compensatory torsion capacity of the spinal segments. When the mobile spine is flexed forward, there is always a degree of related lumbar torsion. However, if the sacroiliac joint is locked, normal torsion is inhibited and axial torsion of the cord and nerve roots occurs.

The greater the degree of sacroiliac fixation, the greater the degree of stress placed upon the lumbosacral and hip joints. Any degree of sacroiliac fixation or hypermobility disturbing reciprocal motion bilaterally can be associated with (1) an adaptive lumbar scoliosis away from the side of pain, leading to biomechanical changes in the thoracic and cervical regions; (2) the direction of excessive rotary forces to the lumbar spine, leading to disc failure; (3) compensatory overstress at the acetabulum, leading to hip pain and arthritis; (4) rotational overstress at the knee to widen the base of support, leading to chronic sprain.

Muscle Fixations

The Lumbar Extensors. Shortening of the lumbar extensors has the opposite effect to that of hamstring shortening. This is a cause and/or effect of hyperlordosis. If the hamstrings are normal and the paravertebral muscles are tight, pelvic motion is free but lumbar flexion is restricted. If motion is forced, abnormal stress is placed upon the hips, sacroiliac joints, and posterior soft tissues of the lumbar region, leading to chronic strain, sprain, avulsion, spurring, and arthritis.

The Hamstrings. Tight hamstrings are common, either bilaterally or unilaterally. As taut hamstrings will prevent pelvic flexion by fixing the ischium and destroying normal lumbosacropelvic rhythm, any motion achieved is forced upon the lumbar segments, often with compensatory stretching of the posterior longitudinal ligaments. If movement is forced, avulsion may occur leading to further degenerative changes.

A supine patient should be able to flex the thigh and fully extend the leg so that the lower extremity is straight and perpendicular to the floor. In attempting this test, many people will be forced to bend their knee—indicating a shortened hamstring. Milne and Mierau[385] have shown that hamstring distensibility appears to occur in the general population beginning at the age of 6 years, and they attribute it to prolonged sitting in school. If the hamstring group fails to elongate properly in the upright position, dysfunction occurs in pelvic and lumbar movements. With stretching exercises, however, a normal degree of extensibility can be attained in time with most cases.

The studies of Hoehler and Tobis[386] concluded that only passive or voluntary straight-leg raising can be strongly recommended for use in the evaluation of spinal manipulative therapy for low-back pain. In contrast, Turner and associates[387] feel that the Activities Discomfort Scale (ADS) is the most promising predictor of patient-rated pain intensity after nonsurgical treatment. Both of these conclusions, however, are obviously moot from a chiropractic viewpoint.

Ligament Fixations[388]

No other area of the axial skeleton is more prone to fixation from ligamentous shortening than the sacroiliac articulations. In fact, Gillet[101] feels that it is almost impossible to find a state of clinical imbalance that does not reflect this state. This is probably because few occupations require pelvic motion throughout the maximum range of possible motion. However, generalized bilateral ligamentous shortening in itself is not necessarily a cause of clinical concern even if a state of mobility is considered ideal. The clinical state of the sacroiliac ligaments is determined by the habitual positions the articulations are required to maintain.

The iliolumbar, sacroiliac, and sacrotuberous ligaments are common sites of ligamentous shortening that affect pelvic dynamics, and they appear to become involved in that order according to Grieve.[389] Gillet,[101] however, reports many cases of iliolumbar and sacrotuberous fixation without involvement of the sacroiliac ligaments.

The Iliolumbar Ligaments. When an iliolumbar ligament becomes shortened, the iliac crest tends to be pulled medially while the ischium is forced outward. In response to the load above, the sacral base is forced anteriorly and the apex is forced posteriorly. Thus, the patient exhibits the normal state of the sitting pelvis while in the standing posture. This same condition may be the result of a fibrotic or reflexly contracted quadratus lumborum.

The Sacroiliac Ligaments. When the posterior ligaments shorten, they tend to push the sacrum anteriorly so that the PSISs appear more prominent and closer together. When the anterior ligaments shorten, the sacrum has a tendency to bulge posteriorly with an unusual mass palpable medial to the PSISs which have spread further apart.

The Sacrotuberous Ligaments. These ligaments have a tendency toward considerable shortening. When shortened, the sacrum is seen displaced deeper between the two ilia like a driven wedge. With the patient in the lateral recumbent position, deep gluteal palpation will reveal the taut cords (Fig. 12.66). Grieve reports that ipsilateral calf and heel numbness is often associated, thus suggesting sciatic nerve involvement.

Dynamic Sacroiliac Palpation[390–392]

The sacroiliac and the lumbosacral joints may be palpated in the standing and sitting positions. Several quick sacroiliac tests are recommended, and each should be conducted bilaterally. The thumbs are usually

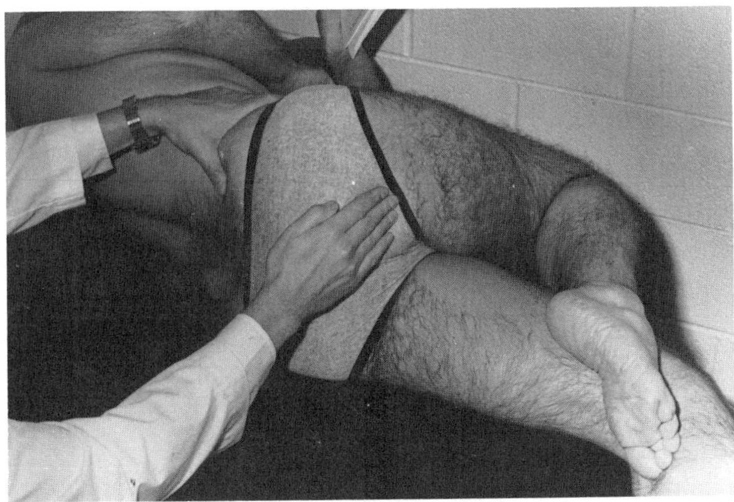

Figure 12.66. Palpation of the right sacrotuberous ligament and ischial bursa.

used for reference because deep pressure is necessary to hold firm contact during the tests. The sites of palpatory contact for the following tests are shown in Figure 12.67.

General Sacroiliac Motion. To screen iliac flexion and extension on the sacrum in the standing position, the examiner's thumbs are placed on the PSISs and the patient is asked to raise the right leg up and down, for example, bending the knee as if in taking a high step. The right PSIS will be felt to move posterior and inferior. After about 20° of leg raise, the left sacroiliac spine also drops posterior and inferior. This is normal sacroiliac motion. Any motion other than this indicates a problem in this joint. If the joint is fixated, the pelvis tends to move as a whole and the ipsilateral thumb will tend to remain level or even rise, rather than drop. These signs of thumb movement can be seen as well as felt.

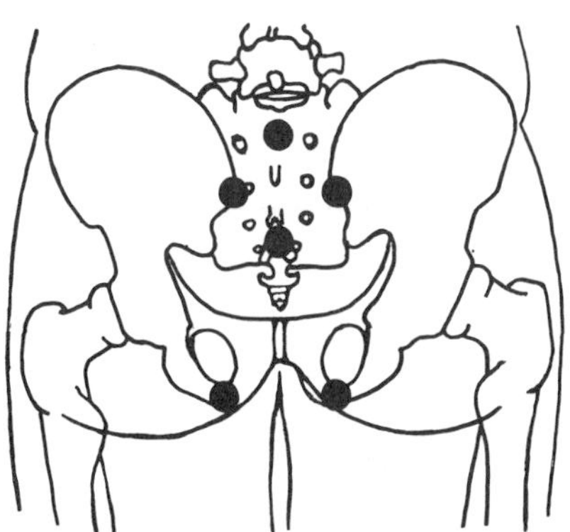

Figure 12.67. Reference points in sacroiliac and sacroischial dynamic palpation.

Standing Superior Joint Motion. One thumb is placed on the sacral base and the other on the right PSIS, for example. The patient is asked to raise the right knee as if taking a high step; the separation of the thumbs is noted. The sacral base will normally be seen and felt to move ¼–½ inch anterior and inferior at the end of flexion. Or, conversely, the PSIS will move posterior and inferior. The sacroiliac tissues should be felt to relax. If the superior sacroiliac joint or the symphysis pubis is locked, the sacrum and ilium will move as a unit, the thumbs will not separate appreciably, and the sacral tissues (ligaments and spinal muscle attachments) will remain taut. This is probably the most common pelvic fixation found. Invariably, there is a degree of forward tilting of the pelvis associated with hyperlordosis.

Standing Inferior Joint Motion. A thumb is placed on the patient's sacral apex, and the other thumb is placed on the ischial protuberance. The patient is asked to raise the knee on the side being tested. A ¼–½-inch excursion should be felt as the ischium moves anterosuperior and lateral on the sacrum. If the inferior sacroiliac joint is locked, the ischium and sacral apex will move as a unit. Fixation of this motion is most often associated with a contralateral sacral base fixation. The direct cause is failure of the muscles acting on the sacral apex to elongate. Piriformis contracture is the common cause, but the iliopsoas or deep glutei may be involved.

Sitting A-P Sacral Apex Motion. To test forward flexion freedom with the patient seated, a thumb is placed on one PSIS and the other thumb is placed on the sacral apex. The PSISs are normally about ¼-inch closer together in the sitting position than the standing position because of ischial spread. Note the separation of the thumbs as the patient flexes forward enough to flatten the lumbar curve. This will normally be about a half inch if the dynamics are normal, and the sacral tissues will be felt to tighten. If either the spinal extensors (multifidi, sacrospinalis) or pelvic extensors (hamstrings, gluteus maximus) fail to elongate during flexion, the sacroiliac joint will be inhibited from above or below, and the lumbars will remain somewhat lordotic. Thus, this type of fixation can be secondary to failure of the lower thoracic and lumbar muscles to elongate. Gluteal length can be further evaluated by flexing the thigh of the supine patient diagonally toward the opposite shoulder. To test A-P motion during extension, the same contacts are taken, and the patient arches his back posteriorly. The distance between the thumbs should shorten and the sacral tissues should relax.

Sacroiliac End-Play Motion. Two tests have been developed to evaluate joint translation freedom and lateral flexion with the patient seated. These are concerned with sacroiliac end play and lateral flexion of the pelvis in the sitting position.

The degree of translatory motion (end play) at the end of voluntary motion can be tested along with test 4, which is an evaluation of ligamentous elasticity suggested by Mennell.[393] The test is made at the end of extension by firm thumb pressure on the sacral apex while the other thumb is on the PSIS. This pressure should elicit further tissue relaxation.

Sitting Lateral Flexion of the Pelvis. Both thumbs are placed on the PSISs so that the fingers firmly grip the crests of the ilia bilaterally. As the patient curves his trunk laterally, the lumbar spine should curve smoothly, the sacrum will normally tilt toward the side of the concavity, but the PSISs should remain relatively level even though there is some bilaterally reciprocal iliac rotation. The sacroiliac tissues on the side of lateral flexion should relax while those on the side of the convexity should tighten. At the end of voluntary motion, added thumb pressure on the sacrum in the direction of its movement should elicit further tissue relaxation. This will not occur if the ligaments have stiffened. If one PSIS raises during lateral flexion, it suggests elongation failure of the lumbar extensors (multifidi, erector spinae) or lateral stabilizers (iliopsoas, quadratus lumborum). If there is bilateral sacroiliac fixation, there will usually be associated lumbar fixation. In the standing position, lateral sacral flexion is most difficult to distinguish from pelvic lateral rotation about the weight-bearing head of the femur.

Position Change Iliac Alterations. Two other tests can be used to evaluate medial and lateral iliac rotation in the horizontal plane. These are concerned with iliac alterations during position changes and horizontal rotation of the ilium while sitting.

The thumbs are placed on the PSISs of a patient seated on a stool. The distance between the contacts is noted. Then the patient stands, and the distance is noted. Upon standing, the PSISs normally open laterally like a book so that the inter-PSIS distance increases. If a firm contact can be held on the ischial spines, a reverse reaction is seen; ie, the ischia tend to close medially when arising to the standing position. If fixation is present, these iliac and ischial motions will not be felt.

Sitting Iliac Horizontal Rotation. With the patient seated, the examiner's thumbs are placed on the PSISs and the patient is asked to fan his knees open and close several times. Normally, as the knees are abducted laterally the PSISs move medially so that they are closer together. Quite frequently, one PSIS will be felt to move less than the other, pinpointing a fixation at the inhibited joint.

Static Palpation

Theoretically, if the thumbs are placed on the PSISs and one thumb is more posterior and inferior or anterior and superior than the other when the patient is either standing or sitting, this would indicate a fixed unilateral pelvic rotation. Likewise, if the thumbs are placed on the PSISs and one thumb is more superior and anterior or inferior and posterior than the other when the patient is prone, this would indicate unilateral pelvic rotation. However, because osseous asymmetry is so common, these signs are frequently misleading. Dynamic tests correlated with other signs and the patient's symptoms are much more reliable during analysis.

Selecting the Side of the Major

As many pelvic distortions are reciprocal in nature, it is often confusing as to which side is the major. There are two general rules emphasized by Stierwalt that are helpful in many cases of pelvic misalignment. (1) The primary subluxation-fixation concern is on the side of most pain, regardless of whether it is on the side of sacral anteroinferiority or posterosuperiority. (2) The side of major misalignment is on the side to which the L5 has rotated, regardless of what direction the ilia have rotated.[394] These rules should always be challenged and confirmed by other tests, however, for there are few clinical rules that are true in every case.

Clinical Implications

Around the sacroiliac articulations are a host of ligaments which, if normal in tension and elasticity, control movements and assure that they remain within normal limits. Unfortunately, most people use a majority of specific and specialized movements instead of maintaining a healthy general mobility. This causes one or several of these ligaments to shorten and tighten, which in turn causes the involved ligament to serve as a new, but abnormal, center of rotation that may restrict mobility in one or several directions. For instance, the pubic articulation may tighten and effectively stop A-P rotation of the ilia. In the sitting position, however, the sacrum will still be able to move between the ilia; in fact, hypermobility of both sacroiliac joints in the sitting position will occur, and the same time, a total fixation of the ilia will be found in the standing knee-lift test.

Anterior Sacral Fixation. In some patients, the anterior sacroiliac ligaments will have shortened, but not the posterior ligaments. These anterior ligaments can be divided into superior and inferior ligaments. If one of these is short, A-P rotation in the knee-lifting test will still take place, but the center of rotation will have changed. Instead of taking place at the femur head, it will be found at the offending ligament and a related hypermobility will exist at the pubic articulation. This A-P mobility can be palpated by putting one thumb on the PSIS and the other thumb on the corresponding part of the sacrum; when the patient lifts his knee, the ilium on the same side will move posteriorly and down. If the contacts are made on the inferior part of the ilium and sacrum, the former will be felt to move anteriorly. Furthermore, both of these movements will be sluggish, quickly reaching their limits and pulling the sacrum into a visible distortion.

Posterior Sacral Fixation. Fixation at the posterior ligaments is more difficult to palpate and demonstrate because the palpating thumbs are on the actual center of rotation, thus registering no perceptible movement. However, if the patient is turned around and the ASISs are contacted, the knee-lifting test will show an abnormally wide mobility. It appears that these forms of sacroiliac fixations also insult the movement of the sacrum itself between the ilia, as tested in the seated patient, making it sluggish or even nonexistent. Bilateral shortening of these ligaments also markedly changes the in- and outflaring of the normal pelvis when either standing or sitting.

Sitting and Standing Pelvic Changes. Keep in mind the various pelvic changes that occur between the sitting and standing postures that vary with different occupations. These changes are essentially controlled by the sacroiliac-ligament complex. If the superior ligaments are tightened, the crests will be pulled together and actually fix the pelvis in the shape characteristic for the sitting position. Such a patient will feel more comfortable when seated, and spinographs taken in the sitting posture appear quite normal. Upon standing, however, the crests of such a pelvis would be incapable of separating and the ischia would not approximate. The opposite may also occur. The inferior sacroiliac ligaments may shorten and pull the ischia toward each other, locking the pelvis in the standing position and making sitting uncomfortable if not painful.

There are many such states of fixation; eg, one ilium may be blocked or one fixed superior on one side and one inferior on the other. Careful analysis is necessary in differentiation.

Pubic Fixations

Pubic fixation offers a clinical dilemma that awaits resolution. The pubic articulation is not a gliding type as seen in the spine, thus one would think it would be prone to only a ligamentous type of fixation. If this were true, a degree of torsion would be possible in spite of fixation. However, motion palpation demonstrates that (1) normal A-P iliac rotation does not take place when the pubis is fixated, and (2) adjustment results in a rapid improvement in mobility. Neither of these characteristics are typical of ligamentous fixation.

ENTRAPMENT SYNDROMES OF THE PELVIS[395,396]

The most common entrapment syndromes related to the pelvis are sciatic nerve compression, lateral femoral cutaneous nerve compression, obturator nerve compression, and adhesive arachnoiditis.

Sciatic Nerve Compression Syndromes[218,302,397–399]

The most common site for the sciatic nerve to become "caught" is at the sciatic notch because the nerve exits the pelvis between the piriformis and sacrotuberous ligament. At this point, it can become compressed against the bony ridge by piriformis spasm, thickened fascia, or adhesions.

Symptoms and Signs. The typical symptom is pain behind the greater trochanter that radiates down the thigh and lateral leg to the foot. This is usually aggravated by walking, and relieved by rest. Numbness and tingling is invariably restricted to below the buttocks. The pain is increased by flexing the knee and hip to right angles and forcing the thigh into internal rotation and adduction (ie, piriformis stress). Tenderness will be most acute near and below the notch. Major signs usually include a positive Lasègue's sign and hypesthesia of the weight-bearing surface of the plantar surface.

Differentiation must be made from disc failure, inflammatory sciatica, and acute sacroiliac sprain, but it may coexist with these disorders. Tumors within the buttocks, a neurofibroma, or a compartment syndrome can also mimic an entrapment syndrome. A fall on the buttocks or a posteriorly dislocated femur head may injure the nerve at the inferior buttock and produce identical signs and symptoms as that of an entrapment syndrome.

Femoral Cutaneous Nerve Syndromes[400]

After the lateral femoral cutaneous nerve leaves the L2–L3 roots, it runs across the lateral border of the psoas muscle before it descends along the posterior wall of the pelvic cavity. Here it enters and travels within the fascia covering the iliacus muscle, pierces the lateral "V" attachment of the inguinal ligament just medial to the ASIS, travels in a fascial tunnel under the ligament, then pierces the fascia lata, and enters the thigh. It offers cutaneous branches to the anterolateral thigh from below the hip to the knee and motor branches to the anterior thigh.

It is at the point where the nerve leaves the subinguinal tunnel and enters the fascia lata that entrapment of the nerve (meralgia paresthetica) usually occurs. At this site, the nerve's sheath is firmly fixed to adjacent tissue. Thigh adduction increases tensile forces on the nerve, and if this occurs simultaneously with severe trunk movements above or thigh movements below, the nerve can become severely stretched. In some cases, just prolonged sitting with the legs crossed can produce a compression syndrome in the upper thigh. An improperly fitted brace may cause compression, and, in obese women, a tight corset may produce compression. In rare cases, the nerve becomes entrapped by a pelvic tumor or encapsulated psoas abscess, hypertrophic arthritis of the upper lumbar spine, a pregnant uterus, or occupational pressure. Visceroptosis may produce a stretch syndrome.

Symptoms and Signs. The typical symptoms are severe unilateral burning pain and paresthesia in the anterolateral thigh. The onset is usually spontaneous. The major signs are aggravation of pain when the nerve is pressed against the medial side of the iliac crest, relief of pain when recumbent, and hyperesthesia of the anterior thigh.

Obturator Nerve Syndromes [401,402]

The obturator nerve leaves the L3–L4 nerve roots, passes through the pelvis, and supplies the gracilis and adductor muscles and the skin of the hip and medial thigh. An obturator hernia or pressure from the edema of osteitis pubis are the common causes of obturator neuritis or neuralgia. Some circulatory impairment may be associated.

Symptoms and Signs. The pain typically radiates from the groin to the medial thigh and is aggravated by any Valsalva maneuver. Cutaneous numbness (infrequent) and paresthesia (frequent) may be associated. As the obturator nerve innervates the adductors of the thigh, the major signs are weakness of the thigh adductors and an unusual gait. The involved leg is brought outward in a wide arc during the swing phase of locomotion. Even in chronic cases there is little or no atrophy because of dual innervation from the sciatic nerve.

Adhesive Arachnoiditis[403]

Adhesive arachnoiditis can produce severe unrelenting sciatica. The common site of entrapment is where the L4 root crosses the L5 transverse process and iliolumbar ligament in the nerve's descent into the pelvis.

SACROILIAC PATHOLOGY[404–407]

Serious visceral pathology and hernias often simulate musculoskeletal dysfunction. It is unexplained why leukemia and other systemic diseases may present only backache as the presenting symptom, but it does occur. Back pain often arises early in visceral disease, long before classic physical signs and hematologic changes are noted. A few pathologies may extend from or affect the sacroiliac joints early that often mimic the symptoms of sprain or chronic subluxation. Confusion exists when related symptoms are brought out after trauma.

The sacroiliac joint in most cases may be only a small part of the systemic picture of a widespread disease process, yet it may be an early focal site. The clinical profiles of pelvic tuberculosis, cancer, Paget's disease, osteoarthritis, rheumatoid arthritis, gout, and the various metabolic and immunologic bone diseases are covered extensively in standard pathology textbooks and need not be repeated here. However, a few major points will be underscored relative to the syndromes of lumbar disc degeneration, sacroiliac infection, spondylitis, and Reiter's syndrome.

Related Disc Degeneration

Sacroiliac fixation to any degree inhibits the compensatory torsion capacity of the spinal segments. Illi's studies show that unilateral or bilateral sacroiliac subluxation predisposes lumbar disc pathology because once the sacroiliac mechanisms are disturbed, the normal dynamics of the lumbar spine overstress the IVDs, articular facets, and paravertebral soft tissues.[354] Degeneration processes follow.

Sacroiliac Infection[408]

Almost any type of bacterial infection may originate in or extend to the sacroiliac joints. Tuberculosis is the first suspicion. The highest incidence is in children regardless of the type of infection.

As the sacroiliac lesion is usually painless, diagnosis must be made by laboratory, roentgenographic, and thermographic evidence when the classical signs of infection arise. Fever and a high sedimentation rate are invariably present. Infrequently, an abscess may appear early. Differentiation must be made from septic arthritis and Ewing's sarcoma.

Buttock Sign. A lower extremity of a supine patient is passively flexed at the hip with the knee extended as in an SLR test. If the flexion of the limb on the trunk is restricted by local or radiating buttock pain (rather than pain in the hip or lower back), it is significant of an inflammatory pelvic lesion such as ischiorectal abscess, osteomyelitis of or near the hip joint, coxa bursitis, sacroiliac septic arthritis, or an advanced pelvic neoplasm.

Hip Abduction Stress Test. The patient

is placed as in Lewin-Gaenslen's test. With the upper limb held straight and extended at the knee, the patient is instructed to attempt to abduct the upper limb while the examiner applies resistance. Pain initiated in the area of the uppermost sacroiliac joint or the hip joint suggests an inflammatory process of that joint.

Spondylitis[409–411]

Ankylosing Spondylitis. This disease resembles spinal rheumatoid arthritis. The latex fixation test is rarely positive in ankylosing spondylitis, but the HLA W27 leukocyte antigen is present in 90% of cases, according to Macnab.[412] The disorder often has a genetic history. The incidence is highest among males 20–40 years of age. Progression to complete or widespread involvement is unpredictable. The sacroiliac joint is the site of the focal lesion in about 80% of cases, with "blurred" sacroiliac joints appearing early on roentgenography. Extension is then made to the costovertebral and manubriosternal joints, and this will exhibit a decrease in normal chest expansion on forced inhalation. Clinical tests will elicit signs of sacroiliitis and rigidity of the lumbar and later the thoracic spine during forward flexion. Later, inflammatory destruction will exhibit widening of the sacroiliac joint space, sclerosis, squaring of the involved vertebral bodies, and anular and paravertebral ossification. When the disorder becomes widespread after several years, cardiovascular and pulmonary signs and symptoms manifest.

Schober's Sign. This test is an excellent method for grossly evaluating lumbar flexion. A mark is placed over the L5 spinous process when the patient is standing erect and a second mark is made on the spine exactly 10 cm above. The patient is then asked to flex forward in the Adams position, and the distance between the two marks is measured. A difference of less than 4–5 cm is a positive sign of spondylitis or something producing severe lumbar spasm.[413,414]

Spondylitis Associated with Psoriasis. Psoriatic arthritis may attack the lumbar spine and sacroiliac joints almost simultaneously. However, it must be kept in mind that a psoriatic patient is subject to the same lumbar and pelvic musculoskeletal dysfunctions as any nonpsoriatic individual. Thus, the examiner should not suspect psoriatic arthritis just because of the presence of the classic skin lesions. Few psoriatic patients with backache are victims of spondylitis. The incidence of psoriatic arthritis is highest in women 20–40 years of age.

Spondylitis Associated with Bowel Disease. Acute spondylitis is sometimes related to ulcerative colitis and Crohn's disease (regional enteritis). Sacroiliac symptoms may appear even before the visceral symptoms, and the joint sacroiliitis may continue to progress after the bowel symptoms subside.

Reiter's Syndrome[415,416]

Reiter's syndrome is a triad of sterile urethritis, arthritis, and conjunctivitis. The cause is unknown. Backache is usually the presenting symptom, but urinary or conjunctival complaints may manifest first. The weight-bearing joints show the first arthritis changes, and later the proximal joints of the fingers and toes become afflicted. In differentiation from ankylosing spondylitis, it is well to mention here that about one in four patients with ankylosing spondylitis will present a degree of iritis. Reiter's syndrome also has its highest incidence among males 20–40 years of age. While associated sacroiliitis is common, progression to spondylitis never occurs early in the disease process.

Sacroiliac Gout[417]

Although not a frequent finding, deposits of urates in the lower spine and sacroiliac joints can be a cause of episodic low-back pain. Evidence of sacroiliitis may or may not be evident on film. Associated signs of hyperostotic spondylosis are more common.

Sacral Tumors[418]

Sacral tumors typically refer pain that mimics a lumbosacral disc syndrome. Tomography is usually necessary for diagnosis because of overlying bowel gas, indistinct sacral anatomy, and the inability to detect moderate demineralization on conventional films.

Other Disorders of Pelvic Bone

Osteitis Condensans Ilii[419–421]

This disorder reflects a disturbance of the normal architecture of the ilium in which increased condensations of bone occur in the auricular portion of the ilium, especially along the lower aspect of the sacroiliac joint, without cartilage space narrowing or erosion. Most accounts describe the phenomenon as a stress-related, sharply marginated sclerotic reaction in the periarticular bone that is frequently unilateral.

There is persistent chronic low-back pain (rarely severe) that radiates to one or both buttocks but never into the lower extremity as does typical sciatica. The symptoms are aggravated by activity and relieved by bed rest. The disorder occurs predominantly in females, especially of childbearing age. It frequently has its onset in the final trimester of pregnancy or immediately after delivery. Symptoms recur or are exaggerated during subsequent pregnancies.

Differential diagnosis should consider Marie-Strumpell's arthritis, Reiter's syndrome, and other inflammatory pathologies of the sacrum or ilium. Osteitis condensans ilii differs from ankylosing spondylitis in that it is rarely seen in males and is usually unilateral.

Additional Concerns

Two other conditions that should be considered in the differential diagnosis of low-back pain are osteomyelitis of the pelvis and calcificationn of the ischiogluteal bursae. Osteomyelitis of the pelvis occurs more frequently than is generally recognized.[422] Calcification of the ischiogluteal bursae (seamstress's bottom, weaver bottom, saddle tumors) is generally the result of prolonged sitting on a hard surface.[423]

REFERENCES

1. Daniels L, Worthingham C: *Therapeutic Exercise*, ed 2. Philadelphia, W.B. Saunders, 1977, p 50.
2. Kendall HO, Kendall FP, Wadsworth GE: *Muscles: Testing and Function*, ed 2. Baltimore, Williams & Wilkins, 1971, pp 201–205.
3. Van Dusen LG: *Chiropractic Relationship to Gravitational Force*. Sodus, NY, published by the author, 1968, pp 91, 93, 97, 103.
4. Smidt G et al: Assessment of abdominal and back extensor function: A quantitative approach and results for chronic low-back patients. *Spine* 8:211–219, 1983.
5. Suzuki N, Endo S: A quantitative study of trunk muscle strength and fatigability in the low-back pain syndrome. *Spine* 8:69–74, 1983.
6. Petty AH: Abdominal injuries. *Annals of the Royal College of Surgeons* 53:169, 1973.
7. Williams JGP, Sperryn PN (eds): *Sports Medicine*, ed 2. Baltimore, Williams & Wilkins, 1976, pp 372–374.
8. Hirata I Jr: *The Doctor and the Athlete*, ed 2. Philadelphia, J.B. Lippincott, 1974, p 181.
9. Scott WN, Nisonson B, Nicholas JA (eds): *Principles of Sports Medicine*. Baltimore, Williams & Wilkins, 1984, pp 236–237.
10. Zuidema GD et al: *The Management of Trauma*, ed 3. Philadelphia, W.B. Saunders, 1979, pp 429–431, 456.
11. Williams JGP, Sperryn PN (eds): *Sports Medicine*, ed 2. Baltimore, Williams & Wilkins, 1976, p 373.
12. Schneider RC, Kennedy JC, Plant ML (eds): *Sports Injuries: Mechanisms, Prevention, and Treatment*. Baltimore, Williams & Wilkins, 1985, p 477.
13. Craig AS: Elements of kinesiology for the clinician. *Physical Therapy* 44:470–473, 1964.
14. Jaskoviak P, Schafer RC: *Applied Physiotherapy*. Arlington, Va, American Chiropractic Association. To be published in 1986.
15. Bolton PM et al: Blunt abdominal injury: A review of 59 consecutive cases undergoing surgery. *British Journal of Surgery* 60:657, 1973.
16. Williams JGP, Sperryn PN (eds): *Sports Medicine*, ed 2. Baltimore, Williams & Wilkins, 1976, pp 372–373.
17. Fisk JW: *The Painful Neck and Back*. Springfield, Ill, Charles C Thomas, 1977, pp 169–172.
18. White AA, Panjabi MM: *Clinical Biomechanics of the Spine*. Philadelphia, J.B. Lippincott, 1978, p 295.
19. Grieve GP: *Common Vertebral Joint Problems*. New York, Churchill Livingstone, 1981, p 200.
20. Cailliet R: *Low Back Pain Syndrome*, ed 3. Philadelphia, F.A. Davis, 1981, pp 107–143.
21. Nash CL, Moe JH: A study of vertebral rotation. *Journal of Bone and Joint Surgery* 51:223, 1969.
22. Roaf R: A study of the mechanics of spinal injuries. *Journal of Bone and Joint Surgery* 42B:810–823, 1960.
23. D'Amico JC: The postural complex. *Journal of the American Podiatry Association* August 1976.
24. Daniels L, Worthingham C: *Therapeutic Exercise for Body Alignment and Function*, ed 2. Philadelphia, W.B. Saunders, 1977, pp 46–47.
25. Barham JN, Wooten EP: *Structural Kinesiology*. New York, Macmillan, 1973, p 274.
26. Burt HA: Effects of faulty posture. *Proceedings of the Royal Society of Medicine* 43:187, 1950.
27. Grice AS: Posture and postural mechanics. *Journal of the Canadian Chiropractic Association* July 1970.
28. Wiles P: Postural deformities of the antero-posterior curves of the spine. *The Lancet* April 17, 1937.
29. Pennal GF et al: Motion study of the lumbar spine: A preliminary report. *Journal of Bone and Joint Surgery* 54B:3, August 1972.
30. Cailliet R: *Low Back Pain Syndrome*, ed 3. Philadelphia, F.A. Davis, 1981, pp 187–225.
31. McKenzie RA: *The Lumbar Spine: Mechanical Diagnosis and Therapy*. Waikanae, New Zealand, Spinal Publications, 1981.

32. Daniels L, Worthingham C: *Therapeutic Exercise for Body Alignment and Function*, ed 2. Philadelphia, W.B. Saunders, 1977, pp 102–103.
33. Charnley J: Acute lumbago and sciatica. *British Medical Journal* 1:344, 1955.
34. Helfet AJ, Gruebel Lee DM: *Disorders of the Lumbar Spine*. Philadelphia, J.B. Lippincott, 1978, pp 3–4.
35. Barge FH: *Tortipelvis*. Davenport, Ia, Bawden Bros, 1980, pp 1–7, 99.
36. Barge FH: *Scoliosis*. Davenport, Ia, Bawden Bros, 1982, pp 119–129, 146, 227–233.
37. Helfet AJ, Gruebel Lee DM: *Disorders of the Lumbar Spine*. Philadelphia, J.B. Lippincott, 1978, pp 5–6.
38. Barge FH: *Tortipelvis*. Davenport, Ia, Bawden Bros, 1980, pp 101–102.
39. Rossman I: *Clinical Geriatrics*. Philadelphia, J.B. Lippincott, 1971, pp 116, 305–306.
40. Cowdry EV, Steinberg FU: *The Care of the Geriatric Patient*, ed 4. St. Louis, C.V. Mosby, 1971, pp 316–319.
41. Helfet AJ, Gruebel Lee DM: *Disorders of the Lumbar Spine*. Philadelphia, J.B. Lippincott, 1978, pp 8–10.
42. Daniels L, Worthingham C: *Therapeutic Exercise*, ed 2. Philadelphia, W.B. Saunders, 1977, pp 50–51.
43. Fisk JW: *The Painful Neck and Back*. Springfield, Ill, Charles C. Thomas, 1977, pp 169–193.
44. White AA, Panjabi MM: *Clinical Biomechanics of the Spine*. Philadelphia, J.B. Lippincott, 1978, pp 166–178, 184.
45. Macnab I: *Backache*. Baltimore, Williams & Wilkins, 1977, pp 19–23.
46. Ruge D, Wiltse LL (eds): *Spinal Disorders: Diagnosis and Treatment*. Philadelphia, Lea & Febiger, 1977.
47. Schmorl G, Junghanns H: *The Human Spine in Health and Disease*, ed 2. New York, Grune & Stratton, 1971.
48. Shephard WD: Subluxation compensation or strain? *The Texas Chiropractor* June 1975.
49. Davis PR et al: Movements of the thoracic and lumbar spine when lifting: A chronocyclophotographic study. *Journal of Anatomy* 99:13–26, 1965.
50. Markolf KL: Deformation of the thoracolumbar intervertebral joints in response to external loads. *Journal of Bone and Joint Surgery* 54A:511–533, 1972.
51. Leskinen TPJ et al: A dynamic analysis of spinal compression with different lifting techniques. *Ergonomics* 26:595–604, 1983.
52. Hviid H: Erect working posture. *Annals of the Swiss Chiropractors' Association* 6:71–90, 1976.
53. Magora A: Investigation of the relation between low back pain and occupation. *Industrial Medicine* 39:11, November 1970.
54. Gracovetsky S, Farfan HF, Lamy C: The mechanism of the lumbar spine. *Spine* 6:249–262, 1981.
55. McNeil TW: The role of spinal fusion in the treatment of problems of the lumbar spine. In Black J, Dumbleton JH (eds): *Clinical Biomechanics: Case History Approach*. New York, Churchill Livingstone, 1981, pp 326–333.
56. Williams PC: *The Lumbosacral Spine*. New York, McGraw-Hill, Blakiston Division, 1965.
57. Finneson BE: *Low Back Pain*. Philadelphia, J.B. Lippincott, 1973, pp 134–138.
58. Turek SL: *Orthopaedics: Principles and Their Application*, ed 3. Philadelphia, J.B. Lippincott, 1977, pp 1350–1353.
59. Nachemson AL: The lumbar spine, an orthopaedic challenge. *Spine* 1(1):59, 1976.
60. Morris JM: Biomechanics of the spine. *Archives of Surgery* 107:418–423, 1973.
61. Olsen GA, Hamilton A: The lateral stability of the spine. *Clinical Orthopaedics* 65:143, 1969.
62. Gunn CC, Milbrandt WE: Early and subtle signs in low-back sprain. *Spine* 3:267–281, September 1978.
63. Neuberger T: Low back pain. *Athletic Journal* 47:10–40, 1966.
64. Turek SL: *Orthopaedics: Principles and Their Application*, ed 3. Philadelphia, J.B. Lippincott, 1977, pp 1356–1358.
65. Brown T et al: Some mechanical tests on the lumbosacral spine with particular reference to the intervertebral discs. *Journal of Bone and Joint Surgery* 39A, 1957.
66. Helfet AJ, Gruebel Lee DM: *Disorders of the Lumbar Spine*. Philadelphia, J.B. Lippincott, 1978, p 13.
67. Schafer RC: *Chiropractic Management of Sports and Recreational Injuries*. Baltimore, Williams & Wilkins, 1982, p 452.
68. Evans FG: Some basic aspects of biomechanics of the spine. *Archives of Physical Medicine and Rehabilitation* 51:214–226, 1970.
69. Durling TF: Low back differential diagnosis. *Florida Chiropractic Association Newsletter* October 1978.
70. Johnson AC: *Postural Correction*. Los Angeles, Chiropractic Educational Extension Bureau (undated).
71. Howe JW: Determination of lumbo-sacral facet subluxations. *Roentgenological Briefs*. Council on Roentgenology of the American Chiropractic Association (undated).
72. Schafer RC: *Chiropractic Management of Sports and Recreational Injuries*. Baltimore, Williams & Wilkins, 1982, pp 447–448.
73. Triano J: Significant lumbar dyskinesia. *ACA Journal of Chiropractic* February 1980.
74. Kirkaldy-Willis WH: Five common back disorders: How to diagnose and treat them. *Geriatrics* December 1978.
75. Helfet AJ, Gruebel Lee DM: *Disorders of the Lumbar Spine*. Philadelphia, J.B. Lippincott, 1978, pp 11–25.
76. McNeil TW: The role of spinal fusion in the treatment of problems of the lumbar spine. In Black J, Dumbleton JH (eds): *Clinical Biomechanics: Case History Approach*. New York, Churchill Livingstone, 1981, pp 317–321, 326–333.
77. Turek SL: *Orthopaedics: Principles and Their Application*, ed 3. Philadelphia, J.B. Lippincott, 1977, pp 1322–1323.

78. Barge FH: *Tortipelvis.* Davenport, Ia, Bawden Bros, 1980, pp 12–17.
79. Rosse C: The vertebral canal and its contents. In Rosse C, Clawson DK (eds): *The Musculoskeletal System in Health and Disease.* Hagerstown, Md, Harper & Row, 1980, p 159.
80. Janse J: Differentiation and interpretation of spinal pain syndromes. *Notes on Correlative Techniques.* Chicago, National College of Chiropractic (undated).
81. Fisk JW: *The Painful Neck and Back.* Springfield, Ill, Charles C Thomas, 1977, pp 13–27.
82. Frymoyer W et al: Risk factors in low-back pain. *Journal of Bone and Joint Surgery* 65:213–218, 1983.
83. Wyke BD: Neural aspects of pain therapy. In Swerdlow IM (ed): *The Therapy of Pain—Current Status of Modern Therapy.* Lancaster, MTP Press, vol 6.
84. Lamb DW: The neurology of spinal pain. *Physical Therapy* 59:971–973, 1979.
85. Calin A: Back pain: Mechanical or inflammatory? *American Family Physician* 20:97–100, 1979.
86. Waddell G et al: Nonorganic physical signs in low back pain. *Spine* 5:117–125, 1980.
87. Kelsey JL, White AA: Epidemiology and impact of low back pain. *Spine* 5:133–142, 1980.
88. Frymoyer JW, Pope MH: The role of trauma in low back pain: A review. *Journal of Trauma* 18:628–633, 1978.
89. Kuo PP, Tang HF: Manipulation as a treatment of low back pain. *The Journal of the Western Pacific Orthopaedic Association* 2:31–34, 1983.
90. Murphy KA, Cornish D: Prediction of chronicity in acute low back pain. *Archives of Physical Medicine and Rehabilitation* 65:334–337, 1984.
91. Schafer RC: *Chiropractic Physical and Spinal Diagnosis.* Oklahoma City, Associated Chiropractic Academic Press, 1980, pp IV-7, IV-10, IV-29.
92. Janse J: *Principles and Practice of Chiropractic.* Lombard, Ill, National College of Chiropractic, 1976, p 116.
93. Ebel JN: Reflex relationships of paravertebral muscles. *American Journal of Physiology* 200(5), May 1961.
94. De Sterno CV: The pathophysiology of TMJ dysfunction and related pain. In Gelb H (ed): *Clinical Management of Head, Neck and TMJ Pain and Dysfunction.* Philadelphia, W.B. Saunders, 1977.
95. Van Dusen LG: *Chiropractic Relationship to Gravitational Force.* Sodus, NY, published by the author, 1968.
96. Travell J: Myofascial trigger points: Clinical view. In Bonica JJ, Albe-Fessard D (eds): *Advances in Pain Research and Therapy.* New York, Raven Press, 1976.
97. Wax M: Procedures in elimination of trigger points in myofascial pain syndromes. *ACA Journal of Chiropractic* October 1962.
98. Finneson BE: *Low Back Pain.* Philadelphia, J.B. Lippincott, 1973, pp 99–100.
99. Grieve GP: *Common Vertebral Joint Problems.* New York, Churchill Livingstone, 1981, p 198.
100. Simons DG, Travell JG: Myofascial origins of low back pain. *Postgraduate Medicine* 73(2):66–108, February 1983.
101. Gillet H, Liekens M: *Belgian Chiropractic Research Notes.* Huntington Beach, Cal, Motion Palpation Institute, 1981.
102. West HG Jr: Physical and spinal examination procedures utilized in the practice of chiropractic. In Haldeman S (ed): *Modern Developments in the Principles and Practice of Chiropractic.* New York, Appleton-Century-Crofts, 1980, p 283.
103. Gitelman R: A chiropractic approach to biomechanical disorders of the lumbar spine and pelvis. In Haldeman S (ed): *Modern Developments in the Principles and Practice of Chiropractic.* New York, Appleton-Century-Crofts, 1980, pp 317–319.
104. Gillet H, Liekens M: A further study of spinal fixations. *Annals of the Swiss Chiropractic Association (Geneva)* 4:41, 1967.
105. Kirkaldy-Willis WH: A more precise diagnosis for low back pain. *Spine* 4(2), March/April 1979.
106. Cassidy JD, Potter GE: Motion examination of the lumbar spine. *Journal of Manipulative and Physiological Therapeutics* 2(3), September 1979.
107. Gillet H: Evolution of a chiropractor. *National Chiropractic Journal* November 1945, January 1949, December 1949, January 1951.
108. Gates D: *Spinal Palpation.* Lakemont, Ga, published by the author, 1981, pp 61–62.
109. Cassidy JD: Roentgenological examination of the functional mechanics of the lumbar spine in lateral flexion. *Journal of the Canadian Chiropractic Association* July 1976.
110. Johnston WL: The role of static and motion palpation in structural diagnosis. In Goldstein M (ed): *The Research Status of Spinal Manipulative Therapy.* NINCDS Monograph, No. 15, DHEW Publication No. (NIH) 76-998, Stock No. 017-049-000607, Washington, DC, U.S. Government Printing Office, 1975.
111. McAndrews JF: Spinal motion examination. *ACA Journal of Chiropractic* May 1969.
112. Stonebrink RD: Palpation for vertebral motoricity. *ACA Journal of Chiropractic* February 1969.
113. Weitz EM: The lateral bending sign. *Spine* 6:388–397, July/August, 1981.
114. Schafer RC: *Chiropractic Management of Sports and Recreational Injuries.* Baltimore, Williams & Wilkins, 1982, p 442–444.
115. Splithoff CA: The lumbosacral junction. *Journal of the American Medical Association* 152:1610–1613.
116. Schoenholtz F: The diagnosis and conservative treatment of the lumbar disc syndrome. *ACA Journal of Chiropractic* April 1978.
117. Crock HV: Normal and pathological anatomy of the lumbar spinal nerve root canals. *Journal of Bone and Joint Surgery (British)* 63:487–490, 1981.
118. Edgelow PI: Physical examination of the lumbosacral complex. *Physicl Therapy* 59:974–977, 1979.
119. Wigh RE: The transitional lumbosacral osseous complex. *Skeletal Radiology* 8:127–131, 1982.
120. Cassidy JD, Potter GE: Motion examination of the lumbar spine. *Journal of Manipulative and Physiological Therapeutics* 3:151–158, 1979.

121. Harriman DG: Lumbosacral instability. *Roentgenological Briefs.* Council on Roentgenology of the American Chiropractic Association (undated).
122. Carmichael SW, Burkart SL: Clinical anatomy of the lumbosacral complex. *Physical Therapy* 59:966–975, 1979.
123. Panjabi MM, Goel VK, Takata K: Physiologic strains in the lumbar spinal ligaments. *Spine* 7:192–203, 1982.
124. Finneson BE: *Low Back Pain.* Philadelphia, J.B. Lippincott, 1973, p 134.
125. Olsen RE: Acute lumbosacral angle. *Roentgenological Briefs.* Council on Roentgenology of the American Chiropractic Association (undated).
126. Vernon H: Static and dynamic roentgenography in the diagnosis of degenerative disc disease: A review and comparative assessment. *Journal of Manipulative and Physiological Therapeutics* 5(4):163–168, December 1982.
127. Finneson BE: *Low Back Pain.* Philadelphia, J.B. Lippincott, 1973, p 138.
128. Sweere JJ: Type II round back deformity. *Orthopedic Brief.* ACA Council on Chiropractic Orthopedics, August 1985.
129. Cailliet R: *Low Back Pain Syndrome,* ed 3. Philadelphia, F.A. Davis, 1981, p 53.
130. Barge FH: *Tortipelvis.* Davenport, Ia, Bawden Bros, 1980.
131. Gitelman R: A chiropractic approach to biomechanical disorders of the lumbar spine and pelvis. In Haldeman S (ed): *Modern Developments in the Principles and Practice of Chiropractic.* New York, Appleton-Century-Crofts, 1980, pp 314–315, 319–320.
132. Drevet JG, Chirossel JP, Phelip X: Lumbago-lumboradiculalgia and posterior vertebral joints. *Lyon Medical* 245:781–787, 1981.
133. Fisk JW: *The Painful Neck and Back.* Springfield, Ill, Charles C Thomas, 1977, pp 28–34.
134. Badgley CE: The articular facets in relation to low back pain and sciatic radiation. *Journal of Bone and Joint Surgery* 23:2, April 1941.
135. Markey LP: The facet syndrome—lumbar instability diagnosis algorithm. Part III. *The Digest of Chiropractic Economics* November/December 1984.
136. Peters RE: The facet syndrome. *Journal of the Australian Chiropractors' Association* 13:15–18, 1983.
137. Yang KH, King AI: Mechanism of facet load transmission as a hypothesis for low back pain. *Spine* 9:557–565, 1984.
138. Schafer RC: *Chiropractic Management of Sports and Recreational Injuries.* Baltimore, Williams & Wilkins, 1982, pp 449–452.
139. Helfet AJ, Gruebel Lee DM: *Disorders of the Lumbar Spine.* Philadelphia, J.B. Lippincott, 1978, pp 3–10, 116, 237–242.
140. Harris RI, Macnab I: Structural changes in the lumbar intervertebral discs. *Journal of Bone and Joint Surgery* 35B:304, 1954.
141. Lenz WF: Spondylolisthesis and spondyloptosis of the lumbar spine. *ACA Journal of Chiropractic* November 1980.
142. Grieve GP: *Common Vertebral Joint Problems.* New York, Churchill Livingstone, 1981, pp 145–147.
143. Finneson BE: *Low Back Pain.* Philadelphia, J.B. Lippincott, 1973, pp 279–287.
144. Macnab I: *Backache.* Baltimore, Williams & Wilkins, 1977, pp 44–63.
145. Turek SL: *Orthopaedics: Principles and Their Application,* ed 3. Philadelphia, J.B. Lippincott, 1977, pp 1362–1366.
146. Rothman RH, Simeone FA (eds): *The Spine.* Philadelphia, W.B. Saunders, 1975, vol 1, pp 229–244, 476.
147. Gehweiler JA Jr, Osborne RL Jr, Becker RF: *The Radiology of Vertebral Trauma.* Philadelphia, W.B. Saunders, 1980, pp 401, 407–425, 429.
148. Kestler OC: Spondylolysis and spondylolisthesis: Updated review. *New York State Journal of Medicine* April 1979, p 700.
149. Penning L, Blickman JR: Instability in lumbar spondylolisthesis: A radiologic study of several concepts. *American Journal of Roentgenology* 134:293–301, 1980.
150. Davis BM: Spondylolisthesis and spondylolysis. *Roentgenological Briefs.* Council on Roentgenology of the American Chiropractic Association (undated).
151. Rehberger LP: Spondylolisthesis. *Roentgenological Briefs.* Council on Roentgenology of the American Chiropractic Association (undated).
152. Fredrickson BE et al: The natural history of spondylolysis and spondylolisthesis. *Journal of Bone and Joint Surgery* 66:699–707, 1984.
153. Meyerling HW: The low backache and sciatic pain associated with spondylolisthesis and protruded intervertebral disc: Incidence and treatment. *Journal of Bone and Joint Surgery* 23:461, 1941.
154. Boxall D et al: Management of severe spondylolisthesis in children and adolescents. *Journal of Bone and Joint Surgery* 61A:479–495, 1979.
155. Cassidy JD, Potter GE, Kirkaldy-Willis WH: Manipulative management of back pain in patients with spondylolisthesis. *Journal of the Canadian Chiropractic Association* 22:15–120, 1978.
156. Cox JM: *Low Back Pain: Mechanism, Diagnosis and Treatment,* ed 4. Baltimore, Williams & Wilkins, 1985.
157. Cox JM: Pre- and post-CT scans on chiropractic treated disc protrusion patients. Parts I and II. *The Digest of Chiropractic Economics* January/February 1985; March/April 1985.
158. Robertson JA: Intermittent lumbar flexion-distraction applied in the treatment of spondylolisthesis: a statistical analysis. *Journal of Manipulative and Physiological Therapeutics* 2(3):159–169, September 1979.
159. Finneson BE: *Low Back Pain.* Philadelphia, J.B. Lippincott, 1973, p 287.
160. Gehweiler JA Jr, Osborne RL Jr, Becker RF: *The Radiology of Vertebral Trauma.* Philadelphia, W.B. Saunders, 1980, pp 446–447.
161. Rothman RH, Simeone FA (eds): *The Spine.* Philadelphia, W.B. Saunders, 1975, vol 1, pp 229–240, 475, 738.
162. Macnab I: *Backache.* Baltimore, Williams & Wilkins, 1977, pp 69–74.

163. Turek SL: *Orthopaedics: Principles and Their Application*, ed 3. Philadelphia, J.B. Lippincott, 1977, pp 1383–1389.
164. Gehweiler JA Jr, Osborne RL Jr, Becker RF: *The Radiology of Vertebral Trauma.* Philadelphia, W.B. Saunders, 1980, pp 401–406, 409, 426–429.
165. Porter RW, Park W: Unilateral spondylolysis. *Journal of Bone and Joint Surgery (British)* 64:344–348, 1982.
166. Finneson BE: *Low Back Pain.* Philadelphia, J.B. Lippincott, 1973, pp 262–268, 277–279.
167. Cyron BM, Hutton WC: Variations in the amount and distribution of cortical bone across the partes interarticularis of L5: A predisposing factor in spondylolysis. *Spine* 4:163–167, 1979.
168. Julkunen H, Knekt P, Aromaa A: Spondylosis deformans and diffuse idiopathic skeletal hyperostosis (DISH) in Finland. *Scandinavian Journal of Rheumatology* 10:193–203, 1981.
169. Eisentein S: Spondylolysis—a skeletal investigation of two population groups. *Journal of Bone and Joint Surgery* 60B:488–494, 1979.
170. Helfet AJ, Gruebel Lee DM: *Disorders of the Lumbar Spine.* Philadelphia, J.B. Lippincott, 1978, pp 38, 42–44.
171. Turner EA: Spondylosis—spondylitis—spondylolysis. *Roentgenological Briefs.* Council on Chiropractic Roentgenology of the American Chiropractic Association (undated).
172. Henderson DJ: Intermittent claudication—with special reference to its neurogenic form as a diagnostic and management challenge. *Journal of the Canadian Chiropractic Association* 23:9, 1979.
173. Buehler MT: Spinal stenosis. *Journal of Manipulative and Physiological Therapeutics* 1(2), June 1978.
174. White AA, Panjabi MM: *Clinical Biomechanics of the Spine.* Philadelphia, J.B. Lippincott, 1978, pp 292–293.
175. Grieve GP: *Common Vertebral Joint Problems.* New York, Churchill Livingstone, 1981, pp 147–150.
176. Finneson BE: *Low Back Pain.* Philadelphia, J.B. Lippincott, 1973, pp 256–272.
177. Helfet AJ, Gruebel Lee DM: *Disorders of the Lumbar Spine.* Philadelphia, J.B. Lippincott, 1978, pp 51–61.
178. Macnab I: *Backache.* Baltimore, Williams & Wilkins, 1977, pp 98–104, 198–200.
179. Nilsson N, Dahl M: Lumbar spinal stenosis in general chiropractic practice. *European Journal of Chiropractic* 33(1):21–23, March 1985.
180. Sweere JJ: Clinical manifestations of lumbar spinal stenosis. *Orthopedic Brief.* ACA Council on Chiropractic Orthopedics, June 1985.
181. Russell AS, Percy JS, Lentle BC: Vertebral sclerosis in adults. *Annals of the Rheumatic Diseases* 37:18–22, 1978.
182. Magnaes B, Hauge T: Rheumatoid arthritis contributing to lumbar spinal stenosis. *Scandinavian Journal of Rheumatology* 7:215–218, 1978.
183. Naylor A: Factors in the development of the spinal stenosis syndrome. *Journal of Bone and Joint Surgery* 61B:306–309, 1979.
184. Porter RW, Hibbert CS, Wicks M: The spinal canal in symptomatic lumbar disc lesions. *Journal of Bone and Joint Surgery* 60B:485–487, 1978.
185. Porter RW, Hibbert C, Wellman P: Backache and the lumbar spinal canal. *Spine* 5:99–105, 1980.
186. Wildenauer JR: A discussion of lumbar disc syndromes and the value of computed axial tomography. *Ortho Briefs.* ACA Council on Chiropractic Orthopedics, April 1984, pp 30–37.
187. Wiehe RJ: Low back injury with pain due to lumbar disc rupture. *The Chiropractic Family Physician* 2(5):9–14, 28, July 1980.
188. Grieve GP: *Common Vertebral Joint Problems.* New York, Churchill Livingstone, 1981, pp 143–145.
189. Janse J: *Principles and Practice of Chiropractic.* Lombard, Ill, National College of Chiropractic, 1976, pp 187–196.
190. Schafer RC: *Chiropractic Management of Sports and Recreational Injuries.* Baltimore, Williams & Wilkins, 1982, pp 448–449.
191. Wyke BD: Articular neurology and manipulative therapy. In *Aspects of Manipulative Therapy.* Proceedings of Multidisciplinary International Conference on Manipulative Therapy, Melbourne. Lincoln Institute of Health Sciences, Carlton, Victoria, Australia, August 1979, pp 67–72.
192. Gehweiler JA Jr, Osborne RL Jr, Becker RF: *The Radiology of Vertebral Trauma.* Philadelphia, W.B. Saunders, 1980, pp 296–299.
193. Finneson BE: *Low Back Pain.* Philadelphia, J.B. Lippincott, 1973, pp 26–35, 263–264.
194. Barge FH: *Tortipelvis.* Davenport, Ia, Bawden Bros, 1980, pp 121–135.
195. Farfan HF et al: The effects of torsion on the lumbar intervertebral joints: The role of torsion in the production of disc degeneration. *Journal of Bone and Joint Surgery* 52A:468, 1970.
196. Jessen AR: The intervertebral discs: Shock absorbers or shock transmitters? *ACA Journal of Chiropractic* 9:S121–S127, October 1975.
197. Farfan HF: Symptomatoogy in terms of the pathomechanics of low-back pain and sciatica. In Haldeman S (ed): *Modern Developments in the Principles and Practice of Chiropractic.* New York, Appleton-Century-Crofts, 1980.
198. Barge FH: *Tortipelvis.* Davenport, Ia, Bawden Bros, 1980, p 27.
199. Helfet AJ, Gruebel Lee DM: *Disorders of the Lumbar Spine.* Philadelphia, J.B. Lippincott, 1978, pp 15, 31.
200. Hadley LA: *Anatomico-Roentgenographic Studies of the Spine.* Springfield, Ill, Charles C Thomas, 1981, pp 230–252.
201. Gehweiler JA Jr, Osborne RL Jr, Becker RF: *The Radiology of Vertebral Trauma.* Philadelphia, W.B. Saunders, 1980, pp 267–273.
202. Sante LR: *Principles of Roentgenological Interpretation.* Ann Arbor, Edwards Brothers, 1961.
203. Sunderland S: Anatomical perivertebral influences on the intervertebral foramen. In Goldstein M (ed): *The Research Status of Spinal Manipulative Therapy.* NINCDS Monograph, No. 15, DHEW Publication No. (NIH) 76-998, Stock No. 017-049-00060-7, Washington, DC, U.S. Government Printing Office, 1975.
204. Sharpless SK: Susceptibility of spinal roots to

compression block. In Goldstein M (ed): *The Research Status of Spinal Manipulative Therapy.* NINCDS Monograph, No. 15, DHEW Publication No. (NIH) 76-998, Stock No. 017-049-00060-7, Washington, DC, U.S. Government Printing Office, 1975.

205. Schaumberg HH, Spencer PS: Pathology of spinal root compression. In Goldstein M (ed): *The Research Status of Spinal Manipulative Therapy.* NINCDS Monograph, No. 15, DHEW Publication No. (NIH) 76-998, Stock No. 017-049-00060-7, Washington, DC, U.S. Government Printing Office, 1975.
206. Sandoz R: New trends in the pathogenesis of spinal disorders. *Annals of the Swiss Chiropractic Association* 5:93, 1971.
207. Sandoz R: Some reflex phenomena associated with spinal derangements and adjustments. *Annals of the Swiss Chiropractic Association* 7:45, 1981.
208. Kellgren JH: Observations on referred pain arising from muscle. *Clinical Science* 3:175, 1938.
209. Armstrong JR: *Lumbar Disc Lesions,* ed 3. Baltimore, Williams & Wilkins, 1965.
210. Farfan HF: *Mechanical Disorders of the Low Back.* Philadelphia, Lea & Febiger, 1973.
211. Leavitt F et al: Low back pain in patients with and without demonstrable organic disease. *Pain* 6:191–200, 1979.
212. Laban MM et al: Aortic aneurysm may be manifested by lumbosacral pain. *American Family Physician* December 19, 1979.
213. Kirkaldy-Willis WH: The relationship of structural pathology to the nerve root. *Spine* 9:49–52, 1984.
214. Kortelainen P et al: Symptoms and signs of sciatica and their relation to the localization of the lumbar disc herniation. *Spine* 10:88–91, 1985.
215. Poole PB: Considerations of neurogenic pain. *Ortho Briefs.* Council on Chiropractic Orthopedics of the American Chiropractic Association, Fall 1982.
216. Blower PW: Neurologic patterns in unilateral sciatica: A prospective study of 100 new cases. *Spine* 6:175–179, 1981.
217. Brewer BJ: Low-back pain. *American Family Physician* 19:114–119, 1979.
218. Finneson BE: *Low Back Pain.* Philadelphia, J.B. Lippincott, 1973, pp 325–326.
219. Triano J, Luttges M; Subtle, intermittent mechanical irritation of sciatic nerves in mice. *Journal of Manipulative and Physiological Therapeutics* 3:75–80, 1980.
220. Bogduk N: Lumbar dorsal ramus syndrome. *Medical Journal of Australia* 2:537–541, 1980.
221. Jabre JF, Bryan RW: Bent-knee pulling in the diagnosis of upper lumbar root lesions. *Archives of Neurology* 39:669–670, 1982.
222. Rosse C: The vertebral canal and its contents. In Rosse C, Clawson DK (eds): *The Musculoskeletal System in Health and Disease.* Hagerstown, Md, Harper & Row, 1980, pp 153–156.
223. Finneson BE: *Low Back Pain.* Philadelphia, J.B. Lippincott, 1973, pp 141–177.
224. Cailliet R: *Low Back Pain Syndrome,* ed 3. Philadelphia, F.A. Davis, 1981, pp 144–171.
225. Macnab I: *Backache.* Baltimore, Williams & Wilkins, 1977, pp 133–207.
226. Turek SL: *Orthopaedics: Principles and Their Application,* ed 3. Philadelphia, J.B. Lippincott, 1977, pp 1323–1333, 1339–1341.
227. Rothman RH, Simeone FA: Lumbar disc disease. In Rothman RH, Simeone FA (eds): *The Spine.* Philadelphia, W.B. Saunders, 1975, vol 2, pp 443–476.
228. Coventry MB: Anatomy of the intervertebral disk. *Clinical Orthopaedics* 67:9, 1969.
229. Cox JM: Mechanism, diagnosis and treatment of lumbar disc protrusion and prolapse: A statistical evaluation. Parts I and II. *ACA Journal of Chiropractic* September 1976; October 1976.
230. Yamada K: The dynamics of experimental posture. *Clinical Orthopaedics* 25:20–31, 1962.
231. Voloshin A, Wosk J: An in vivo study of low back pain and shock absorption in the human locomotor system. *Journal of Biomechanics* 15:21–22, 1982.
232. Hodge CJ, Binet EF, Kieffer SA: Intradural herniation of lumbar intervertebral discs. *Spine* 3:346–350, 1978.
233. Martin G: The role of trauma in disc protrusion. *New Zealand Medical Journal* 22:208–211, 1978.
234. Acute symptomatic disk prolapse: Clinical manifestations and therapeutic considerations. *Physical Therapy* 59:978–987, 1979.
235. Resnick D, Niwayama G: Intervertebral disc abnormalities associated with vertebral metastasis: Observations in patients and cadavers with prostatic cancer. *Investigative Radiology* 13:182–190, 1978.
236. Sweere JJ: A method of physiological testing in the differential diagnosis of acute mechanical low back pain. *Orthopedic Brief.* ACA Council on Chiropractic Orthopedics, September 1984.
237. Rothman RH, Simeone FA: Lumbar disc disease. In Rothman RH, Simeone FA (eds): *The Spine.* Philadelphia, W.B. Saunders, 1975, vol 2, pp 443–461.
238. Postacchini F et al: An ultrastructural study of recurrent disc herniation. *Spine* 7:492–497, 1982.
239. Burkart SL, Beresford WA: The aging intervertebral disk. *Physical Therapy* 59:969–974, 1979.
240. Milgram JW: Osteoarthritic changes at the severely degenerative disc in humans. *Spine* 7:498–505, 1982.
241. Lipson SJ, Muir H: An animal model of intervertebral disc herniation. *Annals of the Rheumatic Diseases* 38:185, 1979.
242. Venner RM, Crock HV: Clinical studies of isolated disc resorption in the lumbar spine. *Journal of Bone and Joint Surgery (British)* 63:491–494, 1981.
243. Park WM et al: Fissuring of the posterior annulus fibrosis in the lumbar spine. *British Journal of Radiology* 52:382–387, 1979.

244. Macnab I: *Backache.* Baltimore, Williams & Wilkins, 1977, pp 101–104.
245. Farfan HF, Sullivan JD: The relation of facet orientation to intervertebral disc failure. *Canadian Journal of Surgery* 10:179, 1967.
246. Hasue M et al: Anatomic study of the interrelation between lumbosacral nerve roots and their surrounding tissues. *Spine* 8:50–58, 1983.
247. Wiltse LL et al: Alar transverse process impingement of the L5 spinal nerve: The far-out syndrome. *Spine* 9:31–41, 1984.
248. Fisk JW: *The Painful Neck and Back.* Springfield, Ill, Charles C Thomas, 1977, pp 91–114, 141–153, 169–193.
249. Macnab I: *Backache.* Baltimore, Williams & Wilkins, 1977, pp 181–184.
250. Finneson BE: *Low Back Pain.* Philadelphia, J.B. Lippincott, 1973, pp 93–132.
251. Helfet AJ, Gruebel Lee DM: *Disorders of the Lumbar Spine.* Phildelphia, J.B. Lippincott, 1978, pp 145–161, 170–182.
252. Rothman RH, Simeone FA: Lumbar disc disease. In Rothman RH, Simeone FA (eds): *The Spine.* Philadelphia, W.B. Saunders, 1975, vol 2, pp 476–506.
253. Goodheart GL: *Collected Published Articles and Reprints.* Montpellier, Oh, Williams County Publishing, 1969, pp 36–37.
254. Cyriax E: Some common postural deformities and their treatment by exercise and manipulation. *British Journal of Physical Medicine* June 1938.
255. Jayson MIV et al: Mobilization and manipulation for low back pain. *Spine* 6:4, July/August 1981.
256. Molloy RD: A correlation between muscle testing and chiropractic treatment. Thesis, Anglo-European College of Chiropractic, 1976.
257. Nickel VL (ed): *Orthopedic Rehabilitation.* New York, Churchill Livingstone, 1981.
258. Kraus H: *Therapeutic Exercise.* Springfield, Ill, Charles C Thomas, 1963.
259. Brunarski DJ: Functional considerations of spinal manipulative therapy. *ACA Journal of Chiropractic* May 1980.
260. Brodin H: Inhibition-facilitation technique for lumbar pain treatment. *Manuell Medizin* 20:95–98, 1982.
261. Triano J: Significant lumbar dyskinesia. *ACA Journal of Chiropractic* February 1980.
262. Free RV: Paravertebral muscle equalization. *The Digest of Chiropractic Economics* January/February 1985.
263. Malik DD et al: Effectiveness of chiropractic and physical therapy to treat spinal subluxation. *ACA Journal of Chiropractic* June 1983.
264. Malik DD et al: Recovery from radiculalgia by chiropractic adjustment and physical therapy. *ACA Journal of Chiropractic* June 1984.
265. Markey LP: Markey distraction technique: New protocol for doctor and patient safety. Part I. *The Digest of Chiropractic Economics* September/October 1985.
266. Farrell JP, Twomey LT: Acute low back pain: Comparison of two conservative approaches. *Journal of the Australian Medical Association* 1:160–164, 1982.
267. Jayson MIV et al: Mobilization and manipulation for low-back pain. *Spine* 6:409–416, 1981.
268. Burton CV: Conservative management of low back pain. *Postgraduate Medicine* 70:168–183, 1981.
269. Grynbaum BB, Belandres PV: Managing low back pain. *Female Patient* 3:43–45, 1978.
270. Jackson CP, Brown MD: Is there a role for exercise in the treatment of patients with low back pain? *Clinical Orthopaedics and Related Research* 179:39–45, 1983.
271. Bell GR, Rothman RH: The conservative treatment of sciatica. *Spine* 9:54–56, 1984.
272. Cailliet R: *Low Back Pain Syndrome,* ed 3. Philadelphia, F.A. Davis, 1981, pp 90–94.
273. Sample JJ: Traction therapy as an aid to the chiropractic profession. Presented at the convention of the National Chiropractic Association, Las Vegas, Nevada, June 1961.
274. Martin RJ: Traction therapy for lumbar disc pressure. *The Chiropractic Family Physician* 2(5):17–20, July 1980.
275. King LM: *Motorized Spinal Traction.* Monograph. Denver, Spears Chiropractic Hospital (undated).
276. Saunders HD: *Orthopaedic Physical Therapy: Evaluation and Treatment of Musculoskeletal Disorders.* Minneapolis, published by the author, 1982, p 146.
277. Schafer RC: *Chiropractic Management of Sports and Recreational Injuries.* Baltimore, Williams & Wilkins, 1982, p 203.
278. Anderson GBJ, Schultz AB, Nachemson AL: Intervertebral disc pressures during traction. *Scandinavian Journal of Rehabilitative Medicine* 9:88–91, 1984.
279. Voss DE et al: Traction and approximation. In *Proprioceptive Neuromuscular Facilitation: Patterns and Techniques*, ed 3. Philadelphia, Harper & Row, 1985, p 294.
280. Mathews JA: The effects of spinal traction. *Physiotherapy* 58:64–66, 1972.
281. Gatterman MI: Contraindications and complications of spinal manipulative therapy. *ACA Journal of Chiropractic* September 1981.
282. Burton AK: Back pain in osteopathic practice. *Rheumatology and Rehabilitation* 20:239–246, 1981.
283. Gottlieb HJ et al: An innovative program for the restoration of patients with chronic back pain. *Physical Therapy* 59:996–999, 1979.
284. Grieve GP: *Common Vertebral Joint Problems.* New York, Churchill Livingstone, 1981, pp 151–158.
285. Fisk JW: *The Painful Neck and Back.* Springfield, Ill, Charles C Thomas, 1977, pp 54–76, 176–187.
286. Barge FH: *Tortipelvis.* Davenport, Ia, Bawden Bros, 1980, pp 104–120.
287. Gitelman R: A chiropractic approach to biomechanical disorders of the lumbar spine and pelvis. In Haldeman S (ed): *Modern Developments in the Principles and Practice of Chiropractic.* New

York, Appleton-Century-Crofts, 1980, pp 297–299.
288. Illi FW: The phylogenesis and clinical import of the sacroiliac mechanism. *Journal of the National Chiropractic Association* September/October 1963.
289. Reynolds HM: Three dimensional kinematics in the pelvic girdle. *Journal of the American Osteopathic Association* 80:4, December 1980.
290. Grice AS, Fligg DB: *Class Notes: Spinal Dynamics.* Department of Biomechanics/Kinesiology, BK202. Toronto, Canadian Memorial Chiropractic College (undated), pp 91–101.
291. Carver W: *Carver's Chiropractic Analysis,* ed 4. Oklahoma City, published by the author; vol 1, 1921; vol 2, 1922.
292. Beal MC: The sacroiliac problem: Review of anatomy, mechanics, and diagnosis. *Journal of the American Osteopathic Association* 81:667–679, 1982.
293. Barham JN, Wooten EP: *Structural Kinesiology.* New York, Macmillan, 1973, pp 273–274.
294. Bosshard R: Spinal hygiene. *Annals of the Swiss Chiropractic Association* 4:163–182.
295. Klein KK: Progression of pelvic tilt in adolescent boys. *Archives of Physical Medicine and Rehabilitation* 54:57–59, February 1973.
296. Greenman PE: Lift therapy: Use and abuse. *Journal of the American Osteopathic Association* December 1979.
297. Goodheart GJ: *Applied Kinesiology.* City of publication not shown, published by the author, privately distributed, 1964.
298. Merriam WF et al: A study revealing a tall pelvis in subjects with low back pain. *Journal of Bone and Joint Surgery* 65B:153–156, 1983.
299. Granger CV: The clinical discernment of muscle weakness. *Archives of Physical Medicine* 44:430–438, 1963.
300. Fisk JW: *The Painful Neck and Back.* Springfield, Ill, Charles C Thomas, 1977, pp 39–43.
301. Logan AL: *Clinical Application of Chiropractic: Low Back and Pelvis.* Westminster, Cal, West-Print, 1977.
302. Pace JB, Nagle D: Piriform syndrome. *Western Journal of Medicine* 124:435–439, 1976.
303. McDonald TS: The balanced psoas. *The Digest of Chiropractic Economics* July/August 1983.
304. Schmidt WH Jr: The psoas sitting test: Key to hidden lumbosacral problems. *The Digest of Chiropractic Economics* September/October 1983.
305. Goodheart GL: The psoas muscle and the foot pronation problem. In *Collected Published Articles and Reprints.* Montpellier, Oh, Williams County Publishing, 1969, pp 72–73.
306. Borrmann WR: Applied kinesiology of the hamstring muscles and related factors. *Wisconsin Chiropractic Association Journal* 28:15, April 1975.
307. Phalen GS, Dickson JA: Spondylolisthesis and tight hamstrings. (From Proceedings of the Association of Bone and Joint Surgeons.) *Journal of Bone and Joint Surgery* 38A:946, 1956.
308. Janse J: *Principles and Practice of Chiropractic.* Lombard, Ill, National College of Chiropractic, 1976, p 181.
309. Retzlaff EW et al: The piriformis muscle syndrome. *Journal of the American Osteopathic Association* 73:799–807, 1984.
310. Ng YS: The significance of psoas myospasm in the lordotic compared to the kyphotic sacrolumbar spine. *ACA Journal of Chiropractic* October 1978.
311. Janse J: *Principles and Practice of Chiropractic.* Lombard, Ill, National College of Chiropractic, 1976, p 151.
312. Nachemson AL: Electromyographical studies of the vertebral portion of the psoas muscle (with special reference to its stabilizing function of the lumbar spine). *Acta Orthopaedica Scandinavica* 37:177–190, 1966.
313. Michelle AA: *Iliopsoas: Development of Anomalies in Man.* Springfield, Ill, Charles C Thomas, 1962.
314. Fairbank J, O'Brien J: The iliac crest syndrome: A treatable cause of low-back pain. *Spine* 8:220–224, 1983.
315. Hirschberg GG, Froetscher L, Naeim F: Iliolumbar syndrome as a common cause of low-back pain: Diagnosis and prognosis. *Archives of Physical Medicine and Rehabilitation* 60:415–419, 1979.
316. Grice AS, Fligg DB: *Class Notes: Spinal Dynamics.* Department of Biomechanics/Kinesiology, BK202. Toronto, Canadian Memorial Chiropractic College (undated), p 97.
317. Pitkin HC, Pheasant HC: Sacroarthrogenetic tekalgia: A study of referred pain. *Journal of Bone and Joint Surgery* vol 18, 1936.
318. Simons DG, Travell JG: Myofascial origins of low back pain. *Postgraduate Medicine* 73(2):66–108, February 1983.
319. Janse J: *Principles and Practice of Chiropractic.* Lombard, Ill, National College of Chiropractic, 1976, p 310.
320. Schafer RC: *Chiropractic Management of Sports and Recreational Injuries.* Baltimore, Williams & Wilkins, 1982, pp 263–264, 286–287.
321. Janse J: *Principles and Practice of Chiropractic.* Lombard, Ill, National College of Chiropractic, 1976.
322. Denton DG: Sacro-occipital technique biomechanics of the pelvis. In ACA Council on Technic: *Biomechanics of the Pelvis.* Denver Conference, June 17–20, 1980, Spears Chiropractic Hospital. Des Moines, Ia, Council on Technic of the American Chiropractic Association, 1982.
323. Ng SY: Sacroiliac lumbar mechanism. *ACA Journal of Chiropractic* April 1983.
324. White AA, Panjabi MM: *Clinical Biomechanics of the Spine.* Philadelphia, J.B. Lippincott, 1978, pp 264–270.
325. Gehweiler JA Jr, Osborne RL Jr, Becker RF: *The Radiology of Vertebral Trauma.* Philadelphia, W.B. Saunders, 1980, pp 379–398.
326. Fisk JW: *The Painful Neck and Back.* Springfield, Ill, Charles C Thomas, 1977, pp 46–47.
327. Grieve GP· *Common Vertebral Joint Problems.* New York, Churchill Livingstone, 1981, pp 328–334.
328. Shunke GB: Anatomy and development of the sacroiliac joint in man. *Anatomical Record* 72:3, 1938.

329. Barham JN, Wooten EP: *Structural Kinesiology.* New York, Macmillan, 1973, p 277.
330. Cassidy JD, Bowen CV: Anatomy and biomechanics of the sacroiliac joint. In ACA Council on Technic: *Biomechanics of the Pelvis.* Denver Conference, June 17–20, 1980, Spears Chiropractic Hospital. Des Moines, Ia, Council on Technic of the American Chiropractic Association, 1982.
331. Milne RA, Mierau DR: Relationship of pelvic and low back stress. *Journal of Manipulative and Physiological Therapeutics* 2:3, September 1979.
332. Macnab I: *Backache.* Baltimore, Williams & Wilkins, 1977, pp 64–69.
333. Mitchell T: Structural pelvic function. *Yearbook of Applied Osteopathy* 1965.
334. Grieve GP: *Common Vertebral Joint Problems.* New York, Churchill Livingstone, 1981, p 153.
335. Janse J: Clinical biomechanics of the sacroiliac mechanism. *ACA Journal of Chiropractic* February 1978.
336. Pinkenburg CA: A study of the sacroiliac articulations. *ACA Journal of Chiropractic* November 1978.
337. Otter R: A review study of the differing opinions expressed in the literature about the anatomy of the sacroiliac joint. *European Journal of Chiropractic* 33(4):221–241, December 1985.
338. Grieve DW: The sacroiliac joint. *Physiotherapy* 62(12):384–400, 1976.
339. DonTigny RL: Function and pathomechanics of the sacroiliac joint: A review. *Physical Therapy* 65:35–44, 1985.
340. Kotheimer WJ: Analysis of the sacroiliac. *The Digest of Chiropractic Economics* July/August 1985.
341. Grieve GP: *Common Vertebral Joint Problems.* New York, Churchill Livingstone, 1981, pp 309, 329.
342. Janse J: *Principles and Practice of Chiropractic.* Lombard, Ill, National College of Chiropractic, 1976, pp 136–140.
343. Hemauer JD: Sacroiliac anatomy, movement, and subluxation. In ACA Council on Technic *Biomechanics of the Pelvis.* Denver Conference, June 17–20, 1980. Council on Technic of the American Chiropractic Association, 1982, p 118.
344. Baltzell LG, Mackey RH (eds): *Firth's Technic Notes.* Publishing data not shown, 1967, pp 28–31. Available from National College of Chiropractic.
345. States AZ: *Spinal and Pelvic Technics,* ed 2. Lombard, Ill, National Chiropractic College, 1968, pp 2, 12–15.
346. Janse J, Houser RH, Wells BF: *Chiropractic Principles and Technic.* Chicago, National College of Chiropractic, 1947, pp 456–487.
347. Logan AL: *Clinical Application of Chiropractic: Low Back and Pelvis.* Westminster, Cal, West-Print, 1977, pp 9–10, 17–39.
348. Reinert OC: *Chiropractic Procedure and Practice,* ed 3. Florissant, Mo, Marian Press, 1972, pp 82–85, 116–118, 144–151.
349. Faucret BH: Introduction to pelvic biomechanics. In ACA Council on Technic *Biomechanics of the Pelvis.* Denver Conference, June 17–20, 1980. Council on Technic of the American Chiropractic Association, 1982, pp 58–75.
350. Logan VF: *Chiropractic Palpation and Analysis.* Chesterfield, Mo, Logan College of Chiropractic (undated) pp 85–91.
351. Levine M: *The Structural Approach to Chiropractic.* New York, Comet Press, 1964, pp 54–62.
352. Grecco MA: *Chiropractic Technic Illustrated.* New York, Jarl, 1953.
353. Logan HB: *Textbook of Logan Basic Methods.* St. Louis, Logan Chiropractic College, 1950.
354. Illi FW: *The Vertebral Column: Life-Line of the Body.* Chicago, National College of Chiropractic, 1951.
355. Grieve GP: *Common Vertebral Joint Problems.* New York, Churchill Livingstone, 1981, pp 151–153.
356. Schafer RC: *Chiropractic Management of Sports and Recreational Injuries.* Baltimore, Williams & Wilkins, 1982, pp 454–456, 458.
357. Williams JGP, Sperryn PN (eds): *Sports Medicine,* ed 2. Baltimore, Williams & Wilkins, 1976, pp 430–435.
358. Hirata I Jr: *The Doctor and the Athlete,* ed 2. Philadelphia, J.B. Lippincott, 1974, pp 191–196, 211.
359. La Ban M et al: Symphyseal and sacroiliac joint pain associated with pubic symphysis instability. *Archives of Physical Medicine and Rehabilitation* 59:470–472, 1978.
360. Schafer RC: *Chiropractic Management of Sports and Recreational Injuries.* Baltimore, Williams & Wilkins, 1982, pp 458–459.
361. Schafer RC: Perineal injuries common to cyclists. *Journal of the ACA Council on Sports Injuries* April 1982, pp 10–14.
362. Janse J, Houser RH, Wells BF: *Chiropractic Principles and Technic.* Chicago, Ill, National College of Chiropractic, 1947, pp 487–492.
363. Postacchini F, Massobrio M: Idiopathic coccygodynia: Analysis of fifty-one operative cases and a radiographic study of the normal coccyx. *Journal of Bone and Joint Surgery* 65:1116–1124, 1983.
364. Noakes T: 120 pelvic stress fractures in long distance runners. *The American Journal of Sports Medicine,* 13(2):120, March/April 1985.
365. McLaughlin HL: *Trauma.* Philadelphia, W.B. Saunders, 1959.
366. Paul LW, Juhl JH: *Essentials of Roentgen Interpretation.* New York, Harper & Row, 1965.
367. Schafer RC: *Chiropractic Management of Sports and Recreational Injuries.* Baltimore, Williams & Wilkins, 1982, pp 459–460.
368. Williams JGP, Sperryn PN (eds): *Sports Medicine,* ed 2. Baltimore, Williams & Wilkins, 1976, pp 428–429.
369. Albers VL: Avulsion fracture of the anterior inferior iliac spine. *ACA Journal of Chiropractic* November 1984.
370. Wild JJ, Hanson GW, Tullos HS: Unstable fractures of the pelvis treated by external fixation. *Journal of Bone and Joint Surgery* 64A:1010–1020, 1982.
371. Pavlov H et al: Stress fractures of the pubic

ramus. *Journal of Bone and Joint Surgery* 64A:1020–1025, 1982.
372. Jackson H et al: The sacral arcuate lines in upper sacral fracture. *Radiology* 145:35–39, 1982.
373. Lourie H: Spontaneous osteoporotic fracture of the sacrum: An unrecognized syndrome of the elderly. *Journal of the American Medical Association* 248:715–719, 1982.
374. Kirkaldy-Willis WH: Five common back disorders: How to diagnose and treat them. *Geriatrics* December 1978, pp 32–33, 37–41.
375. West HG Jr: Physical and spinal examination procedures utilized in the practice of chiropractic. In Haldeman S (ed): *Modern Developments in the Principles and Practice of Chiropractic.* New York, Appleton-Century-Crofts, 1980, pp 281–282, 283–284
376. Gitelman R: A chiropractic approach to biomechanical disorders of the lumbar spine and pelvis. In Haldeman S (ed): *Modern Developments in the Principles and Practice of Chiropractic.* New York, Appleton-Century-Crofts, 1980, pp 299, 304–307.
377. Gillet H: Clinical measurement of sacro-iliac mobility. *Annals of the Swiss Chiropractors' Association* 6:59–70, 1976.
378. Gillet H: Movement palpation—measurements. *Bulletin of the European Chiropractors Union* 23(2), 1974.
379. Grice AS, Fligg DB: Clinical analysis of the sacroiliac joint. In ACA Council on Technic: *Biomechanics of the Pelvis.* Denver Conference, June 17–20, 1980. Council on Technic of the American Chiropractic Association, 1982, pp 105–109.
380. Gatterman B: Motion palpation of the sacroiliac joints. In ACA Council on Technic: *Biomechanics of the Pelvis.* Denver Conference, June 17–20, 1980. Council on Technic of the American Chiropractic Association, 1982, pp 76–80.
381. Gatterman MI: Sacroiliac motion and pelvic tilt. In ACA Council on Technic: *Biomechanics of the Pelvis.* Denver Conference, June 17–20, 1980. Council on Technic of the American Chiropractic Association, 1982, p 91.
382. Wilder DG et al: The functional topography of the sacroiliac joint. *Spine* 5:60, 1980.
383. Wiles MR: Reproducibility and interexaminer correlation of motion palpation findings of the sacroiliac joints. *Journal of the Canadian Chiropractic Association* 24(2), 1980.
384. Gates D: *Spinal Palpation.* Lakemont, Ga, published by the author, 1981, pp 63–66.
385. Milne RA, Mierau DR: Hamstring distensibility in the general population: Relationship to pelvic and low back stresses. *Journal of Manipulative and Physiological Therapeutics* 2(3):146–150, September 1979.
386. Hoehler FK, Tobis JS: Low back pain and its treatment by spinal manipulation: Measures of flexibility and asymmetry. *Rheumatology and Rehabilitation* 21:21–26, 1982.
387. Turner JA, Robinson J, McCreary CP: Chronic low-back pain: Predicting response to nonsurgical treatment. *Archives of Physical Medicine and Rehabilitation* 64:560–563, 1983.
388. Weisl H: Ligaments of the sacro-iliac joint examined with particular reference to their function. *Acta Anatomica* 20:201–213, 1954.
389. Grieve GP: *Common Vertebral Joint Problems.* New York, Churchill Livingstone, 1981, p 284.
390. Weisl H: Movements of the sacro-iliac joints. *Acta Anatomica* 23:80–91, 1955.
391. Weisl H: The articular surfaces of the sacro-iliac joint and their relation to movements of the sacrum. *Acta Anatomica* 22(1)1–14, 1954.
392. Brunarski D: Sacroiliac concomitants of the iliolumbar syndrome: A case report. *Journal of the Canadian Chiropractic Association* 24:19–20, 1980.
393. Mennell JMcM: *Back Pain.* Boston, Little, Brown, 1960, pp 18, 27.
394. Stierwalt DD: *Fundamentals of Motion Palpation.* Davenport, Ia, published by the author, 1977, p 31.
395. Salter RB: *Textbook of Disorders and Injuries of the Musculoskeletal System.* Baltimore, Williams & Wilkins, 1981, pp 257–258.
396. Cyriax J: *Textbook of Orthopaedic Medicine,* Diagnosis of Soft Tissue Lesions, ed 8. London, Bailliere Tindall, 1982, vol 1, pp 297–300.
397. Helfet AJ, Gruebel Lee DM: *Disorders of the Lumbar Spine.* Philadelphia, J.B. Lippincott, 1978, p 24.
398. Taylor RG, Fowler WM Jr: Electrodiagnosis of musculoskeletal disorders. In D'Ambrosia RD (ed): *Musculoskeletal Disorders: Regional Examination and Differential Diagnosis.* Philadelphia, J.B. Lippincott, 1977, p 84.
399. Morris WT: Spinal nerve compression: A cause of claudication. *New Zealand Medical Journal* 88:101–103, 1978.
400. Helfet AJ, Gruebel Lee DM: *Disorders of the Lumbar Spine.* Philadelphia, J.B. Lippincott, 1978, pp 24–25.
401. Finneson BE: *Low Back Pain.* Philadelphia, J.B. Lippincott, 1973, p 326.
402. Mumenthaler M: *Neurology,* ed 2. Translated by EH Burrows. New York, Thieme-Stratton, 1983, p 432.
403. Finneson BE: *Low Back Pain.* Philadelphia, J.B. Lippincott, 1973, p 332.
404. Davis P, Lentle BC: Evidence for sacroiliac disease as a common cause of low backache in women. *Lancet* 2:496–497, 1978.
405. Grieve GP: *Common Vertebral Joint Problems.* New York, Churchill Livingstone, 1981, pp 279–295.
406. Normal GF: Sacroiliac disease and its relationship to lower abdominal pain. *American Journal of Surgery* 116:54–56, 1968.
407. Sashin D: A critical analysis of the anatomy and the pathologic changes of the sacroiliac joints. *Journal of Bone and Joint Surgery* vol 12, 1930.
408. Macnab I: *Backache.* Baltimore, Williams & Wilkins, 1977, pp 78–79.
409. Cohen AS, Cathcart ES, Brandt KD: Arthritis and connective tissue disorders. In Wilkins RW, Levinsky NG (eds): *Medicine: Essentials of Clinical Practice.* Boston, Little, Brown, 1978, 580–583.
410. Rudge SR et al: The clinical assessment of sacroiliac joint involvement in ankylosing spondy-

litis. *Rheumatology and Rehabilitation* 21:15–20, 1982.
411. Inman RD, Mani VJ: Subluxation of the sacroiliac joints in a black female with ankylosing spondylitis. *Journal of Rheumatology* 6:300–304, 1979.
412. Macnab I: *Backache.* Baltimore, Williams & Wilkins, 1977, pp 69–77.
413. Jacobs MD: Demonstration of Schober's test. *ACA Journal of Chiropractic* May 1984.
414. Tran T: Personal communication.
415. Macnab I: *Backache.* Baltimore, Williams & Wilkins, 1977, pp 77–78.
416. Weissman BN: HLA-B27 associated arthritis. In Feldman F (ed): *Radiology: Pathology, and Immunology of Bones and Joints: A Review of Current Concepts,* New York, Appleton-Century-Crofts, 1978, pp 114–115.
417. Jajic I: Gout in the spine and sacro-iliac joints: Radiological manifestations. *Skeletal Radiology* 8:209–212, 1982.
418. Makley JT, Cohen AM, Boada E: Sacral tumors: A hidden problem. *Orthopaedics* 5:996–1003, 1982.
419. Weissman BN: HLA-B27 associated arthritis. In Feldman F (ed): *Radiology, Pathology, and Immunology of Bones and Joints: A Review of Current Concepts,* New York, Appleton-Century-Crofts, 1978, pp 109–110.
420. Anonymous: Osteitis condensans ilii: Ortho-differential diagnosis. *Ortho Briefs.* ACA Council on Chiropractic Orthopedics, Fall 1982, p 4.
421. Nykoliation JW, Cassidy JD, Dupuis P: Osteitis condensans ilii. *Journal of the Canadian Chiropractic Association* 28:209–211, 1984.
422. Osteomyelitis of the pelvis: A diagnostic problem. *American Journal of Diseases of Children* 132:581–582, 1978.
423. Withesty DJ, Chillag SA: Seamstress's bottom. *American Family Physician* 19:85–88, 1979.

SUGGESTED READINGS

Adams MA, Hutton WC: The relevance of torsion to the mechanical derangement of the lumbar spine. *Spine* 6:241–248, 1981.

Bishop B: Pain: Its physiology and rationale for management. *Physical Therapy* 60:13–23, 1980.

Breathnach AS: *Frazer's Anatomy of the Human Skeleton,* ed 5. London, England, J & A Churchill, 1958.

Campbell JR: Gonstead analysis of pelvic biomechanics. In ACA Council on Technic: *Biomechanics of the Pelvis.* Denver Conference, June 17–20, 1980, Spears Chiropractic Hospital. Council on Technic of the American Chiropractic Association, 1982.

Cipriano JJ: *Photographic Manual of Regional Orthopaedic Tests.* Baltimore, Williams & Wilkins, 1985.

Coyle BA, Martinez DP (eds): *Proceedings of the Second Conference on Current Topics in Chiropractic: Reviews of the Literature,* May 4–5, 1985. Sunnyvale, Cal, Palmer College of Chiropractic—West, 1985.

Epstein MC: Causes of low back problems. *Digest of Chiropractic Economics* January/February 1983.

Evans BA, Stevens JC, Dyck PJ: Lumbosacral plexus neuropathy. *Neurology* 31:1327–1333, 1981.

Gardner E et al: *A Regional Study of Human Structure,* ed 4. Philadelphia, W.B. Saunders, 1975.

Grice AS: Radiographic, biomechanical, and clinical factors in lumbar lateral flexion. Part 1. *Journal of Manipulative and Physiological Therapeutics* March 1979.

Hollingshead WH, Jenkins DB: *Functional Anatomy of the Limbs and Back.* Philadelphia, W.B. Saunders, 1981.

Jacobs MD: Preventive spinal hygiene and the human machine. *ACA Journal of Chiropractic* August 1980.

Johnson J: Manipulative body mechanics therapy. *Journal of the American Osteopathic Association* vol 60, June 1961.

Kikuchi S et al: Anatomic and clinical studies of radicular symptoms. *Spine* 9:23–30, 1984.

Krupp MA, Chatton MJ, Werdegar D: *Current Medical Diagnosis and Treatment—1985.* Los Altos, Cal, Lange Medical, 1985.

Krupp MA et al: *Physician's Handbook,* ed 21. Los Altos, Cal, Lange Medical, 1985.

LeBars D, Chitour D: Do convergent neurones in the spinal dorsal horn discriminate nociceptive from non-nociceptive information? *Pain* 17:1–19, 1983.

LeVeau B: *Williams and Lissner: Biomechanics of Human Motion,* ed 2. Philadelphia, W.B. Saunders, 1977.

Markey WJ: The sacrum. *The Digest of Chiropractic Economics* July/August 1984.

Mazion JM: *Illustrated Manual of Neurological Reflexes/Signs/Tests; Orthopedic Signs/Tests/Maneuvers,* ed 2. Arizona City, published by the author, 1980.

Moore KL: *Clinically Oriented Anatomy.* Baltimore, Williams & Wilkins, 1980.

Nachemson AL: The load on lumbar discs in different positions of the body. *Clinical Orthopaedics* 45:107–122, 1966.

Pierce WV: Pelvic technique. *Digest of Chiropractic Economics* January/February 1983.

Sandoz R: Some physical mechanics and effects of spinal adjustments. *Annals of the Swiss Chiropractors' Association* 6:91–142, 1976.

Schafer RC (ed): *Basic Chiropractic Procedural Manual,* ed 4. Arlington, Va, American Chiropractic Association, 1984.

Shaak DL: Low back injuries. *Chiropractic Today* May/June 1985.

Triano JJ, Luttges MW: Nerve irritations: A possible model of sciatic neuritis. *Spine* 7:129–136, 1982.

Walmer HC: A comprehensive, nonsurgical approach to the low back problems. *Osteopathic Annals* 6:522–527, 1978.

Wyke B: Neurological mechanisms in the experience of pain. *Acupuncture and Electro-Therapeutics Research* 4:27–35, 1979.

CHAPTER 13

Scoliosis

In traditional medicine, scoliosis is commonly ignored until gross cosmetic effects or signs of structural destruction are witnessed. In chiropractic, however, even minor degrees of distortion should be considered at the time of spinal analysis because of their subtle biomechanical and neurologic consequences, and to halt potential progression at an early stage. To give a better appreciation of these points, this chapter describes the general structural, examination, and biomechanical concerns that should be considered, along with the highlights of conservative therapy.

GENERAL CONSIDERATIONS

The Spinal Curves[1-9]

A curved column has increased resistance to compression forces. This is just as true in the spine as for a rib or long bone.

Most authorities consider the spine to have four major curves: anteriorly convex curves at the cervical and lumbar areas and anteriorly concave curves at the thoracic and sacral levels. Cailliet considers the coccyx a curve, but this curve is usually considered an extension of the sacral curve. A few authorities consider the atlanto-occipital junction as a separate anteriorly convex curve. Regardless, the spinal curves offer the vertebral column increased inflexibility and shock-absorbing capability while still maintaining an adequate degree of stiffness and stability between vertebral segments (Fig. 13.1).

Structural vs Functional Curves

The adult thoracic and sacral anteriorly concave curves are firm *structural* arcs as the result of their vertebral bodies being shorter anteriorly than posteriorly. The normal kyphosis of the adult thoracic and sacral curves is quite similar to that of the fetal spine. This is not true for the anteriorly convex cervical and lumbar regions where the curves are essentially the result of their soft tissue wedge-shaped IVDs. It is for this reason that the cervical and lumbar curves readily flatten in the supine position, while the thoracic kyphosis reduces only a slight amount.

There is a clinical correlation of disc wedging to disc disease. Most disc lesions are found in the cervical and lumbar regions where the greatest degree of physiologic wedging occurs. This appears to be true in both hyperlordosis and an exceptionally flat cervical or lumbar curve.

Effect of Bipedism

An adult discless spine would resemble that of the newborn. Since animals that walk on four legs and infants prior to assuming the erect position do not have the physiologic curves of the erect adult, it can be assumed that these curves are the result of bipedism. In the erect position, the lower lumbar area is especially subjected to considerable shearing stress.[10, 11]

Overall Balance

Although the spine is often considered as the central pillar of the body, this is only true when the spine is viewed from the anterior or posterior aspect. When viewed laterally, the spine lies distinctly posterior to the thoracic body mass essentially because of the space-occupying heart (Fig. 13.2). It lies much more centrally in the cervical and lumbar regions. An abundance of body mass also lies anterior to the midline in the head, which must be held by erector and check ligament strength if a thoracic "hump" or a flattened cervical curve are to be avoided.

From a balance standpoint, the 7 cervical vertebrae and the 5 lumbar vertebrae arc anteriorly from the central gravity line to compensate for the 12 thoracic vertebrae curved posteriorly from the gravity line. The female spine, below the age of 40 years, arcs

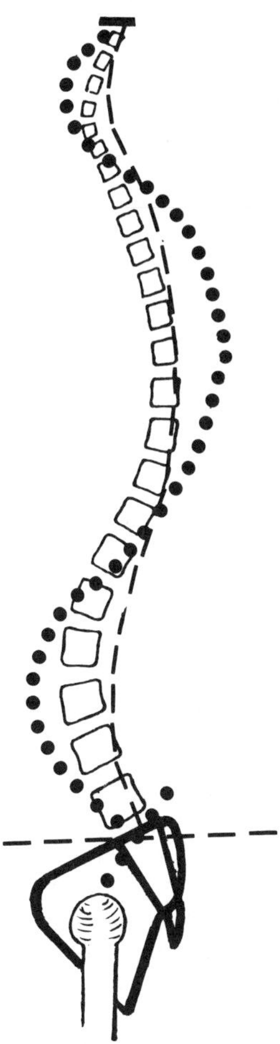

Figure 13.1. Curves of the spine, as viewed from the lateral: normal spine (*squares*), lordosis-kyphosis (*dots*) from increased angles, and "flat back" (*dashes*) from decreased angles.

less than that of the male, and the thoracic arc increases with age regardless of gender.

The extent of deviation from the midline of the cervical and lumbar curves is controlled to a great extent by the strength of the antigravity extensors, the weakness of the flexors, and the ability of the flexors to stretch. Keep in mind that the fetus is curved like a crescent. When the infant gains the erect position, the anterior lumbar curve and pelvic tilt are governed essentially by the strength of the lumbar-pelvic erectors and how far the iliopsoas and iliacus will elongate.

The Base Effect

The greater the S1 or T1 angles, the sharper the lumbar or cervical curves must

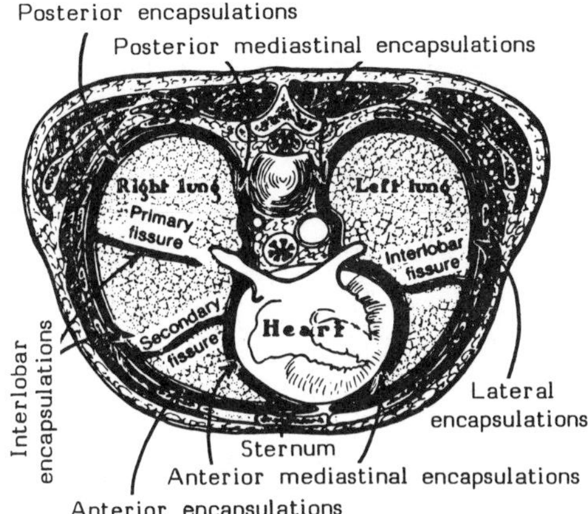

Figure 13.2. Transverse section of the chest showing the relationship of the thoracic viscera and their encapsulations to the spine.

be to bring the spine back toward the center of gravity. Thus, the sacral angle and wedge shape of the L5 disc determine the angles of the lower lumbars and the compensatory upper lumbar angles, and the T1 plane and shape of its disc generally control the cervical curve. Ideally, this base effect would progress up the spine from the sacrum so that the odontoid process would be in line with the gravity line. However, because the thoracic area allows minimum mobility to the anterior or posterior, considerable stress is placed at the L1–T12 and T1–C7 junctions.

Spinal Stability[12–17]

The stability of the spine depends upon a number of factors, but essentially it is maintained by the relationship of the vertical gravity line to the segments. When weight is in balance to the gravity line, muscular activity is minimal. When in a chronic unbalanced state, fatigue and structural deformity are induced (Fig. 13.3). This is readily brought out when vertebral asymmetry horizontally or a short leg produces a lateral tilt that must be compensated by scoliosis. In short time, the muscles on the concave side of the curve become fatigued, the vertebral bodies rotate toward the side of convexity, and the spinous processes rotate toward the side of concavity.

Head and trunk weight is fairly balanced in the frontal plane where the gravity line passes posterior to most of the centers of

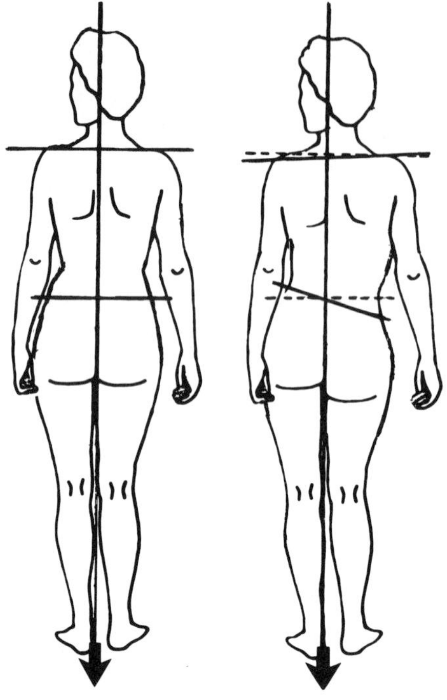

Figure 13.3. *Left*, good spinal alignment, in which the gravity line bisects the spinal column and a horizontal line drawn across the sacral base. *Right*, lateral pelvic tilt from a unilateral short leg, in which the lumbar spine must adapt to the sacral obliquity to return the spine to the midline.

the cervical vertebral bodies, through the bodies at the cervicothoracic junction, anterior to the thoracic body centers, through the bodies at the thoracolumbar junction, and posterior to most of the lumbar body centers.

Because body mass is heavier anteriorly in the thoracic region, the thoracic curvature must arc posteriorly in compensation. This compensatory kyphosis is limited by restricted A-P thoracic motion and the posterior ligament straps. As muscles fatigue rapidly, the erectors have little influence. Most severe thoracic kyphoses result from collapse of the anterior vertebral bodies.

Since the lumbar spine carries more weight than any other region of the spine, it is the responsibility of this area to make major adjustments to load shifts from the gravity line. For example, thoracic kyphosis shifts the line anteriorly so that the lumbar area must increase its lordosis to prevent the body from falling forward. In this regard, the lumbar effect is secondary to the thoracic kyphosis. A similar effect is seen in late stages of pregnancy when a temporary increase in lumbar lordosis develops in adjustment to the increased anterior body mass. On the other hand, any condition that would tend to shift the center of gravity posteriorly would tend to flatten the lumbar curve.

These adjustments are in addition to the adjustments the lumbar vertebrae must make to the normally anteroinferior slant of the sacrum. As the sacrum is usually more oblique in females than in males, due to different pelvic design, lumbar compensations will usually be more pronounced in females.

Terms and Definitions[18–22]

The term scoliosis refers to any combination of lateral curvature from a straight line with twisting of the spine when viewed from the front or the back. *What is grossly viewed in the typical scoliosis from the posterior are the typical spinal curves normally seen from the lateral.* That is, the curves are situated in the wrong plane, frontal rather than sagittal, and the vertical axis rotation is usually in the wrong direction and often exaggerated.[23] Simply, it is often as if the spine were fixed in space and the head and pelvis were rotated ±90° in the same direction (Fig. 13.4). Thus the majority of the distortion seen in scoliosis is the result of rotation. This is the gross effect of scoliosis. The segmental effect is abnormal focal motion-unit disrelationship in which normal rotation, lateral tilting, and A-P facet slip has become fixed, functionally and/or structurally.

Scoliosis is a mechanical disorder when gross, but there are always many biologic influences operating as well as purely mechanical forces. When relatively straight, the spine behaves much like a column. When deformed, it becomes subject to bending loads and behaves more like a bending beam than it does a column. In either case, however, and unlike engineered columns of uniform size and homogenous materials, the effects of spinal loading on a biped are much more complex to understand or to predict by the laws of physics.

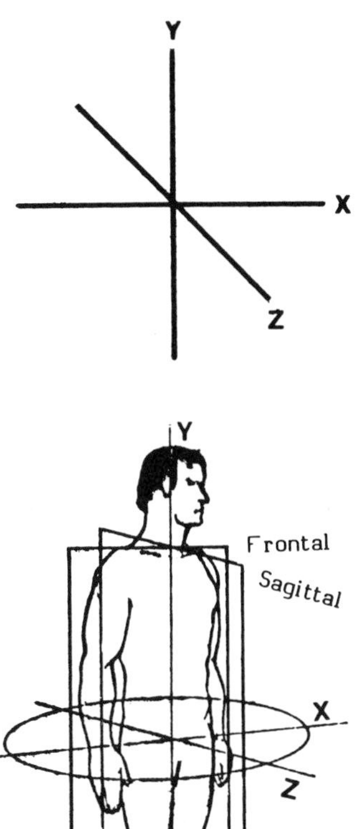

Figure 13.4. The *X*, *Y*, and *Z* planes of the body.

To appreciate the biomechanics involved, an understanding of what comprises good body balance is necessary. This has been discussed in Chapter 4 under the subjects of body alignment, posture, and gait. Our concern here will be those factors that have special importance to the thorax; especially its weight-bearing structure, the thoracic spine.

Clinical Evaluation[24–27]

When a postural distortion is recognized, several clinical questions arise. For example, how severe is the distortion? Is it affecting function? Is the distortion stabilized or progressing? What was the initial cause or causes—congenital, pathologic, acquired, or a combination of factors? Can it be corrected? If so, how? How much correction can be expected? How long will it take? How much patient cooperation will be necessary?

The first step in answering these questions is a thorough postural examination. In slight or doubtful cases, the tips of the spinous processes should be marked with a marking pencil which makes the deviation more readily visible. It is assumed here that the postural analysis will follow a complete case history and standard physical, neurologic, and orthopedic examinations. Joint motion, muscle strength, sensation, and reflexes must be evaluated (see Figs. 13.5 and 13.6).

While not absolutely necessary in all cases, such instruments as a plumb line or grid with a footplate, a measuring tape, a posturometer device, electromyography, contourography, and bilateral or quadrant weight scales offer a distinct advantage in recording changes during analysis and therapy. If pathologic structural changes have occurred, radiographic analysis is a must.

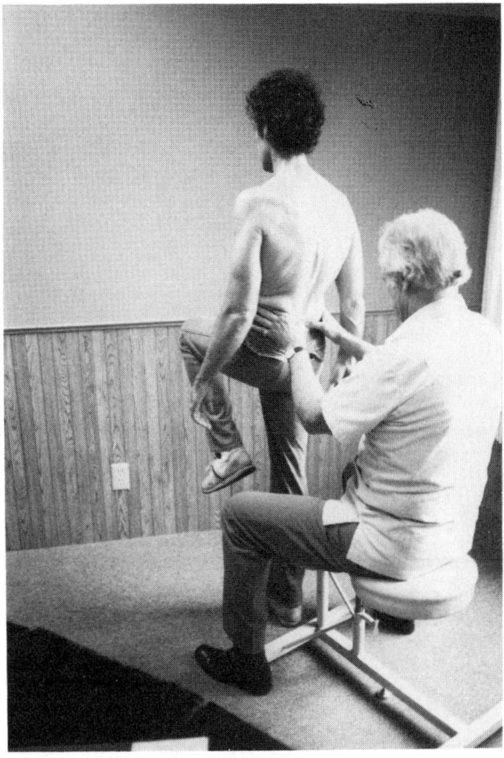

Figure 13.5. Motion palpation of the sacroiliac joints. (Courtesy of the Motion Palpation Institute.)

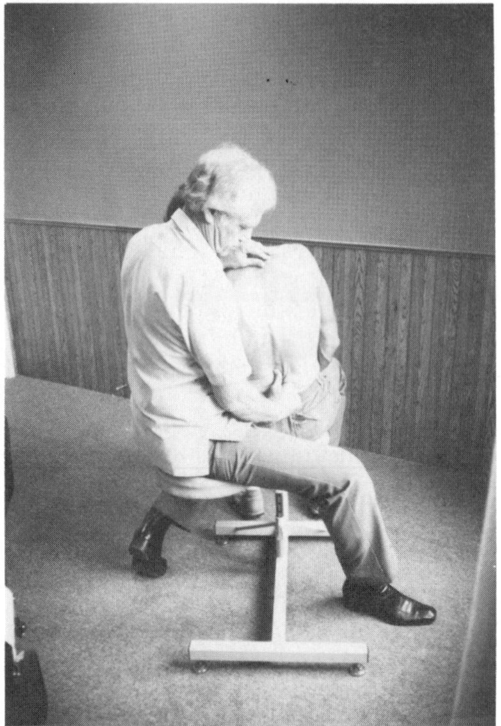

Figure 13.6. Motion palpation of L3 during lateral flexion to the left. (Courtesy of the Motion Palpation Institute.)

Regardless, analysis must be made in all positions of movement as well as in the erect position (ie, flexion, extension, lateral bending, and rotation). Only by such comparisons will inequalities and the effects of other abnormalities be properly observed.

It is impossible to accurately analyze posture through street clothes or the typical female patient gown. If some type of clothing is necessary, it should be similar to a close-fitting nonrestrictive leotard. Unlevel shoulders, belt level, skirt hem length, clothing creases, abnormally worn shoe heels, etc, are screening clues that are often deceiving.

As an aid to differential diagnosis, common posterior thoracic pain syndromes are listed in Table 13.1 and the major trigger points causing posterior thoracic pain are shown in Table 13.2.[28]

Good Posture: What Is It?[29–31]

Postural faults are probably more obvious in the thorax than in other regions. Yet, while poor posture is readily recognized, good posture is difficult to define. Most people think of good posture in the erect position as one in which the overall body is in good balance, the head is held erect, the shoulders are drawn back, the spinal curves are not exaggerated, the abdomen is relatively flat, and movements can be initiated with ease.[32] Note that this common observation fails to consider the lower extremities which are the foundation of body balance.

The picture gets confused when we realize the large variety of subdivisions among "normal" body types. A minority of us have the body type depicted by the models used in "good posture" examples. We are not all lean mesomorphs of an "average" height and weight, nor do we all have occupations that require equal bilateral activity. Add to this the fact that righting and antalgic reflexes do not act upon each body in an identical manner.

For the sake of establishing a basis for discussion, the following definition from a clinical biomechanical standpoint is offered:

> Good posture, in any position, is that physical attitude that allows the segments of the body to be in good biomechanical alignment to cope with gravitational and acceleration forces and one which optimally protects against injury or deformity and allows optimal function.

Types of Curves and Their Terminology[33–40]

A great variety of terms are used in describing the various types of spinal distortion. In each case, however, scoliosis is described as if viewed from the posterior, and exaggerated A-P curves are described as if seen from the side.

Scoliosis. Originally, the term scoliosis meant any abnormal deviation of the spine from the midline, but for many years the term has been restricted to lateral deviation when viewed from the anterior or posterior (Fig. 13.7). As the cervical and lumbar curves are normally lordotic and the thoracic curve is normally kyphotic, the terms for exaggeration of these curves are best referred to as hyperlordosis and hyperkyphosis. Even minor scolioses become apparent in the Adams position (Fig. 13.8).

Direction. Abnormal spinal curves can

Table 13.1.
Posterior Thoracic Pain and Associated Symptoms

Syndrome: posterior thoracic pain +	Primary suspect disorders	
Hematuria	Kidney stone	Pyelonephritis
Neurologic focal signs	Multiple myeloma Spinal cord tumor Spinal tuberculosis	Subluxation complex Vertebral fracture
Pain, local	Aortic aneurysm Carcinoma Multiple myeloma Osteoarthritis	Scoliosis Spinal tuberculosis Spondylitis Sprain/strain
Pain, radiating	Costovertebral subluxation IVD syndrome Pyelonephritis	Radiculitis Rib fracture Spinal cord tumor Trigger point
Pain, upper abdominal	Cholecystitis Duodenal ulcer Gastric ulcer	Hiatal hernia Pancreatic carcinoma Pancreatitis
Pyrexia	Epidural abscess Hodgkin's disease Meningitis Osteomyelitis	Perinephric abscess Poliomyelitis Retrocecal appendicitis Tuberculosis

Table 13.2.
Major Trigger Points Causing Posterior Thoracic Pain

Area of perceived pain	Primary suspect muscles	
Low thoracic area	Iliocostalis thoracis Longissimus thoracis Multifidi	Rectus abdominis Serratus posterior inferior
Middle thoracic area	Iliocostalis thoracis Infraspinatus Latissimus dorsi Levator scapulae Multifidi	Rhomboids Scaleni Serratus anterior Serratus posterior superior Trapezius
Upper thoracic area	Levator scapulae Multifidi Rhomboids	Scaleni Supraspinatus Trapezius

be described according to the direction of the *convexity* of the curve from the midline, such as a right thoracic curve or a left lumbar curve.

Location. Curves can be described according to their anatomical region. Examples are cervical, cervicothoracic, thoracic, thoracolumbar, and lumbar types.

Flexibility or Stiffness Factor. A curve that is corrected by active or passive bending toward the side of convexity is considered a *nonstructural curve*. If the curve remains fixed, it is termed a *structural curve*.

Complexity. Curvatures can be described relative to their number. A *simple curve* is a single "C" curve. A *compound curve* consists of two or more curves that displace to both the right and the left of the vertical axis (eg, an "S" curve).

Etiology. The *primary curve* of a scoliosis is that curve which develops first. It is usually singular but may be double in cases of spinal trauma or the effect of multiple lesions. A *secondary curve*, invariably a compensatory curve to maintain equilibrium, is a curve that develops after the primary curve is established.

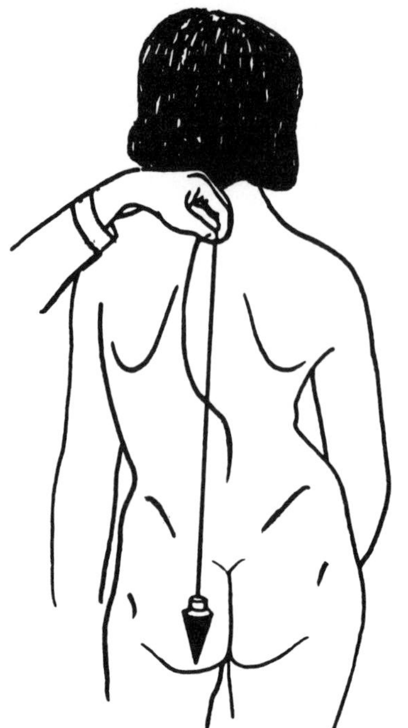

Figure 13.7. Diagram of a left thoracic scoliosis with a plumb dropped from the C7 spinous process. Weight shift can be noted by the plumb line striking the left buttock.

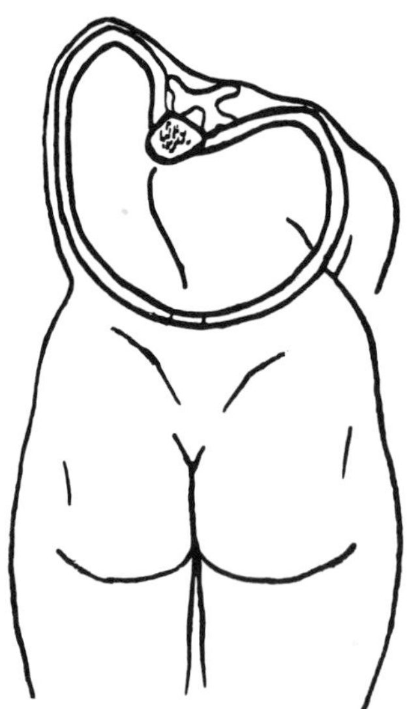

Figure 13.8. Diagram of the same patient shown in Figure 13.7 in the Adams position. Note how the left dorsal curve and rib hump become accentuated.

Various types of scolioses are often referred to by their primary etiology. Several examples are shown in Table 13.3.[41–43]

Biochemical, immunologic, and hormonal imbalances appear to be factors in the development of early scoliosis, especially the secondary congenital varieties.[44] For example, congenital scoliosis has been shown to be an effect within fetal alcohol syndrome[45] and arthrogryposis multiplex congenita[46]. Patients with congenital scoliosis or metastatic lesions of the spine have been found to have a level of cold agglutinins that is 250–1000 times greater than that in the general population.[47] Collagen abnormalities appear to play a role in the etiology of both congenital and idiopathic scoliosis.[48,49] A study of Chinese girls (aged 12–20 years) suggested that girls with idiopathic adolescent scoliosis mature more rapidly in secondary sexual characteristics and bone growth during early adolescence (12–14 years), but their rate of maturity slows down in late adolescence (16–20 years).[50] The studies of Yarom and associates suggest that a calcium-related neuromuscular defect could be an important factor in the genesis of idiopathic scoliosis.[51]

Severity. Curves can be described according to the degree of deviation from the midline. The *major curve* is the one of two or more curves that curves the most from the midline. It is the site of major structural changes, and is usually but not always the primary curve. A major curve usually has compensatory secondary adaptations directed in the opposite direction in the spine or occiput above and in the spine or pelvis below the major curve. In chronic states, there may be more than one major curve; that is, a secondary curve exhibiting equal severity and structural damage. These *double major curves* are sometimes erroneously labeled double primary curves.

Equilibrium. Whenever the occiput is sited over the sacrum, the curvature is considered *compensated* regardless of the deviations between. If the head is lateral to the midline, the curvature is considered *decompensated* (Fig. 13.9). A decompensated curvature indicates structural changes that prohibit weight redistribution to maintain equilibrium, an antalgic position, or a defect in

Table 13.3.
Scolioses Related to Their Cause

Type	Cause
Cicatrical scoliosis	Necrosis
Compensatory scoliosis	Adaptation, usually to a pelvic tilt
Congenital scoliosis	Defective embryonic development
Coxitic scoliosis	Hip disease producing a pelvic tilt
Empyematic scoliosis	Ipsilateral pyemic retraction of thorax
Habit scoliosis	Habitually distorted posture
Hysterical scoliosis	Psychoneurosis
Inflammatory scoliosis	Vertebral or paravertebral inflammation
Ischiatic scoliosis	Hip disease
Myopathic scoliosis	Weakened spinal muscles
Ocular scoliosis	Visual defect producing habitual head tilt
Ophthalmic scoliosis	Visual defect producing habitual head tilt; ocular
Osteopathic scoliosis	Weakened spinal muscles; myopathic
Paralytic scoliosis	Paralyzed spinal muscles
Postural scoliosis	Habitually distorted posture
Rachitic scoliosis	Rickets
Rheumatic scoliosis	Thoracic spinal muscle rheumatism
Sciatic scoliosis	Sciatica
Static scoliosis	Unequal femur height
Traumatic scoliosis	Fracture, surgery, burns, irradiation, etc

the righting mechanism. These structural changes usually begin as muscular mechanisms that progress to degenerative fibrotic and osseous changes.

Pathologic vs Functional Hyperkyphosis. Any gross backward convexity of the spine, if sharply angular, suggests Pott's disease. If the curve is gentle and gradual, it may be due to postural "round shoulders," to hypertrophic arthritis, to emphysema, Paget's disease, or rickets. The rachitic curve is flaccid, simply from muscle weakness, and associated with other evidences of rickets. In emphysema and Paget's disease, the kyphosis goes with the other signs of these diseases. In hypertrophic arthritis, the curve is rigid, irreducible, and usually painless. "Round shoulders" can be straightened by muscular effort and represents a postural habit. In addition to the above, the possibility of neoplastic lesions, spondylitis, osteochondrosis of the vertebral epiphyses (Scheuermann's disease), or an old compression fracture should not be overlooked.

In their study of right thoracic idiopathic scoliosis, DeSmet and associates[52] found that the degree of scoliosis did not correlate with the degree of thoracic kyphosis present. They also found that the apex of the scoliosis was at or below the apex of the thoracic kyphosis in 30 of the 31 female patients studied, and that the degree of displacement of the apical vertebrae had a positive correlation ($r = 0.732$) with the degree of scoliosis.

Hyperlordosis. An exaggeration of the normal forward convexity of the lumbar spine may extend to or be compensated by the thoracic region. It is seen in disc trauma, tuberculosis of the spine, paralysis of the dorsal or abdominal muscles (especially muscular dystrophy), hip disorders, anterior sacral tilting, genu recurvatum, and gastrocnemius weakness, and with abdominal tumors and pregnancy that require counterbalancing by backward bending.

Prominent Scapulae. This condition is usually due to (1) lateral curvature of the spine or (2) serratus paralysis, recognized by the startling prominence of the scapula if the patient pushes forward with both hands against resistance, resulting in a condition called "angel-wing" scapula. In congenital syphilis, the median or vertebral border of the scapula is sometimes markedly concave and called a scaphoid scapula.[53]

Types of Scoliosis Classifications

Scoliosis can be classified from a structural, functional, or clinical viewpoint. In

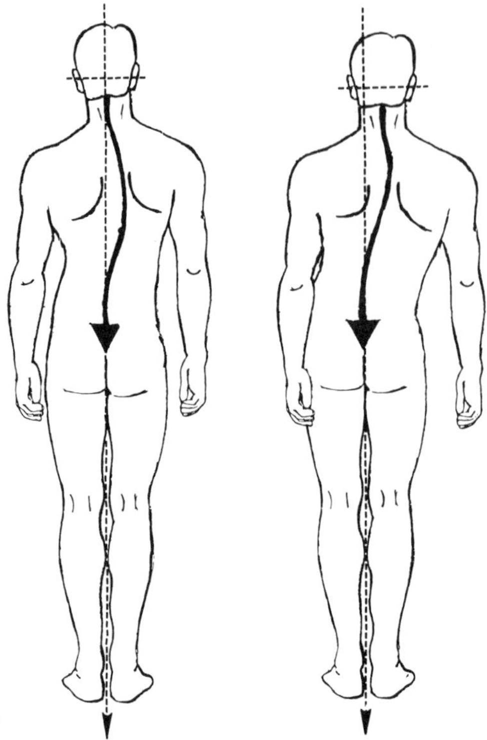

Figure 13.9. Compensated scoliosis shown on *left*, with the occipital protuberance directly above the sacral processes. Decompensated scoliosis shown on *right*, in which poor equilibrium is exhibited by the occipital protuberance located lateral to the midline. A deviation of an inch or more places considerable stress on the contralateral thoracic soft tissues to prevent toppling.

each classification, there is considerable overlapping and no single classification offers answers to all questions. However, we will briefly mention these so that a better appreciation can be developed.

Structural Classification of Scoliosis[54–63]

Scoliosis can be classified into two major structural types (structural and nonstructural), and each has its subdivisions according to its major etiology.

Nonstructural Scoliosis. A nonstructural scoliosis is the effect of gravitational forces on muscles and ligaments of asymmetrical integrity. It will straighten by voluntary effort or in the non-weight-bearing positions. Nonstructural (functional) scolioses are not usually as progressive as structural scolioses.

Nonstructural scoliosis can be of the postural, compensatory, or transient type. *Postural scoliosis* curves are slight, disappear in the Adams and recumbent positions, and usually are first noticed at about 12 years of age. *Compensatory scoliosis* is the typical result of a leg length defect in which the pelvis dips down on the short side. *Transient structural scoliosis* may be of the sciatic, hysterical, or inflammatory type. *Sciatic scoliosis* is not a true scoliosis, but rather a functional antaglic adaptation to pain caused by nerve root pressure or irritation. *Hysterical scoliosis*, most rare, is a manifestation of organ language of psychic origin. *Inflammatory scoliosis* is the result of such processes as a perinephric (eg, psoas) abscess.

Structural Scoliosis. A structural scoliosis will not straighten with voluntary effort in a non-weight-bearing position. It is quite rigid and the result of osseous deformation or fixated soft-tissue changes of related discs, ligaments, muscles, and joint capsules. Structural scoliosis may be of the idiopathic, congenital, neuromuscular, neurofibromatotic, mesenchymal, or traumatic type. Its most common overt sign is a lack of adequate compensatory secondary curvatures; that is, decompensation, in which the head and neck are lateral to the base of support when viewed from the posterior or anterior.

There are two major types of structural curves:

1. Irreversible structural curves that exhibit gross structural asymmetry and/or anomalies. Deformation can be exhibited between, within, and/or around vertebrae. When this occurs, there are two problems: (a) the spinal curves are "out of plane" and (b) there is vertebral motion-unit deformation. The immediate structural defect may be osseous, in the soft tissues, or both.
2. Structural curves that are the result of possible reversible connective tissue changes such as ligament shortening or chronic muscular hypertonicity. This type is usually the first stage of the first type. It is not unusual for a curve to exhibit some degree of functional reduction but not complete reduction; that is, it may be both functional and structural.

Features. Certain generalities can be drawn bilaterally as scoliosis progresses:

1. On the side of concavity, the vertebral bodies rotate anteriorly, the ribs are closer together and projected backward, the intercostal spaces are reduced and the soft tissues are thickened and contracted, the disc spaces are thinned (wedged) and the nucleus shifts toward the opposite side, the vertebral pedicles and laminae shorten and thicken, and the flank rib-ilium distance is reduced.

2. On the side of convexity, the vertebral bodies rotate posteriorly, the ribs are further apart and projected anteriorly, the intercostal spaces are widened and the soft tissues are stretched, the disc spaces are widened, the vertebral canal becomes narrowed, the flank rib-ilium distance is increased, and the intrathoracic viscera become compressed.

Differentiation. The degree of nonstructural scoliosis superimposed upon structural changes can be evaluated by films taken in the standing position and compared to those taken in horizontal traction or hanging traction. However, this will *not* differentiate irreversible changes from areas of possibly reversible fixation.

Prognosis. A fairly accurate prognosis can be made if the natural course of the curve has been followed. However, this is rarely the case, because the typical patient usually seeks professional help only when symptoms appear, the postural defect becomes a social concern, or trauma is superimposed on the disorder. Each patient is an individual who presents many variables. Progression may be fast, slow, and/or intermittent. Related visceral dysfunction varies from mild to severe.[64]

In general, decompensated single major curves are more likely to lead to severe deformity than compensated double major curves. Right thoracic or thoracolumbar major curves appear to be more deforming than left curves, but this is just a statistical conclusion.

Signs of osteoporosis near the apical vertebra and severely thinned, wedged apical IVDs indicate that the problem is severe. Turek feels that a translatory shift in the thoracolumbar transitional area indicates ligament relaxation. When these signs are present, progression to deformity is likely unless immediate corrective care is instituted.

Clinical Classification of Scoliosis[23, 56, 57, 59, 62, 65–69]

A more detailed classification of spinal distortions is appropriate for many clinicians. One is offered in Table 13.4 that has been adapted from data of the Scoliosis Research Society, White and Panjabi, Rothman and Simeone, Cailliet, Keim, Barge, and others.

Idiopathic scoliosis constitutes 70–90% of scoliotic cases, depending upon what reference is used. The term "idiopathic" is not often correct because much of the etiology of such cases can be speculated with considerable accuracy. Because the term is in such general use, we use it reluctantly in those cases where specific pathology is not evident, and hope the reader will do likewise.

Incidence, Prevalence, and Course of Scoliosis[70–72]

Reports of the incidence of scoliosis vary considerably. This is probably due to poor standardization of the criteria, technique, or procedures used. Lonstein and associates report that scoliosis was found in 1.2% of 225,000 school children examined.[73] Willner reported a 2.8% occurrence of a scoliosis measuring 5° or more in children between the ages of 7 and 16 years.[74] During the screening of 10-year-old school children by Willner, positive moire findings were exhibited in 13% of the boys and 16% of the girls.[75,76]

Rogala and associates found a 4.5% incidence of adolescent idiopathic scoliosis in adolescent students.[77] They also reported that a two-year follow-up study showed progression in 6.8% of the students and in 15.4% of skeletally immature girls with a curve of more than 10° at the initial examination. In 20% of the skeletally immature children with curves of 20° at the initial examination, there was no progression. Spontaneous improvement occurred in 3% and was seen more frequently in children with curves of less than 11°.

Bjerkreim and Hassan found that the curves in untreated idiopathic scoliotics in-

Table 13.4.
Clinical Classification of Spinal Deformity

Idiopathic scoliosis

Infantile: Present at birth or before the age of 3 years. An environmental factor is thought to be involved. In over 85% of cases, the curves resolve spontaneously without therapy. Most cases are of a left thoracic scoliosis and are more common in males.

Juvenile: Onset occurs after 3 years but before puberty. Most cases are right thoracic, first recognized at the age of 6 years, and involve males and females equally. They rarely resolve spontaneously, leading to severe deformity if not treated early.

Adolescent: Onset occurs after puberty. A hereditary-familial factor is thought to be involved. Most cases involve a right thoracic structural curve that is progressive, and 85% of cases are females.

Adult: Onset occurs after maturity. A neuromuscular factor is believed to be responsible. Most cases are essentially nonstructural with a large degree of soft-tissue fixation that can be resolved.

Congenital spine deformity

Congenital scoliosis may be of the extravertebral (eg, congenital rib fusions) or vertebral type. The vertebral type may be open and characterized by a posterior spinal defect with a neurologic deficit (eg, myelomeningocele) or without a neurologic deficit (eg, spina bifida occulta); or it may be closed and characterized by no posterior spinal defect with a neurologic deficit (eg, diastematomyelia with spina bifida) or without a neurologic deficit (eg, hemivertebra).

Abnormal bone development: Examples are congenital scoliosis from failure of bone formation, segmentation, or symmetry; Klippel-Feil syndrome; Sprengel's deformity; congenital kyphosis; or congenital lordosis.

Abnormal spinal cord development: Examples are myelodysplasic scoliosis, kyphosis, or lordosis.

Osseous defects associated with neurologic defects: Examples are meningocele, myelomeningocele, and spinal dysraphism.

Neuromuscular

Neuropathic: Examples are distortions as the result of upper motor neuron lesions (eg, cerebral palsy, cord trauma, CNS tumor, syringomyelia) or lower motor lesions (eg, trauma, viral infections, various trophic diseases).

Myopathic: Examples are those types of muscle disorders seen in lumbopelvic malpositions, short-leg syndromes, torticollis, postural syndromes, muscular dystrophy, hypotonic states, amyotonia, visual disturbances, etc. Myopathic forms may be either of the progressive type (eg, muscular dystrophy) or static type (eg, amyotonia congenita).

Psychogenic: Such as seen in hysteria and conversion syndromes.

Miscellaneous: Examples are Friedreich's ataxia and unilateral amelia.

Scoliosis associated with neurofibromatosis

This infrequent familial condition is associated with developmental changes in nerves, muscles, bones, and skin, and marked by the development of tumors of peripheral nerves due to the abnormal proliferation of Schwann cells. It is frequently related to spinal distortion and is often called von Recklinghausen's disease when cafe-au-lait skin pigmentations with smooth borders and severe progressing kyphosis and scoliosis are associated.

Mesenchymal disorders

These rare cases involve either congenital or acquired mesenchymal disorders. Congenital varieties include origin in Marfan's syndrome, Morquio's syndrome, Ehlers-Danlos syndrome, homocystinuria, amyoplasia congenita, and various types of dwarfism. Acquired mesenchymal scoliosis is seen with rheumatoid arthritis and Still's disease. Other forms are seen with Scheuermann's disease and osteogenesis imperfecta.

Trauma

Vertebral: Examples are distortions resulting from fracture, improper dislocation reduction, burn scars (radiologic, thermal, chemical), post-traumatic fibrosis and contractures, or surgery.

Extravertebral: Examples are the same.

Secondary to irritative phenomena

Examples in this classification include such disorders as nerve root or peripheral irritations, noxious viscerosomatic or somatosomatic reflexes, spinal cord tumors, vertebral tumors, bone or renal infection.

Others

Within this miscellaneous classification are placed those distortions that have an endocrine, metabolic, or nutritional etiology such as rickets, osteomalacia, and gout.

creased 3° per year before 20 years of age and 1° per year after this age. Curves below 40° increased significantly less than did the larger curves, and curves of 60–80° increased the most.[78] Single curves increased significantly more than double curves. It was concluded that surgery should be recommended only for adolescent patients with thoracic or thoracolumbar single curves larger than 40°. In congenital scoliosis, however, the rate of deterioration and the ultimate severity of untreated curves are far greater and usually require surgical intervention.[79]

While the incidence was similar, Jackson and associates report that the clinical course of back pain in adults without spinal deformity and in scoliotics was different: 64% improvement in adults without scoliosis vs 83% persistence and progression in adults with scoliosis.[80] Of the adult scoliotics, 51% had significant pain, and the pain increased with age and the degree of scoliotic curvature.

In a study of the elderly, Robin and associates[81] found no direct relationship between the presence or progression of scoliosis and osteoporosis. Nor was there a direct relationship between scoliosis and low-back pain or between scoliosis and degenerative changes in the spine.

Evaluative Procedures

Various visual, palpatory, and roentgenographic features of spinal analysis have been described in several previous chapters of this book. In this section, some of these points will be highlighted and a few additional procedures will be described that are especially pertinent to the clinical evaluation of scoliosis when correlated.

Inspection, Palpation, and Mensuration

Careful inspection should be conducted in the standing and Adams positions. A grid, quadrant weight scales, and/or other types of instrumentation are helpful in gaining objective data. Connoly and Michael[82] report that a relationship exists between the convex side of a scoliotic curvature and the side of a positive asymmetrical tonic neck reflex, regardless of the gender of the patient.

Moire Topography

During school screening of structural scoliosis, Laulund and associates[83] found that moire topography revealed twice as many cases of scoliosis as did conventional clinical screening procedures, even though the method revealed many false positive results. Similar benefits have been reported by Willner.[74–76]

Electromyography

A comparatively higher EMG signal amplitude has been found on the convex side of a scoliosis, which was due to a lower amplitude on the concave side when the scoliosis group was compared to a control group.[84] The amplitude difference was correlated to the degree of scoliosis. A shift in the myoelectric spectrum toward the lower frequencies occurred during loading. There were no differences in this respect between the sides of the scoliosis, nor were there differences between the scoliotic patients and the controls. Secondary adaptation to the higher load demand by the muscles on the convex side in scoliosis appeared to explain the findings.

A study by Reuber and associates also suggested that the asymmetries in muscle actions evidenced by myoelectric measurements were the result of scoliosis. Scoliosis progression does not appear to be caused by asymmetry in muscle contractions; rather, it may be caused by a lack of adequate asymmetry.[85]

Roentgenography

Various systems used in the roentgenographic measurement of scoliotic curves will be described later in this chapter.

Tomography

Tomography provides a method to describe the relationship between the rib hump, the longitudinal axis rotation, the lateral curve, and the kyphosis-lordosis using exceedingly small radiation doses. In a study by Aaro and Dahlborn, vertebral rotation was found to be correlated to the lateral curve but not to the location or the length of the curve.[86] The longitudinal axis rotation of the vertebrae seems to be the most important factor for the development of the rib hump, which is accentuated further by an increased lordosis. With computerized tomography, the spine can be mathematically reconstructed and a scoliotic angle accurately calculated—thus providing an efficient method to evaluate the true shape of the curve.[87]

Computerized spinal analysis utilizing a tomographic top view was found by DeSmet and associates to be an excellent serial method to evaluate scoliotic progression.[88]

SELECTED CLINICAL APPROACHES: SOME OLD, SOME NEW

Thoughts of Willard Carver[89, 90]

During the early years of chiropractic, Willard Carver laid down several basic principles about the management of spinal distortions that are still worthy to note. Following are a few points selected from his 1921 texts that are pertinent to spinal fixations and scoliosis. Although the passages have been summarized, an attempt has been made to retain the author's unique style.

1. *Disrelationship vs displacement concepts.* Disrelation has generally been conceived and expressed by the word "displacement." This has given room for a certain amount of error. Displacement in its basic conception leads the mind to fix upon a *place* from which something has been forcibly ejected, and in a certain abstract sense this is not wholly true of disrelationship. A structure may be responding to the impulsion of force, but not be performing in harmony with the law of its being, and therefore be out of relationship with parts with which it should be related; this situation has too frequently been called, "being out of place" or "displaced." The first error, then, in the use of the word "displacement," comes from the fact that *place* applied to a moving structure is hardly a correct term. A moving structure occupies a relationship, and in that sense a place. Therefore, when it is out of relationship, it should be said to be *disrelated* instead of *displaced*. A vertebra has no place per se, any more than a cell in the biceps has (when the arm is in motion). The vertebra only has place in contemplation of its relationship to its fellows and relative tissues. If it occupies its exact relationship to all such structures (ie, cartilages, ligaments, arteries, veins, lymph vessels, lymph glands, etc), we say it is in place, but we realize that we only mean that it is *in relationship*. "Displacement of a vertebra," then, as it is frequently spoken of in chiropractic terminology, does not mean the removal of the vertebra from a certain place, but it means the change of relationship of the vertebra to its relative structures. It will be seen that the disrelationship of a vertebra is not a trifling matter of local consideration, but presents for consideration a local disrelationship and a disrelating influence that acts upon and produces adverse results of the distortion type in the whole organism.

2. *The scoliotic key.* This is one or two vertebrae (in a great majority of cases only one) that have failed to rotate in harmony with the other vertebrae of a scoliosis. The apical vertebra, which fails to rotate in ratio with its fellows, acts as a keystone in an arch to the scoliosis, preventing reduction of the scoliosis. Before application can be made to the scoliosis for its reduction, the key must be reduced. To reduce a scoliotic key, no force is permitted to go deeply into the body. The application is short, sharp, and quick, and does not project weight upon the body—for it must be remembered that the thrust is being accomplished in a scoliosis, and the only object is to secure the release of a key-like effect by opening a gap, which only requires that the body of the vertebra shall move definitely a short distance.

3. *The lordotic key.* This is found in a lordosis in which the most ventral vertebra forms the bottom of a curve so definite that by approximation of the contiguous vertebrae it forms a keystone, as it were, to the lordotic arch, preventing elevation of the lordosis. The complexity in this relation results from the fact that no force can be applied to a lordotic area, except in such way as to secure a muscular opponent recoil that has the effect of raising the lordosis. It will be plainly seen that a lordosis presents to the operator a situation not dissimilar to a bow definitely strung. The office of the operator is to release the string, not so that the two ends of the bow may fly back leaving the bow straight, but so that the

middle of the bow may be brought dorsally into proper relationship with its two ends. The adjuster's force, therefore, must be applied so that it will go into the opponent musculature headwardly and feetwardly in such a definite way as to result in an instantaneous recoil from both, centering dorsalward under the ventral aspect of the keyed vertebra. To apply force as described will require first the projection that will go both headwardly and feetwardly from the point of contact, thus operating a sufficient gap that when the recoil comes from the opponent musculature, it will be able to raise the keyed vertebra dorsally.

4. *The general curvature.* Having by the means described made the necessary preparation for the reduction of a scoliosis (adjustment of the scoliotic and lordotic keys), the operator is now ready to reduce the general scoliosis.

Applied Kinesiology[91,92]

Applied kinesiology is the branch of chiropractic science that utilizes, in a system-oriented approach, muscle testing as a barometer and monitor of a patient's physiologic, anatomical, and emotional state of health. Analysis (therapy localization and the direction of therapy) is essentially achieved by a complex method of interpreting body language expressing through the muscular system.

Five basic elements are found within the IVF: nerves, blood vessels, lymph vessels, spinal fluid, and the acupuncture meridian connector. The systemic reflections of these elements are challenged during analysis, then therapy is directed to balancing any one or combination of the five basic elements in addition to adjusting specific vertebrae to relieve the dysfunction of the system(s).

Basic Technique[93,94]

Basic technique is a system of body mechanics that is directed to normalizing body structure to maintain normal function, with emphasis on postural alignment of the spine and pelvis and balancing of their associated soft tissues. Certain structural patterns and spinal distortions have been isolated, and their recognition and interpretation guide the direction of therapy.

The primary premise of basic technique states that the body of the lowest freely movable vertebra will rotate to the low side of the sacrum or the vertebral foundation upon which it rests. In other words, the body of the lowest freely movable vertebra will always rotate to the side of least support, which is thought to be the low side of the sacrum in most but not all instances.

Another premise of basic technique is that the sacrum is the mechanical centrum of the body and strategically situated as the foundation of the spinal column. The sacrum is considered the key of the mechanical system of spinal levers; that is, the ligaments and muscles that are attached to the spine, pelvis, and rib cage. Imbalances are treated by a specific contact under the sacrotuberous ligament, the gluteal muscles, or other designated areas of the posterior pelvis. The use of heel and ischial lifts is an integral part of the therapy.

The King Concept[95]

Wallace E. King has developed a concept for roentgenographic interpretation that is based upon the analysis of structural problems, essentially those of the axial skeleton, that are reflected in terms of postural distortions effected by gravitational forces upon the human body's upright position.

The basic model, called the *spinal tetrahedron,* is a schematic displaying a system of six adjacent tetrahedrons in a vertical plane (Fig. 13.10). A positional change (dynamic or static) of any one triangle will reflect itself in adaptive responses throughout the system. It is projected that the five junction points of these triangles are the key locations at which spinal stress is focused; ie, the occiput-atlas, C7–T1, T12–L1, L5–S1 levels, and the sacroiliac joints. In chronic musculoskeletal conditions, a corrective adjustment is directed not only to the area of presenting complaint (usually a stress point at one angle of a regional triangle) but also to stabilization of the other angles influenced.

The Pettibon Approach[96]

This is a system of biomechanical analysis of the spine that considers gravitational

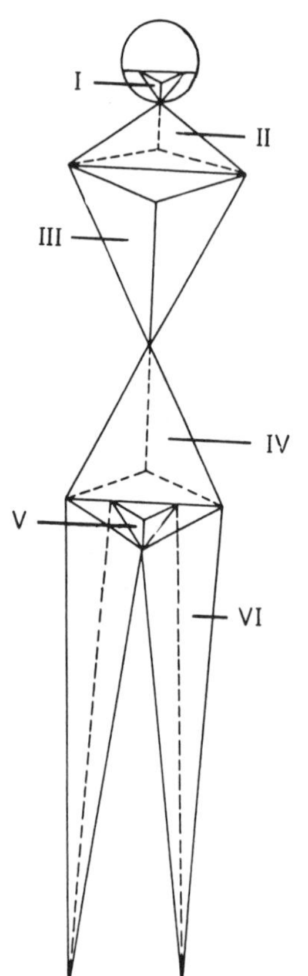

Figure 13.10. The spinal tetrahedron in a balanced vertical body, showing the six triangular regions that provide the mechanics for the strength and mobility of the vertical body. (Courtesy of Wallace E. King, DC.)

forces acting upon abnormal spinal angles or abnormal positions of vertebrae that are thought to produce adverse electromagnetic fields and consequent architectural alterations. It is postulated that extrinsically stressed bone converts the mechanical energy to electrical energy which, in turn, alters the electrical environment of the affected tissues (eg, a stressed vertebra setting up an electromagnetic field in the IVF and around the cord that interferes with the normal field induced in nerves when they fire).

The Pettibon spinal model attempts to explain the interdependence of the cervical, thoracic, and lumbar areas of the spine. In this model, triangles of 30°, 60°, and 90° are the conical building blocks of the Pettibon concept (Fig. 13.11).

CERVICAL SCOLIOSIS[25,97-102]

When viewed from the back, the vertical lateral line of gravity passes through the occipital protuberance and the vertebrae's spinous processes. In cervical scoliosis, the midcervical spinous processes will especially tend to deviate laterally from this line.

Background

Cervical scoliosis is often mechanically predisposed by flattening rather than exaggeration of the cervical lordosis. This is quite common during youth. The posterior joints become relatively lax during flattening of the cervical spine. This encourages retropositioning and posterior subluxations that are frequently the first step toward cervical scoliosis.

In the common rotary cervical scoliosis, the spinous processes tend to rotate toward the *convex* side of the lateral curve, the vertebral bodies rotate toward the *concave* side, and the discs and articular facets become subjected to abnormal stretching forces as they open on the side of convexity and to compressive forces on the side of concavity. This type of cervical scoliosis is usually the compensatory effect of a lower scoliosis to the other side and is a common cause of recurring episodes of nontraumatic torticollis.

Biomechanics

It is important here to review how normal discs react to asymmetrical forces. When a cervical disc is loaded unilaterally, the disc initially becomes wedge-shaped and the normally parallel vertebral plateaus form an angle. This vertically stretches the anular fibers that are opposite the weight-bearing side, but this action is quickly counteracted by forces transmitted laterally from the resilient nucleus to help the disc return to its normal shape. This self-stabilization factor is the product of a healhty nucleus and anulus working as a mechanical couple.

In cervical scoliosis, there are also disc reactions to rotary forces that must be considered. As the apposing layers of anular fibers run alternately oblique in opposite directions, the oblique disc fibers angled toward the direction of twist become stretched when a vertebra rotates, and the

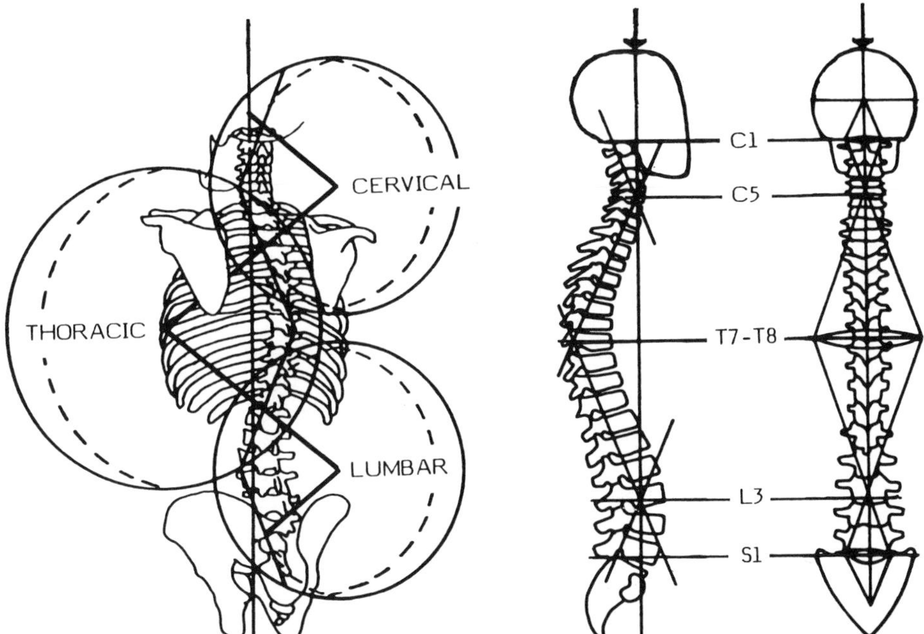

Figure 13.11. Sample Pettibon schematics. *Left*, the major feature of the Pettibon spinal model is that the spinal curves in the lateral view are the strongest when the radius of the curvature equals the chord across the arc. *Middle*, the tangent lines laterally represent the force lines within their cones of motion. *Right*, the cones normally meet at C5, T7–T8, L3, and S1. From an A-P view, the gravity line bisects the 60° angles of the cones into two 30° angles.

oblique fibers running against the direction of rotation tend to relax. The greatest tension from stretch is seen centrally where the fibers are nearly horizontal. This increases nuclear pressure by compression in proportion to the amount of rotation. If severe, the nucleus can be dislodged from its central position.

Cervical scoliotic rotation is also associated with a lateral tilt that increases the distance between the lateral margins of the vertebral bodies on the convex side of the curve. This stretches the lateral anulus, which produces a contraction of that part of the disc and a compensatory bulging of its contralateral (thinned) aspect. If the anular filaments become stretched and weakened, and the disc loses some of its stiffness property, the nucleus may shift from its central position so that the vertebral segment is unable to return to its normal position. A firmly locked rotation subluxation can result.

Thus, vertebral tilting as seen in subluxations with a disc wedging alters the relationship of apposing articular surfaces to produce a change in the direction of compressive forces on these joints and the nucleus of the disc. In addition to tilting, severe rotation produces abnormal jamming compression forces on ipsilateral facets and stretching tension forces on contralateral opened facets.

When continuous compression is applied to any active and mobile joint, cartilaginous erosion followed by arthritis can be expected. When continuous stretching is applied to any active and mobile synovial joint, capsulitis can be expected.

When scoliotic rotation takes place evenly among the cervical segments and the cervical nuclei hold their relatively central position in the discs, the situation is usually asymptomatic even though erosion and arthritis can be demonstrated on roentgenographs. However, if a nucleus fails to hold its central position and shifts laterally away from the point of maximum compression, the superimposed vertebra will be encouraged to present a fixed clinical subluxation.

CONSIDERATIONS IN PRIMARY THORACIC SCOLIOSIS

The treatment of scoliosis has been described in literature that dates as far back as 1500 B.C. Even at that early date, manipulation, traction, exercises, and braces were in common use.

Acquired Factors during Development

Idiopathic functional scoliosis has been a concern in chiropractic ever since the early writing of Carver, later of Logan, and more recently of DeJarnette, Illi, Gillet, Goodheart, Barge, and others. Each in his own way has tried to establish a relationship between the neuromuscular and the osseoligamentous structures of the spinal column.

Some medical writers admit that it has been common in allopathic general practice to "keep an eye on the child's scoliosis to see if it progresses and produces symptoms." As early functional scoliosis is easier to correct than later structural deformity, such an attitude is a clinical sin because irreversible damage can take place at the epiphyseal plates at this time.

I feel that the basic premise in the biomechanical approach to spinal deformities is that *once a focus of spinal curvature has started and been left untreated, it will progress until a new equilibrium design is reached if this is possible.*

Because spinal growth and scoliotic progression are considerably reduced if not halted at maturity, osseous age should be judged by the degree of iliac apophyseal ossification, the degree of fusion of the vertebral apophyseal rings, the maturity level of the carpals, secondary sexual characteristics, anthropometric measurements, and age-height norms.

The Heuter-Volkmann Theory[103–105]

While it can be appreciated that functional scoliosis during youth must be treated early to prevent structural deformity, the biomechanical reason is not as commonly recognized. This explanation, confirmed by Stillwell,[106] is offered in the Heuter-Volkmann theory: *Increased pressure across an epiphyseal plate inhibits growth, while decreased pressure tends to accelerate growth.* The effect is asymmetrical development.[107–109]

Significant Research Findings

A review of some pertinent research findings, some of which are in conflict with common belief, places emphasis on the basic mechanical and biologic processes involved in idiopathic scoliosis. The most significant will be briefly mentioned here.

Unusual Rotational Coupling

Scoliosis frequently begins in the midthoracic area. In lateral flexion of a healthy spine, the upper thoracic vertebral bodies are normally coupled to rotate toward the concavity, the lower bodies rotate toward the convexity, and the transitional midthoracic vertebrae tend to be fixed by the rotary forces above and below. However, there is frequently a normal physiologic curve to the right in the midthoracic area, attributed to the aorta. If this curve becomes exaggerated, there is a tendency for lumbar-like coupling in the midthoracic vertebrae in which rotation is to the *convexity*. This can initiate a series of adverse biomechanical events. The involved epiphyses, end-plates, anuli, nuclei, and apophyseal joints are put under asymmetrical loading, the lateral paravertebral muscles and ligaments become imbalanced, and the effect is progression to distinct scoliosis.

The determining factor of this biomechanical syndrome is when the focal midthoracic vertebra rotates (ie, clinically subluxates) toward the convexity rather than to the concavity of the lateral physiologic curve.[110] *The axial rotation of idiopathic scoliosis appears to invariably be into the convexity of the lateral curve.* The precipitating cause is usually subluxated facets from intrinsic trauma (eg, unilateral muscular stress) whereafter the motion unit becomes fixed, but it could also result from reflex, vascular, lymphatic, or chemical irregularities or myotonic function.

Nuclear Shifting

The nucleus pulposus normally bulges toward the side of convexity and shifts slightly toward the side of concavity during unilateral loading (eg, in lateral bending). In scoliosis, this transverse shift is toward the convexity. Ponsetti[111] and Barge[112] suggest that the initial cause of scoliosis can be a traumatic shifting of the nucleus toward the stretched aspect of a disc; that is, the wide side of lateral disc wedging that is under tensile forces. However, Roaf's comprehensive studies of spinal compression forces showed that, unless a disc is severely degenerated, the tendency is for the nucleus to bulge the thin end-plates axially into adjacent spongiosa rather than to shift peripherally.[113] Traumatic malalignment of vertebral bodies commonly displaces the superior end-plate of the inferior vertebra either anteriorly or laterally with little nuclear displacement. Sharp nuclear shifting in a healthy disc would require violent shearing forces applied at the end of a range of motion.

The Node Theory

Kashimoto and associates[114] studied the range of motion from the atlas to the sacrum in 30 cadaveric spines and found that individual spines had a characteristic level-dependent difference in the capacity for elementary motions at the facet joints. Those segments with restricted motion capacity were called *spinal nodes.* The human spine was found to usually have three or four spinal nodes between the skull and the sacrum. Their location was determined at the C7–T1, T4–T5, T8–T9, and T11–T12 levels. This intrinsic structural character of the human spine is described as "nodal motion structure" by these researchers, who postulated that this state plays an important role in the formation of curve patterns in idiopathic scoliosis and other spinal deformities. It should be noted that Gillet, Illi, King,[115] and Ward[116] have frequently pointed out the high incidence of subluxation-fixation at similar areas.

Neurologic Implications

Kaplan and associates found that a radiculopathic process on the convex side is associated with idiopathic thoracic scoliosis.[117] EMG studies of the erector spinae muscles showed the radiculopathy to be maximal near the apex of the curve. At one time it was thought that a polyneuropathy or polyneuritis was involved in the development of adolescent idiopathic scoliosis. This theory, however, has been shown by nerve conduction velocity studies to be false.[118]

Cord Maladaptation

Recent surveys have shown that idiopathic structural scoliosis of mild degree is generally not progressive, according to Lloyd-Roberts and associates[119] who have proposed a mechanism that may be responsible for deterioration when it is seen. They report that although the spinal cord is displaced toward the concavity of a scoliotic curve, it does *not* rotate in company with the vertebrae. This exposes the involved nerve roots to traction and possible entrapment. It is suggested that progression occurs when the neuraxis is unable to adjust to the change in the anatomy of the vertebral column: a significant increase in degenerated cells was demonstrated in the dorsal root ganglia at the apex on the convex side.

The Effect of Right- or Left-Handedness

The theory that thoracic curves to the right are common in right-handed people and that curves to the left are common in left-handed people, as proposed in several editions of Gray's *Anatomy of the Human Body,* is not confirmed by the 1971 data of McCarver and associates.[120] From personal experience in 1972, I examined the spines of 200 league bowlers in Denver, about 20% of whom were left-handed. There was no correlation between right- and left-hand preference and the side of the lateral thoracic curve if one was present. Although a right scoliosis was far more common, it was just as common in left-handed bowlers.

Anterior vs Posterior Motion Unit Fixation

Animal experiments reported by White and Panjabi have shown that fixation of vertebral bodies in a curved position *sometimes* resulted in the development of scoliosis, while fixation of the spinous processes *always* resulted in severe scoliosis with lordosis and rotation. This indicates that fixation of the posterior elements is more conducive to scoliosis than fixation of the anterior elements.[121]

Effect of Sensory Input Deficit

Experiments on animals have shown that transection of the dorsal root causes a defect in sensory input that produces scoliosis.[122] In each case, the resulting curve was to the side of the disrupted neural elements. Alexander and associates have demonstrated that such a transection also produces a related spinal cord motor impairment.[123]

Postural Stabilization and Questions Unanswered

Postural stabilization is generally considered to be the sum result of several osseous, ligamentous, muscular, and neurologic factors. Bones must be in proper articular alignment, ligaments must be loose enough to allow movement and strong enough to resist overstress, muscles must have good tone and contractability yet not be constantly active, and the righting mechanisms must be alert and true. Most authorities feel that the greatest direct resistance to scoliosis appears to be given by the apophyseal planes, the elastic tension of the ligamentum flava, and balanced muscle tone of the agonists and antagonists.

The Osseous Structures. Signs of bone deformation in vertebrae and ribs follow Wolff's law in that the bone design (internally and externally) in scoliosis is the effect of the intensity and stress to which the bone is subjected.[124] Bone mass reflects the amount of functional forces (gravitational or myogenic) habitually applied. The same principle applies to any tissue containing collagen and polysaccharide (eg, IVDs).

The Spinal Ligaments. Surprisingly, studies have shown that there is no appreciable difference between the physical properties of ligaments and tendons in a scoliotic spine and in a normal spine. However, Scandinavian animal experiments by Michelsson to induce scoliosis surgically have shown that the integrity of the posterior costotransverse ligaments are especially vital to maintain symmetrical growth and lateral balance in the spine.[125]

The Spinal Muscles. As mentioned in earlier chapters, very little muscle activity is necessary to maintain the erect posture if the weight-bearing structures are in good alignment and the ligaments are healthy. It would then appear logical that if distortion exists, greater muscular activity and ligament strength are necessary to maintain balance. Many medical and chiropractic authors emphasize this in scoliosis and exaggerated A-P spinal curves, as well as in hip deformities; genu varum, valgum, and recurvatum; pes planus, etc. In most approaches to scoliosis, it has been presumed that the exhibited distortion is initially muscular in nature; ie, either agonist weakness on the side of the convexity or hypertonicity or spasticity of antagonists on the side of the concavity. Here, attention is upon the strong posterior and intrinsic spinal musculature. This purely kinesiologic approach must be considered against facts brought out by recent research.

1. As pointed out by Cailliet, electromyographic studies on paraspinous muscles in idiopathic scoliosis fail to reveal any significant muscle activity on either side of the curvature.[126]

2. Roaf's experiments have added to the complexity of understanding the etiology in all cases of scoliosis.[127, 128] He shows that the unilateral shortening (eg, abdominal wall hypertonicity) of the prevertebral components of the spine relative to the posterior components results in severe lateral distortion of the spine. This would appear to support but not necessarily confirm the theory of T. J. Bennett, often denounced by orthopedic purists, that many situations of scoliosis are the result of noxious viscerosomatic reflexes.[129]

In idiopathic scoliosis, a significantly large number of Type I fibers are found in the multifidus muscle at the apex of the curve on the convex side.[130] While usually found predominantly in deep muscles, these Type I fibers are also found in the superficial muscles above and below the apex of the curve on the convex side. Why this occurs has not been explained.

Histographic analyses of patients with idiopathic scoliosis have pointed toward specific pathology in the *deltoids*, especially ipsilateral to the concave side of the curvature.[131] The pathology consists of an overall fiber "hypotrophy" and a Type I area decrease, often with frank atrophy. EMG confirmation of this pathology shows a myopathic pattern in all the concave-side deltoids and often in the convex ones as well. It is thought that the cause of the cephalocaudal and side-to-side asymmetry is possibly connected to developmental and neurotrophic factors that may be operative in the complex etiology of the disorder.

To develop an animal model of idiopathic scoliosis, Bagnall and associates produced a deep vertebral muscle imbalance in rabbits by surgically removing the rotatores at one level of the vertebral column on one side only.[132] The effect was the development of curves that progressed in a manner similar to that of idiopathic scoliosis in humans.

A study conducted by Haderspeck and Schultz[133] suggested that if the progression of idiopathic scoliosis results from dysfunction of the trunk neuromuscular system, the dysfunction is more likely to be in the neural systems that control trunk muscle contractions and body-weight support strategies than in the functional capabilities of the muscles themselves.

The major thoracic muscles and the effect of their prolonged hypertonicity on the spine are shown in Table 13.5.[28]

The Righting Reflexes. Independent experiments by Michelsson[125] and Ponsetti[111] have shown that unilateral labyrinthine stimulation or removal has resulted in scoliosis. This points to the delicate relationship between righting reflexes and spinal balance and offers an explanation to how cervical disrelationships with vertebral artery or vasomotor effects can produce scoliosis. Yamada and associates found that 99 out of 100 scoliotic patients studied had an associated equilibrium defect and that the greater the spinal distortion, the greater the dysfunction in the proprioceptive and optic reflex systems.[134] However, this has not been confirmed by research in this country.

Equilibrium Sway Effects. In an analysis of sagittal, lateral, and total postural sway when erect, the patterns of scoliotic children were compared to those of healthy children.[135] Scoliotic patients had significantly poorer postural control, especially in tests in which the proprioceptive functions were most important for maintaining postural equilibrium. Patients with a left convex curve had more pronounced reactions quantitatively than patients with a right convex curve, and patients with small curvatures had significantly increased postural sway compared to patients with more severe deformity. These facts, together with findings in patients with double primary curves, and the results of studies of brace effects, were assumed to indirectly indicate the possibility of postural disequilibrium as a contributory cause in adolescent scoliosis. This observation appears to support reports of those who specialized in upper-cervical techniques.

Subthoracic Considerations

The effects of pelvic tilt, pelvic rotation, the short-leg syndrome, and lower extremity misalignment on thoracic scoliosis, and the use of lifts in therapy are always significant if not primary. The biomechanical implications of these conditions will be discussed later in this chapter.

Biomechanical Considerations in the Therapy of Thoracic Scoliosis

The primary considerations involved in the treatment of any scoliosis are the application of correcting loads and the balancing of asymmetrical forces. In chiropractic, this is usually strived for essentially by corrective segmental adjustments, the freeing of articular fixations, muscle balancing, traction, therapeutic exercises, and the use of corrective lifts and corsets. In more radical medical therapy, the Milwaukee brace, Harrington rod, plaster casts, traction with osseous pinning, brutal manipulation under anesthesia, surgery, and combinations of these are utilized. In either approach, basic biomechanical and bioengineering principles must be applied if the therapy is to be optimally successful.[136]

The Radius of a Scoliotic Curve and Its Implications[137–139]

The larger the radius of a curvature, the less the spine is curved from the midline and vice versa. This can be crudely expressed mathematically by saying that the length of a spinal curvature (l) divided by its radius (r) equals the apical bending moment (M) divided by the area's stiffness (S): $l/r = M/S$. This points out that the radius of a curvature is inversely related to the ap-

Table 13.5.
Selected Effects of Thoracic Area Hypertonicity

Muscle	Effect of hypertonicity
Iliocostalis dorsi	Hypertonicity tends to lift the lower six ribs. If unilateral and chronic, a functional scoliosis will develop. Increased tone, especially if bilateral, also tends to flatten the normal thoracic kyphosis.
Latissimus dorsi	Excessive tone tends to pull the lower half of the spine and the pelvis anterior, lateral, and superior, and to internally rotate the humerus.
Multifidus	Excessive tone tends to place a rotary torque on the involved vertebral motion unit.
Quadratus lumborum	Although this is considered a flank muscle, it has a most significant effect on the lower thoracic spine. Rarely is there a lower thoracic scoliosis that does not have a quadratus component. Increased tone tends to pull L1–L4 inferior, and lateral, and the ilium superior, and medial.
Rhomboid major	Increased tone tends to pull the T2–T4 spinous processes lateral and inferior and the inferior vertebral border up and toward the midline.
Trapezius, lower	Increased tone tends to pull the T6–T12 spinous processes lateral and the shoulder girdle medial and inferior.
Trapezius, upper	Hypertonicity tends to pull the head down and back, the cervical spinal processes lateral, and the shoulder girdle medial.

plied bending moment and inversely proportional to the spine's stiffness properties contributed to by both vertebral and extravertebral tissues (Fig. 13.12).

Thus, progression depends upon the magnitude of the bending moment and the counteracting moments inherent in the spinal and paraspinal tissues. If the bending moment is high and the stiffness resistance to bending is low, collapse results. This is the picture we see in cases of gross, usually irreversible, changes in spinal configuration and segmental structure.

Range of Curvature

We usually think of scoliosis, lordosis, and kyphosis as extending over several vertebrae. While this is usually true, it is not always true.[140] Compensation can occur at a single vertebral motion unit. For example, multisegmental lumbar hyperlordosis is usually compensated by a compensatory multisegmental thoracic hyperkyphosis. However, cases of multisegmental lumbar lordosis are not infrequently seen in which the compensatory kyphosis takes place at a single, highly stressed, thoracic segment in the T10–T12 area. Here we have a patient in relatively good balance when viewed from the side or the back. That is, the occiput is directly over the sacrum and in the midline. There is a distinctly increased sacral angle and "sway back" accompanied by a flattened thoracic area.

This occurrence is frequently seen in female patients during advanced pregnancy and in middle-aged male endomorphs. Increased thoracic stiffness would explain this phenomenon, but it is not always related. Instances of lateral deviations compensated by a single motion unit are also seen in scoliosis. This latter phenomenon appears most commonly at the L4–L5, thoracocervical, and cervico-occipital joints, and is often not symptomatic until sudden trauma causes the already stressed motion unit to "cry for help."

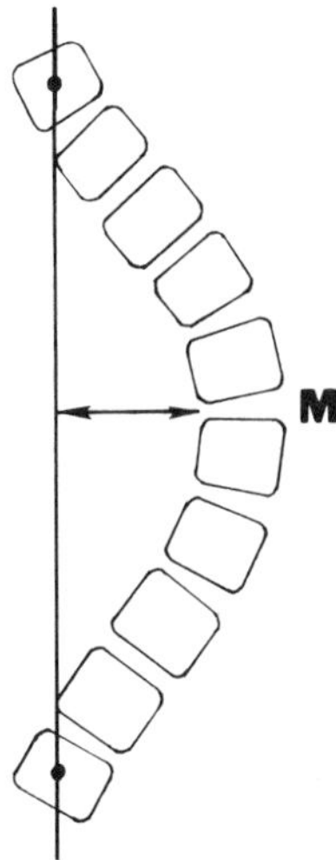

Figure 13.12. The more the spine deviates from the midline, the greater the bending moment of the curve. The larger the radius of a curvature, the less the spine is curved from the midline. A curve's length divided by its radius equals the apical bending moment divided by the area's stiffness.

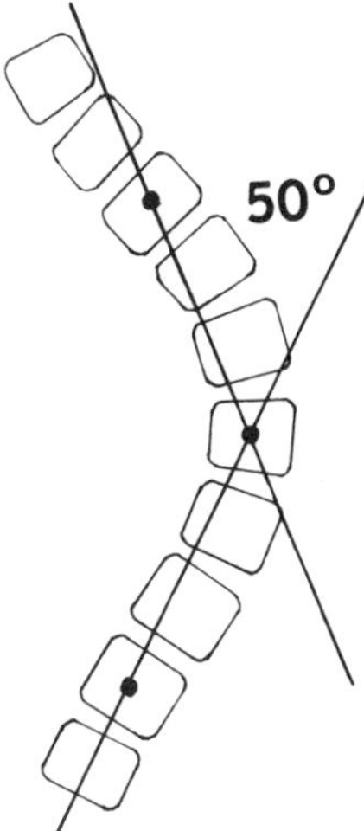

Figure 13.13. The Risser-Ferguson method of measuring spinal curves.

Measuring Scoliotic Curves[138, 141, 142]

There are various roentgenographic methods used in measuring the degree of progressing or improving scoliotic curves. Three of these methods will be described, and each can be used in measuring the degree of scoliotic, lordotic, or kyphotic deformity present.

The Risser-Ferguson Method. The lowest vertebra whose inferior surface tilts the most to the convexity of the curve and the highest vertebra whose superior surface tilts the most toward the concavity are located. Next, the apical vertebra midway between the lowest and highest vertebrae selected is located. A line is drawn from the center of the lowest vertebra to the center of the vertebra at the apex of the curve. The same is done from the highest vertebra to the apex vertebra (Fig. 13.13). The angle formed where the lines intersect at the middle of the apical vertebra is measured.[139, 143]

The Cobb Method. The Risser-Ferguson method has not been generally accepted for several years, but it is well to appreciate if you are reviewing patient films or records that have used the method. The R-F method has been replaced by one originally developed by Cobb, and it has become the most common method used today.[144] It is arrived at by drawing a line through the upper border of the cephalad vertebra that tilts the most to the concavity of the curve, as in the R-F method. The same is done at the inferior border of the caudad vertebra that tilts the most to the convexity of the curve. However, the angle is measured where these two lines transect. The vertebrae from which these measurements are taken are called the "transitional" vertebrae by Cobb, and they should not be confused with the anatomical transitional vertebrae between spinal regions.[145–147]

In most cases, Cobb's angle may be far lateral to the film. When this is the case, a perpendicular line is extended up from the lower line and down from the upper line. The acute angle formed above the intersection of these two lines is Cobb's angle.

As with the R-F method, the exact selection of the transitional vertebrae by Cobb's method is often confusing and quite subjective. In addition, Cobb's angle does not give an accurate picture of the type of curvature present.[148] Two scoliotic curvatures of quite different configuration may have the same Cobb's angle (Fig. 13.14). These inaccuracies can be avoided by using the method of White and Panjabi.

The White-Panjabi Method.[149] To determine the amount of curvature at the ap-

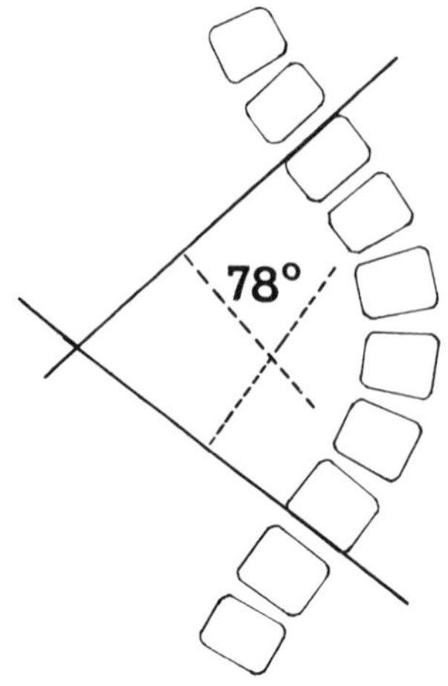

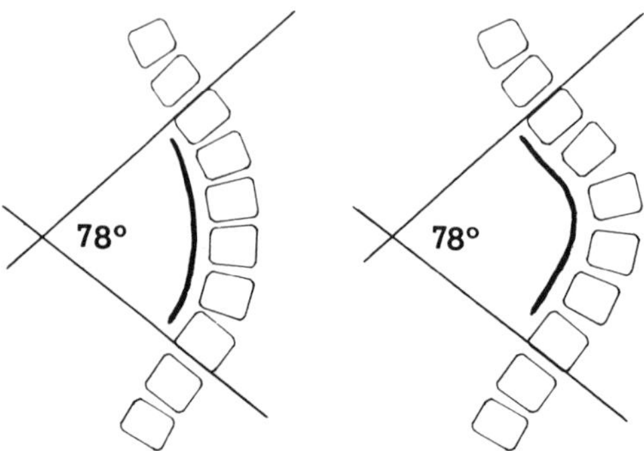

Figure 13.14. *Top*, the Cobb method of measuring spinal curves. Note in the *bottom drawings* that two curves of different design may have the same Cobb angle, thus the angle alone may be deceiving as to the severity of the curve.

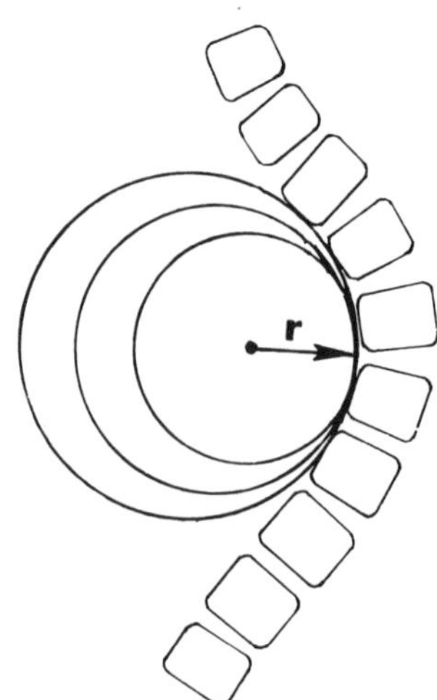

Figure 13.15. The White-Panjabi method of measuring spinal curves. The radius of a curvature is inversely related to the applied bending moment and inversely proportional to the spine's stiffness.

ical vertebra, the site of greatest bending moment, the center of the apical vertebra or disc of the curve to be measured is located first. Next, two points are marked in the center of a cephalad and a caudal vertebra that are equally distant from the apical vertebra. Third, a circle is drawn through these three points. Fourth, the cephalad and caudad points are moved closer to the apical point and a new circle is drawn. This will be a smaller circle within the first circle. Fifth, this procedure is continued until all three points are approximately at the same site. Sixth, the radius of this circle is measured. It will be the radius of the curvature (Fig. 13.15).

Measuring Rib Distortion[150–152]

Spinal rotation in scoliosis occurs posteriorly on the side of convexity of the curve and anteriorly on the side of concavity. This is manifested by rib cage deformity (hump) in the thoracic area and bulging erector spinae in the lumbar area. The intercostal spaces are vertically stretched on the side of convexity and narrowed on the side of concavity. The normal contours of the entire thorax are distorted, appearing as an oblique configuration rather than a relatively ovoid shape when viewed from above. This is produced so that the shoulders and head can be oriented forward–the effect of a biologic mandate rather than a biomechanical need.

Rib hump is readily observed in the Adams position and can be measured by various methods. Ribs do not distort by themselves; the distortion is essentially the result of vertebral rotation coupled with tilting. Thus, rib distortion offers an indirect measurement of spinal rotation.

In measuring in vivo rib cage distortion transverse to the apical vertebra, the doctor can apply the simple carpenter's instrument used for measuring curved surfaces, to which a small line level has been fixed (Fig. 13.16). As the points of the instrument are quite sharp, a thin sheet of pliable plastic is placed on the patient's back. This sheet should be thick enough to protect the patient's skin, yet thin enough to conform

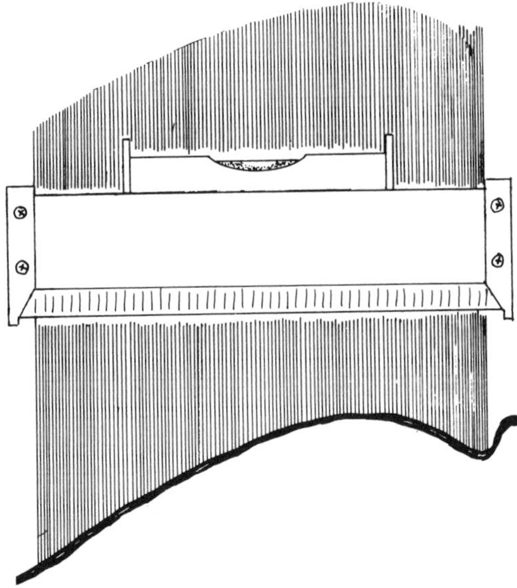

Figure 13.16. A carpenter's instrument used to measure curved cornices, with a line level attached. This is an excellent instrument to use in measuring physical configurations.

exactly to the curvature present. The instrument is applied, then the curve formed is traced on a sheet of paper and made part of the patient's progress record. This method may be used in both the prone and Adams positions if desired. It can be used on any region of the spine and on extremity joints to record progressive changes in skin configuration (eg, swelling reduction).

Traction[153–155]

The clinical objectives of traction in scoliosis, especially during youth, are based upon Wolff's law and the Heuter-Volkmann theory.[105, 156, 157]

Severe Distortions. Several reports have shown that traction can be used as a major tool in the treatment of spinal deformities such as scoliosis.[158–163] Turnbuckle hinge jackets, localizer casts, plaster jackets or vests, and halo casts with traction devices apply corrective forces gradually on a sustained basis. These methods are commonly used presurgically. A halo-apparatus, usually requiring surgical pinning, is widely accepted as an effective method to treat severe cervicothoracic curves. Halo-femoral traction is often indicated in rigid curves greater than 80° and/or those associated with pelvic obliquity and paralytic/neuromuscular curves, but Cotrel's traction is generally considered ineffective in such cases.[164, 165] Halo-pelvic traction is reported to have poor results in "collapsing spines" and has generally been replaced by halo-gravity procedures (eg, circoelectric bed, specialized wheelchair).

A professional traction table is shown in Figure 13.17.

Axial Loading. Continuous and intermittent axial traction has proven helpful in many cases of scoliosis. The typical mechanism is opposite stretching forces that are applied cephally and caudally to elongate the spine. The actual correction of the angular distortion, however, is *not* produced by the axial tensile forces created. It is produced by the bending moments produced at the wedged disc spaces (Fig. 13.18).

Computing Axial Loads. When applying axial stress to the spine, the corrective bending moment at the farthest lateral point of the curve can be computed by multiplying the axial force by its perpendicular distance from the midline to the apex of the curve. Thus, a given axial force that would increase corrective bending moments in a severe deformity would not be as helpful to a mild deformity. This is important to consider when adjusting the magnitude of traction forces.

Transverse Loading. Transverse loading is also beneficial but more difficult to apply. Attempts have been made by using a lateral pad within a spinal corset. Another method is to apply broad transverse pressure by some means during axial traction. A shoe lift creates transverse spinal loading by shifting the body's center of gravity unless these forces are absorbed in lower segments such as in a supple spine. As in applying axial stresses, the corrective forces are the bending moments created at the wedged disc spaces (Fig. 13.19).

Computing Transverse Loads. When applying transverse stress to the spine, the correcting bending moment at the farthest lateral point of the curve can be computed by multiplying *half* of the axial force by its perpendicular distance from the midline to the apex of the curve. In contrast to axial stress, the corrective bending moments in

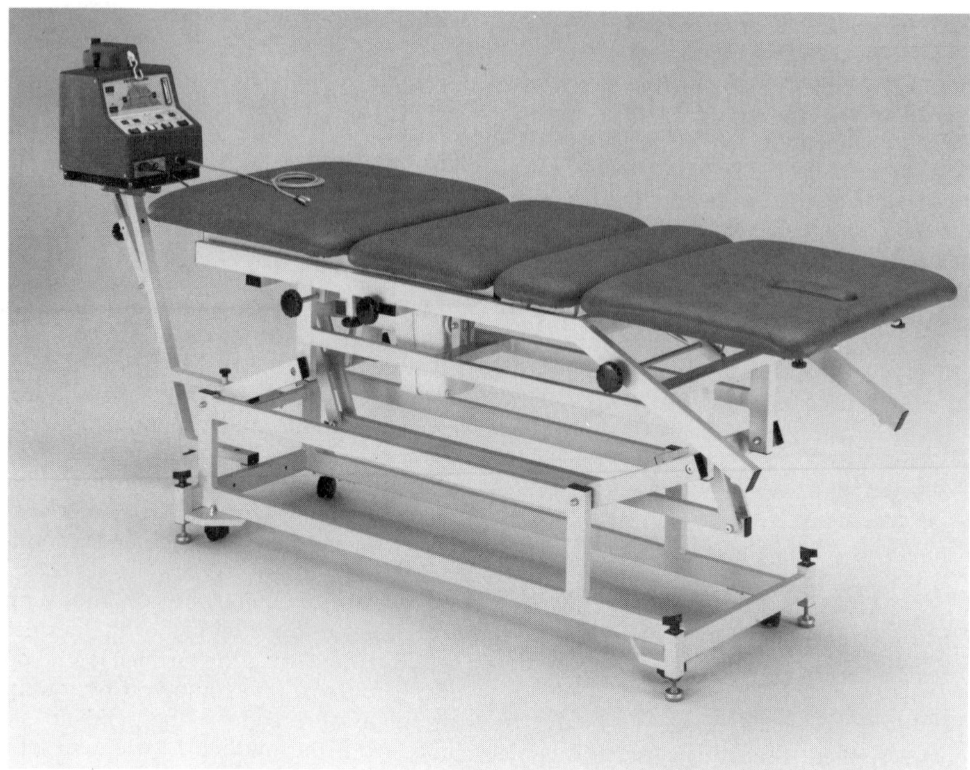

Figure 13.17. Model TRE-24 traction table. (Courtesy of the Chattanooga Corporation.)

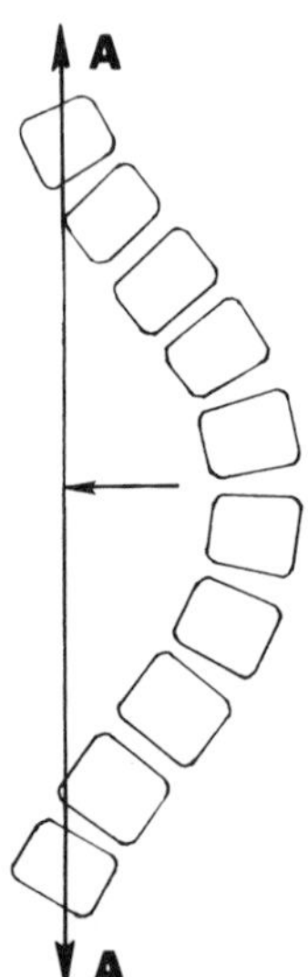

Figure 13.18. A scoliotic spine under two-point load from typical axial traction. *A*, axial forces.

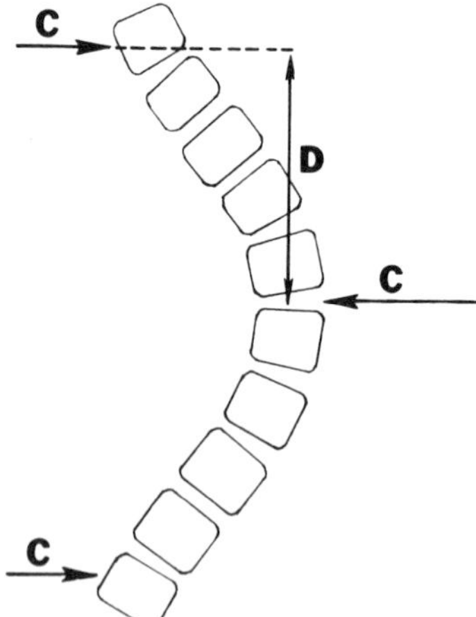

Figure 13.19. A scoliotic spine under three-point transverse loading. *C*, transverse forces; *D*, distance between opposing forces. (Compare with Figure 2.15.) Orthopedic braces are usually designed to provide some transverse forces or to provide cutaneous stimulation to produce corrective intrinsic reactions.

transverse loading decrease as the deformity increases from the midline.

Axial vs Transverse Loading. The basic facts just discussed point out that axial traction is most beneficial in cases of severe deformity and transverse loading is most beneficial in mild deformities. In all instances, however, combined axial and transverse loading is always the ideal biomechanical approach. For example, if axial forces are being applied with the patient supine, some means of applying transverse pressure should be applied laterally to the apex of the curve while contralateral aspects above and below the curve are fixed by some padded device.

Presently, transverse forces must be applied either manually or by using an extra portable traction unit (Fig. 13.20). Possibly some traction equipment company in the future will design a unit that will apply adjustable transverse force simultaneously with axial traction. If for some reason axial and transverse forces cannot be applied simultaneously, it is best to begin therapy with axial loading and then change to transverse loading as the apex of the curve begins to reduce.

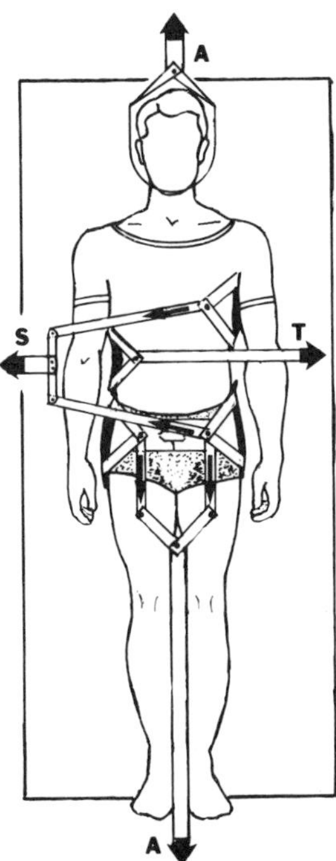

Figure 13.20. A model of axial and transverse loading being applied simultaneously, as viewed from above. *A*, axial forces applied by cephalad and caudad traction units; *S*, stabilizing harness or counterforce applied by lateral traction unit; *T*, transverse force applied at apex of lumbothoracic curve by contralateral unit.

Braces and Casts[166–173]

When using braces, corsets, and other supports in the treatment of scoliosis, at least four objectives should be kept in mind: (1) to prevent progression, (2) to hold the improvement gained by minimizing adverse forces, (3) to apply corrective mechanical forces, and (4) last but not least, to stimulate corrective neuromuscular forces. Success is usually relative to tissue flexibility and plasticity properties and to sensory excitement on the convexity to initiate corrective muscular reactions. This latter point refers to the patient moving away from a site of irritation by straightening the spine, such as with the tracheal and abdominal pads of a Milwaukee brace (Fig. 13.21).

Braces and casts have little effect in idiopathic scoliosis if there is a strong neurologic defect present or if the curve is extreme.[174] If paraspinal muscles cannot respond to the irritation of the appliance, there is no corrective neuromuscular action. The more the spine is curved, the more the spinal segments are subjected to lateral bending moments than to axial forces. In curves greater than 40°, braces have little effect because such curves are invariably associated with severe muscle weakness and frequently exhibit the lack of optimal mechanoreceptor input.

The Milwaukee brace is used, generally, to prevent progression of a mild–moderate curve until maturity is reached or until a more appropriate age for surgery is attained. It is also used to prevent postoperative regression and for some cases of nonoperative scoliosis that do not exceed 40°.[175] To be effective to any degree, it must be worn until bone growth ceases.

Within the conservative treatment of scoliosis, emphasis should be on reducing the lumbar lordosis. Uden and Willner[176] have shown that pure lumbar flexion per se produces a correction of scoliosis of the same degree as does the Milwaukee brace. Bracing in cases of mild idiopathic scoliosis, how-

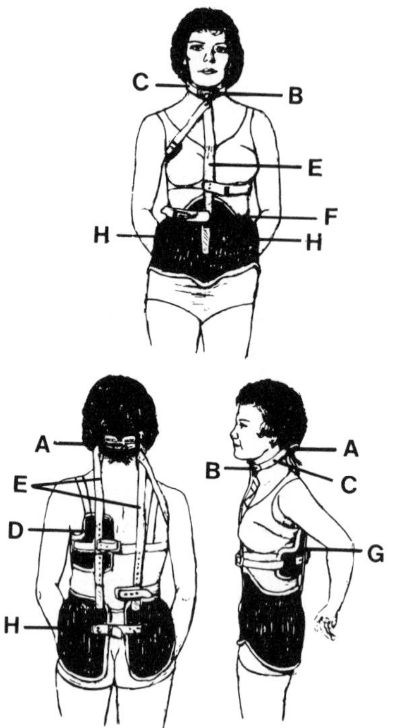

Figure 13.21. Diagram of a Milwaukee brace as viewed from the front, back, and side. *A*, occipital pad, which tends to straighten the cervical and lumbar lordoses; *B*, anterior trachial pad; *C*, cervical ring; *D*, lower thoracic apex transverse pressure pad; *E*, vertical bars; *F*, abdominal pad; *G*, upper lumbar apex transverse pressure pad; *H*, molded pads over the iliac crests.

ever, is probably not necessary in a large proportion of patients who meet current criteria for bracing.[177]

Some common spinal supports, applicable to a large number of stability problems, and the general guidelines for their fitting are shown in Table 13.6.[178]

Electrical Stimulation

While active exercise, helpful in maintaining mobility, has shown little effect in improving even mild forms of adolescent idiopathic scoliosis,[179] lateral electrical surface stimulation (LESS) for reducing the progression of idiopathic scoliosis has become quite popular in resent years.[180,181] During one study, when electrodes were placed over the lateral trunk musculature rather than on the paraspinals, the scoliosis reduction improved threefold.[182] This procedure can often be used as a welcome alternative to bracing.[183] Bradford and associates feel that the effects appear greatest on curves of less than 30° and that, if the curves fail to respond to LESS, it is unlikely that the patient would respond to a Milwaukee brace.[184]

Biomechanical Relaxation and Creep[185,186]

The principles of biomechanical relaxation and creep are most important considerations in the treatment of scoliosis. The combined components of viscosity and elasticity allow for relaxation and creep, and both of these properties are a function of time.

In review, stress relaxation refers to the viscoelastic property of a tissue of retaining a constant deformation after a load is removed. Relaxation, sometimes popularly called "give," is a steady deformation that occurs with less force over a period of time (Fig. 13.22). This is demonstrated in a tissue being stressed at a constant magnitude when the force necessary to maintain the deformation decreases with time.

Creep refers to the viscoelastic property of slowly increasing deformation under a constant load. That is, there is an initial deformation followed by a slowly increasing degree of deformation. Unlike plastic behavior, creep begins even with a minimal force and the recovery is slow. Creep is exhibited in the loss of an individual's height from many hours in the upright position, which is due to the creep phenomena occurring in the intervertebral discs where a constant weight has been borne over a period of time.

When a constant force is applied to viscoelastic substances such as bones, muscles, tendons, cartilage, and ligaments, the property of creep becomes apparent. When a deformation is fixed, stress relaxation becomes apparent.

"The 9-to-5 Syndrome"

The properties of tissue relaxation, creep, and fatigue should be considered whenever articular correction, traction, lifts, or braces are utilized. For example, the soft tissues involved in spinal distortion will always retain a degree of relaxation for some time after adverse forces have been relieved. Thus, some means of rest and support are

Table 13.6.
Common Spinal Supports

Type of support	Measuring guidelines
THORACOLUMBOSACRAL SUPPORTS	
Dorsolumbar corset	Anterior height from hip angle to comfortable clearance below breasts when seated; hip circumference; posterior height from superior angle of shoulder blade to sacrococcygeal joint; waist circumference.
Jewett brace	Anterior height from 1 inch below sternal notch to symphysis pubis; hip circumference; thorax circumference.
Knight-Taylor brace	Posterior height from midsacrum to 1 inch below the superior angle of the shoulder blade; hip circumference.
Taylor brace	Posterior height from midsacrum to 1 inch below the superior angle of the shoulder blade; hip circumference.
LUMBAR AND SACROILIAC SUPPORTS	
Chairback brace	Posterior height to midsacrum to lower thoracic region; according to patient's comfort; hip circumference.
Knight spinal brace	Posterior height to midsacrum to lower thoracic region; according to patient's comfort; hip circumference.
Lumbosacral corset	Anterior height from hip angle to comfortable clearance below breasts when seated; hip circumference; posterior height from lower thoracic area to sacrococcygeal joint; waist circumference.
Sacroiliac girdle	Hip circumference.
Williams brace	Posterior height to midsacrum to lower thoracic region; according to patient's comfort; hip circumference.

necessary until the deformed tissues can adapt to new conditions.

When a pressure brace or a shoe lift is applied, it must be done slowly in increments so that the degree of creep reversal obtained and residual relaxation present can be evaluated. This would not be immediately apparent at fitting. An ideal lift inserted according to good postural balance at 9 a.m., even if confirmed by quadrant scales or other instrumentation, may be far too much or inadequate at 5 p.m. If so, adverse symptoms can be expected to progress. I have coined this progressive effect the "9-to-5 syndrome." When these soft-tissue properties and changes are appreciated, the term "retracing" rarely needs to be used as an excuse for postadjustment adverse symptoms.

Orthopedic Supports. I suggest that whenever a pressure support of any type is first applied it be fitted in the morning and checked later in the day. Checks twice daily should continue for 3–4 days and thereafter at longer intervals. These checks need not take more than 2–3 minutes and can easily be worked in between other patient visits. The extra effort will be well worth the time involved.

Shoe Lifts. Another consideration is that of a heel or sole lift applied to an individual who works constantly upright most of the day. He may feel fine during the morning hours after being in a non-

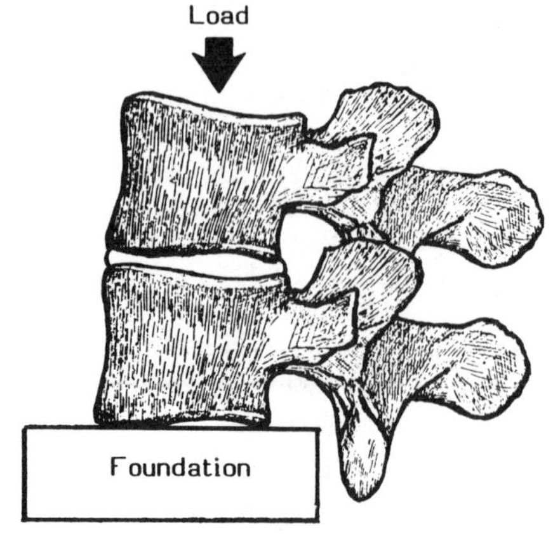

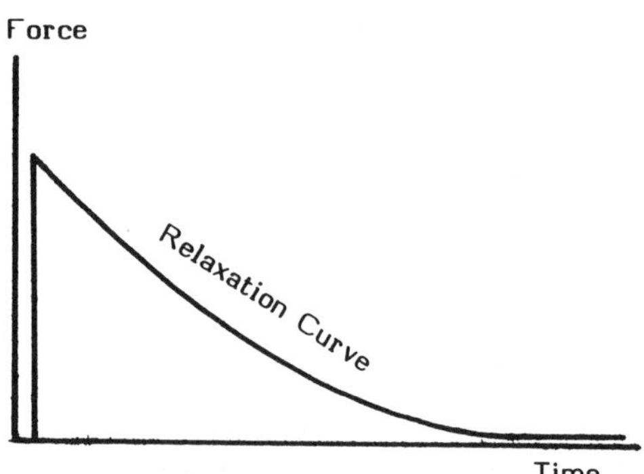

Figure 13.22. *Top*, vertebrae being subjected to a vertical load. *Bottom*, if a constant deformation force is applied to the spine, the force in the motion unit (contiguous vertebrae and disc) slowly decreases with time.

weight-bearing position for several hours, but as time goes on and creep from axial loading takes its effect, symptoms appear and progress. In such a case, a compromise must be made as to the amount of lift prescribed.

Plantar Stabilizers. The same is true for the fitting of plantar stabilizers. The 9 a.m. arch is not necessarily the 5 p.m. arch if the patient is standing or walking for a considerable time.

Corrective Adjustments. In most circumstances that contribute to abnormal soft-tissue stiffness when ankylosis has not occurred, a large degree of functional shortening is superimposed upon structural changes. When adjusting a vertebral motion unit, pelvis, or extremity joint that is obviously fibrotic, I have found that mild traction and a broad contact with mild transverse pressure held in the direction of correction for 30–60 seconds before adjustment helps to "reverse" the established creep and elastic fiber shortening produced by gravity, hypertonicity, etc. This is usually on the side of disc or cartilage thinning. When the adjustment is delivered, it appears to be with further palpable movement and with less discomfort to the patient than would otherwise be achieved. The same mild contact following specific adjustment appears to enhance "holding" of the correction achieved. Postadjustment resting cots in each dressing room offer an excellent means of providing time for the soft-tissue fibers to adapt without fighting gravity and for some corrective disc imbibition. However, this approach is an empirical observation on my part that needs further study to be confirmed.

Visual Subluxation Patterns[187–193]

Any postural pattern is a reflection of an individual's biomechanics that are responsive to underlying processes. The process may be essentially antalgic, muscular, ligamentous, osseous, proprioceptive, or a combination of these factors.

DeJarnette feels that many idiopathic patterns reflect massive movement of structure that is held in a state of fixation by increased myosensory input. Goodheart places emphasis on muscular weakness, usually of a reflex etiology, and Barge feels that the initial distortion is frequently the result of a nuclear shift. B. J. Palmer felt that they were the result of proprioceptive or motor disturbances originating in the upper cervical area, and Hugh Logan felt that they were responsive mechanisms to sacral base inferiorities. Today, few would disagree that all such mechanisms can be involved singularly or in combination.

There is always a danger in describing classic patterns because they lead to such variances in subjective interpretation. There is almost no limit to the possible distortions that may occur and classifications tend to encourage the examiner to try to fit an individual's unique distortion into a certain arbitrary category. This limits thought and leads to frequent error. Patterns only offer visual clues that require challenging by standard diagnostic procedures. With these qualifications in mind, we will portray the most common patterns seen as an exercise in typical coupling mechanisms and/or their commonly associated myotonic forces and equilibrial effects.

For simplicity, these common patterns will be described on one side only, but they may occur just as frequently on the other side, for which the descriptions offered would be reversed. The distortions shown in the drawings are exaggerated from those usually found clinically. Also, they will be described essentially as viewed from the posterior, but keep in mind that a distortion in one plane must have its influences on all planes. Emphasis is placed on the effects of unilateral muscle weakness, but the same postural effect would be produced by antagonistic hypertonicity or spasm.

Muscular Weakness Patterns Manifested as Scoliosis[108, 194–198]

Standard muscle testing and inspection may disclose a pathologic weakness in the absence of palpable or measurable atrophy. This type of relative muscle weakness in comparison to its antagonist is often associated with a palpable trigger point at the origin and/or insertion of affected muscles. For example, a weak quadratus lumborum is frequently found associated on the side of pelvic slant and lumbar rotation (eg, a functional short leg). If this is the case, increasing the muscle's strength tends to normalize the pelvic level and consequent lumbothoracic rotation. Any distortion that is produced by muscular hypo- or hyperactivity is an indication of debilitating postural stress.

Muscular Distortion Pattern 1. In a typical functional "C" scoliosis to the left with level shoulders that are not rotated, the occiput will usually be low on the right with slight rotation and be associated with a weak right splenius and rhomboids. The pelvis will be low on the left and be associated with a weak right psoas and quadratus lumborum (Fig. 13.23). A short leg on the left is often associated, and this may be either functional or structural in nature. This long idiopathic "C" pattern, extending from the pelvis to the occiput, is similar to, but not as severe as, that seen in poliomyelitis, cerebral palsy, syringomyelia, the muscular dystrophies, and Friedreich's ataxia.

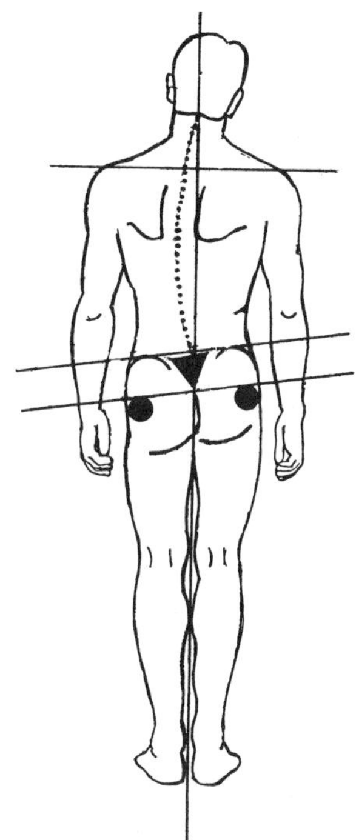

Figure 13.23. Muscular distortion pattern 1.

Muscular Distortion Pattern 2. In time, the idiopathic "C" scoliosis will usually progress into a double major "S" scoliosis of equal magnitude (Fig. 13.24). The majority of these consist of a right thoracic curve and a left lumbar curve.[199] In this example, the left ilium is low and the sacrum tips to the left. Either curve may be primary, and this is usually determined by which curve offers the most stiffness and structural changes. When the distortion fully develops as an attempt to gain better weight distribution, the left shoulder may drop and rotate anterior on the same side as the low and anterior hip. This is not shown in the drawing. The occiput and trochanters will usually be relatively level unless a structural short leg is associated. Invariably, examination will disclose a weak lower latissimus dorsi on the side of concavity of the lower curve, possible hypertonicity or spasm of the quadratus lumborum on the side of convexity of the lower curve, and a weak upper trapezius and deltoid on the side of convexity of the upper curve. The symmetry and balance of

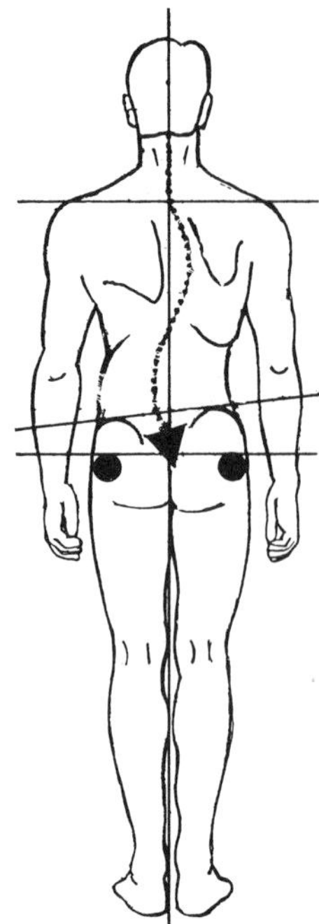

Figure 13.24. Muscular distortion pattern 2.

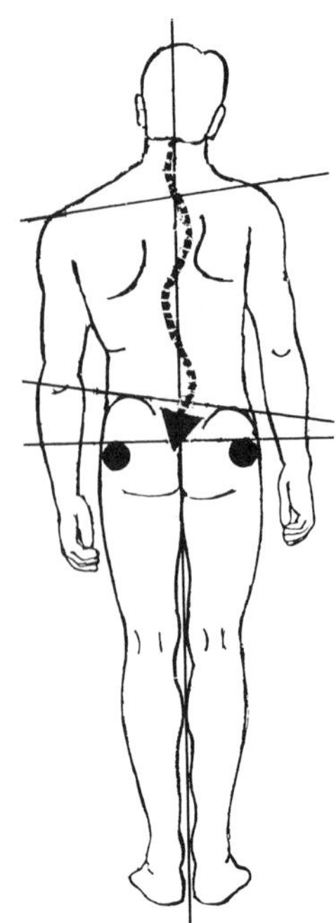

Figure 13.25. Muscular distortion pattern 3.

this type of distortion is usually less deforming from a purely postural point of view than the "C" curve. Keim states that a lumbar major will be to the left in 65% of cases.[200]

Muscular Distortion Pattern 3. Not infrequently, a quadruple curve is presented. For instance, there may be a curve to the right in the lower lumbar and midthoracic areas and a curve to the left in the thoracolumbar and thoracocervical areas. The sacrum and pelvis tip toward the right and anterior, the right shoulder is high and posterior, and the occiput is high on the left and possibly rotated to the right (Fig. 13.25). This situation frequently presents a weak quadratus lumborum, psoas, latissimus dorsi, splenius, and rhomboids on the right and a bilaterally weak upper trapezius. The result is a distinct spinal torsion when viewed from above, with the pelvis and shoulders turned in opposite directions. Quite often, the examiner will find weak glutei associated with a weak psoas or quadratus lumborum and a weak middle deltoid associated with upper trapezius weakness.

Muscular vs Structural Distortions. In addition to the traction tests mentioned previously, DeJarnette feels that a totally muscular scoliosis will be greatly modified when the patient stands on his toes with body weight bilaterally equal, thus offering new stimuli to the higher centers.[201] On the other hand, he feels that a subluxation pattern or one produced by structural changes will not be altered by this "tiptoe" test (Fig. 13.26).

Subluxation Patterns Manifested as Scoliosis[9,93,202–205]

During plumb-line analysis of subluxation patterns, a few basic principles should be remembered.

1. It will be found that an isolated subluxation will strike the line if at all possible. This is the site of antalgic equilibrium that offers the least stress to an already stressed area. However, if splinting is severe, the protective distortion makes visual analysis impossible.

2. From a biomechanical viewpoint, an isolated or focal subluxation can be considered to be in a state of segmental scoliosis (lateral bending and rotation), lordosis (extension), or kyphosis (flexion). When a vertebral segment is in a state of extension (lordosis), the posterior elements of the motion unit are compressed, the facets tend to

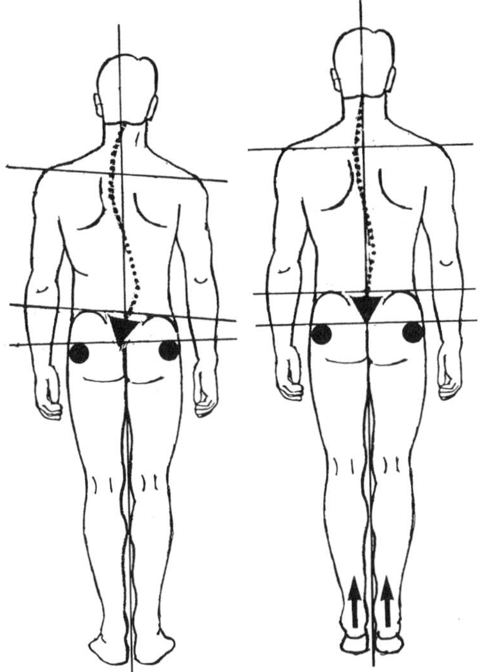

Figure 13.26. *Left*, a double-major scoliosis. *Right*, when the patient stands on his toes, the distortion is greatly reduced. This is a strong indication that this distortion is essentially muscular in nature.

open anteriorly, the anterior elements are under tension, and attached ribs are pushed anteriorly by the transverse processes. During a state of flexion (kyphosis), the posterior elements are stretched, the facets tend to open posteriorly, the anterior elements are compressed, and attached ribs are pulled posteriorly.

3. During lateral flexion of the healthy spine in either the neutral or flexed position, coupled rotation of the upper thoracic vertebral bodies is toward the concavity (cervical coupling) and rotation of the lower thoracic bodies is toward the convexity (lumbar coupling). However, during lateral flexion in the extended posture, the upper thoracic vertebral bodies tend to rotate toward the convexity and rotation of the lower thoracic bodies is toward the concavity. Thus, segmental fixation in the neutral flexed position or the extended position will influence the direction of a scoliosis.

4. When a thoracic vertebra is tipped laterally (as during lateral flexion), an inferior base (increasing shear moments) is provided for the spine above. During lateral tipping of a thoracic vertebra, the inferior facet on the side of concavity arcs down and medially, and the inferior facet gliding up and laterally on the side of convexity tenses the apophyseal capsule. There is no facet jamming or pivoting involved on the side of concavity unless there is considerable extension. The IVD thins and protrudes on the side of concavity because of compressive forces. The IVD widens and contracts on the side of convexity because of tensile forces. The nucleus bulges on the side of convexity.

5. Axial rotation of a thoracic vertebra is always coupled with some degree of lateral bending and takes place with the ribs, not between the ribs.

6. When analyzing spinal distortions, the examiner should determine the type of biomechanical forces and/or muscular weakness or hyperactivity that would be responsible for initially holding the focal subluxation in a fixed position.

Subluxation Pattern 1. This common distortion is a major thoracolumbar curve that usually runs from the T5 area to the upper lumbar area (Fig. 13.27). A short, secondary functional lumbar curve in the opposite direction develops, but compensation above is usually made within one or two of the upper dorsal segments. The occiput, shoulders, and trochanters are usually level, but the ileum is high on the left and the sacrum is tipped to the left when the thoracic major curves to the right. The overall distortion depends on the degree of rotation involved.

Thoracic Subluxation Pattern 2. Structural damage at a lower thoracic segment (eg, wedged vertebra) as the result of a chronic subluxation or structural defect will often present a rapidly developing "C" curve fairly restricted to the thoracic region (Fig. 13.28). According to statistics, most such curves are to the right. This distortion is also one of the most frequently seen idiopathic patterns, thus discussed here. The shoulder will be high on the side of upper thoracic convexity, but the iliac crests, sacrum, and trochanters are usually level. The occiput will usually be level, and the cervical

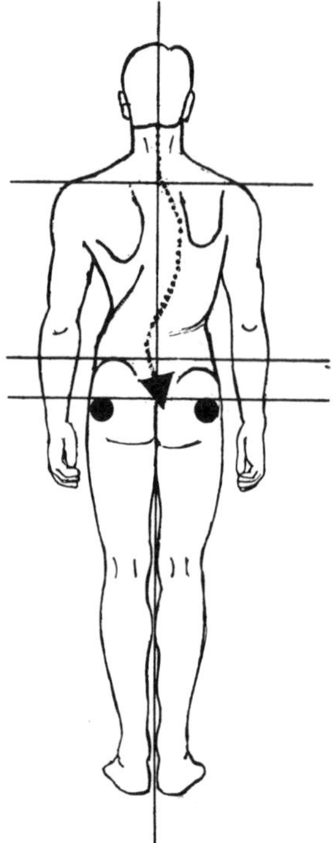

Figure 13.27. Subluxation pattern 1.

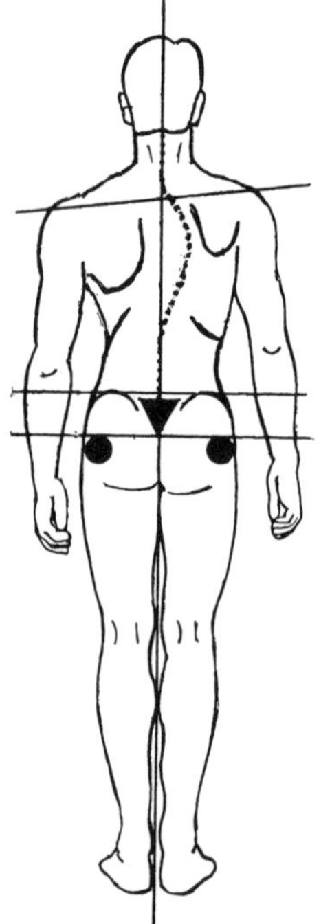

Figure 13.28. Subluxation pattern 2.

segments will be aligned. This "C" curve infrequently progresses to a double-major "S" curve in the thoracic spine with one curve, for example, at the upper spine involving the T1–T6 segments and the lower curve involving the T7–T12 segments. For some unexplained reason, most medical orthopedists always consider the right curve the major. The cervical spine and lower lumbar spine are rarely influenced, and this means that considerable compensation must take place at the thoracocervical and thoracolumbar transitional vertebrae. Regardless of cause, the curve is usually quite stiff and does not reduce much with postural changes. Because there is frequently severe rotation involved, the ribs of the side of convexity become deformed, and this can lead to cardiopulmonary impairment in curves over 60°.

Thoracic Subluxation Pattern 3. These patterns involve a thoracolumbar transitional vertebra that is fixed in both rotation and tipping. The free ribs offer little protection against subluxation. Figure 13.29, *left*, shows the early pattern often seen in a subluxated thoracolumbar transitional vertebra, T10–L1, that has shifted inferior on the right or whose nucleus has shifted lateral to the left, or both. The vertebra is locked in a position where the centrum is rotated to the left and tipped in lateral flexion to the right. Figure 13.29, *center*, shows the same subluxation picture that has become chronic and is over compensated. The "Z" scoliosis is the result of the lumbar spine angling toward the left, abruptly shifting toward the right at the transitional segment, and then the spine returning to the left near the T8 or T9 level. Figure 13.29, *right*, shows the same subluxation pattern that has become well compensated. Although the occiput and shoulders are in the midline, the "Z" distortion is evident but to a much lesser degree.

Thoracic Subluxation Pattern 4. These patterns involve a lower thoracic vertebra that is fixed in a laterally flexed or tipped position inferiorly on the right with minimum or no rotation involved. Figure 13.30, *left*, shows the acute antalgic pattern. Pressure on the involved spinous process toward the left to increase the tilt will increase pain.

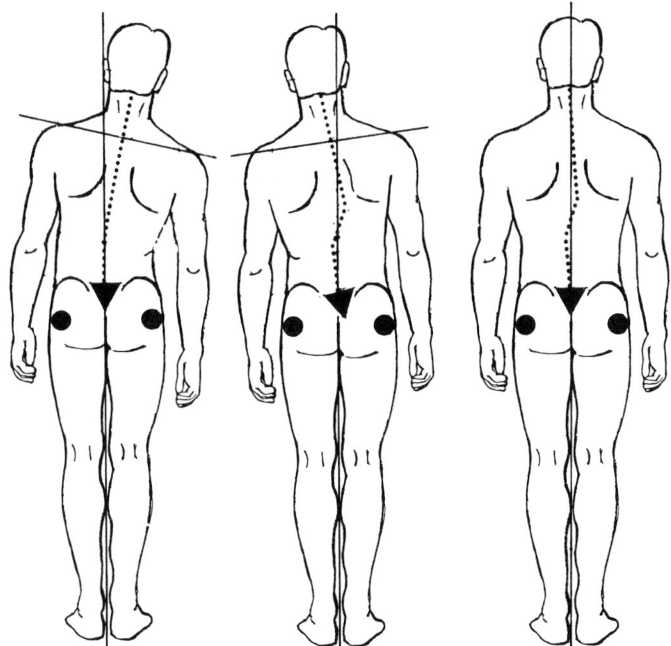

Figure 13.29. Subluxation pattern 3.

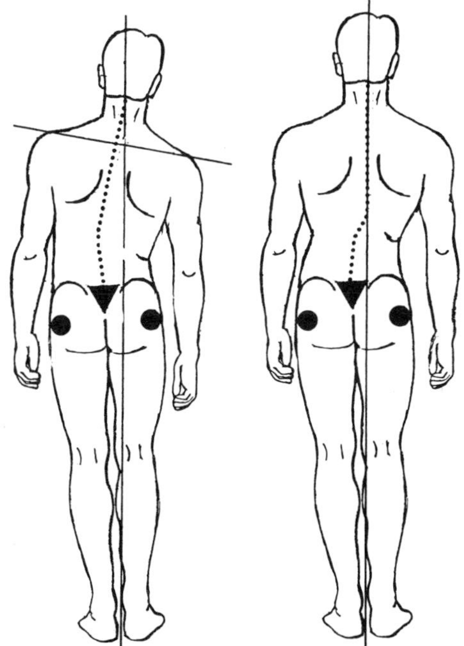

Figure 13.30. Subluxation pattern 4.

Note the lateral shifting of the pelvis to the left and the upper body to the right of the midline. Figure 13.30, *right*, shows the more chronic pattern in which there is still pelvic shifting to the left but the upper body has become well compensated.

Thoracic Subluxation Pattern 5. These patterns involve a lower thoracic vertebra that is fixed in a rotated position with minimal or no tipping involved. Figure 13.31, *left*, shows the acute "Z" pattern in which rotation of the involved vertebra is to the left. This indicates that the vertebra is likely to also be locked in extension. To ease the pain, the lumbar region tries to adapt and the pelvis is shifted to the right of the midline. The right shoulder is high, and the neck is laterally flexed to the right in compensation. Secondary torticollis may be produced. The right drawing shows the more chronic state in which a long "C" curve has developed above the subluxation. Compare the plumb-line position with that of Figure 13.23.

Thoracic Subluxation Pattern 6. These patterns involve a subluxated T9–T11 vertebra. It is frequently a subluxation just superior to the transitional vertebra. Figure 13.32, *left*, depicts the unusual pattern of combined tipping to the right and rotation of the centrum to the left. Note how the pelvis is shifted to the left and the upper

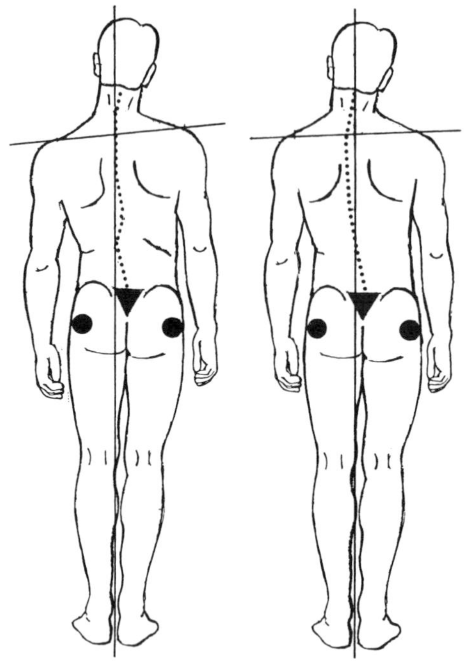

Figure 13.31. Subluxation pattern 5.

body is shifted to the right but parallel to the midline. Figure 13.32, *center,* depicts left rotation of the centrum with minimal or no tipping. Note the absence of pelvic shifting and low occiput on the right. Figure 13.32, *right,* shows a more severe form of left rotation of the centrum with minimal or no tilting. Note that the pelvis is shifted laterally to the right, the shoulder girdle is distorted, and the upper spine fails to return to the midline. Goodheart feels that a unilateral weak left trapezius is indicated by the high occiput and low shoulder.[206]

DeJarnette[207] believes that all these subluxations involve the trapezius to a great extent. The trapezius, supplied by a cranial nerve, plays a major role in corrective righting reflexes for the thoracic spine and shoulder girdle. Over-response from either somatosomatic or viscerosomatic input is characterized by numerous trigger points at the muscle's points of origin and insertion.

Thoracic Subluxation Pattern 7. These patterns involve a subluxated midthoracic vertebra. Figure 13.33, *left,* gives an example in which the vertebra has rotated toward the left and locked in extension, and the right trapezius is hypertonic. Complaints include midthoracic pain extending to the left shoulder and neck. Note the lower-body shift to the left and the high shoulder on the right. Figure 13.33, *right,* portrays the typical pattern of subluxation in which the vertebra is painfully tipped to the left with minimal or no rotation. Note the pelvic shift to the right, the sharp spinal break as the involved area crosses the midline, and the uncompensated neck position.

Thoracic Subluxation Pattern 8. These patterns involve a subluxated upper thoracic vertebra. Figure 13.34, *left,* portrays a vertebra that has subluxated inferior on the right with rotation to the left. Acute tenderness will be found over the left transverse process, and pain is increased by spinous pressure that increases the tilt and rotation. The left shoulder is high, and the occiput is rotated inferior and posterior on the right. Figure 13.34, *center,* shows a vertebra that is subluxated in rotation to the left with minimal tilting. Figure 13.34, *right,* shows a vertebra that is subluxated inferior on the left with minimal rotation.

CONSIDERATIONS IN PRIMARY LUMBAR SCOLIOSIS[208–212]

Traction and DeJarnette's "tip-toe test" to differentiate a fixed spinal distortion from a muscular reaction were described in a previous chapter. If a patient rises bilaterally on his toes and a distortion pattern is greatly modified, it is a clue that the distortion is muscular in nature and not structurally permanent. A fixed pattern would not be altered by such a simple maneuver, but a muscular response would likely be altered by the initiation of new stimuli. The "tip-toe test" can also be utilized unilaterally, first one side and then the other, to note which areas change and which do not. As the heel is elevated, observe the effect upon the total spine and pelvis and especially note actions of the pelvic and shoulder girdles.

Because a curved rod is more flexible than a straight rod, a nonrigid scoliotic spine is much more flexible in axial traction than a normal spine; eg, a coiled spring is more flexible than a straight wire when axial tension is applied.

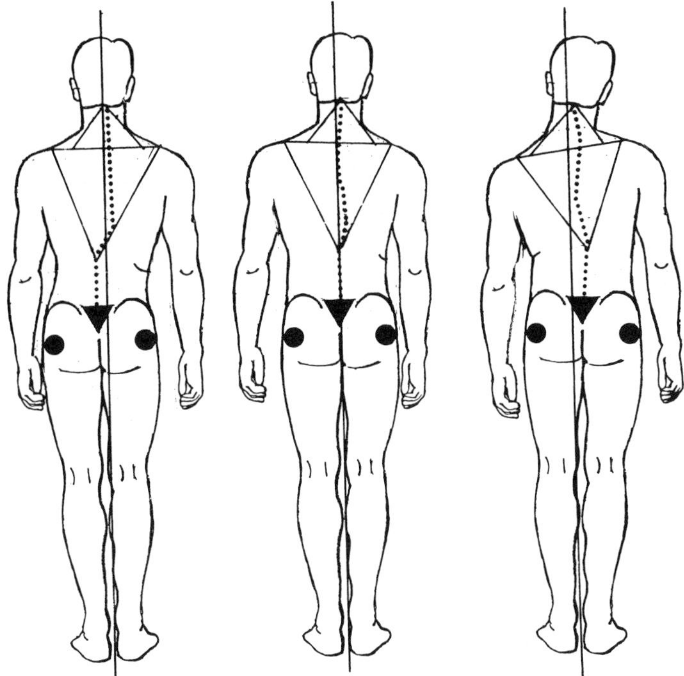

Figure 13.32. Subluxation pattern 6.

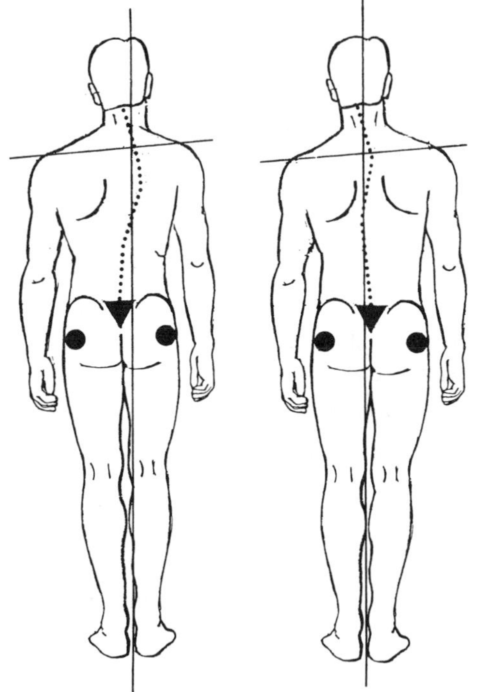

Figure 13.33. Subluxation pattern 7.

Lovett's Principles

An understanding of Lovett's principles and the basic types of lumbar scolioses offers insight into distortion analysis.

Lovett's Rule. This principle states that if the base of a weight-bearing segmented column such as the spine is caused to tilt (eg, unilateral anteroinferior sacral subluxation), the center of weight bearing will shift toward the high side of the base because it is the shortest distance between the point of weight origin and weight reception. The involved segments will then seek to escape the load by shifting and rotating to the opposite side.

Lovett Positive Scoliosis. In a Lovett positive scoliosis, the axis of vertebral rotation in the lumbar area is posterior to the articulating processes. When the segments are asymmetrically loaded, the bodies of the involved segments normally deviate farther from the midline than their spinous processes.

Lovett Excess Scoliosis. If a Lovett positive scoliosis occurs that is far more than that demanded by the base inferiority, the condition is referred to as an excessive Lov-

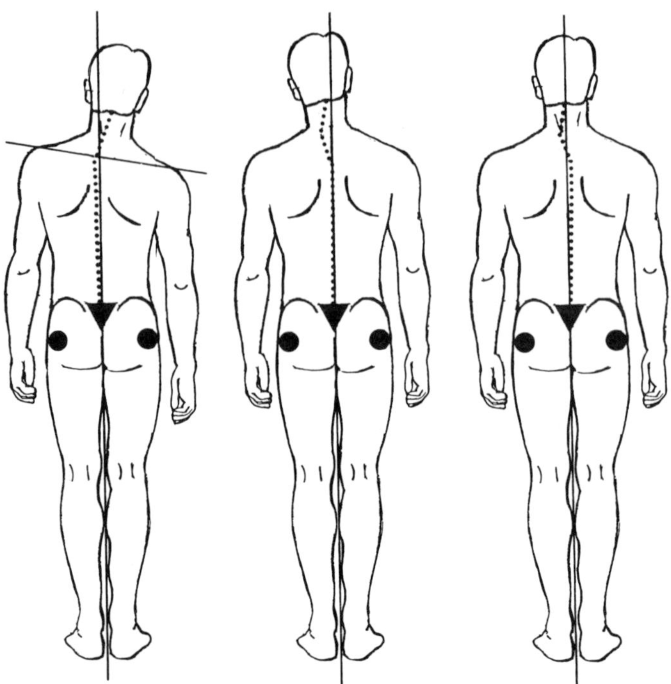

Figure 13.34. Subluxation pattern 8.

ett positive. This state is usually attributed to an iliopsoas spasm on the side of concavity that accentuates the curve beyond the norm.

Lovett Negative Scoliosis. If a lumbar scoliosis shows that the spinous processes have deviated from the midline further than the vertebral bodies, the condition is said to be atypical (negative). A negative scoliosis is indicative of marked muscle involvement. The common causes of this muscle involvement are: (1) muscle spasm associated with facet irritation (eg, jamming, instability); (2) disturbed or incompatible movement dynamics (eg, subluxation, fixation); (3) local unilateral muscle contraction as the result of noxious viscerosomatic reflexes (eg, viscera pathology); (4) antalgic splinting, resulting in scoliotic deviations whose transverse planes are almost completely horizontal. If left uncorrected, such antalgic curves will eventually produce a secondary sacroiliac distortion that will compromise normal lumbopelvic dynamics.

Alteration of Curves Secondary to Muscular Imbalance

This deformity features scoliosis and/or alteration of the normal A-P curves for which there is no apparent structural basis. The distortion is associated with muscular weakness or spasticity such as of the psoas in the lumbar spine or the sternocleidomastoideus in the cervical spine; postural imbalance and interference to normal locomotive effort; muscular soreness and fatigue; irritative microtrauma to all involved vertebral motion units; compensatory curvatures; and biomechanical impropriety transmitted throughout the entire spinal column (Fig. 13.35).

Alteration of Curves Secondary to Structural Asymmetries

This type of distortion is characterized by unleveling of spinal support due to anomaly, trauma, or pathology in which structural unleveling of the spine above tends to portray a normal compensatory response if the motion units are functional. The situation signifies general postural incompetence and interference to the normal locomotive effort; muscular tension, soreness, and fatigue; irritation of the involved motion units; compensatory curvatures; and a biome-

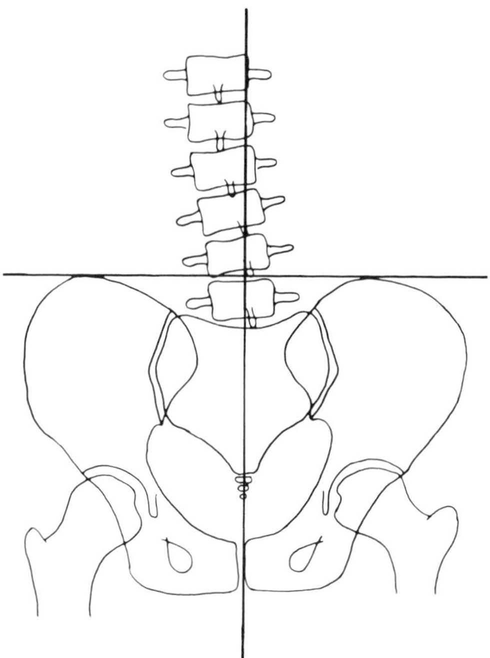

Figure 13.35. Film tracing showing alteration of lumbar region secondary to muscular imbalance.

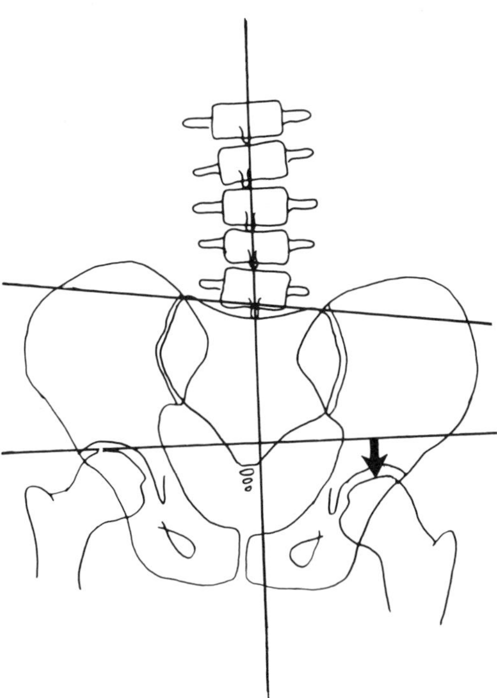

Figure 13.36. Film tracing showing alteration of lumbar region secondary to structural asymmetry. A Lovett positive scoliosis is seen. *Arrow* points to leg length deficiency.

chanical insult transmitted throughout the entire spinal column (Fig. 13.36).

Decompensation of Adaptational Curves

This Lovett negative deformity features an absence or reversal of compensatory curvatures that should be present because of structural unleveling and a tendency for the vertebral bodies to rotate in a direction opposite to that which would normally occur. The situation points toward acute muscular contractions, pain associated with movement, a frequently associated acute disc syndrome, strained effort in the erect posture with compensatory voluntary torsion of the spine above, radicular neurologic involvement, and biomechanical insults transmitted throughout the entire spinal column (Fig. 13.37).

Illi[213,214] describes three basic types of Lovett negative scolioses:

1. A scoliotic state with very little rotation of the vertebral segments, as shown by the midline position of the spinous processes. In the lumbar spine, it frequently indicates unilateral shortening (ie, spasm, hypertonicity, or contracture) of the iliopsoas on the

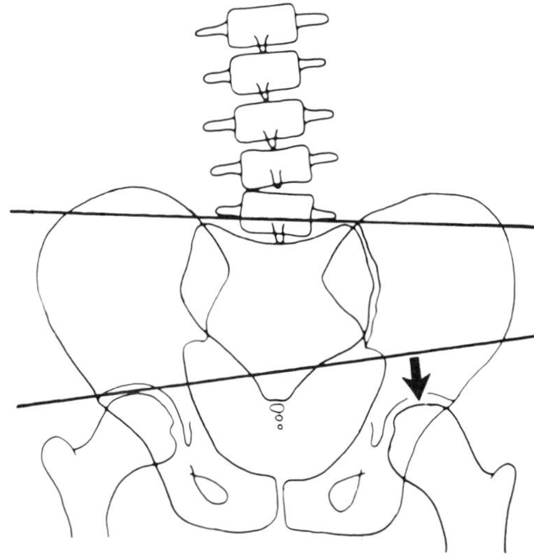

Figure 13.37. Film tracing showing decompensation of adaptational curve. Adaptation is made solely at the L4–L5 joint. *Arrow* points to leg length deficiency.

side of convexity or of the contralateral multifidi.

2. A scoliotic state in which the lumbar spinous processes have deviated farther from the midline than the vertebral bodies. This is indicative of acute muscle contraction, usually involving the multifidi and/or rotatores on the side of convexity.

3. A scoliotic state in which the spine is relatively axially aligned when a compensatory scoliotic deviation should be expected because of an inferiority. This abnormal state may be in the thoracic-lumbar relationship, lumbar-pelvic relationship, or both. Janse gives the example of a right lumbar scoliosis in which there is a failure of a left compensatory dorsal scoliosis to develop because of hypertonicity of the deep right thoracic musculature resulting from chronic reflex irritation arising from an inflamed gallbladder or some other viscerosomatic reflex. A scoliotic state is sometimes seen in which the degree of scoliotic lumbar deviation is far less than that which would be expected by the degree of pelvic tilt. The usual cause for this is an antalgic lumbar splinting, but a viscerosomatic reflex (eg, iliocecal syndrome, ovarian cyst) should not be overlooked.

Abnormal Motion of a Spinal Section

Here we have a deformity that is characterized by restriction of movement of two or more vertebral motion units, with the regions above or below possibly exhibiting excessive compensatory movement. This type of distortion is associated with muscular soreness, fatigue, and other muscle dysfunctions, possible ossification of the longitudinal ligaments, possible degenerative joint disease with concomitant ankylosis, microtrauma to all involved vertebral motion units, and biomechanical insult to all associated motion units (Fig. 13.38).

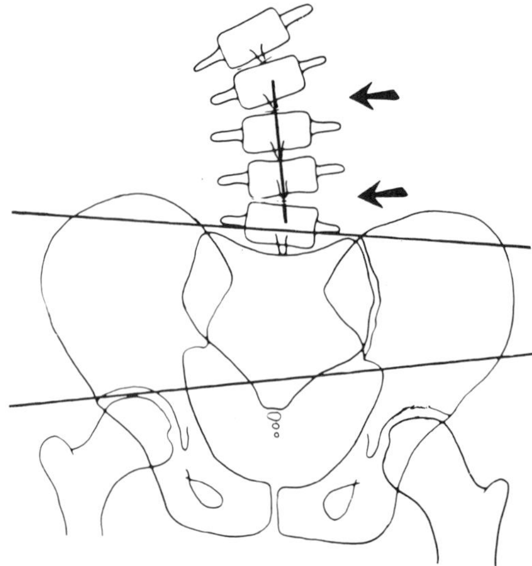

Figure 13.38. Abnormal motion of the lumbar region. In this example, *arrows* point to areas of excessive motion at L2–L3 and L4–L5 to compensate for locking at the L3–L4 joint.

Scoliosis Presenting with Severe Low-Back Pain

The incidence of low-back pain appears to be the same in patients with or without obvious spinal deformity.[215, 216] However, the degree of pain experienced may vary. Jackson and associates found that patients with major lumbar curves had more pain, and the area of complaint was frequently below the site of the major deformity. The most painful and disabling patterns were the compensatory lumbosacral curves. It appeared that the pain originated from the concavity side of the curve and included discogenic, facet joint, and radicular origins. Kostuik and Bentivoglio also found that as the degree of curvature increased, the severity of pain increased, especially for curves of 45° or larger. They also reported that (1) the presence of facet scoliosis correlated with a history of pain in 64% of the cases, and (2) there was a high correlation between radiologic changes and the incidence of pain.

Prophylactic surgery to prevent future back pain in patients who have abnormal lumbar curves is not generally justified.[217] Nachemson reports that whether severe low-back pain occurs more often in patients who have distorted lumbar curves than in those whose spines are straight is open to question, since calculations show approximately the same incidence of surgery for back pain in scoliotic patients and in those whose spines are straight. Because surgery for scoliosis in the adult carries a high risk and long-term efficacy is unproved, he recommends that all types of conservative measures be tried before considering an operation. However, if unremitting pain from room entrapment occurs (eg, foraminal compression, pedicular kinking) or a painful degenerative scoliosis develops in the elderly, referral for surgical decompression may be the only alternative.[218–220]

LUMBOPELVIC CONSIDERATIONS

Unilaterally Low Pelvis[9, 223–237]

Underlying most physical activity is the maintenance of upright posture, which is essentially a continuous contest between the individual and gravitational forces. In just opposing gravity to achieve and maintain posture, a person consumes approximately 40% of his total energy. If one lower extremity is short, additional muscular effort is necessary to avoid toppling.

During maturation, the long bones do not appear to lengthen simultaneously. One side grows faster than the other for a few months. Then the process changes to the other side. Why this occurs has not been explained, but it does explain how a "missed phase" results in one extremity being shorter than its counterpart. When recognized to be severe, orthopedic surgeons frequently place pins within epiphyseal plates of the femoral head to retard growth "until the other side catches up." Unilateral genu varum or valgum, surgical or fracture trauma, atrophy, or a flattened arch will have the same ultimate effect on pelvic level.

Mensuration

Anatomical shortening may be the result of linear retardation anywhere from the height of the plantar surface to the depth of the acetabulum. Because the head of the femur cannot be palpated, the anatomical lower extremity length is measured by custom in the supine position from the ASIS to a point on the medial malleolus (Fig. 13.39).

An apparent leg length inequality is frequently detected after true leg lengths have been found to be symmetrical. Physiologic shortening can come from asymmetrical iliac rotation, abnormal femoral neck angulation, knee or ankle joint distortions, a longitudinal arch flattened by prolonged unilateral weight bearing (eg, occupational), or any factor affecting unilateral pelvic rotation. The functional lower extremity length is measured in the supine position from the navel or xiphisternal junction to the same point used on the medial malleolus. It only offers a clinical impression.

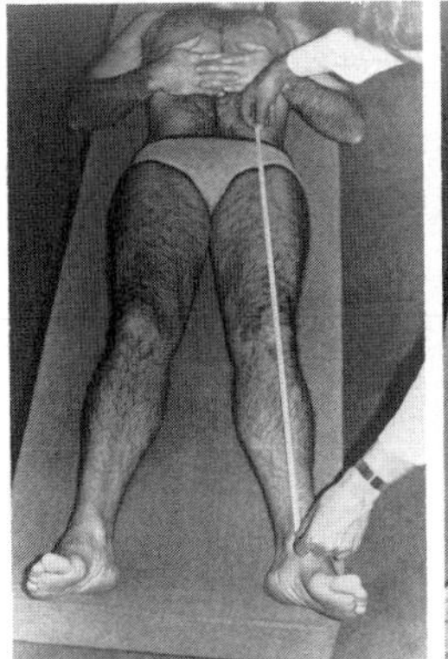
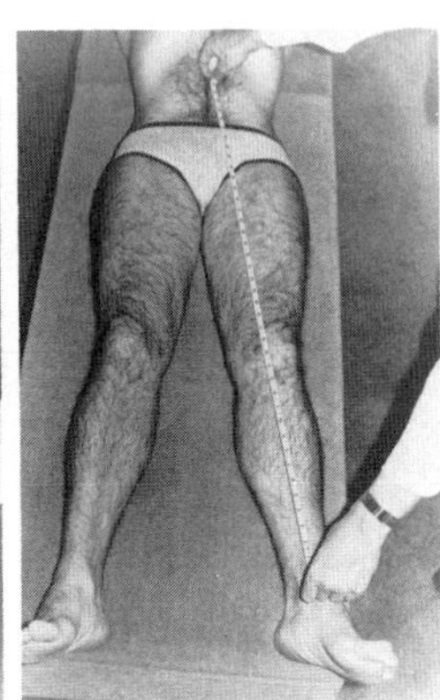

Figure 13.39. Measuring anatomical (*left*) and physiologic (*right*) leg length deficiency.

Ischial deficiency can be screened by noting the level of the iliac crests in the sitting position. This is as accurate as standard roentgenographic techniques unless the films are exposed with an extremely long tube-subject distance to reduce image distortion.

Structural Patterns during Adulthood

An anatomical or functional short leg, or both, will show that:

1. Upon fully extending the legs of the supine patient with a leg deficiency, the extremity on the side of involvement will be retracted shorter than its mate on the opposite side because the posterior innominate rotation causes the acetabulum to be carried superior and anterior: the superior position producing the retraction of the limb. However, upon bringing the extremities upward to an extended position of right angles to the body, the short leg will appear to be the longest because the acetabulum of the posterior innominate has been carried superior and anterior and the anterior position now produces the added length.

2. If a standing patient with a short leg seeks to rest his back by shifting from one foot to the other, he will come to rest by bearing most weight on the side on which the leg is short, the sacrum has gravitated anterior, and inferior, and the low iliac crest

has rotated posterior and inferior. Using dual weight scales, it is clear that the patient habitually carries the most weight on the side of the short leg. When posterior iliac rotation, sacral inferiority, or weight dominance is on the side of the long leg, a biomechanical complication is involved.

3. The pelvis normally tends to rotate as a whole anteriorly on the low side during stance. If this does not occur, a complication is involved. With the patient in the flexed Adams position, the pelvis slants anteriorly and inferiorly on the side of extremity deficiency. The lumbar spine gravitates into scoliotic deviation to the low sacral side, which establishes a state of reverse rotation between L5 and the sacrum. If the pelvis horizontally rotates backward on the low side or the lumbar curve is toward the high extremity, a biomechanical complication is involved. A common exception to this is an acutely inflamed sacroiliac lesion on the low side, the patient will attempt to maintain weight on the high side to relieve pain. This would cause the lumbar scoliosis to straighten or possibly reverse to the high side. If the lower lumbar region is fixed, adaptation will not occur until the first freely movable segment is reached (eg, T12) and the shift will be made sharply (Fig. 13.40).

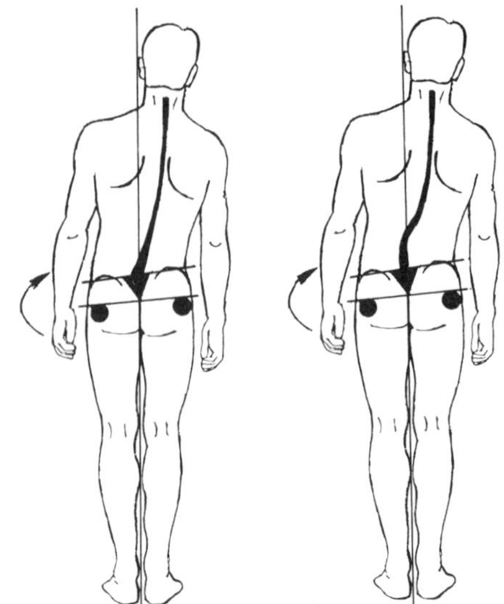

Figure 13.40. *Left*, antalgic posture of acute left sacroiliac lesion. Note eccentric curve to the right as an attempt to shift weight from the irritation. *Right*, same condition with L3–S1 fixation.

Structural Adaptations during Growth

A unilateral short lower extremity during early development produces a pelvic dip and possible anterior pelvic rotation on the low side during stance. This initiates a series of slow compensatory changes in childhood to maintain equilibrium in the most efficient manner.

The Early Stage. The low ilium tends to rotate anteriorly and the high ilium posteriorly. This is an attempt to relatively raise the acetabulum on the low side and lower it on the high side. The lateral aspects of the sacrum are carried with the ilia without subluxation. While this shifting affords 1–2 mm of equalization, the sacrum is forced into an abdominal position of accommodation where its base is tipped anteroinferior on the low side and posterosuperior on the high side.

The Late Stage. The sacrum then tends to laterally tilt upward on the low side and downward on the high side between the ilia in an attempt to level its weight-bearing base, but because of its jammed position between the iliam movement is restricted. As L5 follows the sacral base, tilting and rotation of the remaining supple lumbar vertebra must be made to return the spine to the midline. The midlumbar region is displaced laterally as the lumbar region curves toward the low side. This lateral lumbar sway moves greater body mass toward the low side, which must be restricted by (1) hypertonicity on the contralateral loin, pelvic, hip, and thigh muscles and (2) a laterally reverse sway of the relatively stiff dorsal spine to move body mass on the other side of the midline to assist equilibrium.

If these stages occur prior to maturity when the musculoskeletal system is quite flexible, the picture is asymptomatic. However, if it occurs later in life when the spine is less adaptable, we will witness various patterns of distortion in the body's attempt to maintain level semicircular canals and bilateral body mass distribution.

In the healthy spine, the picture described above in stance should disappear in the sitting position if the pelvis is structurally symmetrical. This ideal situation is infrequently seen clinically because ligaments will tend to shorten in time on the concave side so that the distortion will be in a chronic state of fixation leading to structural changes.

Superimposed on both early and late attempts at adaptation will be the effects of trauma, structural anomalies, poor nutrition, lack of exercise, stresses of daily living, and noxious reflexes. This is the clinical spine examined every day in practice, and accurate analysis of these variables and their effects is what differentiates the physician from the therapist.

Pelvic Subluxation Patterns Exhibiting Scoliosis[9, 93, 204, 208, 209, 238–242]

As with primary thoracic patterns, primary pelvic distortions reflect an individual's biomechanics that are responsive to underlying processes.

Basic Considerations

Logan's Rule.[93] In studying spinal distortion patterns, it is well to keep in mind Logan's rule: "The body of the lowest freely movable vertebra always rotates toward the lowest side of the sacrum or the foundation upon which it rests." This gravitational effect has a mechanical advantage in that, as the thicker anterior aspect of the lower lumbar vertebrae and their discs rotate away from the midline, there is a mechanical compensation created axially to make up mass height for the sacral inferiority to where the apical segment becomes horizontal. Above the apex where the increase in mass has created a superiority, the vertebrae tip toward the concavity and rotate "uphill." This in turn produces an inferior base for the lower dorsal vertebrae on the contralateral side, and a secondary curve develops.

Static vs Dynamic Scolioses. Scoliotic distortions that result from a structural deficiency such as an anatomically short femur, tibia, or flattened longitudinal arch while standing, an axially short ischium while sitting, or a wedged vertebral segment, produce distortions referred to as *static curvatures.* Curvatures arising from locomotion dysfunctions (eg, pelvic subluxation-fixations, contractures, paralysis) are called curvatures of disturbed motion or *dynamic curvatures.* Illi's studies[209] have shown that most scolioses classified by allopaths as primary lumbar scolioses have their origin in sacroiliac dysfunction, but any disturbance in movement may give rise to such a curvature.

Reference Points. The primary points of reference in visual analysis are trochanter level (marked); sacral level; iliac crest level; direction of pelvic rotation; direction of lumbar, thoracic, and cervical scoliosis; shoulder girdle level and its direction of rotation; and occipital tilt.

Unequal-Limb Effects on the Lumbar Spine. Through precision postural roentgenography, Giles and Taylor have shown that leg length inequality of 9 mm or more is often associated with asymmetrical facetal joint angles of the posterior facets.[243] A leg length difference of 1 cm or more is associated with changes in joint cartilage and subchondral bone in the apical and lumbosacral apophyseal joints of the spine in postural scoliosis.[244, 245] It was also shown that leg length inequality is associated with concavities in the end-plates of lumbar vertebrae, wedging of L5, and vertebral traction spurs.[246]

Pelvic Distortion. There is also a distortion of the pelvis as a whole in sacroiliac misalignment. For example, if the sacral base slips anteroinferior on the right with the right ilium rotating posterior on the sacral base, the pelvis as a whole will tend to rotate anteriorly on the right to keep weight centered over the head of the femur because the acetabulum has translated superiorly.

The number of possible patterns that could be shown are almost endless. A few of the basic and unusual patterns will be discussed. Many individual alterations to these examples will be presented clinically because of asymmetry, the effects of superimposed trauma on established patterns, conditioned responses to pain, muscle weakness and soft-tissue shortening from lack of exercise, variable progressing degenerative changes, nutrition, etc. However, it is only from recognizing the normal and the typical that the abnormal and atypical can be appreciated.

Some Pelvic Subluxation Patterns with Level Femurs

Pelvic Subluxation Pattern 1. Hugh B. Logan[204] referred to this acute pattern as exhibiting the primary subluxation. He called it the "leaning tower." It either corrects itself spontaneously or transcends into a more stable state. In the example shown in Figure 13.41, the trochanters are level. The sacral base is slightly subluxated anteroinferior on the right, and the sacral apex is left of the midline. The iliac crests are level. The lower lumbar region is tilted to the right as it follows the sacral base but breaks sharply in the lower or midthoracic area. The spinous processes are well aligned from the lower or midthoracic region upward but slightly lateral to the midline so that the head is level but to the right. The shoulder is slightly low on the side of midline deviation. The iliopsoas and lumbar erector spinae are tense on the right, but the flank muscles are often flaccid. The right sacroiliac ligament is tense and tender. Why is the upper body carried to the right of the midline? The first suspicions should be pain in the left lumbopelvic region or psoas shortening on the right.

Pelvic Subluxation Pattern 2. This S-shaped distortion typically presents a primary and secondary rotary scoliosis. In the example shown in Figure 13.41, the trochanters are level. The sacrum is severely subluxated anteroinferior on the right. The right iliac crest is high, thus exhibiting eccentric innominate rotation, and the sacral apex is deviated to the left of the midline. The whole pelvis is rotated anterior on the right. The lower lumbar bodies are tipped to the right and rotated posterior on the right side of the low sacrum. The thoracic spine is curved to the left, and the left shoulder is high. The cervical region may be aligned or carried to the left depending on upper thoracic compensation. The occiput is usually either high on the left or level, depending upon cervical compensation. The buttock muscles and right sacroiliac ligament are usually tense and tender. The first question to answer is why the right iliac crest is high. The first suspicions should be left flank weakness, right psoas contracture, or a superior right iliac subluxation superimposed on a basic distortion. Iliac position is typically high on the side of pain in lumbar strain and sprain and low on the side of pain in IVD protrusions.

Pelvic Subluxation Pattern 3. This is a compensated triple-curve distortion that is often a progression of pattern 2. In the example shown in Figure 13.42, the lumbar and cervical curves are to the right and the thoracic curve is to the left. The trochanters are level. The sacrum is subluxated anteroinferior on the right, and the sacral apex is deviated to the left of the midline. The right

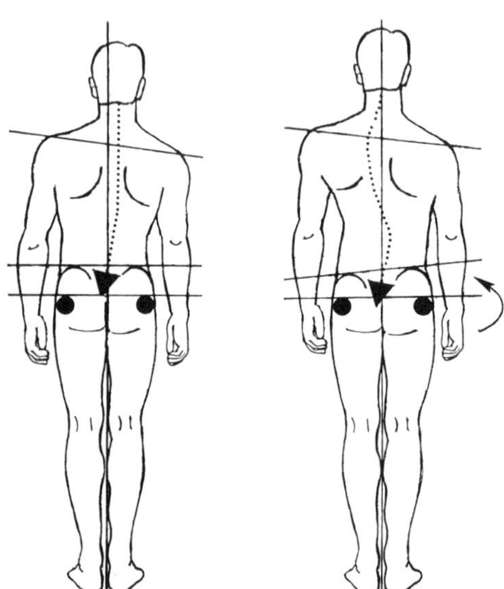

Figure 13.41. *Left*, pelvic subluxation pattern 1; *right*, pelvic subluxation pattern 2.

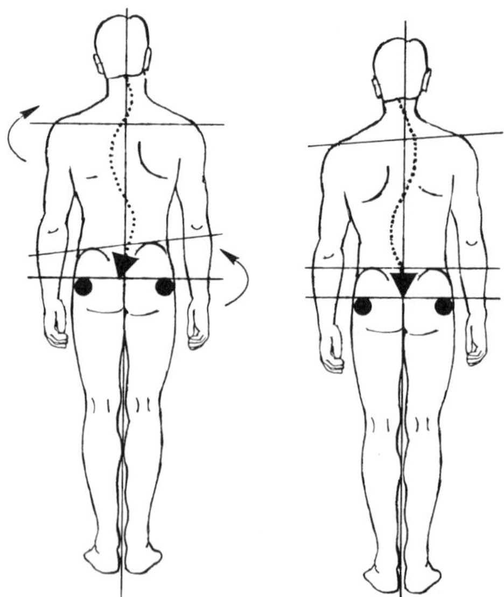

Figure 13.42. *Left*, pelvic subluxation pattern 3; *right*, pelvic subluxation pattern 4.

iliac crest is eccentrically high and rotated posterior. The right sacral dimple will be distinct. The pelvis as a whole is rotated anterior on the right. The lower lumbar bodies are tipped to the right and rotated posterior on the right. The shoulders are either level or tipped to one side, depending upon the site of the thoracocervical transition. The left shoulder in this example is anterior on the right. The occiput is usually tipped low on the left because of the right cervical scoliosis. The lumbar erector spinae and sacroiliac ligament are usually tense and tender on the right. More weight will be carried on the right side, and the patient will tend to flex the right knee or raise the left heel to level the iliac crests. Here there are two priority problems: why the right ilium is high and why the lumbar extensors are spastic on the right. The first things to eliminate would be pelvic pathology (eg, prostate, ovarian) and a lumbar IVD prolapse.

Pelvic Subluxation Pattern 4. This pattern is the effect of structural wedging at L5 or L4. In the example shown in Figure 13.42, the trochanters are level, the sacrum is well aligned with the ilia, and the crests are level. The lumbar region presents a rotary scoliosis on the side of the slanted vertebral body, and a compensatory thoracic scoliosis to the other side develops to bring the head to the midline. The left shoulder in this example would be low and posterior. There are usually few abnormal signs in the lumbar or pelvic soft tissues.

Some Pelvic Subluxation Patterns with Femur Deficiency

Pelvic Subluxation Pattern 5. This distortion is somewhat similar to that of pattern 3, with an added factor of a functional short leg on the right. In the example shown in Figure 13.43, the thoracic curve is shorter, and the tendency is for the shoulder girdle to rotate anterior on the right. The right trochanter is low. The sacrum is rotated anteroinferior on the right, and the sacral apex is to the left of the midline. The iliac crests are level, and the whole pelvis has rotated anterior on the right. The sacral dimple is distinct on the right. The lower lumbar bodies are tipped to the right and rotated posterior on the right. The lower thoracic region is rotated to the left, and the upper thoracic and cervical regions present a right scoliosis. The left shoulder is high, and the occiput is carried low on the left. The lumbar erector spinae, gluteal muscles, and sacroiliac ligament are usually tense and tender on the right. As in pattern 3, more weight will be carried on the right side. Are the crests level because of a short ilium on the left? The muscles on the right should not be tense and tender in a chronic compensated scoliosis. The cause of this acute reaction should be sought.

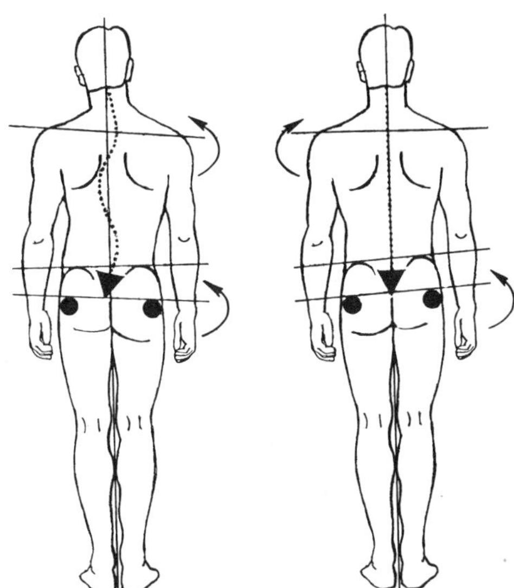

Figure 13.43. *Left*, pelvic subluxation pattern 5; *right*, pelvic subluxation pattern 6.

Pelvic Subluxation Pattern 6. This chronic distortion presents a paradox in that an anteroinferior sacral subluxation on the right is associated with a congenital leg deficiency on the left. In the example shown in Figure 13.43, the left trochanter is low. This pattern often disguises the sacral subluxation in visual analysis because the sacrum appears level but is subluxated anteroinferior on the right. The pelvis as a whole is rotated anterior on the right. The right iliac crest is high, but because more weight is shifted to the right, compressive forces are increased on the right that, in time, tend to push the right innominate inferior and medial. There is also joint compression at the right hip, knee, ankle, and longitudinal arch. When this occurs, the sacrum that appeared level in the first stage will now appear slightly lower on the right and the crests will be level. The lumbar, thoracic, and cervical regions are well aligned, and the shoulders and occiput are level. The lower lumbar erector spinae and sacroiliac ligament are usually taut on the right.

Pelvic Subluxation Pattern 7. This pattern is always the result of acute trauma producing a functional leg deficiency. It grossly appears somewhat like pattern 1, with subtle differences created by the short leg. In the example shown in Figure 13.44, the trochanter and iliac crest are low on the right. The sacrum has reciprocally rotated with the ilia and the sagging pelvis. The entire spine leans to the right of the midline, and the right shoulder is low. The problem here is usually a posterior ilium on the right or an anterior ilium on the left, which may or may not be associated with a contralateral fixation. This is typical, but why is the head held to the right of the midline? This can be easily explained by left sacroiliac pain, but if pain is on the right, seek a proprioception disturbance related to an upper cervical subluxation. If left uncorrected, later compensation will probably produce a long smooth thoracic "C" or "S" curve.

Long-Leg Sciatica

A study by Maxwell revealed that patients with a presenting complaint of sciatica affecting the high side of pelvic inequality did not respond as well to chiropractic therapy as did those with sciatica on the low side.[247] Re-evaluation of patients who did not respond initially revealed the presence of a *piriformis muscle syndrome* on the side of the long extremity.

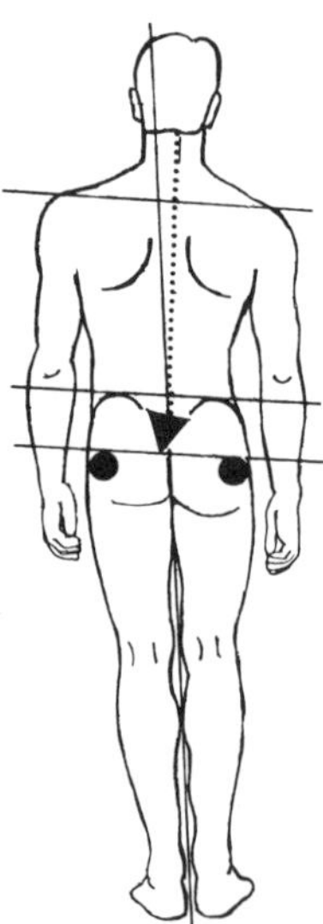

Figure 13.44. Pelvic subluxation pattern 7.

Instrumentation

After six years of research, M. A. Sabia has developed a "Scoliometer" that accurately measures six areas to detect even slight degrees of scoliosis and three measurements to detect abnormal A-P curves. Measurements can be recorded in degrees or centimeters-millimeters.[248] Horizontal control of the instrument is maintained by a "Lev-O-Gage" that records from 0° to 45° (Figs. 13.45 and 13.46).

The Use of Lifts[93, 249–256]

A lift should be considered a clinical brace, with all its implications. It is not only an adjunct to basic therapy but often an important modality. Functional leg deficiencies and pelvic distortions, like myopia, should never be corrected 100% by a mechanical appliance if disuse atrophy is to be avoided. The body should always be allowed to make some correction (eg, 20–50%) by itself. The neuromusculoskeletal system readily adapts to its requirements and outside stimuli unless there are mechanical restrictions. If prolonged standing or walking does not aggravate a low-back pain syndrome, it is unlikely that a small difference in femur height is a significant factor in the syndrome.

The 1:2:4 Ratio

Extensive studies by Logan,[204] Steinbach,[9] and others have shown that a 1:2:4 ratio, from above downward, exists between the lumbar spine, the sacrum, and the plantar heel. That is, a 1/4-inch heel lift will raise the ipsilateral sacral base 1/8 inch and the lumbar spine 1/16 inch (Fig. 13.47). This general rule has been applied within chiropractic with excellent results since the 1930s, with adaptations taken for an unusually narrow male pelvis or unusually wide female pelvis. Other investigators report an average 3:1 ratio between leg shortness and L5 tilt; ie, a

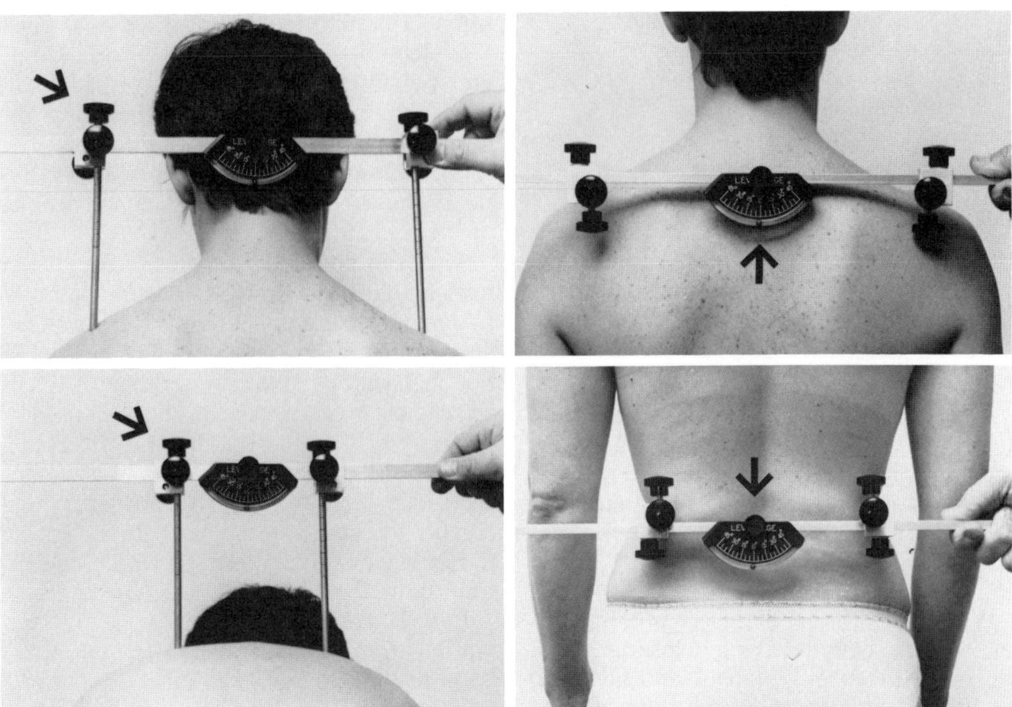

Figure 13.45. Sample applications of Dr. Sabia's Scoliometer. *Top left*, position for measuring shoulder tilt in centimeters; *top right*, measuring shoulder tilt in degrees; *bottom left*, measuring thoracic deviation in degrees or centimeters; *bottom right*, measuring pelvic tilt in degrees. (With the permission of M. A. Sabia, Ph.D., D.C., Little Silver, N. J.)

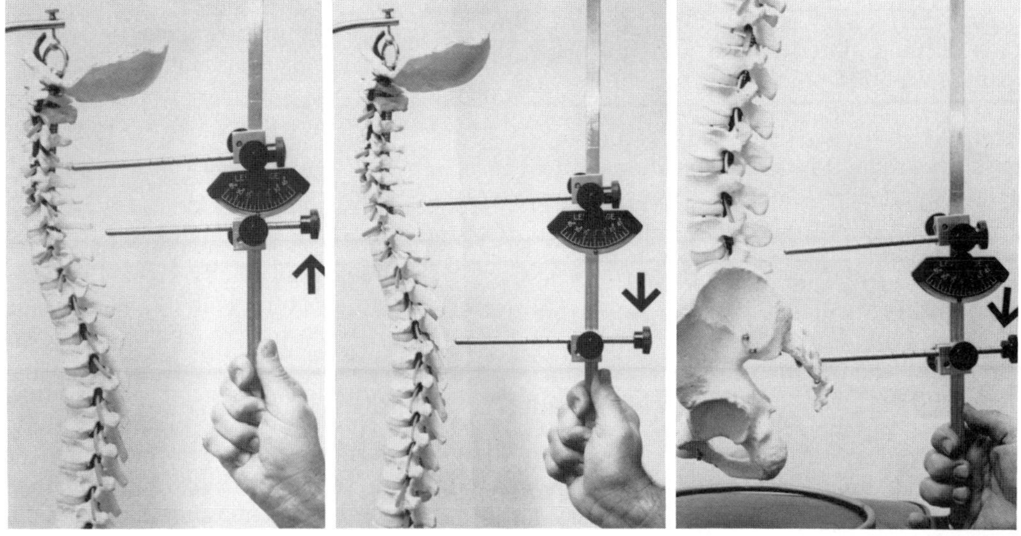

Figure 13.46. A few other uses of Dr. Sabia's Scoliometer. *Left*, position for measuring the lower cervical curve in centimeters; *center*, measuring the upper thoracic curve; *right*, measuring the A-P angulation between L5 and the sacral apex. (With the permission of M. A. Sabia, Ph.D., D.C., Little Silver, N. J.)

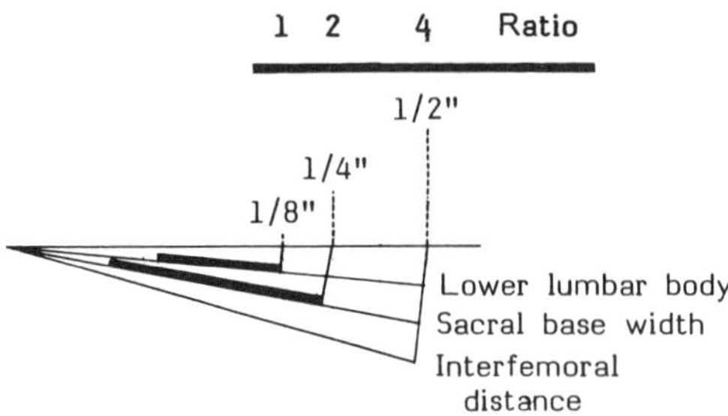

Figure 13.47. The 1:2:4 ratio between lower lumbar level and unilateral heel lift.

9-mm femoral head height deficiency would be related to a 3-mm L5 slanting that averages a 10–15° Cobb's angle. The difference between these two ratios is clinically insignificant unless a severe anatomical deficiency is involved (eg, over 1½ inches).

Common Types of Lifts

When shoe lifts are discussed in this chapter, we are usually referring to inserts within the patient's shoes (bilateral or unilateral) because their use is usually temporary. When a relatively permanent shoe lift is necessary, it is best done exteriorly by shoe reconstruction: ipsilateral heel lengthening or contralateral heel shortening. A heel drop (shortening) has the same effect as a heel lift on the opposite side or an ipsilateral sole lift.

Heel Lifts. A heel-only lift physically does nothing more than raise the heel, yet its biomechanical and biological effects are registered as far as the atlanto-occipital joint. When the heel is raised, the pelvis is raised *and* rotated anterior. The ilium rotates anterosuperior and lateral and the ischium posteroinferior and medial. As the sacrum is lifted and rotated anterior, the base of support for L5 is altered accordingly. Thus, the body of L5 will tend to rotate away from the side of lift.

Bilateral heel lifts increase the lumbar lordosis and this is compensated for by an increase in the thoracic kyphosis. This may be beneficial in cases of lumbar flattening or the rigid "military spine." They also remove stress from minor cases of sprained posterior lumbar ligaments (sprung back).

Sole Lifts. A unilateral or bilateral sole-only lift or a reduction in shoe heel height is sometimes applied. This has no effect upon extremity length, but it tends to place a stretch on the posterior ankle, calf, thigh, and pelvic extensors. When applied bilaterally, they are beneficial in reducing the lumbosacral angle in cases of anterior pelvic rotation, lumbar hyperlordosis, thoracic hyperkyphosis, or "kissing" spinous processes of the lumbar spine.

To avoid possible tendinitis, a sole lift or heel-height reduction is contraindicated in patients whose Achilles tendons have shortened and stiffened. Gradual reduction in heel height, along with progressive stretching exercises of the calf, has been beneficial in many of these cases. Heel height reduction would also be inadvisable in any condition in which stretching the posterior musculature, posterior rotation of the pelvis, or flattening the lumbar lordosis would be contraindicated.

Full Plantar Lifts. A plantar lift extending from the heel to the toe within or without the shoe tends to raise the femoral head without altering pelvic rotation. This is most helpful when it is desirable to shift weight laterally but not alter ipsilateral iliac posture.

Ischial Lifts. If the axial measurements of the ischia are asymmetrical and aggravating a sacroiliac dysfunction or lumbar scoliosis in the sitting position, a lift under the deficient ischium is sometimes advisable (Fig. 13.48). This is especially true with patients whose occupations require prolonged sitting on a firm surface (eg, typists, computer operators, students).

Heel Lift Indications and Contraindications

When used correctly, heel lifts are beneficial in aiding faulty body mechanics, improving static balance, creating a corrective force, and supporting the benefits gained from articular or soft-tissue adjustments. Once structural changes have occurred, full correction cannot be expected. In applications where the biomechanics involved are not fully appreciated or individual reactions are not carefully monitored, lifts can increase symptomatology.

Indications. There are four basic reasons for the use of temporary unilateral heel lift.

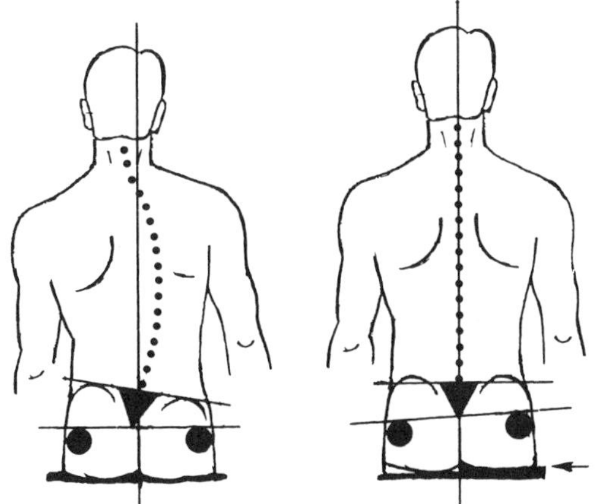

Figure 13.48. *Left*, sitting functional scoliosis due to structural deficiency in length of the right side of the pelvis. *Right*, postural correction through use of a right ischial lift. Correction would not be this ideal if structural changes in the spine had taken place.

1. To raise the ipsilateral pelvis up and forward.

2. To raise an inferoposteriorly rotated lumbar segment that is contributing to a lumbar scoliosis. If there is inferiority without posteriority (wedge tilt), a plantar lift would be more appropriate.

3. To shift body weight contralaterally with the goal of balancing body weight or shifting weight temporarily away from the side of acute irritation. Application in the latter example is for the same reason that the acute sciatic or hip case will lift the heel and stand on the toe of the painful side.

4. *To force mobility of a contralateral fixated area. In this case, enough lift must be provided to shift more weight contralaterally as judged by dual weight scales.*

Contraindications. Due to the mechanics involved, a heel lift would be inadvisable whenever a shift in body weight contralaterally or an ipsilateral anterior rotation of the ilium on the same side would be contraindicated.

The use of a lift without articular correction and comprehensive chiropractic care can lead to an increase in symptoms. This may have effects similar to temporarily casting an unreduced fracture of a weight-bearing structure.

Prescription of Lifts

Shoe inserts should always be provided by and fitted by the doctor. Periodic assessment of biomechanical changes must be evaluated and the applied forces altered as necessary for the particular situation at hand. For general reference, lift applications related to common distortions are outlined in Table 13.7.

The exact amount of initial lift is a clinical judgment based upon patient adaptability as exhibited by signs and symptoms. Thus, a degree of trial and error is always involved even by the experienced practitioner. Acute and minimal conditions can usually adapt to immediate 50% correction. Chronic and gross distortions, undoubtedly with fibrosis, require progressive changes of no more than 1/8-inch at a time. Some patients will respond dramatically to a 1/8-inch lift, while others will show little change with an immediate 3/8-inch correction.

A lift should never be prescribed and its effects left unchecked. By the same token, the effects of a lift cannot be appreciated immediately. This is essentially due to the biomechanical creep, relaxation, and fatigue phenomena involved, as well as the new patterns of mechanoreceptor excitation produced.

Overcorrection should be avoided unless there is a special clinical reason for its employment. In a flexible spine, overcorrection can lead to instability. On rare occasions, it may be desirable for a few days to move gravitational forces away from an ipsilateral irritation. In a stiff spine, overcorrection may be carefully employed to stretch contralateral tissues that have shortened (eg, scoliotic concavity) if pain or new symptoms are not produced. When in doubt, it is always better to undercorrect rather than overcorrect.

Permanent Applications. The only time a permanent heel lift is necessary is in cases of anatomical or stubborn functional shortening over 1/4 inch. Keep in mind that a functional deficiency may be superimposed on an anatomical deficiency, and the degree must be differentiated before a permanent lift is prescribed. If a permanent heel lift of over 3/8 inch is necessary, it is best to have half the required amount added to the ipsi-

Table 13.7.
Common Distortions and Related Shoe Lift Applications

Lateral Distortions		
Type	Ipsilateral application	Contralateral application
Lumbar scoliosis (convexity)	Heel lift	Sole lift or heel drop
Sacral anteroinferiority	Heel lift	Sole lift or heel drop
Sacral posterosuperiority	Sole lift or heel drop	Heel lift
Iliac anterosuperiority	Sole lift or heel drop	Heel lift
Iliac posteroinferiority	Heel lift	Sole lift or heel drop
Unilateral pelvic anteriority	Sole lift or heel drop	Heel lift
Unilateral pelvic posteriority	Heel lift	Sole lift or heel drop
Unilateral low femur head	Plantar lift	
Unilateral short ischium	Ischial lift	

Anterior-Posterior Distortions	
Type	Application
Sprung back (lumbar)	Bilateral heel lifts
Kissing spines (lumbar)	Bilateral sole lifts or heel drops
Lumbar hyperlordosis	Bilateral sole lifts or heel drops
Lumbar flattening	Bilateral heel lifts
Fixed pelvic anterior tilt	Bilateral sole lifts or heel drops
Fixed pelvic posterior tilt	Bilateral heel lifts

lateral heel and half the requirement removed from the contralateral heel.

Examples of Application

In uncomplicated cases, lift prescription offers little difficulty if initially undercorrected and the effects are carefully monitored. Unfortunately, many cases seen in practice are complicated and present eccentric manifestations.

Pelvic Subluxation Pattern 1. In this distortion, the basic inferiority is at the sacrum. If the pelvis has rotated posteriorly on the right, a heel lift should be applied on the right (Fig. 13.49). If the pelvis has rotated anterior on the right, apply a right plantar lift.

Pelvic Subluxation Pattern 2. In this distortion, the sacrum has shifted anteroinferior on the right, the pelvis has rotated anterior on the right, the ilium has rotated posterosuperior on the right, and there is a right lumbar scoliosis. This presents a dilemma. A heel lift on the right would help level the sacrum but increase the iliac superiority and pelvic rotation. The decision would depend upon the patient's symptoms, indicating the acute major. In most cases, a plantar lift on the right would be beneficial (Fig. 13.50). If the sacrum has been displaced anteroinferior only because of being carried by a severe anterosuperior rotation of the right ilium, a heel lift on the left may be indicated.

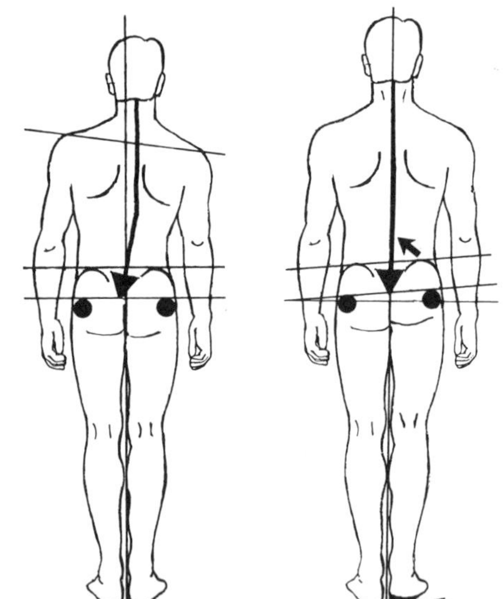

Figure 13.49. *Left*, pelvic subluxation pattern 1; *right*, postural change with the application of a right heel lift.

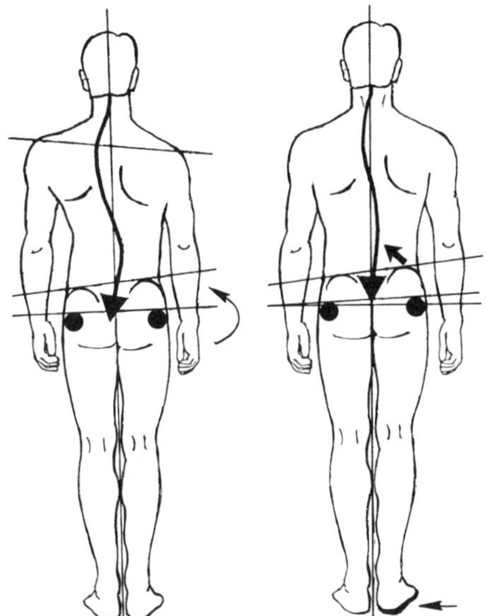

Figure 13.50. *Left*, pelvic subluxation pattern 2; *right*, postural change with the application of a right plantar lift.

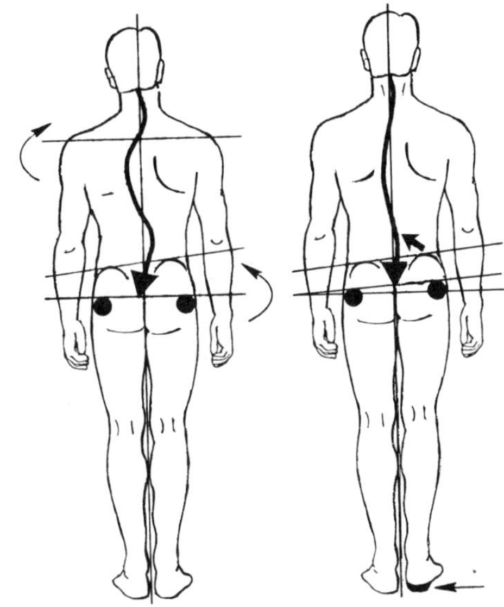

Figure 13.51. *Left*, pelvic subluxation pattern 3; *right*, postural change with the application of a right heel lift.

Pelvic Subluxation Pattern 3. In this example, the sacrum is anteroinferior on the right, the pelvis has rotated anterior on the right, the right ilium is high and rotated posterior, and there is a right lumbar scoliosis. This is another problem case because a heel lift on the right would level the sacrum and posteriority of the right ilium but aggravate the anterior pelvic rotation and the iliac superiority. Again, the decision must be based on the patient's symptoms and clinical judgment of the major. Quite possibly, the superiority of the right ilium is due to hypertonicity of the right psoas and the pelvic anteriority is compensatory to the thoracic scoliosis. If this is the situation, a right heel lift would be indicated (Fig. 13.51).

Pelvic Subluxation Pattern 4. In this distortion, the sacrum and pelvis are well aligned. The cause of the lumbar scoliosis to the left is vertebral wedging, a congenital defect, or degenerated lumbar facets that resemble thoracic articulations. A heel lift on the left will help inhibit the progression of the "S" scoliosis (Fig. 13.52).

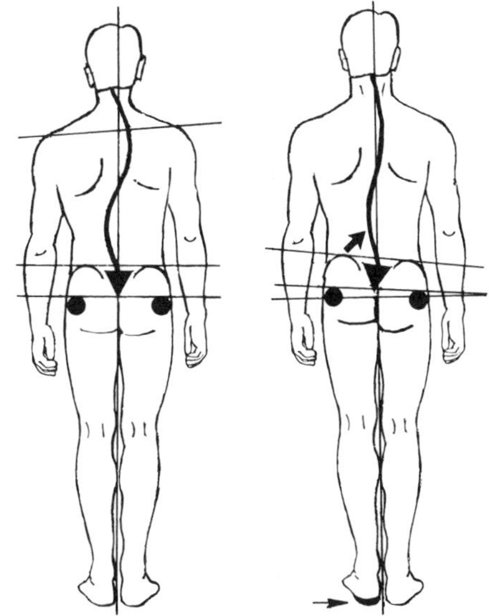

Figure 13.52. *Left*, pelvic subluxation pattern 4; *right*, postural change with the application of a left heel lift.

Pelvic Subluxation Pattern 5. Here the sacrum is anteroinferior on the right, the pelvis is rotated anterior on the right, the iliac crests are level, the right trochanter is low, and there is a right lumbar scoliosis. In this example, a plantar lift on the right would be indicated (Fig. 13.53). Normally, the right ilium would be low and posterior on the side of the low leg. Its level position in the example is most likely from psoas

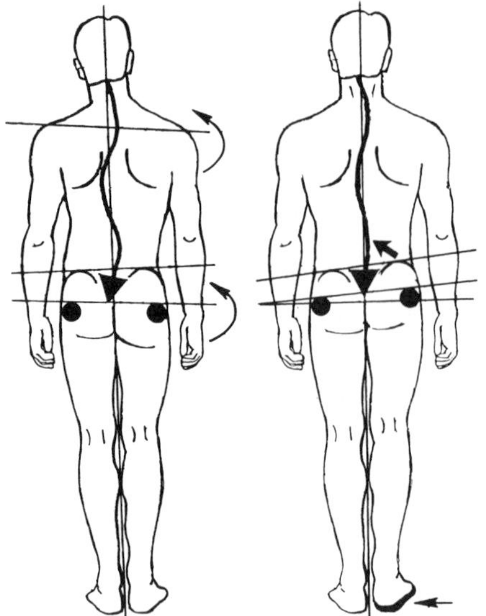

Figure 13.53. *Left*, pelvic subluxation pattern 5; *right*, postural change with the application of right plantar lift.

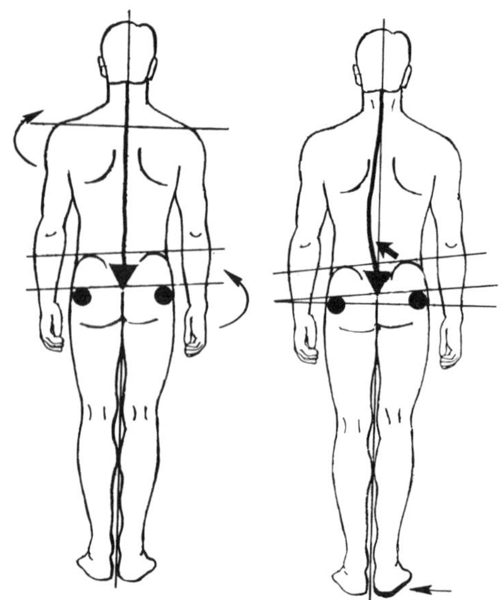

Figure 13.54. *Left*, pelvic subluxation pattern 6; *right*, postural change with the application of a right plantar lift to relieve pain and support adjustment.

contracture, which would not be aggravated by the right plantar lift.

Pelvic Subluxation Pattern 6. In this paradoxical distortion, the sacrum is anteroinferior on the right, the pelvis is rotated anteriorly on the right, and the left trochanter is low, which drops the left ilium. In most cases such as this, the sacral subluxation is an overcompensation to make up for the inferiority of the left femur with possible fixation at the left sacroiliac joint. If pain is severe on the right, a plantar lift should be placed on the side of pain to shift weight to the left to relieve the right sacroiliac irritation and help mobilize the fixation on the left (Fig. 13.54). Once the acute right area is relieved and strengthened, the femur deficiency can be considered. If pain is presented on the left, a heel lift on the left would be indicated.

Pelvic Subluxation Pattern 7. In this decompensated distortion, the entire pelvis appears to drop on the right because of a posterior ilium on the right. It is obvious that a heel lift on the right would correct body balance (Fig. 13.55). If the pelvis as a whole shows exaggerated anterior rotation on the right, a right plantar lift would be indicated.

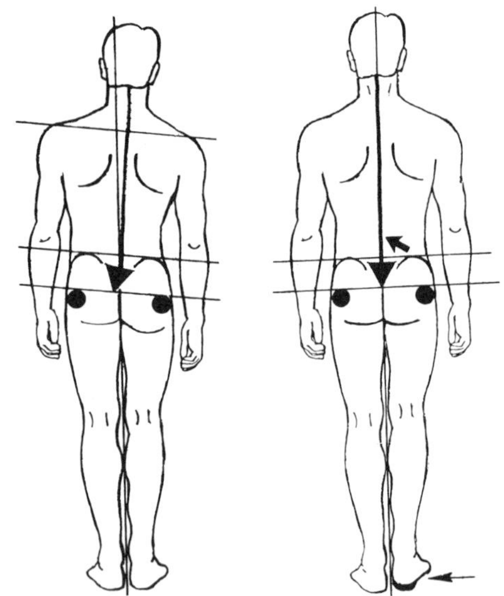

Figure 13.55. *Left*, pelvic subluxation pattern 7; *right*, postural change with the application of a right heel lift.

EFFECTS OF CHRONIC PRONATION[257–262]

In-roll of the talocalcaneal articulation is a common disorder. A weak foot is usually hypermobile. An associated shin-splint syndrome often arises in the flexor group, which is often isolated within the posterior tibial muscle. The most common cause of excessive pronation is foot fatigue.

Subotnick reports that limb length inequality is often associated with functional abnormalities such as overpronation of one foot in contradistinction to the other or imbalances within the pelvis itself.[263] Likewise, anatomical (true shortness) may be present or a combination of anatomical and functional discrepancies may be found. There appears to be a high correlation of injury on the short leg side of athletes and weakness associated with the short side. Conversely, utilizing a heel lift for a functional problem may cause contralateral symptoms.

Basic Biomechanics

Abnormal pronation is characterized by the superior aspect of the calcaneus tilting and rolling toward the midline carrying the talus with it. This releases the navicular from its arthrodial articulation with the talus, permitting it to roll toward the midline. As the navicular is the keystone of the medial longitudinal arch, its downward subluxation results in collapse of the arch and the beginning of a progressive distortion that may extend onto the occiput. When viewed from the rear, observation of the exposed Achilles tendon shows deviation with the inward tilting of the calcaneus. An associated tendon inflammation may be associated with abduction strain, characterized by motion restriction, pain, tenderness behind the medial malleolus, and crepitus on rare occasions.

As the inward tilting of the foot includes the talus which supports the tibia, unusual and downward tilting of the articulating surface of the talus causes an inward rotation of the tibia which extends onto the femur. This brings the greater trochanter forward and outward, stretching the piriformis muscle. The piriformis muscle inserts into the apex of the trochanter and is placed on a windlass-type stretch. As this muscle's origin is at the anterolateral aspect of the sacrum, the sacrum may be pulled into a subluxated anterior and inferior position. In compensation, the gluteus maximus muscle contracts to resist the downward and forward pelvic tilt. Because this muscle finds its origin on the outer lip of the posterior third of the iliac crest, the ilium rotates posteriorly to produce a typical pelvic distortion. With the sacrum thus drawn into an anteroinferior position, the L5 vertebral body gravitates and rotates toward the low side according to Lovett's law and establishes the beginning of a structural scoliosis. Thus, the biomechanical effects of pronation can be witnessed as high as the occiput.

Signs and Symptoms

The basic problem manifests essentially as an inward roll of one foot or both that results in lengthening of the foot involved with an automatic stretching of the plantar muscles. This produces many reflex patterns that evidence themselves as sciatic pain, numbness, tingling and various other paresthesias—all of reflex origin. But as the foot pronates and rolls inward, it also produces an inward roll of the talus, and this inward roll continues to have an inward torque on the tibia. Ordinarily, the fibula follows suit with the torque continuing through the knee joint, producing a sustained torque to the femur which then allows the lesser trochanter to move in a rotary fashion backward and laterally. This produces a microavulsion at the trochanteric attachment of the iliopsoas muscle. Thus, if the psoas tests weak, a foot pronation problem is frequently associated.

The thigh abductors and neck flexors will usually test weak on the side of a weak iliopsoas, and a lower inner longitudinal arch will usually be found on the side of the weak iliopsoas. When the arch rolls inward (pronates), the tibia twists, the knee strains, the femur rotates, the pelvis tilts forward, and the curves of the spine are affected.

Associated foot and ankle signs include lateroinferior cuboid, medioinferior navicular, posterocalcaneal torque, internally rotated tibia, inferior tarsals, inferior 2nd–4th metatarsals, superior 1st and 5th metatarsals, lateral deviation of the Achilles tendon during weight bearing, and flattening of the longitudinal arch. A corn at the 2nd metatarsal head, a tailor's bunion on the lateral 5th metatarsal head, Haglund's deformity, and bunion are typical findings.

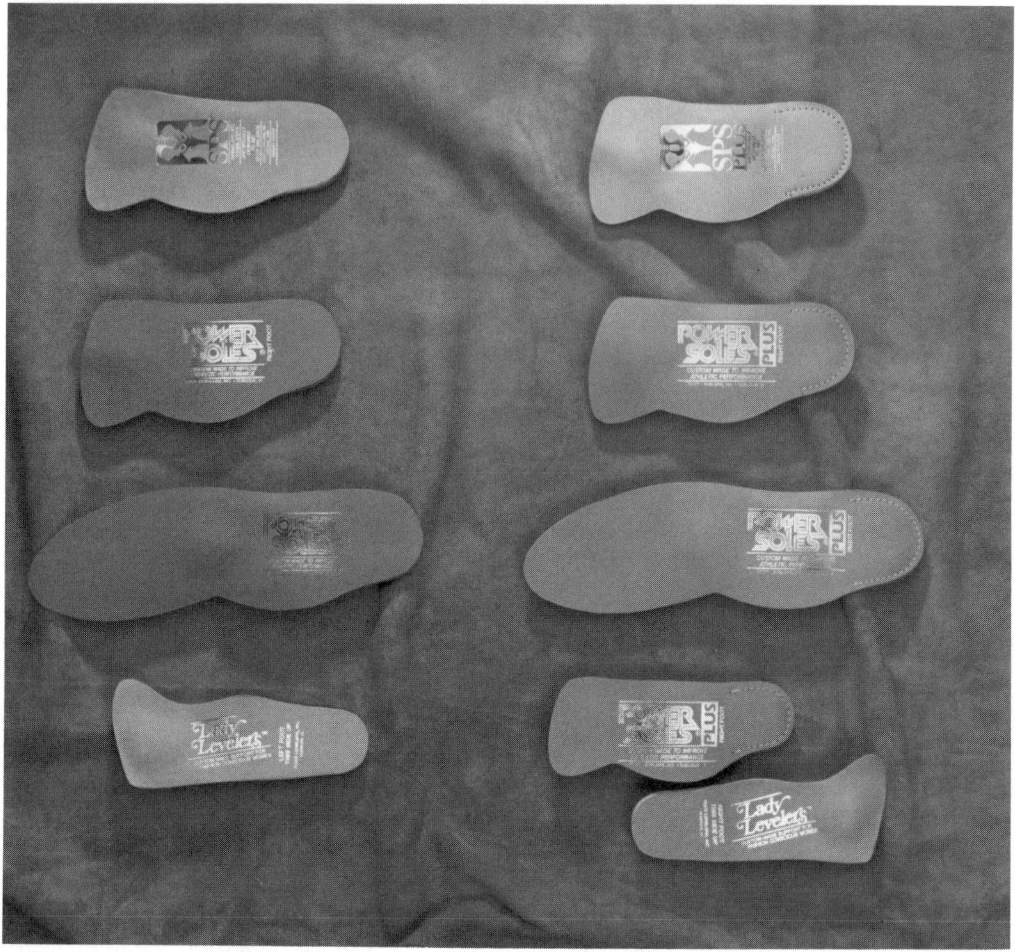

Figure 13.56. A wide variety of custom-made orthotic appliances is available for the management of postural deficits that are initiated by improper foot balance. (Courtesy of Foot Levelers, Inc.)

Management

A wide variety of problems of the feet, ankles, knees, pelvis, and spine contribute to leg length inequalities. To mechanically control pronation and other musculoskeletal imbalance disorders, Foot Levelers, Inc has developed a wide assortment of orthotics that have been designed to reduce or eliminate postural deficits initiated by improper foot balance (Fig. 13.56).

A study of changes in biomechanics after placing 10 individuals in Spinal Pelvic Stabilizers showed significant improvement in femoral head height equality, sacrovertebral angle, and lumbosacral disc angle.[264] Further information can be requested from Foot Levelers, Inc, 1901 Rockdale Road, P.O. Box 272, Dubuque, Iowa 52004-0272.

REFERENCES

1. Keith A: Man's posture: Its evolution and disorders. Hunterian Lectures. *Clinical Orthopaedics* 62:5–14, 1969.
2. Jaquet P: The upright position of man: Its phylogenetic and psychological aspects and some therapeutic considerations of interest. *Annals of the Swiss Chiropractic Association* 4:185–195, 1969.
3. Gehweiler JA Jr, Osborne RL Jr, Becker RF: *The Radiology of Vertebral Trauma.* Philadelphia, W.B. Saunders, 35–36, 41.
4. Basmajian JV (ed): *Grant's Method of Anatomy*, ed 9. Baltimore, Williams & Wilkins, 1975, pp 14–15.
5. Kapandji IA: *Physiology of the Joints: Lower Limbs*, ed 2. New York, Churchill Livingstone, 1981, vol 3, pp 14–17, 20–21.
6. Cailliet R: *Low Back Pain Syndromes*, ed 3. Philadelphia, F.A. Davis, 1981, pp 12–25.

7. Moore KL: *Clinically Oriented Anatomy.* Baltimore, Williams & Wilkins, 1980, p 608.
8. Morehouse LE, Cooper JM: *Kinesiology.* St. Louis, C.V. Mosby, 1959, pp 41, 43.
9. Steinbach LL: *Spinal Balance and Spinal Hygiene.* Pittsburgh, published by the author, 1957.
10. Janse J: The Waldo Poehner memorial lecture. *ACA Journal of Chiropractic* 9:93–94, August 1975.
11. Brennan MJ: Adaptations to bipedalism. *ACA Journal of Chiropractic* pp 24–31, November 1980.
12. Walters RL, Morris JM: An in vitro study of normal and scoliotic interspinous ligaments. *Journal of Biomechanics* 6:343, 1973.
13. Evans DC: Biomechanics of spinal injury. In Gonzna ER, Harrington IJ (eds): *Biomechanics of Musculoskeletal Injury.* Baltimore, Williams & Wilkins, 1982, p 217.
14. White AA, Panjabi MM: *Clinical Biomechanics of the Spine.* Philadelphia, J.B. Lippincott, 1978, pp 191–195.
15. Cailliet R: *Low Back Pain Syndrome,* ed 3. Philadelphia, F.A. Davis, 1981, pp 31–37.
16. Hollingshead WH, Jenkins DB: *Functional Anatomy of the Limbs and Back.* Philadelphia, W.B. Saunders, 1981, pp 207–210.
17. Johnson AC: *Postural Correction.* Los Angeles, Chiropractic Educational Extension Bureau (undated).
18. Turek SL: *Orthopedics: Principles and Their Application,* ed 3. Philadelphia, J.B. Lippincott, 1977, pp 1413–1419.
19. Keim HA: *Scoliosis.* Summit, NJ, Ciba Pharmaceutical Company, 1978, Clinical Symposia, vol 30(1), pp 2–4.
20. Schafer RC: *Chiropractic Physical and Spinal Diagnosis.* Oklahoma City, American Chiropractic Academic Press, 1980, pp I-17, X-29, XIII-20.
21. Schafer RC (ed): *Basic Chiropractic Procedural Manual,* ed 4. Arlington, Va, American Chiropractic Association, 1984, pp 26–28, 239.
22. Cailliet R: *Scoliosis.* Philadelphia, F.A. Davis, 1975, pp 5–19.
23. White AA, Panjabi MM: *Clinical Biomechanics of the Spine.* Philadelphia, J.B. Lippincott, 1978, p 94.
24. Schafer RC: *Chiropractic Physical and Spinal Diagnosis.* Oklahoma City, American Chiropractic Academic Press, 1980, pp I-19, IV-47, IV-48.
25. Triano JJ: The use of instrumentation and laboratory examination procedures by the chiropractor. In Haldeman S (ed): *Modern Developments in the Principles and Practice of Chiropractic.* New York, Appleton-Century-Crofts, 1980, pp 232–233.
26. Schafer RC: *Chiropractic Management of Sports and Recreational Injuries.* Baltimore, Williams & Wilkins, 1982, pp 66–67, 156–157, 278–279.
27. Barge FH: *Scoliosis.* Davenport, Ia, Bawden Bros, 1982, pp i–x.
28. Schafer RC: *Symptomatology and Differential Diagnosis.* Arlington, Va, American Chiropractic Association. To be published in 1986.
29. Schafer RC: *Chiropractic Physical and Spinal Diagnosis.* Oklahoma City, American Chiropractic Academic Press, 1980, pp I-21, I-22, I-28, IV-54–IV-56, IIV-34.
30. Johnson AC: *Postural Correction.* Los Angeles, Chiropractic Educational Extension Bureau (undated), pp 5–19.
31. Steinbach LL: *Spinal Balance and Spinal Hygiene.* Pittsburgh, published by the author, 1957.
32. Rogers MH: Basic body mechanics: An interpretation. *Journal of Health, Physical Education, and Recreation* 32:12–20, 1961.
33. Wiles P: Postural deformities of the antero-posterior curves of the spine. *Lancet* April 17, 1937.
34. Cureton TK: The validity of antero-posterior spinal measurements. *Research Quarterly* 2:101–113, 1931.
35. Turek SL: *Orthopedics: Principles and Their Application,* ed 3. Philadelphia, J.B. Lippincott, 1977, pp 1416–1421.
36. Cailliet R: *Scoliosis.* Philadelphia, F.A. Davis, 1975, pp 21–28.
37. Keim HA: *Scoliosis.* Summit, NJ, Ciba Pharmaceutical Company, 1978, Clinical Symposia, vol 30(1), pp 4–7.
38. Teranel JG: *Chiropractic Orthopedics and Roentgenology.* Newark, NJ, Medusa Press, 1953, pp 412, 416–420.
39. Johnson AC: *Postural Correction.* Los Angeles, Chiropractic Educational Extension Bureau (undated), pp 37–48.
40. Zaoussis AL, James JIP: The iliac apophysis and the evaluation of curves in scoliosis. *Journal of Bone and Joint Surgery (British)* 40:422, 1958.
41. Thomas CL: *Taber's Cyclopedic Medical Dictionary,* ed 14. Philadelphia, F.A. Davis, 1981, pp 1286–1287.
42. *Stedman's Medical Dictionary,* ed 24. Baltimore, Williams & Wilkins, 1984, p 1265.
43. Keim HA: *Scoliosis.* Summit, NJ, Ciba Pharmaceutical Company, 1978, Clinical Symposia, vol 30(1), p 6.
44. Shapiro F, Eyre D: Congenital scoliosis: A histopathologic study. *Spine* 6:107–117, 1981.
45. Aragona J, Lee CK: Scoliosis in fetal alcohol syndrome: A case report. *Orthopaedics* 4:1141–1143, 1981.
46. Drummond DS, Mackenzie DA: Scoliosis in arthrogryposis multiplex congenita. *Spine* 3:146–151, 1978.
47. McKinley LM et al: Occurrence of cold agglutinins in congenital scoliosis. *Spine* 3:157–159, 1978.
48. Uden A, Nilsson IM, Willner S: Bleeding time and scoliosis. *Acta Orthopaedica Scandinavica* 53:73–77, 1982.
49. Uden A, Nilsson IM, Willner S: Collagen changes in congenital and idiopathic scoliosis. *Acta Orthopaedica Scandinavica* 51:271–274, 1980.
50. Low WD et al: The development of Southern Chinese girls with adolescent idiopathic scoliosis. *Spine* 3:152–156, 1978.
51. Yarom R, Robin GC, Gorodetsky R: X-ray fluorescence analysis of muscles in scoliosis. *Spine* 3:142–145, 1978.

52. DeSmet AA et al: Three-dimensional analysis of right thoracic idiopathic scoliosis. *Spine* 9:377–381, 1984.
53. Cabot RC: *Physical Diagnosis*. New York, William Wood, 1919, pp 59–60.
54. Bradford DS, Moe JH, Winter RB: Sciolosis. In Rothman RH, Simeone FA (eds): *The Spine*. Philadelphia, W.B. Saunders, 1975, vol 1, pp 281–282.
55. Cailliet R: *Scoliosis*. Philadelphia, F.A. Davis, 1975, pp 41–44.
56. Turek SL: *Orthopedics: Principles and Their Application*, ed 3. Philadelphia, J.B. Lippincott, 1977, p 1416.
57. Johnson AC: *Postural Correction*. Los Angeles, Chiropractic Educational Extension Bureau (undated), pp 37–38.
58. Schafer RC: *Chiropractic Management of Sports and Recreational Injuries*. Baltimore, Williams & Wilkins, 1982, pp 421–422.
59. Teranel JG: *Chiropractic Orthopedics and Roentgenology*. Newark, NJ, Medusa Press, 1953, pp 412–413.
60. Keim HA: *Scoliosis*. Summit, NJ, Ciba Pharmaceutical Company, 1978, Clinical Symposia, vol 30(1), pp 4, 6–7.
61. Barge FH: *Scoliosis*. Davenport, Ia, Bawden Bros, 1982, pp 97–118.
62. Mawhiney RB: *Scoliosis Manual*. Waukesha, Wis, published by the author, 1982, pp 6–7.
63. Hildebrandt RW: *Synopsis of Chiropractic Postural Roentgenology*, ed 2. Lombard, Ill, National-Lincoln School of Postgraduate Chiropractic Education, Division of the National College of Chiropractic, 1974, p 147.
64. Ponsetti IV, Friedman B: Prognosis in idiopathic scoliosis. *Journal of Bone and Joint surgery* 32A:381, 1950.
65. Goldstein LA, Waugh TR: Classification and terminology of scoliosis. *Clinical Orthopaedics and Related Research* 93:10–22, 1973.
66. Bradford DS, Moe JH, Winter RB: Scoliosis. In Rothman RH, Simeone FA (eds): *The Spine*. Philadelphia, W.B. Saunders, 1975, vol 1, pp 281–283.
67. Cailliet R: *Scoliosis*. Philadelphia, F.A. Davis, 1975, pp 1, 19, 41–48.
68. Keim HA: *Scoliosis*. Summit, NJ, Ciba Pharmaceutical Company, 1978, Clinical Symposia, vol 30(1), pp 6–7.
69. Barge FH: *Scoliosis*. Davenport, Ia, published by the author, 1981, vol 3, pp 97–98.
70. Hassan I, Bjerkreim I: Progression in idiopathic scoliosis after conservative treatment. *Acta Orthopaedica Scandinavica* 54:88–90, 1983.
71. Kane WJ et al: Scoliosis and school screening for spinal deformity. *American Family Physician* 17:123–127, 1978.
72. Cailliet R: *Scoliosis*. Philadelphia, F.A. Davis, 1975, pp 1–3, 99–105.
73. Lonstein JE et al: Voluntary school screening for scoliosis in Minnesota. *Journal of Bone and Joint Surgery* 64:481–488, 1982.
74. Willner S, Uden A: A prospective prevalence study of scoliosis in southern Sweden. *Acta Orthopaedica Scandinavica* 53:233–237, 1982.
75. Willner S: Prevalence study of trunk asymmetries, structural scoliosis in 10-year-old school children. *Spine* 9:644–647, 1984.
76. Willner S: A comparative study of the efficiency of different types of school screening for scoliosis. *Acta Orthopaedica Scandinavica* 53:769–774, 1982.
77. Rogala EJ, Drummond DS, Gurr J: Scoliosis: Incidence and natural history. *Journal of Bone and Joint Surgery* 60A:173–176, 1978.
78. Bjerkreim I, Hassan I: Progression in untreated idiopathic scoliosis after end growth. *Acta Orthopaedica Scandinavica* 53:897–900, 1982.
79. McMaster MJ, Ohtsuka K: The natural history of congenital scoliosis. *Journal of Bone and Joint Surgery* 64A:1128–1147, 1982.
80. Jackson RP, Simmons EH, Stripinis D: Incidence and severity of back pain in adult idiopathic scoliosis. *Spine* 8:749–756, 1983.
81. Robin GC et al: Scoliosis in the elderly. *Spine* 7:355–359, 1982.
82. Connoly BH, Michael BT: Early detection of scoliosis. A neurological approach using the asymmetrical tonic neck reflex. *Physical Therapy* 64:304–307, 1984.
83. Laulund T, Sojbjerg JO, Horlyck E: Moire topography in school screening structural scoliosis. *Acta Orthopaedica Scandinavica* 53:765–768, 1982.
84. Zetterberg C et al: Electromyography of the paravertebral muscles in idiopathic scoliosis: Measurements of amplitude and spectral changes under load. *Acta Orthopaedica Scandinavica* 55:304–309, 1984.
85. Reuber M et al: Trunk muscle myoelectric activities in idiopathic scoliosis. *Spine* 8:447–456, 1983.
86. Aaro S, Dahlborn M: The longitudinal axis rotation of the apical vertebrae: The vertebral spine and rib cage deformity in idiopathic scoliosis studies by computer tomography. *Spine* 6:567–572, 1981.
87. Jeffries BF et al: Computerized measurement and analysis of scoliosis: A more accurate representation of the shape of the curve. *Radiology* 134:381–387, 1980.
88. DeSmet AA et al: The top view for analysis of scoliosis progression. *Radiology* 147:369–372, 1983.
89. Carver W: *Carver's Chiropractic Analysis*, ed 4. Oklahoma City, published by the author, 1921, vol 1, pp 212–213.
90. Carver W: *Carver's Chiropractic Analysis*, ed 4. Oklahoma City, published by the author, 1922, vol 2, pp 6–9.
91. Goodheart G: Applied kinesiology. In Kfoury PW (ed): *Catalog of Chiropractic Techniques*. Chesterfield, Mo, Logan College of Chiropractic, 1977, pp 117–119.
92. Stoner F: Kinesiology. In Kfoury PW (ed): *Catalog of Chiropractic Techniques*. Chesterfield, Mo, Logan College of Chiropractic, 1977, pp 107–111.
93. Coggins WN: *Basic Technique: A System of Body*

Mechanics. Creve Coeur, Mo, published by the author, 1983.
94. Gabel RA: Basic technique. In Kfoury PW (ed): *Catalog of Chiropractic Techniques.* Chesterfield, Mo, Logan College of Chiropractic, 1977, pp 7–11.
95. King WE: *The King Concept: The Spinal Tetrahedron,* ed 4. Grand Forks, ND, published by the author, 1985.
96. Pettibon Bio-Mechanics Institute: *Pettibon Spinal Bio-Mechanics: Theory and Implications,* ed 2. Vancouver, Wash, Pettibon Bio-Mechanics, 1976.
97. White AA, Panjabi MM: *Clinical Biomechanics of the Spine.* Philadelphia, J.B. Lippincott, 1978, pp 93, 212.
98. Barge FH: *Torticollis.* Davenport, Ia, Bawden Bros, 1979, pp 7–10, 18–20, 99.
99. Jeffreys E: *Disorders of the Cervical Spine.* London, Butterworths, 1980, pp 5, 14.
100. West HG Jr: Physical and spinal examination procedures utilized in the practice of chiropractic. In Haldeman S (ed): *Modern Developments in the Principles and Practice of Chiropractic.* New York, Appleton-Century-Crofts, 1980, pp 277–279.
101. Grieve GP: *Common Vertebral Joint Problems.* New York, Churchill Livingstone, 1981, pp 5, 38–47, 322–324.
102. Cailliet R: *Neck and Arm Pain.* Philadelphia, F.A. Davis, 1974, pp 47–59.
103. Turek SL: *Orthopedics: Principles and Their Application,* ed 3. Philadelphia, J.B. Lippincott, 1977, p 1417.
104. Barge FH: *Scoliosis.* Davenport, Ia, Bawden Bros, 1982, pp 4, 119–123, 126, 175.
105. Mawhiney RB: *Scoliosis Manual.* Waukesha, Wis, published by the author, 1982, p 31.
106. Stillwell DL: Structural deformities of vertebrae: Bone adaptation and modeling in experimental scoliosis and kyphosis. *Journal of Bone and Joint Surgery* 44A:611, 1962.
107. Arkin AM: The mechanism of the structural changes in scoliosis. *Journal of Bone and Joint Surgery* 31:519–528, 1949.
108. Moe JH, Kettleson DN: Idiopathic scoliosis. *Journal of Bone and Joint Surgery* 52A:1509, 1970.
109. Cailliet R: *Scoliosis.* Philadelphia, F.A. Davis, 1975, pp 45, 63.
110. White AA: Kinematics of the normal spine as related to scoliosis. *Journal of Biomechanics* 4:405–411, 1971.
111. Ponsetti IV et al: Biomechanical analysis of intervertebral discs in idiopathic scoliosis. *Journal of Bone and Joint Surgery* 54:1993, 1972; 56A, 1973.
112. Barge FH: *Scoliosis.* Davenport, Ia, published by the author, 1981, vol 3, pp 17–18.
113. Roaf R: A study of the mechanics of spinal injuries. *Journal of Bone and Joint Surgery* 42B:810–823, 1960.
114. Kashimoto T, Yamamuro T, Hatakeyama K: Anatomical and biomechanical factors in the curve pattern formation of idiopathic scoliosis. *Acta Orthopaedica Scandinavica* 53:368–371, 1982.
115. King WE: *The King Concept: The Spinal Tetrahedron,* ed 4. Grand Forks, ND, published by the author, 1985, p 7.
116. Ward LE: *The Dynamics of Spinal Stress.* Long Beach, Cal, SSS Press, 1980.
117. Kaplan PE et al: Neuropathy in thoracic scoliosis. *Acta Orthopaedica Scandinavica* 51:263–266, 1980.
118. Sahlstrand T, Sellden U: Nerve conduction velocity in patients with adolescent idiopathic scoliosis. *Scandinavian Journal of Rehabilitation Medicine* 12:25–26, 1980.
119. Lloyd-Roberts GC et al: Progression in idiopathic scoliosis: A preliminary report of a possible mechanism. *Journal of Bone and Joint Surgery* 60B:451–460, 1979.
120. McCarver C et al: Left thoracic and related curve patterns in idiopathic scoliosis. *Journal of Bone and Joint Surgery* 53A:196, 1971.
121. White AA et al: The clinical biomechanics of kyphotic deformities. *Clinical Orthopaedics* 128:8–17, 1977.
122. MacEwen GD: Experimental scoliosis. In Zorab, PA (ed): *Proceedings of the Second Symosium on Scoliosis: Causation.* Edinburgh, E & S Livingstone, 1969.
123. Alexander MA et al: Can experimental dorsal rhizotomy produce scoliosis? *Journal of Bone and Joint Surgery* 54A:1509, 1973.
124. Albright JA, Brand RA (eds): *The Scientific Basis of Orthopaedics.* New York, Appleton-Century-Crofts, 1979, pp 69, 174.
125. Michelsson JE: The development of spinal deformity in experimental scoliosis. *Acta Orthopaedica Scandinavica* Supplement 81, 1965.
126. Cailliet R: *Scoliosis.* Philadelphia, F.A. Davis, 1975, p 47.
127. Roaf R: The basic anatomy of scoliosis. *Journal of Bone and Joint Surgery* 480:786, 1966.
128. Roaf R: Rotation movements of the spine with special reference to scoliosis. *Journal of Bone and Joint Surgery* 40B:312–332, 1958.
129. Bennett TJ: *A New Clinical Basis for the Correction of Abnormal Physiology.* Burlingame, Cal, published by the author, 1960.
130. Ford DM et al: Paraspinal muscle imbalance in adolescent idiopathic scoliosis. *Spine* 9:373–376, 1984.
131. Yarom R, Wolf E, Robin GC: Deltoid pathology in idiopathic scoliosis. *Spine* 7:463–470, 1982.
132. Bagnall K, Draganiuk J, Secord D: Experimentally induced scoliosis in rabbits. *Physiotherapy Canada,* 35:126–132, 1983.
133. Haderspeck K, Schultz A: Progression of idiopathic scoliosis: An analysis of muscle actions and body weight influences. *Spine* 6:447–455, 1981.
134. Yamada K et al: A neurological approach to the etiology and treatment of scoliosis. *Journal of Bone and Joint Surgery* 53A:197, 1971.
135. Sahlstrand T, Ortengren R, Nachemson A: Postural equilibrium in adolescent idiopathic scoliosis. *Acta Orthopaedica Scandinavica* 49:354–365, 1978.
136. Evans DC: Biomechanics of spinal injury. In Gonza ER, Harrington IJ (eds): *Biomechanics of*

Musculoskeletal Injury. Baltimore, Williams & Wilkins, 1982, pp 165–172.

137. White AA, Panjabi MM: *Clinical Biomechanics of the Spine.* Philadelphia, J.B. Lippincott, 1978, pp 100–104, 493.
138. Turek SL: *Orthopedics: Principles and Their Application,* ed 3. Philadelphia, J.B. Lippincott, 1977, pp 1425–1426.
139. Keim HA: *Scoliosis.* Summit, NJ, Ciba Pharmaceutical Company, 1978, Clinical Symposia, vol 30(1), pp 18–19.
140. Barge FH: *Scoliosis.* Davenport, Ia, Bawden Bros, 1982, pp 188, 189.
141. Teranel JG: *Chiropractic Orthopedics and Roentgenography,* Newark, NJ, Medusa Press, 1953, pp 415–416.
142. Reinert OC: *Fundamentals of Chiropractic Techniques and Practice Procedures.* Chesterfield, Mo, Marian Press, 1983, pp 303–304.
143. D'Ambrosia RD: *Musculoskeletal Disorders: Regional Examination and Differential Diagnosis.* Philadelphia, J.B. Lippincott, 1977, p 304.
144. Barge FH: *Scoliosis.* Davenport, Ia, published by the author, 1981, vol 3, pp 131–132.
145. Bradford DS, Moe JH, Winter RB: Scoliosis. In Rothman RH, Simeone FA (eds): *The Spine.* Philadelphia, W.B. Saunders, 1975, vol 1, p 276.
146. Cailliet R: *Scoliosis.* Philadelphia, F.A. Davis, 1975, pp 28, 54, 73–74.
147. Mawhiney RB: *Scoliosis Manual.* Waukesha, Wis, published by the author, 1982, p 27.
148. White AA, Panjabi MM: *Clinical Biomechanics of the Spine.* Philadelphia, J.B. Lippincott, 1978, p 494.
149. White AA, Panjabi MM: *Clinical Biomechanics of the Spine.* Philadelphia, J.B. Lippincott, 1978, pp 493–494.
150. Cailliet R: *Scoliosis.* Philadelphia, F.A. Davis, 1975, pp 1–2, 28–29, 76, 78, 90.
151. Barge FH: *Scoliosis.* Davenport, Ia, Bawden Bros, 1982, pp 140–143, 229–230.
152. White AA, Panjabi MM: *Clinical Biomechanics of the Spine.* Philadelphia, J.B. Lippincott, 1978, pp 45–46.
153. Dumbleton JH, Black J: Principles of mechanics. In Black J, Dumbleton JH (eds): *Clinical Biomechanics: Case History Approach.* New York, Churchill Livingstone, 1981, pp 360–362.
154. Bradford DS, Moe JH, Winter RB: Scoliosis. In Rothman RH, Simeone FA (eds): *The Spine.* Philadelphia, W.B. Saunders, 1975, vol 1, pp 302–304.
155. Blout WP, Bolinski J: Physical therapy in the nonoperative treatment of scoliosis. *Journal of Physical Therapy* 47:10, 1966.
156. Cailliet R: *Low Back Pain Syndrome,* ed 3. Philadelphia, F.A. Davis, 1981, pp 90–94.
157. Cyriax J, Russell G: *Textbook of Orthopaedic Medicine,* ed 9. Baltimore, Williams & Wilkins, 1977, vol 2, pp 286–296.
158. Moe JH et al: *Scoliosis and Other Spinal Deformities.* Philadelphia, W.B. Saunders, 1978, p 467.
159. Dewald A, Ray RD: Skeletal traction for the treatment of severe scoliosis. *Journal of Bone and Joint Surgery* 52A:233–238, 1970.
160. Garrett A et al: Stabilization of the collapsing spine. *Journal of Bone and Joint Surgery* 43A:474–484, 1961.
161. Cotrel Y: Proceedings: Traction in the treatment of vertebral deformity. *Journal of Bone and Joint Surgery* 57B:260, 1975.
162. Letts RM, Bobechko WP: Preoperative skeletal traction in scoliosis. *Journal of Bone and Joint Surgery* 57A:616–619, 1975.
163. White AA, Panjabi MM: *Clinical Biomechanics of the Spine.* Philadelphia, J.B. Lippincott, 1978, p 108.
164. Lawson SM, Crawford AH: Traction in the treatment of spinal deformity. *Orthopedics* 6(4):447–451, April 1983.
165. Bjerkreim I, Carlsen B, Korsell E: Preoperative Cotrel traction in idiopathic scoliosis. *Acta Orthopaedica Scandinavica* 53:901–905, 1982.
166. Cochran GVB, Waugh TR: The external forces in correction of idiopathic scoliosis. Proceedings of the Scoliosis Research Society. *Journal of Bone and Joint Surgery* 51:201, 1961.
167. Yamada K: Equilibrium function in scoliosis and active corrective plaster jacket for the treatment. *Journal of Experimental Medicine* 16:1, 1969.
168. Lindh MA: The effect of sagittal curve changes on brace correction of idiopathic scoliosis. *Spine* 5:26–36, 1980.
169. Turek SL: *Orthopedics: Principles and Their Application,* ed 3. Philadelphia, J.B. Lippincott, 1977, pp 1434–1442.
170. White AA, Panjabi MM: *Clinical Biomechanics of the Spine.* Philadelphia, J.B. Lippincott, 1978, pp 105–112.
171. Bradford DS, Moe JH, Winter RB: Scoliosis. In Rothman RH, Simeone FA (eds): *The Spine.* Philadelphia, W.B. Saunders, 1975, vol 1, pp 287–301.
172. Cailliet R: *Scoliosis.* Philadelphia, F.A. Davis, 1975, pp 62–75.
173. Barge FH: *Scoliosis.* Davenport, Ia, Bawden Bros, 1982, pp 303–307.
174. Black J, Dumbleton JH (eds): *Clinical Biomechanics.* New York, Churchill Livingstone, 1980, p 337.
175. Turek, SL: *Orthopedics: Principles and Their Application,* ed 3. Philadelphia, J.B. Lippincott, 1977, pp 1433, 1436.
176. Uden A, Willner S: The effect of lumbar flexion and Boston thoracic brace on the curves in idiopathic scoliosis. *Spine* 8:846–850, 1983.
177. Miller JAA, Nachemson AL, Schultz AB: Effectiveness of braces in mild idiopathic scoliosis. *Spine* 9:632–635, 1984.
178. Jaskoviak P, Schafer RC: *Applied Physiotherapy.* Arlington, Va, American Chiropractic Association. To be published in 1986.
179. Stone B et al: The effects of an exercise program on change in curve in adolescents with minimal idiopathic scoliosis. *Physical Therapy* 59:759–763, 1979.
180. Brown JC, Axelgaard J, Howson DC: Multicenter trial of a noninvasive stimulation method for idiopathic scoliosis. A summary of early treatment results. *Spine* 9:382–387, 1984.

181. Axelgaard J, Nordwall A, Brown JC: Correction of spinal curvatures by transcutaneous electrical muscle stimulation. *Spine* 8:463–481, 1983.
182. Schultz A, Haderspeck K, Takashima S: Correction of scoliosis by muscle stimulation. *Spine* 6:468–476, 1981.
183. Eckerson LF, Axelgaard J: Lateral electrical surface stimulation as an alternative to bracing in the treatment of idiopathic scoliosis. *Physical Therapy* 64:483–490, 1984.
184. Bradford DS, Tanguy A, Vanselow J: Surface electrical stimulation in the treatment of idiopathic scoliosis: Preliminary results in 30 patients. *Spine* 8:757–764, 1983.
185. White AA, Panjabi MM: *Clinical Biomechanics of the Spine*. Philadelphia, J.B. Lippincott, 1978, pp 99, 108, 465.
186. Cochran GVB: *A Primer of Orthopaedic Biomechanics*. New York, Churchill Livingstone, 1982, pp 92–93, 117, 121–122.
187. DeJarnette MB: *Subluxation Patterns*. 1975 Seminar Notes. Nebraska City, published by the author, 1975, pp 3–44, 64–66.
188. DeJarnette MB: *Sacro Occipital Technic*. Nebraska City, published by the author, 1977, pp 226–231.
189. Walther DS: *Applied Kinesiology*. Pueblo, Colo, Systems DC, 1981, vol 1, pp 29–39.
190. Mawhiney RB: *Scoliosis Manual*. Waukesha, Wis, published by the author, 1982, pp 11–20, 38–57.
191. Levine M: *The Structural Approach to Chiropractic*. New York, Comet Press, 1964, pp 52–80.
192. Loomis RC, Steinbach LJ: *Examination of the Spinal Column for Defects of Balance and Subluxation*. Pittsburgh, Universal Chiropractic College, 1930.
193. Keim HA: *Scoliosis*. Summit, NJ, Ciba Pharmaceutical Company, 1978, Clinical Symposia, vol 30(1), pp 9–10.
194. MacEwen GD: A look at the diagnosis and management of scoliosis. *Orthopaedic Review* 3:9, 1974.
195. Roaf R: The basic anatomy of scoliosis. *Journal of Bone and Joint Surgery* 480:786, 1966.
196. Risser JC: Scoliosis: Past and present. *Journal of Bone and Joint Surgery* 46:167, 1964.
197. Farkas A: The pathogenesis of idiopathic scoliosis. *Journal of Bone and Joint Surgery* 36:617, 1954.
198. James JIP: Idiopathic scoliosis. *Journal of Bone and Joint Surgery* 36B:36, 1954.
199. Turek SL: *Orthopaedics: Principles and Their Application*, ed 3. Philadelphia, J.B. Lippincott, 1977, pp 1416–1419.
200. Keim HA: *Scoliosis*. Summit, NJ, Ciba Pharmaceutical Company, 1978, Clinical Symposia, vol 30(1), p 9.
201. DeJarnette MB: *Subluxation Patterns*. 1975 Seminar Notes. Nebraska City, published by the author, privately distributed, 1975, p 3.
202. Janse J: *Principles and Practice of Chiropractic*. Lombard, Ill, National College of Chiropractic, 1976, pp 59–60, 138–139.
203. Johnson AC: *Postural Correction*. Los Angeles, Chiropractic Educational Extension Bureau (undated), pp 5–10, 15–16, 36–38.
204. Logan VF, Murray FM (eds): *Textbook of Logan Basic Methods* (from the original manuscript of Hugh B. Logan). St. Louis, Logan Chiropractic College, 1950.
205. Barge FH: *Tortipelvis*. Davenport, Ia, Bawden Bros, 1980, pp 19–68.
206. Goodheart, GJ: *Applied Kinesiology*. City of publication not shown, published by the author, privately distributed, 1964, pp 3–10.
207. DeJarnette MB: *Subluxation Patterns*. 1975 Seminar Notes. Nebraska City, published by the author, privately distributed, 1975, p 52.
208. Janse J: *Principles and Practice of Chiropractic*. Lombard, Ill, National College of Chiropractic, 1976, pp 59–60.
209. Janse J: The concepts and research of Dr. Fred W. Illi. *Notes on Correlative Techniques*. Chicago, National College of Chiropractic (undated).
210. Phillips RB: The use of x-rays in spinal manipulative therapy. In Haldeman S (ed): *Modern Developments in the Principles and Practice of Chiropractic*. New York, Appleton-Century-Crofts, 1980, pp 196–199.
211. Arkin AM: The mechanism of the structural changes in scoliosis. *Journal of Bone and Joint Surgery* 31:519–528, 1949.
212. Schafer RC (ed): *Basic Chiropractic Procedural Manual*, ed 4. Arlington, Va, American Chiropractic Association, 1984, pp 239–240.
213. Janse J: The concepts and research of Dr. Fred W. Illi. *National College Journal of Chiropractic* 28(1), June 1956.
214. Illi FW: *The Vertebral Column: Life-Line of the Body*. Chicago, National College of Chiropractic, 1951.
215. Jackson RP, Simmons EH, Stripinis D: Incidence and severity of back pain in adult idiopathic scoliosis. *Spine* 8:749–756, 1983.
216. Kostuik JP, Bentivoglio J: The incidence of low-back pain in adult scoliosis. *Spine* 6:268–273, 1981.
217. Nachemson A: Adult scoliosis and back pain. *Spine* 4:513–517, 1979.
218. Simmons EH, Jackson RP: The management of nerve root entrapment syndromes associated with the collapsing scoliosis of idiopathic lumbar and thoracolumbar curves. *Spine* 4:533–541, 1979.
219. Epstein JA, Epstein BS, Jones MD. Symptomatic lumbar scoliosis with degenerative changes in the elderly. *Spine* 4:542–547, 1979.
220. Benner B, Ehni G: Degenerative lumbar scoliosis. *Spine* 4:548–552, 1979.
221. Olsen GA, Hamilton A: The lateral stability of the spine. *Clinical Orthopaedics* 65:143, 1969.
222. Mitchell T: Structural pelvic function. *Yearbook of Applied Osteopathy*, 1965.
223. Gatterman MI: Sacroiliac motion and pelvic tilt. In ACA Council on Technic: *Biomechanics of the Pelvis*. Denver Conference, June 17–20, 1980. Council on Technic of the American Chiropractic Association, 1982.
224. Janse J: *Principles and Practice of Chiropractic*.

Lombard, Ill, National College of Chiropractic, 1976, pp 139–140.
225. Sweere JJ: Factors to consider in the determination of relative leg-length "differences." *Orthopedic Brief* ACA Council on Chiropractic Orthopedics, November 1984.
226. Bailey HW: Theoretical significance of postural imbalance, especially the "short leg". *Journal of the American Osteopathic Association* vol 7, February 1978.
227. Fisk JW: *The Painful Neck and Back.* Springfield, Ill, Charles C Thomas, 1977, pp 56–65.
228. West HG Jr: Physical and spinal examination procedures utilized in the practice of chiropractic. In Haldeman S (ed): *Modern Developments in the Principles and Practice of Chiropractic.* New York, Appleton-Century-Crofts, 1980, pp 286–287.
229. Grieve GP: *Common Vertebral Joint Problems.* New York, Churchill Livingstone, 1981, pp 270–273.
230. Schafer RC (ed): *Basic Chiropractic Procedural Manual,* ed 4. Arlington, Va, American Chiropractic Association, 1984, p 80.
231. Schafer RC: *Chiropractic Physical and Spinal Diagnosis.* Oklahoma City, American Chiropractic Academic Press, 1980, p IV-48.
232. Schafer RC: *Chiropractic Management of Sports and Recreational Injuries.* Baltimore, Williams & Wilkins, 1982, pp 452–453.
233. Kendall HO, Kendall FP, Wadsworth GE: *Muscles: Testing and Function,* ed 2. Baltimore, Williams & Wilkins, 1971, p 22.
234. D'Ambrosia RD: The hip. In D'Ambrosia RD (ed): *Musculoskeletal Disorders: Regional Examination and Differential Diagnosis.* Philadelphia, J.B. Lippincott, 1977, pp 404, 405–407.
235. Barge FH: *Scoliosis.* Davenport, Ia, Bawden Bros, 1982, pp 109, 126, 180, 182.
236. Barge FH: *Tortipelvis.* Davenport, Ia, Bawden Bros, 1980, pp 69–81.
237. Klein KK: Progression of pelvic tilt in adolescent boys. *Archives of Physical Medicine and Rehabilitation* 54:57–59, February 1973.
238. DeJarnette MB: *Sacro Occipital Technic.* Nebraska City, published by the author, privately distributed, 1977, pp 1–162, 201–217.
239. DeJarnette MB: *Subluxation Patterns.* 1975 Seminar Notes. Nebraska City, published by the author, privately distributed, 1975, pp 3–44.
240. Mawhiney RB: *Scoliosis Manual.* Waukesha, WI, published by author, 1982, pp 11–20, 38–56.
241. Phillips RB: The use of x-rays in spinal manipulative therapy. In Haldeman S (ed): *Modern Developments in the Principles and Practice of Chiropractic.* New York, Appleton-Century-Crofts, 1980, pp 192–198.
242. Cook GE: The anterior ilium subluxation—a clinical impression. *PCC Research Forum* 1(4):126, Summer 1985.
243. Giles LGF: Lumbosacral facetal "joint angles" associated with leg length inequality. *Rheumatology and Rehabilitation* 10:223–238, 1981.
244. Giles LGF, Taylor JR: The effect of postural scoliosis on lumbar apophyseal joints. *Scandinavian Journal of Rheumatology* 13:209–220, 1984.
245. Giles LGF, Taylor JR: Low-back pain associated with leg length inequality. *Spine* 6:510–521, 1981.
246. Giles LGF, Taylor JR: Lumbar spine structural changes associated with leg-length inequality. *Spine* 7:159–162, 1982.
247. Maxwell TD: The piriformis muscle and its relation to the long-legged syndrome. *Journal of the Canadian Chiropractic Association* July 1978, pp 51–53.
248. *Dr. Sabia's Scoliometer: Handbook of Instruction.* Little Silver, NJ, Dr. Sabia's Scoliometer, Inc, 1983.
249. Janse J: Prescription of heel and sole lifts and heel drops. *Notes on Correlative Techniques.* Chicago, National College of Chiropractic (undated).
250. Davidson MS: Investigation into the influence of bilateral heel height variations on posture. Thesis, Anglo-European College of Chiropractic, 1977.
251. Greenman PE: Lift therapy: Use and abuse. *Journal of the American Osteopathic Association* 79:238–250, December 1979.
252. Janse J: *Principles and Practice of Chiropractic.* Lombard, Ill, National College of Chiropractic, 1976, pp 66, 97–99, 125–126, 167.
253. Mawhiney RB: *Scoliosis Manual.* Waukesha, Wis, published by the author, 1982, pp 28–29.
254. Barge FH: *Scoliosis.* Davenport, Ia, Bawden Bros, 1982, pp 177–226.
255. Janse J, Houser RH, Wells BF: *Chiropractic Principles and Technic.* Chicago, National College of Chiropractic, 1947, pp 327, 492–493.
256. Reinert OC: *Fundamentals of Chiropractic Techniques and Practice Procedures.* Chesterfield, MO, Marian Press, 1983, pp 293–296.
257. Greenawalt MH: *Spinal Pelvic Stabilization,* ed 2, Dubuque, Ia, Foot Levelers, 1978.
258. Janse J: *Principles and Practice of Chiropractic.* Lombard, Ill, National College of Chiropractic, 1976, pp 116–118.
259. Daniels L, Worthingham C: *Therapeutic Exercise for Body Alignment and Function,* ed 2. Philadelphia, W.B. Saunders, 1977, pp 18, 96–97.
260. Chistensen K: Spinal pelvic stabilizers: Their influence on spinal biomechanics. *The Digest of Chiropractic Economics* May/June 1982.
261. D'Amico JC: The postural complex. *Journal of the American Podiatry Association* August 1976.
262. Carolusson CS: Investigation of the possible effect of shoes on the lumbar and thoracic anterior-posterior curvatures. Thesis, Anglo-European College of Chiropractic, 1974.
263. Subotnick SI: Limb length discrepancies of the lower extremity (The Short Leg Syndrome). *Journal of Orthopaedic and Sports Physical Therapy* 3:11–16, 1981.
264. Christensen K: Spinal pelvic stabilizers and their effect upon spinal biomechanics: A preliminary report. Research Bulletin No. 516. Dubuque, Ia, Foot Levelers, Inc.

SUGGESTED READINGS

Briard JL, Jegou D, Cauchoix: Adult lumbar scoliosis. *Spine* 4:526–532, 1979.

DeJarnette, MB: *Chiropractic Manipulative Technique,* 1975 Seminar Notes. Nebraska City, published by the author, 1975.

Farady JA: Current principles in the nonoperative management of structural adolescent idiopathic scoliosis. *Physical Therapy* 63:512–523, 1983.

Goldthwait JE et al: *The Essentials of Body Mechanics in Health and Disease,* ed 5. Philadelphia, J.B. Lippincott, 1952.

Griesse R: *The Crooked Shall Be Made Straight.* Atlanta, John Knox, 1979.

Hierholzer E, Luxmann G: Three-dimensional shape analysis of the scoliotic spine using invariant shape parameters. *Journal of Biomechanics* 15:583–598, 1982.

Hosek RS: Computerized leg check: A computer-aided gravity weight line analyzer. *Chiropractic Today* January/February 1985.

James JIP et al: *Scoliosis,* revised ed 2. New York, Churchill Livingstone, 1976.

Kendall HO et al: *Posture and Pain.* Baltimore, Williams & Wilkins, 1952.

Kostuik JP: Decision making in adult scoliosis. *Spine* 4:521–525, 1979.

Logan AL: *Clincal Application of Chiropractic: Low Back and Pelvis,* Westminster, Cal, West-Print, 1977.

Logan VF: *Chiropractic Corrections.* Chesterfield, Mo, Logan College of Chiropractic (undated).

Mazzarelli JP (ed): *Chiropractic Interprofessional Research.* Torino, Italy, Edizioni Minerva Medica, 1983. Reprinted in the United States by the International Chiropractors Association, Washington, DC 1985.

Reuben JD et al: In vivo effects of axial loading on double-curve scoliotic spines. *Spine* 7:440–447, 1982.

Robin GC (ed): *Scoliosis.* New York, Academic Press, 1973.

Robin GC: *Scoliosis and Neurologic Disease.* New York, Halsted Press, 1975.

States AZ: *Spinal and Pelvic Technics,* ed 2. Lombard, Ill, National Chiropractic College, 1968.

Toftness IN: *A Look at Chiropractic Spinal Correction,* Cumberland, Wis, published by the author, 1977.

Truscott LL, Frisbie GK: *Truscott System of Angular Analysis and Controlled Adjusting,* ed 2. San Jose, Cal, Rosicrucian Press, 1948.

Zorab PA (ed): *General Medical Aspects of Scoliosis.* New York, Academic Press, 1977.

Zorab PA: Scoliosis and muscle. *Clinics in Developmental Medicine.* Research Monographs, vol 4A, 1974.

Part 3

CLINICAL BIOMECHANICS OF THE EXTREMITIES

CHAPTER 14
The Upper Extremity

CHAPTER 15
The Lower mExtremity

CHAPTER 14

The Upper Extremity

This chapter considers forces acting within and upon the shoulder girdle, arm, forearm, and hand, and their related clinical problems, with emphasis on the related musculoskeletal disorders. Therapy can be directed efficiently when the mechanisms of injury are appreciated and correction is applied in harmony with proven biomechanical principles.

THE SHOULDER GIRDLE AND ARM

A kinematic chain extends from the cervical and upper thoracic spine to the fingertips. Only when certain multiple segments are completely fixed can these parts possibly function independently in mechanical roles.

Basic Functional Anatomy[1-6]

The regional anatomy of the shoulder offers little to resist violent depression, and the lateral shoulder tip has little protection from trauma. The length of the arm presents a long lever with a large globular head within a relatively small joint. This allows a great range of motion with little stability. The stability of the shoulder is derived entirely from its surrounding soft tissues, capsule, muscles, and ligaments.

The Shoulder Girdle[7-9]

The scapula, clavicle, and the humerus function as a biomechanical unit. Forces generated from or upon one of the three segments will affect the other two segments. Thus, in this chapter, they will be discussed as a functional unit.

The Scapula. The scapula is frequently underrated clinically. Morehouse calls it one of the most outstanding engineering miracles of the human body.[10] The blade of the shoulder, resembling an inverted right triangle, lies at the posterior T2–T7 rib level and attaches to the thorax only by muscles and fascia. Its medial border is about 2 inches lateral from the spinous processes, and its laterosuperior aspect articulates with the clavicle and the humerus in a rocking and gliding action. Its design allows it to function as a base for humeral motion and at the same time to move independently of arm action.

The Clavicle. This bony brace offers mechanical support to the anterosuperior thorax and cervical spine. It forms a mechanical link with the scapula and protects the vital vessels at the anterolateral aspect of the base of the neck. The clavicle is necessary in all animals that either climb, swim, or fly.[10] It serves as a strut to hold the shoulder joint outward so that the range of motion of the upper extremity is increased and the pull of the brachiating muscles is mechanically improved. The clavicle articulates medially with the manubrium of the sternum and cartilage of the 1st rib (sliding joint), and laterally with the acromion (sliding joint) and coracoid process (syndesmoses) of the scapula.

The Sternoclavicular Joint. This joint is supported by a capsule and reinforcing anterior and posterior ligaments. It is the *sole* point where the shoulder girdle articulates with the thorax. An interclavicular ligament crosses the jugular notch, connects the manubrium with both clavicles, and tends to restrict sternoclavicular motion. A costoclavicular ligament straps the inferomedial clavicle to the 1st rib below (Fig. 14.1).

The Acromioclavicular Joint. The articulation between the acromion and the lateral clavicle is supported by a capsule that is reinforced superiorly by the acromioclavicular ligament. An incomplete articular disc is sometimes found at the upper aspect of the joint.

The Coracoclavicular and Coracoacromion Unions. The clavicle is strapped to the coracoid process of the scapula by the conoid and trapezoid ligaments. The coracoacromial ligament extends between the coracoid process and acromion (Fig. 14.2).

The Shoulder Joint. This highly mobile

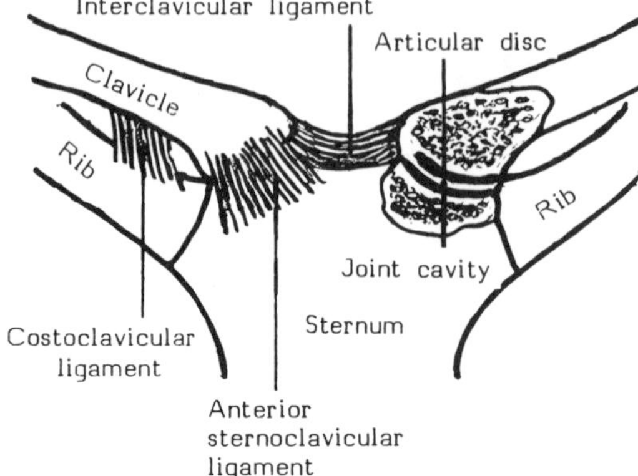

Figure 14.1. Schematic of the sternoclavicular joints and related ligaments.

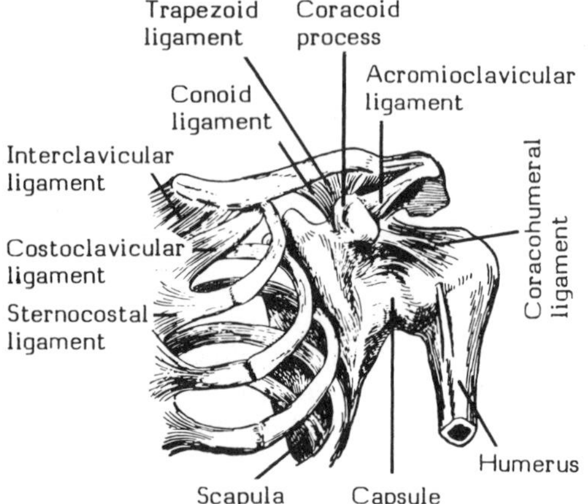

Figure 14.2. The ligaments of the lateral clavicle and shoulder joint.

joint is aided somewhat by a narrow fibrocartilaginous rim around the glenoid fossa. A surrounding joint capsule extends loosely from the lateral scapula and clavicle to attach firmly at the anatomical neck and shaft of the humerus. A series of anterior glenohumeral ligament bands and tendon fibers reinforce the articular capsule, and the transverse humeral ligament forms a canal for the long tendon of the biceps brachii within the bicipital groove. The arm rotates about a point that is considered to be in the center of the head of the humerus.

Shoulder Movements[11-16]

The versatile shoulder girdle consists of the sternoclavicular, acromioclavicular, and glenohumeral joints, along with the scapulothoracic union. These allow, as a whole, universal mobility by way of the shallow glenoid fossa, the joint capsule, and the suspension muscles and ligaments. The shoulder, a ball-and-socket joint, lacks the close connection between its articular surfaces that is seen in weight-bearing joints.

Joint motions of the shoulder and shoulder girdle, along with the prime movers and major accessories, are listed in Table 14.1. Almost all shoulder muscles have the same triangular design—broadly fanned fibers at their origins that narrow and converge at their tendinous insertions (Fig. 14.3). Because of overlapping innervation, portions of these muscles are capable of functioning separately and in harmony with portions of other muscles acting on the shoulder joint.

Active and Passive Range of Motion[17,18]

Complete patient relaxation is necessary to obtain an accurate judgment of the range of motion. Tension will cause considerable motion restriction. As in all range of motion tests, passive motion should not be attempted if there is any possibility of fracture, dislocation, severe tears, advanced bone pathology, etc. If active motion is normal, there is usually no need to test passive motion unless unusual circumstances exist that make active motion difficult. It is important during all tests that the examiner form a mental picture of the underlying anatomy and normal motion.

Spasm, contractures, fracture, and dislocation are the common causes of motion restriction and muscle weakness. In uncomplicated muscle weakness, a joint may move through its normal range passively but not actively. Active and passive restriction is likely from a bony or soft-tissue blockage, and the atrophy present will be most likely from disuse. Upon passive movement, bone blocks will feel as abrupt inflexible stops in motion, while extra-articular soft-tissue blocks will be less abrupt and slightly flexible upon additional pressure.

Shoulder Motion[19,20]

Elevation, depression, abduction (180°), adduction (45°), extension (45°), flexion (90°), internal rotation (55°), and external rotation (45°) are the basic movements of the shoulder girdle. Other movements normally tested are scapular retraction (military

Table 14.1.
Shoulder Girdle and Shoulder Motion

Joint motion	Prime movers	Accessories
Shoulder Girdle		
Elevation	Trapezius, upper	
	Levator scapulae	
	Rhomboids, major and minor	
Depression	Trapezius, lower	
	Latissimus dorsi	
	Pectoralis major, sternal head	
	Pectroalis minor	
Abduction	Serratus anterior	
	Pectoralis major and minor	
Adduction	Trapezius, upper and lower	
	Rhomboids, major and minor	
Upward rotation	Serratus anterior	
	Trapezius, upper and lower	
Downward rotation	Levator scapulae	Latissimus dorsi
	Rhomboids, major and minor	
	Pectoralis minor	
Shoulder		
Flexion	Deltoid, anterior	
	Coracobrachialis	
	Pectoralis major, clavicular head	
Extension	Deltoid, posterior	Infraspinatus, lower fibers
	Teres major	Teres minor
	Latissimus dorsi	Triceps, long head
	Pectoralis major, sternal head	
Abduction	Deltoid, middle	Deltoid, anterior and posterior
	Supraspinatus	
Horizontal abduction	Deltoid, posterior	Infraspinatus
		Teres minor
Adduction	Pectoralis major	Triceps, long head
	Teres major	Coracobrachialis
	Latissimus dorsi	Biceps brachii, short head
Horizontal adduction	Pectoralis major	Biceps brachii, short head
	Deltoid, anterior	Coracobrachialis
External rotation	Infraspinatus	Deltoid, posterior
	Teres minor	
Internal rotation	Subscapularis	Deltoid, anterior
	Pectoralis major	
	Latissimus dorsi	
	Teres major	

position of attention) and shoulder protraction (reaching). The patient may be in either the standing of sitting position during testing.

Elevation and depression are checked by having the patient hunch the shoulders and return to the normal position.

Active external rotation and abduction are easily tested by having the patient reach up and over the shoulder and attempt to touch the spinal border of the opposite scapula. External rotation and abduction can be tested bilaterally at the same time by having the patient place both hands behind the neck with interlocking fingers, then the elbows, which are initially pointing forward, are moved laterally and posteriorly in an arc.

If the examiner wishes to check solely glenohumeral joint passive abduction, the stabilizing hand should firmly anchor the scapula while the examiner's active hand passively abducts the patient's arm with the forearm horizontal. The shoulder blade will

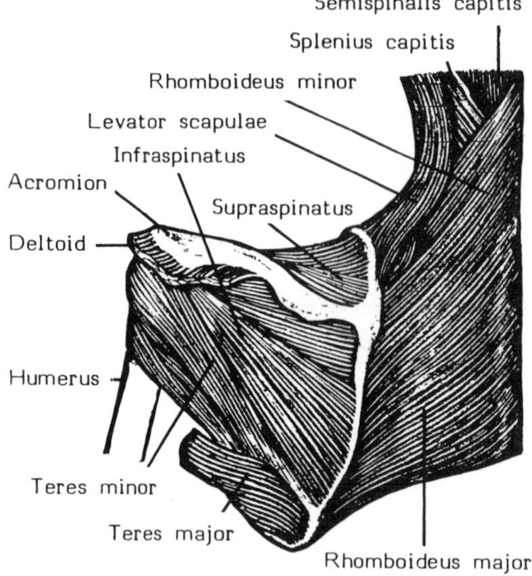

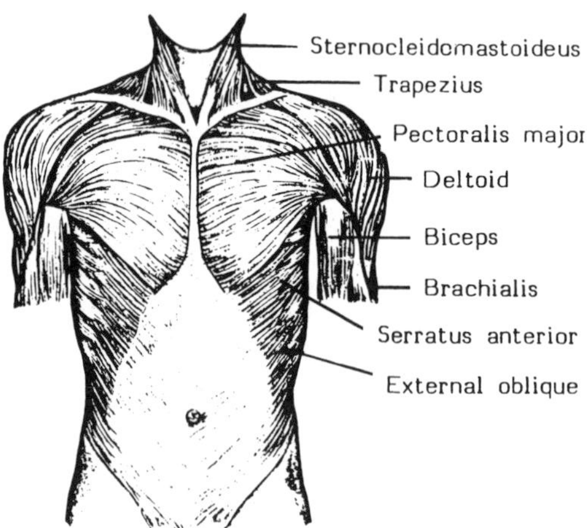

Figure 14.3. *Top*, major muscles of the posterior shoulder girdle; *bottom*, major superficial muscles of the anterior trunk.

normally not be felt to move until about 20° of abduction has occurred. Abduction should normally continue in this position to about 120° where the surgical neck of the humerus meets the tip of the acromion. The examiner should next turn the patient's forearm to externally rotate the humerus and move the surgical neck away from the acromion, then continue abduction to its maximum. For every 3° of humeral abduction, 1° occurs at the scapulothoracic articulation for every 2° at the glenohumeral joint.

Internal rotation and adduction are checked by having the patient reach across his chest, keeping the elbow as close to the chest as possible, and touch the opposite shoulder tip. A more extreme method is to have the patient reach behind the back and attempt to touch the bottom angle of the opposite shoulder blade. In each of these tests, both upper limbs may be tested at the same time, if desired, to compare bilateral action.

Test full active bilateral abduction by having the patient abduct the arms horizontally to 90° while keeping the elbows straight and the palms turned upward, then continuing abduction in an arc until the hands meet in the middle over the head.

Kinesiology of the Shoulder Girdle[21-26]

The major muscles of the shoulder, their primary function, and their innervation are listed in Table 14.2.

Flexion. Shoulder flexion is conducted primarily by the anterior deltoid (C5–C6) and coracobrachialis (C5–C6) with assistance by the clavicular head of the pectoralis major (C5–T1) and biceps (C5–C6). Strength of flexion can be tested from the back of the patient by placing the stabilizing hand on the patient's shoulder so that the anterior deltoid may be palpated during testing. The examiner's active hand grips the patient's anterior lower arm. With the patient's elbow flexed to 90°, resistance is increased as the patient is asked to flex the shoulder. Muscle strength is recorded by grade or in a percentage and compared bilaterally (Fig. 14.4).

Extension. Extension of the shoulder is controlled by the latissimus dorsi (C6–C8), teres major (C5–C6), and posterior part of the deltoid (C5–C6). Assistance is offered by the teres minor (C5–C6) and long head of the triceps (C7–C8). Strength of extension is judged from the back of the patient with the stabilizing hand in nearly the same position so as to palpate the posterior deltoid while the palm of the active hand grips the patient's lower arm at the posterior. The patient's elbow is again flexed, and he or she is asked to slowly extend the shoulder against increasing resistance.

Abduction. When the hand is abducted horizontally, the forces created at the shoulder joint have been calculated to approxi-

Table 14.2.
Major Muscles of the Shoulder

Muscle	Major function	Spinal segment
Biceps brachii	Flexion, adduction (short head)	C5–C6
Coracobrachialis	Flexion, adduction	C5–C6
Deltoid		C5–C6
Anterior fibers	Flexion, internal rotation, abduction, horizontal adduction	C5–C6
Dorsal fibers	Extension, external rotation, horizontal abduction	C5–C6
Middle fibers	Abduction	C5–C6
Infraspinatus	External and lateral rotation, extension (lower fibers), horizontal abduction	C5–C6
Latissimus dorsi	Extension, adduction, medial rotation, depression, downward rotation	C6–C8
Levator scapulae	Elevation, downward rotation	C3–C5
Pectoralis major	Adduction, flexion, depression	C5–T1
Clavicular head	Flexion, medial rotation, adduction	C5–C7
Sternal head	Extension, depression, medial rotation	C6–T1
Pectoralis minor	Adduction, medial/downward rotation, flexion, depression, extension	C7–C8
Rhomboids	Retraction, elevation, adduction, downward rotation	C5
Serratus anterior	Protraction, abduction, upward rotation, depression (lower fibers)	C5–C7
Subscapularis	Medial rotation and adduction	C5–C6
Supraspinatus	Abduction	C5–C6
Teres major	Extension, adduction, medial rotation	C5–C6
Teres minor	External/lateral rotation, extension, horizontal abduction	C5
Trapezius	Retraction	C3–C4, XI
Upper fibers	Elevation, adduction, upward rotation	
Lower fibers	Depression, adduction, upward rotation	
Triceps	Adduction, extension (long head)	C7–C8

Spinal innervation varies somewhat in different people. The spinal nerves listed here are averages and may differ in a particular patient; thus, an allowance of a segment above and below those listed in most text tables should be considered.

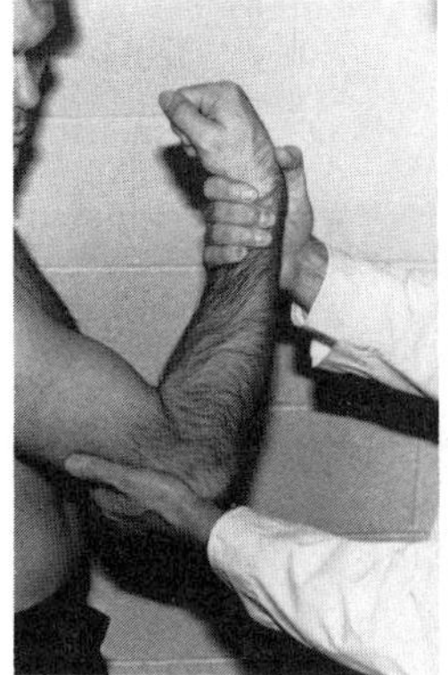
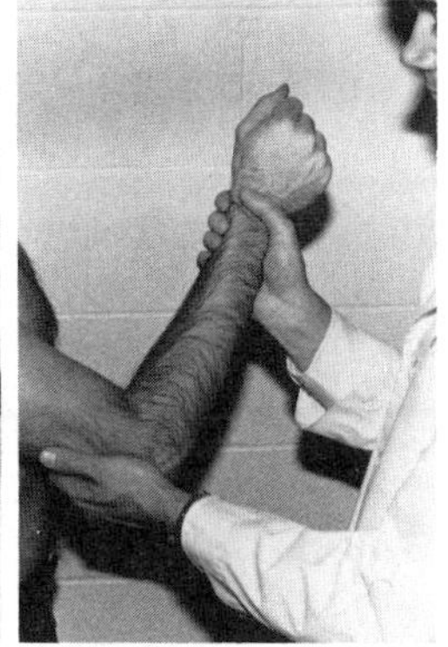

Figure 14.4. *Left*, testing shoulder flexion strength against resistance; *right*, testing extension strength.

mate total body weight. Shoulder abduction is conducted by the middle deltoid (C5–C6) and supraspinatus (C5–C6) with assistance by the serratus anterior (C5–C7). Strength of abduction can be tested at the side of the patient by placing the stabilizing hand on the lateral shoulder tip so that the middle of the deltoid may be palpated. The examiner applies increasing resistance laterally above the flexed elbow of the patient as abduction is attempted (Fig. 14.5).

Adduction. Adduction of the shoulder is controlled by the pectoralis major (C5–T1) and latissimus dorsi (C6–C8). Assistance is offered by the teres major (C5–C6) and anterior deltoid (C5–C6). Strength of adduction is measured from behind the patient with the stabilizing hand still on the shoulder tip. The patient's arm is abducted and the elbow is flexed. The examiner then applies increasing resistance medially above

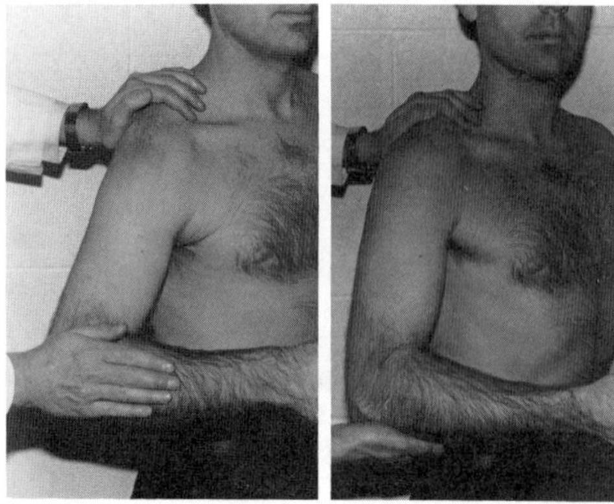

Figure 14.5. *Left*, testing the strength of shoulder abduction against resistance; *right*, testing strength of shoulder adduction.

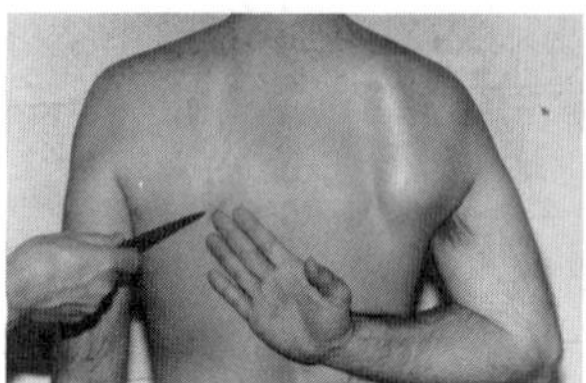

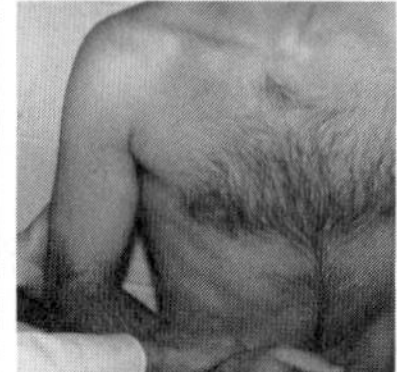

Figure 14.6. *Left*, evaluating internal rotation and adduction motion of the right shoulder joint; *right*, testing the strength of shoulder internal rotation against resistance.

the flexed elbow of the patient as the patient attempts adduction.

Internal Rotation. Internal rotation of the shoulder is controlled by four muscles: the subscapularis (C5–C6), pectoralis major (C5–T1), latissimus dorsi (C6–C8), and teres major (C5–C6). The anterior deltoid assists. Strength of the internal rotators is tested with the examiner's stabilizing hand and active hand in the same position. An increasing pulling resistance is applied to the patient's wrist as the patient attempts internal rotation of the arm by moving the hand toward the abdomen (Fig. 14.6).

External Rotation. External rotation of the shoulder is conducted by the infraspinatus (C5–C6) and teres minor (C5), with assistance by the posterior part of the deltoid. Strength of external rotation is judged at the side of the patient by placing the stabilizing hand on the patient's flexed elbow with the examiner's thumb in the angle of the patient's elbow. The active hand, gripping the patient's wrist, applies an increasing pushing resistance to the patient's attempt to externally rotate the arm by moving the hand away from his body (Fig. 14.7).

Scapular Elevation. Shoulder elevation is conducted by the trapezius (XI, C3–C4) and levator scapulae (C3–C5) with assistance from the major and minor rhomboids (C5). Strength is judged by the examiner standing behind the patient and applying increasing resistance with both palms on the patient's shoulders as the patient attempts to shrug his shoulders (Fig. 14.8).

Scapular Depression. Shoulder retraction is controlled by the major and minor rhomboids, both of which are usually innervated solely by C5. The trapezius assists. To evaluate the strength of scapular depression, the examiner stands in front of the patient with his hands grasping the patient's shoulder tips over the upper deltoids. The doctor's thumbs are braced under the patient's clavicles, and the fingers are behind the deltoids. The patient is instructed to slowly "throw his shoulders back and down" while the examiner applies increasing resistance; ie, forward toward the thumbs.

Shoulder Protraction. Protraction of the shoulder is conducted by the serratus anterior (C5–C7). In determining strength of protraction, with the examiner behind the patient, the patient is asked to flex the arm so that it is parallel to the floor with the elbow at a right angle to the arm. The examiner's stabilizing hand is placed in the midscapular area to stabilize the patient's spine from rotating, and the active hand is cupped around the patient's flexed elbow.

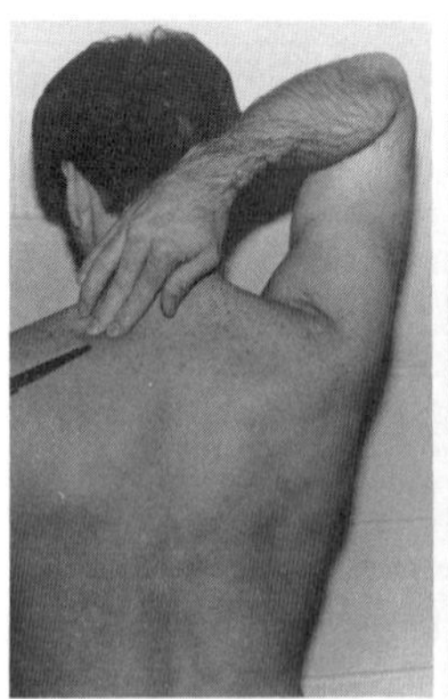

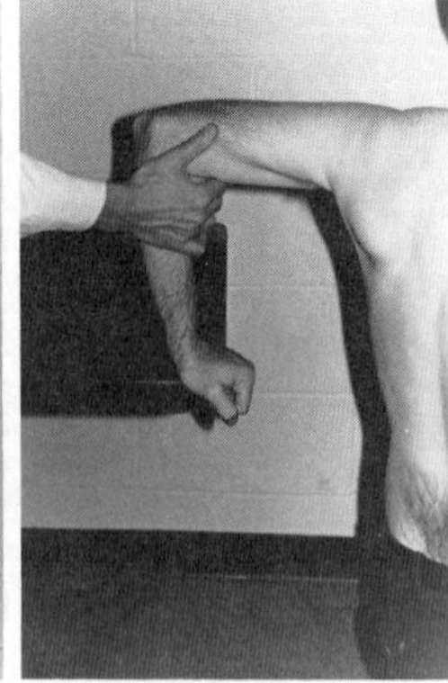

Figure 14.7. *Left*, Apley's scratch test to evaluate humeral abduction and external rotation motion; *right*, testing shoulder adduction strength against resistance.

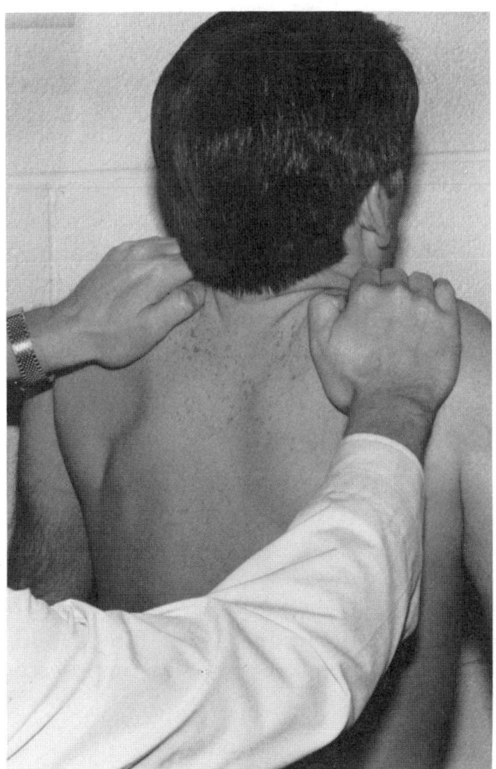

Figure 14.8. Testing the integrity of the spinal accessory nerve and shoulder girdle elevation strength. The patient shrugs his shoulders against the examiner's resistance.

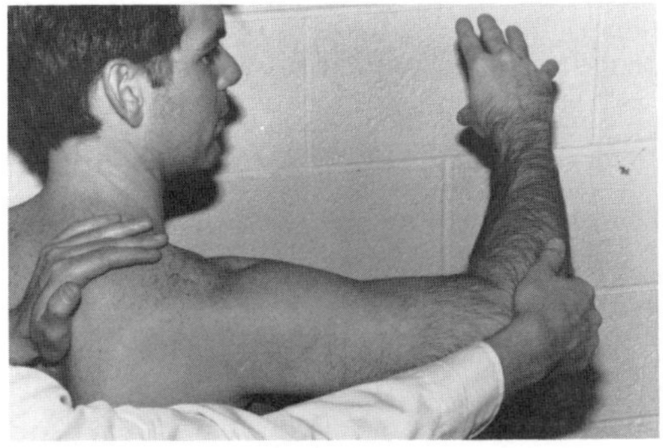

Figure 14.9. Testing the strength of scapular protraction against resistance.

Increasing resistance is applied as the patient attempts to slowly thrust the arm forward as if to touch a forward wall. During this movement, the examiner observes the scapula for possible winging (Fig. 14.9).

"The troublesome fifth cervical area" was discussed in Chapter 9. In this context, note in the above that shoulder girdle flexion, extension, abduction, adduction, internal rotation, external rotation, scapular elevation, scapular depression, and shoulder protraction are all subject to function of the C5 root.

Reactive Muscle Patterns

When the neuromuscular spindle cell is influencing a remote muscle, the remote muscle is called a *reactive muscle*.[27] Goodheart has reported that when 46 volunteers were screened for the reactive phenomenon in an EMG study of reactive muscle pairs, 14 were found with a positive deltoid-rhomboid reactivity. The deltoid could lift a 25-lb weight and hold it for 10 seconds from a neutral position. However, when the deltoid contraction followed contraction of the rhomboids, the weight could not be held by the reactive subjects. In all 14 subjects, a proprioceptor technique to both muscles of the reactive pair normalized function.[28]

Goniometry of the Shoulder[29, 30]

Restricted Forward Elevation. The patient is placed in the neutral position, the goniometer is centered next to the patient's shoulder, then the neutral reading with the goniometer arm along the patient's upper arm axis is recorded. The patient elevates both arms as far as possible; then the arm readings are recorded at the end of the motion.

Restricted Backward Elevation. The patient is placed in the neutral prone position, the goniometer is centered next to the patient's shoulder, and the neutral reading with the goniometer arm along the axis of the patient's upper arm is recorded. The patient elevates both arms as far as possible; then the arm being tested is recorded at the end of the motion.

Restricted Abduction or Adduction Motion. The patient is placed in the neutral position, and the goniometer is centered over the patient's shoulder. With the goniometer arm along the axis of the patient's arm, the neutral reading is recorded. The patient abducts both arms, and the readings at the end of the motions are recorded. Then the goniometer base is rotated, the patient abducts the arm to be tested, and the reading is recorded at end of the motion.

Restricted External or Internal Rotation Motion. The patient is placed in the neutral position, the goniometer is centered next to the patient's elbow, and the neutral reading (90°) is recorded with the goniometer arm along the axis of the patient's forearm. The patient attempts to touch the back of his hand and forearm to the top of the examining table. The reading for external rotation is recorded at the end of the motion. After returning to the neutral position, the patient attempts to touch his palm and volar surface of his forearm to the table top. The reading for internal rotation is recorded at the end of the motion.

Ankylosis. When taking the above measurements in ankylosis, any deviation from the neutral position should be measured.

SELECTED CLINICAL PROBLEMS OF THE SHOULDER GIRDLE[31-35]

A general classification of musculoskeletal and related disorders of the upper extremity is shown in Table 14.3.

Upper Extremity Pain: Clues within the History[36-38]

Shoulder pain has a high incidence. Cailliet states that it is second only to low-back and neck pain. Upper extremity pain may be the result of any structural disorder of the limb or a disturbance elsewhere in which the sensory phenomena are referred to the limb. Pain situated in various parts of the extremities will often reveal the point of origin by its peculiar location and quality. The pain may be of mechanical, chemical, thermal, toxic, nutritional, metabolic, or circulatory origin, or a combination of some of these factors, depending upon the nature of the pathologic process involved. The most important clues toward determining cause—type of pain, its distribution, and its associated symptoms—are the result of a carefully taken case history.

Peripheral nerve disease frequently indicates a history of entrapment neuropathy. The origin of nerve root lesions may be traced to trauma, a herniated disc, compression, hypertrophic changes in the vertebrae, neoplasms, or inflammation of the nerve root. Differentiation should be made from rare nutritional disorders resulting in a polyneuropathy because of unfavorable metabolic activities within the nerve cells. Peripheral neuritis, less common than peripheral neuropathy, can be classified into one of three types: infectious, allergic, or idiopathic.

Postural Disorders of the Upper Extremity[39-42]

Shoulder girdle pain and discomfort are often seen in typists, assembly-line workers, and laborers who work overhead with repetitive motions for long durations with little postural change. Many authorities believe the cause can usually be traced to muscular overuse leading to lower cervical or upper thoracic subluxations. Fixated misalignments may be found in the shoulder girdle itself, especially when the scapulae are chronically affected. Acute or chronic fibrositis of the trapezius and rhomboids with trigger points is often superimposed or consequential.

Muscle Strengthening

In the therapeutic alignment of the thoracic spine and the shoulder girdle, the common muscles to be strengthened are the scapular adductors and rotators; eg, trapezius, rhomboid major and minor, infraspinatus, and teres minor. Invariably, an associated weakness will be found in the gluteals and abdominals inducing pelvic misalignment.

Muscle Stretching

The common muscles to be stretched in postural misalignment of the thoracic spine and shoulder girdle are the shoulder adductors and medial rotators; eg, the latissimus dorsi, teres major, subscapularis, and pectoralis major and minor. When these muscles are stretched, the scapula should be firmly stabilized.

Spasm within the Shoulder Girdle[43-45]

Selected Effects of Hypertonicity in the Shoulder Girdle

Excessive hypertonicity of a muscle, confirmed by palpatory tone and soreness, will tend to subluxate its site of osseous attach-

Table 14.3.
Classification of Musculoskeletal and Related Disorders of the Upper Extremity

- **Lesions producing neck and shoulder pain**
  - Cervical subluxations
  - Cervical spondylosis
  - Postural strains
  - Fibrositis
  - Snapping scapula
  - Diseases of the abdominal or thoracic viscera
- **Lesions producing pain predominantly in the shoulder**
  - Local subluxations
  - Subdeltoid bursitis
  - Bicipital tenosynovitis
  - Tears of the rotator cuff
  - Arthritis of the glenohumeral, acromioclavicular, and sternoclavicular joints
  - Tumors
  - Abdominal pathology
  - Thoracic pathology
- **Lesions producing shoulder pain with radiation into the arm**
  - Cervical root syndrome
  - Neurovascular compression syndromes
  - Shoulder-hand syndrome
  - Angina
  - Miscellaneous diseases
- **Shoulder problems in children**
  - Birth trauma
  - Congenital deformities
  - Infections
- **Trauma**
  - Sprain/strain
  - Subluxation
  - Fracture
  - Dislocation
- **Congenital deformities below the shoulder**
  - Radial club hand
  - Floating thumb
  - Radioulnar synostosis
  - Finger deformities
    - Polydactyly
    - Syndactyly
    - Cinarthrosis
  - Constrictions
  - Megalodactyly
  - Arthrogryposis
  - Congenital trigger thumb
- **Bone and joint swelling**
  - Infectious arthritis
    - Pyogenic arthritis
    - Nonpyogenic arthritis
    - Tuberculous tenosynovitis
  - Acute and chronic osteomyelitis
  - Noninfectious arthritis
    - Rheumatoid arthritis
    - Psoriatic and lupus arthritis
    - Gouty arthritis
    - Primary hypertrophic arthritis
    - Post-traumatic arthritis
    - Avascular necrosis
    - Osteochondritis dissecans
    - Kienböck's disease
    - Preiser's disease
    - Fracture complications
- **Soft-tissue pain or swelling**
  - Infection
    - Olecranon bursitis
    - Perionychium infection
    - Felon
    - Tendon sheath suppuration
    - Hand space infections
    - Collar button abscess
    - Web space infection
  - Inflammation
    - de Quervain's syndrome
    - Triger or snapping finger
    - Tennis elbow
- **Nerve compression syndromes**
  - Median nerve
    - Pronator syndrome
    - Anterior interosseous nerve syndrome
    - Carpal tunnel syndrome
  - Ulnar nerve
    - Cubital tunnel syndrome
    - Guyon's canal compression
  - Radial nerve
    - Complete radial palsy
    - Posterior interosseous nerve syndrome
- **Tumor and tumor-like conditions**
  - Dupuytren's contracture
  - Ganglion
  - Xanthoma
  - Epidermoid systs
  - Chondroma
  - Epithelioma
  - Carcinoma of the nailhead

ment. Below is a listing of common problem areas in the upper extremities.

Trapezius. Increased tone tends to pull the shoulder girdle medial, the occiput posterioinferior, and the involved spinous processes lateral (Fig. 14.10).

Levator Scapulae. Increased tone tends to pull the scapula medial and superior and

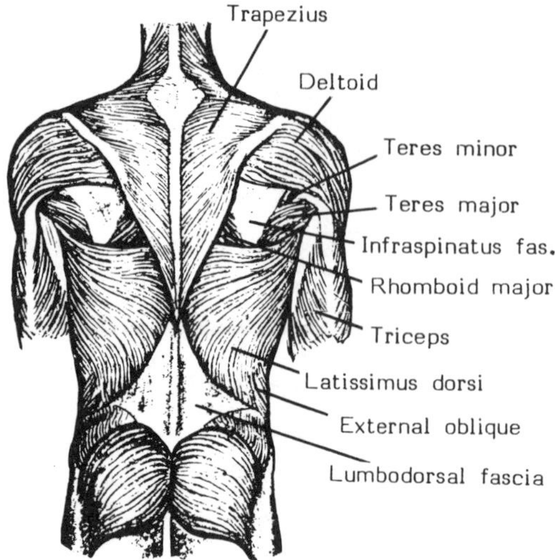

Figure 14.10. Superficial muscles of the posterior trunk.

the involved transverse processes inferior, lateral, and posterior.

Rhomboid Major. Increased tone tends to pull the scapula medial and superior and the spinous processes lateral and inferior.

Rhomboid Minor. Increased tone tends to pull the scapula medial and superior and the spinous processes lateral and inferior.

Many authorities feel that the excessive hypertonicity commonly witnessed is the result of overstress. However, Nelson[46] doubts the muscular "overuse" concept and offers this thought: "The more a muscle is used, the stronger it gets. Certainly, there may be a subluxation, but it would be the *result* of the muscle spasticity. The *cause* then must be a nervous or circulatory defect wherein the muscle cannot do sustained work without spasticity. A normal muscle merely tires."

Spasm Management[47–50]

Spasm management is usually necessary prior to articular correction and following articular correction to hold the adjustment in alignment.

Passive Stretch. Mild passive stretch is an excellent method of reducing spasm in the long muscles, but heavy passive stretch destroys the beneficial reflexes. In rhomboid spasm, for example, the prone patient should place his hand on the involved side behind his back to "wing" the scapula. This slightly stretches the muscle fibers by pulling the scapula from the midline. This may be assisted by the doctor offering a slight tug upward on the scapular angle. The muscle should relax within 2–3 minutes. Thumb pressure, placed on a trigger area, is directed toward the muscle's attachment and held for a few moments until relaxation is complete. Resisting active antagonist contraction is also helpful, especially if the disorder is highly acute.

Therapeutic Exercises. When pain has subsided, two beneficial home progressive exercises are (1) gravity-assisted pendulum exercises holding a weight or iron while prone and (2) holding a broomstick in front with both hands and doing elevations. Isotonic exercises are useful in improving circulation and inducing the stretch reflex when done supine to reduce exteroceptive influences on the central nervous system.

Modalities. Other adjunctive therapies may also be helpful. Peripheral inhibitory afferent impulses can be generated to partially close the presynaptic gate by acupressure, acupuncture, or transcutaneous nerve stimulation. An acid-base imbalance from muscle hypoxia and acidosis may be prevented by supplemental alkalinization. In chronic cases, high-voltage galvanic, relaxation training, and biofeedback therapy are beneficial.

Myofascial Shoulder Syndrome

In most cases of posttraumatic shoulder pain, its origin can generally be localized to a small area by palpation or reproduced at some point in active or passive motion. This is typical of many common disorders—capsulitis, bicipital tendinitis, dislocations, impingement syndromes, rotator cuff strains, subacromial bursitis, and supraspinatus injuries, for example.

Trigger point pain differs from pain associated with most structural injuries in that the physical findings are few. Rather than being localized, the pain is described over a broad area that does not coincide with specific segmental patterns. Associated paresthesias are described in extremely vague expressions. Range of motion tests and muscle strength grading offer little help, even after referred pain from the cervical spine, lungs, or viscera is ruled out. While trauma may be involved, it may be only a precipitating rather than a causative factor.

The muscles of the shoulder girdle are highly susceptible to trigger point formation because they are anatomically susceptible to fatigue, easy victims of the stresses of poor posture and biomechanical faults, and the target for many psychosomatic reflexes. Michelle and Eisenberg[51] state that no less than one-third of their middle-aged patients with shoulder pain had the myofascial pain syndrome.

The focal point of pain in a myofascial syndrome will be found as one or more small areas of muscle fiber degeneration that feel fairly firm and ropey to the touch. Further probing will usually elicit the characteristic involuntary "jump sign" as the patient reacts and the physiologic "twitch sign" which is the result of a brief contraction of the surface fibers near the trigger point.

Sites

Although a trigger point may develop in any muscle, certain sites appear to be favored. A point in the superior medial aspect of the scapula, near the insertion of the levator scapulae, is a common site, as are points in the supraspinatus and trapezius. Weed[52] describes frequently occurring points over the heads of the 2nd, 3rd, or 4th ribs, just lateral to the spinous processes.

A common source of many shoulder pains sited in the anterolateral shoulder will be found at the insertions of the infraspinatus and supraspinatus muscles at the scapula (Fig. 14.11). In other cases, a localized trigger point may be found in the anterior deltoid, with pain referred to the subdeltoid bursa, or in the sternalis, whch refers pain across the chest and down the medial arm (Fig. 14.12).

Other common trigger point sites in should pain occur at the lesser tuberosity at the insertion of the subscapularis, at the greater tuberosity at the insertion of the supraspinatus tendon, at the glenohumeral joint space, within the bicipital groove, at the acromioclavicular joint, or at the sternoclavicular joint. The levator scapulae, scaleni, pectoralis major and minor, and serratus anterior are less common sites.

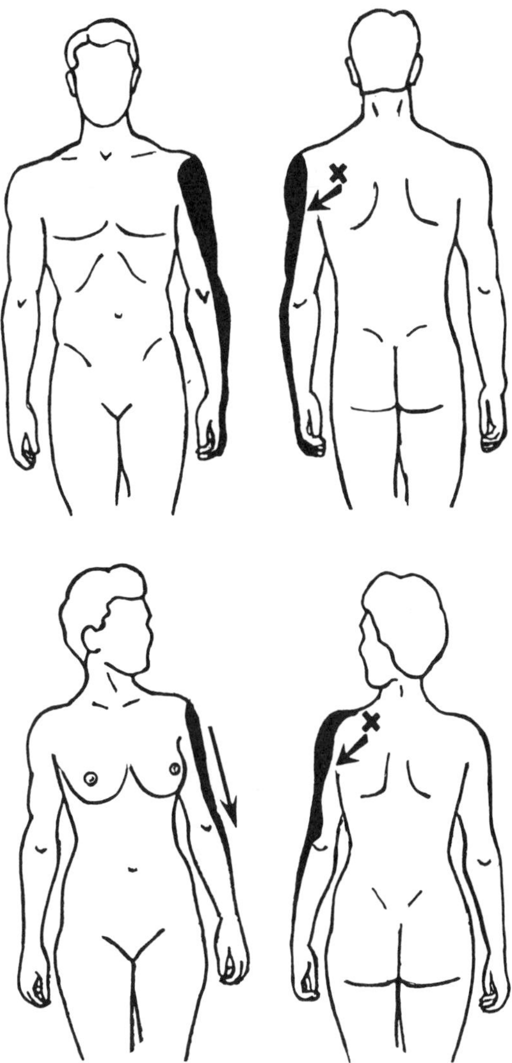

Figure 14.11. *Top*, infraspinatus trigger point; *X*, common site. *Blackened areas* indicate typical sites of referred pain. *Bottom*, supraspinatus trigger point.

Management

As in other areas, goading, acupuncture, high-volt stimulation, spray-and-stretch, and deep percussion/vibration are generally the conservative therapies of choice in trigger point therapy.

Painful Shoulder Syndromes[53–57]

Tendon inflammation is not as common in the shoulder as it is in the elbow and wrist. However, because tendons are relatively avascular, they are subject to chronic

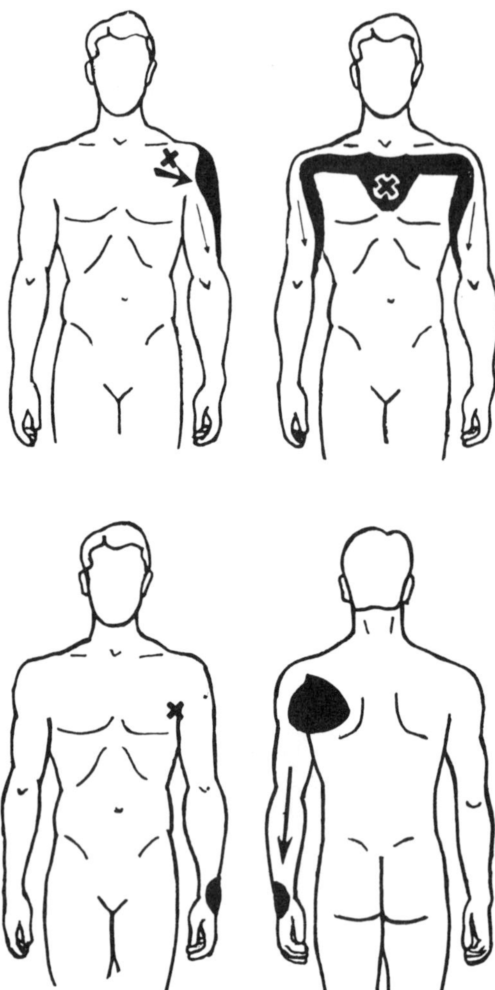

Figure 14.12. *Top left*, deltoid trigger point; *X*, common site. *Blackened areas* indicate typical sites of referred pain. *Top right*, sternalis trigger point. *Bottom*, subscapularis trigger point.

trauma, microtears, slow repair, and aging degeneration in the shoulder.

Most shoulder syndromes involve a degree of either overuse or underuse:

1. Overuse of poorly conditioned tissues is the common cause. The shoulder tendons are wide bands of collagen fibers. If stress roughens a tendon, its tensile strength decreases. This leads to fibrinoid degeneration in and between the collagen fibers and later fibrosis. With necrosis and the initial inflammatory reparative process, the local tissues become akaline, which induces precipitation of calcium salts. This deposition may invade an overlying bursa.

2. Excessive postinjury immobilization leads to muscle atrophy and loss of capsular elasticity, a predisposing factor to capsulitis and periarthritis. Lack of joint movement fosters retention of metabolites, edema, venous stasis, and ischemia leading to fibrous adhesions and trigger point development.

Supraspinatus Tendinitis[58–60]

Inflammation of paratendinous supraspinatus tissues is often a part of subdeltoid or subacromial bursitis. It is also frequently a part of rotator cuff injury and a complication of severe supraspinatus strain. An ache is present on rest which is aggravated by abduction. Pain may be referred as far distal as the deltoid insertion. The distinguishing feature is that pain is restricted to movement only within a certain point of the arc (painful arc syndrome). This is because the acromion process affects the tendon area only during part of its excursion. Point tenderness will be found over the site of inflammation. The patient will complain that it is painful to sleep on the affected side. Treatment is similar to that of bicipital tendinitis.

Supraspinatus Press Test. With the patient in the relaxed seated position, the examiner applies strong thumb pressure directed toward the midline in the soft tissues located superior to the midpoint of the scapular spine. The production of pain signifies an inflammatory process in the supraspinatus muscle (eg, strain, rupture, tendinitis).

Apley's Scratch Test. This is a two-phase test: (1) The patient (seated or standing) is asked to raise the arm on the involved side overhead, flex the elbow overhead, and then place the fingers as far down on the opposite shoulder blade as possible. (2) The patient is then asked to relax the arm at the side, then place the hand behind the back and attempt to touch as far up on the opposite scapula as possible. If either of these maneuvers increases shoulder pain, inflammation of one of the rotator cuff's tendons is indicated. The supraspinatus tendon is most commonly involved. Restricted motion without sharp pain points to osteoarthritis or shortened soft tissues.

Shoulder Abduction Stress Test. The seated patient is asked to abduct the arm laterally to the horizontal position with the elbow extended while the examiner applies resistance. If this causes pain in the area of the insertion of the supraspinatus tendon, acute or degenerative tendinitis should be suspected.

Codman's Sign. This is a variation of the shoulder abduction stress test and the arm drop test. If the patient's arm can be passively abducted laterally to about 100° without pain, the examiner then removes support so that the position is held actively by the patient. This produces sudden deltoid contraction. If a rupture of the supraspinatus tendon or strain of the rotator cuff is present, the pain elicited will cause the patient to hunch the shoulder and lower the arm.

Bicipital Tendinitis[60–62]

The synovia of the bicipital groove is a common site of chronic paratendinous inflammation. It is frequently a complication of bicipital rupture (long head) or subluxation of the tendon from the groove. Pain is aggravated on abduction and extension, and tenderness is localized over the inflamed tendon. Most symptoms mimic supraspinatus tendinitis, but the pain is referred distally in the area of the biceps insertion to the radius. Tenderness is found along the anterior shoulder in the bicipital groove, and pain is increased if the patient abducts, flexes, and internally rotates the shoulder. When the patient flexes his arm and supinates his wrist against resistance, a positive sign is pain within the anterior medial upper humerus area. Bicipital tendinitis will greatly affect flexion and extension strength.

Lippman's Test. In the relaxed seated position, the patient is asked to flex the elbow on the involved side and rest the forearm in the lap. The examiner palpates for the tendon of the long head of the biceps about 3 inches distal from the glenohumeral joint. An attempt is made to displace the tendon laterally or medially from its groove. Pain, reduplication of other symptoms, and a palpable displacement of the tendon from its groove signifies tenosynovitis with instability.

Gilcrest's Sign. The patient is instructed to lift a 5-lb weight (eg, dumbbell) overhead and then to externally rotate the arm and slowly lower it to the lateral horizontal position. Pain and/or reduplication of symptoms during this maneuver (with or without tendon displacement from the groove) are said to indicate instability of the long head of the biceps and probable tenosynovitis.

Biceps Stability Test. The seated patient is asked to flex his elbow so that the forearm is held forward and horizontal. As the patient attempts to externally rotate the arm, the examiner applies resistance. Localized pain indicates an inflammatory instability of the long head of the biceps and/or displacement of the tendon from the bicipital groove.

Booth-Marvel's Test. The examiner abducts the patient's arm laterally to the horizontal position, flexes the elbow to a right angle, and deeply palpates the bicipital groove as the humerus is passively rotated internally and externally. If the transverse humeral ligament has been stretched, a painful and palpable snap will be felt as the tendon of the long head displaces from the bicipital groove.

Hueter's Sign. If pain and/or reduplication of other symptoms appear when the patient's supinated forearm is flexed against resistance, partial rupture of the biceps is suggested.

Subdeltoid Bursitis[63, 64]

Of the 140 bursae of the body, none have more trouble than the subdeltoid bursa (Fig. 14.13). When it becomes inflamed, the patient presents acute, severe, deep-seated local pain. There is weakness with shoulder movement in any plane but especially on abduction. Quite frequently, bursitis will usually limit flexion, extension, and both internal and external rotation. The entire bursa and paratendinous tissues will be swollen and readily palpable. This swelling prevents the greater tuberosity from sliding under the acromion during abduction. Dysfunction of the rotator, bicipital, and subscapularis tendons (which pass through the bursa) will commonly be demonstrated. The initial attacks are localized in the vicinity of the greater tubercle. The chronic stage is characterized by subdeltoid tenderness, restricted motion in abduction and external rotation, and associated capsular contraction and adhesions.

Shoulder bursitis is rarely a primary condition. Degenerative changes in the rotator

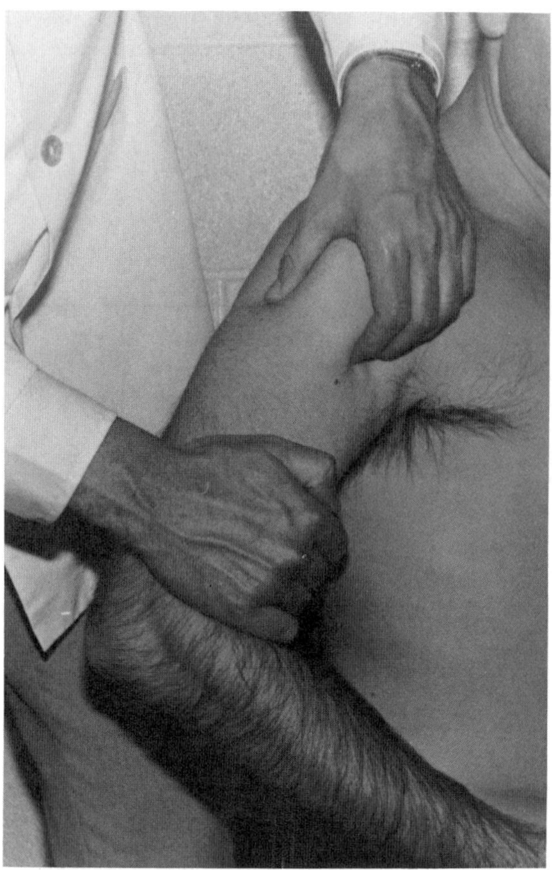

Figure 14.13. Palpating the right deltoid and the lesser tuberosity area.

cuff at the floor of the subdeltoid bursa lead to calcific deposits resulting in acute inflammation of the bursa. When a calcium deposit breaks into the bursa, it absorbs water. This enlarges the bursal space, resulting in increased pressure that exhibits severe pain and some warmth and redness of the overlying skin.

Subacromial Bursitis[65, 66]

A painful, faltering abduction arc is also characteristic of subacromial bursitis. To differentiate, the coracoid process is palpated under the pectoralis major. It is found by circumducting the humerus, and it is normally tender. Once the process is found, the finger is slid slightly laterally and superiorly until it reaches a portion of the subacromial bursa. If the same palpation pressure here causes greater tenderness than at the process, it is a positive sign of subacromial bursitis.

Subacromial Button Sign. The examiner stands behind the seated patient, cups a palm over the involved shoulder, and applies finger pressure over the subacromial bursa. If this produces pain or unusual tenderness, subacromial bursitis is suggested.[67]

Dawbarn's Test. The examiner stands behind the seated patient and deeply palpates the area just below the acromion process to determine symptoms of focal tenderness or referred pain. Then, while still maintaining this palpatory pressure to patient tolerance, the examiner grasps the patient's wrist with the other hand and brings the arm to the lateral extended position so that it is abducted to about 100°. If subacromial bursitis exists, the pain elicited on initial palpation should decrease substantially when the arm is raised because the deltoid will cover the spot below the acromion during abduction. If the pain remains unaltered or is increased by this abduction maneuver, subacromial bursitis can usually be ruled out.[68]

Supraspinatus Calcification[58, 69]

Tendon calcification is commonly found in the supraspinatus tendon, near its insertion at the greater tuberosity of the humerus. Symptoms arise suddenly. Pain is usually severe and aggravated by shoulder movement, but the pain is less severe and movements more tolerated than in supraspinatus tendinitis. Tenderness is localized over the bursa. A painful arc syndrome may be noted, similar to that seen in supraspinatus tendinitis. Associated bursitis may be present, which is responsible for much of the acute symptoms.

Deposits may appear in shoulder tendons, ligaments, or aponeuroses, and especially within the rotator cuff. They may be chronic, silent, or extremely acute. Spontaneous absorption may occur relatively fast. The calcification is viewed in roentgenography as a large dense opacity above the outer head of the humerus. It is most frequently related to middle age with no definite history of trauma, but it is only occasionally seen in the young. In the well-developed person, symptoms from calcification may not appear for many months after injury.

Triceps Brachii Calcification[65, 70]

Repetitive stretching of the posterior elements of the shoulder from throwing frequently causes an inflammation of the posterior capsule tissues of the shoulder. This may result in an osteotendinous calcification at the infraglenoid area where the long head of the triceps originates. Once calcification forms, the follow-through in throwing is quite painful.

Capsulitis[71]

Capsulitis of the shoulder is often the result of a sprain attended by a spontaneously reduced subluxation or of prolonged overuse. Joint pain is aggravated by movement. Tenderness and other symptoms are generalized within the whole joint area rather than being localized. Motion limitation may be considerable in adhesive capsulitis (frozen shoulder) in which the head of the humerus is "glued" to the glenoid cavity.

Periarthritis[72–74]

Periarthritis of the shoulder—commonly called "frozen shoulder" or Duplay's syndrome—is often a challenge because it is usually near the terminal stage when the patient is first seen. A combination of several chronic, diffuse, degenerative shoulder disorders are usually involved. Loss of scapulohumeral rhythm is a characteristic feature. This is readily noted when viewed from the posterior. During the early stage, shoulder motion stiffens at the extreme ranges of abduction and internal rotation.

Differentiation must be made from the early stage of capsulitis. Humeral motion restriction is exhibited in all planes in periarthritis, but adduction and rotation are especially affected. Scapulothoracic motion, however, will be normal. Atrophy is readily noted and proportionate to the chronicity of the condition. Tenderness is diffuse throughout the upper arm with the possible exception of the posterior and medial aspects. The capsule becomes thick and contracted, which contributes to motion limitation. The rotator cuff also becomes thick and inelastic, and the tendon becomes cemented within the groove.

In time, the adhesions and soft tissues thicken and become tightly fixed, binding capsule to bone. As the joint cavity "dries," the head of the humerus is pulled tightly against the glenoid fossa. Arm use aggravates the condition, and symptoms are more acute at night after a day's activity. Rest offers relief, so improvement is seen in the morning. The accessory muscles overwork in an attempt to compensate for primary shoulder muscle deficiency, causing aching posterior shoulder and neck muscles. A superiorly subluxated 1st rib or a lower cervical subluxation is usually a common and important contributing factor. Roentgenography is often negative with the exception of an obliterated joint space.

Traumatic Arthritis[75]

Osteoarthritis of the shoulder is seen more in literature than in actual practice. Usually, the case is a periarthritis in which degenerative changes have occurred within the soft tissues. The characteristic picture is one of pain, tenderness on pressure, and rarely some swelling. Passive motion is comparatively painless, but active motion induces severe pain. Differentiation must be made from supraspinatus rupture, subdeltoid bursitis, and inflammation of other bursae about the shoulder.

Other Syndromes

Cervical pathology and subluxation syndromes, traumatic brachial plexus traction, cervical ribs, and neurovascular compression syndromes frequently involve or refer pain to the upper extremity. These disorders have been discussed previously in Chapter 9. Upper rib and upper thoracic syndromes may also involve or refer pain to the upper extremity, and these have been described in Chapter 10.

The examiner should also keep in mind that both referred pain and tenderness may be of a visceral nature, especially from the liver, gallbladder, and right diaphragm to the right shoulder and from the stomach, left diaphragm, and heart to the left shoulder.[76] Referred pain and tenderness, however, are not always predictable. It is *not* true that visceral reflexes do not affect local joint function. They may or may not produce musculoskeletal symptoms and signs.

INJURIES OF THE SHOULDER JOINT[77-82]

The shoulder girdle is a common site of minor injury and not infrequent site of serious disability. It is second only to the knee as a site of chronic prolonged disability. Most shoulder injuries are not single-entity injuries. They are composed of a variety of contusions, strains, and sprains, and possible avulsion and fracture. Fixed dislocations, spontaneously reduced dislocations, and subluxations also complicate the picture. Thus, any painful shoulder syndrome requires careful differentiation.

Shoulder Sprains and Strains[83, 84]

The shoulder is at the forefront of high-incidence injuries. Tears of the rotator cuff, usually without humeral displacement, are common. Most are the result of throwing injuries, falls on the shoulder point, and vertical forces directed along the humerus. Careful evaluation of the soft tissues is necessary (Fig. 14.14). Subclavian and axillary vessel injury may be the result of direct trauma or a sudden and violent shoulder movement. Rarely, just muscular hypertrophy may produce venous insufficiency or thrombosis. Brachial plexus and coracoid injuries are sometimes related in anterior blows. Epiphyseal injuries of the proximal humerus are rare, heal well, and are usually treated conservatively (closed).

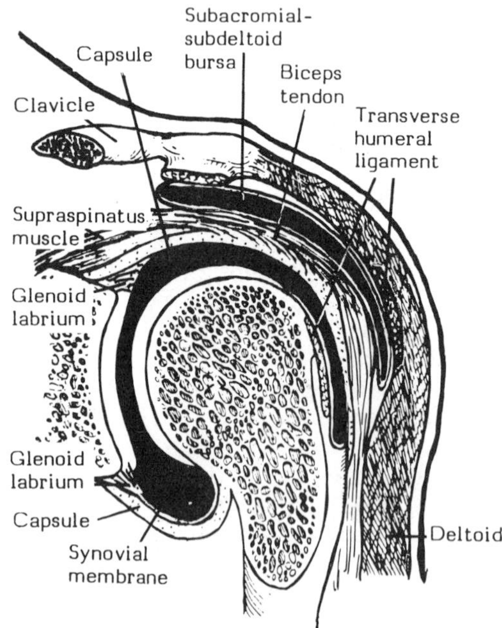

Figure 14.14. Coronal section of the shoulder joint showing some clinically significant structures.

Mechanics of the Arm during Elevation

The poise of the clavicle and the suspension of the upper extremity are determined by the integrity of the capsule of the sternoclavicular joint and its associated ligaments, while the vertical stability of the upper extremity at the glenohumeral joint is determined by the strength of the capsule's superior aspect and the coracohumeral ligament.[85] During the first half of arm abduction, all components of the rotator cuff are active and with the deltoid they produce compressive and shear forces at the surface of the glenoid cavity. These forces are maximal at 90° of elevation; at 150° of elevation, they are usually absent. During the last phase of elevation, EMG studies show that the infraspinatus and teres minor tendon maintain their high level of activity to provide the necessary external rotation for complete elevation of the arm.

Mechanisms in Throwing Injuries

The shoulder girdle is a multiaxial, intricately synchronized joint complex that has considerable power and an extreme range of motion. The anterior, superior, and posterior shoulder muscles provide the great power, and the collateral ligaments do not appreciably limit motion in any plane. Thus, stability must be provided by the musculature: essentially the rotator cuff and subscapularis muscles, which are aided somewhat by the glenohumeral ligaments. Muscle forces must act through four relatively unique joints (glenohumeral, scapulothoracic, acromioclavicular, sternoclavicular) to achieve the normally graceful coordination required of shoulder motion. Because of this, alterations of the throwing mechanism about the shoulder produce a clinical picture that is often difficult to diagnosis and effectively treat.

For the purposes of analysis, Tullos and King[86] divide the throwing mechanism into three separate, independent stages, each of which is associated with specific shoulder injuries:

1. *The Cocking Phase.* During windup, the shoulder is brought into extreme external rotation, abduction, and extension. The biceps, triceps, and internal and external rotators are highly tensed. For this reason, a professional baseball pitcher will invariably exhibit abnormal external humeral rotation and subnormal internal rotation. Overstress makes the proximal arm vulnerable to biceps tendinitis, triceps tendinitis, and humeral subluxation.

2. *The Acceleration Phase.* The actual throwing phase is a two-stage process: (a) With the forearm and hand stationary, the shoulder is brought forward, the elbow is placed into extreme valgus strain as the muscular forces multiply on the shaft of the humerus, and the elbow is stabilized by the flexors of the forearm. (b) In the second stage, the forearm is rapidly whipped forward by internal shoulder rotation produced by severe contraction of the pectoralis major and latissimus dorsi. This stage ends when the hand is near ear level and the ball is released. Overstress makes the shoulder complex vulnerable to pectoralis and latissimus tendinitis, along with the effects of the mechanical forces upon the humerus.

3. *The Follow-Through Phase.* The last phase begins as the ball is released near head level and ends when the pitch is completed. Its major function is involved with deceleration of the arm and forearm and, usually, some type of ball rotation. Great stress is applied to the glenohumeral joint and its adjacent tissues.

General Shoulder Sprains

The major symptoms and signs of shoulder sprain are pain, tenderness on pressure, and, rarely, swelling. Passive motion is comparatively painless, but active motion induces severe pain. Differentiation must always be made from rupture of the supraspinatus tendon, subdeltoid bursitis, fracture, and inflammation of other bursae about the shoulder.

The Lax Shoulder Joint[87]

Repeated subluxations without clinical dislocation often produce a loose joint. The history will reveal frequent episodes of mild trauma, each incorporating a period of pain and limited motion, followed by an audible "click" as the head of the humerus slips painfully back into the fossa. After reduction, examination reveals few signs except residual tenderness and a lax capsule.

Shoulder Stability.[88] Stability in the shoulder is mainly dependent upon muscle tone and not ligament strength. This becomes readily apparent in paralysis. The weakest part of the shoulder joint is at the anterolateral aspect of the capsule, thus the greatest stress is applied to the joint when the arm is abducted to the horizontal and the humerus is externally rotated. The strongest position of the joint is when the arm is held downward and rotated internally. Note that this is the position instinctively used both in active shoulder "blocking" and when the arm is placed in a sling for rest.

The Lax Capsule Test.[89] To determine a lax capsule, have the patient clasp his fingers behind his head and laterally abduct his elbows. Palpate high in the axilla over the glenohumeral capsule while applying posterior force on the patient's flexed elbow. While laxity of the anterior capsule can always be demonstrated by this maneuver, care must be taken not to dislocate the humerus within a loose capsule. If episodes of pain from the instability are frequent, some form of external support should be provided, and the patient should be advised of the risks involved in repeated subluxation.

The Bicipital Syndrome[90, 91]

In shoulder injury, after possible dislocation and fracture have been eliminated, special attention should be given to the bicipital muscle (Fig. 14.15). The biceps is the most powerful flexor of the elbow and a strong supinator. Within the shoulder area, proximal strains and tears along the long head's course within the bicipital groove to the glenoid rim are frequently seen.

Acute rupture of the biceps tendon occurs as a result of forceful contraction of the biceps muscle or forceful movement of the arm with the biceps contracted. The injury may be avulsion of the tendon from the muscle belly anywhere along its course or the tendon's pulling free from its glenoid

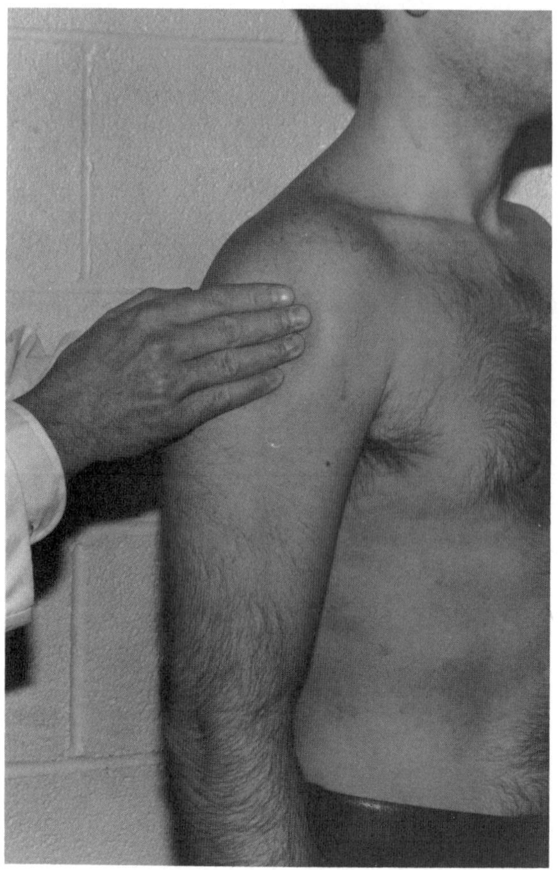

Figure 14.15. Palpating the right bicipital groove and related tissues.

attachment. It is often a crippling problem and usually accompanied by tenosynovitis.

Signs and Symptoms. An acute tendon tear is often felt by the patient as a "snap," followed by swelling, tenderness, and ecchymosis over the bicipital groove and bulging of the biceps near the antecubital fossa at the lower half of the humerus. Pain is usually felt on the anterior shoulder about 2 inches below the humeral head at the site of the thecal tunnel. If the long head is torn, the contracted muscle belly moves distally and bulges even if the short head is intact. This is an important sign in differentiating a proximal biceps problem from other shoulder problems. A hollow in the upper humeral area can usually be both seen and felt. Flexion and supination, especially against resistance, increases the bulging at the lower half of the upper arm. Strength of forearm supination is decreased.

Yergason's Stability Test.[92, 93] The seated patient flexes the elbow, pronates the forearm, and attempts elbow flexion, forearm supination, and humeral external rotation against the resistance of the examiner. The doctor stabilizes the patient's elbow with one hand while offering resistance in the patient's distal forearm with his other hand during the maneuver (Fig. 14.16). Severe pain in the shoulder during this test is usually a positive indication of a bicipital tendon lesion, a tear of the transverse humeral ligament, or bicipital tendinitis.

Loose-Tendon Syndrome.[94] In some chronic bicipital disorders, the tendon may appear slack and actually glide from side to side on palpation during repeated adduction and external rotation. To further evaluate, the patient's affected forearm is placed on the examiner's knee. The bicipital groove is palpated with one hand while the other hand moves the patient's elbow lateral and anterior while the patient resists the movement. If the tendon is slack, it will be felt to "jump" during the motion. Injury to the transverse humeral ligament is often involved.

Bicipital Tendon Dislocation[62, 95]

A bicipital tendon may be found to be dislocated or at least partially subluxated from its groove and express symptoms. This is due to rupture or loosening of the transverse ligament which holds the tendon of the long head within the bicipital groove. The mechanism of injury is usually heavy lifting, "Indian" arm wrestling, or a slip while carrying a heavy object. Injury occurs, especially in young adults, when the contracted biceps meets an overload.

Signs and Symptoms. A subluxated tendon will be felt and/or heard to snap as the patient forward flexes and abducts his arm, then returns it to its natural position. The patient is unable to place the ipsilateral hand on the sacrum. As time passes, motion restrictions indicate cuff degeneration. Yergason's and Abbott-Saunders' tests are positive. Extreme tenderness will be found at the superior aspect of the bicipital groove, with some tenderness along the groove distally. A slack tendon will be found on palpation of the upper groove as the humerus is abducted and internally rotated. A "jump-

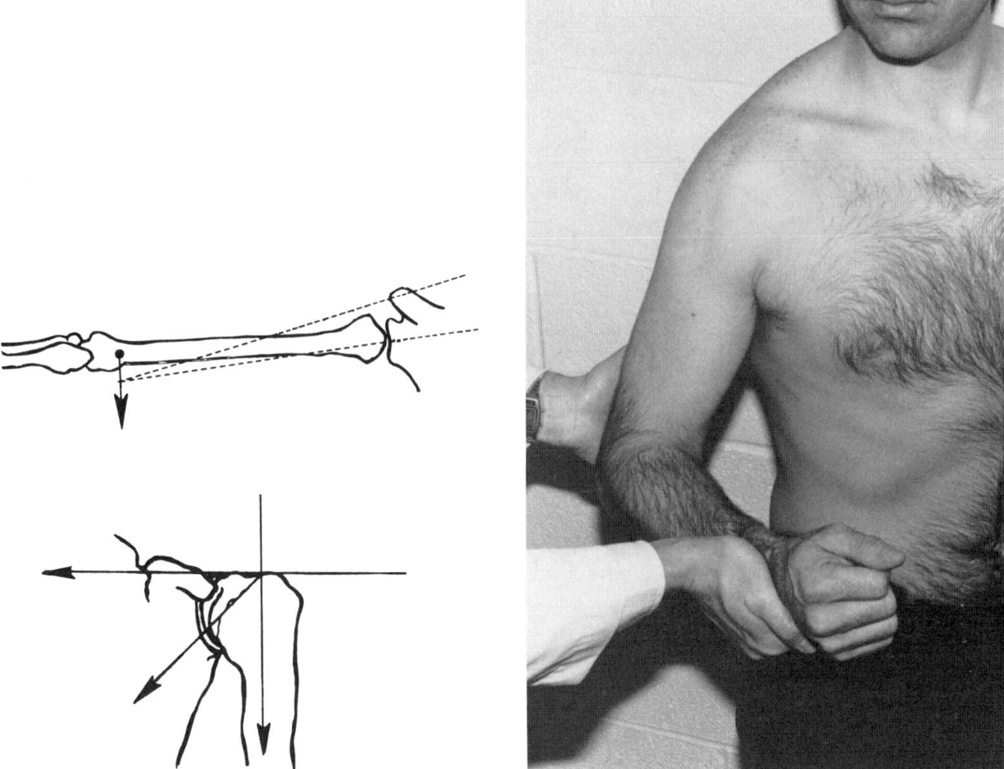

Figure 14.16. *Top left*, schematic of forces supporting the upper limb during abduction. *Bottom left*, forces acting upon the shoulder to stabilize humerus within the glenoid fossa. *Right*, Yergason's test to evaluate the stability of the long head of the biceps tendon within the bicipital groove.

ing" sensation from the tendon is felt if the transverse ligament is partially torn. A gliding sensation is felt if the ligament is completely torn.

Abbott-Saunders' Test.[96, 97] This is a modification of Yergason's test that forces the biceps tendon against the lesser tuberosity which will stress an instable tendon. The arm of the seated patient is brought into full abduction, rotated externally, and the lowered to the patient's side. A "click" felt or heard, frequently accompanied by pain and a reproduction of symptoms, is a positive sign of subluxation or dislocation of the biceps tendon.

Locking Position Test. The patient's arm is extended and internally rotated. If a painful reduplication of the patient's symptoms occurs on this maneuver, an impingement syndrome of the supraspinatus and/or bicipital tendon is suggested.

Impingement Syndrome Test. The patient is placed supine with the arms resting loosely at the sides. The elbow on the involved side is then flexed to a right angle and the arm is rotated internally so that it rests comfortably on the patient's upper abdomen. The examiner places one hand on the patient's shoulder and the other hand on the patient's elbow. A compressive force is then applied, which pushes the humerus against the inferior aspect of the acromion process and the glenohumeral fossa. Pain and/or a reduplication of symptoms indicates an impingement syndrome of the supraspinatus and/or bicipital tendon.

Rotator Cuff Strains[98–100]

Five deep muscles lying around the glenohumeral joint comprise the rotator cuff. The infraspinatus and teres minor work as external rotators of the humerus. The subscapularis and teres major rotate the humerus medially. The supraspinatus pulls the humerus into the glenoid fossa and abducts the humerus initially (10–15°) before the deltoid becomes effective. In further abduction, the supraspinatus stabilizes the humerus as the deltoid, during full abduction, tends to diplace the humerus from the glenoid. The mechanism of injury may be a fall on an outstretched hand, a blow on the shoulder, throwing, or heavy lifting.

The Role of the Rotator Cuff. The intrinsic rotators of the shoulder are active during abduction and external rotation. When the horizontal arm is loaded to produce anterior dislocation of the humerus, the subscapularis has proved to be the primary muscle responsible for preventing displacement. The supraspinatus, infraspinatus, and teres minor contract to stabilize the head of the humerus in the glenoid fossa. If the horizontal arm is also extended backward about 30° and loaded so that the complete rotator cuff is at full contraction, the anterior shear force is about quadrupled. Because the shallow glenoid fossa offers almost no protection, this force must be counteracted by the capsule and associated ligaments to prevent anterior displacement.

Force Couples.[101-103] The upward pull on the humerus by the supraspinatus and deltoid must be counterbalanced by the weight of the arm and the oblique, somewhat downward, pull of the subscapularis and teres minor. If these forces are not balanced, the humerus will not be stabilized in the glenoid fossa. These force couples explain why rotator cuff tears seriously impair the initial 20–30° of humeral abduction, when the supraspinatus tendon is active but the deltoid has yet to become fully active.

When the arm is hanging loosely at the side, the slope of the glenoid fossa, the horizontal pull of the supraspinatus, and the tightening of the superior aspect of the joint capsule prevent downward subluxation of the humerus even without the aid of the deltoid. The plane of the glenoid fossa and the weight of the individual's arm (plus added weight) determine the necessary force of the supraspinatus and joint capsule to prevent inferior subluxation of the humeral head.

Signs and Symptoms. On examination, the patient's arm is held to the side and cannot be abducted and externally rotated actively without pain; however, a nearly full range of passive movement can be obtained with care. The arc of pain is generally located between 45° and 90° as the tuberosity of the humerus passes under the acromion process. Pain may also be noticed during adduction from 120° to 170° with subacromial crepitus, varying amounts of weakness, and recurrent "bursitis" episodes. When the patient is asked to raise his arm, the shoulder hunches in support, a short motion may be made, but the arm quickly collapses to the side in pain. While passive motions of the shoulder are unrestricted, pain may be felt when the humeral head presses under the acromial arch. When the shoulder is extended, the front and back of the humerus will be tender but not as acute as at the greater tubercle. Extreme tenderness is found where the cuff inserts into the tuberosities. A superior subluxation of the humerus is often associated. Pain is increased when active internal rotation is resisted.

Arm Drop Test. The patient's arm is held horizontally at 90° abduction, and then he is asked to hold that position without assistance. If this cannot be done actively for a few moments without pain, it is a positive indication of a torn rotator cuff. In lesser tears, the patient may be able to hold the abduction (a slight tap on the forearm will make it drop) and slowly lower it to his side, but the motion will not be smooth.[104]

Subacute Cases. Tenderness will be found over the lesser tuberosity. An important sign in 1–2 weeks after injury is an area of thinning or depression at the fossae of the supraspinatus and infraspinatus (especially) muscles. If this is the site of rupture, a "catch" and clicking sound may be felt and heard at the site during passive movements if swelling is minimal.

Stages. Three stages of trauma are commonly recognized and can often be related to age. (1) Edema and hemorrhage resulting from overuse are characteristically seen in the young before 25 years, but may be seen at any age. (2) With repeated episodes, the subacromial bursa becomes fibrotic and thickened. The patient is usually 25–40 years old. (3) This stage is characterized by wearing of bone and rupture of the tendon in individuals over 40 years, associated with anterior acromial erosion and spurs. However, as Nelson points out, these stages fail to recognize the effect of a reflex-produced ischemia so often seen in practice.

Supraspinatus Ruptures.[105] A supraspinatus tear is characterized by a dull ache on rest which is aggravated by initial abduction. It is usually sited in the rotator cuff or common tendinous insertion rather than within the tendon itself. Complete ruptures are rare in comparison to partial tears. The tendon of the supraspinatus may be the site of paratendinitis or ectopic calcification.

The degree of injury is determined by the degree of pain or weakness on passive motion or active motion against resistance. Differentiation must be made from bicipital tenosynovitis by a positive Yergason's sign and severe pain on palpation. Roentgenographs are usually negative; but in chronic cases, the anterior edge of the acromion may show spur formation or a displaced fracture of the tuberosity.

Ischemic Sites

A hypovascular area has been identified in the area of the supraspinatus tendon. This is referred to as the "critical zone," and it occurs between the anastomosis of the vascular supply from the humeral tuberosity and the longitudinally directed vessels arriving from the muscle's belly. Tullos and Bennett[106] report that this relatively avascular area of the supraspinatus corresponds to the most common site of rotator cuff tendinitis, calcification, and spontaneous rupture.

Two other "critical zones" of hypovascular phenomena are found at the insertion of the infraspinatus tendon and at the intracapsular aspect of the biceps tendon. These areas of avascularity seem to expand with age, enhancing the potential for tendon rupture. Other factors can be added to this. For example, prolonged abduction such as seen in the common side-lying sleeping posture also produces compression or impingement under the acromion process or coracoacromial ligament. In the early stages, this leads to an inflammatory response and scar tissue development. Later, the avascularity leads to a breakdown of the tendon and encourages rotator cuff rupture in the middle-aged individual.[107]

Deltoid Strains[108, 109]

This powerful abductor is a frequent site of acute and chronic disability. Injury may be from intrinsic forces; eg, powerful contraction of the deltoid has been known to fracture its attachment from the clavicle or humerus. Anterior, middle, or posterior deltoid strain can be associated with acute subdeltoid bursitis, but the clinical picture is quite different.

Anterior Deltoid Strain. This strain is often seen following a posteriorly directed force on a horizontally extended arm. Symptoms arise slowly, often peaking 6–8 hours after injury. Pain and weakness increase on forward abduction. Evidence of swelling and tenderness appear in the anterior third of the muscle.

Middle Deltoid Strain. This strain follows forceful abduction against resistance in the lateral plane. Symptoms arise slowly. Pain and weakness increase on lateral abduction. Evidence of swelling and tenderness appear in the middle third of the muscle.

Posterior Deltoid Strain. This strain is the result of a posteriorly directed strain. Symptoms arise slowly. Pain and weakness increase on posterior abduction. Evidence of swelling and tenderness appear in the posterior third of the muscle.

Brachialis Strain[110]

In sprain of the proximal radioulnar joint, there is often a related injury to the brachialis anticus muscle with contracture, or, especially in children, a strip of periosteum may be torn from the anterior aspect of the humerus, followed by callus formation and blocked joint motion. The athlete or manual laborer may present a highly developed muscle belly on the anterolateral aspect of the upper arm which is easily found between the deltoid and the lateral head of the triceps.

Subluxations of the Shoulder[111–115]

Most shoulder subluxations are not acute and exhibit little or no swelling, but they usually present chronic (often episodic) pain, movement stiffness or "blocks," and other signs of local tissue fibrosis and joint "gluing." Mild to moderate local muscle weakness and possible atrophy are characteristic. Postural distortions of the lower cervical and upper dorsal spine and musculoskeletal abnormalities of some aspect of the shoulder girdle are invariably related.

Shoulder subluxations may be primary conditions after injury, or they may occur weeks or months after reduction of a primary dislocation. Thus, in cases of chronic shoulder pain, the history should be probed for possible shoulder dislocation with spontaneous reduction.

During articular correction of a shoulder subluxation, dynamic thrusts should be reserved for nonacute, fixated situations. When subluxation accompanies an acute sprain, attempts at correction should be more in line with gentle traction pressures after the musculature has been relaxed. Obviously, the probability of fracture fragments, osteoporosis, abscess, etc, must be eliminated prior to any form of manipulation.

Orthopedic Subluxation of the Humeral Head

This acute condition is probably a dislocation that has partially reduced itself spontaneously. It usually occurs when the greater tuberosity has been displaced upward as a whole to lie between the humeral head and the glenoid. The capital part is rotated to a degree but has not completely escaped from its capsular envelope. The outer border of the shaft is impacted firmly into the cancellous tissue of the head of the humerus.

Superior Humerus Subluxation

Because of its bony arch, the humerus cannot dislocate much superiorly unless there is severe traction involved. However, several authorities believe that superior subluxation can often be demonstrated on bilateral roentgenography. Schultz feels that this is the most common shoulder subluxation seen.[116] This writer, however, believes the term to be a misnomer because the suprahumeral joint is not an articulation in the true sense of the word but is solely a structure that serves as a protective and supportive mechanism. Most likely what is referred to as a superior humeral subluxation is the result of contractures within the superior humeral area that prevent the greater tuberosity from gliding smoothly under the coracoacromial ligament during abduction. The result is chronic compression and irritation of the enclosed tissues. It should be kept in mind that the acromioclavicular meniscus progressively thins with age. It is quite thick in the young but may be completely gone by the 5th or 6th decade.

Anterior Humerus Subluxation

This is a frequent type of shoulder subluxation in which the mechanism of injury is similar to that of anterior humeral dislocation. There is difficulty in raising the arm overhead. Fullness will be noted on the upper anterior arm that will be tender on palpation. The deltoid will feel taut and stringy. A sensitive coracoid process will be found higher than the head of the humerus. Signs of acute or chronic sprain will be found depending upon the history. The infraspinatus, teres minor, and rhomboid major muscles should be checked for possible strain.

Posterior Humerus Subluxation

The physical signs of this infrequently seen disorder are usually negative, and bilateral roentgenography is required for confirmation. In a few cases, the posterior area may feel fuller than the unaffected side. An unusually prominent coracoid process may be felt, and a slight hollow may be felt above the humerus. Signs of taut tissues on the posterior aspect of the humeral head and lax tissues on the anterior aspect are often found. The integrity of the pectoralis major muscle should be evaluated.

Inferior Humerus Subluxation

A slight hollowness may be found at the joint space, indicating that the humeral head has dropped from its normal position. The deltoid will often feel firm and stringy, indicating a chronic disorder. The integrity of the supraspinatus, long head of the triceps, deltoid, coracobrachialis, and clavicular division of the pectoralis major should be evaluated. Signs are often vague and should be confirmed by bilateral roentgenography.

Internal Humerus Subluxation

This type of malposition is frequently associated with a fixation that restricts external rotation of the humerus. Rotator cuff tendinitis and inferior humerus subluxation may be associated.

External Humerus Subluxation

An external subluxation of the humerus is often related to restricted internal rotation of the humerus. Supraspinous tendinitis, bicipital tendinitis, tendon displacement from the bicipital groove, and inferior humerus subluxation are common complications.

Fixations of the Humerus

It is common in most life-styles and occupations that the humerus is frequently used in flexion and abduction, but it is less frequently used in adduction and rarely used in backward extension. Likewise, internal rotation of the humerus is made much more frequently than is external rotation. Such lack of exercise can readily lead to uncomfortable or painful motion restriction when unaccustomed movements are made with or without external loading. Mobilizing such points of restriction often relieves functional shoulder complaints as well as referred symptoms (Fig. 14.17).

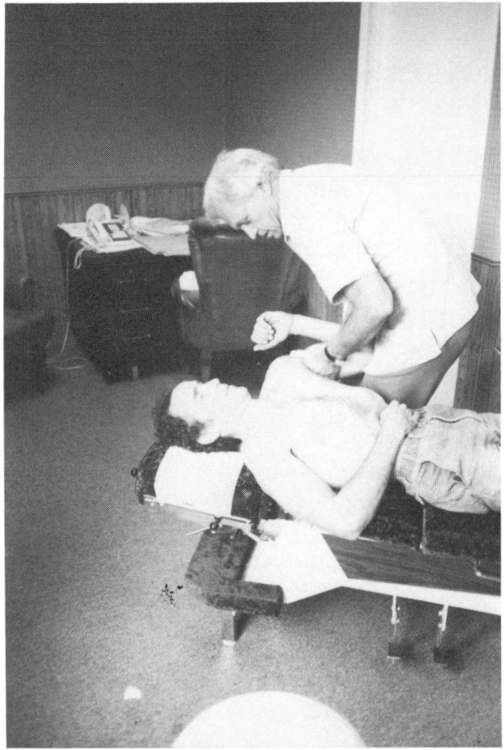

Figure 14.17. Position for testing the left shoulder for lateral joint play. (Courtesy of the Motion Palpation Institute.)

Dislocations of the Shoulder[117–125]

Most dislocations are anterior dislocations of the glemohumeral joint (85%), followed by acromioclavicular dislocations (10%), sternoclavicular dislocations (3%), and posterior dislocations (2%). True dislocations must be differentiated from pseudo-subluxations in which the humerus is displaced inferiorly by hemarthrosis. Poor muscle tone is usually related. The typical mechanism is an extension force against an abducted arm that is externally rotated.

The glenoid cavity covers only a small part of the head of the humerus. In extreme degrees of abduction, extension, and flexion, any force transmitted through the humeral shaft is applied obliquely to the body surface and directly on the capsule of the joint, through which the head of the bone is then forced. In fracture dislocations, the humeral fracture is invariably displaced with the articular surface outside the joint.

The primary stabilizers of the shoulder under passive loading are the abductors, the glenohumeral capsule, and ligament complex of the shoulder joint. The subscapularis and capsule provide the major dynamic stability anteriorly during external rotation. Once these tissues are torn, stretched, or weakened, less force is necessary for subsequent dislocations. If this is the case, surgical shortening of the subscapularis may be necessary.

Clinical Tests[60, 126, 127]

Apprehension Test. If chronic shoulder dislocation is suspected, slowly and gently abduct and externally rotate the patient's arm with the elbow flexed toward a point where the shoulder might easily dislocate. If shoulder dislocation exists, the patient will become quite apprehensive, symptoms may be reproduced, and the maneuver is resisted as further motion is attempted.

Dugas' Test. The patient places his hand on his opposite shoulder and attempts to touch his chest wall with his elbow and then raise his elbow to chin level. If it is impossible to touch the chest with the elbow or to raise the elbow to chin level, it is a positive sign of a dislocated shoulder (Fig. 14.18).

Calloway's Sign. The circumference of the proximal arm of a seated patient is measured at the shoulder tip when the patient's arm is laterally abducted. This measurement is compared to that of the noninvolved side. An increase in the circumference on the affected side suggests a dislocated shoulder.

Bryant's Sign. A post-traumatic ipsilateral lowering of the axillary folds (anterior and posterior pillars of the armpit), but level shoulders, is indicative of dislocation of the glenohumeral articulation.

Hamilton's Ruler Sign. Normally, a straight edge (eg, a yardstick) held against the lateral aspect of the arm cannot be placed simultaneously on the tip of the acromion process and the lateral epicondyle. If these two points do touch the straight edge, it signifies a dislocated shoulder.

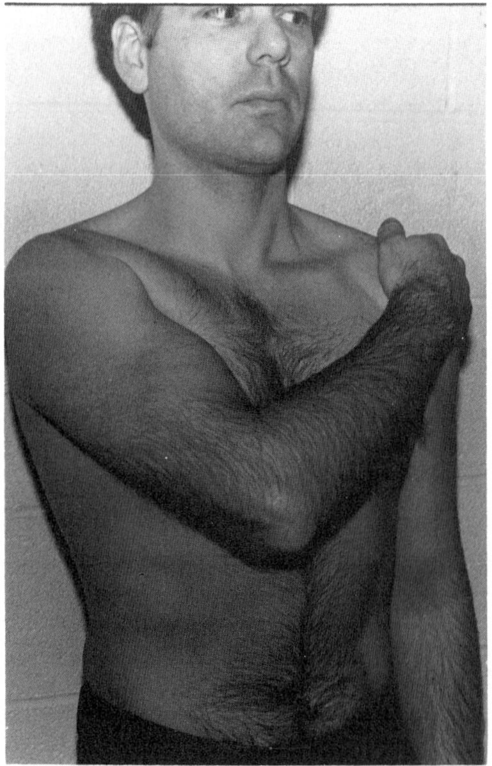

Figure 14.18. Dugas' test to evaluate the integrity of the right shoulder joint.

Varieties

Symptoms may be severe in primary dislocation, even if the soft tissues and capsule are not greatly damaged. Heroic reductions from misguided compassion should be avoided.

Four types of dislocations may be classified according to the direction in which the humeral head leaves the socket, and these can be subclassed according to the point at which the head of the humerus comes to rest or according to limb position; anterior, inferior, posterior, or superior displacement.

Anterior Dislocations.[128] Subcoracoid (common), intracoracoid, and subclavicular types may be found. The typical mechanism involves a combination of abduction, extension, and external rotation of the shoulder. The common means are: (1) a fall on the outstretched arm in which the trauma drives the humeral head forward against the anterior capsule; (2) abduction with the humerus in internal rotation or forward flexion when the humerus in external rotation becomes limited by the acromial arch; if forceful elevation is applied when this point of impingement is reached, the arch is used as a fulcrum to dislocate the proximal head anterior and inferior; (3) a fall or blow to the lateral shoulder from the rear.

In *subcoracoid luxation,* the head of the humerus lies under the coracoid process—either in contact with it or at a finger's breadth distance at most below it. The humeral head may be displaced inward until three-fourths of its diameter lies to the medial side of the process or be simply balanced on the anterior edge of the glenoid fossa. The humeral axis passes to the medial side of the fossa. The elbow hangs away from the side, the lateral deltoid bulge is flat, the acromion is prominent, and the glenoid cavity is empty. Palpation reveals the absence of the usual bony resistance below the lateral aspect of the acromion and the presence of abnormal resistance below the coracoid process or in the axilla. Active movement is lost, and passive abduction is strongly resisted by the patient. Dugas' test is positive. The arm can be passively adducted but not to the degree that the elbow can touch the chest with the fingers resting on the opposite shoulder. Measurement in abduction shows shortening.

In *intracoracoid dislocations*, the humeral head is displaced further medially. The symptoms and signs are those of the subcoracoid type except that the head of the humerus is felt further displaced and the shoulder is more flattened. The arm may be fixed in horizontal abduction. Severe capsule laceration is usually involved, which allows for the greater displacement.

Complications of Anterior Dislocations. When the humerus dislocates anteriorly, its posterolateral margin is often forced against the rim of the glenoid to produce a compression fracture (Hill-Sachs deformity). The malpositioned humerus frequently tears the cartilaginous labrum and capsule from the glenoid rim (Bankhart's lesion) with an avulsed fragment of bone. If the anatomical neck has fractured, the humeral head will not participate in passive movement of the shaft. Crepitus can usually be felt. Fracture of the greater tuberosity, tears of the rotator cuff, and recurrent dislocation are common complications. Anterior fracture dislocations are usually related with displacement of the greater tuberosity, but the capsule is not displaced. Any anterior luxation can do great harm to the brachial artery, vein, or nerves. Circulation must always be checked before reduction is attempted.

Inferior Dislocations. Subglenoid and luxatio erecta types are infrequently seen in which the humeral head lies below the glenoid fossa. The common cause is forcible abduction followed by rotation or impulsion. The mechanism of injury is usually a leverage force on an abducted arm such as in an arm tackle. There is severe pain and disability. The arm is fixed at about 45° in abduction. A hollowness will be found at the joint space, with the humeral head inferior to its normal position and often palpable within the axilla. The deltoid is flattened and extremely spastic. In *subglenoid luxation*, the symptoms are those of subcoracoid flattening, but abduction and flattening of the shoulder are more marked. The upper part of the greater tuberosity is usually torn. In the rare instances of *luxatio erecta*, forcible elevation of the arm causes the head of the humerus to be displaced far downward so that the arm becomes locked in a vertically erect position.

Posterior Dislocations. This is often a diagnostic challenge in the young, well-muscled individual because all joint motions may be unrestricted, yet disability is acute. Two types are seen which differ only in the extent of displacement; ie, subacromial and subspinous types. The cause is direct lateral and posterior pressure, or pressure exerted in the same direction along a flexed, adducted, and internally rotated humerus. It is sometimes produced during a convulsive attack. The patient's arm is abducted and rotated internally, and the elbow is directed slightly forward. The shoulder is flat in front and full behind, where the head of the humerus may be felt. The coracoid is prominent. The head of the humerus lies on the outer edge of the glenoid fossa or further to the posterior under the scapular spine or on the infraspinatus. These features are not as obvious as those of anterior dislocation. Passive abduction and external rotation motions are restricted. In severe cases, the lateral side of the capsule is usually torn. There may be an associated cuff tear or an avulsion fracture of the greater tuberosity resulting in persistent pain. The internal and external scapular muscles are usually lacerated or contain fragments of the torn tuberosities.

Superior Dislocations. A supraglenoid luxation is very rare except in rough sports or accidents with unusual force mechanisms. A routine anteroposterior (A-P) x-ray view may show narrowing of the space between the head of the humerus and the acromion, indicating a tear. Referral for arthrography may be necessary. Care should be taken not to confuse the growth plate of the proximal humerus with that of a fracture line.

Roentgenographic Considerations

Careful evaluation of the glenohumeral articulation is necessary to judge alignment congruity. In approximately 20% of cases of shoulder dislocation, fractures of the glenoid are associated. Lesser tuberosity fractures are often related to a posterior dislocation of the shoulder. Vigorous contractions of the triceps muscle, as seen in throwing excesses, may produce avulsion injuries to the inferior aspect of the glenoid.

Fractures of the Humerus[129–131]

Fractures of the proximal humerus are not common. They are usually seen in mature women with a degree of osteoporosis. The mechanism is often a fall on the outstretched pronated upper extremity. About 85% of these fractures are of the simple type, usually involving the surgical neck and greater tuberosity of the humerus. A scapula fracture may be associated. In most cases, early mobilization, without compromising long-term effects, is beneficial.

Roentgenographic Considerations

Fragments are usually displaced less than 1 cm, are angulated less than 45°, and are held in place by an intact rotator cuff and periosteum. Displacement of the greater tuberosity of more than 1 cm indicates a torn rotator cuff. Fractures through the surgical neck, frequently associated with brachial plexus injuries, are usually displaced anteriorly and medially due to the pull of the pectoralis major. Fractures through the head or anatomical neck of the humerus are rare. When present, they have a high incidence of avascular necrosis. In the area of the subacromial or subdeltoid bursae, calcification may simulate a fracture of the greater tuberosity. A calcification shadow appears more dense and irregular than that of bone and is not trabeculated.

As with the elbow joint, the epiphyseal lines in the shoulder make interpretation difficult unless contralateral views are taken. The epiphysis for the lateral end of the acromion process does not unite until about 20 years of age. In the young, the upper humeral epiphysis may be damaged from excessive throwing ("Little League shoulder").

Injuries of the Scapular Area

Chronic shoulder girdle pain and discomfort are often seen in people who work overhead with repetitive motions for long durations with little postural change. Trigger points will inevitably be found along the vertebral borders of one or both scapulae. Most authorities feel that the cause can usually be traced to muscular overuse leading to lower cervical or upper thoracic subluxations. Subluxations may be found in the shoulder girdle itself, especially when the scapulae are chronically affected. Acute or chronic fibrositis of the trapezius and rhomboids with trigger points is often superimposed or inconsequential.

Acute Trapezius Strains[132]

Most trapezius injuries will be seen at the proximal portion, rarely distal to the scapular spine. That aspect between the occiput and the shoulder is the only significant muscle that can resist forceful shoulder depression.

Fibrositis[51, 133, 134]

Fibrositis is a generalized term which refers to a syndrome featuring spasm, stiffness through the range of motion without limitation, a dull gnawing ache at rest which is aggravated by exercise, localized tenderness, possible soft-tissue crepitus, and one or more palpable trigger points. Strains and associated fibrositis are often seen in the musculature attachments to the vertebral border of the scapula from throwing heavy objects. The initial trauma may not be remembered.

The disorder is most often seen in the rhomboids and trapezius (Fig. 14.19). However, the levator scapulae, scalene group, or erector spinae are often involved. Fibrofatty nodules herniate through the superficial fascia of the involved muscles. Palpation and movements may cause pain to radiate up the posterior neck and/or over the shoulder and sometimes down the arm. Cervical motions cause a vague soreness in the affected tissues. This is usually worse in the morning after arising and during cold, damp weather.

Scapular Fixations[135–137]

Restricted movements are commonly found in the scapular area. They affect both performance and posture. Their usual causes are (1) the consequence of injury, (2) trigger point spasm, or (3) viscerosomatic reflexes. The local source of the difficulty may be local, at the spine, or at the shoulder. The common sites to search are a costovertebral or upper dorsal subluxation, or contraction of any muscle that has a scapular attachment such as the rhomboids, trape-

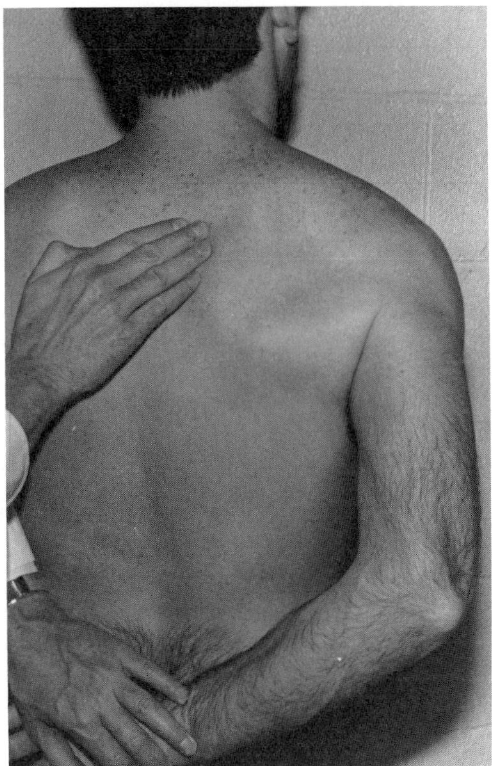

Figure 14.19. Palpating the right rhomboid area. Note position of patient's right forearm.

zius, levator scapulae, supraspinatus, infraspinatus, and/or teres major and minor muscles.

Management. Scapular joint play should be found in all directions: superiorly, laterally, inferiorly, medially, and slightly clockwise and counterclockwise. If not, corrective manipulation is usually necessary. The adjustive procedure is conducted with the patient prone. Pressure is made with the base of the contact hand, the stabilizing hand is positioned on the wrist of the contact hand as in a toggle recoil, and the direction of trust is into the fixation (restriction) on an almost horizontal plane so that the underlying thoracic cage is not greatly disturbed. To inhibit recurrence, therapeutic exercises should be prescribed that will stretch the shoulder in flexion, extension, adduction, and horizontal abduction.

Scapular Fractures[138, 139]

Scapular fractures are not frequently seen, but in severe trauma, fractures of the scapular body and spine can occur. Strong muscular attachments usually prevent significant displacement. All that is usually required in therapy is rest in a sling until acute pain subsides, then early mobilization. Infrequently, the brachial plexus or axillary nerve may be injured. Fractures of the scapular neck (uncommon) are usually impacted and present little displacement. Acromion fractures are the result of a downward blow on the shoulder, often leading to avulsion of the brachial plexus roots. Fractures of the coracoid process, easily confused with an ununited epiphysis, are uncommon. When they occur, they are usually associated with acromioclavicular separations.

Injuries of the Clavicle[140, 141]

At the acromioclavicular and sternoclavicular joints, a wide range of injury and displacement may occur. The tip of the shoulder, near the lateral aspect of the clavicle, is a common site of extremely painful and tender contusions to the trapezius. Localized swelling is easily seen and palpable. The patient will depress the entire shoulder girdle in an attempt at relief. Care must be taken not to confuse this contusion with acromioclavicular separation.

Acromioclavicular Sprain[142–145]

The acromioclavicular joint is relatively weak and inflexible, yet must bear constant stress in contact sports. Those who expose the joint to excessive and repeated trauma risk contusion, sprain, and separation. Posttraumatic arthritis is a typical consequence. Any force which tends to spring the clavicle from its attachments to the scapula is bound to cause severe sprain to the acromioclavicular, coronoid, and trapezoid ligaments unless the clavicle fractures beforehand. Keep in mind that the acromioclavicular ligament can be considered a part of the acromioclavicular joint capsule, thus severe sprain must involve a degree of capsule tear.

Major sprain consists of a degree of severe stretching and tearing of the tough coracoclavicular ligaments. The doctor should carefully palpate for evidence of conoid or trapezoid sprain. Acute tenderness and possible swelling will be found in the area of the coracoclavicular ligament below the clavicle. There is distinct abnormal mobility of the clavicle relative to the acromion process. After a week or more, a subcutaneous discoloration may appear. An aftermath of an old injury may be exhibited by laxity of the acromioclavicular joint without localized tenderness.

Acromioclavicular Separation[146–148]

The acromioclavicular joint serves as a roof for the head of the humerus. It is one of the weakest joints of the body but is assisted by the strong coracoclavicular ligament. The ends of the joint are bound loosely so the scapula can raise the glenoid fossa. During shoulder injury, the scapula often rotates around the coracoid, which acts as a fulcrum. The intrinsically weak superior and inferior acromioclavicular ligaments give way and the joint dislocates. In other instances, a downward force of great intensity lowers the clavicle onto the 1st rib which acts as a fulcrum, tearing the acromioclavicular and coracoacromial ligaments, resulting in complete acromioclavicular separation. Continued force can fracture the clavicle. Incomplete luxation can tear the intra-articular meniscus and lead to degenerative arthritis of the joint.

Initial Evaluation. Sternoclavicular sprains vary from minor to complete dislocation, either posterior (retrosternal) or anteroinferior to overlap the 1st rib. In any acute separation, the most significant sign is that of demonstrable and significant false motion of the acromioclavicular joint from joint laxity. If examination of the seated patient can be made before swelling develops, good evaluation can be made by pivoting the joint after the scapula has been stabilized by the nonpalpating hand. The swollen joint may give a false impression of a tender but stable joint.

Schultz's Test.[149] Standing behind the sitting patient, the examiner faces the affected side. One hand of the examiner is placed under the patient's flexed elbow and pushes up while the other hand placed over the acromioclavicular joint applies firm pressure. The more "give" that is felt in the joint, the greater the separation.

Chronic Cases. Signs of posttraumatic arthritis may appear, such as pain over the shoulder region with little or no radiation to the arm, tenderness over the acromioclavicular joint, and pain-free movement until the scapula begins to move. Shrugging the shoulders usually elicits pain.

The Costoclavicular Syndrome

This syndrome is due to the neurovascular bundle being compressed between the 1st rib and the clavicle at the point where the brachial plexus joins the subclavian artery and courses over the 1st rib. Symptoms are similar to those of the scalenus anticus syndrome and reproduced by the costoclavicular maneuver.

Sternoclavicular Disc Injury

In some injuries to this joint that are just below the severity of a dislocation, the articular disc may be pulled from its sternal attachment in a manner similar to a semilunar tear of the knee. The patient will complain of localized pain on movement. A "catch" may be felt by the patient, especially during ipsilateral shoulder flexion and circumduction. As in the knee if the cartilage is fragmented, referral for surgery may be required if conservative measures fail.

Subluxations of the Clavicle[150–152]

During correction of a subluxation, even mild dynamic thrusts should be reserved for nonacute, fixated situations. When subluxation accompanies an acute sprain, correction should be more in line with gentle traction pressures after the musculature has been relaxed. Obviously, the probability of fracture fragments, infection, osteoporosis, etc, must be eliminated prior to any form of manipulation.

Anterior Medial Clavicular Subluxation

The typical mechanism of force is one of a posterolateral impact which drives the shoulder anterior and medial. If sternoclavicular subluxation does not occur in the young, a green-stick midshaft fracture often results. Acute disability ensues, and sometimes false joint motion can be palpated. Pain is acute and aggravated by joint motion. There is severe tenderness at the sternoclavicular joint. Secondary capsule injury may be expressed by intracapsular swelling, edema, and generalized tenderness. Exhibited crepitus suggests attending fracture fragments or articular comminution, thus making adjusting procedures contraindicated.

Evaluate the integrity of the pectoralis major and subclavius muscles. In older cases, a degree of fixation will inevitably be present. This is easily determined by placing two finger pads upon the sternoclavicular joint and widely circumducting the patient's abducted arm.

Clavicular Fixations

Gillet[153] feels that clavicular fixations, especially at the sternal joint, are frequently related to readily palpable fixated ligamentous and muscular tissues in the C7–T1 area that extend laterally from the spine. Immobility at either the medial or lateral joint of the clavicle can be easily determined by placing a thumb firmly upon the joint and moving the patient's shoulder back and forth in an A-P direction. Then the patient's ipsilateral elbow is cupped with the examiner's stabilizing hand, and the shoulder is moved in a superior-inferior direction.

Dislocations of the Clavicle[154, 155]

Clavicular dislocations are common but not as frequently seen as clavicular fractures. Analysis of complications should be made by roentgenography prior to considered reduction.

Acromioclavicular Dislocation

In injuries of the lateral clavicle, the clavicle is usually elevated, which increases the distance between the clavicle and the coracoid process. Thus, a distinct palpable and visible "step" will be noted in the supraspinatus region. If the prominent lateral clavicle is depressed, it will spring back to its elevated position once pressure is released. The scapula falls away from the clavicle, and the acromion lies below and anterior to the clavicle. Fracture of the coracoid process is often associated.

Dalinka[156] states that in roentgenography, an increase of the coracoclavicular distance by 5 mm or greater than 50% of the contralateral side indicates a true acromioclavicular dislocation. Complete dislocation cannot occur unless the conoid and trapezoid ligaments are severely torn. The soft tissues within this area frequently ossify after injury. After chronic injury, signs of erosion or tapering may be observed, along with indications of soft-tissue calcification subsequent to an old hematoma.

Anterior Sternoclavicular Dislocation

The sternoclavicular joint is the least stable major joint of the body, although complete dislocations are rare. Shoulder girdle movement at the sternoclavicular joint is slight but essential. At the medial end of the clavicle, displacement may occur either anterior, as is more common, or posterior in relation to the sternum. The latter is often associated with dyspnea and cervical edema from vasculature compression. When dislocations occur and are reduced, a deformity often persists. The displacement of the clavicle in anterior dislocation is typically anterior, superior, and medial.

Posterior Sternoclavicular Dislocation

These luxations are often hidden by soft-tissue swelling. In chronic cases, a distinct depression is palpable. Acute posterior dislocations can be a medical emergency requiring the attention of a thoracic surgeon. Pure dislocations should be reduced by a specialist because of possible weakening of the vital tissues behind the sternum.

Fractures of the Clavicle[157–159]

Fractured ends sometimes can be felt under the skin. The involved shoulder may be lower than the other, and the patient is unable to raise the involved arm above the shoulder. Characteristically, the patient will support the elbow of the involved side with the contralateral palm.

The most common site of clavicular fracture is near the midpoint, but both ends also deserve careful evaluation. In midshaft fracture, there is sometimes inferior, anterior, and medial displacement of the lateral section. Fractures of the inner third are uncommon and often represent an epiphyseal injury because the medial clavicular epiphysis does not close until about the age of 25 years. Most fractures (66%) of the outer third of the clavicle present intact ligaments with no significant displacement. About 30% of outer-third fractures present detached ligaments medially and attached ligaments distally, with displacement inferior and medial on the trapezius muscle. Early active shoulder movements should be encouraged.

If this injury is due to a fall on an outstretched hand, the impact is transferred from the palm to the carpals, to the radius and ulnar, to the elbow and humerus, to the scapula and clavicle, and to the spine and thoracic cage (Fig. 14.20). Thus, all structures involved in the line of impact deserve careful evaluation, not just the immediate area of obvious fracture.

THE ELBOW AND FOREARM[160, 161]

The proximal ulna forms the most important articulation in the elbow, while the distal radius forms the most important articulation in the wrist.

Basic Functional Anatomy[162–166]

The arm and forearm are joined by a trochoginglymus joint—a hinge and a pivot. The semilunar notch of the ulna is hinged with the hyperboloid trochlea of the humerus. The proximal head of the radius pivots with the spherical capitulum of the humerus and also glides against both the proximal and distal ends of the ulna. Because the distal humerus curves slightly forward, its articulating surface faces somewhat posteriorly. This places the forearm in slight flexion in its resting position, which increases the mechanical advantage of the flexor muscles.

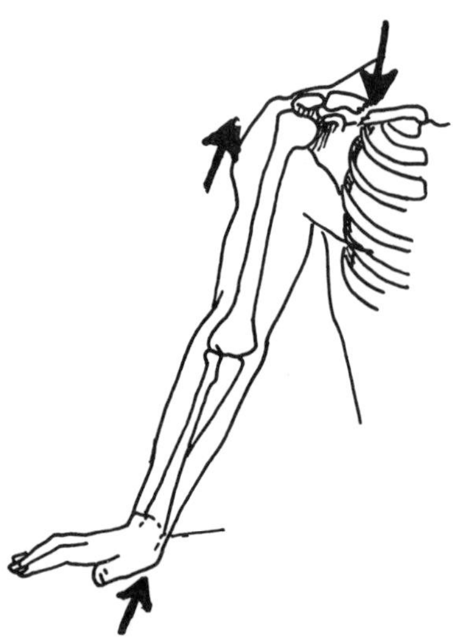

Figure 14.20. Typical mechanism of shoulder injury and lateral clavicle fracture.

The distal aspect of the humerus presents an articular surface that is cylindrical and smooth except for about 35° of its circumference. The distal end of the humerus can be viewed as two columns, larger medial one (trochlea) that articulates with the semilunar notch of the ulna and a smaller lateral one that articulates with the head of the radius. The pulley-like trochlea apparatus has (1) a depression at the front that lodges the coronoid process of the ulna and (2) a depression at the rear that holds the olecranon process of the ulna when the elbow is extended. The olecranon process restricts hypertension of the elbow and protects the ulnohumeral articulation posteriorly. The concave head of the radius glides against the spherical capitulum of the humerus. The capitulum and trochlea are separated by a bony crest that fits into the opening between the proximal ulna and the radius and serves as a fixed rudder to guide elbow motion. The elbow flexors originate from the medial epicondyle, and the extensors originate from the lateral epicondyle.

Elbow and Radioulnar Movements[167–172]

The basic range of elbow joint motion involves elbow flexion (135°) and extension (0°), and forearm supination (90°) and pronation (90°). The patient may be examined in either the standing or sitting position. If a blockage is obtained in active motion, passive motion should be checked and the type of block and degree of restriction noted.

During extension, the elbow functions as a first-class lever. The mechanical advantage is poor because of the short lever arm between the insertion of the triceps and the center of the joint. During flexion, the elbow functions as a third-class lever. Force from the biceps and brachialis act between the fulcrum and weight of the forearm.

Elbow Motion[173–176]

Flexion and Extension. The excursion of the head of the radius over the capitulum in full flexion is about 140°. Active flexion is judged by having the patient touch an ipsilateral shoulder with the supinated hand, and extension is checked by the patient straightening the elbow as far as possible. Some females normally reach 5° of hyperextension. The easiest testing maneuvers is to have the patient flex and extend both elbows at the same time in one continuous movement. Flexion is limited normally by the biceps muscle mass, and extension is limited when the olecranon touches the olecranon fossa.

Pronation and Supination. During forearm pronation, the ulna remains fixed and the radius crosses over it. In supination, the bones merely uncross. Active pronation and supination is checked with the patient's elbow 90° in flexion and firmed against the waist. The patient is then instructed to turn the closed fist first downward so that the palmar surface is parallel with the floor (pronation) and then upward so that the dorsal surface is parallel with the floor (supination). Restriction in pronation suggests pathology at the elbow, radioulnar articulation at the wrist, or within the forearm; restriction in supination is associated with a disorder of the elbow or radioulnar articulation of the wrist.

Kinesiology of the Elbow[177–179]

Flexion. Elbow flexion is controlled by the brachialis (C5-C6) and biceps brachii (C5-C6) with assistance offered by the brachioradialis (C5-C6) and supinator (C6). (See Tables 14.4 and 14.5.) Strength is tested with the examiner in front of the patient. The stabilizing hand is cupped under the patient's elbow, which is flexed 90°, and the active hand grips the patient's wrist. Increasing resistance is added as the patient attempts to flex the elbow.

Extension. Extension of the elbow is provided by the triceps (C7-C8) with help from the anconeus (C7-C8). The examiner's stabilizing and active hands are in the same position, and increasing resistance is offered as the patient attempts elbow extension.

Supination. Forearm supination is conducted by the biceps (C5-C6) and supinator (C6), which are aided by the brachioradialis (C5-C6). The examiner's stabilizing hand remains cupped under the elbow, and the active hand grips the patient's pronated wrist. Increasing resistance is applied as the patient attempts to turn the forearm from pronation to supination.

Pronation. Pronation of the forearm is provided by the pronator teres (C6-C7) and pronator quadratus (C8-T1), with assistance from the flexor carpi radialis (C7-C8). The examiner's stabilizing hand remains in place as above, and the active hand grips the patient's supinated wrist. Increasing resistance is applied as the patient attempts to turn the forearm from supination to pronation.

Goniometry of the Elbow[180, 181]

Restricted Flexion or Extension Motion of the Elbow. The supine patient is placed in the neutral position, the goniometer is centered next to the elbow, and the neutral reading is recorded with the goniometer arm along the axis of the patient's forearm. Any extension loss is noted, and the deviation from the neutral is recorded. Then the pa-

Table 14.4.
Elbow and Forearm Motion

Joint motion	Prime movers	Accessories
Elbow		
Flexion	Biceps brachii Brachialis Brachioradialis	Flexor carpi radialis Flexor digitorum superficialis Pronator teres Extensor carpi radialis longus Palmaris longus
Extension	Triceps	Anconeus
Forearm		
Supination	Supinator Biceps brachii	
Pronation	Pronator teres Pronator quadratus	

Table 14.5.
Major Muscles of the Forearm

Muscle	Major function	Spinal segment
Anconeus	Extension	C7–C8
Biceps brachii	Flexion,supination	C5–C6
Brachialis	Flexion	C5–C6
Brachioradialis	Flexion, supination	C5–C6
Extensor carpi radialis	Extension	C6–C7
Extensor carpi ulnaris	Extension	C7
Flexor carpi radialis	Flexion	C7–C8
Flexor carpi ulnaris	Flexion	C8–T1
Palmaris longus	Flexion	C7–C8
Pronator quadratus	Pronation	C8–T1
Pronator teres	Pronation, flexion	C6–C7
Supinator	Supination, flexion	C6
Triceps	Extension (long head)	C7–C8

Spinal innervation varies somewhat in different people. The spinal nerves listed here are averages and may differ in a particular patient; thus, an allowance of a segment above and below those listed in most text tables should be considered.

tient flexes his arm, and the end of the motion is recorded.

Restricted Rotation Motion of the Elbow. The patient is placed in the neutral supine position. The goniometer is not used to evaluate rotation. The patient supinates and pronates his forearm; then each estimated arc is recorded at the end of the motions.

Trigger Points[182]

The most common trigger points in the forearm are those of the supinator, the extensor carpi radialis, and the extensor of the middle finger. These are shown in Figure 14.21.

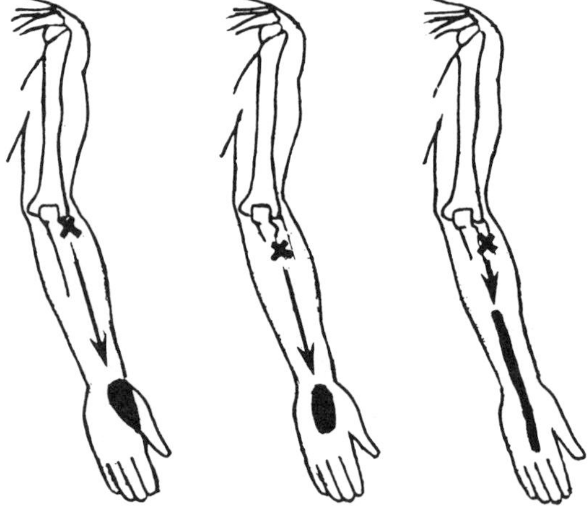

Figure 14.21. Posterior aspect of upper extremity trigger points; *X*, common sites. *Blackened areas* indicate typical areas of referred pain. *Left*, supinators; *center*, extensor carpi radialis; *right*, middle finger extensor.

SELECTED CLINICAL PROBLEMS OF THE ELBOW AND FOREARM[183–187]

Most forearm injuries are the result of direct blows or falls. Commonly seen are avulsion-type injuries of the elbow as a result of acute or chronic strain at a site of tendon or ligament attachment (Fig. 14.22).

Roentgenographic Considerations[188]

As a consequence of avulsion injury, bone fragments may be seen in the area of the epicondyles or olecranon process, and epicondyle spurs may point to chronic stress.

The Soft Tissues

Displacement of fat pads is often found at the elbow after injury. It can occur in any injury that distends the joint capsule. A pad appears as a thin strip of radiolucent fat density. The anterior fat pad is normally seen on lateral views, but the posterior humeral pad is hidden by the epicondyles' posterior extensions. However, as Bowerman[189] points out, the posterior pad will become visible at the posterior edge of the humerus on lateral views if effusion causes displacement of the pad. The most important complication is ischemia of the forearm, which may cause an irreversible contracture deformity.

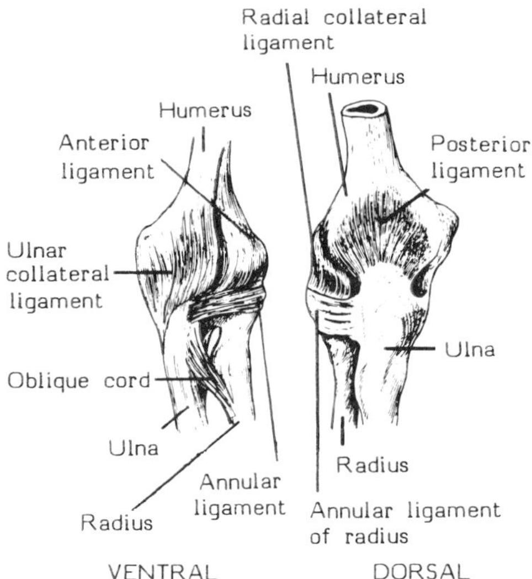

Figure 14.22. Major ligaments of the elbow joint.

Growth Centers

Normal ossification of distal humeral epiphyses is not an even process, especially during the periods of rapid growth and development; thus knowledge of secondary ossification centers of the elbow is necessary in dealing with children or teenagers. One or more bony centers may remain uneven in density and irregular on the margins, especially the trochlea and olecranon epiphyses. Because of this irregularity, careful differentiation must be made from osteochondrosis and epiphysitis. The trochlear center is irregularly mineralized and always develops from several small foci. The lateral epicondyle does not fuse directly with the humerus as the medial epicondyle does; rather, it fuses first with the neighboring epiphyseal ossification center, the capitelum, then the fused mass joins the end of the shaft of the humerus. After injury, the position of various centers must be evaluated for possible displacement and incarceration into the joint.

Elbow Strains[190]

There may be an injury to the upper radioulnar articulation by sudden overpronation or oversupination followed by pain over the articulation with limitation of rotation (Fig. 14.23). Trigger points are commonly found just below the horizontal midline of the antecubital fossa over the proximal radius and ulna. When the joint proper is involved, motion is limited chiefly in extension and may persist indefinitely. An associated injury to the brachialis anticus muscle with contracture is common. In children, a strip of periosteum may be torn from the anterior humerus, followed by bone formation and blocked joint motion. Local myositis ossificans may also develop in the tendon of the brachialis anticus. Some cases will be complicated by ulnar neurapraxia.

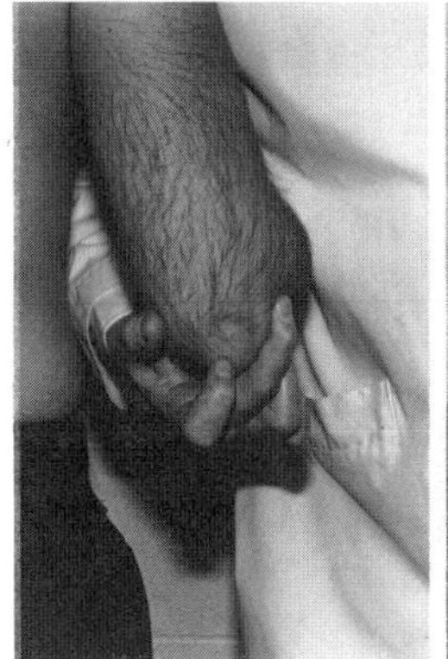
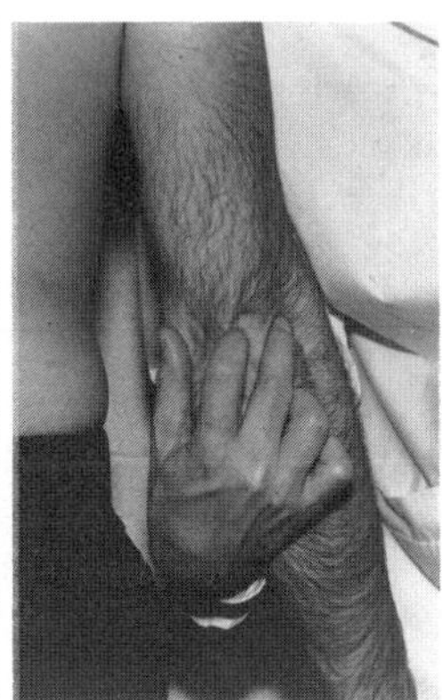

Figure 14.23. During elbow palpation, general bony relationships of the elbow are checked by placing the thumb on the medial epicondyle, index finger on the olecranon, and middle finger on the lateral epicondyle. When the patient's elbow is fully extended, the tips of all three fingers should be level. During 90° flexion, the tips of the three fingers form an inverted triangle. This will offer a general appraisal of alignment. *Left*, the olecranon and the medial and lateral epicondyles form a triangle when the elbow is flexed at a right angle. *Right*, when the elbow is extended, the points at the olecranon and epicondyles lie in a straight line.

Strains of the bicipital attachment to the ulna are not common. They occur in elbow hyperextension injuries. The course of the tendon will be tender on palpation. Management consists of rest in a sling for a few days along with standard sprain therapy.

Elbow Sprains[191, 192]

Articular or extra-articular injuries to the elbow without fracture are not uncommon and are peculiarly resistant to treatment. There may be a primary or secondary injury to the upper radioulnar articulation by sudden overpronation or oversupination, followed by pain over the articulation and limited rotation. Overlooking radial head dislocation is a common orthopedic error.

Forced joint movement beyond full extension, abduction, or adduction causes ruptures within the capsular apparatus and its reinforcing ligaments from their attachment to the humerus, radius, and ulna. The capsule is tender and frequently distended with blood. Movement in the direction of injury aggravates the pain, and there is some restriction at extreme ranges.

Trauma in Extension[193–195]

The proximal forearm, elbow joint, and distal humerus are frequently injured when the mechanism of trauma is a fall on the outstretched hand (Fig. 14.24). When the elbow is extended, the upper extremity acts as a mechanical brace that transmits force from the point of hand contact to the torso. The axial compression combined with a bending moment to sharply dorsiflex the wrist produces a force couple that compresses the wrist dorsally and stretches the ventral soft tissues. If a portion of this strut is weakened by age, for instance, and bone is weaker than the involved ligaments and tendons, this weakness will determine the type of injury. It is for this reason that falls on the outstretched hand usually involve the wrist of the elderly and the distal humerus of the young.

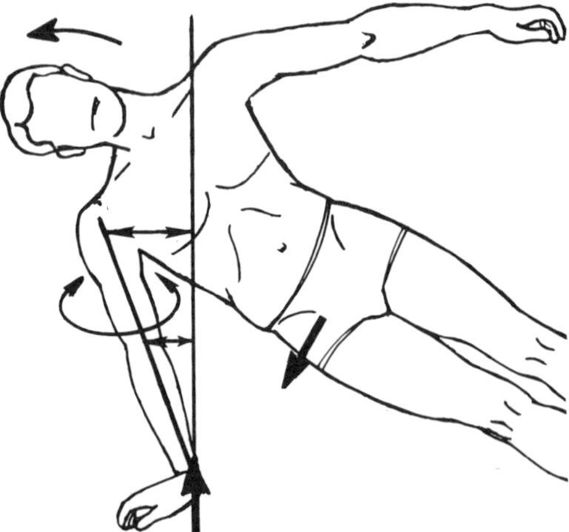

Figure 14.24. A heavy fall on the outstretched hand produces a bending moment to the wrist, elbow, and shoulder. Excessive flexion, extension, abduction, or adduction, with or without torque, may occur at any one of these joints, depending on the direction of the impact force from the ground. Excessive lateral flexion of the cervical region is usually associated.

When a fall is made on the outstretched hand, several mechanisms are effected: (1) axial compression forces throughout the limb; (2) bending moments at the wrist, elbow, and shoulder joints; (3) torsion about the long axis of the limb; and (4) violent lateral flexion of the cervical spine. The moment of axial loading (impact force × lever arm) must be resisted by the elbow tissues to prevent failure. If the elbow holds, the force not absorbed is transmitted to the shoulder.

Common Types of Elbow Sprain[196]

Hyperextension Sprain. Hyperextension sprains strongly mimic posterior dislocation of the elbow. Swelling and tenderness will be found at the joint capsule posteriorly, bicipital tendon, olecranon fossa, lateral and medial collateral ligaments, and attachments of the flexors at the medial condyle. Pain is relieved by flexion and increased on attempted extension. If the joint proper is involved, extension is chiefly limited, and it may persist for weeks or years.

Hyperabduction Sprain. Tenderness is found below the lateral epicondyle, indicating sprain of the ulnar collateral ligament. Pain is increased by forcing the elbow into valgus stress.

Hyperadduction Sprain. Tenderness is exhibited below the medial epicondyle, indicating sprain of the radial collateral ligament. Pain is increased by forcing the elbow into varus stress.

Ligamentous Stability Test[127,197]

To roughly judge the stability of the medial and lateral collateral ligaments of the elbow, the patient's wrist is held with one hand and the stabilizing hand is cupped under the patient's distal humerus. As the patient is directed to slightly flex his elbow, the examiner (1) pushes medially with his active hand and laterally with his stabilizing hand, then (2) pushes laterally with his active hand and medially with his stabilizing hand. With the fingers of the stabilizing hand, any joint gapping felt during either the valgus or varus stress maneuver should be noted (Fig. 14.25).

Other Elbow Stress Tests. Besides elbow abduction and adduction, stability and range of motion should also be tested in extension, flexion, pronation, and supination. These motions should be carefully attempted when the elbow joint is as relaxed as possible. Pain or motion restriction will be found if contractures, acute tendinitis, and/or acute joint pathology are present. If negative, the tests should be repeated against patient resistance. Pain or instability will then be found if sprain, acute or chronic tendinitis, and/or chronic joint pathology are present.

Tennis Elbow[198–200]

"Tennis elbow" is a painful condition of traumatic origins not limited to tennis that occurs about the external epicondyle of the humerus. The term incorporates a group of conditions, especially epicondylitis or radiohumeral bursitis. It is caused by repeated violent elbow extension combined with sharp twisting supination or pronation of the wrist against resistance. The result is severe contraction of the extensor-supinator muscles of the forearm.

The clinical picture is one of synovitis, subperiosteal hematoma, fibrositis, or partial rupture of the fibrous origin of muscles and ligaments at the affected epicondyle with some associated periostitis. Radial nerve entrapment may be involved. If the medial epicondyle is sore, the flexor-pronator muscles and medial ligaments are involved. The lateral epicondyle area is affected seven times more often than the medial epicondyle.

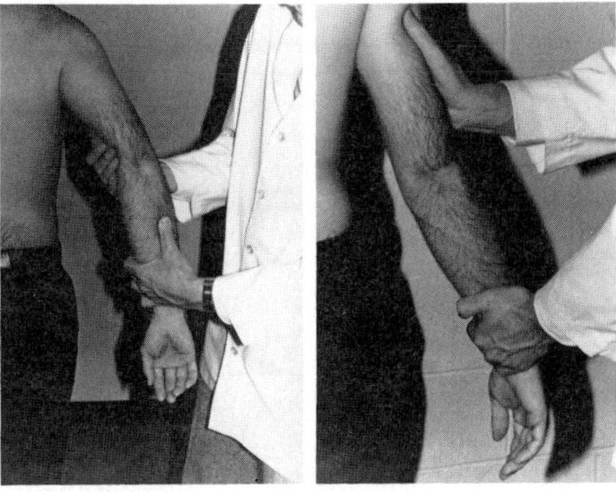

Figure 14.25. Maneuvers for testing for ligamentous stability of the elbow joint.

Roentgenographic Considerations[201]

The x-ray features in the elbow may include soft-tissue calcification at the margin of the lateral joint, lateral epicondyle and capitellum erosion and fragmentation, and spur development at the coronoid process of the ulna. A medial slope deformity of the lateral condyle of the humerus is frequently related. Strenuous unilateral use of the active upper extremity (eg, tennis) often leads to hypertrophy of muscle and bone in the forearm and hands in comparison to the nondominant side. Increased radial length and width is frequently found.

Typical Physical Signs

Hasemeir[202] describes the typical symptomatic picture as pain over the outer or inner side of the elbow, distal to the affected epicondyle. Pain may be severe and radiate when the patient extends his arm. The pain is usually sharp and lancinating on exertion, but it may be dull, aching, and constant. Squeezing an object with the fingertips is usually painful (writer's cramp). Tenderness, heat, and swelling are found over the affected epicondyle, and limited passive movement on extension may be found. This syndrome is the result of microscopic and macroscopic tears at the common origin of the extensor and flexor muscle groups, occurring as a consequence to overstress of tendon fibers. The supinator has its tendinous origin just behind the common extensor tendon. Grip strength as well as supination and pronation strength are affected.

Tests

The easiest and surest test is to have the patient put forward his relaxed limb (flexed about 30°) and attempt supination against resistance. Moderate fingerpressure resistance will produce pain at the lateral epicondyle.

Cozen's Test. With the patient's forearm stabilized, he makes a fist and extends his wrist. The patient's elbow is gripped with the examiner's stabilizing hand, and the top of the patient's fist is gripped with the active hand. The examiner attempts to force the patient's wrist into flexion against resistance (Fig. 14.26). A sign of tennis elbow is a severe sudden pain at the lateral epicondyle area.[203,204]

Mills' Test. The patient makes a fist; flexes the forearm, wrist, and fingers; pronates the forearm, and then attempts to extend the forearm against the examiner's resistance. This stretches the extensors and supinators attached to the lateral epicondyle. Pain at the elbow during this maneuver is an indication of radiohumeral epicondylitis.[205,206]

Kaplan's Test. This is a two-phase test. (1) The seated patient is given a hand dynamometer and instructed to extend the involved upper limb straight forward and squeeze the instrument as hard as possible. Induced pain and grip strength are noted. (2) The test is then repeated as before except that this time the examiner firmly encircles the patient's forearm with both hands (placed about 1–2 inches below the antecubital crease). Induced pain and grip strength are noted. If the second phase of the test shows increased induced pain and increased grip strength when the muscles of the proximal forearm are compressed, lateral epicondylitis is indicated.[207]

Medial Epicondyle Test. On the side of involvement, the patient is instructed to flex the elbow about 90° and supinate the hand. If severe pain arises over the medial epicondyle when the patient in this position attempts to extend the elbow against resistance, medial epicondylitis (golfer's elbow) is suggested.

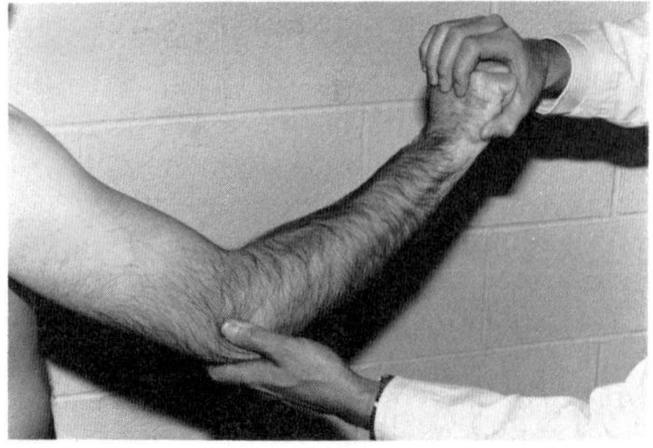

Figure 14.26. Position for Cozen's tennis elbow test.

Olecranon Bursitis[208,209]

Smooth mobility of the elbow is provided by this fluid-filled bursa, which is exposed to injury when the elbow is fixed on a firm surface. It is subject to direct impact and indirect mechanisms that may cause chronic inflammation, thickening of synovium, and formation of excessive fluid. The mechanism of injury is usually one of repetitive direct injury, constant friction of extensor tendons as in tennis elbow, and/or repetitious local injuries with synovial irritation. Local pain, tenderness, swelling, and movement restrictions are exhibited. Secondary infection readily converts the inflammation into an abscess.

Subluxations of the Elbow[210–215]

Most subluxations in the elbow area will offer dramatic relief upon correction. Generally, the adjustment is made with a quick, short thrust to minimize the pain (and time) of relocation. It is essential that the patient's muscles be relaxed or correction will be inhibited and extremely painful. Naturally, quick thrusts are contraindicated in arthritic and advanced fibrotic conditions.

Posterior-Medial Radial Head Subluxation

This "pulled elbow" injury results when the radial head is jerked from the annular ligament. Pain and tenderness in the area of the radial head result. Motion is severely limited in pronation and supination, but flexion and extension are normal. The arm is held in a pronated position, and pain is fairly localized at the elbow. X-ray films are negative. This type of subluxation is commonly associated with tennis elbow or wrist trauma, lateral elbow pain, and restricted anterolateral radial-head motion.

Olecranon Subluxations

Anterior Olecranon Subluxation. Subluxation of the olecranon anteriorly is seen in relation to hyperextension sprains and restricted posterior olecranon motion.

Posterior Olecranon Subluxation. This type of subluxation is associated with elbow or wrist trauma, epicondyle and bursa tenderness, triceps dyskinesia, and restricted anterior olecranon movement.

Medial Olecranon Subluxation. Subluxation of the olecranon medially is often seen in association with ulna nerve paresthesias, wrist or elbow trauma, medial elbow pain, triceps dyskinesia, decreased distance between olecranon and medial epicondyle, and restricted lateral olecranon joint motion.

Lateral Olecranon Subluxation. This type of subluxation is related to elbow or wrist trauma, lateral elbow pain, triceps dyskinesia, decreased distance between olecranon and lateral epicondyle, and restricted medial olecranon motion.

Superior Ulna Subluxation

Subluxation of the ulna superiorly is usually related to elbow or wrist trauma—often a consequence of a falling person catching himself with an outstretched hand. This results in the ulna being jammed upward toward the shoulder.

Fractures and Dislocations of the Elbow Area[216–219]

Fractures in the area of the elbow frequently involve the joint. In the order of frequency, the most common fractures are supracondylar humeral, olecranon, radial head, and coronoid process. Olecranon fractures result from a fall on the elbow or excessive triceps action. Displacement may be severe because of the strong pull of the triceps. Olecranon stress fractures are usually seen after overuse throwing injuries.

The radial head at the elbow transmits the force of a fall on the hand to the shoulder; this explains why the radial head is a common site of fracture in the elbow area. Subtle impaction fractures of the distal humerus and radial head are common, but they are often not witnessed on x-ray films until after a week or two. Acute signs are local swelling, tenderness about the radial head, and severe pain increased on pronation or supination. Severe displacement is not typical.

Physical Assessment

If obvious deformity and crepitus are not present, the range of motion should be checked and the radial pulse determined. Sensation is assessed by light touch and distal motion function by having the patient appose his thumb and forefinger. Elbow fractures and dislocations should be reduced by an orthopedist; they should be splinted in the "as is" postion, placed in a sling, and referred immediately. Delay in referral can easily result in massive heterotopic bone formation.

Myositis ossificans, nerve damage, brachial arterial compression, contractures, abnormal carrying angle, and joint stiffness may complicate recovery from any severe elbow injury. Poorly reduced supracondylar fractures, resulting in cubitus valgus, readily lead to ulnar neuritis.

Roentgenographic Considerations[220,221]

Elbow dislocations are usually the result of excessive hyperextension in which the olecranon and radial head are displaced posteriorly. Severe soft-tissue damage is associated, usually resulting in subperiosteal hematoma. Comminuted or marginal fracture fragments from the radial head are frequently related with elbow dislocations. In uncomplicated cases, gentle forward traction on the forearm with the humerus stabilized can be conducted to ease pain prior to referral. Roentgenography is required to analyze possible complications prior to considering even simple dislocation reduction.

Especially in the adolescent, trochlea, capitellum, and epicondyle growth centers may be enlarged, fragmented, displaced, or prematurely fused. Epiphyseal lines cause the most errors in interpretation of this area. Epiphyseal cartilage may be lacerated and the ossification centers displaced, sometimes into the articular cavity.

The most common fracture is a line running from the anterior to the posterior surface of the humeral shaft (supracondylar) with the proximal fragment shifted anteriorly. A fracture line between the condyles (intercondylar) or through one or both of the condyles (diacondylar) may be seen. Fracture of the ulnar shaft with dislocation of the radial head (Monteggia injury) and fracture of the radial head may also be present.

Nerve Compression Injuries[222,223]

Radial Nerve Compression at the Elbow

This nerve compression syndrome features pain and disturbed sensation in the area of distribution on the superficial branch and is thus frequently confused with de Quervain's disease. If the deep branch is involved, pain is at or below the lateral epicondyle. On palpation, the nerve trunk is tender near the origin of the extensors, and active extension of the fingers initiates or aggravates pain. If the elbow is extended and the 3rd finger is actively extended against resistance, pain is acutely increased because the extensor carpi radialis inserts at the base of the 3rd metacarpal.

Ulnar Nerve Compression at the Elbow

The ulnar nerve is often injured, just slightly less in incidence than the radial nerve. The injuries are usually at the inner side of the elbow where it is quite vulnerable in its superficial position along the elbow's posteromedial aspect. After damage, a characteristic "claw hand" results, with sensory loss of the medial side of the hand.

Ulnar nerve compression is often called cubital tunnel syndrome or tardy ulnar nerve palsy. It is the result of trauma or compression of the ulnar nerve at the elbow when the medial ligament ruptures during elbow dislocation. It may also be involved if the medial epicondyle becomes fractured. Disability and pain occur along the ulnar aspect of the forearm and hand. Early signs are inability to separate the fingers and disturbed sensation of the 4th and 5th digits. Interosseous atrophy is usually evident, and light pressure on the cubital tunnel initiates or aggravates pain. Nerve conduction studies help to confirm the diagnosis.

THE WRIST[224]

The carpals articulate with the ulna only during extreme wrist abduction. The distal radius enlarges to form the seat of the articulation of the proximal row of carpals.

Basic Functional Anatomy[225–231]

The radial facet is concave and sheathed with a triangular cartilage. The convexity of the transverse proximal carpal surface is sharper than the concavity of the radioulnar surfaces to afford a good range of joint motion. The proximal carpals rock and glide toward the ulna during wrist abduction and toward the radius during adduction. Adduction is slightly greater in pronation because the styloid process of the ulna restricts motion when the hand is supinated. During adduction, the styloid swings backward out of the way. Because the A-P curve of the proximal carpals is more acute than the transverse curve, greater excursion is allowed in wrist flexion and extension than in lateral motion, but the exact degree of wrist motion varies considerably from patient to patient. It appears that the more delicate the bone structure, the greater the mobility.

The distal row of carpals form a complex joint with the proximal row. Because they are loosely connected, the navicular and trapezium spread during wrist abduction and approximate during adduction. The volar surfaces of the carpals present eminences that serve as attachment points, allowing increased mechanical advantage for the muscles and ligaments of the hand. They also guide tendon passages.

Wrist Movements[232–236]

The intricate anatomical architecture of the wrist allows flexion (80°), extension (70°), radial deviation (15°), ulnar deviation (35°), supination and pronation of the forearm.

Wrist Motion[237–240]

Active flexion, extension, ulnar deviation, and radial deviation are tested simply by having the patient flex and extend the wrist, then deviating the wrist medially and laterally (Fig. 14.27). Supination and pronation tests have been discussed previously in conjunction with the forearm. (See Tables 14.6 and 14.7.)

Kinesiology of the Wrist[241–243]

Flexion. Flexion of the wrist is provided by the flexor carpi radialis (C7–C8) and flexor carpi ulnaris (C8–T1) (Fig. 14.28). To judge strength, the patient makes a fist, the examiner stabilizes the wrist, and the patient flexes the closed fist. At the end of flexion, the examiner applies increasing extension resistance to the patient's fist with the active hand.

Extension. Wrist extension is controlled by the extensor carpi radialis longus (C6–C7), extensor carpi radialis brevis (C6–C7), and extensor carpi ulnaris (C7) (Fig. 14.29).

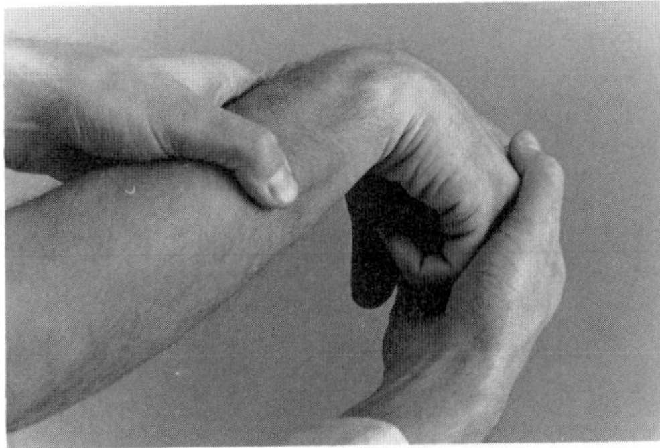

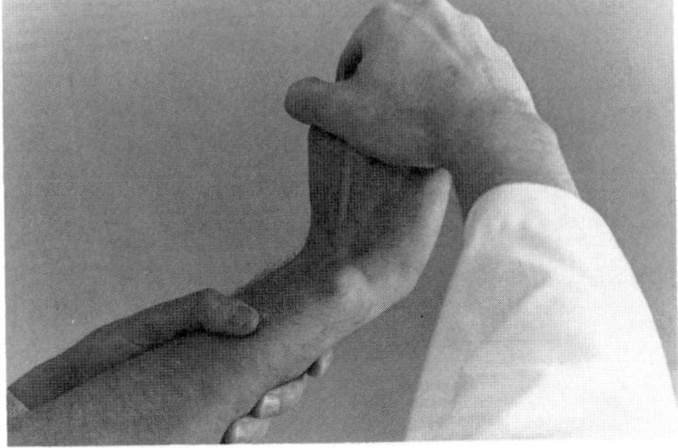

Figure 14.27. *Top*, testing wrist extension strength against resistance; *bottom*, evaluating wrist flexion strength.

Strength is tested by having the examiner stabilize the patient's forearm by firmly grasping the patient's wrist with one hand and applying increasing flexion pressure against the dorsum of the patient's hand after motion has reached maximum extension.

Wrist supination and pronation strength has been discussed previously with the forearm.

Coupled Wrist and Finger Dynamics

The muscles of the wrist are placed obliquely to the parts to be moved. This requires coordination with other muscles whenever the wrist is moved. Wrist strength in flexion is nearly double that in extension, and the power of extension is greatly lessened when the wrist is flexed. During extreme flexion of the wrist, it is impossible to strongly curl the fingers in full flexion because the flexor tendons are slackened. When the wrist is hyperextended, the extensors become slackened and the fingers cannot fully hyperextend.

Goniometry of the Wrist[244,245]

Restricted Dorsal and Palmar Flexion Motion of the Wrist. The patient is placed in the neutral position, the goniometer is centered under the patient's wrist, and the neutral reading is recorded with the goniometer arm between the patient's ring and middle fingers. The patient dorsiflexes the wrist as far as possible, and the reading is recorded at the end of the motion. To evaluate palmar flexion, the patient palmarflexes his wrist as far as possible, and the end of the motion is recorded.

Restricted Abduction and Adduction of the Wrist. The patient is placed in the neutral position with his hand and forearm pronated, the goniometer is centered over the patient's wrist with the goniometer arm

Table 14.6.
Wrist Motion

Joint motion	Prime movers	Accessories
Flexion	Flexor carpi radialis Flexor carpi ulnaris	Palmaris longus Flexor digitorum superficialis Flexor digitorum produndus Flexor pollicis longus Abductor pollicis longus
Extension	Extensor carpi radialis longus Extensor carpi radialis brevis Extensor carpi ulnaris	Extensor digitorum Extensor indicis Extensor digiti minimi Extensor pollicis longus
Radial deviation	Flexor carpi radialis Extensor carpi radialis longus	Extensor pollicis longus Extensor pollicis brevis Abductor pollicis longus
Ulnar deviation	Extensor carpi ulnaris Flexor carpi ulnaris	

Table 14.7.
Major Muscles of the Wrist

Muscle	Major function	Spinal segment
Abductors pollicis	Flexion, radial deviation	C8–T1
Extensor carpi radialis	Extension, radial deviation	C6–C7
Extensor carpi ulnaris	Extension, ulnar deviation	C8–T1
Extensor digiti minimi	Extension	C7–C8
Extensor digitorum	Extension	C6–C8
Extensor indicis	Extension	C7–C8
Extensor pollicis longus	Extension, radial deviation	C7–C8
Extensor pollicis brevis	Radial deviation	C7–C8
Flexor carpi radialis	Flexion, radial deviation	C6–C7
Flexor carpi ulnaris	Flexion, ulnar deviation	C8–T1
Flexor digiti profundus	Flexion	C8–T1
Flexor digiti superficialis	Flexion	C7–T1
Flexor pollicis longus	Flexion	C8–T1
Palmaris longus	Flexion	C7–C8

Spinal innervation varies somewhat in different people. The spinal nerves listed here are averages and may differ in a particular patient; thus, an allowance of a segment above and below those listed in most text tables should be considered.

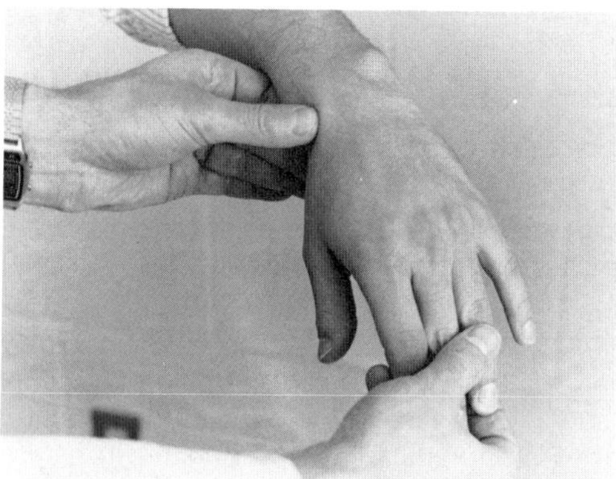

Figure 14.29. The tendons of the extensor carpi radialis longus and brevis are located on the radial side of the radial tubercle.

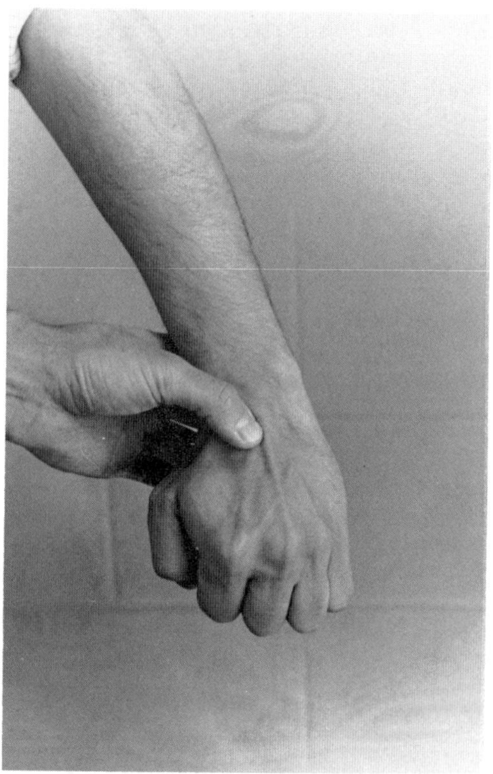

Figure 14.28. When the fist is clenched, palpation of the extensor carpi radialis longus and brevis is enhanced.

over the third metacarpal, and the neutral reading is recorded. The patient radially deviates the wrist as far as possible, and the reading is recorded at the end of the motion. Then the patient ulnar deviates the wrist as far as possible, and the reading at the end of the motion is recorded.

SELECTED CLINICAL PROBLEMS OF THE WRIST AREA

Restriction in pronation suggests pathology at the elbow, radioulnar articulation at the wrist, or within the forearm (Fig. 14.30). Restriction in supination is associated with a disorder of the elbow or radioulnar artic-

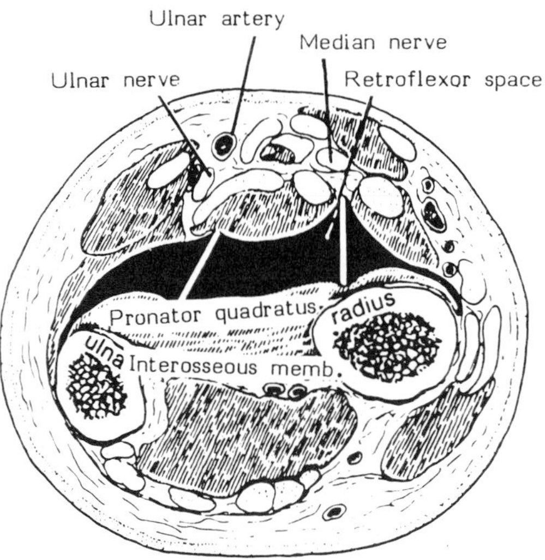

Figure 14.30. Cross section of forearm just proximal to wrist. In this drawing, the retroflexor space lying above the pronator quadratus and interosseous membrane and beneath the flexor muscles and tendons is invaded by an infectious process following rupture of the radial or ulnar bursae.

ulation at the wrist. Thickened tissues may cause compression symptoms, and nerve injury is often secondary to epicondylar fracture or severe trauma.

Biomechanical Considerations[246]

Trauma of the wrist should never be taken lightly. An improperly diagnosed and treated case can readily lead to severe arthritis. Good management rests on a thorough knowledge of the underlying anatomy of the carpal bones and fibrocartilage complex.

The wrist complex is far more than eight bones arranged in two horizontal rows between the forearm and hand. Three vertical columns must also be considered. The wrist is essentially a biaxial joint that is capable of motion in two planes: (1) radial and ulnar deviation and (2) palmar flexion and extension. The patterns of movement between the two horizontal carpal rows are reciprocal to each other. In radial deviation, the distal row moves toward the radius, while the proximal row moves toward the ulnar. In ulnar deviation, these movements are reversed; ie, the distal row moves ulnarly, while the proximal row moves radially.

The most important ligaments of the wrist are the volar and intercapsular groups. The weaker dorsal ligaments are arranged in laminar bands. As the proximal carpal row lacks tendon support, the integrity of the volar ligament intracapsular supporting system is vital.

Trauma of the Wrist Area[247–249]

Tenderness over the medial collateral ligament as it arises from the medial epicondyle is a sign of valgus sprain. Muscle tenderness in the wrist flexor-extensor group is characteristic of flexor-pronator strain (Fig. 14.31). Tenderness in the 1st tunnel on the radial side is a common site for stenosing tenosynovitis associated with a positive Finkelstein's sign. Rupture of the tendon should be sought in the 3rd tunnel, which often results from a healed Colles' fracture defect at the dorsal radial tubercle or arthritis causing tendon wearing. Tenderness in the 5th or 6th tunnel is characteristic of synovitis, dorsal carpal subluxation, dislocation of the ulnar head, or rheumatoid

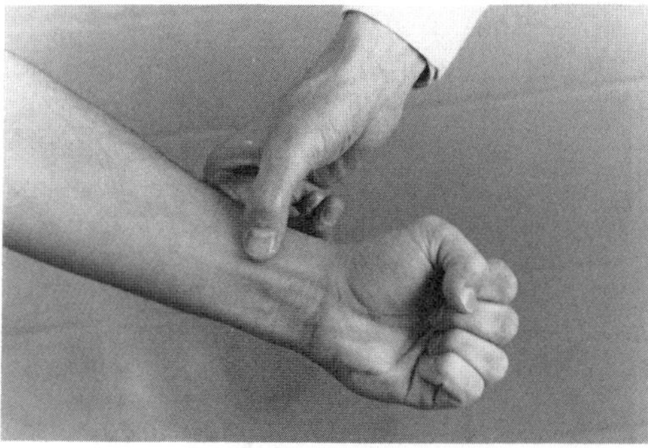

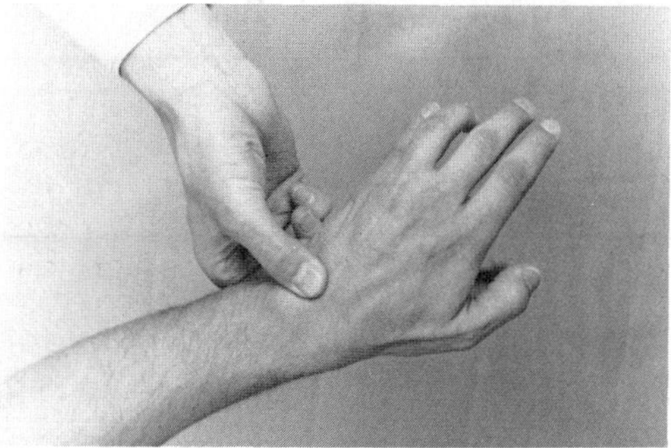

Figure 14.31. *Top*, palpation of the flexor carpi radialis tendon, aided by clenching of the fist. *Bottom*, ulnar deviation of the wrist makes the tensor carpi ulnaris tendon more prominent during palpation.

arthritis. The easily fractured scaphoid should be checked by sliding it out from under the radial styloid with ulnar deviation of the wrist. The wrist is radially deviated, and the triquetrum, a common site of fracture is checked. Pain, tenderness, and swelling about the ulnar styloid process suggest a Colles' fracture or a local pathology such as arthritic erosion.

Forearm Strains

These usually affect the flexors. Simple strains such as from overenthusiastic weight lifting respond quickly to rest and standard strain management, but chronic strain can develop into a frustrating problem if the patient insists on continuing irritating activities. Avulsion at the bicipital tubercle and stress fracture of the olecranon are sometimes associated.

Contractures

After cerebral lesions involving the arm center and in almost any spinal or peripheral nerve lesion that involves one set of muscles and spares another, healthy muscles contract (or overact) and permanent deformities result. In trauma-related hysteria, similar contractures occur. Contractures have in themselves little or no diagnostic value but indicate a late and stubborn stage of whatever lesion is present.

Brachialis Calcification

Following brachialis strain, a local myositis ossificans may develop in the brachialis anticus tendon. This is usually the result of recurrent bruising and bleeding.

Unilateral Wasting

Rapid atrophy occurs in all types of neuritis, as well as in poliomyelitis and progressive muscular atrophy. In the latter, it occurs without complete paralysis, though the wasted muscles are, of course, weak. Progressive muscular atrophy usually begins in the muscles at the base of the thumb and between it and the index finger. Less often, the process begins in the deltoid. In either case, the rest of the arm muscles become involved later. In the atrophies just mentioned, a lack of the trophic or nourishing functions that should flow down the nerve is assumed to explain the trophic wasting. From this, we can distinguish atrophy due simply to disuse of the muscles without nerve lesions. Slow atrophy of disuse occurs in the arm in hemiplegia (infantile or adult) and in other cerebral lesions involving the arm center or the fibers leading down from it. A cervical rib disorder occasionally leads to wasting as well as pain in the corresponding arm.

Wrist Sprains and Related Disorders[250-252]

Wrist Sprain

Wrist sprain (eg, a jammed wrist) is quite common and may be associated with fractures and dislocations of the carpals, elbow, or shoulder girdle. Consequently, all severe wrist joint injuries should include roentgenography of the elbow and shoulder. The symptoms of wrist sprain are the same as in any other extremity joint sprain and may be associated with tenosynovitis. Severe wrist sprains are frequently accompanied by carpal and/or radial subluxations (Fig. 14.32).

On the dorsal aspect of the wrist, the

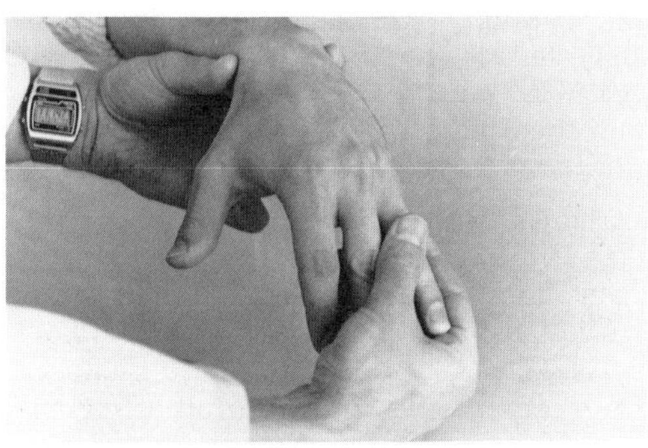

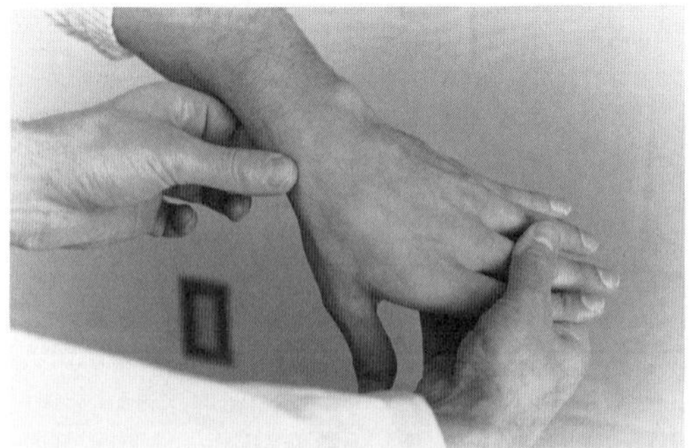

Figure 14.32. *Top*, the radial and ulnar styloid processes are the basic reference points to be palpated in the wrist. *Bottom*, ulnar deviation of the wrist helps in palpation of the navicular carpal.

scaphoid is the common carpal problem; on the ventral aspect, it is the lunate, hamate, and pisiform. Extension sprain with radial deviation is characterized by tenderness along the ulnarmetacarpal collateral ligament. Dorsiflexion sprain features tenderness along the volar aspect of the wrist and distal radius. In either case, pain is short of fracture and crepitus is absent. Palpation of the anterior wrist is greatly hampered by the tendon bulk of the area and useless on either aspect after swelling has taken place. It should be noted that scaphoid fracture, a dangerous situation, is often mistaken for a sprain (Fig. 14.33).

Flexion/Extension Stress Tests. The examiner moves the wrist firmly into flexion and extension. If pain is induced, wrist fracture, subluxation, sprain, acute tendinitis, or pathology are suggested. If negative, the movements are repeated against patient resistance. Induced pain then indicates wrist strain, rupture, acute or chronic tendinitis, or pathology.

Radial/Ulnar Stress Tests. The examiner moves the wrist firmly into radial and ulnar deviation (abduction and adduction). If pain is induced, sprain, acute tendinitis, joint pathology, fracture, or subluxation are suggested. If negative, the movements are repeated against patient resistance. Induced pain then indicates acute or chronic tendinitis, strain, rupture, or joint pathology.

Tenosynovitis

The extensor muscles of the forearm are often affected in tenosynovitis. The clinical picture is one of pain along the dorsal forearm, crepitus along the extensor tendons, swelling (palpable and visible), and possible hypertrophy of the extensors and abductors of the thumb.

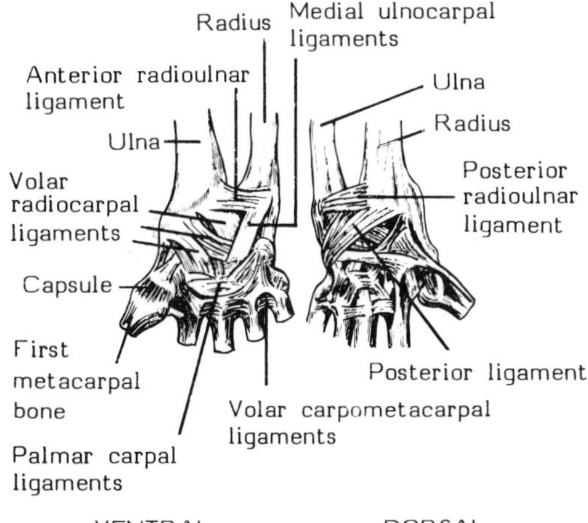

Figure 14.33. Major ligaments of the wrist.

Ganglion[253]

A ganglion is a cystic swelling occurring in association with a joint or tendon sheath, apparently formed as a defense mechanism when the wrist is repeatedly twisted and strained. It has a fibrous outer coat and an inner synovial layer containing a thick gelatinous fluid. A common site is in the wrist or hand; they are rarely found in the ankle or foot. A firm localized swelling and possibly weakened grip strength are found. Aching or sometimes pain from pressure on adjacent structures is typically exhibitied.

Subluxations of the Wrist[254-258]

As in any adjustive procedure, fracture, dislocation, and pathology must be ruled out prior to adjustment.

Distal Forearm Subluxations

Separated Distal Radius and Ulna. This type of subluxation is commonly seen in association with carpal tunnel syndrome, chronic wrist pain, and after wrist trauma.

Approximated Distal Radius and Ulna. Jamming of the distal radius and ulna are often seen in chronic wrist pain or following wrist and hand trauma.

Inferior Radius Subluxation. An inferiorly subluxated radius is often a consequence of wrist sprain from a fall on the outstretched hand.

Common Carpal Subluxations.

Anterior Carpal Subluxation. Subluxation of a carpal anteriorly is related to carpal tunnel syndrome, chronic wrist pain, extension sprain, and restricted posterior wrist flexion. The lunate is commonly involved (Fig. 14.34).

Posterior Carpal Subluxation. This type of subluxation is frequently associated with wrist trauma, chronic pain upon motion, carpal tunnel syndrome, and restricted wrist extension.

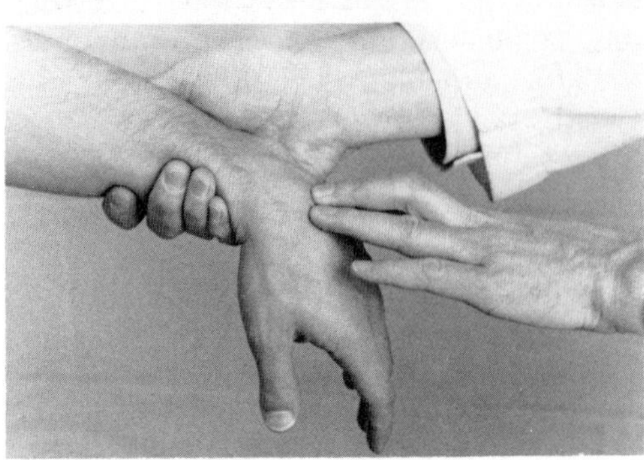

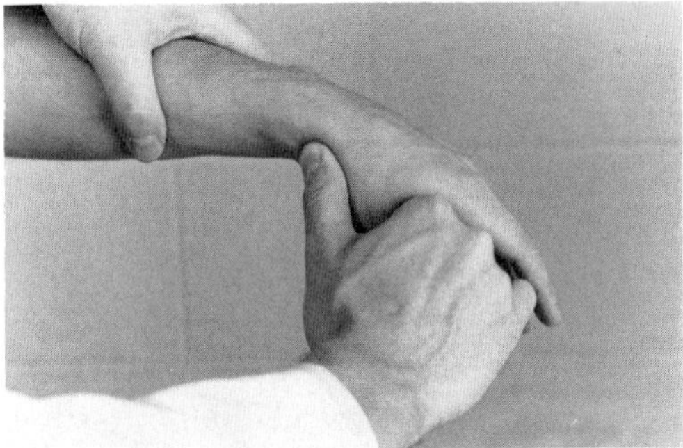

Figure 14.34. *Top*, wrist flexion aids in palpation of the lunate. *Bottom*, the navicular tubercle is palpated proximally while the trapezium and 1st metacarpal are palpated radially in this position.

Metacarpal Base Posterior Subluxation

A metacarpal base subluxated posteriorly is associated with pain especially increased by wrist flexion, excessive wrist flexion sprain, wrist ganglion, and restricted wrist extension.

Fractures and Dislocations of the Wrist Area[259-263]

Uncomplicated distal-forearm fractures and dislocations should immediately be aided somewhat by steady axial traction. Motor and sensory function of the hand should be assessed and circulation by capillary filling of the fingernails noted with finger pressure. Such injuries should be padded, splinted in the position of function, and referred. Roentgenography is required to analyze possible complications prior to considered reduction.

Roentgenography of Injuries of the Forearm[264,265]

Fractures of the bones in the forearm usually involve both bones. Sometimes, however, these bones do not fracture at the same level. The bulk of forearm bone injuries are from falls or direct blows. When a midarm blow fractures the radius or ulna, both ends of each bone must be evaluated for possibly associated subluxation, dislocation, and rotational abnormality. Dislocation of the proximal radius accompanies midulna fracture in Monteggia injury, while midradius fracture is accompanied by distal ulnar subluxation in Galeazzi's fracture. The ulna is usually displaced posteriorly when the distal ulna is subluxated. In radial or ulnar fractures, ulnar rotational abnormalities may be a complication. Malposition of the bicipital tubercle proximally and the ulnar styloid distally are helpful clues to rotational abnormalities. Comparison should be made with views of the contralateral (uninjured) arm.

If a fracture of the distal radius is difficult to view on film, careful inspection of the pronator muscle fat pad should be made just proximal to the wrist. It may be the only radiographic sign present. This fat pad, which separates the pronator quadratus muscle and tendons of the flexor digitorum profundus, is normally viewed on lateral films of the wrist. Blurring, bowing, or obliteration of the fat pad may be seen as a consequence of injury or disease of the radius or volar soft tissues.

Fracture of the distal radius (Colles') is the first consideration in wrist injuries, but the close relationship of both forearm and wrist bones and all articulations must be carefully evaluated (Fig. 14.35). The joint spaces between the carpal bones are normally uniform. Epiphyseal fractures and fractures through the growth plate with or without shifting are not uncommon in youth. The typical deformity in this injury is a compression of the posterior margin of the radius, resulting in a backward tilting of the anterior surface as viewed in the lateral view. The articular margin of the radius will be disturbed, and the distal radius may be fragmented and impacted. Old fractures are differentiated from recent ones by the presence of rarefaction and the absence of a distinct fracture line.

On the lateral view, the radiocarpal articulation should be carefully evaluated. The radial longitudinal axis normally extends

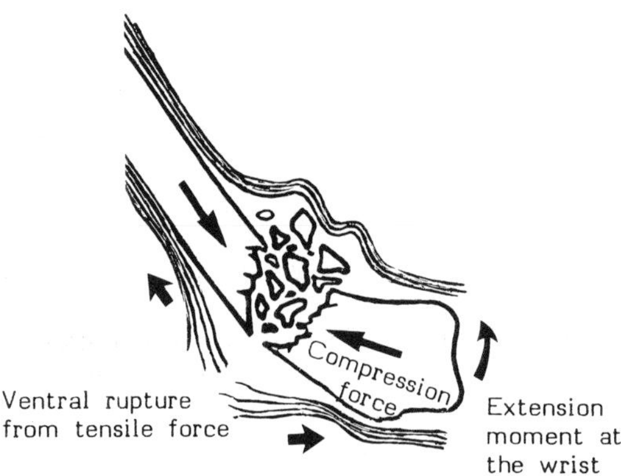

Figure 14.35. The force mechanisms involved in Colles' fracture of the wrist. There is a combined wrist hyperextension moment and axial compression forces that crush the posterior cortex and spongiosa, with tensile forces disrupting the anterior ligaments and periosteum.

through the lunate's midpoint. On the P-A view, disruption of the distal radioulnar articulation is seen as joint widening or narrowing. During an impacted fracture of the radius, bone fragments are frequently telescoped and both styloid processes are seen at the same but more distal level; ie, the radial styloid is normally seen 1 cm distal to the ulnar styloid process.

Maisonneuve's Sign. Normal extension of the wrist rarely exceeds 75°. Marked hyperextension (near 90°) is a sign of Colles' fracture.

Carpal Fracture-Dislocations[266]

Any carpal may be a potential fracture or dislocation site. A common predisposing factor to fracture is general osteoporosis. In order of frequency, the bones usually involved are the scaphoid, lunate, and capilate—all of which may be associated with injuries of the radius or ulna. Of the carpals, the lunate is the most frequently dislocated; the scaphoid is the most frequently fractured. The scaphoid is the most lateral of the four bones in the proximal row of carpals; the lunate, second from thumb side.

Even slight tenderness in the anatomical "snuffbox" around the scaphoid and swelling obliterating the space between the thumb's extensor tendons suggest the danger of scaphoid fracture, which may not appear on film for 10–14 days. Axially directed percussion on the knuckle of the patient's index finger when his fist is closed will usually elicit scaphoid pain if it is fractured. Bone necrosis and nonunion are always a danger, because the bone is poorly nourished in a third of the population.

Lunate Injury[267]

This dislocation-fracture may be seen after a fall on the outstretched hand but is most common in boxers whose hands are carelessly wrapped. Damage to the median nerve is a complication. The clinical picture is one of anterior wrist swelling, with stiff and semiflexed fingers. Carpal dislocations, especially lunate or paralunate, are frequently missed during evaluation. These are often associated with a trans-scaphoid fracture and necrosis.

The lunate usually dislocates posteriorly or anteriorly, disrupting its relationship with the neighboring carpals and the distal radius. Anterior displacement is the common mechanism, in which the bone rests deep in the annular ligament and may affect the median nerve. The lunate is loosely stabilized by anterior and posterior ligaments that contain small nutritive blood vessels. A torn ligament thus interferes with the lunate's nutrition, resulting in necrosis. On a P-A view, the lunate's normal quadrilateral shape becomes triangular, and the 3rd metacarpal and capitate usually move proximally. With paralunate dislocation, the lunate keeps normal alignment with the radius but the distal carpals become displaced from their normal position with associated changes in intercarpal joint spaces.

Finsterer's Test. This is a two-phase test for Kienbock's disease. (1) If when clenching the fist firmly the normal prominence of the 3rd knuckle is not produced, the test is initially positive. (2) If percussion of the 3rd metacarpal just distal to the dorsal aspect of the midpoint of the wrist elicits abnormal tenderness, the test is confirmed.[268]

Compression Syndromes[269,270]

Median Nerve Entrapment at the Wrist[60,222,271–274]

The median nerve is commonly injured in trauma of the anterior wrist. Consequently, sensation and motion of the fingers should be carefully studied. It is difficult to injure any of the flexors of the medial anterior wrist without damaging the median nerve. When severely bruised, the characteristic "flat hand" deformity results. Median nerve paresthesias may have their cause in the spine, but they are just as common from interference in the thoracic outlet, the shoulder, the elbow, or at the wrist. Correction must be directed to where the interference is located and not where it *should be* located.

Carpal Tunnel Syndrome. This is a nerve compression syndrome featuring median nerve entrapment at the carpal tunnel resulting in symptoms in the hand and fingers, often extending up the arm to the elbow. The cause may be either an increase of structural volume within the tunnel or any condition that tends to narrow the tunnel. The history will often indicate an old scaphoid fracture, paralunar dislocation, or tendinitis at the wrist. Frequently, the history tells of a fall stopped abruptly by the palm of the hand when the wrist was sharply dorsiflexed or of overstress in people who strongly manipulate their wrists. A syndrome may also be produced by radial or ulnar arterial impairment since these arteries also pass beneath the transverse carpal ligament. Such symptoms may be aggravated by pressure of the sphygmomanometer cuff during blood pressure evaluation.

Signs and Symptoms. There is a history of pain, numbness, and tingling, which worsen at night and with wrist compression, in the first two or three digits and/or the area proximal to the wrist. Weakness is exhibited by a history of dropping light objects and difficulty in holding a pen or pencil while writing. Venous engorgement and a bulge may be seen of the flexor mass in the distal wrist, which is chracteristic of tenosynovitis or hypertrophied muscles. The first sign is swelling at the volar wrist. Later, thenar atrophy and sensation impairment of the thumb, forefinger, middle finger, and medial half of the ring finger exhibit. In many cases, there is distinct difficulty in pronating or supinating the forearm. Compression or percussion of the carpal ligament usually initiates or increases pain. Electromyogram and nerve conduction studies offer confirmative data for a diagnosis. Misdiagnosis is sometimes made by attributing a unilateral or bilateral syndrome to slight arthritic changes of the midcervical vertebrae.

Phalen's Test. The patient places both flexed wrists into opposition and applies slight pressure for 30–45 seconds (Fig. 14.36). A positive sign of carpal tunnel syndrome is the production of symptoms (eg, pain, tingling).

Tinel's Wrist Test. With the patient's elbow flexed and the hand supinated, the volar surface of the wrist is tapped with the broad end of a triangular reflex hammer. If this induces pain in all fingers of the involved hand except the little finger, carpal tunnel syndrome is indicated.

Wrist Tourniquet Test. A sphygmomanometer cuff is wrapped around the involved wrist of a seated patient. The cuff is inflated to a point just above the patient's systolic blood pressure level and maintained for 1–2 minutes. If an exacerbation of pain is exhibited, carpal tunnel syndrome is indicated.

Ochsner's Clasping Test. The patient is

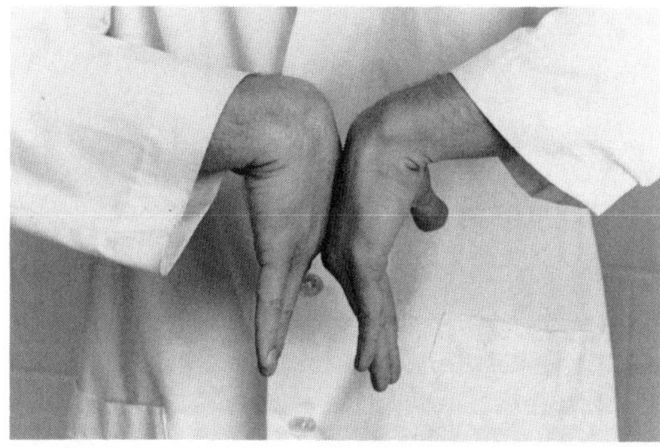

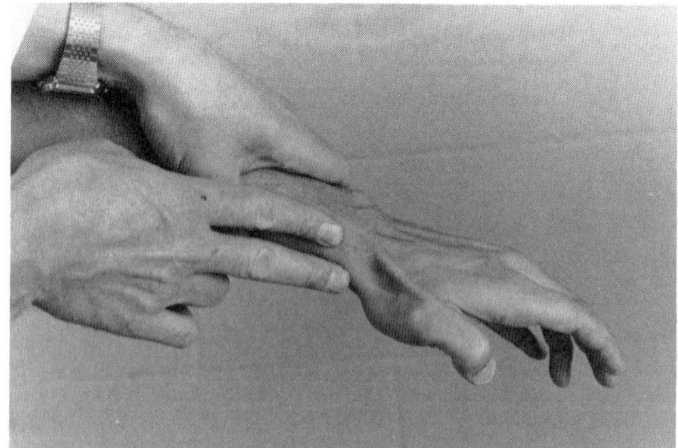

Figure 14.36. *Top*, Phalen's test to elicit signs of carpal tunnel syndrome. *Bottom*, the abductor pollicis longus and the extensor pollicis brevis tendons define the radial border of the carpal "snuffbox."

instructed to clasp the hands together and interlock the fingers. If the index finger on the involved side fails to flex, median nerve paralysis is indicated—with the lesion at or above the level where the nerve to the flexor digitorum superficialis branches.

Wartenburg's Oriental Prayer Sign. The patient is instructed to fully extend the adducted fingers and the thumb of each hand so that the palms are flat and then to move both hands so that the thumbs and index fingers touch. In median nerve palsy, the thumbs will not touch because of paralysis of the abductor pollicis brevis.

The Ulnar Tunnel Triad. If inspection and palpation over the ulnar tunnel in the wrist determines the three signs of (1) tenderness, (2) clawing of the ring finger, and (3) hypothenar wasting, ulnar compression in the tunnel of Guyon is indicated.

Bracelet Test. The examiner surrounds the patient's wrist with the thumb and forefinger and applies from mild to moderate compression to the distal ends of the radius and ulna. If acute pain arises in the wrist and/or radiates to the forearm or hand, rheumatoid arthritis should be suspected.

Ulnar Nerve Entrapment At the Wrist[275,276]

This compression syndrome features ulnar nerve entrapment, usually in the canal of Guyon. Entrapment may be of the superficial or the deep branch of the ulna nerve, but the superficial branch is rarely affected by itself. The pisiform-hamate tunnel syndrome is similar to but less frequently seen than that of carpal tunnel syndrome.

Signs and Symptoms. Entrapment of the deep branch produces a motor loss exhibited by a weak pinch, weak little finger and thumb abduction, inability to actively flex the metacarpophalangeal joints, and interosseous atrophy. Compression of the superficial branch features burning sensations in the 4th and 5th digits. Palpation of the pisiform-hamate tunnel initiates or aggravates pain. In roentgenography, a hamate fracture or pisiform dislocation may be found in tangential views.

Froment's Test. In paralysis of the ulnar nerve, there is an inability to approximate the tips of fingers to the thumb to form a cone (*cone sign*) or to make an "O" with the thumb and index finger.

THE HAND AND THUMB[277-280]

The metacarpal of the thumb conforms to the articular surface of the trapezium. This saddle joint allows a wide range of mobility in all directions so that the pad of the thumb can appose any finger pad. The two sesamoids of the flexor pollicis brevis ride upon two eminences on the volar surface of the 1st metacarpal. These protect the joint between the thumb's 1st metacarpal and proximal phalanx.

Thumb Movements[281-286]

The thumb is capable of metacarpophalangeal flexion (50°) and extension (0°) and interphalangeal flexion (90°) and extension (20°). Abduction (70°) and adduction (0°) occur at the carpometacarpal joint. (See Tables 14.8 and 14.9.)

Thumb Motion[287,288]

Active overall thumb flexion, extension, abduction and adduction are tested by having the patient touch the tip of his thumb to the base of his little finger, to each fingertip, and then to extend the thumb as far as possible laterally. If joint restriction is noted, both joints should be checked passively.

Kinesiology of the Thumb[289,290]

Extension. Thumb extension is provided essentially by the extensor pollicis brevis (C7–C8) at the metacarpophalangeal joint and the extensor pollicis longus (C7–C8) at the interphalangeal joint. Strength is tested by stabilizing the patient's wrist and having him extend the thumb as far as possible. Increasing flexion resistance is applied by the examiner, and the degree is recorded.

Flexion. Flexion of the thumb is controlled by the medial (C8, ulnar) and lateral (C6–C7, median) flexor pollicis brevis at the metacarpophalangeal joint and by the flexor pollicis longus (C8–T1) at the interphalangeal joint. Strength is tested by having the patient touch the tip of the thumb firmly against the pad below his little finger. The power it takes the examiner to pull the patient's thumb out of flexion should be noted (Fig. 14.37).

Abduction. Thumb abduction is pro-

Table 14.8.
Thumb Motion

Joint motion	Prime movers	Accessories
Metacarpophalangeal flexion	Flexor pollicis brevis	Flexor pollicis longus Abductor pollicis brevis
Interphalangeal flexion	Flexor pollicis longus	
Metacarpophalangeal extension	Extensor pollicis brevis	Abductor pollicis longus Extensor pollicis longus
Interphalangeal extension	Extensor pollicis longus	
Adduction	Adductor pollicis	Flexor pollicis brevis, deep head
Abduction	Abductor pollicis brevis Abductor pollicis longus	
Opposition	Opponens pollicis Opponens digiti minimi	

Table 14.9.
Major Muscles of the Thumb

Muscle	Major function	Spinal segment
Abductor pollicis brevis	Thumb metacarpophalangeal flexion, abduction	C8–T1
Abductor pollicis longus	Thumb abduction and metacarpophalangeal extension	C6–C7
Adductor pollicis	Thumb adduction	C8–T1
Extensor pollicis brevis	Thumb metacarpophalangeal extension	C7–C8
Extensor pollicis longus	Thumb metacarpophalangeal and interphalangeal extension	C7–C8
Flexor pollicis brevis	Thumb adduction, metacarpophalangeal flexion	C8–T1
Flexor pollicis longus	Thumb metacarpophalangeal and interphalangeal flexion, abduction	C8–T1
Opponens digiti minimi	Opposition	C8–T1
Opponens pollicis	Opposition	C6–C7

Spinal innervation varies somewhat in different people. The spinal nerves listed here are averages and may differ in a particular patient; thus, an allowance of a segment above and below those listed in most text tables should be considered.

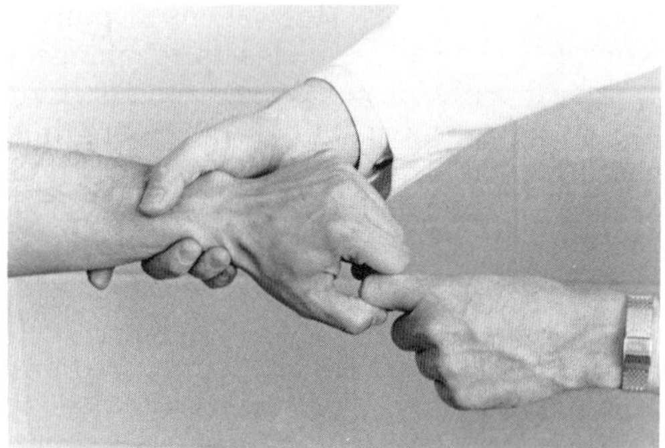

Figure 14.37. Testing pinch strength.

vided by the abductor pollicis longus (C6–C7, radial) and abductor pollicis brevis (C8–T1, median). Strength is tested by stabilizing the patient wrist, especially on the ulnar side. The patient fully abducts his thumb, and, at the end of motion, the examiner increasingly applies reverse pressure (Fig. 14.38).

Adduction. Adduction of the thumb is controlled by the adductor pollicis (C8–T1, ulnar). Strength is tested by stabilizing the patient's wrist along the ulnar border and having the patient adduct the thumb against the examiner's increasing resistance.

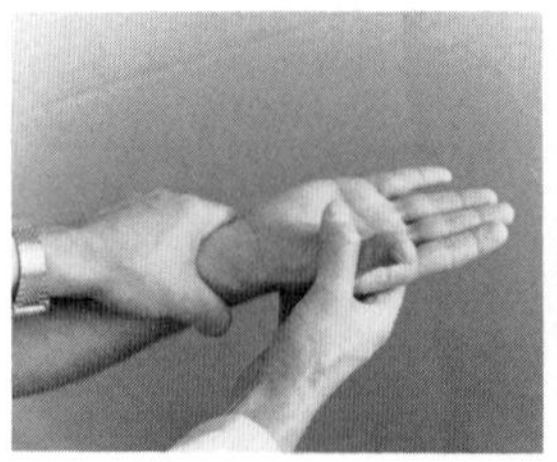

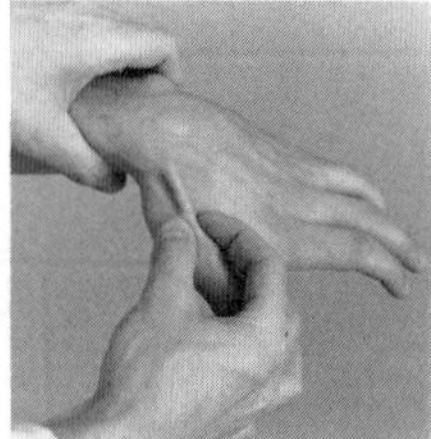

Figure 14.38. *Left*, testing thumb abduction strength against resistance. *Right*, when the thumb is extended, palpation of the tendons of the abductor pollicis longus and brevis is enhanced.

Goniometry of the Thumb[291,292]

Restricted Motion of the Interphalangeal Joint of the Thumb. The patient's hand is placed in the neutral position, the goniometer is centered over the dorsum of the patient's interphalangeal joint, and the neutral position is recorded. The patient flexes the interphalangeal joint as far as possible; the end of the motion is then recorded.

Restricted Motion of the Carpometacarpal Joint of the Thumb. The patient's hand is placed in the neutral position with the goniometer next to his carpometacarpal joint, and the neutral position reading is recorded. The patient flexes his thumb, then the reading at the end of the motion is recorded. Next, the patient extends his thumb from the index finger in the palm's plane, and the reading at the end of the motion is recorded.

Trigger Points

The most common trigger point found in the hand is that of the adductor pollicis. This is shown in Figure 14.39.

Dislocation of the Thumb[293]

A fracture of the 4th and/or 5th metacarpal, especially at the neck of the bone, is often referred to as a "fighter's" dislocation-fracture. The bone's head and neck are sometimes pushed into the palm. This is most often seen in the bare-knuckled fighter or during riots rather than with the gloved boxer who more often presents a fracture at the proximal third of the 1st metacarpal.

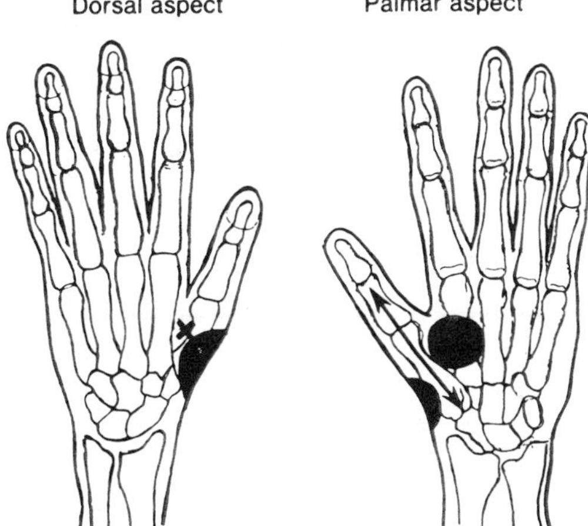

Figure 14.39. Adductor pollicis trigger point; *X*, common site. *Blackened areas* indicate typical sites of referred pain.

SELECTED CLINICAL PROBLEMS OF THE HAND AND THUMB[294–296]

Direct Trauma

The hand, being the least protected and most active part of the upper etremity, is easily hurt. From a structural standpoint, the hand is made for grasping, not for hitting.

Sprained Thumb[297]

A severe injury can occur to the inner thumb ligaments from a fall on a thumb directed outward or when caught in someone's clothing. This often results in a complete tear which requires surgery. The thumb is also often jammed, and the medial or lateral ligaments sprained, when hitting with the closed fist.

Ulnovolar neuroma (bowler's thumb) is the result of trauma to the digital nerve from the edge of the thumb hole in the ball. After repeated bowling, fibrous proliferation and enlargement of the 3rd and 2nd fingers are frequently seen. Bony callus formation may be evident on roentgenography.

A rupture to the ulnar collateral ligament of the thumb may occur during a fall when the leather loop of a woman's purse or the handle strap of a ski pole is wrapped around the thumb. Chronic sprain associated with forearm supinator strain is becoming quite common among video game players.

THE FINGERS[298,299]

Finger motion is versatile because of the dynamic balance between muscles and tendons that creates an equilibrium of static and dynamic forces. This is an excellent example of viscoelastic forces that resist tendon unit lengthening. The components involved are the fascia, tendon sheath, perimyseum, joint capsule, and joint inertia. If the viscoelastic forces on the anterior aspect exceed those on the posterior aspect and the extensors relax, for example, the digit will flex.

Basic Functional Anatomy[300]

In the fingers, the carpal-metacarpal articulations are fortified by a complex ligamentous apparatus that surrounds the joints in all directions. This tends to greatly restrict carpometacarpal motion. All reciprocally concave-convex metacarpophalangeal joints are freely movable with the exception of abduction and adduction. The convex metacarpal heads fit snugly against the shallow sockets of the proximal phalanges. The interphalangeal joints are true hinge joints that allow considerable flexion but only slight hyperextension.

Finger Movements[301–305]

There is a distinct relationship between finger joint position and the position of more proximal joints, ie, joint motion is the effect of involuntary viscoelastic forces in addition to normal active contraction. Active wrist flexion, for example, increases the viscoelastic forces on the posterior of the digit. The result is finger extension even without active contraction of the finger extensors.[306] Likewise, active wrist extension affects finger flexion.

Finger Motion[288, 307–309]

Gross movements of the fingers are regulated by the extrinsic muscles of the hand, while the intrinsics control the finer movements and tend to counterbalance the extrinsics. Finger extension is associated with finger spreading, and flexion tends to draw the fingers together.

Finger motion involves flexion and extension at the metacarpophalangeal and interphalangeal joints. Abduction and adduction occur at the metacarpophalangeal joints. Active metacarpophalangeal motion is tested by stabilizing the patient's wrist and having him extend (30–45°) and flex (90°) with the digits straight. Active proximal interphalangeal motion is checked by stabilizing the metacarpophalangeal joints and having the patient extend (0°) and flex (100°) the proximal interphalangeal joints. Active distal interphalangeal movement is judged by stabilizing the proximal interphalangeal joints and having the patient extend (10°) and flex (90°) the distal interphalangeal joints. Inspect finger abduction (20°) and adduction by having the patient place his hand flat and spread his fingers apart and then tight. Individual joint motion restriction is tested actively in all normal directions, and passively if necessary.

Kinesiology of the Fingers[310–313]

During contraction of the flexor digiti group, for example, their tendons move proximally, and this exerts a pull on the attached phalanges. The degree of tendon excursion decreases distally with each joint for about 4 cm at the wrist to less than 1 cm at the metacarpophalangeal joint, thus determining the movement of the joint involved.

Flexion. Flexion of the fingers is controlled essentially by the lateral (C7, median) and medial (C8, ulnar) lumbricals for the metacarpophalangeal joint, the flexor digiti superficialis (C7–T1) for the proximal interphalangeal joint, and the flexor digiti profundus (C8–T1) for the distal interphalangeal joint (Fig. 14.40). (See Tables 14.10 and 14.11.) To test the strength of the flexors as a whole, the patient tightly flexes the fingers with the wrist pronated. The examiner stabilizes the patient's wrist with one

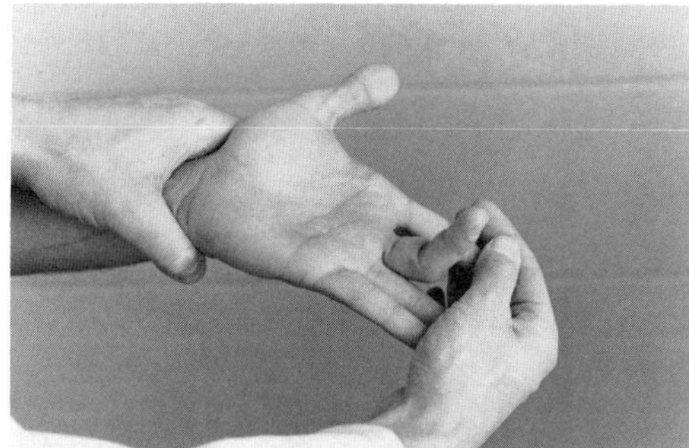

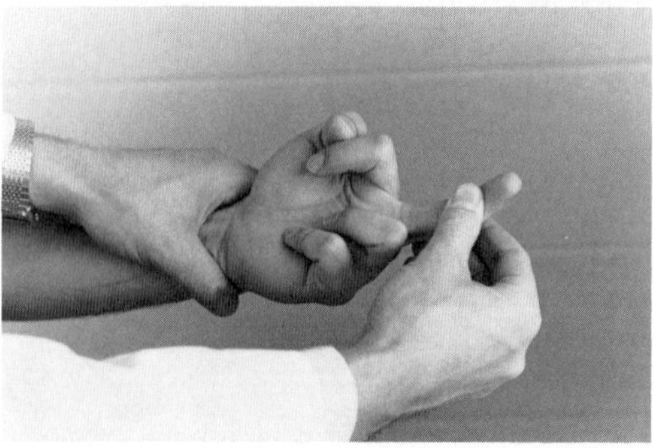

Figure 14.40. Testing the integrity of the flexor digitorum profundus tendon.

Table 14.10.
Finger Motion

Joint motion	Prime movers	Accessories
Metacarpophalangeal flexion	Interossei, dorsal Interossei, volar Lumbricales Flexor digiti minimi	Flexor digitorum profundus Flexor digitorum superficialis
Proximal interphalangeal flexion	Flexor digitorum superficialis	Flexor digitorum profundus
Distal interphalangeal flexion	Flexor digitorum profundus	
Extension	Extensor digitorum Extensor digiti minimi Extensor indicis Lumbricales Interossei, dorsal and volar	
Abduction	Interossei, dorsal Abductor digiti minimi	
Adduction	Interossei, volar	

Table 14.11.
Major Muscles of the Fingers

Muscle	Major function	Spinal segment
Abductor digiti minimi	Abduction, flexion	C8–T1
Dorsal interossei	Abduction, flex proximal, extend mid and distal phalanges	C8–T1
Extensor digiti minimi	Extension	C6–C8
Extensor digitorum	Extension	C6–C8
Extensor indicis	Extension	C7–C8
Flexor digiti minimi	Flex metacarpophalangeal joint	C8–T1
Flexor digiti profundus	Flex metacarpophalangeal, proximal, and distal interphalangeal joints	C8–T1
Flexor digiti superficialis	Flex metacarpophalangeal and proximal interphalangeal joints	C7–T1
Lumbricales	Flex metacarpophalangeal joints, extend mid and distal phalanges	C7–C8
Palmar interossei	Adduction, flex proximal, extend mid and distal phalanges	C8–T1

hand, and with his active supinated hand curls his fingertips under those of the patient's, then grasps the patient's fingers in the palm, and increasingly applies extension pressure (Fig. 14.41).

Extension. Primary finger extension is provided by the extensor digitorum (C6–C8), extensor indicis (C7–C8), and extensor digiti minimi (C8–T1). Strength is tested by stabilizing the patient's wrist in the neutral position, having the patient extend the metacarpophalangeal joints while he flexes the proximal interphalangeal joints. The examiner then places his active hand on the back of the patient's proximal phalanges and increasingly applies flexion pressure (Fig. 14.42).

Abduction. Finger abduction is produced by the dorsal interossei (C8–T1) and the abductor digiti minimi (C8–T1). Strength is tested by having the patient extend and fan the fingers. The examiner, with his thumb and first finger, applies increasing pressure to force together any two fingers being measured.

Adduction. Adduction of the fingers is controlled by the palmar interossei (C8–T1). Strength is tested by having the patient extend his fingers, keeping them together. A sheet of paper is slipped between any two fingers being tested, the patient applies maximum pressure, and the slip of paper is pulled out by the examiner, with resistance being noted.

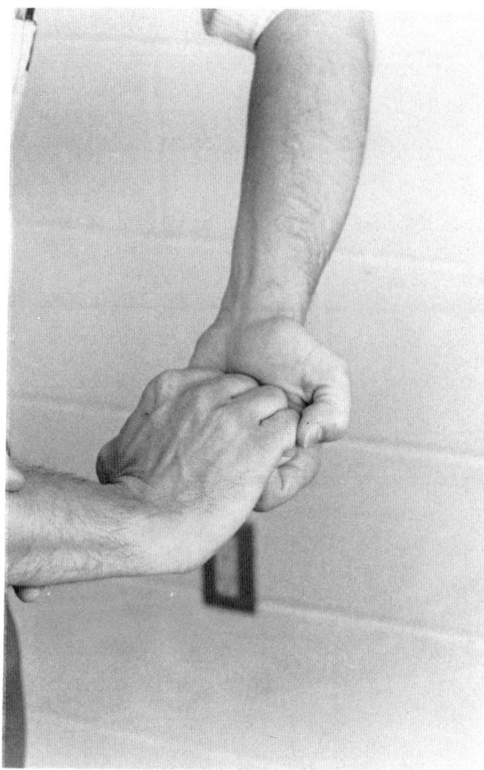

Figure 14.41. Testing grip strength against resistance.

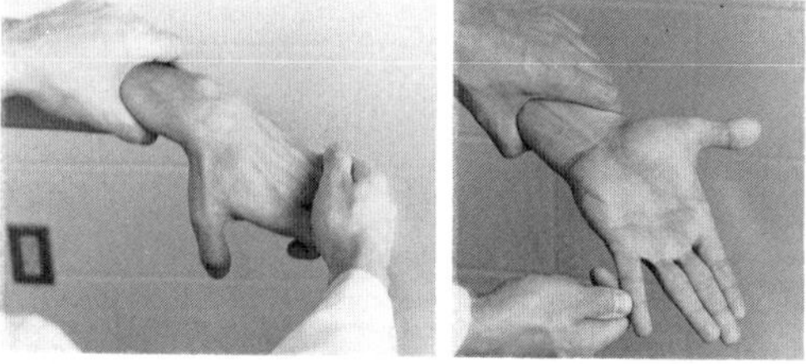

Figure 14.42. *Left*, muscle test for finger extension; *right*, muscle test for finger abduction.

Bilateral grip strength is best tested with a dynamometer and pinch strength by a pinch meter if objective data records are necessary.

Basic Finger Mechanics[306]

Finger motion is less difficult to appreciate when the proximal bone of the joint is stabilized while the distal bone moves about it. For example, the axis of flexion for an interphalangeal joint is considered to be at that point which does not move in relation to either involved digit.

The digit's flexor tendon lies close to the axis when the finger is extended, but it moves further from the axis during flexion. This creates better mechanical advantage because of the longer moment arm produced. From a biomechanical viewpoint, each tendon is considered to exert tension on the end of a lever whose vector extends from the joint axis perpendicular to the tendon.

Each tendon is held in a sling of fibrous tissue to create a series of pulleys parallel along the finger bones. If these pulleys were absent, the tendons would bowstring between the joints during flexion and fingertip control would be lost. Another important effect of these pulleys is that when the tendon changes direction across a pulley, there is an equal and opposite reaction force at the pulley that establishes a state of equilibrium; ie, the sum of the plus and minus factors is zero.

Goniometry of the Fingers[315,315]

Restricted Motion of the Metacarpophalangeal Joint of Any Finger. The patient's hand is placed in the neutral position, the goniometer is centered over the dorsum of the patient's metacarpophalangeal joint, and the neutral reading is recorded. The patient attempts to make a fist, and the reading is recorded. The patient attempts to make a fist, and the reading at the end of the motion is recorded.

Restricted Motion of the Proximal Interphalangeal Joint of Any Finger. The patient's hand is placed in the neutral position, the goniometer is centered over the dorsum of the patient's proximal interphalangeal joint, and the neutral reading is recorded. The patient flexes his proximal interphalangeal joint as far as possible, and the reading at the end of his motion is recorded for the joint being measured.

Restricted Motion of the Distal Interphalangeal Joint of Any Finger. The patient is placed in the neutral position, the goniometer is centered over the dorsum of the patient's distal interphalangeal joint, and the neutral reading is recorded. The patient flexes the distal interphalangeal joint of the finger being tested. After flexion is made as far as possible, the reading is recorded.

Trigger Points

The most common area of referred trigger-point pain in the hand is found at the distal 2–4 metacarpal area. This shown in Figure 14.43.

Structural Fixations in the Hands

Gillet[316] feels that extraspinal fixations in the hands are second in frequency only to those found in the feet. It has been his experience that these fixations are common in "hand laborers" who must grasp their tools tightly for extended periods. This tends to form a "claw hand" even during rest. If this is the case, extension will be resisted at the involved joints. Gillet reports that release of these fixations, for some unknown reason, appears to have an influence on upper midthoracic fixations, especially in the T4–T6 area.

SELECTED CLINICAL PROBLEMS OF THE FINGERS[317–324]

Finger subluxations are often left untreated by the unaware, resulting in long-term disability and, possibly, permanent deformity. Capsulitis and later arthritis are common complications.

Metacarpophalangeal and Interphalangeal Sprains[297,325]

The mechanism of metacarpophalangeal injury is one of sudden hyperextension or a severe lateral force. Subluxation, pain, and disability are often severe, and recovery is slow until the involved ligaments tighten to prevent recurring subluxation.

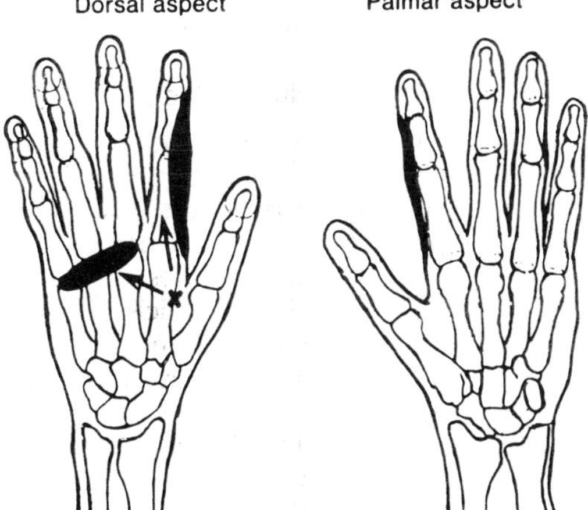

Figure 14.43. First interosseous trigger point; *X*, common site. *Blackened areas* indicate typical sites of referred pain.

The interphalangeal joints are easily sprained, torn, and dislocated. This is due to their thin capsule, delicate collateral ligaments, and slender articulations. In acute sprain, the ligament tears and allows the bone ends to subluxate and disrupt the integrity of the joint structure. Local pain, tenderness, swelling, and motion restriction are exhibited. A previously torn ligament may predispose a joint to recurring luxation because of laxity of the stabilizers.

Mallet Finger[326,327]

A hard object may strike a finger resulting in an extensor digitorum tendon injury in which the tendon avulses from its insertion at the posterior base of the terminal phalanx. The jammed distal phalanx assumes a position of about 70°. It appears "dropped" and is rigidly flexed with active distal interphalangeal extension severely limited. In such an injury, small bone fragments may be seen at the distal interphalangeal joint's posterior aspect on roentgenography. Both phalangeal fractures and extensor tendon abnormalities may produce mallet finger.

Trigger Finger[328,329]

This is an entrapment syndrome produced by scar tissue compressing an extensor tendon, often a consequence of de Quervain's disease (Fig. 14.44). Squeezing action by the constricted sheath tends to develop a pea-like mass distal to the thickening. It is most often seen in the thumb, but several fingers are sometimes affected.

Contractures[330–332]

The metacarpophalangeal joint is held in slight extension, and an attempt is made to flex the patient's proximal interphalangeal joint of any finger being tested. If the joint cannot be flexed in this position, it is a sign that the intrinsic muscles are tight or capsule contractures exist.

Retinacular Test. To distinguish between intrinsic muscle tightness and capsule contractures, the involved metacarpophalangeal joint is flexed slightly, relaxing the intrinsics, and the proximal interphalangeal

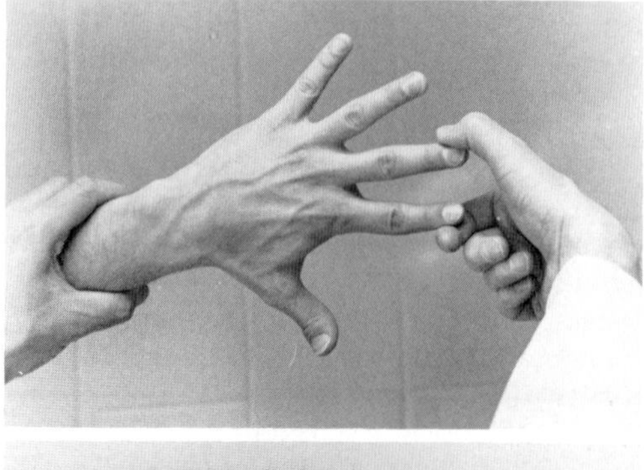

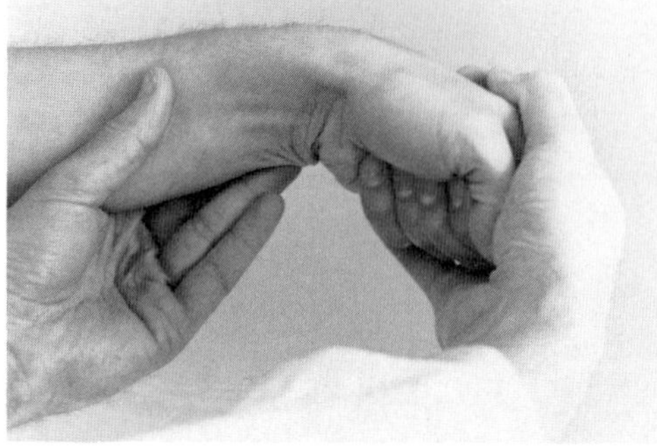

Figure 14.44. *Top*, testing the strength of the intrinsic muscles of the hand by the patient attempting to maintain the fingers spread against resistance. *Bottom*, Finkelstein's test.

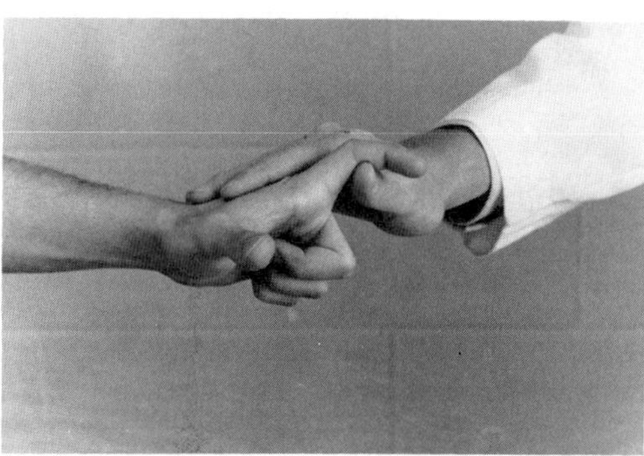

Figure 14.45. The Bunnel-Littler test to evaluate the tightness of the hand intrinsics. The examiner attempts to flex a proximal interphalangeal joint with the metacarpophalangeal joint extended a few degrees. Inability to flex a joint points to either tight intrinsics or joint capsule contracture.

joint is moved into flexion. Full flexion of the joint shows tight intrinsics; limited flexion indicates probable contracture of the interphalangeal joint capsule. This procedure is often called the Bunnel-Littler test (Fig. 14.45).

Fractures and Dislocations of the Fingers[333-335]

All severe hand traumas have a high incidence of metacarpal fractures, but severe displacement is not common.

Finger Fractures

The incidence of metacarpophalangeal thumb joint fracture-dislocation is quite high. A fracture of a proximal phalanx tends to displace anteriorly in an angular fashion because of lumbrical pull. A rotated phalanx, often noted by a fingernail's relationship with its neighbors, is an indication of fracture. It is cautioned that fracture symptoms mimic severe sprain plus abnormal bone or joint contour. Crepitus is not always exhibited in finger fractures.

Finger Dislocations

Many finger dislocations often spontaneously reduce themselves. Dislocation of the proximal interphalangeal joint usually entails severe injury of the collateral ligaments and is likely to heal with an unstable, swollen, stiff joint.

Bone length of a suspected fracture or dislocation is judged by comparing it with the uninjured hand. Abnormal motion is checked by applying axial and leverage pressure to patient tolerance. It should be kept in mind that incomplete and impacted fractures may be present, yet associated tendon, nerve, and vascular damage are not common. Comparative x-ray views of the sound limb are frequently helpful.

Miscellaneous Clinical Tests[60, 127]

Pollicis Longus Tests. The examiner stabilizes the proximal phalanx of the patient's thumb, and the patient is instructed to flex and extend the distal phalanx. Inability to flex the phalanx indicates an injury to the tendon of the flexor pollicis longus. Inability to extend the phalanx indicates an injury to the tendon of the extensor pollicis longus.

Extensor Digitorum Communis Test. The patient is instructed to first make a fist, and then to extend all fingers. Inability to extend any finger indicates an injury to that particular tendon of the extensor digitorum communis.

Kleist's Hooking Sign. The patient is instructed to place both supinated hands forward, with the elbows moderately flexed. The examiner grasps the fingers and gently moves them into extension. If the patient's fingers react into flexion rather than passively going into extension, this pathologic reflex is thought by several authorities to indicate a frontal or thalamic lesion.

Klippel-Weil's Test. The examiner quickly pries open the flexed fingers of the spastic limb. A reflex response of automatic thumb flexion and adduction indicates a pyramidal tract lesion.

Palmomental Reflex. The examiner strokes the palm of the patient with a moderately blunt instrument. In pyramidal tract disease, the ipsilateral mentalis muscle will often contract so that the lower lip will protrude and rise and the skin of the chin wrinkles so that a facial expression of contempt or scorn is produced.

REFERENCES

1. Rosse C: The shoulder region and the brachial plexus. In Rosse C, Clawson DK (eds): *The Musculoskeletal System in Health and Disease*. Hagerstown, Md, Harper & Row, 1980, pp 179–181, 183–186.
2. Basmajian JV (ed): *Grant's Method of Anatomy*, ed 9. Baltimore, Williams & Wilkins, 1975, pp 75–115, 152–155.
3. Cailliet R: *Shoulder Pain*, ed 2. Philadelphia, F.A. Davis, 1981, pp 1–37.
4. Hollingshead WH, Jenkins DB: *Functional Anatomy of the Limbs and Back*. Philadelphia, W.B. Saunders, 1981, pp 67–97.
5. Cailliet R: *Soft Tissue Pain and Disability*. Philadelphia, F.A. Davis, 1980, pp 149–154.
6. Basmajian JV: Recent advances in the functional anatomy of the upper limb. *American Journal of Physical Medicine* 48:165–177, 1969.
7. Barham JN, Wooten EP: *Structural Kinesiology*. New York, Macmillan, 1973, pp 283–296.
8. Morehouse LE, Cooper JM: *Kinesiology*. St. Louis, C.V. Mosby, 1950, pp 51–57.
9. Esch D, Lepley M: *Musculoskeletal Function: An Anatomy and Kinesiology Laboratory Manual*. Minneapolis, University of Minnesota Press, 1974, pp 13–14.
10. Morehouse LE, Cooper JM: *Kinesiology*. St. Louis, C.V. Mosby, 1950, p 44.
11. Rosse C: The shoulder region and the brachial plexus. In Rosse C, Clawson DK (eds): *The Musculoskeletal System in Health and Disease*. Hagerstown, Md, Harper & Row, 1980, pp 181–183, 186–190, 193.
12. Kapandji IA: *Physiology of the Joints: Upper Limb*, ed 2. New York, Churchill Livingstone, 1980, vol 1, pp 10–77.
13. Basmajian JV (ed): *Grant's Method of Anatomy*, ed 9. Baltimore, Williams & Wilkins, 1975, pp 155–156, 160–161.
14. Hollingshead WH, Jenkins DB: *Functional Anatomy of the Limbs and Back*. Philadelphia, W.B. Saunders, 1981, pp 97–108.
15. Riggins RS: The shoulder. In D'Ambrosia RD: *Musculoskeletal Disorders: Regional Examination and Differential Diagnosis*. Philadelphia, J.B. Lippincott, 1977, pp 320–328.
16. Inman VT et al: The function of the shoulder joint. *Journal of Bone and Joint Surgery* 26A:1–30, 1944.
17. Mennell JMcM: *Joint Pain*. Boston, Little, Brown, 1964, pp 78–90.
18. Barham JN, Wooten EP: *Structural Kinesiology*. New York, Macmillan, 1973, pp 305–315.
19. Gowitzke BA, Milner M: *Understanding Scientific Basis of Human Movement*, ed 2. Baltimore, Williams & Wilkins, 1980, pp 33–36.
20. Hoppenfeld S: *Physical Examination of the Spine and Extremities*. New York, Appleton-Century-Crofts, 1976, pp 20–25.
21. Daniels L, Worthingham C: *Muscle Testing: Techniques of Manual Examination*, ed 4. Philadelphia, W.B. Saunders, 1980, pp 90–118.
22. Kendall HO, Kendall FP, Wadsworth GE: *Muscles: Testing and Function*, ed 2. Baltimore, Williams & Wilkins, 1971, pp 102–133.
23. Hoppenfeld S: *Physical Examination of the Spine and Extremities*. New York, Appleton-Century-Crofts, 1976, pp 25–32.
24. Esch D, Lepley M: *Musculoskeletal Function: An Anatomy and Kinesiology Laboratory Manual*. Minneapolis, University of Minnesota Press, 1974, pp 73–87.
25. Bennett RL: Muscle testing: A discussion of the importance of accurate muscle testing. *Physiotherapy Review* 27:242–243, 1947.
26. Goodheart GJ: *Applied Kinesiology*. City of publication not shown, published by the author, privately distributed, 1964, pp 44–53, 58, 59–62.
27. Walther DS: *Applied Kinesiology*. Pueblo, Colo, Systems DC, 1981, vol 1, p 146.
28. Goodheart, GJ: Reactive muscle patterns in athletes. Presentation at Biomechanics and Kinesiology in Sports, an Olympic Sports Medicine Conference, Colorado Springs, January 1984. Sponsored by the U.S. Olympic Committee.
29. Esch D, Lepley M: *Evaluation of Joint Motion: Methods of Measurement and Recording*. Minneapolis, University of Minnesota Press, 1974, pp 14–17.
30. Schafer RC (ed): *Basic Chiropractic Procedural Manual*, ed 4. Arlington, Va, American Chiropractic Association, 1984, pp 301–304.
31. Grieve GP: *Common Vertebral Joint Problems*. New York, Churchill Livingstone, 1981, pp 324–325.
32. Cailliet R: *Soft Tissue Pain and Disability*. Philadelphia, F.A. Davis, 1980, pp 154–167.
33. Hirata I Jr: *The Doctor and the Athlete*, ed 2. Philadelphia, J.B. Lippincott, 1974, pp 135–137.
34. Schoenholtz F: Conservative management of se-

lected shoulder problems. *ACA Journal of Chiropractic* October 1979.

35. Kane WJ (ed): *Current Orthopaedic Management.* New York, Churchill Livingstone, 1980.
36. Hadler NM: *Medical Management of the Regional Musculoskeletal Diseases.* New York, Grune & Stratton, 1984, pp 105–136.
37. Rosse C: The shoulder region and the brachial plexus. In Rosse C, Clawson DK (eds): *The Musculoskeletal System in Health and Disease.* Hagerstown, Md, Harper & Row, 1980, p 192.
38. Mills KLG: *Guide to Orthopaedics.* New York, Churchill Livingstone, 1981.
39. Kendall HO, Kendall FP, Wadsworth GE: *Muscles: Testing and Function,* ed 2. Baltimore, Williams & Wilkins, 1971, pp 135–139.
40. Daniels L, Worthingham C: *Therapeutic Exercise for Body Alignment and Function,* ed 2. Philadelphia, W.B. Saunders, 1977, pp 66–72.
41. Riggins RS: The shoulder. In D'Ambrosia RD: *Musculoskeletal Disorders: Regional Examination and Differential Diagnosis.* Philadelphia, J.B. Lippincott, 1977, pp 331–332.
42. Basmajian JV (ed): *Grant's Method of Anatomy,* ed 9. Baltimore, Williams & Wilkins, 1975, p 157.
43. Van Dusen LG: *Chiropractic Relationship to Gravitational Force.* Sodus, NY, published by the author, 1968, pp 109, 119, 105, 107.
44. Craig AS: Elements of kinesiology for the clinician. *Physical Therapy* 44:470–473, 1964.
45. Brunnstrom S: Muscle group testing. *Physiotherapy Review* 21:3–21, 1941.
46. Nelson WA: Personal communication, 1980.
47. Schafer RC: *Chiropractic Management of Sports and Recreational Injuries.* Baltimore, Williams & Wilkins, 1982, pp 370–371.
48. Ng SY: Skeletal muscle spasm: various methods to relieve it. *ACA Journal of Chiropractic* February 1980.
49. Stierwalt DD: Effective usage of heat and cold for back and extremity injuries. *The Digest of Chiropractic Economics* May/June 1983.
50. Wood KW: Myospasm, myostrain, and myalgia. *The Digest of Chiropractic Economics* May/June 1985.
51. Michelle AA, Eisenberg J: Scapulocostal syndrome. *Archives of Physical Medicine and Rehabilitation* 49:383–387, 1968.
52. Weed, ND: When shoulder pain isn't bursitis. *Postgraduate Medicine* 73(3):97–104, September 1983.
53. Rocks JA: Intrinsic shoulder pain syndrome. *Physical Therapy* 59:153–159, 1979.
54. Jacobs RC: Painful shoulder. In Friedman HH (ed): *Problem-Oriented Medical Diagnosis,* ed 2. Boston, Little, Brown, 1979, pp 261–264.
55. Wilson FC (ed): *The Musculoskeletal System: Basic Processes and Disorders,* ed 2. Philadelphia, J.B. Lippincott, 1983, pp 257–272.
56. Hart FD (ed): *French's Index of Differential Diagnosis,* ed 12, Bristol, England, Wright, 1985, pp 764–767.
57. Goodheart GL: *Collected Published Articles and Reprints.* Montpellier, O, Williams County Publishing, 1969, pp 14–16.
58. Williams JGP, Sperryn PN (eds): *Sports Medicine,* ed 2. Baltimore, Williams & Wilkins, 1976, p 392.
59. Iverson LD, Clawson DK: *Manual of Acute Orthopaedic Therapeutics.* Boston, Little, Brown, 1977, pp 140–141.
60. Mazion JM: *Illustrated Manual of Neurological Reflexes/Signs/Tests, Orthopedic Signs/Tests/Maneuvers,* ed 2. Arizona City, published by the author, 1980.
61. Riggins RS: The shoulder. In D'Ambrosia RD: *Musculoskeletal Disorders: Regional Examination and Differential Diagnosis.* Philadelphia, J.B. Lippincott, 1977, pp 334–335.
62. Scott WN, Nisonson B, Nicholas JA (eds): *Principles of Sports Medicine.* Baltimore, Williams & Wilkins, 1984, p 120.
63. Hirata I Jr: *The Doctor and the Athlete,* ed 2. Philadelphia, J.B. Lippincott, 1974, pp 146–147.
64. Riggins RS: The shoulder. In D'Ambrosia RD: *Musculoskeletal Disorders: Regional Examination and Differential Diagnosis.* Philadelphia, J.B. Lippincott, 1977, pp 333–334.
65. Schafer RC: *Chiropractic Management of Sports and Recreational Injuries.* Baltimore, Williams & Wilkins, 1982, p 382.
66. Schneider RC, Kennedy JC, Plant ML (eds): *Sports Injuries: Mechanisms, Prevention, and Treatment.* Baltimore, Williams & Wilkins, 1985, pp 565–566, 703.
67. Cipriano JJ: *Photographic Manual of Regional Orthopaedic Tests.* Baltimore, Williams & Wilkins, 1985, p 117.
68. Mazion JM: *Illustrated Manual of Neurological Reflexes/Signs/Tests; Orthopedic Signs/Tests/Maneuvers,* ed 2. Arizona City, published by the author, 1980, p 255.
69. Cyriax J: *Textbook of Orthopaedic Medicine. Vol 1, Diagnosis of Soft Tissue Lesions,* ed 8. London, Bailliere Tindall, 1982, p 166.
70. Schneider RC, Kennedy JC, Plant ML (eds): *Sports Injuries: Mechanisms, Prevention, and Treatment.* Baltimore, Williams & Wilkins, 1985, p 709.
71. Williams JGP, Sperryn PN (eds): *Sports Medicine,* ed 2. Baltimore, Williams & Wilkins, 1976, pp 390–391.
72. Rizk TE, Pinals RS: Frozen shoulder. *Arthritis and Rheumatism* 11:440–452, 1982.
73. Schafer RC: *Chiropractic Management of Sports and Recreational Injuries.* Baltimore, Williams & Wilkins, 1982, pp 382–383.
74. Hadler NM: *Medical Management of the Regional Musculoskeletal Diseases.* New York, Grune & Stratton, 1984, p 118.
75. Schafer RC: *Chiropractic Management of Sports and Recreational Injuries.* Baltimore, Williams & Wilkins, 1982, p 383.
76. Bennett TJ: *A New Clinical Basis for the Correction of Abnormal Physiology* (Formerly, *Autonomic Nerve Control*). Burlingame, Cal, published by the author, 1960.
77. Slocum DB: The mechanics of some common injuries to the shoulder in sports. *American Journal of Surgery* 98:394–400, 1959.
78. Harrington IJ: Biomechanics of joint injuries. In

Gonzna ER, Harrington IJ: *Biomechanics of Musculoskeletal Injury*. Baltimore, Williams & Wilkins, 1982, pp 67–70, 75–79.

79. Rosse C: The shoulder region and the brachial plexus. In Rosse C, Clawson DK (eds): *The Musculoskeletal System in Health and Disease*. Hagerstown, Md, Harper & Row, 1980, pp 196–197.
80. Barham JN, Wooten EP: *Structural Kinesiology*. New York, Macmillan, 1973, pp 315–316.
81. Elftman H: Biomechanics of muscle. *Journal of Bone and Joint Surgery* 48A:363–377, 1966.
82. Frankel VH, Nordin M: *Basic Biomechanics of the Skeletal System*. Philadelphia, Lea & Febiger, 1980.
83. Cailliet R: *Shoulder Pain*, ed 2. Philadelphia, F.A. Davis, 1981, pp 38–47, 74–76, 82–85.
84. Scott WN, Nisonson B, Nicholas JA (eds): *Principles of Sports Medicine*. Baltimore, Williams & Wilkins, 1984, pp 118–121, 125–128.
85. Sarrafian SK: Gross and functional anatomy of the shoulder. *Clinical Orthopaedics and Related Research* 173:11–19, 1983.
86. Tullos HS, King JW: Throwing mechanism in sports. *Orthopedic Clinics of North America* 4:709–720, 1973.
87. Hirata I Jr: *The Doctor and the Athlete*, ed 2. Philadelphia, J.B. Lippincott, 1974, pp 156–157.
88. Rosse C: The shoulder region and the brachial plexus. In Rosse C, Clawson DK (eds): *The Musculoskeletal System in Health and Disease*. Hagerstown, Md, Harper & Row, 1980, pp 190–191.
89. Schafer RC: *Chiropractic Management of Sports and Recreational Injuries*. Baltimore, Williams & Wilkins, 1982, p 379.
90. Cailliet R: *Shoulder Pain*, ed 2. Philadelphia, F.A. Davis, 1981, pp. 137–139.
91. Hirata I Jr: *The Doctor and the Athlete*, ed 2. Philadelphia, J.B. Lippincott, 1974, pp 159–160.
92. Hoppenfeld S: *Physical Examination of the Spine and Extremities*. New York, Appleton-Century-Crofts, 1976, p 32.
93. Mazion JM: *Illustrated Manual of Neurological Reflexes/Signs/Tests, Orthopedic Signs/Tests/Maneuvers*, ed 2. Arizona City, published by the author, 1980, p 376.
94. Schafer RC: *Chiropractic Management of Sports and Recreational Injuries*. Baltimore, Williams & Wilkins, 1982, p 365.
95. Turek SL: *Orthopaedics: Principles and Their Application*, ed 3. Philadelphia, J.B. Lippincott, 1977, p 834.
96. Schafer RC: *Chiropractic Management of Sports and Recreational Injuries*. Baltimore, Williams & Wilkins, 1985, p 133.
97. Cipriano JJ: *Photographic Manual of Regional Orthopaedic Tests*. Baltimore, Williams & Wilkins, 1985, p 133.
98. Hirata I Jr: *The Doctor and the Athlete*, ed 2. Philadelphia, J.B. Lippincott, 1974, pp 147–149.
99. Scott WN, Nisonson B, Nicholas JA (eds): *Principles of Sports Medicine*. Baltimore, Williams & Wilkins, 1984, pp 118–121.
100. Schneider RC, Kennedy JC, Plant ML (eds): *Sports Injuries: Mechanisms, Prevention, and Treatment*. Baltimore, Williams & Wilkins, 1985, 699, 702, 704–707.
101. Rosse C: The shoulder region and the brachial plexus. In Rosse C, Clawson DK (eds): *The Musculoskeletal System in Health and Disease*. Hagerstown, Md, Harper & Row, 1980, pp 188–189.
102. LeVeau B: *Williams and Lissner: Biomechanics of Human Motion*, ed 2. Philadelphia, W.B. Saunders, 1977, pp 115–117, 130–131.
103. Basmajian JV (ed): *Grant's Method of Anatomy*, ed 9. Baltimore, Williams & Wilkins, 1975, p 161.
104. Hoppenfeld S: *Physical Examination of the Spine and Extremities*. New York, Appleton-Century-Crofts, 1976, p 33.
105. Williams JGP, Sperryn PN (eds): *Sports Medicine*, ed 2. Baltimore, Williams & Wilkins, 1976, pp 391–392.
106. Tullos HS, Bennett JB: The shoulder in sports. In Scott WN et al (eds): *Principles of Sports Medicine*. Baltimore, Williams & Wilkins, 1984, pp 110–138.
107. Brewer BJ: Aging and the rotator cuff. *American Journal of Sports Medicine* 7:102–110, 1979.
108. Hirata I Jr: *The Doctor and the Athlete*, ed 2. Philadelphia, J.B. Lippincott, 1974, pp 144–146.
109. Schafer RC: *Chiropractic Management of Sports and Recreational Injuries*. Baltimore, Williams & Wilkins, 1982, pp 368–369.
110. Hirata I Jr: *The Doctor and the Athlete*, ed 2. Philadelphia, J.B. Lippincott, 1974, pp 160–161.
111. Schultz AL: *The Shoulder, Arm, and Hand Syndrome*. Stickney, SD, Argus, 1969, pp 152–161, 186–192, 200–203, 206–214.
112. Janse J, Houser RH, Wells BF: *Chiropractic Principles and Technic*. Chicago, National College of Chiropractic, 1947, pp 523–546.
113. Gertler L: *Illustrated Manual of Extravertebral Technic*, ed 2. Bayside, NY, published by the author, 1978, pp 64–87.
114. Riggins RS: The shoulder. In D'Ambrosia RD: *Musculoskeletal Disorders: Regional Examination and Differential Diagnosis*. Philadelphia, J.B. Lippincott, 1977, p 336.
115. Maitland GD: *Peripheral Manipulation*. Boston, Butterworths, 1976, pp 25–51.
116. Schultz AL: *The Shoulder, Arm, and Hand Syndrome*. Stickney, SD, Argus, 1969, p 154.
117. Cailliet R: *Shoulder Pain*, ed 2. Philadelphia, F.A. Davis, 1981, pp 125–136.
118. Bowerman JW: *Radiology and Injury in Sport*. New York, Appleton-Century-Crofts, 1977, pp 61–64.
119. Williams JGP, Sperryn PN (eds): *Sports Medicine*, ed 2. Baltimore, Williams & Wilkins, 1976, pp 387–390.
120. Gertler L: *Illustrated Manual of Extravertebral Technic*, ed 2. Bayside, NY, published by the author, 1978, pp 88–95.
121. Schultz AL: *The Shoulder, Arm, and Hand Syndrome*. Stickney, SD, Argus, 1969, pp 127–136, 146–152.
122. Janse J, Houser RH, Wells BF: *Chiropractic Principles and Technic*. Chicago, National College of Chiropractic, 1947, pp 546–552.
123. Stierwalt DD: *Extremity Adjusting*. Davenport, Ia, published by the author, 1975, pp 13–15.

124. Hirata I Jr: *The Doctor and the Athlete*, ed 2. Philadelphia, J.B. Lippincott, 1974, pp 152–156.
125. Holmes GW, Robbins LL: *Roentgen Interpretation*, ed 7. Philadelphia, Lea & Febiger, 1947, p 48.
126. Hoppenfeld S: *Physical Examination of the Spine and Extremities*. New York, Appleton-Century-Crofts, 1976, p 34.
127. Cipriano JJ: *Photographic Manual of Regional Orthopaedic Tests*. Baltimore, Williams & Wilkins, 1985.
128. Riggins RS: The shoulder. In D'Ambrosia RD: *Musculoskeletal Disorders: Regional Examination and Differential Diagnosis*. Philadelphia, J.B. Lippincott, 1977, pp 343–344.
129. Teranel JA: *Chiropractic Orthopedics and Roentgenology*. Newark, NJ, Medusa Press, 1953, pp 31, 392–394.
130. Bowerman JW: *Radiology and Injury in Sport*. New York, Appleton-Century-Crofts, 1977, pp 64–65, 150, 155–158.
131. Riggins RS: The shoulder. In D'Ambrosia RD: *Musculoskeletal Disorders: Regional Examination and Differential Diagnosis*. Philadelphia, J.B. Lippincott, 1977, pp 342–343.
132. Hirata I Jr: *The Doctor and the Athlete*, ed 2. Philadelphia, J.B. Lippincott, 1974, pp 137–138.
133. Riggins RS: The shoulder. In D'Ambrosia RD: *Musculoskeletal Disorders: Regional Examination and Differential Diagnosis*. Philadelphia, J.B. Lippincott, 1977, p 332.
134. Williams JGP, Sperryn PN (eds): *Sports Medicine*, ed 2. Baltimore, Williams & Wilkins, 1976, p 395.
135. Maitland GD: *Peripheral Manipulation*. Boston, Butterworths, 1976, pp 51–54.
136. Stierwalt DD: *Extremity Adjusting*. Davenport, Ia, published by the author, 1975, pp 16.
137. Schultz AL: *The Shoulder, Arm, and Hand Syndrome*. Stickney, SD, Argus, 1969, pp 183–186.
138. Teranel JA: *Chiropractic Orthopedics and Roentgenology*. Newark, NJ, Medusa Press, 1953, p 395.
139. Riggins RS: The shoulder. In D'Ambrosia RD: *Musculoskeletal Disorders: Regional Examination and Differential Diagnosis*. Philadelphia, J.B. Lippincott, 1977, p 343.
140. Bowerman JW: *Radiology and Injury in Sport*. New York, Appleton-Century-Crofts, 1977, pp 53–61.
141. McLaughlin HL: *Trauma*. Philadelphia, W.B. Saunders, 1959.
142. Schultz AL: *The Shoulder, Arm, and Hand Syndrome*. Stickney, SD, Argus, 1969, pp 110–112.
143. Hirata I Jr: *The Doctor and the Athlete*, ed 2. Philadelphia, J.B. Lippincott, 1974, pp 140–143.
144. Maitland GD: *Peripheral Manipulation*. Boston, Butterworths, 1976, pp 54–56.
145. Stierwalt DD: *Extremity Adjusting*. Davenport, Ia, published by the author, 1975, p 12.
146. Riggins RS: The shoulder. In D'Ambrosia RD: *Musculoskeletal Disorders: Regional Examination and Differential Diagnosis*. Philadelphia, J.B. Lippincott, 1977, pp 344–345.
147. Schultz AL: *The Shoulder, Arm, and Hand Syndrome*. Stickney, SD, Argus, 1969, p 117.
148. Bjerneld H, Hovelius L, Thorling J: Acromioclavicular separations treated conservatively: A five year follow up study. *Acta Orthopaedica Scandinavica* 54:743–745, 1983.
149. Schultz AL: *The Shoulder, Arm, and Hand Syndrome*. Stickney, SD, Argus, 1969, p 111.
150. Gertler L: *Illustrated Manual of Extravertebral Technic*, ed 2. Bayside, NY, published by the author, 1978, pp 96–99.
151. Stierwalt DD: *Extremity Adjusting*. Davenport, Ia, published by the author, 1975, pp 8, 11.
152. Janse J, Houser RH, Wells BF: *Chiropractic Principles and Technic*. Chicago, National College of Chiropractic, 1947, p 560.
153. Gillet H, Liekens M: *Belgian Chiropractic Research Notes*. Huntington Beach, Cal, Motion Palpation Institute, 1981, pp 90–91.
154. Iverson LD, Clawson DK: *Manual of Acute Orthopaedic Therapeutics*. Boston, Little, Brown, 1977, pp 129–133.
155. Turek SL: *Orthopaedics: Principles and Their Application*, ed 3. Philadelphia, J.B. Lippincott, 1977, pp 854–855, 857–858.
156. Dalinka MK: Ankle fractures and fractures and dislocation about the shoulder. In Feldman F (ed): *Radiology, Pathology, and Immunology of Bones and Joints*. New York, Appleton-Century-Crofts, 1978.
157. Williams JGP, Sperryn PN (eds): *Sports Medicine*, ed 2. Baltimore, Williams & Wilkins, 1976, p 384.
158. Riggins RS: The shoulder. In D'Ambrosia RD: *Musculoskeletal Disorders: Regional Examination and Differential Diagnosis*. Philadelphia, J.B. Lippincott, 1977, p 342.
159. Teranel JA: *Chiropractic Orthopedics and Roentgenology*. Newark, NJ, Medusa Press, 1953, p 394.
160. Hollingshead WH, Jenkins DB: *Functional Anatomy of the Limbs and Back*. Philadelphia, W.B. Saunders, 1981, pp 112–124, 127–157.
161. Barham JN, Wooten EP: *Structural Kinesiology*. New York, Macmillan, 1973, pp 323–325, 326–327, 331–335.
162. Kapandji IA: *Physiology of the Joints: Upper Limb*, ed 2. New York, Churchill Livingstone, 1980, vol 1, pp 78–89, 106–111.
163. Rosse C: The arm, forearm, and wrist. In Rosse C, Clawson DK (eds): *The Musculoskeletal System in Health and Disease*. Hagerstown, Md, Harper & Row, 1980, pp 199–201, 202–210, 212.
164. Morehouse LE, Cooper JM: *Kinesiology*. St. Louis, C.V. Mosby, 1950, pp 57–66.
165. Basmajian JV (eds): *Grant's Method of Anatomy*, ed 9. Baltimore, Williams & Wilkins, 1975, pp 109–124, 161–165.
166. Esch D, Lepley M: *Musculoskeletal Function: An Anatomy and Kinesiology Laboratory Manuel*. Minneapolis, University of Minnesota Press, 1974, p 15.
167. Rosse C: The arm, forearm, and wrist. In Rosse C, Clawson DK (eds): *The Musculoskeletal System in Health and Disease*. Hagerstown, Md, Harper & Row, 1980, pp 210–212.
168. Kapandji IA: *Physiology of the Joints: Upper Limb*,

ed 2. New York, Churchill Livingstone, 1980, vol 1, pp 90–101, 112–121.
169. Daniels L, Worthingham C: *Muscle Testing: Techniques of Manual Examination*, ed 4. Philadelphia, W.B. Saunders, 1980, pp 118–127.
170. Hollingshead WH, Jenkins DB: *Functional Anatomy of the Limbs and Back*. Philadelphia, W.B. Saunders, 1981, pp 124–125.
171. Gowitzke BA, Milner M: *Understanding Scientific Basis of Human Movement*, ed 2. Baltimore, Williams & Wilkins, 1980, p 23.
172. Gillet H, Liekens M: *Belgian Chiropractic Research Notes*. Huntington Beach, Cal, Motion Palpation Institute, 1981, p 92.
173. Barham JN, Wooten EP: *Structural Kinesiology*. New York, Macmillan, 1973, pp 351–352.
174. Hoppenfeld S: *Physical Examination of the Spine and Extremities*. New York, Appleton-Century-Crofts, 1976, pp 50–51.
175. Chuinard RG: The upper extremity: Elbow, forearm, wrist and hand. In D'Ambrosia RD: *Musculoskeletal Disorders: Regional Examination and Differential Diagnosis*. Philadelphia, J.B. Lippincott, 1977, p 360.
176. Mennell JMcM: *Joint Pain*. Boston, Little, Brown, 1964, pp 68–77.
177. Esch D, Lepley M: *Musculoskeletal Function: An Anatomy and Kinesiology Laboratory Manual*. Minneapolis, University of Minnesota Press, 1974, pp 88–91.
178. Kendall HO, Kendall FP, Wadsworth GE: *Muscles: Testing and Function*, ed 2. Baltimore, Williams & Wilkins, 1971, pp 96–102.
179. Hoppenfeld S: *Physical Examination of the Spine and Extremities*. New York, Appleton-Century-Crofts, 1976, pp 51–53.
180. Esch D, Lepley M: *Evaluation of Joint Motion: Methods of Measurement and Recording*. Minneapolis, University of Minnesota Press, 1974, pp 18–19.
181. Schafer RC (ed): *Basic Chiropractic Procedural Manual*, ed 4. Arlington, Va, American Chiropractic Association, 1984, pp 304–308.
182. Schafer RC: *Chiropractic Management of Sports and Recreational Injuries*. Baltimore, Williams & Wilkins, 1982, p 389.
183. Cailliet R: *Soft Tissue Pain and Disability*. Philadelphia, F.A. Davis, 1980, pp 168–178.
184. LeVeau B: *Williams and Lissner: Biomechanics of Human Motion*, ed 2. Philadelphia, W.B. Saunders, 1977, pp 130–134.
185. Rosse C: The arm, forearm, and wrist. In Rosse C, Clawson DK (eds): *The Musculoskeletal System in Health and Disease*. Hagerstown, Md, Harper & Row, 1980, pp 222–224.
186. Barham JN, Wooten EP: *Structural Kinesiology*. New York, Macmillan, 1973, pp 363–364.
187. Parkes JC: Common injuries about the elbow in sports. In Scott, WN et al (eds): *Principles of Sports Medicine*. Baltimore, Williams & Wilkins, 1984, pp 140–154.
188. Bowerman JW: *Radiology and Injury in Sport*. New York, Appleton-Century-Crofts, 1977, p 67.
189. Bowerman JW: *Radiology and Injury in Sport*. New York, Appleton-Century-Crofts, 1977, p 5.
190. Hirata I Jr: *The Doctor and the Athlete*, ed 2. Philadelphia, J.B. Lippincott, 1974, pp 162–166, 167–168.
191. Williams JGP, Sperryn PN (eds): *Sports Medicine*, ed 2. Baltimore, Williams & Wilkins, 1976, p 403.
192. Hirata I Jr: *The Doctor and the Athlete*, ed 2. Philadelphia, J.B. Lippincott, 1974, p 162.
193. Harrington IJ: Biomechanics of joint injuries. In Gonzna ER, Harrington IJ: *Biomechanics of Musculoskeletal Injury*. Baltimore, Williams & Wilkins, 1982, pp 71–75.
194. Black J, Dumbleton JH (eds): *Clinical Biomechanics: Case History Approach*. New York, Churchill Livingstone, 1981, pp 62–69.
195. Miller DI, Nelson RC: *Biomechanics of Sport*. Philadelphia, Lea & Febiger, 1973.
196. Schafer RC: *Chiropractic Management of Sports and Recreational Injuries*. Baltimore, Williams & Wilkins, 1982, pp 386–387.
197. Hoppenfeld S: *Physical Examination of the Spine and Extremities*. New York, Appleton-Century-Crofts, 1976, p 56.
198. Chuinard RG: The upper extremity: Elbow, forearm, wrist and hand. In D'Ambrosia RD: *Musculoskeletal Disorders: Regional Examination and Differential Diagnosis*. Philadelphia, J.B. Lippincott, 1977, pp 384–385.
199. Williams JGP, Sperryn PN (eds): *Sports Medicine*, ed 2. Baltimore, Williams & Wilkins, 1976, pp 404–410.
200. Morehouse LE, Rash PJ: *Sports Medicine for Trainers*, ed 2. Philadelphia, W.B. Saunders, 1963.
201. Bowerman JW: *Radiology and Injury in Sport*. New York, Appleton-Century-Crofts, 1977, pp 251–254.
202. Hasemeir RR: The elbow. Part 3. *Roentgenological Briefs*, Council on Roentgenology of the American Chiropractic Association (undated).
203. Hoppenfeld S: *Physical Examination of the Spine and Extremities*. New York, Appleton-Century-Crofts, 1976, p 57.
204. Mazion JM: *Illustrated Manual of Neurological Reflexes/Signs/Tests, Orthopaedic Signs/Tests/Maneuvers*, ed 2. Arizona City, published by the author, 1980, p 253.
205. Schafer RC: *Chiropractic Management of Sports and Recreational Injuries*. Baltimore, Williams & Wilkins, 1982, p 388.
206. Cipriano JJ: *Photographic Manual of Regional Orthopaedic Tests*. Baltimore, Williams & Wilkins, 1985, p 141.
207. Mazion JM: *Illustrated Manual of Neurological Reflexes/Signs/Tests, Orthopedic Signs/Tests/Maneuvers*, ed 2. Arizona City, published by the author, 1980, p 296.
208. Chuinard RG: The upper extremity: Elbow, forearm, wrist and hand. In D'Ambrosia RD: *Musculoskeletal Disorders: Regional Examination and Differential Diagnosis*. Philadelphia, J.B. Lippincott, 1977, pp 381–382.
209. Hirata I Jr: *The Doctor and the Athlete*, ed 2. Philadelphia, J.B. Lippincott, 1974, pp 166–167.
210. Schultz AL: *The Shoulder, Arm, and Hand Syn-*

drome. Stickney, SD, Argus, 1969, pp 215–219, 222–227.
211. Janse J, Houser RH, Wells BF: *Chiropractic Principles and Technic*. Chicago, National College of Chiropractic, 1947, pp 552–554.
212. Stierwalt DD: *Extremity Adjusting*. Davenport, Ia, published by the author, 1975, pp 17–20.
213. Maitland GD: *Peripheral Manipulation*. Boston, Butterworths, 1976, pp 59–80.
214. Gertler L: *Illustrated Manual of Extravertebral Technic*, ed 2. Bayside, NY, published by the author, 1978, pp 57–63.
215. Teranel JA: *Chiropractic Orthopedics and Roentgenology*. Newark, NJ, Medusa Press, 1953, p 308.
216. Holmes GW, Robbins LL: *Roentgen Interpretation*, ed 7. Philadelphia, Lea & Febiger, 1947, p 47.
217. Chuinard RG: The upper extremity: Elbow, forearm, wrist and hand. In D'Ambrosia RD: *Musculoskeletal Disorders: Regional Examination and Differential Diagnosis*. Philadelphia, J.B. Lippincott, 1977, pp 389, 390.
218. Teranel JA: *Chiropractic Orthopedics and Roentgenology*. Newark, NJ, Medusa Press, 1953, pp 307, 389–392.
219. Hirata I Jr: *The Doctor and the Athlete*, ed 2. Philadelphia, J.B. Lippincott, 1974, pp 161–162.
220. Williams JGP, Sperryn PN (eds): *Sports Medicine*, ed 2. Baltimore, Williams & Wilkins, 1976, pp 397–401.
221. Bowerman JW: *Radiology and Injury in Sport*. New York, Appleton-Century-Crofts, 1977, pp 67, 70, 153.
222. Chuinard RG: The upper extremity: Elbow, forearm, wrist and hand. In D'Ambrosia RD: *Musculoskeletal Disorders: Regional Examination and Differential Diagnosis*. Philadelphia, J.B. Lippincott, 1977, pp 385–387.
223. Cyriax J: *Textbook of Orthopaedic Medicine. Vol 1, Diagnosis of Soft Tissue Lesions*, ed 8. London, Bailliere Tindall, 1982, pp 175–177.
224. Cailliet R: *Hand Pain and Impairment*. Philadelphia, F.A. Davis, 1975, pp 1–14.
225. Basmajian JV (eds): *Grant's Method of Anatomy*, ed 9. Baltimore, Williams & Wilkins, 1975, pp 165–168.
226. Kapandji IA: *Physiology of the Joints: Upper Limb*, ed 2. New York, Churchill Livingstone, 1980, vol 1, pp 122–135, 152.
227. Barham JN, Wooten EP: *Structural Kinesiology*. New York, Macmillan, 1973, pp 325–326, 328–329.
228. Hollingshead WH, Jenkins DB: *Functional Anatomy of the Limbs and Back*. Philadelphia, W.B. Saunders, 1981, pp 166–171.
229. Rosse C: The arm, forearm, and wrist. In Rosse C, Clawson DK (eds): *The Musculoskeletal System in Health and Disease*. Hagerstown, Md, Harper & Row, 1980, pp 201–202, 216–222.
230. Morehouse LE, Cooper JM: *Kinesiology*. St. Louis, C.V. Mosby, 1950, pp 67–68.
231. Esch D, Lepley M: *Musculoskeletal Function: An Anatomy and Kinesiology Laboratory Manual*. Minneapolis, University of Minnesota Press, 1974, p 16.
232. Daniels L, Worthingham C: *Muscle Testing: Techniques of Manual Examination*, ed 4. Philadelphia, W.B. Saunders, 1980, pp 128–131.
233. Hollingshead WH, Jenkins DB: *Functional Anatomy of the Limbs and Back*. Philadelphia, W.B. Saunders, 1981, pp 158–165.
234. Rosse C: The arm, forearm, and wrist. In Rosse C, Clawson DK (eds): *The Musculoskeletal System in Health and Disease*. Hagerstown, Md, Harper & Row, 1980, pp 212–214.
235. Kapandji IA: *Physiology of the Joints: Upper Limb*, ed 2. New York, Churchill Livingstone, 1980, vol 1, pp 136–145.
236. Morehouse LE, Cooper JM: *Kinesiology*. St. Louis, C.V. Mosby, 1950, p 72.
237. Barham JN, Wooten EP: *Structural Kinesiology*. New York, Macmillan, 1973, pp 353–355.
238. Hoppenfeld S: *Physical Examination of the Spine and Extremities*. New York, Appleton-Century-Crofts, 1976, pp 88–89, 91.
239. Chuinard RG: The upper extremity: Elbow, forearm, wrist and hand. In D'Ambrosia RD: *Musculoskeletal Disorders: Regional Examination and Differential Diagnosis*. Philadelphia, J.B. Lippincott, 1977, pp 360–362.
240. Mennell JMcM: *Joint Pain*. Boston, Little, Brown, 1964, pp 43, 44–67.
241. Esch D, Lepley M: *Musculoskeletal Function: An Anatomy and Kinesiology Laboratory Manual*. Minneapolis, University of Minnesota Press, 1974, pp 92–95.
242. Kendall HO, Kendall FP, Wadsworth GE: *Muscles: Testing and Function*, ed 2. Baltimore, Williams & Wilkins, 1971, pp 90–95.
243. Hoppenfeld S: *Physical Examination of the Spine and Extremities*. New York, Appleton-Century-Crofts, 1976, pp 93–94.
244. Schafer RC (ed): *Basic Chiropractic Procedural Manual*, ed 4. Arlington, Va, American Chiropractic Association, 1984, pp 308–311.
245. Esch D, Lepley M: *Evaluation of Joint Motion: Methods of Measurement and Recording*. Minneapolis, University of Minnesota Press, 1974, pp 20–21.
246. Posner MA: Wrist injuries. In Scott, WN et al (eds): *Principles of Sports Medicine*. Baltimore, Williams & Wilkins, 1984, pp 156–177.
247. Harrington IJ: Biomechanics of joint injuries. In Gonzna ER, Harrington IJ: *Biomechanics of Musculoskeletal Injury*. Baltimore, Williams & Wilkins, 1982, pp 70–71.
248. Barham JN, Wooten EP: *Structural Kinesiology*. New York, Macmillan, 1973, p 364.
249. Bowerman JW: *Radiology and Injury in Sport*. New York, Appleton-Century-Crofts, 1977, pp 69–70, 70–81.
250. Hirata I Jr: *The Doctor and the Athlete*, ed 2. Philadelphia, J.B. Lippincott, 1974, pp 169–170.
251. Schafer RC: *Chiropractic Management of Sports and Recreational Injuries*. Baltimore, Williams & Wilkins, 1982, pp 396–397.
252. Bowerman JW: *Radiology and Injury in Sport*. New York, Appleton-Century-Crofts, 1977, pp 70–77, 210.
253. Schultz AL: Disorders of the wrist and hand.

Part 3, ganglion. *The Digest of Chiropractic Economics* January/February 1984.
254. Gertler L: *Illustrated Manual of Extravertebral Technic*, ed 2. Bayside, NY, published by the author, 1978, pp 54–56.
255. Stierwalt DD: *Extremity Adjusting*. Davenport, Ia, published by the author, 1975, pp 21–24.
256. Schultz AL: *The Shoulder, Arm, and Hand Syndrome*. Stickney, SD, Argus, 1969, pp 228–233.
257. Janse J, Houser RH, Wells BF: *Chiropractic Principles and Technic*. Chicago, National College of Chiropractic, 1947, pp 554–558.
258. Maitland GD: *Peripheral Manipulation*. Boston, Butterworths, 1976, pp 80–91.
259. Chuinard RG: The upper extremity: Elbow, forearm, wrist and hand. In D'Ambrosia RD: *Musculoskeletal Disorders: Regional Examination and Differential Diagnosis*. Philadelphia, J.B. Lippincott, 1977, pp 389, 391.
260. Teranel JA: *Chiropractic Orthopedics and Roentgenology*. Newark, NJ, Medusa Press, 1953, pp 307, 385, 386.
261. Williams JGP, Sperryn PN (eds): *Sports Medicine*, ed 2. Baltimore, Williams & Wilkins, 1976, pp 417–422.
262. Grilliot JR, Staines MJ: Isolated rotary subluxation of the carpal navicular. *ACA Journal of Chiropractic* February 1985.
263. Belinghausen H et al: Post-traumatic palmar carpal subluxation. *Jounral of Bone and Joint Surgery* 65:998–1006, 1983.
264. Bowerman JW: *Radiology and Injury in Sport*. New York, Appleton-Century-Crofts, 1977, pp 67–81.
265. Holmes GW, Robbins LL: *Roentgen Interpretation*, ed 7. Philadelphia, Lea & Febiger, 1947, p 46.
266. Cailliet R: *Hand Pain and Impairment*. Philadelphia, F.A. Davis, 1975, pp 110–115.
267. Bowerman JW: *Radiology and Injury in Sport*. New York, Appleton-Century-Crofts, 1977, p 77.
268. Mazion JM: *Illustrated Manual of Neurological Reflexes/Signs/Tests, Orthopedic Signs/Tests/Maneuvers*, ed 2. Arizona City, published by the author, 1980, p 273.
269. Cailliet R: *Soft Tissue Pain and Disability*. Philadelphia, F.A. Davis, 1980, pp 179–188.
270. Cailliet R: *Hand Pain and Impairment*. Philadelphia, F.A. Davis, 1975, pp 68–81.
271. Rosse C: The hand. In Rosse C, Clawson DK (eds): *The Musculoskeletal System in Health and Disease*. Hagerstown, Md, Harper & Row, 1980, pp 242–243.
272. Goodheart GL: *Collected Published Articles and Reprints*. Montpellier, O, Williams County Publishing, 1969, pp 33–35.
273. Grant JM: Carpal tunnel syndrome: a new concept in conservative chiropractic management. *ACA Journal of Chiropractic* February 1979.
274. Kamerud BJ: Diagnostic considerations in median nerve paresthesia. *ACA Journal of Chiropractic* February 1979.
275. Rosse C: The hand. In Rosse C, Clawson DK (eds): *The Musculoskeletal System in Health and Disease*. Hagerstown, Md, Harper & Row, 1980, pp 243–244.
276. Cyriax J: *Textbook of Orthopaedic Medicine. Vol 1, Diagnosis of Soft Tissue Lesions*, ed 8. London, Bailliere Tindall, 1982, p 197.
277. Rosse C: The hand. In Rosse C, Clawson DK (eds): *The Musculoskeletal System in Health and Disease*. Hagerstown, Md, Harper & Row, 1980, pp 227–228, 245–248.
278. Kapandji IA: *Physiology of the Joints: Upper Limb*, ed 2. New York, Churchill Livingstone, 1980, vol 1, pp 146–151, 178–180.
279. Morehouse LE, Cooper JM: *Kinesiology*. St. Louis, C.V. Mosby, 1950, pp 68–72.
280. Barham JN, Wooten EP: *Structural Kinesiology*. New York, Macmillan, 1973, pp 330, 335–336.
281. Daniels L, Worthingham C: *Muscle Testing: Techniques of Manual Examination*, ed 4. Philadelphia, W.B. Saunders, 1980, pp 142–151.
282. Kendall HO, Kendall FP, Wadsworth GE: *Muscles: Testing and Function*, ed 2. Baltimore, Williams & Wilkins, 1971, pp 66–73.
283. Chuinard RG: The upper extremity: Elbow, forearm, wrist and hand. In D'Ambrosia RD: *Musculoskeletal Disorders: Regional Examination and Differential Diagnosis*. Philadelphia, J.B. Lippincott, 1977, p 362.
284. Rosse C: The hand. In Rosse C, Clawson DK (eds): *The Musculoskeletal System in Health and Disease*. Hagerstown, Md, Harper & Row, 1980, p 240.
285. Kapandji IA: *Physiology of the Joints: Upper Limb*, ed 2. New York, Churchill Livingstone, 1980, vol 1, pp 154–165, 182–196, 202.
286. Hollingshead WH, Jenkins DB: *Functional Anatomy of the Limbs and Back*. Philadelphia, W.B. Saunders, 1981, pp 176–177.
287. Hoppenfeld S: *Physical Examination of the Spine and Extremities*. New York, Appleton-Century-Crofts, 1976, pp 90–91, 92–93.
288. Barham JN, Wooten EP: *Structural Kinesiology*. New York, Macmillan, 1973, pp 355–357.
289. Esch D, Lepley M: *Musculoskeletal Function: An Anatomy and Kinesiology Laboratory Manual*. Minneapolis, University of Minnesota Press, 1974, pp 101–105.
290. Hoppenfeld S: *Physical Examination of the Spine and Extremities*. New York, Appleton-Century-Crofts, 1976, pp 97–98.
291. Schafer RC (ed): *Basic Chiropractic Procedural Manual*, ed 4. Arlington, Va, American Chiropractic Association, 1984, p 313.
292. Esch D, Lepley M: *Evaluation of Joint Motion: Methods of Measurement and Recording*. Minneapolis, University of Minnesota Press, 1974, pp 25–29.
293. Schultz AL: *The Shoulder, Arm, and Hand Syndrome*. Stickney, SD, Argus, 1969, pp 254–256.
294. Maitland GD: *Peripheral Manipulation*. Boston, Butterworths, 1976, pp 99–101.
295. Barham JN, Wooten EP: *Structural Kinesiology*. New York, Macmillan, 1973, pp 364–365.
296. Gertler L: *Illustrated Manual of Extravertebral Technic*, ed 2. Bayside, NY, published by the author, 1978, p 53.
297. Chuinard RG: The upper extremity: Elbow, fore-

arm, wrist and hand. In D'Ambrosia RD: *Musculoskeletal Disorders: Regional Examination and Differential Diagnosis*. Philadelphia, J.B. Lippincott, 1977, p 388.
298. Rosse C: The hand. In Rosse C, Clawson DK (eds): *The Musculoskeletal System in Health and Disease*. Hagerstown, Md, Harper & Row, 1980, pp 228–234.
299. Kapandji IA: *Physiology of the Joints: Upper Limb*, ed 2. New York, Churchill Livingstone, 1980, vol 1, pp 166–170.
300. Barham JN, Wooten EP: *Structural Kinesiology*. New York, Macmillan, 1973, pp 330–331, 336–338.
301. Hollingshead WH, Jenkins DB: *Functional Anatomy of the Limbs and Back*. Philadelphia, W.B. Saunders, 1981, pp 190–195.
302. Morehouse LE, Cooper JM: *Kinesiology*. St. Louis, C.V. Mosby, 1950, pp 72–73.
303. Rosse C, Clawson DK (eds): *The Musculoskeletal System in Health and Disease*. Hagerstown, Md, Harper & Row, 1980, pp 214–216, 235–239, 240.
304. Kapandji IA: *Physiology of the Joints: Upper Limb*, ed 2. New York, Churchill Livingstone, 1980, vol 1, pp 172–176.
305. Basmajian JV (ed): *Grant's Method of Anatomy*, ed 9. Baltimore, Williams & Wilkins, 1975, pp 19–171.
306. Black J, Dumbleton JH (eds): *Clinical Biomechanics: Case History Approach*. New York, Churchill Livingstone, 1981, pp 18–22.
307. Mennell JMcM: *Joint Pain*. Boston, Little, Brown, 1964, pp 32–39, 40–42.
308. Hoppenfeld S: *Physical Examination of the Spine and Extremities*. New York, Appleton-Century-Crofts, 1976, pp 89–90, 91–92, 93.
309. Chuinard RG: The upper extremity: Elbow, forearm, wrist and hand. In D'Ambrosia RD: *Musculoskeletal Disorders: Regional Examination and Differential Diagnosis*. Philadelphia, J.B. Lippincott, 1977, pp 362–363.
310. Esch D, Lepley M: *Musculoskeletal Function: An Anatomy and Kinesiology Laboratory Manual*. Minneapolis, University of Minnesota Press, 1974, pp 96–100.
311. Daniels L, Worthingham C: *Muscle Testing: Techniques of Manual Examination*, ed 4. Philadelphia, W.B. Saunders, 1980, pp 132–141.
312. Kendall HO, Kendall FP, Wadsworth GE: *Muscles: Testing and Function*, ed 2. Baltimore, Williams & Wilkins, 1971, pp 74–89.
313. Hoppenfeld S: *Physical Examination of the Spine and Extremities*. New York, Appleton-Century-Crofts, 1976, pp 94–95.
314. Esch D, Lepley M: *Evaluation of Joint Motion: Methods of Measurement and Recording*. Minneapolis, University of Minnesota Press, 1974, pp 22–24.
315. Schafer RC (ed): *Basic Chiropractic Procedural Manual*, ed 4. Arlington, Va, American Chiropractic Association, 1984, pp 313–317
316. Gillet H, Liekens M: *Belgian Chiropractic Research Notes*. Huntington Beach, Cal, Motion Palpation Institute, 1981, pp 88–89.
317. Hirata I Jr: *The Doctor and the Athlete*, ed 2. Philadelphia, J.B. Lippincott, 1974, pp 170–174.
318. Schultz AL: *The Shoulder, Arm, and Hand Syndrome*. Stickney, SD, Argus, 1969, pp 240–245, 253, 261, 263.
319. Bowerman JW: *Radiology and Injury in Sport*. New York, Appleton-Century-Crofts, 1977, pp 82–84.
320. Williams JGP, Sperryn PN (eds): *Sports Medicine*, ed 2. Baltimore, Williams & Wilkins, 1976, pp 411–417, 422–424.
321. Maitland GD: *Peripheral Manipulation*. Boston, Butterworths, 1976, pp 92–99.
322. Stierwalt DD: *Extremity Adjusting*. Davenport, Ia, published by the author, 1975, p 25.
323. Janse J, Houser RH, Wells BF: *Chiropractic Principles and Technic*. Chicago, National College of Chiropractic, 1947, pp 558, 560.
324. Burnside JW: *Adams' Physical Diagnosis*, Baltimore, Williams & Wilkins, 1974, pp 94–103.
325. Cailliet R: *Soft Tissue Pain and Disability*. Philadelphia, F.A. Davis, 1980, pp 189–190.
326. Teranel JA: *Chiropractic Orthopedics and Roentgenology*. Newark, NJ, Medusa Press, 1953, p 302.
327. Chuinard RG: The upper extremity: Elbow, forearm, wrist and hand. In D'Ambrosia RD: *Musculoskeletal Disorders: Regional Examination and Differential Diagnosis*. Philadelphia, J.B. Lippincott, 1977, pp 387–388.
328. Cailliet R: *Soft Tissue Pain and Disability*. Philadelphia, F.A. Davis, 1980, p 188.
329. Chuinard RG: The upper extremity: Elbow, forearm, wrist and hand. In D'Ambrosia RD: *Musculoskeletal Disorders: Regional Examination and Differential Diagnosis*. Philadelphia, J. B. Lippincott, 1977, p 384.
330. Teranel JA: *Chiropractic Orthopedics and Roentgenology*. Newark, NJ, Medusa Press, 1953, pp 301–302.
331. Hoppenfeld S: *Physical Examination of the Spine and Extremities*. New York, Appleton-Century-Crofts, 1976, pp 101–102.
332. Chuinard RG: The upper extremity: Elbow, forearm, wrist and hand. In D'Ambrosia RD: *Musculoskeletal Disorders: Regional Examination and Differential Diagnosis*. Philadelphia, J.B. Lippincott, 1977, p 363.
333. Cailliet R: *Hand Pain and Impairment*. Philadelphia, F.A. Davis, 1975, pp 101–109.
334. Teranel JA: *Chiropractic Orthopedics and Roentgenology*. Newark, NJ, Medusa Press, 1953, pp 381–384.
335. Chuinard RG: The upper extremity: Elbow, forearm, wrist and hand. In D'Ambrosia RD: *Musculoskeletal Disorders: Regional Examination and Differential Diagnosis*. Philadelphia, J.B. Lippincott, 1977, pp 389–390, 391–393.

SUGGESTED READINGS

Aston JN: *A Short Textbook of Orthopaedics and Traumatology*, ed 2. London, Hodder & Stoughton, 1978.

Cyriax J: *Textbook of Orthopaedic Medicine. Vol 2, Treatment by Manipulation, Massage and Injection*, ed 11. London, Bailliere Tindall, 1984.

Dolan JP, Holladay LJ: *First-Aid Management: Athletics,*

Physical Education, Recreation, ed 4. Danville, NY, Interstate Printers & Publishers, 1974.

Gardner E et al: *A Regional Study of Human Structure*, ed 4. Philadelphia, W.B. Saunders, 1975.

Hains G: *Post-Traumatic Neuritis*. Trois-Rivieres, Quebec, published by the author, 1978.

Johnson AC: *Chiropractic Physiological Therapeutics*. Palm Springs, Cal, published by the author, 1977.

Kuorinka I, Viikari J: Prevalence of neck and upper limb disorders (NLD) and work load in different occupational groups. Problems in classifications and diagnosis. *Human Ergology* 11:65–72, 1982.

O'Donoghue DH: *Treatment of Injuries to Athletes*, ed 3. Philadelphia, W.B. Saunders, 1976.

Radin EL et al: *Practical Biomechanics for the Orthopaedic Surgeon*. New York, John Wiley & Sons, 1969.

Robertson WE, Robertson HF: *Diagnostic Signs, Reflexes, and Syndromes*, ed 3. Philadelphia, F.A. Davis, 1947.

Salter RB: *Textbook of Disorders and Injuries of the Musculoskeletal System*. Baltimore, Williams & Wilkins, 1970.

Schafer RC: "Hot shots" and brachial plexus traction. *Journal of the American Chiropractic Association* September 1982.

Schoenholtz F: *Chiropractic Orthopedics*. Los Angeles, The Los Angeles College of Chiropractic, 1976.

Straus RH: *Sports Medicine and Physiology*. Philadelphia, W.B. Saunders, 1979.

Zuidema GD, Rutherford RB, Ballinger WF (eds): *The Management of Trauma*, ed 3. Philadelphia, W.B. Saunders, 1979.

CHAPTER 15

The Lower Extremity

Biomechanical disorders of the lower extremities are quite common, both as primary and secondary disorders. Any physician may be faced with the problems involved in such cases, thus it is vital to have an understanding of the principles involved for accurate diagnosis and efficient case management. This concluding chapter discusses the hip, knee, ankle, and foot, which have a direct influence on both adjacent segments and body structure as a whole.

A wide variety of strains, spasms, sprains, contractures, fixations, subluxations, dislocations, and fractures is discussed. Emphasis is placed on the biomechanical mechanisms involved in segmental misalignment from either postural or traumatic forces. Some static and dynamic disorders are similar to those found in the upper extremity; however, many are unique because of the weight-bearing function of the lower extremities.

THE HIP AND THIGH

Basic Functional Anatomy[1–5]

The Hip Joint[6–8]

Stability of the hip joint is provided by its structural design and ligaments. The major structures at the proximal femur are the head and neck of the femur, the greater and lesser trochanters, and the intertrochanteric crest (Fig. 15.1). The shaft of the femur attaches to the pelvis at an approximate 130° angle via its superomedially slanted neck. The neck ends in the large globe-like head of the femur, which articulates within the deep acetabulum, while the shaft proper ends cephalad in the greater trochanter. The articulating surface of the head of the femur is more than half a sphere, yet a fibrocartilaginous labrum surrounds the acetabulum to even further deepen the articular cavity. The femoral shaft bows inferiorly and twists obliquely anterior and medial to bring the knee joint in pump with the hip joint. This spiral of shaft of the femur gives it increased resistance to bending forces and shear stress (Fig. 15.2).

Unlike the shoulder, the capsule of the hip is quite strong and is closely associated with four ligaments: the iliofemoral, ischiofemoral, pubofemoral, and interarticular. The strong triangular iliofemoral ligament covers the front of the joint capsule and connects with the ilium below the anterior inferior iliac spine (AIIS). It attaches to the femur at two insertions (the inverted "Y" ligament of Bigelow) on the anterior aspects of the greater and lesser trochanters, and thus is able to restrict excessive extension of the joint imposed by body weight in the erect posture. The ischiofemoral ligament covers the posterior aspect of the capsule. It spans relatively horizontal between the ischial rim of the acetabulum and the greater trochanter. The spiral design of its fibers gives extra stability to the joint during extension. The pubofemoral ligament spans from the pubic aspect of the acetabulum to the medial aspect of the femoral neck, thus covering the medial aspect of the capsule. This position allows the pubofemoral ligament to strap excessive abduction of the femor and helps to check severe extension. These three ligaments tend to tighten on internal rotation and relax on external rotation and flexion. This forces the hip muscles to provide stability during external rotation and flexion.

The flat interarticular band is frequently referred to as the ligament of the femur head, ligamentum teres, or the round ligament of the hip. It spans from the pit of the femur head, through the capsule, to the nonarticular surface of the acetabulum.

The Thigh Muscles

The thigh consists of three major muscle groups, some of which cross both the hip and the knee joints. In general, the anterior group controls hip flexion and knee exten-

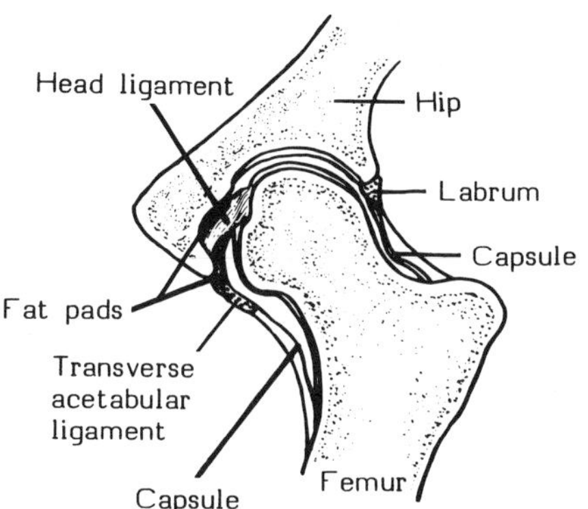

Figure 15.1. Frontal section of the hip depicting the major structures associated with the head of the femur.

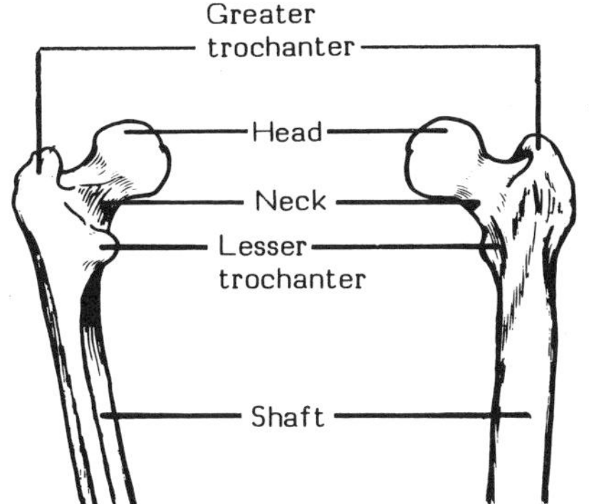

Figure 15.2. Anterior and posterior views of the femur.

sion and is innervated by the femoral nerve. The anteromedial group governs adduction of the thigh and is supplied by the obturator nerve. The posterior group (hamstrings) controls extension of the hip and flexion of the knee and is innervated by the sciatic nerve.

Hip Movements

Joint Motion[9–13]

All hip maneuvers should be tested bilaterally. Hip motion, prime movers, and accessories are outlined in Table 15.1.

Flexion. The supine patient should be placed in a straight line with his trunk square to the pelvis so that a line drawn between the ASISs strikes the midline at right angles. The examiner places a stabilizing hand under the patient's lumbar spine and flexes the patient's hips by bringing both thighs toward the abdomen as far as possible with the knees flexed. The thighs should normally rest against the patient's abdomen and almost touch the chest.

Extension. Extension is judged with the patient prone with ankles on a small roll to relax his hamstrings. The examiner stabilizes the pelvis by placing an arm horizontally across the upper pelvic area about the level of the iliac crests. The examiner's active hand is placed under the patient's thigh above the knee and an upward lifting motion is made to extend the hip with the patient's knee kept extended. The hip should normally extend about 30°; if not, a flexion contracture should be the first suspicion.

Abduction. To test hip abduction passively, the supine patient is placed in the neutral position and the examiner stands at the patient's side. He places his stabilizing forearm across the patient's pelvis. The examiner's active hand grasps one leg of the patient and slowly abducts the limb as far as possible (normally about 45°). At the end of abduction, the pelvis under the stabilizing arm will begin to move.

Adduction. The range of hip adduction is tested in the same manner, by bringing the patient's limb horizontally across the other limb (normally about 20–30°). Upper thighs that are quite muscular or fat will restrict the degree of adduction.

Rotation in Extension. To test passive internal and external rotation in extension, the patient is placed supine in the neutral position and a dot is made with a marking pencil in the center of each patella. The examiner stands at the foot of the examining table and grasps each leg just above the ankle. The legs are rotated internally and externally, and the movement of the dot on each patella is noted to judge the range of motion (Fig. 15.3). Excessive rotation can usually be traced to anteversion or retroversion of the femoral neck. Anteversion will result in excessive toe-in, while retroversion will have the opposite effect. In young children, excessive external rotation and restricted internal rotation may be the result of a slipped capital upper femoral epiphysis that has moved inferior and posterior.

Rotation in Flexion. To test passive hip rotation in hip flexion, the patient sits upright with knees hanging from the edge of

Table 15.1.
Hip Motion

Joint motion	Prime movers	Accessories
Flexion	Iliopsoas Sartorius Rectus femoris	Tensor fascia latae Pectineus Adductor brevis and longus Adductor magnus, oblique fibers Gluteus medius, anterior fibers Gluteus minimus
Extension	Gluteus maximus Hamstrings	Gluteus medius, dorsal fibers Adductor magnus, vertical fibers
Abduction	Gluteus medius Gluteus minimus Tensor fascia latae	Sartorius
Adduction	Adductor longus Adductor brevis Adductor magnus Pectineus Gracilis	
External rotation	Obturator internus Obturator externus Gemelli Quadratus femoris Piriformis	Gluteus maximus Gluteus medius, dorsal fibers Sartorius
Medial rotation	Gluteus medius, anterior fibers Gluteus minimus Tensor fascia latae	Adductor magnus, vertical fibers

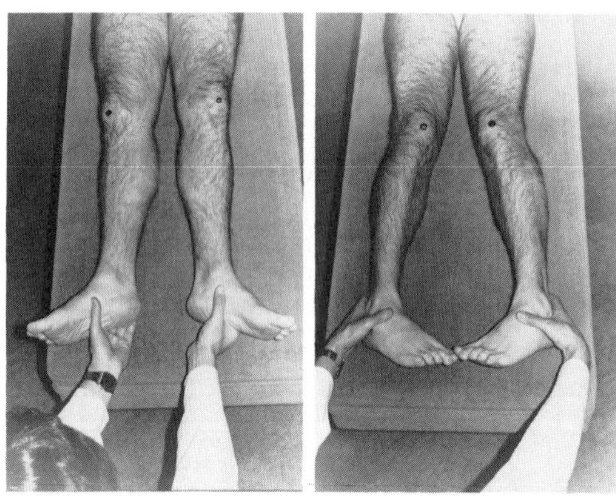

Figure 15.3. Testing the limits of external and internal rotation of the neutral femur with the patient supine.

the table. The examiner stabilizes the patient's thigh (femur) with one hand while his active hand, placed just above the ankle, moves the limb laterally and medially in an arc to test hip internal and external rotation (Fig. 15.4).

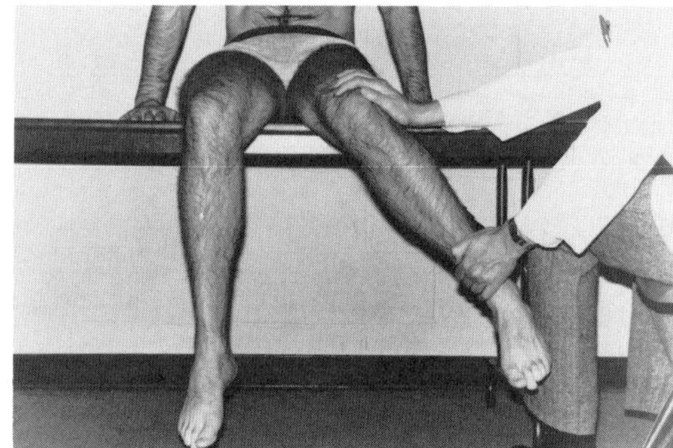

Figure 15.4. Testing the limit of internal hip rotation in the sitting position (flexed femur).

Kinesiology[14–21]

Evaluation should be made of muscle groups controlling flexion, extension, abduction, and adduction to evaluate integrity of the muscles and their nerve supply. (See Table 15.2.) The same system of grading muscle strength is used as mentioned previously. All muscles should be tested bilaterally. Only in unusual situations is it necessary to test the internal and external rotators.

Flexion. Hip flexion is provided essentially by the iliopsoas, innervated by the femoral nerve (L1–L5), with assistance from the rectus femoris and sartorius (Fig. 15.5).

Table 15.2.
Major Muscles of the Hip and Thigh

Muscle	Major functions	Spinal segment
Adductor brevis	Adduction, flexion, external rotation	L2–L4
Adductor longus	Adduction, flexion, external rotation	L2–L3
Adductor magnus	Adduction	L3–L4
Oblique fibers	Flexion	L3–L4
Vertical fibers	Extension, weak medial rotation	L3–L4
Gemelli	External rotation	L4–S2
Gluteus maximus	Extension, external rotation	L5–S2
Gluteus medius	Abduction, rotation	L4–S1
Anterior fibers	Flexion, internal rotation	L4–S1
Dorsal fibers	Extension, external rotation, abduction	L4–S1
Gluteus minimus	Abduction, medial rotation, flexion	L4–S1
Gracilis	Adduction	L2–L4
Hamstrings	Extension	L5–S2
Semitendinosus	Extension	L5–S2
Semimembranosus	Extension	L5–S1
Biceps femoris	Extension	L5–S2
Iliacus	Flexion	L2–L3
Obturators	External rotation	L3–L4
Pectineus	Adduction, flexion	L2–L3
Piriformis	External rotation	L5–S2
Psoas major	Flexion	L1–L5
Quadratus femoris	External rotation	L4–S1
Rectus femoris	Flexion	L2–L4
Sartorius	Flexion, abduction, external rotation	L2–L3
Tensor fasciae latae	Abduction, medial rotation, flexion	L2–S1

Spinal innervation varies somewhat in different people. The spinal nerves listed here are averages and may differ in a particular patient; thus, an allowance of a segment above and below those listed in most text tables should be considered.

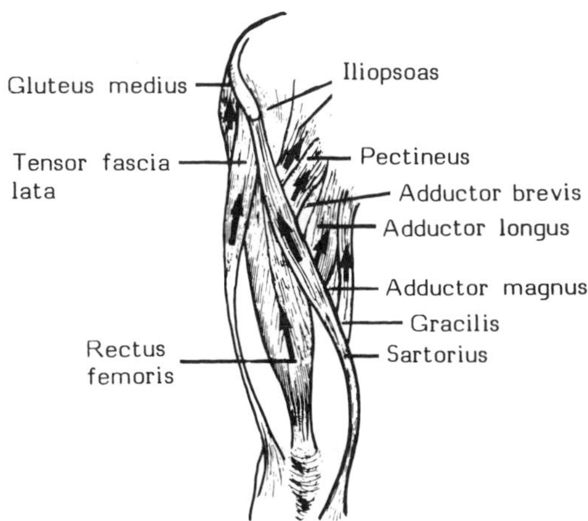

Figure 15.5. The major flexors of the thigh.

To test active hip flexion, the sitting or supine patient is asked to draw each knee up to his chest as far as possible without bending the back. The knee should normally come near the thorax (about 135°).

Extension. Extension of the hip is primarily offered by the gluteus maximus, supplied by the inferior gluteal nerve (L5–S2), with secondary effort by the hamstrings (Fig. 15.6). Active extension can be tested roughly in the sitting position by having the patient fold his arms across his chest keeping his back straight while he rises from the chair.

Abduction. Hip abduction is provided for the most part by the gluteus medius, innervated by the superior gluteal nerve (L4–S1), with assistance by the gluteus minimus and tensor fascia lata (Fig. 15.7). For a quick test, the patient standing in the neutral position is asked to spread his legs as far apart as possible. Each leg should normally be able to be actively abducted at least 45° from the midline. A better test is to place the patient in the side position. The examiner's stabilizing hand is placed on the iliac crest to fix the pelvis. The patient is asked to abduct his uppermost thigh while the

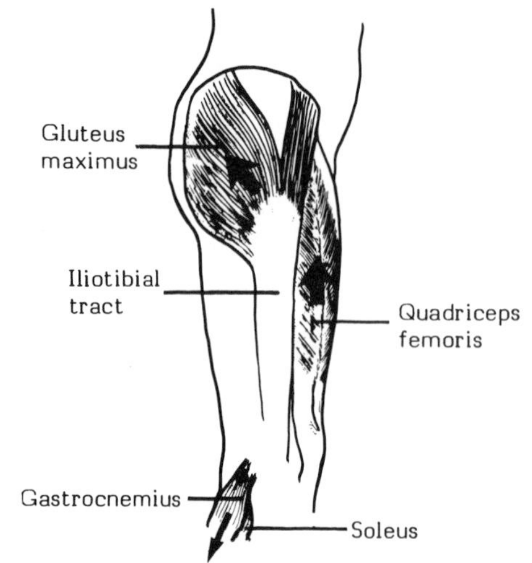

Figure 15.6. Extensor action of the thigh and leg.

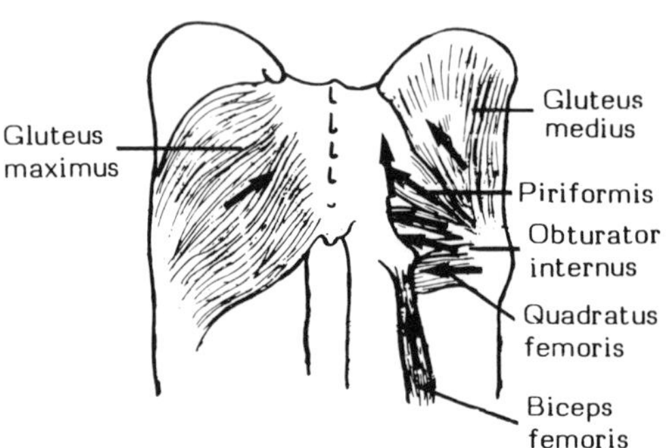

Figure 15.7. Major external rotators of the thigh.

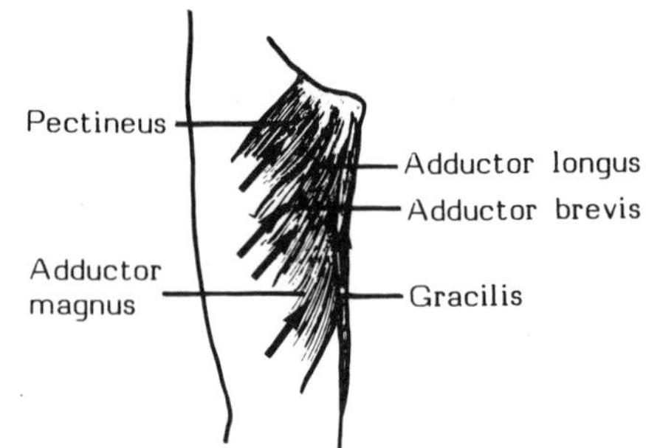

Figure 15.8. Major anterior adductors of the thigh.

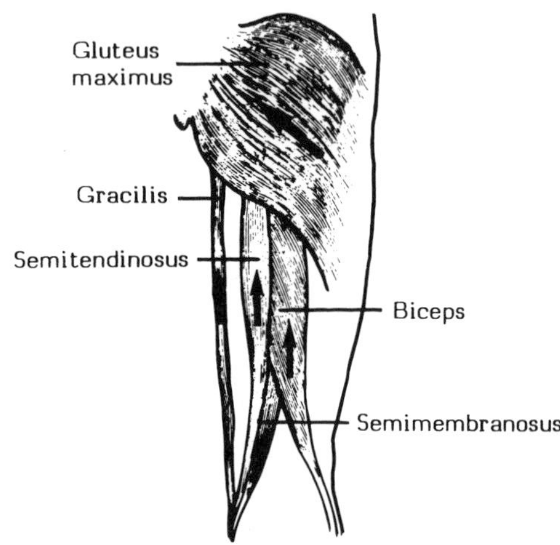

Figure 15.9. Major posterior adductors of the thigh.

doctor applies increasing resistance to the lateral knee area. The fingers of the examiner's stabilizing hand can be used to palpate the origin of the gluteus medius muscle.

Adduction. Adduction is primarily offered by the adductor longus, supplied by the obturator nerve (L3–L4), with help from the adductor brevis, adductor magnus, pectineus, and gracilis (Figs. 15.8 and 15.9). To test active motion in the standing position, the patient in the neutral position is requested to alternately cross the left leg in front of the right and then the right leg in front of the left. Normally, at least a 20° active adduction from the midline should be achieved. A better method to test adduction strength is for the examiner to slip his active hand under the medial aspect of the patient's knee and apply increasing resistance as the patient adducts his thigh toward the midline.

Another method to test hip abduction and adduction is to place the patient supine with his legs abducted about 20°. The examiner, at the foot of the table, grasps the patient's legs above the ankles and applies increasing resistance as the patient attempts first to abduct his legs laterally and then to adduct his lower limbs medially.

Goniometry of the Hip[22, 23]

When taking the following hip measurements, deviation from the neutral position in cases of ankylosis should be measured.

Restricted Hip Flexion. The patient is placed in the supine neutral position. The opposite hip should be flexed and held by the examiner to lock the patient's pelvis. The hip being tested is extended in a relaxed position. The goniometer is placed next to the hip joint, and the reading is taken for the neutral position. With the hip to be tested flexed, the goniometer arm follows the range of motion until the iliac crest begins to move. This is the end of motion which should be recorded.

Restricted Hip Extension. The patient is placed in the prone neutral position, and the goniometer is centered over the hip joint with its arm extended along the thigh. The patient's pelvis is stabilized as the patient extends the thigh while keeping the knee straight. The reading is recorded at the end of the motion.

Restricted Hip Abduction/Adduction. The patient is placed in the supine neutral position, with the opposite hip flexed and the knee held by the patient in a locked position against his abdomen. The goniometer is centered over the upper anterior thigh with its arm extended down the midline of the thigh to be tested. The limb to be tested is extended and relaxed, and the neutral reading is recorded. Then the patient abducts the thigh of the extended limb as far as possible, and the reading at the end of the motion is recorded (when the pelvis begins to move). The patient then adducts the thigh as far as possible, and the reading at the end of hip motion is recorded.

Restricted Hip Rotation. The patient is placed in the supine neutral position with the goniometer centered over the midheel, and the neutral reading is recorded with the goniometer's arm at the level of the 2nd and 3rd toes. (Neutral is considered to be 90%.) The patient externally rotates the hip as far as possible, and the reading at the end of the motion is recorded. The same maneuver is repeated toward the midline to check internal rotation.

Hip Load and Its Resolution[24–28]

The hip joint operates as a first-class lever. Any applied force multiplied by its lever arm equals the weight of the object multiplied by its lever arm, the distance from the fulcrum to the weight. The mechanical advantage is related to the ratio of the lever-arm lengths extending from the fulcrum. During normal gait, forces across the hip joint are from 3–5 times the imposed body weight. These forces multiply considerably during running or jumping.

The load on the hips varies according to body weight, body position, and applied external load (Fig. 15.10). In the erect posture that is bilaterally balanced, the load on the femoral heads is essentially vertical (compression). Thus, there is no need for much action by the joint muscles. Body weight is balanced over the hip joint by the thigh abductors acting through the greater trochanter. In other words, the abductors create an equal and opposite turning effect to counteract the forces of body weight acting through the center of gravity that tend to rotate the trunk toward the midline.

The line of action extends from the femoral head to the medial condyle of the distal femur. Thus, when standing, the trabeculae of the femur are subjected to compression forces medially and tensile forces laterally. This produces a degree of lateral femoral bending. These compression and tensile forces in the shaft produce their greatest shear forces in the subtrochanteric area of the shaft.

In a 200-lb individual, a horizontal line through the joint axis of the femurs is perpendicular to the pull of gravity if the extremities are of equal length. The force of body weight above the hips passes an equal distance between the two hip joints (about 6 inches laterally from the midline) in a parallel force system. As the average lower limb weight of such an individual is 31.2% of total body limb weight, the femoral head load can be calculated by subtracting the weight of the lower extremities from total body weight to arrive at a total force of 137.6 lb or 68.8 lb on each hip. This force exerts a moment about the apex of the fem-

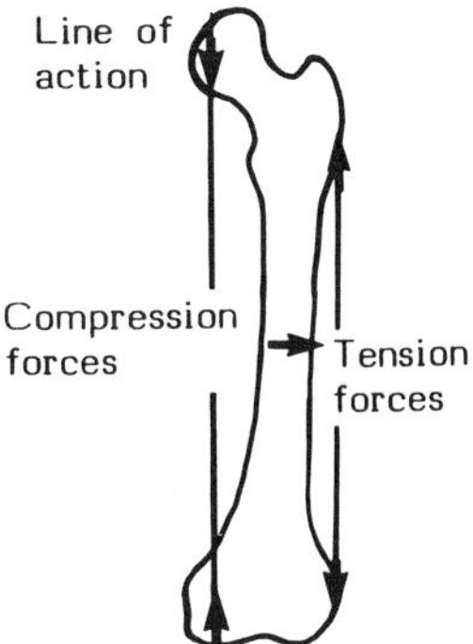

Figure 15.10. Normal loading forces within the femur.

oral angle. The longer the distance of this line of force to the apex of the femoral angle (eg, coxa varum), the greater the bending moment on the femoral neck.

The femoral neck is usually set at a 130° angle to the shaft. The anatomical axis of the femur is at a 5° angle to a vertical line. With these norms, the femoral neck forms a 50° angle to a vertical line. As mentioned above for a 200-lb person, the reaction force is 68.8 lb on each hip. Using trigonometric functions and the known angle of the femoral shaft, it can be computed that the compression force is 44.2 lb and the shearing force acting along the epiphysis is 52.7 lb. It can therefore be anticipated that epiphyseal slippage is a danger in an obese child with coxa varum.

SELECTED CLINICAL PROBLEMS OF THE HIP AND THIGH[29–34]

Conditioning Problems[35, 36]

The hip, knee, and ankle work as a functional unit (kinematic chain). Thus, all three joints must be considered when correcting an obvious postural distortion of any one joint.

The common muscles to be strengthened in postural distortions of the hip are the lateral and medial hip rotators, hip adductors, knee extensors and flexors, foot invertors, metatarsophalangeal flexors, and the abductors, flexors, and extensors of the toes. The common muscles to be stretched in lower extremity postural distortions are the flexors, medial rotators, and adductors of the thigh; the ankle plantar flexors; and the foot evertors and invertors.[37]

Biomechanical Adaptation to Hip Abductor Weakness[38, 39]

When one foot is removed from the floor (eg, in walking), the center of mass of above body weight plus the weight of the lifted limb sits on the supporting hip medial to the femoral head. This force, which tends to force the pelvis downward on the unsupported side, is counteracted by contraction of the hip abductors on the supported side so that the pelvis is relatively stabilized in the frontal plane. These two forces are opposed by the force of the femoral head acting upward.

If the hip abductors are weak, the patient must laterally abduct his trunk from the supporting side so that the gravity line falls laterally over the supporting femoral head to stabilize the hip in the frontal plane. This gross shifting moves the center of mass of the supported weight nearer the femoral fulcrum to reduce the moment of superimposed weight on the supporting hip and thus reduce the need for abductor stabilization. Such a limp is often attributed to the gluteus medius, but the gluteus minimus, upper gluteus maximus, and tensor fascia lata are just as important considerations.

Biomechanical Factors in Cane Use[40–42]

If a cane is used, the base of support is increased to assist a weakness. If the crane is carried in the hand contralateral to the hip involvement, the distance from the cane to the contralateral hip is far greater than the distance from the femoral head to the action line of the adjacent abductors. Slight leaning on the cane greatly reduces the superincumbent weight of the hip. However, if the cane is held in the ipsilateral hand, the involved hip has a less favorable lever arm and a much greater force must be placed on the cane to offer the same amount of hip relief.

Traumatic Disorders[43–45]

The majority of injuries involving the hip and thigh are those of a musculotendinous unit. For accurate diagnosis, careful palpation of bone and soft tissues, evaluation of the active and if necessary the passive range of joint motion, and testing muscle action against resistance will usually quickly pinpoint the site of trauma.

General Muscle Spasm

Limitations of motion due to muscular spasm are seen with special frequency in joint disease and spinal dyskinesias, but may occur in almost any form of joint trouble, particularly in the larger joints. In the hip joint, two forms of spasm are important: (1) that which is due to irritation of the psoas alone, and (2) that in which all muscles moving the joint are more or less contracted. General spasm of the hip muscles is tested by Patrick's test.

Patrick's F-AB-ER-E Test.[46–48] This test

helps to confirm a suspicion of hip joint pathology (Fig. 15.11). The patient lies supine, and the examiner grasps the ankle and the flexed knee. The thigh is flexed (F), abducted (AB), externally rotated (ER), and extended (E). Pain in the hip during the maneuvers, particularly on abduction and external rotation, is a positive sign of coxa pathology.

Strains and Related Disorders[49–55]

Hamstring Strains. The posterior thigh is a common site of strain (Fig. 15.12). These strains have myriad variations and are difficult to treat. It is difficult to prevent recurrence if a faulty biomechanical style persists. Injury is usually the result of deficient reciprocal actions of opposing hamstrings and quadriceps, poor muscle flexibility, inadequate warmup, fatigue, or sudden violent contraction or stretching. The features of severe hamstring strain include acute pain, generally at the origin of the short head of the biceps femoris, restricted motion, hamstring dyskinesia, loss of strength, discoordination, and an altered gait (Fig. 15.13). Symptoms develop slowly with progressive disability. Bleeding is usually mild, but general spasm is common. Tenderness is found at the ischial origins and attachments at the

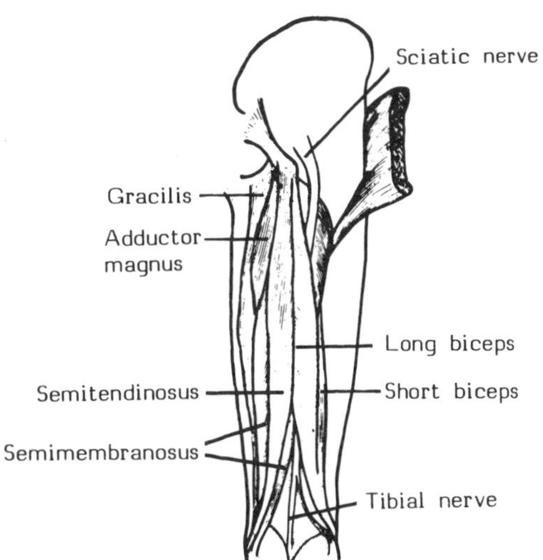

Figure 15.12. The major muscles of the posterior thigh.

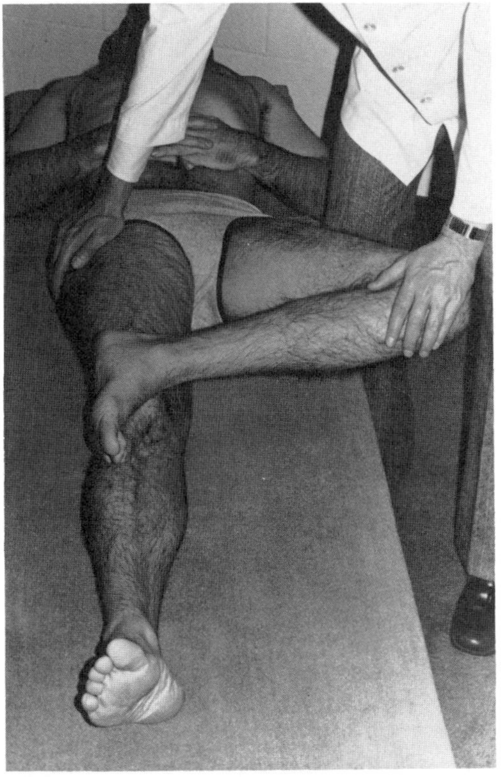

Figure 15.11. Patrick's F-AB-ER-E test.

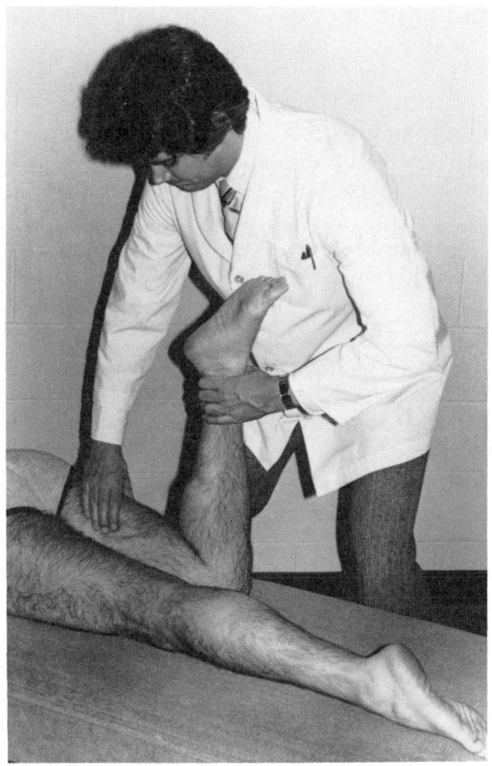

Figure 15.13. Hamstring palpation during muscle strength test.

musculotendinous junctions. A palpable, compensatory, fibrous thickening may be exhibited. Care must be taken to differentiate bicipital strain from knee sprain of the lateral ligaments or lateral meniscus tear.

Hamstring Ruptures. Hamstring tears often involve the long head of the biceps, the semimembranosus, or semitendinosus. Bicipital tendinitis is a frequent complication of distal bicipital strain. Symptoms may be exaggerated at either the hip or the knee. Roentgenographs may show avulsion fracture at the fibular head. In contrast to a severe stretch, a tear features a history of bursting pain during activity and a highly tender mass at the site of hemorrhage (Fig. 15.14). The size of the mass varies from that of a walnut to a melon and parallels the degree of spasm and weight-bearing disability. During recovery, a startling ecchymosis usually appears in the popliteal fossa and slowly extends caudadly.

Hamstring Contractures. Tight, scarred hamstrings result from improperly treated strains and tears. They are a common factor of prolonged immobility. In some cases, the cause can be traced to excessive exercise that has produced a horizontal tear across the muscle's belly. Recurring episodes are typical. A program of graduated activity must be undertaken because prolonged rest encourages tightening and functional disability.

General Groin Strains. Severe groin strains are often difficult to manage and are usually associated with the sedentary patient with muscle shortening in the groin. These strains are also common from slips on a slick surface during which severe hip abduction or adduction overstress might occur. A wrenching-type disability arises slowly rather than suddenly as in a quickly torn muscle.

Specific Sartorius Strains and Tears. This often mild but persistent disability is often seen with activities that require excessive and unaccustomed "squatting" or rowing positions. Discomfort is aggravated by abduction and extension, and eased after warmup (Fig. 15.15).

Adductor Strains. Painful groin strains may involve either the gracilis, abductor longus, or iliopsoas, but differentiation is usually not necessary in management (Fig. 15.16). Interfiber bleeding is always a problem. Healing is slow, often taking 2–3

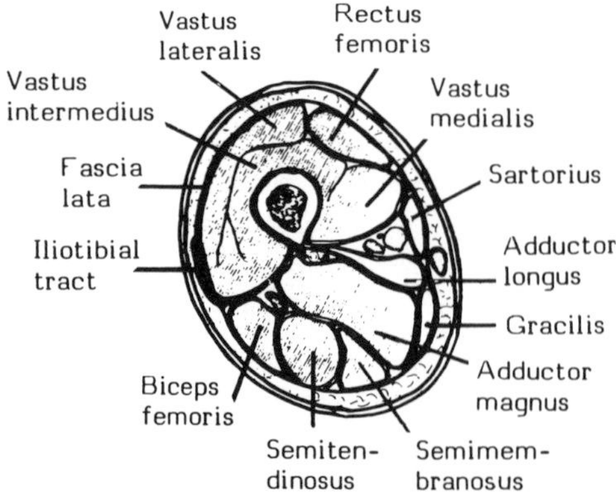

Figure 15.14. Transverse section of midthigh showing musculature relationships.

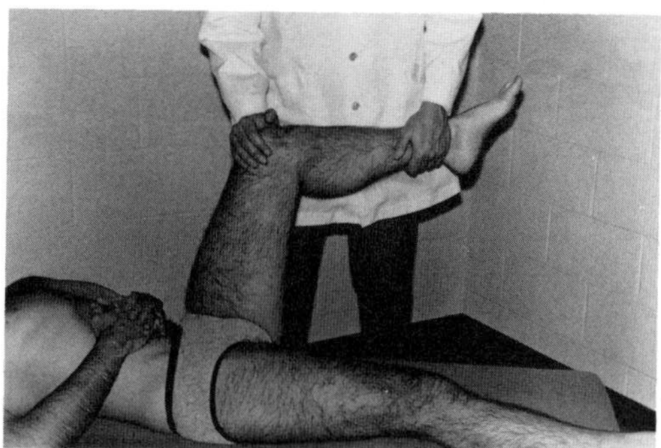

Figure 15.15. Testing sartorius strength by resisting flexion, abduction, and lateral rotation of the hip.

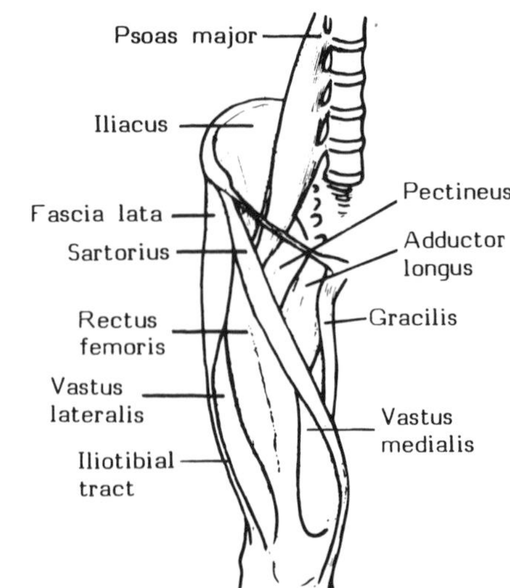

Figure 15.16. Some major muscles of the anterior upper thigh and related structures.

months for full recovery. Low adductor strains, contusions, and bone bruises seen on the medial femoral epicondyle often mimic knee joint injury. Such strains result from a fall on the adducted knee, causing overadduction and avulsion stress to the adductor tendon which may lead to periosteal calcification (Pellegrini-Stieda disease). Fortunately, severe posttraumatic disability is rarely a factor except with the aged and severely unconditioned patient.

Quadriceps Strains. Quadriceps injuries are often a management problem because healing is especially slow. Poor warmup or overstrain is a common factor. Symptoms may be exaggerated at either the hip or the knee, and may not appear for several hours in mild strains (Fig. 15.17). Pain is aggravated by movement, especially going down stairs. Swelling is usually mild, but spasm is always present to some degree depending upon the extent of injury. Quadriceps flexion will reveal a distinct degree of limitation. It is almost impossible to have a strong knee and weak quadriceps, and the quadriceps are the first to show atrophy after knee injury (Fig. 15.18).

Quadriceps Flexion Test. Scars within muscle tissue following trauma always limit the working length of all muscles in the group. Quadriceps contracture is simply tested by placing the patient prone, flexing the leg toward the buttocks to tolerance, and measuring the distance from heel to buttock. Once the point of tolerance is measured, the lumbosacral spine will arch and the buttocks will rise to prevent further stretch. This test may prove a lesion too deep to palpate as well as evaluate progress during therapy. Activity should be restricted until flexion exceeds 90°. All squatting activities must be avoided until full healing is demonstrated. Premature postinjury activity may easily tear a weakened muscle.

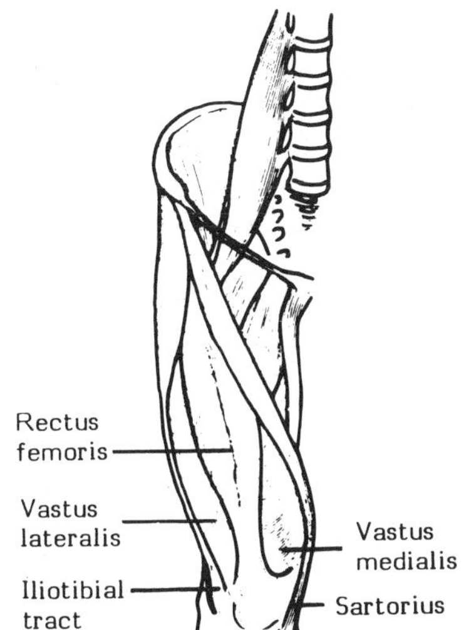

Figure 15.17. Major muscles of the anterior lower thigh.

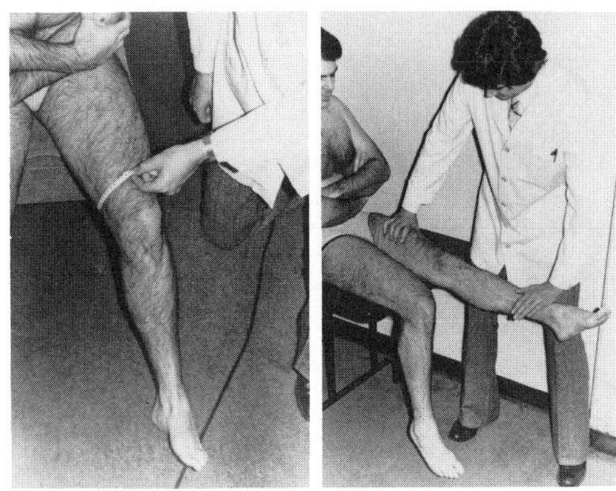

Figure 15.18. *Left*, measuring for quadriceps atrophy; *right*, evaluating quadriceps strength against resistance.

Fibrotic Masses. Fibrotic masses, as well as bony lesions in muscles and connective tissue, often develop within the quadriceps muscle or hamstrings after rupture of some muscle fibers. They are palpable in the relaxed muscle, usually circumscribed, and often visible. The mechanism is intrinsic; ie, one of uncoordinated forceful activity without a direct blow to the muscle.

Muscular Shortening

Muscle shortening may be the result of lack of exercise or pathology. However, it is more often an effect of chronic strain leading to structural misalignment.

Selected Effects of Hypertonicity in the Thigh. Excessive hypertonicity of a muscle, confirmed by palpatory tone and soreness, will tend to subluxate its site of osseous attachment. Below is a listing of common problem areas in the lower extremities.[56]

Biceps femoris. Increased tone tends to rotate the pelvis posterior and externally rotate the leg.

Rectus femoris. Increased tone tends to rotate the pelvis anterior and subluxate the patella to the superior.

Semitendinosus. Increased tone tends to pull the pelvis posterior and internally rotate the leg.

Sartorius. Increased tone tends to rotate the ilium anterior, inferior, and medial, and internally rotate the leg.

Gracilis. Increased tone tends to pull the pelvis anterior and internally rotate the leg.

Iliotibial Band Contracture: Ober's Test. This is the standard test for iliotibial band contractures.[57, 58] The patient is placed directly on his side with the unaffected side next to the table (Fig. 15.19). The examiner places one hand on the pelvis or under the thigh to steady it and grasps the patient's ankle with the other hand, holding the knee flexed at a right angle. The thigh is abducted and extended in the coronal plane of the body. In the presence of iliotibial band contracture, the leg will remain abducted, the degree of abduction depending upon the amount of contracture present.

Ober points to the frequency of a negative roentgenograph in the presence of clinical signs and symptoms of irritation of the sacroiliac or lumbosacral joints, and refers to the importance of the iliotibial band as a factor in the occurrence of lame backs, with or without associated sciatica. In differentiation, (1) pain on extension and abduction points to sacroiliac lesion; (2) pain when the knee is released suggests lumbosacral strain; and (3) contraction of the iliotibial band is indicated when the thigh does not return to the table on being released. Many report that Ely's test will pinpoint femoral nerve (L3–L4) involvement; Lasègue's test will differentiate lumbosacral from lumbar involvement. Biomechanically and neurologically, these tests are not that specific.

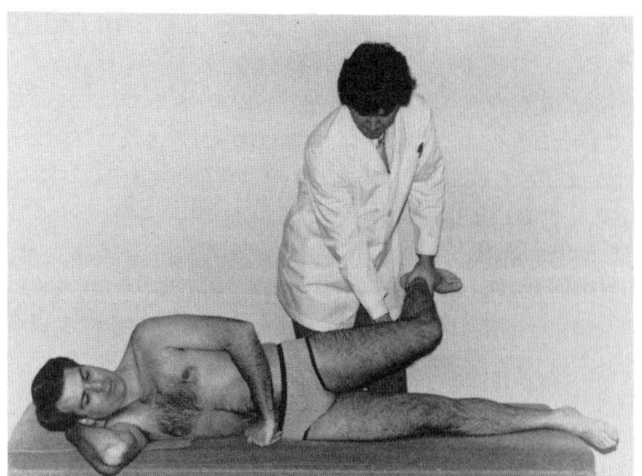

Figure 15.19. Conducting Ober's test.

Beery's Sign. This test is positive if a patient with a history of lower-trunk discomfort and fatigue is fairly comfortable when sitting with the knees flexed but experiences discomfort in the standing position. Beery's sign is typically positive in spasticity or contractures of the posterior thigh and/or leg muscles.

Lewin's Knee Sign. If quick extension of a knee in the standing position produces pain and a sharp flexion response, hamstring spasm should be suspected.

Neri's Bowing Sign. This sign is positive when a patient can flex the trunk further without low-back discomfort when the ipsilateral leg is flexed than when both knees are held in extension. A positive sign suggests hamstring spasm, contractures of the posterior thigh and/or leg muscles, sciatic neuritis, a lumbar IVD lesion, or a sacroiliac subluxation syndrome.

Tripod Sign. The patient is placed prone with the knees flexed over the edge of the table as in Huntington's test, and active and passive muscle strength and range of motion of knee extension are evaluated. If the patient must lean back (extend the trunk on the pelvis) and grasp the table to support body weight on the arms when the knees are bilaterally extended, hamstring spasm is indicated. This may be the result of any lower motor irritation located between the midthoracic area and the lower sacrum.

Quadriceps Hyperthyroidism Test. The patient sits well forward on the edge of a straight chair and attempts to hold his legs out at right angles to the trunk. A strong healthy person can usually hold this position for a minute or more, but a person with hyperthyroidism or taut hamstrings has difficulty holding this position for a few seconds.

Phelp's Test. The patient is placed in the prone position with both lower limbs extended in the relaxed position. The patient's thighs are then abducted just short of the patient's threshold of pain, and then the examiner flexes the patient's knees to 90° angles with the thighs. If this flexion allows greater abduction of a thigh on the hip without undue discomfort, a contracture of the gracilis muscle is suggested.

Hip Sprains[59, 60]

The hip articulation is situated beneath heavy muscles, fat, and fascia which protect the joint but often obscure physical signs. In the young, sprains of this joint frequently injure the upper femoral epiphysis; in adults, trauma more frequently causes injury to the muscles about the joint than to the hip joint itself.

After severe hip strain, motion is restricted and pain is often referred to the medial aspect of the knee. A limp is invariably present. A lateral fixation of the hip joint is not an uncommon finding. On the involved side, internal rotation will be restricted and the psoas muscle will test weak. In hip sprain, the mechanism is usually a twisting or wrenching motion. Occasionally, a stubborn case will show pus on aspiration.

Kinematic Tests. Laguere's, Ely's, Patrick's F-AB-ER-E, and Ober's tests should be used to support the diagnosis. Thomas' sign is positive in hip contracture; Trendelenburg's sign in hip dislocation; and Allis' knee sign in hip fracture. Trendelenburg's sign and Allis' knee sign will be described later in this chapter.

Laguere's Test. With the patient supine, the thigh and knee are flexed and the thigh is abducted and rotated outward. This forces the head of the femur against the anterior portion of the coxa capsule. Increased groin pain and spasm are usually positive signs of a lesion of the hip joint, iliopsoas muscle spasm, or a sacroiliac lesion. It can help to differentiate from a lumbar disorder.

The Iliotibial Band Syndrome[61, 62]

When flexed, the knee essentially depends on muscular support rather than that of its ligamentous elements. This is performed laterally by the iliotibial band (ITB) and biceps femoris; medially by the combined action of the semitendinosis, semimembranosus, gracilis, and sartorius; anteriorly by the quadriceps femoris; and posteriorly by the action of the popliteus. Because the ITB crosses the knee joint, its effect on the knee varies according to the position of the hip. Evans, as reported by Hazel, believes that this band greatly assists rest in the standing position.[63]

Function during Gait. During the walking cycle, the knee is in full extension at the moment of heelstrike—this is the only time in the cycle when this occurs. At all other phases of the cycle, the knee is in various degrees of flexion. When running on flat terrain, the knee does not accomplish full extension at heelstrike. However, it is close enough that lateral stability is satisfactorily accomplished by the ligamentous straps. This situation changes when running on hills, particularly during up-hill running when flexion of the knee reduces the support contributed by the ligaments and places more emphasis on dynamic muscle tissue.[64]

Etiology. Three factors will alter the functional system sufficiently to produce symptoms:

1. The first factor occurs during semiflexion of the knee. During this action, as mentioned above, the dynamic muscle groups must perform the stabilization. When performed repetitively, this can precipitate the formation of trigger points in the stressed tissues, especially when even slight biomechanical faults are associated. The ITB is victimized often since it has such a high connective tissue content. The resulting trigger points cause aberrant control of the leg during performance, and they also produce pain.

2. The second factor involves contracture and inelasticity of the hamstrings—a common finding in the entire populace and especially in the athlete. Hamstring shortening disallows full extension of the knee at heelstrike, which precipitates the same negative situation that is seen in hill running.

3. The third factor is related to contracture of the triceps surae, which alters normal gait by causing pushoff before the full stride is accomplished—thus producing the characteristic knee posture and semiflexion at heelstrike. The result is the same as described in factors 1 and 2.

Subluxations of the Hip[65–68]

Internally Rotated Femur. This subluxation is commonly associated with anterior pelvic tilting, external tibia rotation, and subtalar pronation. A degree of genu valgum and hip pain are presented.

Externally Rotated Femur. This subluxation is related to internal tibia rotation and subtalar pronation. A degree of genu varum and hip pain are associated.

Superior Femur Subluxation. This situation is usually seen when nagging hip pain complicates low-back pain. A degree of fixed internal or external rotation is often involved.

Anteriorly Subluxated Femur. Occasionally one comes upon a lesser degree of an anterior (obturator) dislocation. The cause is usually a severe fall or being forced backward against an obstacle. On the involved side, the patient exhibits hip pain and an externally rotated limb that is lengthened. The head of the femur lies near the obturator foramen.

Posteriorly Subluxated Femur. When the femur is subluxated backward, the patient has difficulty in extending his thigh. Measurement indicates limb shortening. The mechanism of injury is usually a fall, long jump, or severe upper-thigh blow from the anterior.

Sciatic Displacement. This is a chronic postural disorder associated with pelvic tilt in which weight balance is decidedly unilateral on the involved side. Acute trauma is rarely involved, but it may be in the patient's history. The patient presents hip pain, internal limb rotation, and a shortened limb. The head of the femur is found near the lesser sciatic notch.

Hip Fractures[69–71]

Hip pain mandates careful physical and roentgenographic evaluation of the soft tissues on the lateral and medial aspects of the hip. A hip dislocation with or without fracture should be considered a major injury and referred immediately without attempts at reduction. X-ray films will never indicate all soft-tissue damage present. Severe pain on motion is typical in both hip dislocations and fracture.

Allis' Knee Sign. With the patient supine, knees flexed, and soles of feet flat on table, the examiner observes heights of knees superiorly from the foot of the table. If one knee is lower than the other, it is indicative of a unilateral hip dislocation, a severe coxa disorder, or a short femur.

Langoria's Sign. Relaxation of the extensor muscles of the thigh is an indication of intracapsular fracture of the femur.

Hennequin's Sign. The patient is placed supine with the knees extended. A positive sign is found if deep palpation just inferior to Poupart's ligament and lateral to the large inguinal vessels produces deep tenderness, pain, and crepitation—signs of femoral neck fracture.

Anvil Test. If a fracture of the leg or femur is suspected, the patient is placed supine and the examiner grasps the ankle of the involved side in one hand and strikes the patient's heel with the fist of the other hand, sending a shock wave up the extremity. The result may be localized pain that will help to locate the site of fracture or pathologic focus.

Gauvain's Sign. With the patient in the sidelying position, the examiner stabilizes the patient's uppermost iliac crest with the heel of the hand and the fingerpads are fixed against the patient's lower abdomen. With the patient's uppermost knee extended, the examiner grasps the patient's upper ankle with the other hand, moderately abducts the limb, and firmly rotates it internally and externally. With the patient's knee locked in extension, these rotary maneuvers will affect the entire limb, as far superiorly as the head of the femur. A positive sign is seen when a strong abdominal contraction occurs, indicating a somatosomatic reflex spasm that is usually attributed to a hip lesion (eg, fracture, coxa tuberculosis).

Roentgenographic Considerations[72–74]

Hip dislocations and fractures are quite common, especially in the elderly, and they may lead to avascular necrosis of the femoral head. Femur fractures occurring above the intertrochanteric line are within the joint capsule. They usually heal without the formation of visible callus.

Shenton's Line. This diagnostic line is frequently disturbed in hip fracture: a gracefully arching line is drawn connecting the inferior margin of the superior pubic ramus with the medial margin of the neck of the femur (Fig. 15.20). With minimal hip displacement, landmarks will be altered when compared bilaterally.

Impactions. It is often difficult to locate a fracture of the margin of the head of the femur following severe impaction. When

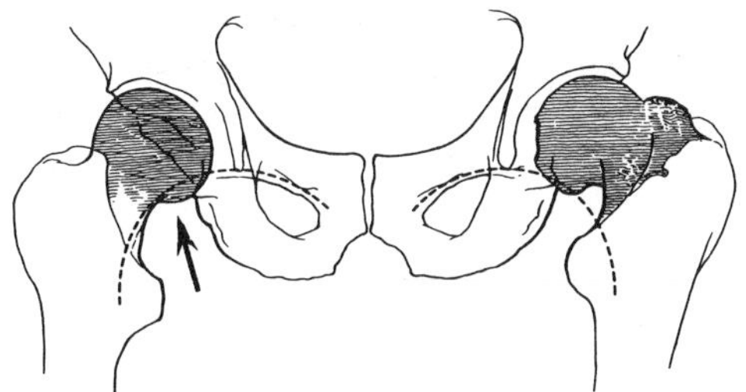

Figure 15.20. Shenton's line is represented by the dotted line drawn at the right hip along the medial margin of the femoral neck, smoothly arching to connect with the inferior margin of the superior pubic ramus. Points of reference on the left are altered because of a fractured neck of the femur, causing the femoral neck to protrude into the arch to cross Shenton's line.

visible, it is shown by slight contour changes and unusual densities.

Avulsions. The trochanteric areas should be checked for possible injury of the gluteal insertion at the greater trochanter or avulsion of the iliopsoas insertion at the lesser trochanter. Hip pain should invite careful evaluation of the soft-tissue structures in the area of the obturator internus.

Epiphyseal Slips. It is not unusual for patients in late midlife to exhibit degenerative disease of the hip, suggesting evidence of an old slipped capital femoral epiphysis. Even in minimal slip of this epiphysis, a chronic "tilt deformity" may result which exhibits the femoral head sitting eccentrically on its neck in a drooped or tipped position. When swelling and ecchymosis appear at the base of Scarpa's triangle and the patient is unable to raise the thigh while in the sitting position, traumatic separation at the epiphysis of the lesser trochanter is suggested (Ludloff's sign). Evidence is clear that there is an association of certain forms of degenerative hip disease, often with osteophytic flanges on the femoral head, secondary to a rearranged femoral-acetabular articulation. Thus, recognition during the early years is most helpful. Slippage of the femoral capital epiphysis often occurs 1–2 years earlier in females because the most rapid growth in that area comes earlier.

Fractures of the Proximal Femur. Femoral neck fractures are rare in the young; usually a degree of osteoporosis is predisposing. However, a stress fracture of the femoral neck may become a complete fracture following later torsional stress. In anterior dislocations, a shear fracture of the superior aspect of the femoral head is usually associated. The limb will usually be externally rotated without leg shortening. In posterior dislocations, the inferior aspect of the head may be fractured. Severe trauma may result in comminuted femoral head fractures. Relaxation of the fascia between the crest of the ilium and the greater trochanter is a sign of fracture of the neck of the femur (Allis' hip sign).

Hip Dislocations[75, 76]

Trendelenburg's Hip Test. If the hip and its muscles are normal, the iliac crest and sacral dimple will be slightly low on the weight-bearing side and high on the leg-elevated side when one leg is lifted. To test, have the patient with a suspected hip involvement stand on one foot, on the side of involvement, and raise the other foot and leg in hip and knee flexion. If there is hip joint involvement and muscle weakness, the iliac crest and sacral dimple will be markedly high on the standing side and low on the side the leg is elevated. A positive sign suggests that the gluteus medius muscle on the supported side is weak. The gait will exhibit a characteristic lurch to counteract the imbalance caused by the descended hip.

Posterior Dislocations. The most common hip luxation is posterior dislocation of the femoral head, exhibiting thigh adduction and internal rotation at the hip and leg shortening on the affected side. When dislocation takes place, the head of the femur may be driven into the posterior or central acetabulum creating acetabular comminution fragments. But posterior displacement may also be seen without fracture, with a single major posterior acetabular fragment, or with femoral head fracture. The cause is usually a force against the flexed knee with the hip in flexion and slight adduction. Common complications are sciatic nerve stretching causing foot drop and numbness of the lateral calf.

Anterior Dislocations. Anterior dislocation is relatively rare because Bigelow's ligament offers considerable protection. The limb will be externally rotated and abducted, without leg shortening. Obturator, iliac, and pubic displacement may be seen, as well as those associated with femoral head fractures. These usually occur from a blow to the back while squatting, a fall in which forced abduction occurs, or forced abduction of the extended hip.

Central Dislocations. These injuries feature (1) displacement toward the inner wall only with partial dome fractures or (2) central displacement with comminution of the dome. This type of dislocation-fracture commonly results from a severe force to the lateral trochanter and pelvis directed through the femoral head. Occasionally, they are produced by a force on the long axis of the femur when the hip is abducted.

Trigger Points

There is only one common trigger point in the thigh, and that is of the vastus medialis (Fig. 15.21).

Fixations[77]

Hip Fixations. The head of the femur is a common site of functional fixations, especially the ligamentous type, as well as pathologic fixations. Occupations that require prolonged sitting frequently produce, over many months or years, shortening of "Y" ligament. This produces a lordosis-type spinal distortion when erect that disappears when sitting. Another type of common fixation is that of a lateral fixation of the hip joint. On the involved side, internal rotation will usually be restricted and the psoas muscle will test weak.

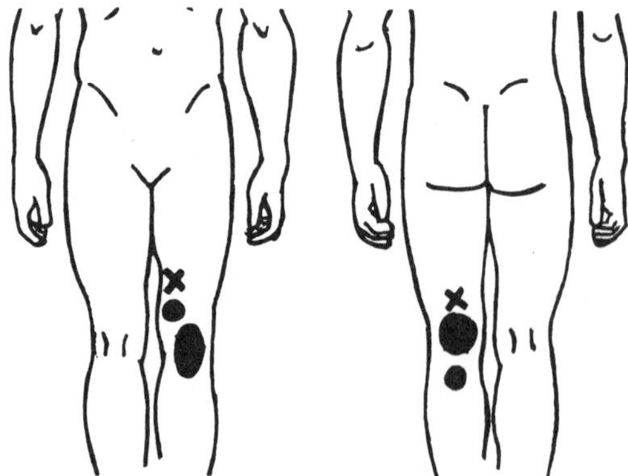

Figure 15.21. *Left*, vastus medialis trigger point; *X*, common site. *Blackened areas* indicate typical sites of referred pain. *Right*, biceps femoris trigger point.

Thigh Fixations. Hypomobility of the thigh's long muscles from intrinsic hypertonicity decreases the mobility of the knee and patella. Gillet feels that this state is often secondary to a site of pelvic fixation.

Meralgia Paresthetica[78–80]

This syndrome, often referred to as lateral femoral cutaneous neuropathy, features a patch of anesthesia, paresthesia, or hyperesthesia, with or without pain, on the anterior surface of one or both thighs in the distribution of the lateral femoral cutaneous nerve.

Background. The lateral femoral cutaneous nerve arises from the posterior divisions of L1–L3, appears at the lateral border of the psoas, passes obliquely across the iliacus to the anterior superior iliac spine, and then travels under the inguinal ligament to enter the anterolateral aspect of the thigh.

Etiologic Considerations. Most authorities feel that the syndrome has its origin in some form of inflammatory process involving the lateral femoral cutaneous nerve or its roots. This focus of irritation may often be found (1) at the L1–L3 IVFs from subluxation encroachment or arthritic hyperplasia or (2) in the pelvis from repetitive trauma as seen in athletic injuries and late pregnancy. Nevertheless, pathology lying anywhere along the course of the nerve may be responsible, whether it be intraspinal, intersegmental, paraspinal, retroperitoneal, pelvic, or, rarely, abdominal.

Differential Diagnosis. The typical patient reports a sense of numbness or burning in the anterolateral aspect of the thigh, which is rarely painful until the late stages. Care must be taken to differentiate this syndrome from trochanteric or iliopectineal (iliopsoas) bursitis, both of which refer pain to the anterolateral thigh. It should also be kept in mind that pronation or supination of the ankle, genu varum, genu valgum, genu recurvatum, flexion contracture, etc, can cause or contribute to anterosuperior thigh pain.

Management. Associated lumbar subluxations should be freed immediately. Aiken[81] reports that low-wattage ultrasound applied paraspinally at the L2 level for 3 minutes and at the area where the nerve leaves the pelvis for 2 minutes may be of value. High-voltage stimulation in the area of L2 and again in the anterolateral aspect of the thigh may also assist recovery. Massage and muscle stripping of the involved thigh is recommended in the postgraduate notes of Northwestern College of Chiropractic, as is moist heat. Weight reduction should be recommended if obesity is a factor.

THE KNEE

The knee is the largest joint in the body. In the normal erect relaxed posture, the support of body weight and stability of the knee joint is provided strictly through the bony design and ligaments of the joint. No muscle action is involved.

Basic Functional Anatomy[82-86]

The Patella[87, 88]

The triangular knee cap, the largest sesamoid of the body, has its apex directed caudally. Its posterior surface is smooth for articulation with the femur. The patella lies within the tendon of the quadriceps, tending to hold the tendon anterior from the femur. This improves quadriceps extension ability about 30%. In this sense, the patella can be considered a movable pulley.

The Knee Joint[89-92]

The major osseous structures of the knee joint, a typical hinge joint, are the lateral and medial condyles of the distal femur and the superior articular surfaces of the tibia. The head of the fibula at the upper leg can be considered a part of the knee joint complex. On rare occasions, the simple synovial joint of the tibial-fibular articulation communicates with the knee joint proper.

The synovial joint capsule of the knee is supported laterally to the patella by the inferior fibers of the fascia lata and quadriceps. The posterior capsule is supported by the semimembranosus tendon and the oblique popliteal ligament, but the major ligamentous structures of the knee are the collateral ligaments, the capsule, the menisci, the cruciate ligaments, and coronary ligaments (Fig. 15.22).

Collateral Ligaments. The broad medial (tibial) collateral ligament spans from the medial epicondyle of the femur to the

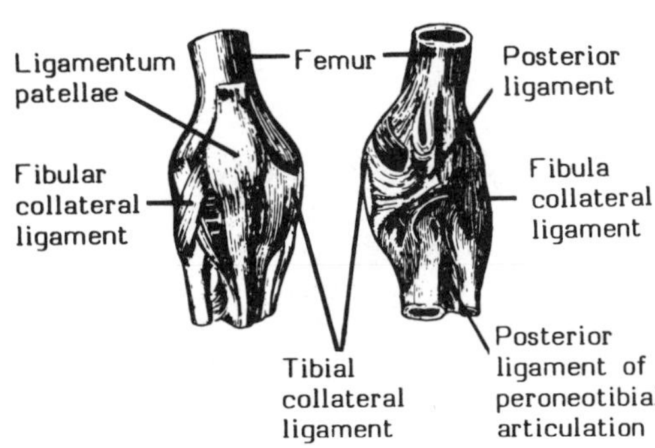

Figure 15.22. Some major superficial ligaments of the knee area. *Left*, anterior view; *right*, posterior view.

medial aspect of the superior tibia, supporting the posterior aspect of the capsule. These fibers relax on knee flexion and tighten on extension, rotation, and lateral motions. The lateral (fibula) collateral ligament extends from the lateral epicondyle of the femur to the head of the fibula, offering no support to the capsule. These fibers relax on knee flexion and tighten on extension, rotation, and lateral motions.

Cruciate Ligaments. The cross-shaped anterior and posterior cruciate ligaments lie within the joint capsule but are separated from the joint cavity by synovial tissue. They attach between the menisci in the intercondylar area. The anterior cruciate spans between the anterior tibial condyle and the back of the medial surface of the lateral condyle of the femur. The posterior cruciate extends from the posterior intercondylar area to the lateral side of the medial condyle of the femur. Both of these ligaments are tense in all positions but are especially so during extreme flexion, extension, and rotation. Their main function is to restrict shear forces across the knee joint.

The Menisci and Coronary Ligaments. The two wedged-shaped internal and external menisci communicate only anteriorly. These crescents deepen the joint, cushion axial forces between the femur and tibia, and help to smooth the distribution of synovial fluid. The medial and lateral coronary ligaments, extensions of the capsule, attach the borders of the menisci to the tibia and femur. The popliteus muscle pierces the capsule but is separated from the cavity by a synovial membrane (Fig. 15.23).

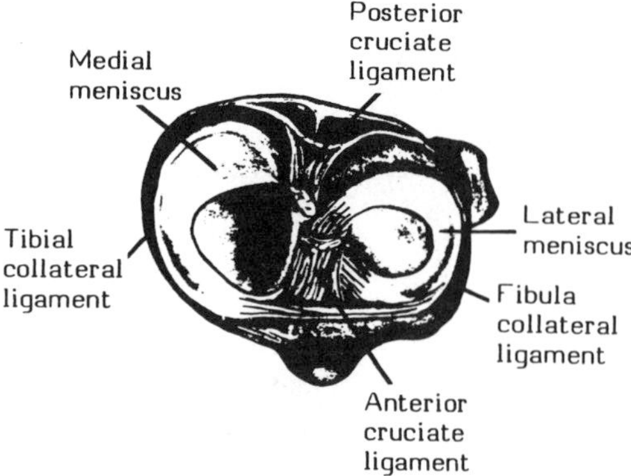

Figure 15.23. Schematic of the superior surface of the tibia.

Knee Movements[93–102]

Joint Motion[103, 104]

Basic movements of the knee joint are flexion, extension, internal rotation, and external rotation (Table 15.3). Flexion and extension occur essentially between the femur and tibia. Rotation during slight flexion, internal and external, occurs between the tibia and femur and from displacement of the menisci.

Flexion and Extension. Active flexion (135°) is tested by having the patient squat in a deep knee-bent position. Active extension (0°) is tested by having the patient arise from this position to the standing position. Dominance of one knee over the other and the smoothness of movement should be noted, especially of the last 10° of extension. Flexion and extension should be tested passively if necessary, with the patient prone. The popliteal space is stabilized with one hand, and the patient's ankle grasped with the other hand. The leg is flexed as far as possible on the femur, noting the distance from the heel to the buttock. The leg should normally extend to 0° in a smooth arc.

The Bounce Home Test. Hoppenfeld[105] describes an evaluation of full knee extension which he calls the "bounce home" test. The patient is placed supine. The examiner cups one hand under the patient's heel and fully flexes the knee with the other hand. While the patient's heel is grasped, the patient's knee is allowed to passively drop toward the tabletop in full extension, normally with an abrupt stop. If this full extension is not achieved and passive pressure elicits a "rubbery" resistance to extension, a blockage is indicated. This lack of full extension points to a torn meniscus, intracapsular swelling, or a loose fragment within the knee joint.

Because of its anatomical design, the leg cannot be fully extended without a degree of external tibial rotation on the femur. A maximal rotation of 6° of lateral rotation occurs during the last 10° of extension and the reverse during the first 10° of flexion. This has been called the "screw-home" mechanism. A simple test to be described later, the Helfet test, determines the integrity of the knee relative to the presence of this normal motion.

Table 15.3.
Knee Motion

Joint motion	Prime movers	Accessories
Flexion	Hamstrings Semimembranosus Semitendinosus Biceps femoris	Sartorius Gracilis Gastrocnemius Plantaris Popliteus
Extension	Rectus femoris Vastus lateralis Vastus medialis Vastus intermedius	
External rotation	Biceps femoris	Tensor fasciae latae
Internal rotation	Semimembranosus Semitendinosus Gracilis Popliteus Sartorius	

Internal and External Rotation. To test active knee rotation, the patient slightly flexes his knee and rotates his foot laterally and medially. About 10° either way is normal. Passive rotation is tested with the patient supine. The examiner places a stabilizing hand just above the knee and rotates the tibia internally and externally with his active hand. It is helpful to have the stabilizing hand simultaneously palpate the tibial tubercle to note the amount of movement.

Kinesiology of the Knee[106–110]

Extension. Knee extension is provided essentially by the rectus femoris (L2–L4) and quadratus femoris (L4–S1), with help from the vastus group (L2–L4). To test with the patient seated, the stabilizing hand of the examiner is placed above the patient's knee and the femur is fixed. Then increasing resistance is applied on the patient's tibia above the ankle as he attempts to extend his knee. It is helpful to palpate the prime movers with the stabilizing hand during the test.

Flexion. Knee flexion is under the control of the hamstring group (semitendinosus, semimembranosus, and biceps femoris), supplied by the sciatic nerve (L5–S2). Help is provided by the sartorius, gracilis, gas trocnemius, plantaris, and popliteus (Table 15.4). To evaluate with the patient supine, test the group by stabilizing the thigh above the knee. Grasp the patient's leg above the ankle with the other hand, and offer increasing resistance as the patient attempts to flex the knee. If the patient rotates his leg externally during the test, more work is forced upon the biceps femoris, and upon the semitendinosus and semimembranosus when the leg is rotated internally.

Rotation. During internal rotation, power is provided medially by the reciprocal action of the semitendinosus, semimembranosus, sartorius, popliteus, and gracilis. The biceps femoris controls external rotation.

Goniometry of the Knee[111,112]

As in other readings, deviation from neutral should be measured in situations of ankylosis.

Flexion and Extension. To record restricted knee flexion and extension, the patient is placed in the supine neutral position. The goniometer is centered over the lateral aspect of the patient's knee joint, and the reading recorded. The base of the goniometer should be along the axis of the femur, and the goniometer arm should be along the axis of the leg. If there is extension loss, the deviation from the neutral position should be recorded. The patient flexes the knee as far as possible, and the reading at the end of the motion is recorded. Then the test is repeated with the patient in the sitting position.

Table 15.4.
Muscles of the Knee

Muscle	Major functions	Spinal segment
Gastrocnemius	Flexion	S1–S2
Gracilis	Flexion, medial rotation	L2–L3
Hamstrings	Flexion, rotation	L5–S2
Biceps femoris	Flexion, external rotation (long head)	S1–S2
Semimembranosus	Flexion, medial rotation	L5–S1
Semitendinosus	Flexion, medial rotation	L5–S2
Plantaris	Flexion	L5–S1
Popliteus	Flexion, medial rotation	L4–S1
Quadratus femoris	Extension	L4–S1
Rectus femoris	Extension	L2–L4
Sartorius	Flexion, medial rotation	L2–L3
Tensor fasciae latae	External rotation	L4–S1
Vastus muscles	Extension	L2–L4

Spinal innervation varies somewhat in different people. The spinal nerves listed here are averages and may differ in a particular patient; thus, an allowance of a segment above and below those listed in most text tables should be considered.

Measuring the Q Angle.[113] A clinical measurement associated with extensor mechanism alignment is that of the quadriceps (Q) angle between the long axis of the femoral shaft and a line from the middle of the patella to the tibial tubercle (Fig. 15.24). The Q angle, normally 10° in men and 15° in women, is measured by placing a dual-arm goniometer on the center of the patella. One arm is aimed at the anterior superior iliac spine (ASIS) and the other is placed in line with the center of the patellar tendon. In external tibial rotation, the Q angle may be markedly increased. The angle increases as the tibial tubercle is displaced laterally when the tibia is externally rotated.

Biomechanics of the Knee[114–120]

The knee, like the hip, operates as a first-class lever, in which the fulcrum is at the point of weight-bearing contact. During gait, body weight acts medial to the knee so that the center of rotation (fulcrum) is centered over the medial condyle when viewed from the A-P. Equilibrium is maintained by the collateral ligaments, fascia lata, and tendon of the biceps femoris. As in the hip during normal gait, forces across the knee joint are from 3–5 times the imposed body weight. Most of the resultant joint forces are located in the medial compartment of the healthy knee.

The line of action extends from the medial condyle of the distal femur through the tibia. The fibula has no weight-bearing function. When loaded, the knee joint and the tibia are subjected to medial compressive forces and lateral tensile forces that tend to shift the tibia laterally relative to the femur. These forces, exaggerated during normal gait, must be counteracted by the medial ligaments of the knee. However, in a Trendelenburg gait, for instance, weight is shifted to the lateral component of the knee and there is a tendency toward medial shifting of the tibia, causing the lateral ligaments to be stressed.

Muscle and compression forces increase rapidly in the knee when deep knee bending is assumed. When erect, no quadriceps activity is necessary because the line of force of body weight is slightly in front of the knee's axis of rotation and the compression force at the articular surface of the knee and the shearing force of the femur on the tibia are due to the stabilizing structures at the posterior aspect of the knee (Fig. 15.25). During squatting, the moment produced by body weight greatly increases, and increased muscular force is necessary to maintain equilibrium. This in turn increases the joint reaction force that places a greater burden of shear on the joint ligaments and compression on the menisci. Squatting exercises are thus contraindicated, even for the athlete.

Knee Stability and Its Evaluation[121–128]

The normal knee joint is provided with strong ligaments, a large joint capsule, and adjacent muscles and tendons that offer great stability. Severe sprain, especially that in hyperextension, readily leads to functional instability with chronic "giving way."

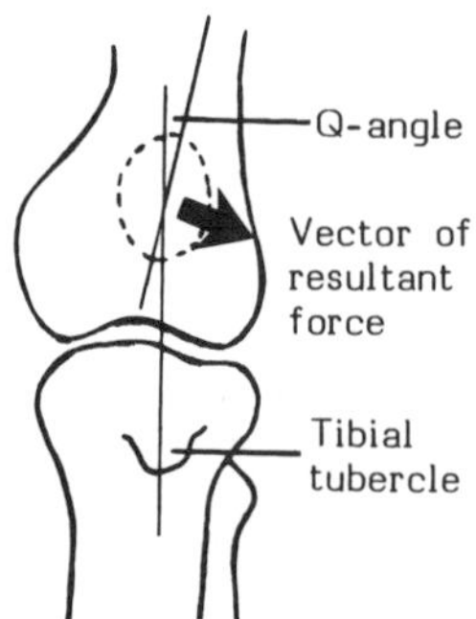

Figure 15.24. Q angle in patella subluxation.

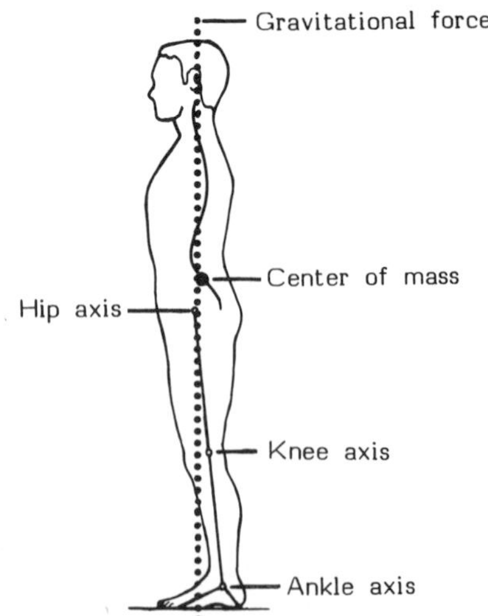

Figure 15.25. The line of gravity normally falls posterior to the hip joint, slightly anterior to mid-knee, and anterior to the ankle joint.

Undoubtedly, a large degree of proprioception loss and loss of quadriceps power will be involved. In partial ligament tears, sprain symptoms are more pronounced, but there is little or no instability involved. Complete tears exhibit marked laxity upon stress movements but may present little pain. Several clinical tests that have been devised to evaluate stability will be described.

General Tests of Knee Integrity

Knee Hyperflexion Stress Test. With the patient in the supine position, the examiner places one hand on the involved knee and the other on the ipsilateral ankle. The knee is moderately flexed, the thigh is brought toward the patient's abdomen, and the patient's heel is slowly pushed toward the patient's buttock. Unless the patient is considerably obese, the normal knee can be flexed without pain so that it touches the buttock. If knee pain or severe discomfort is induced on this maneuver, a subtle localized knee lesion may be brought out.

Knee Hyperextension Stress Test. The patient is placed prone with the knees extended in the relaxed position. The examiner places a fist under the distal thigh of the involved side, flexes the knee to about 30° with the other hand, and then allows the leg to drop without assistance when the muscles are relaxed. Most knee lesions limit extension to some degree. Thus, if extension is limited or the rebound is abnormal during this "knee drop" test (when compared to the contralateral knee), some type of knee disorder should be suspected and may possibly be localized.

External Rotation-Recurvatum

To test for external rotation-recurvatum, the patient is placed supine. The heel is grasped with one hand, and the calf is supported with the other hand. The knee is allowed to pass from about 10° flexion into full extension. A positive sign occurs when the knee assumes a position of slight recurvatum, the tibia rotates externally, and there is increased tibia vara. Such a sign indicates injury to the arcuate complex or lateral half of the posterior capsule, or a degree of injury to the posterior cruciate ligament.

Anterolateral Rotary Instability[129,130]

McIntosh's Test. The patient is placed supine, the lower extremity is supported at the heel with one hand, and the other hand is placed laterally over the proximal tibia just distal to the patella. The caudad hand applies valgus stress and internally rotates the tibia as the knee is gradually moved from full extension into flexion. During flexion of the knee, the lateral tibial plateau can be felt to subluxate anteriorly in relation to the lateral condyle. Lateral crepitation may be felt, and a slight resistance to flexion may be perceived. When the knee is at about 35° flexion, the iliotibial band tightens and passes behind the transverse axis of rotation, and the tibial plateau is suddenly reduced, often with a "clunking" sensation that can often be both felt and heard.

Hughston's Jerk Sign. This is a modification of McIntosh's test. With the patient supine, the foot is grasped with one hand while the other hand rests over the proximal lateral aspect of the leg just distal to the patella. The knee is flexed at 90°, and valgus stress is applied as the tibia is rotated internally. The knee is then gradually extended. The lateral tibial plateau is initially in a reduced position to the femoral condyle; however, as the knee is extended to about 35° of flexion, the lateral tibial plateau suddenly subluxates forward in relation to the femoral condyle with a jerking sensation. The lateral plateau slowly obtains its reduced position, which completes on full extension as the knee is extended.

Slocum's Test.[131] This is another modification of McIntosh's test. The patient is placed in the lateral recumbent position with the involved knee uppermost. The under extremity is flexed at 90° at both the hip and knee. The pelvis is rotated slightly posterior about 30°, and the weight of the extremity is supported by the inner aspect of the foot and heel. This position causes valgus stress at the knee and a slight internal rotation of the leg. The examiner then grips the distal thigh with one hand and the proximal leg with the other hand and presses back of the fibula and femoral condyle with the thumbs. The knee is then gently pushed from extension into flexion and again, as the iliotibial tract passes behind the transverse axis of rotation at about 35°, the lateral tibial plateau, which has subluxated forward, is reduced with a palpable "clunk" or "giving way" sensation.

Losee's Test. With the patient supine and the knee flexed, the examiner applies valgus stress to the tibia with one hand while the head of the fibula is pushed anteriorly with the other hand. If an anterior subluxation occurs at the lateral tibial plateau when the knee approaches full extension, anterolateral rotary instability is indicated.

Anteroposterior Instability

Anterior Drawer Sign.[132,133] The anterior and posterior cruciate ligaments provide A-P stability to the knee joint. These intracapsular ligaments originate from the tibia and insert onto the inner aspects of the femoral condyles. To examine A-P stability, the patient is placed supine and the involved knee is flexed to 90° so that the foot is flat on the table. The examiner should sit sideways so that his hip can keep the patient's foot from moving during the tests. The examiner positions his hands around the knee being examined similar to but lower than the bony palpation starting position; ie, thumbs pointing superiorly over the lateral and medial joint lines with fingers wrapped around the lateral and medial insertions of the hamstrings. In this position, the examiner pulls the tibia forward (Fig. 15.26). When a distinct sliding forward of the tibia from under the femur is noted, it is indicative of a torn anterior cruciate ligament (Lachman's test). A positive sign is called an "anterior drawer sign." Slight anterior sliding, however, is often normal.

A positive anterior drawer sign should be confirmed by repeating the maneuver with the patient's leg internally rotated 30° and externally rotated 15°. The reason for this is that even if the anterior cruciate ligament is torn, external rotation should reduce forward movement of the tibia; if it does not, both the anterior cruciate and the posteromedial joint capsule may be torn. Likewise, even if the anterior cruciate ligament is torn, internal rotation should reduce forward movement of the tibia. If it does not, both the anterior cruciate and the posterolateral joint capsule may be torn. The medial collateral ligaments may also be involved in loss of A-P stability.

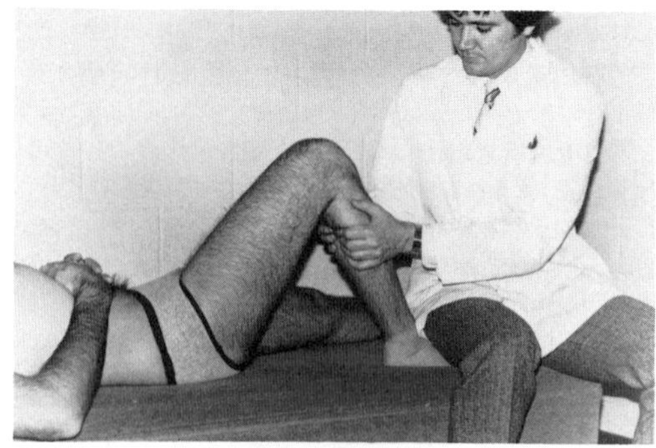

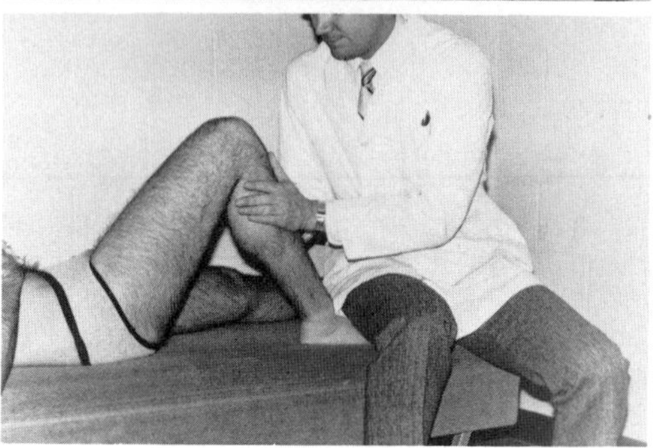

Figure 15.26. *Top*, position for eliciting the anterior drawer sign; *bottom*, position for the posterior drawer sign.

Posterior Drawer Sign. The stability of the posterior cruciate ligament is tested in the same manner as the anterior cruciate, except the tibia is pushed backward rather than pulled forward. Thus, it can be done in one continuous movement with the anterior drawer test. When a distinct sliding backward of the tibia from under the femur is noted, it is indicative of a torn posterior cruciate ligament. A positive sign is called a "posterior drawer sign" and is less common than the anterior sign.

Management. Injuries resulting in anterior or posterior instability may be treated conservatively if a complete rupture has not occurred. Initial cryotherapy and pressure support followed by a carefully supervised regimen of articular correction, massage, crutch walking, guarded weight bearing with the knee in 30° flexion, physiotherapy to enhance circulation and promote healing, and quadriceps strengthening exercises are often successful in returning an athlete to competition in 3–6 weeks.

Posterolateral Rotary Instability

Posterolateral rotary instability results from a posterior subluxation of the lateral tibial plateau in relation to the lateral femoral condyle, accompanied by abnormal external tibial rotation. To test for posterolateral rotary instability, perform the external rotation-recurvatum test and the posterior drawer test. Note excessive posterior sag of the lateral tibial plateau with external tibial rotation. This instability results from laxity of the arcuate complex, the lateral half of the posterior capsule, and a degree of failure of the posterior cruciate ligament.

SELECTED CLINICAL PROBLEMS OF THE KNEE[134–141]

Injuries due to excessive stress appear especially on the short arm of a first-class lever joint such as the elbow and knee. This can be witnessed with the mechanism of injury to the medial collateral ligament when the valgus knee is overstressed. During extension, a force (body weight) is applied at a distance from the fulcrum that is several times that occurring between the fulcrum and the ligament.

Because it is a strong joint yet relatively unstable (a clinical paradox), sprain of the knee may be complicated by derangement of the intra-articular structures and precautions must be taken to carefully examine for possible displacement of the cartilages and rupture of related stabilizing ligaments. Biomechanically, the knee is far more than a simple hinge joint.

Functional Distortions of the Knee[142–148]

Genu Valgum[149]

If there is more than a few centimeters distance between the knees when the subject is standing with the knee caps straight ahead, a degree of genu valgum (knock knees) is present that may be more marked on one side than the other. There is (1) excessive internal rotation of the femur and external rotation restriction, (2) excessive external rotation of the tibia and internal rotation restriction, and (3) medial patella deviation due to femur rotation. This results in a short leg causing pelvic imbalance if the condition is unilateral. Be aware, however, that people with a large degree of joint flexibility can hyperextend their knees along with femoral rotation which gives a false appearance of structural deformity. Postural knock knees should be differentiated from that due to severe obesity or secondary to rickets, rheumatoid arthritis, and myelomeningocele.

Genu Varum[150]

If the medial malleoli are touching and the knees are not, the space between the knees determines the degree of genu varum (bow legs). There is (1) excessive external rotation of the femur and internal rotation restriction, (2) excessive internal rotation of the tibia and external rotation restriction, and (3) lateral patella deviation due to rotation of the femur (Fig. 15.27). Postural bowed legs should especially be differentiated from achondroplasia, osteogenesis imperfecta, spondyloepiphyseal dysplasia, rickets, and Blount's disease.

Genu Recurvatum[151]

This mark of hyperextensibility is sometimes associated with a joint disorder involving A-P instability. Any activity that may induce anterior leg trauma or strenuous "take offs" from a locked knee would be contraindicated.

Lateral Tibial Rotation and Torsion[152]

If the knee caps are facing straight ahead and the feet point distinctly outward, this is a positive sign of lateral rotation of the tibia on the femur and usually more pronounced on one side than the other. If the feet appear normally positioned but the patellae appear

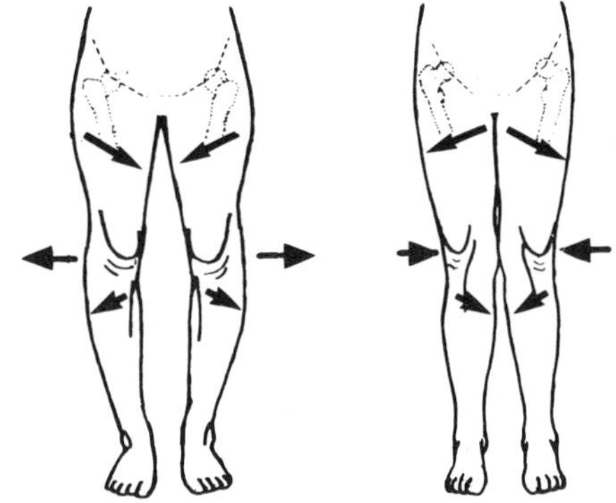

Figure 15.27. *Left*, genu varum; *right*, genu valgum.

rolled medially inward, it is a positive sign of tibial torsion.

Traumatic Disorders of the Patella[153–157]

Rupture or tendinitis of the patella tendon, quadriceps rupture or tendinitis, and stress fractures of the tibia have a high incidence of injury. In tendinitis, the pain may be perceived either during and shortly after activity or be chronic. Forceful jumping may result in an avulsion fracture of the patella.

Soft-Tissue Injuries[158–160]

Infrapatellar Fat Pad Hypertrophy. Repeated stress to the knee joint may cause the infrapatellar fat pad or the synovial villi to become hypertrophied. The symptoms are joint weakness or definite locking, joint effusion when acute, pain on the medial aspect of the knee, and tenderness distal and medial to the patella. Positive diagnosis, however, can only be made upon exploratory surgery.

Intracapsular Pinches. A sudden joint stress, usually rotational, may cause some soft tissue to be pinched within articular structures during jumping, changing direction in running, kicking, etc. This is most frequently seen in the knee in which the infrapatellar fat pad is nipped, resulting in a degree of effusion and possible hemorrhage.

In these disorders, diagnosis is essentially by exclusion. There is no history of external trauma, nor are there signs of joint line tenderness or instability. Discomfort is felt directly behind the patella. A slight effusion may be present and be associated with a slight loss in full extension. The sides of the patella and its tendon will feel thick and firm. This mass will be tender, and it will be the only site of tenderness if ligament and fibrocartilage involvement can be excluded.

Referral for surgery may be necessary if the superior portion of the tibia cuts off a large portion of the infrapatellar pad or if the tag later becomes calcified and causes trouble. Immediate surgery is required in some cases in which a pedunculated part may become strangled by adhesions resulting in torsion gangrene associated with joint locking and hemarthrosis.

Acute Bursitis. Bursitis of the prepatellar bursa is commonly called "housemaid's knee." Fluctuation, with or without heat and tenderness, that is limited to the prepatellar space is usually diagnostic (Fig. 15.28). Conservative management of an acutely swollen bursa is not difficult if undertaken immediately. On rare occasions, referral may be necessary if swelling does not begin to subside within 24 hours. Graduated activity may begin as soon as the acute phase has resolved.

Knee Effusion Test. If a joint is greatly swollen from a major effusion, the patient should be placed in a relaxed supine position. The limb is relaxed, and the knee is slowly extended. Then the patella is pushed into the trochlear groove and released quickly. This will force fluid under the patella to the sides of the joint and then to return under the patella. This rebound is referred to as a "ballottable patella." Minimal effusion, however, will not ballot the patella. In cases of minor effusion, it is necessary to "milk" the fluid from the suprapatellar pouch and lateral side to the medial side of the joint. Once the fluid has been moved medially, tapping over the fluid will return it to the lateral side.

Patella Tendon Strain. The patella tendon is often subject to partial tears, complete rupture (rare), peritendinitis, and focal degeneration. Chronic strain has a high incidence in certain laborers and professional

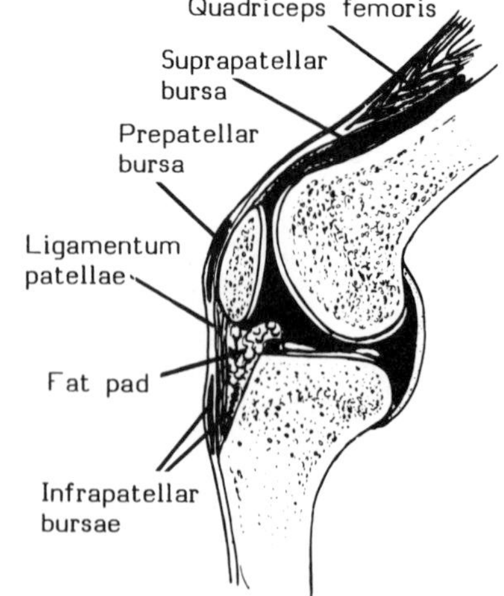

Figure 15.28. Schematic of the knee joint depicting the bursae and their structural relationships.

athletes. Partial tears are often misdiagnosed as strain. The picture is one of pain on forced knee extension and during activity, point tenderness, possible extension block and weakness, thickened adjacent tissues, and roentgenographic soft-tissue changes. Differentiation from peritendinitis can only be made during surgery.

Patella Wobble Sign. A patient in the sitting position is instructed to extend a knee while the examiner cups a palm over the patella. If erratic patellar motion is felt during the last phase of extension, an irregular retropatellar growth or some type of incomplete obstruction is indicated (eg, hypertrophied infrapatellar synovial folds, hardened fat pad).

Popliteal Swelling

There are numerous and variable bursae in the popliteal fossa, and they often fuse to form a large bursa (eg, gastrocnemiosemimembranous bursa). Blits[161] brings out that this is the most common bursa of which the popliteal (Baker's) cyst is a distention. To differentiate this type of swelling in the popliteal fossa from others, aneurysms, hemangiomas, and neoplasms should also be considered.

Baker's Cyst. This is recognized as a soft, nontender collection of synovial fluid that has escaped from the knee joint or a bursa and has formed a new synovial-lined sac in the popliteal space (typically the posteromedial or posterolateral aspect). It is often associated with degenerative and other joint diseases.

Aneurysm. This pulsating mass exhibits a bruit synchronous with the pulse. Diagnosis is confirmed by arteriography.

Hemangioma. This is characterized by a painful, tender, soft swelling; increased local temperature with superficial vessels dilated; and multiple opacities of calcification confirmed by roentgenography.

Neoplasm. Benign tumors are soft, mobile, and well localized. A malignant fibrosarcoma is painful, firm, tender, and fixed to surrounding tissues. The regional lymph nodes may be involved. Diagnosis is confirmed by biopsy.

Patella Subluxations, Fractures, and Dislocations[162–168]

In knee injuries, the incidence of patella subluxation is second only to collateral ligament and meniscus injuries.[169]

Superior Patella Subluxation. Indications include superior displacement, patellar tendinitis, quadriceps spasm, chondromalacia patellae, and restricted inferior patella motion.

Inferior Patella Subluxation. This type of displacement is typically associated with chondromalacia of the patella, blocked superior joint play, suprapatellar tendinitis, and restricted extension of the knee.

Superomedial or Superolateral Patella Subluxations. The major features are diagonal displacement, patellar tendinitis, quadriceps spasm, and chondromalacia patellae. Genu varum and restricted inferolateral patella motion are often associated with superomedial subluxations, while genu valgum and restricted inferomedial patella motion are associated with superolateral subluxations.

Patella Fractures and Dislocations. In patella dislocation, a fixed tilt or malposition of the patella or an osteochondral fracture may be noted. Motion will be restricted, and the surrounding tissues will be stressed. Secondary infection may occur. The most common patella dislocation is sideward, especially laterally, but proximal shifting may occur. In association with traumatic dislocations, fractures of the medial patellar margin and osteochondral fracture of the femoral condyles are quite common. The cause may be a congenital or traumatic decrease in the femoral intrapatellar groove, especially at the lateral lip; trauma tearing the ligamentous attachments; inflammation (traumatic or infectious) in the intrapatellar pad that produces an increase in synovial fluid; vastus medialis dystonia; torn collateral or cruciate ligaments; or femoral or tibial dislocation. The typical acute case presents point tenderness, erythema, mild fever, edema, pain aggravated by motion, joint block, patella restriction, limping, and obvious displacement. The patella apprehension and bounce home tests are positive.

Dreyer's Sign. The patient is placed supine with the legs extended in the relaxed position and asked to raise the involved thigh while keeping the knee extended. If the patient is unable to do this, the examiner grasps the large quadriceps tendon just above the knee to anchor it against the femur and the patient is asked to try to lift the limb again. If the patient is then able to lift the limb when the quadriceps tendon is stabilized, a fractured patella should be suspected. The reason for this is that the rectus femoris (a primary hip flexor) attaches to the patella by way of the quadriceps tendon.

Patella Apprehension Test. The patella displaces laterally with vigorous quadriceps contraction. When a person strongly extends the flexed knee with the leg externally rotated, the patella may dislocate if its attachments are weakened. If a patella is prone to dislocation, any attempt by the examiner to produce such a dislocation will be met with by sharp patient resistance. In testing, the patient is placed in the relaxed neutral supine position, and the examiner applies increasing pressure against the patella. If a chronic weakness exists, the patient will become increasing apprehensive as the patella begins to dislocate.

A recurring dislocation is most common when the patella is small or there is a degree of postural valgus. Each recurrence becomes more difficult to manage even if the dislocation is spontaneously reduced. Rehabilitation should emphasize vastus medialis reeducation and active flexion-extension exercises. When tearing is severe, surgery is necessary.

Traumatic Disorders of the Knee[170–176]

Roentgenographic Considerations[177,178]

The most common type of soft-tissue injury in the knee area is the result of effusion at the suprapatellar joint space in which adjacent fat pads are displaced. The fatty tissue above the patella, anterior to the femur, and posterior to the quadriceps tendon near the superior aspect of the patella is somewhat lucent in the normal knee. If effusion exists, fatty areas are replaced by fluids matching the density of the thigh muscles, and normal signs become obliterated.

Knee effusion may be shown in the A-P view by soft-tissue density medial to the tibia below the joint line. This is usually attributed to paratibial synovial cysts progressing posteriorly and medially which may extend via bursae connections to the popliteal space or to the posterior aspect of the upper calf. It rarely extends to the posterior thigh.

The residual epiphyseal cartilage of the distal femur should be of rather uniform thickness. No displacement of its margins should be noted. The articular margins of the femoral condyles are normally smooth, but fragmentations will be noted in osteochondritis dissecans and osteochondral fractures. Evidence of swelling at the site of insertion of the quadriceps tendon at the apophysis of the tibial tubercle suggests Osgood-Schlatter disease.

Strong, sudden muscle contractions may also cause fracture avulsions in the lateral knee area. Small bone fragments may be found in an A-P view at the lateral edge of the proximal tibia upon iliotibial band injury.

In partial tendon tears, calcification may be found in the patellar tendon following hemorrhage. If joint dislocation has occurred, signs of deposition may be found in the soft tissues. After blunt trauma to a limb soft tissues may show evidence of heterotopic bone formation. Such ossification involves not only the muscle tissue but also occurs within the fascial planes. The typical history is one of trauma, muscle pain and soreness, and hemorrhage into the soft tissues, with signs of poorly defined ossification developing in 2–5 weeks.

Collateral Ligament Injury[179–182]

Collateral ligament sprain presents the same symptoms of localized pain, tenderness, and swelling as does capsule sprain. Stress tests help in differentiation. Typically, pain is progressively severe the aggravated by the motion of injury, swelling is localized, point tenderness is demonstrable, muscles are spastic, and hemarthrosis may be present. Drawer signs are negative. Postinjury x-ray films may show elongated amorphous shadows near the affected femoral condyle, evidence of hematoma resolution, and possible displacement of the fibula or tibia.

Mild Sprains. Minor sprains usually

have a history of a sudden or unexpected movement, especially when the knee is in a valgus position from an internally rotated thigh, a pronated or flat foot, or abduction during foot strike in gait. These injuries are produced by a sudden rotational sprain such as during stumbling, a misstep off a curb or stair, and stepping into a hole or on an object.

Severe Sprains. Rupture of the lateral ligaments is produced by trauma in which the internal lateral ligament is ruptured by overabduction of the leg or the external ligament is ruptured by overadduction. Excessive lateral motion during complete extension indicates laceration of lateral ligaments. The internal lateral ligament is impaired if abduction is excessive; the external ligament, if adduction is excessive.

Medial (Tibial) Collateral Ligament Sprain. An external twisting overstress with the valgus knee in partial flexion frequently produces partial tearing of the long anterior fibers (Fig. 15.29). Complete rupture may occur from violent abduction while the knee is extended or in external rotation and abduction while the knee is partially flexed. Hematoma usually results, especially if the mechanism of injury is a severe blow.

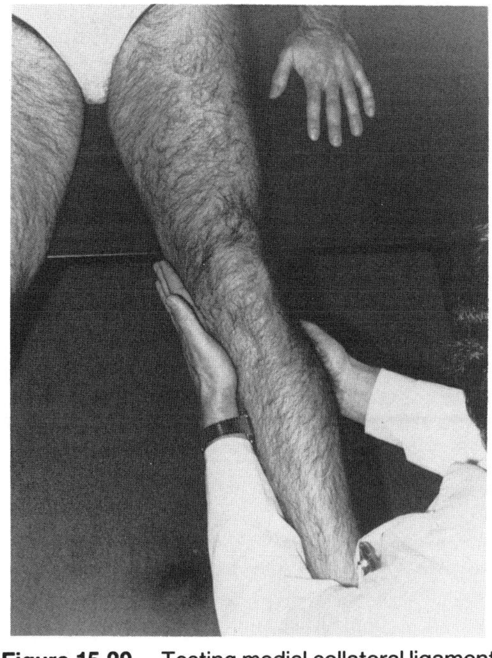

Figure 15.29. Testing medial collateral ligament by applying stress to open the knee joint medially.

In minor sprains, effusion is slight and rapidly disappears with rehabilitative activity.

Lateral (Fibular) Collateral Ligament Sprain. These ligament tears are caused by violent adduction and are often associated with knee dislocation. The mechanism is usually one of partial flexion, varus position, and internal rotation stress. In minor lateral ligament sprains, signs of effusion are rare.

Collateral Ligament Stability Tests. To screen sideward stability, the patient is placed supine and the knee is flexed just enough to free it from extension. To test the integrity of the medial ligament, valgus stress is applied to open the knee joint on the medial side. The lateral ligament is tested by applying stress to open the knee joint on the lateral side (Fig. 15.30). In these maneuvers, the ankle is secured by the examiner with one hand, the other hand is placed on the opposite side of the knee of the ligaments being tested, and pressure is applied toward the ligament being tested. More knowledge can be gained, however, if the examiner locks the patient's ankle between his arm and chest and uses this hand

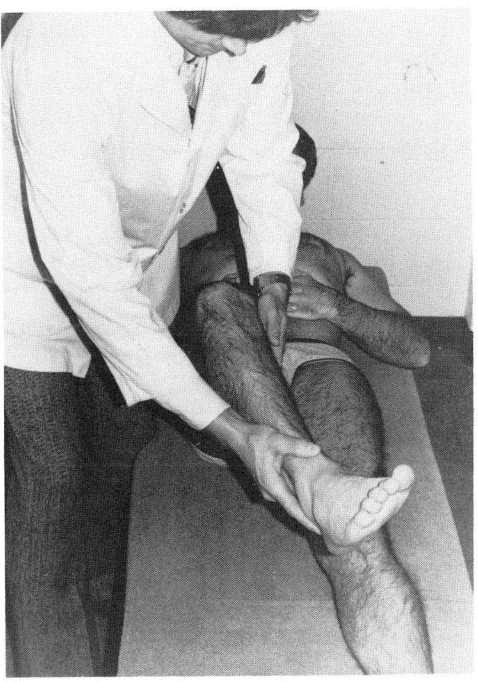

Figure 15.30. Testing lateral collateral ligament by applying stress to open the knee joint laterally.

to palpate the ligament in question and the underlying joint gap during the test.

Capsule Sprains[183]

As the knee is a superficial joint and also the largest joint in the body, symptoms after severe trauma become readily apparent. Any forced movement beyond the normal range of movement can produce symptoms. Tenderness may be immediate, but effusion and stiffness are usually slow in development. Fluctuation and ballottement of the patella from joint distention may be present, and hemarthrosis may be associated. Pain and motion limitation are usually constant symptoms.

Traumatic Synovitis[184]

Even a mild trauma can produce extensive knee swelling if the alar folds of the synovial fringes are pinched between the tibial and femoral condyles. Movement quickly becomes limited and maintained in about 20° flexion, pain is severe, and tenderness is acute. Note that swelling is less severe in complete rupture because the fluid is able to escape through the tear.

Upper calf swelling and pain should be differentiated from and are often confused with thrombophlebitis. Long-standing post-traumatic effusion may be so great as to distend the semimembranosus-gastrocnemius-bursal complex in the popliteal area to produce Baker's cyst. Synovial cysts are frequent complications of knee injuries and meniscus tears, as they are in various arthritides (especially rheumatoid). A firm, mildly tender meniscus cyst may occur; it is usually on the anterolateral aspect of the knee and nonfluctuating. Uncommon tears of the posterior capsule, characterized by extension instability, may produce painful swelling and bleeding into the popliteal fossa.

General Menisci and Related Ligament Injuries[185–188]

Almost any sprain that involves rotation will overstress the menisci and one or both central cruciate ligaments. However, recent research has shown that the vast majority of knee injuries *do not* involve severe cartilage damage as once supposed. Several tests help in differentiating true meniscus injury.

Apley's Compression Test. The patient is placed prone with one leg flexed to 90°. The examiner stabilizes the patient's thigh with his knee and grasps the patient's foot. Downward pressure is applied to the foot to compress the medial and lateral menisci between the tibia and femur. The examiner then rotates the tibia internally and externally on the femur, holding downward pressure. Pain during this maneuver indicates probable meniscal or collateral damage. Medial knee pain suggests medial meniscus damage; lateral pain, lateral meniscus injury. The incidence of medial cartilage damage is far more common than lateral injury.

Apley's Distraction Test. Apley designed this test to follow the compression test as an aid in differentiating meniscal from ligamentous knee problems (Fig. 15.31). With the patient and the examiner in the same position as in the compression test, traction is applied (rather than compression) while the leg is rotated internally and externally. This maneuver reduces

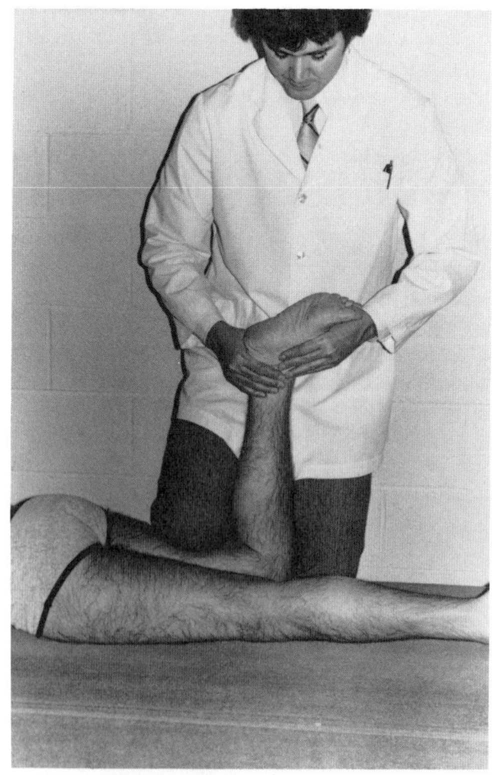

Figure 15.31. Conducting Apley's distraction test on the right knee.

pressure upon the menisci but stretches the medial and lateral ligaments of the knee.

McMurray's Test. In this test, the patient is placed supine with the thigh and leg flexed until the heel approaches the buttock. The examiner's one hand is on the patient's knee; the other hand is on the patient's heel. The examiner internally rotates the leg, then slowly extends the leg (Fig. 15.32). Then the examiner externally rotates the leg, then slowly extends the leg. The test is positive if at some point in the arc a painful click or snap is heard. This sign can be significant of meniscus injury. The point in the arc where the snap is heard locates the site of injury of the meniscus; eg, if noted with internal rotation, the lateral meniscus will be involved. The higher the leg is raised when the snap is heard, the more posterior the lesion is in the meniscus. If noted with external rotation, the medial meniscus will usually be involved. Unfortunately, false positive and false negative signs are not uncommon.

Steinmann's Sign. In meniscus disorders, tenderness moves posteriorly when the knee is flexed and anteriorly when the knee is extended. This displacement of tenderness is said to not occur in degenerative osteoarthrosis.

Payr's Sign. The patient is asked to sit flat on the floor with the legs crossed and folded in so that the femurs are internally rotated, the knees are flexed and abducted, and the feet are plantar-flexed. If pain occurs on the medial side of a knee when the examiner applies downward (valgus) pressure on the knee, a lesion at the posterior horn of the medial meniscus is suggested.

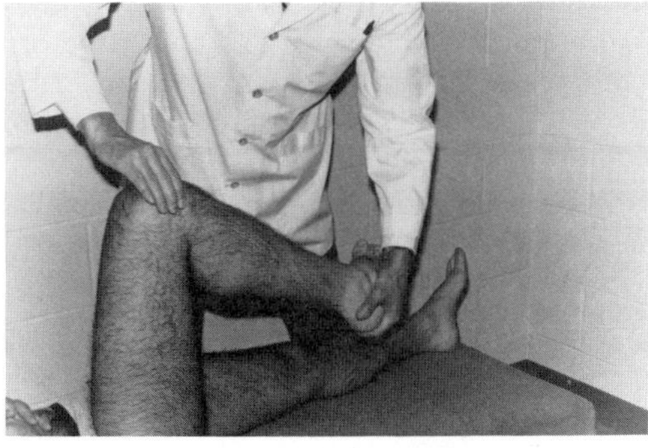

Figure 15.32. Conducting McMurray's test on the right knee.

Childress' Duck Waddle Test. This is a two-phase test: (1) The patient is asked to stand with the feet about 12–18 inches apart, assume a "knock-kneed" position by rotating the thighs inward, and then attempt to squat as low as possible. Pain, joint restriction, or a clicking sensation suggest a lesion of the medial meniscus. (2) The test is then conducted with the patient assuming a "bowed-leg" position by rotating the thighs outward. Pain, joint restriction, or a clicking sensation when attempting to squat suggest a lesion of the lateral meniscus.

Internal Semilunar Cartilage Injury[189–194]

A large number of pathologic factors may produce mechanical derangement within a joint, but trauma is the most common causative agent. The anatomical construction of the knee joint predisposes it to attacks of impingement or instability. Injury to either semilunar cartilage may occur at any age. The injury is most often seen in young adults.

Symptoms reflect the amount of meniscus damage and impingement. The joint may be locked, swollen, and extremely painful. Frequently, there is inability to fully extend the knee, indicating joint locking. The infrapatellar fat pad may be hot and enlarged. Either or both lateral ligaments may be stretched or ruptured. Sometimes swelling does not develop for several hours, upon which tenderness increases over the involved ligament. After recurrent displacement, the picture is not so acute except on rare occasions. A low-grade inflammatory process is related to recurrent displacements associated with proliferative changes in the synovial membrane. Diagnosis is aided by the history, along with physical and roentgenographic findings to differentiate arthritis, anomalies, and other causes for the internal derangement and clinical picture.

Structural Factors Involved in Injury. The internal semilunar cartilage is injured 15 times more frequently than the external meniscus. This is because the internal semilunar cartilage is longer than the external, is crescent in shape, and bifurcates at the anterior extremity with the anterior portion of the bifurcation passing across to attach to the external semilunar cartilage (Fig. 15.33). The coronary ligaments that

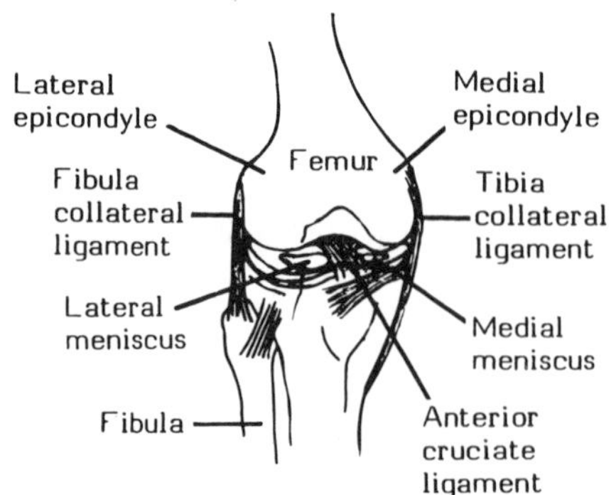

Figure 15.33. Schematic of the major anterior structures of the interior of the knee.

hold the meniscus to the tibia are much shorter than those of its mate and do not permit free play. The external semilunar cartilage is more circular and thicker than the internal. It is tied to the tibia by coronary ligaments, as is the internal, but these fibers are much longer and permit more free play than is allowed to the internal cartilage. The external cartilage conforms to the articular surface of the tibia when the bone is extended, but the internal meniscus does not fit snugly in any joint position.

Mechanisms of Injury. The mechanism of injury that causes internal semilunar stress is also more common: a sudden inward twist of the femur upon the fixed tibia, producing tension and torsion on the anterior border of the meniscus, which may be ruptured or stretched. Tibial abduction is often associated with torsion and, when present, the middle part of the cartilage may be sucked outward and caught between the femur's inner condyle and tibial tuberosity. Also, abduction widens the medial aspect of the articulation, allowing nipping of the internal meniscus. The posterior border of the internal cartilage may be pinched between the articular surfaces by outward rotation of the femur when the tibia is fixed in extreme flexion (eg, the squatting position). During injury, the meniscus may be contused, subluxated, dislocated, or fractured. Fractures and luxations may be combined during the initial injury or occur after cartilage impingement.

Menisci Malpositions. Dislocation of the anterior horn is most common because this part of the meniscus is loosely bound to the internal lateral ligament. After displacement, the anterior border is readily caught between the articulations and may be rolled posteriorly within the joint to cause further displacement or tear. The posterior horn may be loosened and nipped between the back part of the articular surfaces in flexion, preventing full flexion. The central portion may be pulled into the joint when the peripheral attachment is torn. Rarely, the whole cartilage may be detached and avulsed within the joint.

Menisci Fractures. Cartilaginous fractures in the knee may be longitudinal, transverse, oblique, or irregular. Bifurcation of the cartilage's anterior border makes this portion particularly easy to split. When the anterior horn is ripped loose and retracted within the joint, the transverse ligament locks the outer edge of the meniscus while traction upon the displaced horn tears the cartilage. The central portion of the meniscus may be jammed between the articulations, causing a longitudinal split and displacement of the inner half of the cartilage within the joint (bucket-handle type). A similar tear of the posterior horn (posterior tag) may be caused by the same mechanism as dislocation. Transverse menisci fractures are most common where the anterior third of the cartilage joins with the posterior two-thirds. A horizontal "T" or oblique fracture may occur at this point by the cartilage bending without detachment.

External Semilunar Cartilage Injury[195, 196]

The mechanism of injury to the external semilunar cartilage is the reverse of that producing internal cartilage damage. In this type of injury, the foot has usually been fixed upon the ground, the femur rotated outwardly upon the tibia, while the knee was simultaneously adducted. The posterior border of the lateral meniscus ruptures, and the cartilage is avulsed within the anterior compartment. The external lateral ligament may also be stretched or torn. The same type of lesions found in internal malpositions are found, but here the whole cartilage is most often displaced because it is thicker and heavier than its medial mate.

The symptoms are identical, but sometimes milder than those of medial injury, except that they are located at the lateral aspect: locking, local tenderness, and inability to make full extension. Sometimes pain and tenderness are referred medially if the lateral ligament is severely stretched.

Cruciate Ligament Sprain[182,197,198]

The cruciates may be ruptured by the same mechanisms that produce meniscus displacements.

Mechanism of Injury. The anterior cruciate ligament is commonly disrupted when internal rotation of the femur with the knee slightly flexed produces a relaxation of the cruciate ligaments as they untwist. The cruciate ligaments retense with forced external rotation of the femur, and the anterior cruciate gives way because it is weaker than the posterior. Posterior tears are caused by sudden external rotation of the femur with the foot fixed while the knee is forced into abduction, flexion, or by forceful displacement of the tibia backward on the femur with the knee flexed. Another mechanism is a fall onto the knee with the force received on the proximal tibia. Because knee twisting disrupts the meniscus, the coincidence of meniscus and anterior ligament sprain is often seen. Pure A-P shearing stress to the cruciates is rare. Crucial sprain is often involved in "the unhappy triad" of (1) medial collateral ligament sprain, (2) medial fibrocartilage sprain, and (3) anterior cruciate sprain.

Clinical Picture. If the anterior crucial ligament is torn, the tibia can be glided forward on the femur (drawer sign) and the knee can be hyperextended. However, this sign must be elicited early before reflex hamstring spasm obscures a possibly positive sign. If the posterior crucial ligament is torn, the tibia can be glided posteriorly on the femur. Both the anterior and the posterior crucial ligaments may be torn. Laxity of the anterior cruciate is especially common, but it is unimportant if functional stability is maintained. There will be no lateral instability unless the collateral ligaments are also involved. After rupture, the subject is quite apprehensive and insecure. The history is one of the knee "giving way" with slight locking, similar to that seen with stretching of a lateral ligament. In full rupture, severe avulsion or fracture at the bony attachment is usually associated. Stress films exhibit excessive joint motion.

Types. There are three general types: mild, moderate, and severe. In mild cruciate strain, pain is elicited by passive stress, and point tenderness and local swelling are exhibited. The joint is stable, and there is no locking or effusion. In moderate strain, there is local swelling, some effusion, constant pain aggravated by passive stress, and locking if a meniscus rupture is related. There may be hemarthrosis. In severe strain, complete tear with or without avulsion is present. There is severe disability, instability, extensive swelling, agonizing pain, protective spasms, locking if a meniscus is involved, and probable hemarthrosis. Referral for surgery should be considered within 24 hours.

Coronary Ligament Injury[199]

It is not difficult to confuse meniscus tear with an excessively mobile meniscus that results from lax coronary ligaments. The symptoms of coronary sprain mimic mild meniscus sprain with the exceptions that there is no joint locking and point tenderness at the joint line may be more acute. A negative McMurray's sign and Apley's compression sign are typically found.

The Meniscus-Coronary Ligament Relationship[61,200–202]

The menisci of the knee are held firmly at their peripheral boundary to the plateaus of the tibia. This is accomplished by a series of short fibers (the coronary ligaments). Normally, these fibers perform in such a manner that positional stability is afforded the menisci without interference to the shifting that is mandated by the functional design of the articular surfaces.

Meniscus Shifting

Normal menisci must be able to shift posterior during flexion, anterior during extension, and concentrically during rotation. During medial rotation of the tibia, the medial meniscus shifts slightly anterior and the lateral meniscus moves posterior. Opposite reactions occur during lateral rotation.

This shifting effect is actively performed by the bilateral reflection of the extensor retinaculum (via the meniscopatellar ligament) that attaches to each of the horns of the anterior meniscus. The quadriceps, whose tendon fibers form the extensor retinaculum, performs the extension action at the knee and simultaneously shifts the menisci to ready them for the anterior rolling of the femoral condyles.

In the same manner, the posterior meniscus horns are influenced during the posterior shift that occurs when the knee flexes. The responsible structures are the semimembranosus reflection to the posterior horn of the medial meniscus and the popliteus reflection to the posterior horn of the lateral meniscus. These two knee flexors assist in the posterior directional roll of the femoral condyles during flexion and simultaneously shift the menisci in the proper direction, posterior.

If this shifting action should fail to occur, the rolling action of the femoral condyles would traumatize the faulty menisci. Normally, this action just alternately pumps the menisci as an inhibitory influence. This mechanism of shift is therefore responsible for the integrity of the menisci; but, in an altered state during activity, it is responsible for their demise through dessication and traumatic compaction.

The Clinical Picture

The failure of menisci to shift properly is often encountered in patients who complain of knee pain that has no accompanying swelling and is precipitated by an increase in activity. With knowledge of the shifting mechanisms in mind, the examiner must thoroughly evaluate the patient for any weakness, contracture, coordinative aberration, or nonendurant quality of the dynamics of the knee, leg, ankle, or foot that would discourage normal knee mechanics. The examination will usually demonstrate negative signs during meniscus and ligamentous tests.

An increased activity pattern may be related to either the intensity or duration of effort. It is frequently reported by the novice exerciser who has just started an exercise program or the trained athlete who has recently accelerated his training. The obvious commonality in each of these cases would be the recent increase in the duration or intensity of activity.

Careful palpation will reveal single or multiple trigger points that are exquisitely tender. Topographically, they are found immediately below the joint line on the tibial plateau. Either the lateral or medial aspects of the knee may be involved, with the medial aspect affected more than the lateral. The painful sites represent a fibrous scarring reaction in a portion of the delicate coronary ligaments, produced by some minor repetitive biomechanical overstress that appears symptomatically only with the superimposed insult of accelerated activity (duration or intensity).

Management

Treat as any acute sprain during the acute stage. However, to treat the coronary ligaments without regard for the causative entity would merely pacify the problem and result in placing the athlete back into competition where he would be vulnerable to identical or possibly greater damage.

Nash[61] describes the treatment of associated trigger points on the coronary ligaments as deep transverse friction over the painful points for 3–4 minutes, followed by an application of negative high-volt therapy. In the patient with a low threshold of pain, this treatment should be preceded by 15–20 minutes of ice massage. This regimen will usually accomplish its purpose of re-elasticization and cessation of pain in 1–2 weeks if the therapy is applied three times a week.

Subluxations[203–209]

When a subluxation exists between the distal femur and the proximal tibia, it may be attributed to either bone. We have elected the tibia in the following descriptions, and the reader should realize that this has been an arbitrary decision. Thus, a listing for an externally rotated tibia may be described by another as an internally rotated femur, for example, or a lateral tibia subluxation may be rightfully described as a medial femur subluxation.

Because the articulation between the femur and tibia is so complex, an array of subluxation possibilities exist. The tibia may be translated solely in one direction; eg, medially, laterally, posteriorly, or anteriorly in relation to the femur. In addition, rotary instability may produce a displacement in the anteromedial, anterolateral, posteromedial, or posterolateral direction. Therefore, astute evaluation of these displacement possibilities and the integrity of the associated soft tissues must be made before a proper adjustment can be made.

Proximal Tibial Subluxations

Externally Rotated Tibia Subluxation. Indications are medial capsular pain and tenderness, genu valgum, a prominent medial tibial condyle and plateau, tightness of the pes anserine tendons, chondromalacia patellae, and restricted internal tibial rotation.

Internally Rotated Tibia Subluxation. Typical signs are lateral capsular pain and tenderness, genu varum, a prominent lateral tibial condyle and plateau, tightness of the iliotibial band and lateral hamstring tendons, chondromalacia patellae, and restricted external tibial rotation.

Posterior Tibia Subluxation. Indications include popliteal fossa tenderness, posterior cruciate ligament tenderness, posterior drawer sign, patella tendon hypotonicity and depression, and restricted anterior tibia motion. A history of anterior tibial trauma is usually involved.

Anterior Tibia Subluxation. Features include patellar tendon tenderness, an anterior drawer sign, anterior cruciate tenderness, patellar tendon hypertonicity or tendinitis, and restricted posterior tibial motion. The history often involves a blow to the back of the upper leg or falling backward over a low obstacle.

Medial Tibia Subluxation. Subluxation is frequently consequent to medial collateral ligament sprain with restricted lateral motion. Trauma to the lateral upper tibia is usually involved.

Lateral Tibia Subluxation. Subluxation is frequently consequent to lateral collateral ligament sprain with restricted medial motion. Trauma to the medial upper tibia is frequently associated.

Proximal Fibular Subluxations

Superior Fibula Subluxation. Subluxation is often consequent to eversion sprain. Features include tenderness about the fibular collateral ligament due to jamming, restricted inferior fibula motion, and a possible slight foot-drop sign.

Inferior Fibula Subluxation. This subluxation can be the result of inversion sprain and is often associated with tenderness about the collateral ligament of the fibula and restricted superior fibula motion.

Posteroinferior Fibula Subluxation. Indications include pain at the fibula head, lateral collateral ligament pain at the ankle, lateral hamstring complaints, and restricted anterosuperior fibula motion. Subluxation is often the result of inversion ankle sprain.

Posteromedial Fibula Subluxation. This subluxation is often consequent to inversion sprain, violent hamstring pull, trauma to the anterolateral knee, and genu valgum. Severe anterolateral fibula motion is usually associated.

Anterolateral Fibula Subluxation. Subluxation is often the result of lateral hamstring strain, eversion sprain, or trauma to the posterolateral aspect of the knee, characterized by lateral hamstring tendon tenderness, genu varum, excessive pronation, and restricted posteromedial fibula motion.

Joint Locking[210,211]

Meniscus tears and lax coronary ligaments may be exhibited in joint locking, but there are frequently other causes such as free bodies within the joint which cause a blockage. Transient locking is often the result of recurrent nipping of the alar folds which produces pedunculated tags that are easily caught. Hemarthrosis is typically associated.

Helfet's Test[212]

This test is designed to detect the presence of an intra-articular "loose body" that disturbs the normal biomechanics of the joint. To test normal knee locking, place a dot with a skin pencil in the center of the patella and another over the tibial tubercle when the knee is flexed. The knee is then passively extended, and the motion of the dot relative to the patella is observed. A positive Helfet test occurs when there is lack of full lateral movement of the dot. Palpation of the tibial tubercle during this passive tests allows for more subtle determination of disturbed joint mechanics.

Aside from intra-articular bodies, both a

lack of rotational joint play at the tibiofemoral articulation, and imbalance in the tone of the internal and external rotators of the tibia could promote the pathomechanics observed during the test. It should also be noted that all but two of these muscles find their origin in the pelvis.

Peroneal Nerve Injuries[213-215]

Contusion

The peroneal nerve, a terminal branch of the sciatic nerve, is exposed to injury especially as it winds about the neck of the fibula. In addition to lacerations, it is frequently injured in fracture of the neck of the fibula and occasionally by pressure of poorly padded supports. A typical "foot-drop" results.

Compression

This is an entrapment syndrome of the common peroneal nerve near the head of the fibula or as the nerve enters the anterior compartment. There is usually a history of recurrent ankle and/or foot injury. The typical complaint is pain on the lateral aspect of the leg and foot that is initiated or aggravated by direct pressure over the trunk of the common peroneal nerve. This pressure pain usually radiates into the sensory distribution of the nerve. Neurologic tests indicate motor loss characterized by weak ankle and toe dorsiflexion and weak foot eversion. As in any case of nerve compression, the cause must be determined and corrected. If conservative therapy fails, referral for surgical exploration is indicated.

Lust's Sign

When the external branch of the sciatic nerve, the peroneus communis, is struck with a percussion hammer, the reflex produces dorsal flexion and abduction of the foot. This is best accomplished by following the nerve below the bifurcation of the great sciatic nerve, especially in an oblique position outwardly along the outer portion of the popliteal space. This pathologic reflex is indicative of spasmophilia.

Fractures and Dislocations of the Knee Area[216-219]

The mechanism of injury is usually a sideways blow just above the knee or a direct anterior blow when the knee is fully flexed. This impact can be so traumatic that it frequently results in a fracture, ruptured collateral ligament and meniscus, or severe contusions and hemorrhaging of infra- and suprapatellar synovial sacs and tendinous attachments (Fig. 15.34).

Fractures of the Knee Area[220,221]

If fracture is suspected, great care must be made to avoid soft-tissue damage during movement. Supracondylar or intracondylar fractures are rare in the young but are quite frequent in the elderly with minimal trauma. The fracture site may be stable, displaced, or comminuted.

Distal Femur Fractures. Comminuted lower femoral osteochrondral fractures may result from jumping compression forces which produce bony fragments that are difficult to view on x-ray films. On axial or tangential views, ossicles of the tibial tubercle may project over the femoral margins or patella and be confused with an osteochondral fracture or a loose body of bone.

Proximal Leg Fractures. After a violent

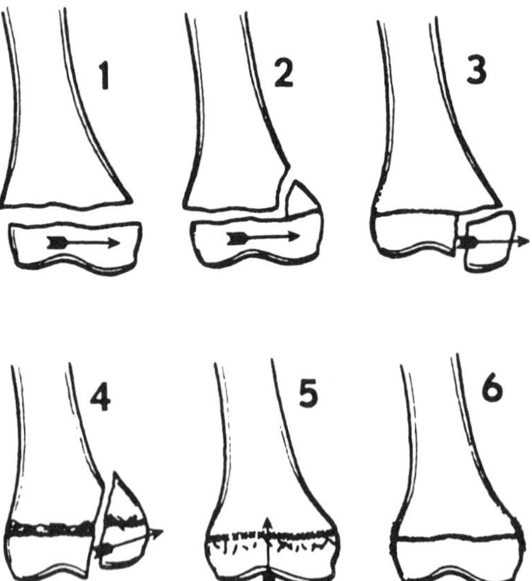

Figure 15.34. Salter-Harris[222] classification of growth plate fractures: *1*, fracture through the growth plate only; *2*, fracture through part of the metaphysis and growth plate; *3*, fracture through the epiphysis and growth plate; *4*, fracture through the epiphysis, growth plate, and metaphysis; *5*, comminuted fracture of the growth plate; *6*, perichondral fracture. Types *3* and *4* are intra-articular injuries.

twisting of the knee followed by pain localized near the proximal fibula, fracture and upper fibula dislocation should be anticipated. Chronic subluxations or post-traumatic arthritis of the proximal tibiofibular joint are frequent complications. As in the forearm, fractures of the bones in the leg often involve both bones. Sometimes, however, these bones do not fracture at the same level. When an x-ray of the leg does not include the entire length of the bones, there is a possibility that a fracture may be missed. When a fracture is seen in only one of the paired bones at a given level, one must be certain to seek other levels for fracture of the other bone. Tibial fractures are rarely seen; when they are, they are usually the result of running into a low obstacle.

Dislocations of the Knee[223]

Dislocations of the knee are rarely seen except in vehicular accidents or falls from great heights, although a few cases have been reported in football and from slight missteps. The diagnosis is usually obvious when a dislocation of the knee is encountered. Unfortunately, only in rare cases will a completely dislocated knee regain complete A-P motion, according to Sisto and Warren.[224]

Because of the severe pain involved and the probability of associated ligamentous and capsule tears, popliteal artery damage, and/or peroneal nerve injury, the patient should be referred to an orthopedic surgeon immediately for reduction under anesthesia and continuous evaluation of vascular and nerve status. Vascular repair is often unsuccessful if delayed for more than 8 hours.

Trigger Points

The five common trigger points of the leg concern the peroneus longus, tibialis anticus, extensor digitorum longus, soleus, and gastrocnemius (Fig. 15.35).

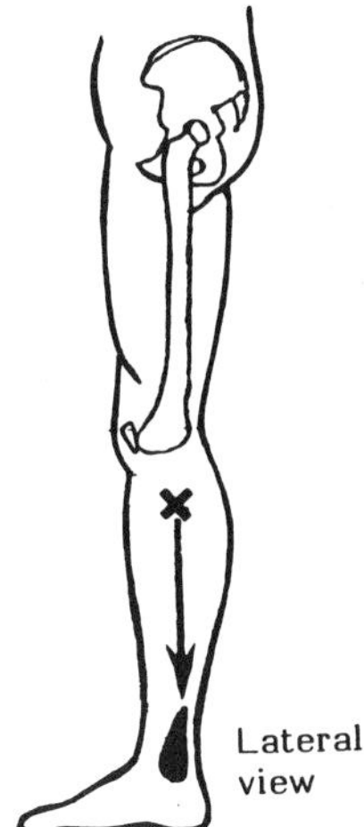

Figure 15.35. Peroneus longus trigger point (*X*). *Blackened area* indicates typical site of referred pain.

Fixations

Gillet[225] reports that tibiofibular fixation is quite common. Normally, the joint between the proximal heads of the tibia and fibula opens slightly when the foot is inverted. This gap can be palpated just inferolateral to the patellar tendon. In addition, the head of the fibula will shift slightly cephalad when the foot is actively dorsiflexed. These movements will not be felt if the joint is locked. Gillet feels that fixation at this joint is linked to an L5 or sacral subluxation.

Related Pathology and Deformities[226–229]

Chronic Effusion[230,231]

In this state of chronic "water on the knee," the original trauma may not be remembered. The effect is from an inflamed synovial membrane of the knee with escape of fluid into a synovial sac. Causes include trauma, atheroslcerosis, flat feet and/or genu valgum, and lymphatic congestion. In some cases, the cause can be traced to psoas dyskinesia from an anterior pelvic tilt and abducted feet producing an increased torque of the knee.

The clinical picture is one of prepatellar or infrapatellar bursitis with a locally inflamed knee presented. There is little pain except on motion, mild to extensive swelling, and obvious quadriceps atrophy. Knee instability tests may not be strongly positive, yet there may be signs of inhibitions of the neuromuscular mechanisms of the knee and signs of recurrent subluxation of the patella over the lateral condyle.

Chondromalacia Patellae[232–235]

This syndrome features rapid erosion and fragmentation of the cartilage of the patella.

Incidence is highest in the young adult (ages 7–25 years), and genu recurvatum is the typical cause; ie, hyperextension during single-leg stance and the pushoff phase of gait.

The cartilage becomes opaque and soft, cracks and fissures appear, and the cartilage becomes thinned. This exposes underlying bone which becomes sclerotic. The exact cause of the syndrome is unknown, although trauma is associated in two-thirds of the cases. In extreme flexion, subpatella pressure may rise to 20 times that of body weight. It may be secondary to recurrent subluxation, quadriceps wasting (especially that of the vastus medialis), pronated or flat feet, Morton's syndrome, postural instability, or a short-leg syndrome.

Pain arises from the posterior aspect of the patella and is increased by patella compression against the femoral condyles and by strong quadriceps contraction. Tenderness is found at the posteromedial and posterolateral aspects of the patella. Clarke's sign is positive, and a sensation of "giving way," locking, or chronic joint clicking is typical. Stiffness arising after sitting long periods with the knee flexed is relieved by activity. Squatting and ascending or descending stairs are aggravating. During active knee motion but not passive motion, grating is palpable and usually audible, and accentuated with patella compression. Joint effusion and quadriceps atrophy are typical findings. Early x-ray films are negative, but the inner aspect of the patella exhibits sclerosis, roughening, irregularity, a narrowed patellofemoral space, and spurring in the late stage.

Clarke's Sign. The supine patient extends the knee and relaxes the quadriceps. The examiner places the web of a hand against the superior aspect of the patella and depresses it distally. The patient then actively contracts the quadriceps as the examiner compresses the patella against the condyles of the distal femur. The sign is positive if the patient cannot maintain contraction without producing sharp pain.

Fouchet's Test. The patient is placed supine with the limbs extended in the relaxed position. If firm pressure on the patella produces pain and focal tenderness at the margin of the patella, chondromalacia of the patella should be suspected.

Perkin's Patella Grinding Test. With the patient supine as in Fouchet's test, the examiner places a firm double hand contact over the anterior knee, leans over the limb, and displaces the patella from side to side while simultaneously applying pressure from the anterior to the posterior. Induced pain or grating (palpable or audible) during this maneuver suggests retropatella arthritis or chondromalacia of the patella.

Sinding-Larsen-Johannson Disease[236, 237]

A complaint of knee pain and joint tenderness at the lower pole (rare at the upper pole) of the patella can be attributed to Sinding-Larsen-Johannson disease (Fig. 15.36). Point tenderness is the main feature. Symptoms mimic chondromalacia; eg, pain on kneeling, lower pole thickening and tenderness. It is a self-limited, benign, temporarily disabling, focal tendinitis seen more often in young boys than girls. It is apparently the result of a traction irritation of the tendon at its patella attachment.

Osteochondromatosis[238, 239]

Osteochondromatosis is a noninflammatory condition in which pedunculated or loose bodies are formed from the synovial membrane within the joint cavity or in the bursae and tendon sheaths. Traumatic, infectious, and neoplastic etiologies have been put forth. The exact cause is controversial, but the facts tend toward trauma being the primary causative agent.

While true joint locking can occur from a displaced fragmented cartilage, a false locking may occur in which there is stiffening on extension which gives way with persist-

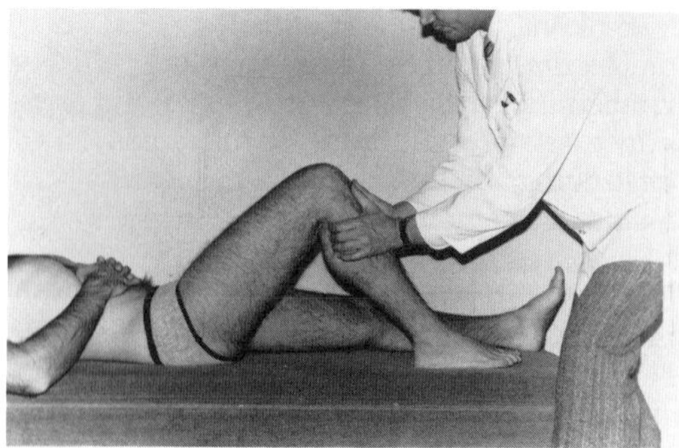

Figure 15.36. Palpation of the infrapatellar region.

ence. It is more of a painful arc than a true block.

Osteochondritis Dissecans[240–243]

A bony defect of the articular margin of the femur at the lateral aspect of the medial condyle is referred to as osteochondritis dissecans. This is, however, a misnomer in that the disorder is a form of compression fracture rather than a dissecting inflammatory lesion.

The process is essentially an affection of adolescence and young adults, rarely seen in middle age, and almost unknown in later life. It occurs most frequently between the ages of 12 and 25 years, and males are more frequently affected than females in a ratio of 15:1. Usually one joint is affected, sometimes bilaterally; and, in 90% of the cases, it is the knee. The elbow is next in frequency.

The Clinical Picture. Osteochondritis dissecans occurs in the knee (or elbow) at the point of greatest impact; ie, the lateral portion of the surface of the internal condyle adjacent to the intercondylar notch. The cause is unknown, but there are many theories; eg, traumatic, embolic, and constitutional. Many authorities feel that trauma is at least a predisposing agent if not the causative factor. Trauma may act in three ways: (1) by direct force at the point of greatest contact; (2) by direct pull on the anterior attachment of the posterior ligament; and (3) by injury to the arterial supply. Fat embolism or bacterial embolism may also be involved. Aseptic necrosis due to embolism, low-grade bacterial infection, and congenital predisposition of the femoral epiphysis are other typical factors. The presenting complaint is usually one of intermittent and mild joint disability. There is usually a low-grade inflammatory process associated with slight effusion, swelling, and joint clicking or locking. Before fragment separation, the pain is dull and aching.

Roentgenographic Considerations. Whatever the cause, a somewhat crater-like, rarefied, conical-shaped depression on the border of the condyle involving subchondral bone is characteristic. This may require months or years to develop. Giammarino reports that the most frequent site of the lesion is in the medial femoral condyle near the intercondylar notch.[244] On the surface of the condyle, a punched-out irregular triangular notch of varying size appears. The loose body or sequestra may be seen in the crater or within the joint space. If the body is not completely detached, it may be seen lying in the cavity and separated from the underlying bone by a clear-cut line of demarcation. If detached, it will appear as an oval shadow in the joint. If it is cartilaginous, it may not be visible. As a line of cleavage is formed, the cavity and loose body are covered with fibrocartilage, becoming rough and irregular. It later releases and falls into the joint cavity where it is ground into small fragments by weight pressure, each of which usually continues to increase in size. The fragments may be small, large, round, oval, or irregular.

Wilson's Sign. The patient is placed supine with the legs in an extended, relaxed position. This is a two-phase test: (1) The knee of the involved side is flexed to a right angle, the leg is firmly rotated internally, and then the knee is slowly extended while maintaining the leg in internal rotation. If osteochondritis of the knee is present, the patient will complain of pain in front of the medial condyle of the distal femur. (2) However, if the leg is then externally rotated, the pain will subside.

Bipartite Patella[244, 245]

A bipartite patella is a congenital deformity characterized by development of the patella as two or more fragments. Two fragments are most frequently seen, usually bilateral. The condition may be discovered incidentally during roentgenography. It is usually asymptomatic unless the components are disrupted. Features usually include a segmented patella with a large crescent-shaped segment located in the superior-lateral quadrant on the A-P view. The lateral view may reveal overlapping anomalous segments rather than the normal smooth outline of the patella.

As there may be a history of trauma, features distinguishing between such an anomaly and a patella fracture should be recognized. An anomaly usually presents an indefinite history of trauma. A uniform space exists between the surfaces of a fragment throughout its length, and the outline of the fragment is smooth and consists of cortical bone. On the other hand, a fracture presents a definite history of trauma accompanied by clinical manifestations of bone injury. It is usually unilateral. There is an absence of uniform space between fragments. The outline of a fragment usually shows serrated edges, and it involves cancellous bone. A fracture less frequently involves the outer-upper quadrant.

THE LEG AND ANKLE[246–255]

The ankle joint operates as a second-class lever. Body weight is imposed between the applied force and the fulcrum at the forefoot. In the normal erect relaxed posture, the support of body weight and stability of the ankle joint are provided through the bony design and the ligaments of the joint, and slight intermittent muscle action is involved to balance normal body sway (Fig. 15.37). This slight muscular action is necessary because body weight does not fall through the center of the joint but slightly anterior to the center.

Ankle Movements[256–259]

Ankle Joint Motion[260–266]

Normal ankle and foot movement utilizes a combination of (1) ankle motion of dorsiflexion (20°) and plantar flexion (50°), (2) subtalar motion of inversion (5°) and eversion (5°), (3) midtarsal motion of forefoot adduction (20°) and abduction (10°), and

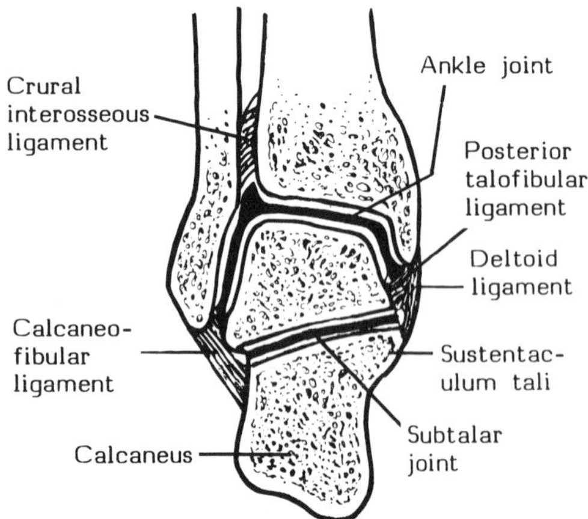

Figure 15.37. Coronal section through the ankle joint.

(4) toe motion of flexion (45°) and extension (80°). (See Table 15.5.)

Dorsiflexion and Plantar Flexion. To passively test ankle dorsiflexion and plantar flexion, the patient's heel and hindfoot are firmly stabilized with the examiner's one hand and the forefoot is gripped with the other hand. The examiner then pushes the foot into dorsiflexion and plantar flexion with his active hand. Ligamentous shortening, pain, or swelling commonly restrict passive motion of the ankle.

Subtalar Inversion and Eversion. In testing passive subtalar inversion and eversion, the distal end of the patient's tibia is stabilized with the examiner's one hand and the heel is firmly gripped with the active hand. Alternately invert and evert the heel. Pain during this maneuver suggests subtalar arthritis, possibly from an old fracture.

Kinesiology of the Ankle and Foot[267–271]

The major muscles of the ankle, foot, and toes are listed in Table 15.6. Grade strength as previously described for other joints.

Quick Tests. Screening for active range of motion and strength can be made by toe walking to test plantar flexion and toe motion, heel walking to test dorsiflexion, lateral-sole walking to test inversion, and walking on the medial borders of the feet to test eversion.[272]

Dorsiflexion. Dorsiflexion is provided by the tibialis anterior (L4–L5), the extensor hallucis longus (L5–S1), peroneus tertius (L4–S1), and the extensor digitorum longus (L4–S1). All are supplied by the deep peroneal nerve. Tibialis anterior strength is tested by applying increasing resistance when the patient attempts to dorsiflex and invert his foot. It is helpful to palpate the tibialis anterior muscle with the stabilizing hand during testing (Fig. 15.38). Strength of the extensor hallucis longus is tested by resisting active dorsiflexion of the great toe with increasing pressure on the nail.

Ankle Dorsiflexion Test for Contractures. Limitation of the gastrocnemius or soleus muscle restricting ankle dorsiflexion can be differentiated by the ankle dorsiflexion test. The patient sits on the examining table with his knees flexed and relaxed. The examiner grasps the foot and flexes the knee to slacken the gastrocnemius, then dorsi-

Table 15.5.
Ankle and Foot Motion

Joint motion	Prime movers	Accessories
Ankle		
Dorsiflexion	Tibialis anterior	
	Extensor hallucis longus	
	Extensor digitorum longus	
	Peroneus tertius	
Plantar flexion	Gastrocnemius	Flexor hallucis longus
	Soleus	Flexor digitorum longus
	Plantaris	Tibialis posterior
		Peroneus longus and brevis
Foot		
Inversion	Tibialis posterior	Flexor digitorum longus
	Tibialis anterior (weak)	
Eversion	Peroneus longus	
	Peroneus brevis	
	Peroneus tertius	
	Extensor digitorum longus	

Table 15.6.
Muscles of the Ankle, Foot, and Toes

Muscle	Major functions	Spinal segment
The Ankle and Foot		
Extensor digiti longus	Dorsiflexion	L4–S1
Extensor hallucis longus	Dorsiflexion	L5–S1
Flexor digiti longus	Plantar flexion, foot inversion	L5–S1
Flexor hallucis longus	Plantar flexion	L5–S2
Gastrocnemius	Plantar flexion	S1–S2
Peroneus brevis, longus	Plantar flexion, foot eversion	L5–S1
Peroneus tertius	Dorsiflexion, foot eversion	L4–S1
Plantaris	Plantar flexion	L5–S1
Soleus	Plantar flexion	S1–S2
Tibialis anterior	Dorsiflexion, weak foot inverter	L4–L5
Tibialis posterior	Plantar flexion, foot inversion	L5–S1
The Toes		
Abductor digiti quinti	Small toe abduction	S1–S2
Adductor hallucis	Hallux adduction-flexion of great toe	L5–S2
Dorsal interossei	Abduction-flexion of toes 2–4	S1–S2
Extensor digiti brevis	Toe extension	L5–S1
Extensor digiti longus	Toe extension of lateral 4 toes	L4–S1
Extensor hallucis longus	Hallux extension	L5–S1
Flexor digiti	Flexion of lateral toes	L5–S2
Flexor hallucis brevis	1st metatarsophalangeal flexion	L5–S1
Flexor hallucis longus	Hallux flexion	L5–S2
Interossei	1st metatarsophalangeal flexion	S1–S2
Lumbricales	Flexion of toes	L5–S2
Plantar interossei	Abduction-flexion of lateral 3 toes	S1–S2
Quadratus plantae	Assist flexion of lateral 4 toes	S1–S2

Spinal innervation varies somewhat in different people. The spinal nerves listed here are averages and may differ in a particular patient; thus, an allowance of a segment above and below those listed in most text tables should be considered.

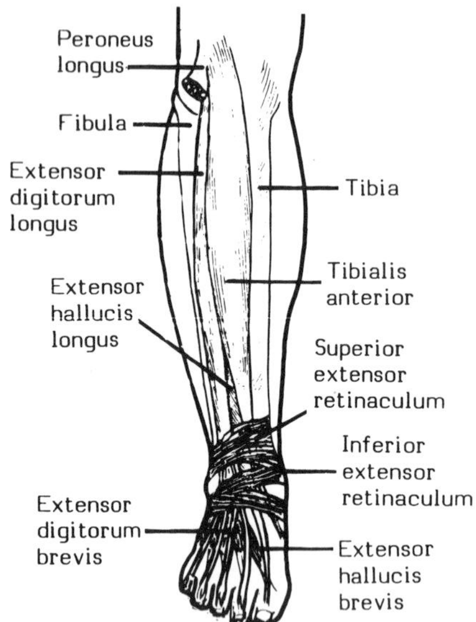

Figure 15.38. Some major anterior muscles of the leg.

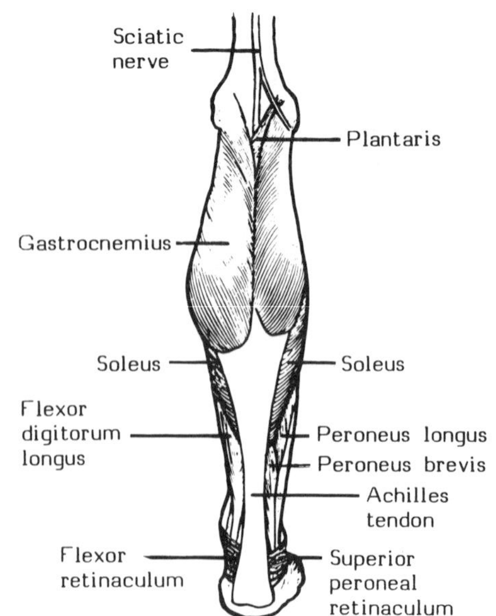

Figure 15.39. Some major posterior muscles of the leg.

flexes the ankle. If this can be achieved, the gastrocnemius is the cause of the restriction. If the soleus is at fault, it will not be affected by knee flexion; ie, it will be the same in either knee flexion or extension.

Plantar Flexion. Plantar flexion is provided by the peroneus longus and brevis (L5–S1), gastrocnemius (S1–S2), soleus (S1–S2), flexor hallucis longus (L5–S2), flexor digitorum longus (L5–S2), plantaris (L5–S1), and tibialis posterior (L5–S1). The peroneus longus and brevis are innervated by the superficial peroneal nerve, all the rest by the tibial nerve. To test the peronei, plantar flexion and eversion of the foot are opposed. The first two tendons posterior to the lateral malleolus are palpated with the stabilizing hand (Fig. 15.39).

Goniometry of the Ankle[273, 274]

Dorsiplantar Flexion

In recording restricted ankle dorsiplantar flexion, the patient is placed in a neutral supine position, and the examiner centers the goniometer over the patient's lateral malleolus, with the base along the tibial axis. The neutral reading is recorded. The patient dorsiflexes the ankle as far as possible, and the reading at the end of the motion is recorded. The patient plantar flexes the ankle as far as possible, and the reading at the end of the motion is recorded. Next, both motions are re-tested with the patient in the sitting position and the knee flexed at 45°. Findings are recorded.

Inversion and Eversion

To record restricted ankle inversion/eversion, the patient is placed in the supine neutral position. The patient actively inverts and everts the foot while the examiner estimates by sight the arc described by the bottom of the foot as it turns. The goniometer is not used.

When mechanical elasticity is impaired, muscle tissue does not yield to passive stretch. After injury, this "contracture tiegel" is frequently the effect of spasm or prolonged immobilization, or both. Thus, it is helpful to conduct goniometry in the weight-bearing position. For example, an ankle or knee may record a full range of motion while supine but be severely restricted in the squatting or kneeling position because of residual muscle shortening without actual fibrous contracture.

Circulatory Tests[275–277]

Low-back pain is one of the most common complaints to be heard in a chiropractic office. Because of this, Wiehe points out the importance of recognizing associated problems of neurovascular stenosis in the large arteries of the leg due to L4–L5 irritation and differentiating them from other factors that can produce circulatory insufficiency. For example, thrombosis of the femoral artery can produce the same symptomatic picture as sciatic neuritis. Thus, diagnostic procedures might include, when indicated, plethysmography, unilateral/vertical and bilateral/horizontal blood pressure comparisons, Doppler ultrasound readings, and reactive hyperemia tests in addition to the clinical tests described below.

Homan's Sign. The patient is placed supine with the knees extended in a relaxed position. The examiner, facing the patient from the involved side, raises the involved leg, sharply dorsiflexes the ankle with one hand and firmly squeezes the calf with the other hand. If this induces a deep-seated pain in the calf, a strong indication of thrombophlebitis is present.

Buerger's Test. The patient is placed supine with the knees extended in a relaxed position, and the examiner lifts a leg with the knee extended so that the lower limb is flexed on the hip to about a 45° angle. The patient is then instructed to move the ankle up and down (dorsiflex and plantar flex the foot) for a minimum of two minutes. The limb is then lowered, the patient is asked to sit up, the legs are allowed to hang down loosely over the edge of the table, and the color of the exercised foot is noted. Positive signs of arterial insufficiency are found if (1) the skin of the foot blanches and the superficial veins collapse when the leg is in the raised position and/or (2) it takes more than one minute for the veins of the foot to fill and for the foot to turn a reddish cyanotic color when the limb is lowered.

Claudication Test. If claudication is suspected, the patient is instructed to walk on a treadmill at a rate of 120 steps/min. If cramping, and sometimes a skin color change, occurs, the approximate level of the local lesion can be identified. The time span between the beginning of the test and the occurrence of symptoms is used to record the "claudication time," which is usually recorded in seconds.

Perthe's Tourniquet Test. This is an excellent test to use in differentiating the extent of superficial and deep lower limb varicosities. An elastic bandage is applied to the upper thigh of a standing patient sufficient to compress the long saphenous vein, and the patient is instructed to walk briskly around the room for approximately 2 minutes. The varicosities are then examined. This exercise with the thigh under pressure should cause the blood in the superficial (long saphenous) system to empty into the deep system via the communicating veins. Thus:

1. If the varicosities increase in their distention (become more prominent) and possibly become painful, it is an indication that the deep veins are obstructed and the valves of the communicating veins are incompetent.
2. If the superficial varicosities remain unchanged, the valves of both the long saphenous and communicating veins are incompetent.
3. If the superficial varicosities disappear, the valves of the long saphenous and the communicating veins are normal.

Pratt's Tourniquet Test. This variation of Perthe's test is used to evaluate the integrity of specific communicating veins. The patient is placed in the supine position with the knees extended. The limb is raised to about 45° to empty the veins, and an elastic bandage is applied to the upper thigh sufficient to compress the long saphenous vein. A second elastic bandage is wrapped about the limb from the foot to the tourniquet on the thigh. The patient is then instructed to stand, and the examiner carefully observes the varicosities of the leg as the lower bandage is slowly unwrapped from above downward. The tourniquet on the thigh is left in place. As the lower bandage is untwined, the site of an incompetent communicating vein will be indicated by the appearance of a prominently bulging varicosity (blowout). When the first blowout is found, the spot is marked, and the upper bandage is extended to that point. Another bandage is then applied from that site downward, and the test is repeated again and again until all blowouts have been marked. Caution should be taken in this test because severe pain and swelling may arise in the calf if the deep veins are obstructed.

Moskowicz's Tourniquet Test. The patient is placed supine with the knees extended in a relaxed position. The straight limb is then elevated by the examiner to about 45°, an elastic bandage is wrapped around the limb in an overlapping fashion from the ankle to the midthigh, and the elevated limb is supported in this position for 5 minutes. At the end of this time, the examiner quickly untwirls the bandage from above downward and notes how rapidly the skin blushes when the obstruction to the collateral circulation has been removed. If the normal blush is absent or lags far behind the unbandaged area, something (eg, an arteriovenous fistula) interfering with the collateral circulation is indicated.

SELECTED CLINICAL PROBLEMS OF THE LEG AND ANKLE[278-281]

The most common injuries in this area are bruises, muscle strains, tendon lesions, postural stress, anterior and posterior compression syndromes, and tibia and fibula fractures. Bruises of the lower leg are less frequent than those of the thigh or knee, but the incidence of intrinsic strain, sprain, and stress fractures is much greater.

Biomechanical Effects of Trauma[282-284]

The lower leg, ankle, and foot work as a functional unit. Total body weight above is transmitted to the leg, ankle hinge, and foot in the upright position, and this force is greatly multiplied in locomotion. Thus the ankle and foot are uniquely affected by trauma and static deformities infrequently seen in other areas of the body.

Jogging has become increasingly popular in most age groups. The result is often strengthening of the antigravity muscles at the expense of the gravity muscles—producing a dynamic imbalance unless both gravity and antigravity muscles are developed simultaneously. An anatomical or physiologic short leg as little as 1/8 inch can affect a stride and produce an overstrain in long-distance running activities.

Common Strains of the Leg[285]

General Leg Strains[286]

With the increased public interest in exercise and physical fitness, musculoskeletal injury is common but usually minor. During middle age, the most common injury is calf muscle strain, but knee, ankle, and foot sprain, and shin splints do occur frequently. Occasionally, stress fractures will be associated. A tear of the musculotendinous junction of the medial belly of the gastrocnemius sometimes occurs (Fig. 15.40). At the site of tenderness, a palpable gap in the muscle is usually found. It is identified in a radiographic lateral view as an indentation of the soft-tissue margins.

Fatigue may increase contractures and produce pain. Fatigue spasms are treated biomechanically by (1) warming the muscle with limbering movements; (2) stretching the muscle by resistance to the tightened muscle and its antagonist; (3) active stretching in an attempt to fulfill the entire possible range of motion; and then by (4) passive stretching to fulfill the possible range of motion. The stretching force must be a careful balance between that of easy performance and that of excessive misuse.

Gastrocnemius and Soleus Strains[287, 288]

Strain of the gastrocnemius is a common strain of the leg and often misdiagnosed as a ruptured plantaris tendon. The onset is usually characterized by immediate calf cramping, generalized calf spasm, and extreme tenderness at the site of strain. Strain

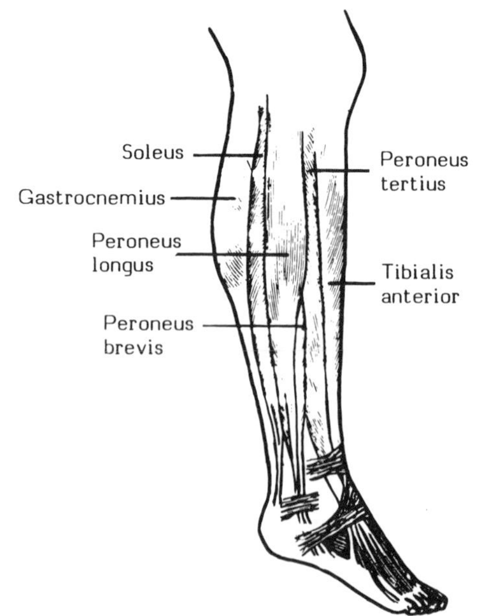

Figure 15.40. Lateral view of some major muscles of the upper leg.

nearer the Achilles tendon is usually attributed to running on the balls of the feet. Occasionally, strain occurs at the gastrocnemius heads and is confused with knee injury after a snapping overextension. If this is the case, tenderness will be found deep in the popliteal fossa when the knee is flexed.

Strain of the soleus independent of the gastrocnemius is rare, but it does occur. It is characterized by a palpably tight and tender soleus but relaxed and nontender gastrocnemius (Fig. 15.41).

Repetitive Heel Raise Test. The standing patient is asked to raise the heels (ie, toe stand) repetitively several times. If this induces ankle pain, instability, a posterior compartment syndrome, or a subluxation complex should be suspected. If this exercise cannot be performed because of weakness and ankle pain is absent, a gastrocnemius weakness or neurologic deficit should be suspected.

Shin Splints[289-292]

Lower-leg pain and discomfort after running or walking overstress characterize this syndrome. It is associated with an aseptic inflammation of the injured muscle-tendon unit. It should be kept in mind that the anterior shin muscles warm slowly and cool rapidly because they are squeezed tightly between bone and skin by fascia. The blood supply of the interosseous membrane is quite limited.

The nondiagnostic term "shin splints" is a general phrase for any discomfort in the anterior leg on exercise. The common cause may be better classified as tibialis anterior or posterior syndrome, tendoperiostosis, or stress fracture. Differentiation is made by mode of onset, site of tenderness, and late roentgenography. Tenderness is usually acute over the posterior tibialis muscle, but it is frequently found at the attachment of the anterior tibial muscle to the lateral border of the tibia. The pain is usually throbbing, deep seated, relieved with rest but increased at night. A poorly responding case of shin splints with pain even on rest suggests a compartment syndrome.

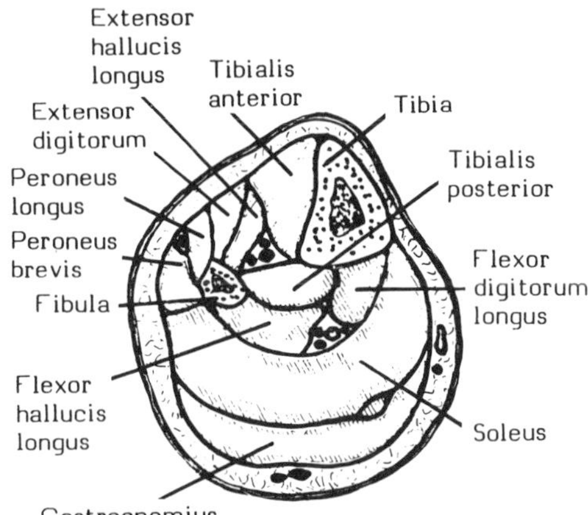

Figure 15.41. Transverse section of the leg showing the relationship of some major musculature.

Cortical thickening of the medial tibia or a minimal periosteal reaction is the roentgenographic feature of shin splints—the result of muscle/fascial attachments of the anterior middle or lower leg being torn or stretched. In uncomplicated cases, no evidence may be visible except for slight cortical thickening. The possibility of a stress fracture must always be eliminated.

Once the actual cause has been found, which may be as high as the lower back or as low as the foot, treat as a severe strain with accompanying subluxations. After the acute stage, emphasis should be on structural alignment and muscle therapy. An anatomical short leg is often involved that requires a permanent heel lift moderately under actual need. It is not unusual that a weak longitudinal arch and a pronated ankle are also involved.

Tibialis Anterior Syndrome[293]

In this syndrome, intramuscular tension (engorgement) is exaggerated by the unyielding surrounding tissues to a degree that local infraction may occur. It can easily lead to local massive necrosis or Volkmann's contracture. Anterior tibial syndrome is essentially a disabling form of muscular stiffness (Fig. 15.42).

Alternately raised muscle fiber tension so alters the muscle's internal frictional resistance that rapid movements are impossible and muscle tearing develops if the whole muscle does not go into spasm. The engorged muscle becomes trapped within its fascial compartment and tends to strip from its bony attachments. Circulation of the anterior tibial artery becomes impaired. Most

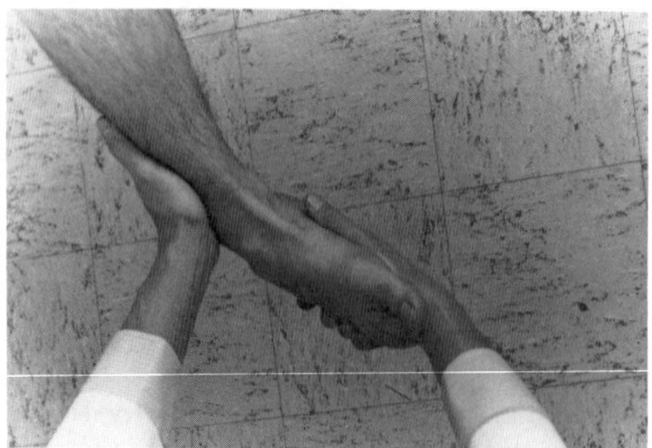

Figure 15.42. Evaluating the strength of the tibialis anterior.

authorities do not attribute any part of the disorder to a local accumulation of lactic acid. On rare occasions, prolonged overuse may produce muscle hypertrophy of the lower fibers of the tibialis anterior that causes blocking of the upper extensor retinaculum of the ankle. This "space-occupying" lesion effect produces local symptoms. A blow to the lower leg will have the same effect.

The major features include gradually increasing anterolateral leg pain increased on activity, swelling, and restricted motion. It should be noted, however, that all muscles swell after exercise, and this is particularly true of unconditioned muscles. During the acute stage, and unlike other shin splints, rest offers little relief. Flat feet, tight calves producing plantar flexion, and imbalance between the anterior and posterior muscles groups are commonly associated. That is, the anterior leg muscles are often weaker than the posterior group and this produces a biodynamic imbalance which requires special consideration in rehabilitation.

Posterior Tibial Compartment Syndrome[294]

In this syndrome, the cause is similar to that of the anterior tibial compartment syndrome or a crushing injury. Pain, entrapped swelling, and numbness are often severe. The engorged muscle becomes trapped within its fascial compartment and tends to strip from its bony attachments. Signs of tendinitis behind the medial malleolus, deep calf myositis, tenderness in the posteromedial angle of the tibia, pain on use, and foot pronation are commonly associated. A difficult complication is widespread tendoperiostitis that terminates in severe scars and adhesions. Referral for surgical decompression is often required.

Popliteus Tendon Rupture

An individual makes a jump, lands, feels a "pop" in the calf, a sudden sharp pain develops, and incapacity ensues. This is the typical picture of popliteus tendon rupture which is often confused with meniscal injury, phlebitis, and Achilles rupture or tendinitis. It occurs most often in the middle aged.

Plantaris Rupture[295]

Although termed "tennis leg" because of its association with overstress during serving, this disorder is related to many physical activities. It is sometimes confused with soleus or gastrocnemius strain in that the plantaris's function is to assist these two muscles. In actual plantaris strain, which is not common, there is pain with an explosive onset, tenderness, and an area of indurated tissues located deep at midcalf and lateral to this site when the palm palpates from the popliteal space to the heel. The pain is increased by dorsiflexing the foot against resistance. Bleeding and a deep thrombophlebitis are often associated. Signs of ecchymosis on each side of the Achilles tendon often appear in a few days. Quite frequently, an Achilles sprain and separation of calf fascia are associated. There is always a danger of tendinitis ossificans. Recurrent symptoms can often be traced to a degree of myositis ossificans.

Achilles Tendon Lesions[296–299]

The Achilles tendon firmly inserts into the calcaneus and is formed by the common tendon of the gastrocnemius and soleus muscles (Fig. 15.43). It can be readily palpated in the lower third of the calf. Signs of tenderness, swelling, tenosynovitis, or crepitation should be noted. Rupture or tear results in lack of pushoff during gait.

Achilles tendon pain is frequently associated with plantar fascitis, leg or ankle tendinitis, peritendinitis, tendon rupture, or local inflammation. Also frequently associated, and often overlooked, are stress fractures of the 2nd metatarsal and fibula. Other

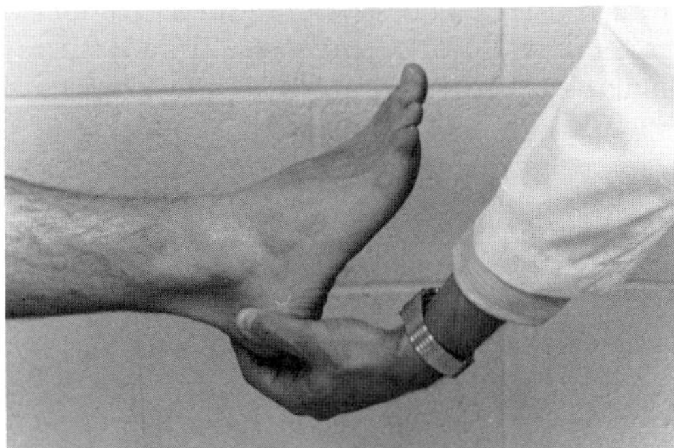

Figure 15.43. Palpating the insertion area of the Achilles tendon.

sites of related fatigue fractures include the calcaneus, tarsal navicular, tibia, and femur.

Ruptures

Because of the great tensile strength of the nomal Achilles tendon, femoral or calcaneus fractures invariably occur before the tendon ruptures. This may not be true, however, when excessive force is applied to a previously injured or diseased tendon. The cause is usually traced to overuse, direct violence during stretch, or a poorly placed injection.

The lateral x-ray view of the normal ankle shows a lucent triangle of fatty tissue bounded below by the calcaneus, posteriorly by the smooth margins of the Achilles, and anteriorly by the posterior tibial muscles. Upon tendon rupture, the smooth margin of the tendon becomes altered at the site of rupture as edema and hemorrhage occur within the tendon and the fatty triangle. Signs of fluid filling the triangle appear.

Rupture may be present even if the patient can extend the foot against resistance. A gap or area of extreme tenderness in the Achilles is greater evidence. The site of tear is invariably about 2 inches above its attachment at the heel. Care must be taken to differentiate rupture from a partial tear.

Rupture. Complete separation is characterized by sharp pain, often accompanied by perception of an abrupt "thud" at the site. The sharp pain soon subsides, but ankle weakness produces a flat-footed gait. Plantar flexion is usually but not always impossible, and passive dorsiflexion is restricted. The onset is always sudden, a tendon deficit is usually palpable, and Thompson's test is positive. The calf muscles retract to a higher position than normal.

Partial Tear. Less common than complete rupture, a partial tear is characterized by acute pain during activity which persists until stress can be avoided. When activity is resumed, severe pain returns. A tender swelling is inevitably noted when the site is palpated. The onset of symptoms is usually sudden. The soleus and gastrocnemius test weak during weight bearing. Thompson's test may be positive or negative. Tenderness is often more severe than that in complete rupture.

Thompson's Test. To detect a rupture of the Achilles tendon, the patient is placed in the prone position or he kneels on a chair with his feet extended over the edge. The middle third of the calf is squeezed by the examiner. If the Achilles tendon is ruptured, especially the soleus portion, the squeeze will not cause the normal plantar flexion response.

Simmond's Test. With the patient prone, the knee is flexed to a 90° angle and the foot is plantar flexed and then relaxed. The examiner grasps the upper calf strongly and squeezes the muscles against the tibia and fibula. A slight loss in plantar flexion is seen when the Achilles tendon is ruptured.

Achilles Tap Test. With the patient prone, flex the knee to a right angle and tap, with a reflex hammer, the Achilles tendon about 1 inch above its insertion into the calcaneus. If pain is induced or the normal plantar flexion reflex of the foot is absent, a rupture of the Achilles tendon should be suspected.

Tendon Inflammation and Related Disorders[300]

Tendinitis. The onset of achillodynia in tendinitis is insidious. There is severe swelling, tenderness, crepitus, and disability. Thompson's test is negative. The cause can sometimes be traced to tape or a support applied too tightly over the tendon.

Peritendinitis. In acute peritendinitis, the onset is rapid, there is swelling, little tenderness, and crepitus may or may not be present. Chronic peritendinitis presents a gradual onset, swelling may or may not be present, and a thickened nontender para-tendon is palpable. Thompson's test is negative in both acute and chronic cases.

Tenosynovitis. Tenosynovitis of the Achilles tendon often produces pain in the tendon area which is increased by use and sometimes associated with palpable crepitus. Other symptoms include pain on motion, tenderness, and a distinct limp.

Dry Sheath. This disorder of unknown cause is the result of diminished lubricating fluid within the sheath of the Achilles tendon. Adhesions form, binding the tendon to its sheath. Symptoms include a burning pain during and after strenuous activity, inability to raise the heel from the ground during weight bearing, tenderness, mild swelling, and restricted ankle motion. Crepitus is often present.

Focal Stress Degeneration

A common site of central tendon degeneration is at the midpoint between the musculotendinous junction and insertion of the Achilles tendon—the site of poorest blood supply in the tendon. Ischemia appears to be the triggering mechanism. Pain is felt only during early warmup and disappears with activity during the early stages. Later, pain becomes persistent and increases in severity. The onset is gradual. Swelling is characteristic, and tenderness is severe. Somewhere in the range of motion, a painful point in the arc is manifested. Thompson's test is negative.

Ossification

Ossification may be found in the patellar tendon during roentgenography following hemorrhage in partial tendon tears. The typical picture is one of trauma, muscle pain and soreness, and hemorrhage into the soft tissues, with poorly defined ossification developing in 2–5 weeks. If joint dislocation has occurred, signs of ossification may be found in the soft tissues. After blunt trauma, the soft tissues may show evidence of heterotopic bone formation. Such ossification involves not only the muscle tissue but also occurs within the fascial planes.

Fractures and Dislocations of the Lower Leg[301,302]

The direction of displacement in lower tibia or fibula fractures is usually posteromedial due to the strong action of the gastrocnemius and soleus (Fig. 15.44). Care must be taken not to mistake an incomplete fracture of the distal-medial tibia (Pott's fracture) for a severely inversion-sprained ankle.

Basic Biomechanical Factors of Long Bone Fractures[303]

Whenever a long bone fracture is noted on an x-ray film, it is well to remember that five variable factors have been involved: (1) the type of load, (2) the load rate, (3) the magnitude of the force, (4) the structural properties (size, design) of the patient's bone, and (5) the material (physical) properties of the specific patient's bone. With these factors in mind, an estimate can be made of the degree of osseous and soft-tissue injury involved.

While some features of a particular fracture will represent a particular patient's bone structure and composition, many features can be explained strictly through biomechanical principles from their pattern and site (Fig. 15.45). For example, torsional forces produce spiral fractures, bending forces produce transverse fractures, and axial compression produces diaphyseal impactions. Bending and torsion fractures require relative low energy forces, while comminuted fractures reflect high energy forces

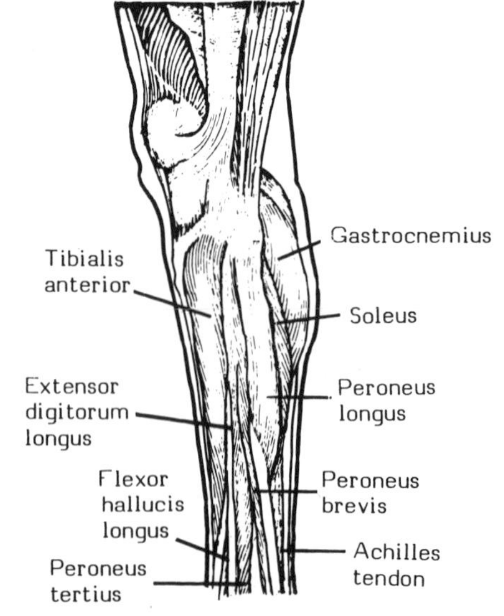

Figure 15.44. Lateral view of some major muscles of the lower leg.

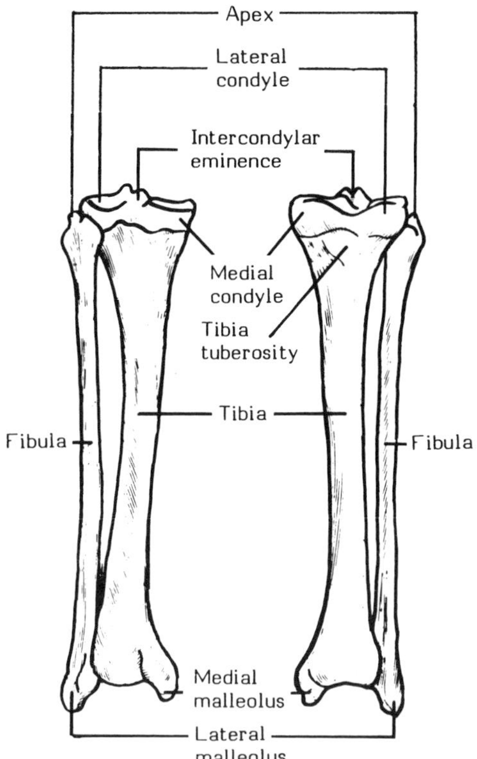

Figure 15.45. *Left*, the anterior leg; *right*, the posterior leg.

because cortical bone is much stronger in tension or compression than torsion. Forces may also be combined such as in oblique fractures resulting from combined bending, axial compression, and torsion forces. Oblique or butterfly patterns result from combined bending and axial compression forces.

Lower Tibia Fractures

Because the tibial epiphysis does not ossify until a person is in his early twenties, epiphyseal fractures are not uncommon in adolescents. Fatigue fractures are characterized by a dull gnawing pain following a run, which increases in severity with time and weight bearing.

Hueter's Fracture Sign. Being relatively dense, bone readily transmits sound waves. Thus, if a fracture of a long bone is suspected (eg, the tibia), the examiner can use a stethoscope to auscultate 2–3 inches proximal to the suspected site while the skin over the bone is tapped with a percussion hammer or a supported index finger 2–3 inches distal to the suspected site. If the percussion sounds are not transmitted in the involved bone, but are in the contralateral limb, a fracture line inhibiting the flow of the vibration is indicated. A variant of this test is to use a 512-c tuning fork rather than percussion. In addition, either procedure can be used effectively to judge the state of healing of a fractured long bone when roentgenography is not available or ill-advised.

Lower Fibula Fractures[304]

Most fibula injuries occur at its distal portion. Minor fractures are often missed because the symptomatic picture often resembles a bruise or mild sprain. As the fibula does not carry direct body weight, a person may continue activity long after fracture has occurred and complicate the original injury. Uncomplicated fractures rarely require more than support followed by progressive exercise unless the medial ligaments of the ankle or tibiofibular supports are ruptured.

Fatigue Fractures

With repeated, forceful contractions of leg muscles, lower leg stress fractures are sometimes seen as the result of tibia or fibula "wobble." These are common whenever a force exceeds the bone's structural strength. Progressive pain during physical activity is the typical symptom.

Roentgenographic Signs. An early sign is that of a linear periosteal reaction which rarely exceeds 1 cm and may present a local bony tenderness. However, bony tenderness is not common. In time, resorption of the fracture margin produces a lucent linear defect on roentgenography. Fatigue fractures of the legs are usually horizontal but occasionally are longitudinal. The first roentgenographic signs are (1) a minute radiolucent tunneling of the cortex as a result of osteoclastic resorption, followed by cortical resorption in a fracture line of one cortex, and (2) a localized haze on the bone surface representing callus or periosteal new bone development. Within the endosteal bony surface, a line of condensation may be seen. Later, an abundant callus may be confused with a neoplasm.

Common Strains and Sprains of the Ankle Area[305,306]

Most ankle strains will involve the peroneus or posterior tibial muscle units. Symptoms often arise a day or two after injury. Strains must be differentiated from sprain, referred trigger-point pain, and stress fractures.

Strains[307,308]

Peronei Strain and Inflammation. The peronei tendons pass behind the lateral malleolus. They are best palpated during active eversion and plantar flexion. The peronei are the primary foot everters and help in plantar flexion. An aseptic tendon inflammation is often involved after overstress. If stenosis of the tunnel in which the tendons run occurs, the peroneal tubercle will feel tender and thick. Tenderness here also suggests bursitis or fracture of the styloid process in severe sprain. When an associated peroneal tenosynovitis or tendovaginitis is associated with strain, it is characterized by acute tenderness, pain, motion restriction, swelling of the sheath, a probable squeaking crepitus on joint movement, and possible ecchymosis.

Peroneoextensor Spasm. Peroneoextensor spasm produces a spastic flat foot characterized by pain at the lower lateral leg and ankle, especially after long runs. There is little or no area tenderness, but dorsiflexion and inversion are restricted. Spasm in eversion may become quite marked and may indicate an eversion subluxation.

Posterior Tibial Tendon Strain. While tendons of the peronei run behind the lateral malleolus, the tendon of the posterior tibial muscle passes behind the medial malleolus. The clinical picture is similar to that of peronei strain and inflammation: tenderness, sheath swelling, crepitus, possible ecchymosis.

Trigger-Point Ankle Pain. Pain referred chiefly to the front of the ankle and big toe is frequently caused by a trigger point located in the upper anterolateral aspect of the leg in the tibialis anticus muscle (Fig. 15.46). Firm sustained pressure at this trigger point sets off an aggravating ache. At other times, a trigger area just lateral to this located in the extensor digitorum longus muscle will refer pain more laterally in the ankle and to the dorsum of the foot in the area of the 4th metatarsal bone.

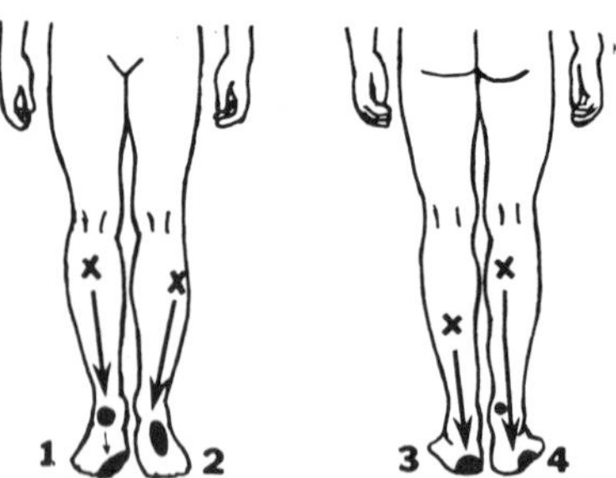

Figure 15.46. Trigger points of the ankle area. *1*, tibialis anticus trigger point; *X*, common site. *Blackened areas* indicate typical sites of referred pain. This point refers pain chiefly to the front ankle and great toe. *2*, extensor digitorum longus trigger point. This point refers pain more laterally in the ankle and to the dorsum of the foot in the area of the 4th metatarsal. Points *1* and *2* are common trigger areas in ankle pain. *3*, soleus trigger point. *4*, gastrocnemius trigger point.

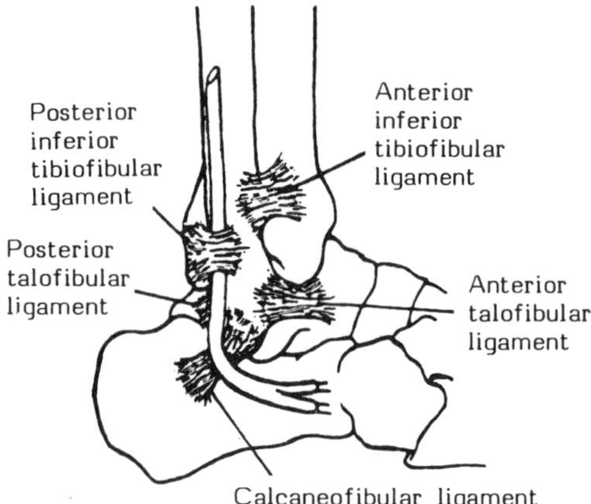

Figure 15.47. Schematic of some major anterior and posterior ankle ligaments.

Sprains[309–313]

As with knee sprain, ankle sprain produces a wide variety of damage depending upon which ligaments are stretched and the degree of tear (Fig. 15.47). Isolated tears are rare, and many severe ruptures are associated with lower leg fracture.

The most common form of tarsotibial sprain is created by twisting the leg in varus; ie, inversion with internal rotation, especially when the foot is plantar flexed with the heel off the ground. This injures the talofibular bundle of the lateral ligament. Tears are usually at attachments, with or without avulsion, rather than at the middle of the ligament. Isolated tenderness may be most acute over the anterior talofibular ligament or less often over the calcaneofibular ligament if stress occurs when the ankle is at a right angle. During inversion stress, we see a first-class lever amplifying the external force (5 or 6 times) far above the resistance limit supplied by the bones and ligaments.

Lateral sprain often produces an indirect tenderness in the deltoid ligament area from impaction. After eversion sprain, this area will exhibit primary tenderness with secondary tenderness from impaction on the lateral aspect. Hyperextension sprain exhibits lateral, medial, and sometimes posterior tenderness and swelling.

Inversion Sprains. The symptoms and local manifestations are mild to severe pain and swelling beneath the affected tendons and ligaments, tenderness, possible ecchymosis, hypermobile inversion, and spastic functional impairment. The lateral malleolus, talus, and cuboid will palpate as prominent. The talus is usually subluxated from the ankle mortise (Fig. 15.48). In mild cases, only the lateral sulcus is filled with effusion. To support the diagnosis, the draw sign should be sought, lateral and medial instability should be judged, and Thompson's test should be used. Acute traumatic arthritis of the ankle following severe sprain is produced by rupture or stretching of the ligaments of the joint by direct or indirect violence.

Dias[314] has shown that complete rupture of the anterior fibulotalar ligament is the first lesion to occur in lateral ankle sprains. However, if a supination force is applied to the neutral-positioned ankle, an incomplete rupture of the fibulocalcaneal ligament may precede the total rupture of the anterior fibulotalar ligament. A partial tear of the deep anterior fibers of the deltoid ligament can occur in extreme degrees of internal rotation or plantar flexion.

Eversion Sprains. In this trauma, low fibula bone damage is more the rule than isolated medial ligament tears because of the strength of the deltoid ligament. If the inferior tibiofibular ligament tears, the fibula and tibia will separate at the ankle mortise. This widening produces instability leading to degenerative changes. Local manifestations include pain, tenderness, swelling, possible ecchymosis, eversion hypermobility, and inversion motion restrictions.

Ankle Instability following Sprain[315,316]

Ankle instability results when inversion or eversion sprains stretch or rupture supporting ligaments. Always test and compare bilaterally. Pain during testing maneuvers suggests subtalar arthritis that is possibly from an old fracture.

The Draw Sign. Tenderness along the course of the anterior talofibular ligament points to sprain damage (Fig. 15.49). Tears in this ligament allow the talus to slide forward (subluxate) on the tibia. To test for instability and subluxation of the tibia and talus, the examiner's one hand is placed on the anterior aspect of the sitting patient's lower tibia and the heel is gripped within

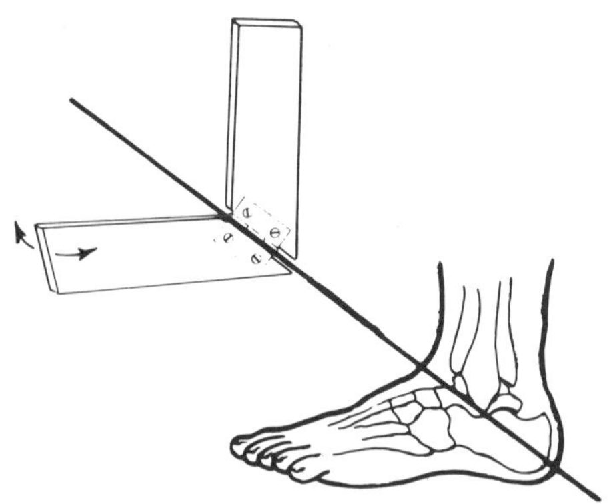

Figure 15.48. The subtalar joint can be likened to a mitered hinge joint.

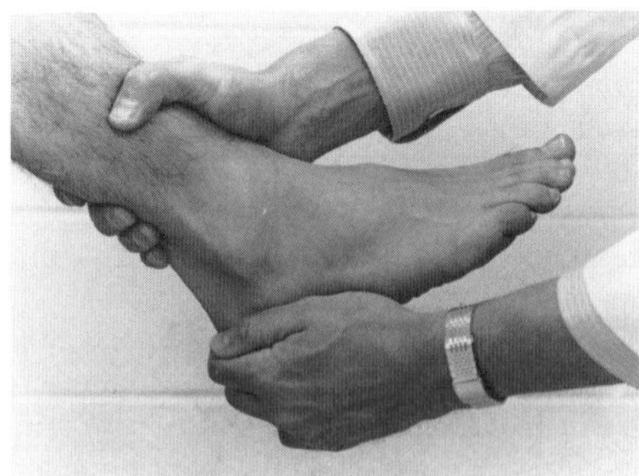

Figure 15.49. Position for eliciting the anterior draw sign.

the other palm. When the calcaneus and talus are pulled anteriorly and the tibia is simultaneously pushed posteriorly, the anterior talofibular ligament should allow no forward movement of the talus on the tibia. The test is positive if the talus slides anteriorly from under cover of the ankle mortise. Sometimes the abnormal bone movement can be heard as well as felt during the maneuver.

Lateral or Medial Instability. Gross lateral instability results when both the anterior talofibular and calcaneofibular ligaments are torn. To test lateral instability, the patient's leg is stabilized and the heel is inverted back and forth. Note if the talus rocks loosely in the ankle mortise. Medial instability results in a tear or stretch of the deltoid ligament. To test medial instability, the patient's leg is stabilized and the heel everted back and forth. Note any gapping at the ankle mortise.

Talar Slide Test. This test evaluates ankle joint play (translation) in the horizontal plane. With the patient in either the prone or supine position, the doctor stands to the side and faces the ankle to be tested. The examiner's cephalad hand grasps the patient's lower leg just above the malleoli and the caudad hand grasps the heel just below the malleoli. A pull is made with the upper hand on the lower leg while the lower hand pushes the heel horizontally. Then a push is made with the upper hand while the lower hand pushes the heel. Excessive lateral or medial motion with pain indicates ligamentous instability.

Subluxations, Fractures, and Dislocations of the Ankle[317,318]

Subluxations[319,320]

Lateral Talus Subluxation. The characteristics associated with this subluxation are inversion ankle sprain, excessive pronation, pain anterior to lateral malleolus, and anterior talofibular ligament tenderness.

Medial-Inferior Talus Subluxation. This subluxation is often found in association with eversion ankle sprain exhibiting tenderness at the deltoid ligament.

Anterior Talus Subluxation. Indications include pain and tenderness at the anterior aspect of the ankle, inversion sprain that occurs with plantar flexion, exostosis of the dorsal talonavicular articulation, and excessive pronation.

Fractures and Dislocations[321–325]

The ankle is subjected to external rotation, abduction, adduction, and vertical compression forces. The patterns of ankle injuries can be classified according to direction of these primary and secondary forces.

External Rotation Injuries. The most common mechanism involved in ankle injury is that of external rotation with abduction. The classic fracture is an oblique fibular line directed from the anterior-inferior to the posterior-superior aspect that is frequently comminuted along the posterior cortex. Foot pronation in weight bearing is the usual injury mechanism, associated with a deltoid tear (Fig. 15.50). The interosseous ligaments are often spared if the foot is in supination rather than pronation. An oblique transverse fracture of the medial

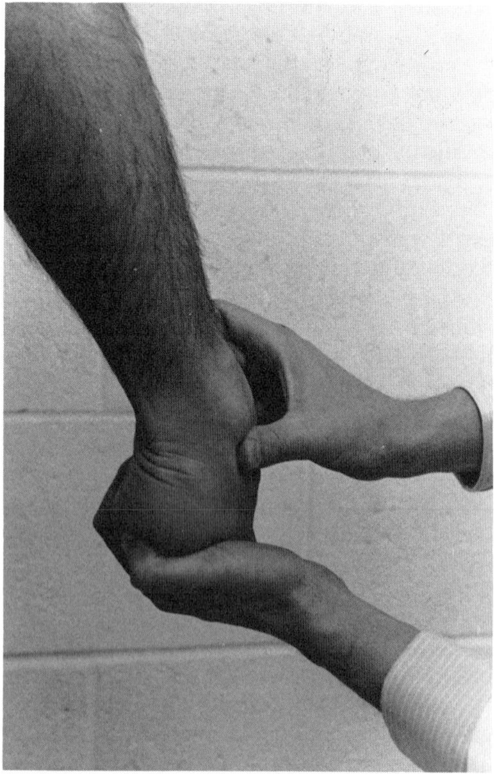

Figure 15.50. Palpating the deltoid ligament area.

malleolus may also occur at or beneath the tibial articular surface, with fragments displaced inferiorly by the pull of the deltoid ligament and tearing of the anterior tibiofibular ligament. A small posterior malleolar fracture may result from the rotating fibula.

Abduction Injuries. An abduction fibula fracture is typically oblique, short, often with comminution of the lateral cortex. As in external rotation injuries, abduction injuries produce transverse malleolar fractures or deltoid tears. This fibula fracture usually occurs below or within the syndesmosis. It may occur above the syndesmosis if it ruptures. When external rotation is a secondary force added to abduction, the fracture is usually higher on the fibula and/or more oblique. The lateral fibular cortex may be comminuted and small posterior tibial and fibular avulsions may be noted. Diastasis is more common because the syndesmosis is ruptured. A horizontal fracture of the medial malleolus, a torn deltoid, a high fibula fracture, or a complete rupture of the syndesmosis (a Dupuytren fracture-dislocation) is an unstable injury resulting from abduction and lateral rotation.

Adduction Injuries. Adduction ankle injuries frequently result in distal fibular horizontal fractures at or below the articular surface. Frequently associated is a vertical fracture of the medial malleolus projecting above the articular surface that is often related with a fracture of the lateral aspect of the talar dome. Diastasis is not associated with adduction injuries, but posttraumatic arthritis may result from comminution of the articular surface. Fractures to the posterior margin are not common.

Vertical Compression Injuries. Vertical compression injuries are subdivided by Dalinka[326] into posterior marginal fractures, anterior marginal fractures, and supramalleolar fractures:

1. *Posterior marginal fractures.* These types may occur (1) with significant vertical compression of the articular margin or (2) without vertical compression. External rotation injuries, with or without an abduction factor, may produce small posterior marginal fractures. Vertical compression with external rotation force is more likely to produce large fragments. When the posterior articular fragment is large, the incidence of posttraumatic arthritis and chronic instability is high. Posterior marginal fractures seldom occur as isolated injuries, thus the proximal fibula must also receive careful evaluation. Tears of the anterior tibiofibular ligament are frequently associated.

2. *Anterior marginal fractures.* These fractures are frequently isolated, but they may be comminuted. They usually occur when the foot is dorsiflexed.

3. *Supramalleolar fractures.* These types, invariable associated with fracture of the fibula, are of the distal 4 cm of the tibia above the ankle (Malgaine fracture). They are typically open, severely comminuted, and related to high-impact forces in the direction of axial compression.

Roentgenographic Considerations in Ankle Trauma[327–329]

Severe Ankle Injuries in Children. The area of greatest weakness in children during ankle trauma is at the growth plate. Epiphyseal separations are more common than fractures because the ligaments attach to the epiphysis. The Salter-Harris classification is widely applied to ankle injuries in childhood:

Type I: Fracture occurs through the zone of provisional calcification where the entire epiphysis may be separated or the growth plate widened. Although views may appear normal, the periosteum may be either intact or torn on one surface. Swelling and tenderness are frequent. The mechanism is usually one of inversion or abduction force. This type of injury is uncommon to the tibia, but common to the fibula. Because the germinal layer is intact, prognosis is excellent. Diagnosis is confirmed in two weeks after injury by noting periosteal new bone formation.

Type II: Epiphyseal separation plus a small metaphyseal fragment (Thurston-Holland sign) is seen. Plantar flexion and eversion result in fracture produced by lateral displacement. The periosteum is intact on the side of the metaphyseal fragment, and ischemia of the foot may be noted if the fracture is severely displaced. With this tibial injury, a green-stick fibula fracture is frequently associated. Prognosis is excellent because the germinal layer remains with the epiphysis and the separation is through the zone of provisional calcification.

Type III: An intra-articular epiphyseal fracture is seen at the lateral aspect of the tibial epiphysis. The mechanism is one of lateral rotation or shearing injury (Tillaux fracture). The lateral part of the tibial epiphysis is attached to the fibular metaphysis by the anterior tibiofibular ligament, and it is the pull of this ligament that avulses the lateral or anterolateral part of the tibial epiphysis. The medial part of the tibial epiphysis fuses at 13–14 years. There is usually no or little displacement. In spite of damage to the growth plate, prognosis is good if growth has ceased.

Type IV: This is a rare fracture across the epiphysis and the growth plate with a small metaphyseal fragment. Premature growth cessation in the fracture area may result.

Type V: A rare compression injury of the growth plate exists, usually medially, which does not exhibit abnormality in the ossified epiphysis. Premature growth cessation in the fracture area results.

Severe Ankle Injuries in Adults. Ankle fractures are frequently associated with severe ligament injury. One report states that rupture of one or more syndesmotic ligaments occurs in more than 90% of malleolar fractures. Ligamentous injury is always indicated in displaced malleolar fractures. One of the more common fracture sites occurs when the talus is displaced in the ankle mortise, shifting the talus and fibula laterally. When this happens, a slight widening of the distal interosseous space between the tibia and fibula (indicating interosseous membrane rupture) will be noted.

Fractures of the calcaneus are the most frequent. They usually result from falls in which the victim lands stiff-legged on his heels. Fracture of the calcaneus may be obvious with a widely separated fracture line and grossly disturbed positioning of fragments or it may be quite discrete with little obvious visible change. Frequently, normal structure is disturbed consequent to crushing of the spongy bone and deformity of outline. The x-ray survey should include the posterior halves of both heels. In later views, the fracture line is seldom seen. These injuries are frequently accompanied by compression fractures in the lumbar or lower thoracic regions from force traveling up the legs to the spine. Thus, it is a good rule to x-ray the thoracolumbar region when crushing fractures of the heel are found.

For accurate diagnosis, the utilization of *Boehler's angle* is recommended (Fig. 15.51). For the normal calcaneus, Boehler's angle results from a line drawn first from the posterosuperior margin of the talocalcaneal joint through the posterosuperior margin of the calcaneus, making an angle of approximately 35–40° with a second line drawn from the posterosuperior margin of the talocalcaneal joint to the superior articular margin of the calcaneocuboid joint. Less than 28° is considered definitely abnormal and poor position from a functional standpoint.

Fractures of the talus and cuboid are next in frequency to those of the calcaneus. Bilateral films are helpful to rule out a trigonum, the posterior extension of the talus occasionally occurring as a separate bone. Another anatomical variation that sometimes leads to interpretative error is the presence of a separate ossification center at the base of the 5th metatarsal that is usually bilateral.

Fractures also commonly occur in the posterior or middle region of the talus. This area may be the site of avascular necrosis, viewed as a lucent crescent under the articular margin of the talus. In advanced cases, the superior portion of the talus may show collapse of its articular margins. Care must

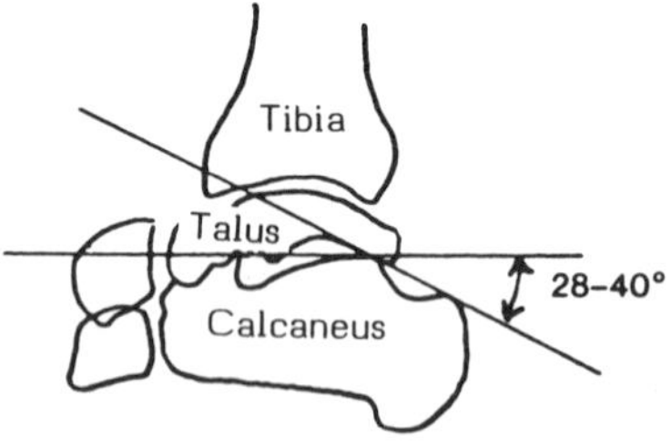

Figure 15.51. Boehler's angle. For the normal calcaneus, a line drawn from the posterosuperior margin of the talocalcaneal joint through the posterosuperior margin of the calcaneous makes an angle of about 32–40° with a second line drawn from the posterosuperior margin of the talocalcaneal joint to the superior articular margin of the calcaneocuboid joint. Boehler's angle of less than 28° is definitely abnormal and indicates poor position from a functional standpoint.

be taken not to confuse a sharp or rough-edged fracture fragment at the posterior talus with a rounded-edged accessory ossicle (os trigonum). Fractures secondary to impact of the talus are oblique and frequently comminuted, while those secondary to ligamentous avulsion are horizontal. The obliquity of the fracture line is determined by the direction of force. As little as 1 mm of lateral displacement reduces the area of tibial-talar contact by 42%.

Effects of Chronic Pronation

This topic is also discussed in Chapter 13.

Evaluation and Mensuration[330, 331]

The patient's shoes should be removed. A-P and P-A foot posture and the degree of inward pronation or outward supination should be inspected. An index finger is inserted under the inner longitudinal arch to a point midway under the foot, and the plantar fascia is palpated for tension. The foot is rotated to its outer border, the knee is rotated laterally, then plantar palpation is repeated. Tenderness on pressure and "fiddle string" fascia that disappear when the foot is rotated to its outer border indicate a degree of pronation in an apparently normal foot.

When a plumb line is dropped from the center of each patella, the bob will normally be in the approximate midline of the ankle. In pronation, the bob will be near the medial malleolus. To record the effects of foot pronation, the amount of knee rotation is measured. A mark is placed with a skin pencil in the middle of each patella, and the distance between the marks is measured. Then the feet are rolled to their outer borders, and the distance between the patella marks is measured: pronation causes inward rotation of the knees.

Related Pathology and Deformities

The Ankle Pulse[332]

Circulatory impairment is always a concern. The pulse of the posterior tibial artery is often difficult to locate, even when the ankle is relaxed. This artery lies between the tendons of the flexor digitorum longus and the flexor hallucis longus muscles. If the pulse is noted, it should be compared bilaterally. The tibial nerve follows the course of the posterior tibial artery and is located just behind and lateral to the artery. A ligament binds the neurovascular bundle to the tibia creating the tarsal tunnel which has the same implications as the carpal tunnel in the wrist.

Tarsal Tunnel Syndrome[277, 333, 334]

This is a nerve compression syndrome of the neurovascular bundle under the medial malleolus. The disorder is characterized by burning sensations in the toes and on the plantar surface. Pain is often referred along the posterior tibial nerve as high as the buttocks. Deep palpation posterior to the medial malleolus initiates or aggravates pain in the sensory distribution of the nerve. When the neurovascular bundle is percussed, a positive Tinel's sign is elicited with radiating pain. In the chronic stage, claw toes develop that restrict extension.

The cause of the compression must be found. This may be traced to the effects of chronic subluxation, scar and adhesion formation, tenosynovitis, venous engorgement, valgus deformity of the foot, etc. Recurrent trauma is usually involved. If symptoms fail to respond to conservative care, referral for exploratory surgery is indicated.

Tinel's Foot Sign. With the patient prone, flex the knee to a right angle and tap, with a reflex hammer, the tibial nerve as it passes just behind the medial malleolus. If paresthesias arise that radiate to the foot, a tarsal tunnel syndrome is suggested.

Ankle Tourniquet Test. The patient is placed supine in a relaxed position, a sphygmomanometer cuff is wrapped around the ankle of the affected side, and the cuff is inflated to just above the systolic level and maintained for 90 seconds. An exacerbation of pain in the ankle or foot is indicative of tarsal tunnel syndrome.

Ankle Spurs[335]

Two common post-traumatic abnormalities are talonavicular spurs and narrowing of the subtalar joint. These are most common from chronic overstress to the talonavicular ligament.

Degenerative changes or fracture may result in spur formation of the posterior talus that may irritate the posterior margin of the tibia's inferior articular surface. It has a high incidence in bowlers. Once formed, the spur becomes constantly irritated by forced ankle flexion. Conservative care is often frustrating when activity is continued, and referral for surgery to remove spurs or loose bodies may be required. Progression into osteoarthrosis is a common complication.

The second disorder consists of a traumatic osteitis that is sometimes confused with chronic sprain. There is general ankle pain, minimal swelling, and soreness which is aggravated by kicking an object such as a football. Roentgenography shows new bone formation on the margins of the inferior articular surface of the tibia, but the joint surfaces are not involved as in osteoarthrosis. Conservative care incorporating rest and graduated active exercises will usually suffice. If not, the spurs must be removed surgically.

THE FOOT[336–340]

Foot Movements[341–347]

Joint Motion[258, 348–351]

When the ankle is stabilized, the major joint motions of the foot are pronation, supination, and toe dorsiflexion and plantar flexion. (Refer to Table 15.5.)

Forefoot Pronation and Supination. To passively test forefoot inversion and eversion, the patient's heel and ankle are stabilized by the examiner with one hand and the forefoot is gripped firmly in the active hand. Then the forefoot is manipulated medially and laterally to test passive range of motion and forefoot adduction (supination) and abduction (pronation).

Flexion and Extension of the Toes. In testing flexion and extension toe motion, the great toe is tested first. To test motion of the 1st metatarsophalangeal joint, the patient's foot is stabilized by the examiner with one hand while the active hand flexes and extends the joint. Restricted movement in this joint frequently produces a protective gait restricting pushoff. Flexion is the only motion of the great toe's proximal interphalangeal joint. In the lesser toes, flexion and extension occur at the proximal and distal interphalangeal joints and the metatarsophalangeal joints. Restricted extension of the proximal and distal interphalangeal joints and restricted flexion of the metatarsophalangeal joints are a feature of claw toes. Restricted flexion of the distal interphalangeal joint and metatarsophalangeal joint with restricted extension of the proximal interphalangeal joint are features of a hammer toe.

Kinesiology[352–355]

Flexion of the toes is controlled by the dorsal interossei, flexor digiti, interossei, plantar interossei, lumbricales, quadratus plantae, adductor hallucis, and flexor hallucis brevis and longus. Extension of the toes is goverened by the extensor digiti brevis and longus, and the extensor hallucis longus. (Refer to Table 15.6)

Testing the strength of the flexor hallucis longus is done simply by opposing flexion of the great toe; that of the flexor digitorum longus by offering resistance to curling toes in flexion (Fig. 15.52). Resistance tp plantar flexion amd inversion tests the strength of the tibialis posterior muscle.

Goniometry of the Foot[356, 357]

The patient sits on the examining table with the knee flexed at 45° and the foot at 90° to the leg.

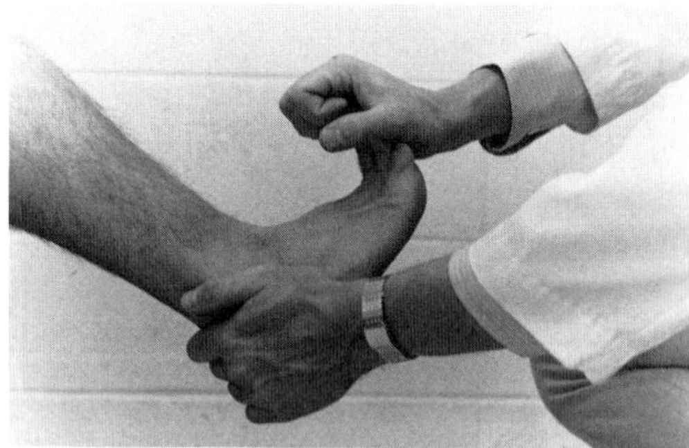

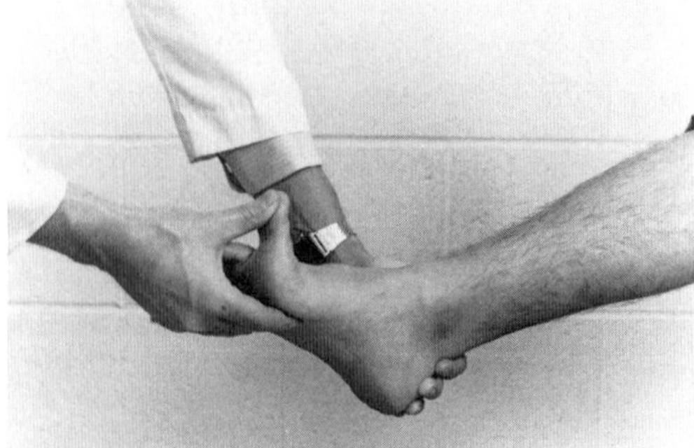

Figure 15.52. *Top*, testing the strength of the digitorum longus against resistance; *bottom*, testing the strength of the great toe.

Restricted Flexion or Extension. To record restricted flexion/extension motion of the interphalangeal joint of the great toe, the goniometer is centered next to the interphalangeal joint and the neutral reading recorded. The patient plantar flexes the great toe as far as possible, and the reading at the end of the motion is recorded.

Restricted Dorsiflexion or Plantar Flexion. In recording restricted dorsiflexion or plantar flexion of the metatarsophalangeal joint of the great toe, the goniometer is centered over the metatarsophalangeal joint and the neutral reading is recorded. The patient dorsiflexes the great toe, and the reading at the end of the motion is recorded. Then the patient plantar flexes the great toe, and the reading at the end of the motion is recorded.

Restricted dorsiplantar flexion of the distal and proximal interphalangeal joints of the 2nd through the 5th toes is not measurable. Ankylosis, however, can be measured from the neutral position.

To record restricted dorsiplantar flexion of the metatarsophalangeal joints of the 2nd through the 5th toes, the goniometer is centered beneath the metatarsophalangeal joint being tested. The neutral reading is recorded. The patient dorsiflexes the toe as far as possible, and the reading at the end of the motion is recorded. For plantar flexion, the goniometer is centered on top of the joint being tested, the patient plantar flexes the toe as far as possible, and the reading at the end of the motion is recorded.

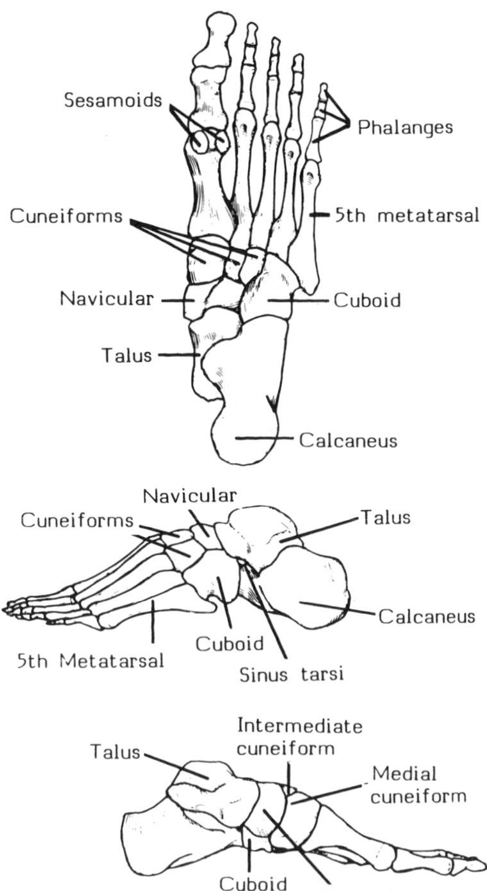

Figure 15.53. *Top*, bones of the foot and ankle as viewed from above; *center*, view of the lateral foot; *bottom*, view of the medial foot.

Loading Considerations in the Foot[358–366]

Bone design conforms to the habitual mechanical stress that exists at its every point. In each case, nature seeks to provide maximum strength with minimal material to support the weight above and to assist the body to maintain equilibrium to the body center line of gravity. *Each articulation is designed to allow its component parts the best possible range of motion to allow normal balance against gravitational force* (Fig. 15.53). This principle is true throughout the skeleton.

Structure[367–372]

The foot presents a series of transverse arches in addition to its longitudinal arch. These arches are strengthened by (1) the interosseous, plantar, and posterior ligaments, and (2) the short muscles of the 1st and 5th toes, especially the transverse head of the adductor hallucis, and the tendon of the peroneus longus which stretches between the arch piers. A complete arch is seen at the posterior part of the metatarsals and the anterior aspect of the tarsus. In the area of the midtarsus, these structures present a half dome in which the concavities are directed downward and medial.

When both feet are placed side by side, a dome-shaped structure can be seen that resembles a short-shanked, wide-mouth, inverted cone. Weight placed upon such a cone is distributed equally along its outer surface from the tip to the base. Thus, the center of the cone's tip can be considered to be directly above the area of greatest weight concentration on the cone and thus be equidistant between the medial malleoli. The apex of the cone, when viewed laterally, is at the cuboid calcaneal junction. Thus, it is at this point where the center line of gravity is located and where the greatest concentration of stress is located within the longitudinal arch. *For this reason, the cuboid is the most frequently subluxated bone of the foot. Unfortunately, this fact is rarely appreciated clinically.*

Weight Distribution[373–375]

The foot is caught between forces from both above and below. When running on a level surface, the force on the support foot is about three times body weight. This increases to four times body weight during downhill runs. Added to this stress is the effect of unyielding surfaces. Even minor traumatic disturbances can greatly inhibit optimal function.

Studies have shown that 25% of body weight is distributed bilaterally to each calcaneus and 25% to the heads of the five metatarsals of each foot. The distribution is fairly even among metatarsals 2–5, with a lesser amount on the 1st metatarsal. The majority of tension stress is borne by the plantar ligaments of the longitudinal arch, and only from 12–20% by the tibialis posterior and the peronei muscles.

SELECTED CLINICAL PROBLEMS OF THE FOOT[376–379]

One study has shown that while 99% of all feet are normal at birth, 8% develop trouble by the first year of age, 41% by 5 years, and 80% by 20 years.

A progressive distortion frequently begins in the foot and moves upward or is reflected into the foot from above. Alterations in foot biomechanics frequently produce and maintain far-reaching effects both in pelvic and spinal distortions as well as distant somatic or visceral disturbances. When these changes are overlooked, symptoms referred to other parts of the body continue because their cause, being in the feet, has failed to be properly diagnosed and corrected.

Postural Realignment[380–382]

A painful foot results in a protective posture and gait, but the foot does not necessarily have to be painful to be the cause of postural imbalance and the resulting nerve and muscular tensions in other parts of the body.

Weight-bearing distortions in time may produce such symptoms as generalized fatigue, dull leg and knee aches, and back pain at any vertebral level. To evaluate the relationship between foot and pelvic mechanics, palpate the greater trochanters while rolling the foot medially and laterally. Femur rotation can be felt with minimal foot rotation.

Flattened Arch[383–388]

The feet of the same patient may vary to an amazing degree. One foot may have a good arch and be in a straight-line position while the other foot is flattened and toed-out. From a biomechanical standpoint, the "arches" of the feet act more like springs than they do rigid mechanical arches (Fig. 15.54). A patient with an apparently short leg frequently has a greater pronation or inward roll on that leg, and the arch may be lessened. A postural flattened arch must also be differentiated from that associated with benign hypotonia, spastic flat foot, congenital tarsal abnormalities, spina bifida occulta, and cerebral palsy.

A "flat foot" is a breaking down or weakening of the normal arch of the foot. The cause may be congenital, atrophic, traumatic, or from obesity or ill-fitting shoes. There may or may not be changes in the sole print. There may be pain and tenderness near the attachment of the ligaments and often higher up on the leg, but many cases appear symptomless.

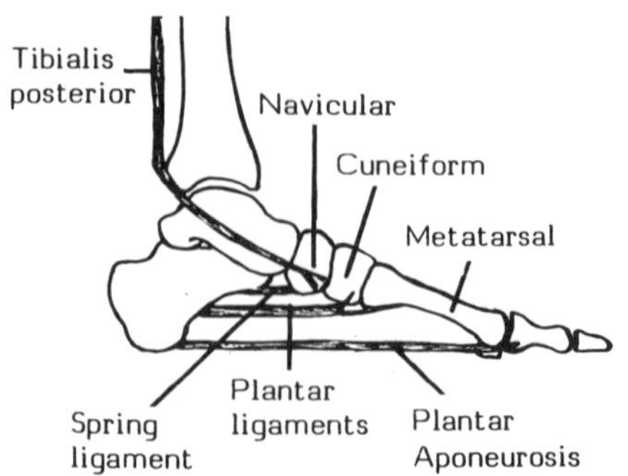

Figure 15.54. Schematic showing the major structures responsible for maintaining the longitudinal arch of the foot.

Evaluation. A convex medial border of the foot is a sign of an extremely flattened arch (Fig. 15.55). Check for foot pronation that may be associated with a fallen arch but is a separate deviation. Note the existence of hammer toes or marked deviation of the large toe toward the midline of the foot (hallux valgus). In a flattened arch, the head of the talus drops down and medially from under the navicular and stretches the tibialis posterior and spring ligament which obliterates the longitudinal arch and causes a callus to form under the talar head. There is usually a pronated gait, joint stiffness, loss of spring in the step, disability during gait, excessive eversion during weight bearing, and peroneal muscle spasm. Related pain may be local in the arch or extend to the medial malleolus, knee, hip, or lumbar area.

Arch Supports. A longitudinal arch that is dropped in both the standing and non-weight-bearing position is rigid and may be aggravated by arch supports. A longitudinal arch that is absent in the weight-bearing position, but present in the non-weight-bearing position may be aided by longitudinal arch supports. The human foot can be held up in an arched position only by the power of the muscles acting coordinately the instant weight is borne. This is anticipating that there is nothing to hinder the bones of the arch from taking their normal position and that the Achilles tendon is not pathologically short.

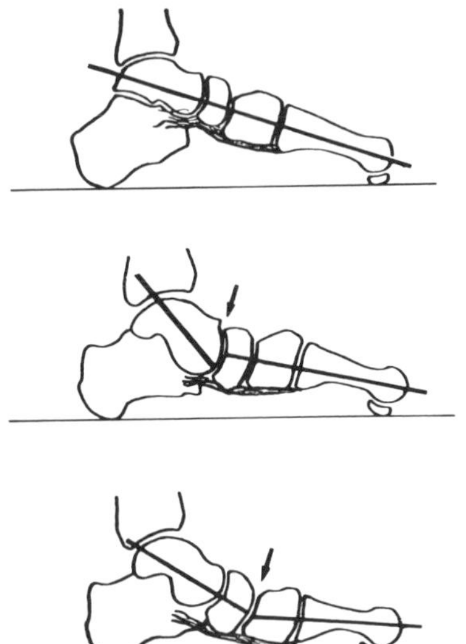

Figure 15.55. *Top*, the normal longitudinal arch; *center*, flattened arch due to talonavicular subluxation; *bottom*, flattened arch due to naviculocuneiform subluxation.

Compensatory Fallen Arch. One might think that a lowered longitudinal arch would be a common cause of a physiologic short leg. Gillet[389] has not found this to be the case. His work has shown that while most deficiencies in femur height are of several millimeters, the influence of a flattened arch on femoral height does not usually exceed 1 millimeter. On the contrary, he found most flattened arches on the side of the long leg. When a heel lift was added to the short side, the fallen arch would correct itself in a few days. The supposition is that such a fallen arch is a product of the hip of the long leg being rotated outward (producing foot eversion) to cause the line of force to fall more medially over the arch and/or is an innate biomechanical attempt to reduce the discrepancy in limb length. If either of these theories is true, an arch support or a heel wedge on the side of the long leg would be contraindicated.

Toe-In[390]

Excessive toe-in, especially in children, may be the result of excessive internal rotation of the tibia caused by a fixed point at either end of the tibia. Common points of fixation are at the malleoli in the ankle or the tibial tubercle below the knee. The ankle mortise normally faces 15° externally; but in internal tibial torsion, the ankle mortise faces anteriorly or internally.

Traumatic Disorders of the Foot and Toes[391,392]

Gait Clues[364,393]

Inability of a foot to heelstrike is an indication of a heel spur and associated bursitis. Pain in a foot during midstance may be caused by corns, callosities from a fallen transverse arch, rigid pes planus, or subtalar arthritis. Sharp pain on pushoff is often caused by corns between the toes or metatarsal callosities. Pushing off with the lateral side of the front of the foot is usually seen in disorders involving the great toe.

Plantar Strains and Fascitis[394–396]

The plantar aponeurosis should feel smooth without areas of tenderness during palpation of the plantar surface of the foot. These strong bands of fascia have their origin at the medial tubercle of the calcaneus, spray across the sole, and insert near the metatarsal heads (Fig. 15.56). True plantar fascitis is rare, but when it occurs, it is often confused with sprain of the spring ligaments in the arch. It is usually the result of chronic pronation or fascial tears from dorsiflexion overstress, or is associated with calcaneal stress fractures. The cause can usually be attributed to chronic pronation, landing hard on the ball of the foot, or injury during quick running starts or stops.

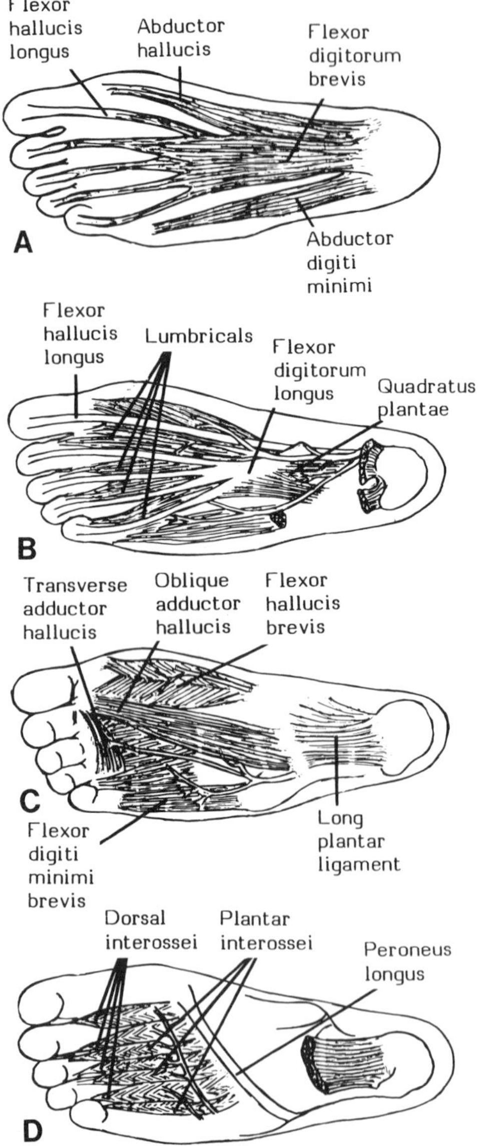

Figure 15.56. *A*, superficial muscles of the foot; *B*, second layer of muscles; *C*, third layer of muscles; *D*, deepest layer of muscles.

The typical clinical picture presents pain upon running due to plantar-fascial stretch, with tenderness found just distal to the calcaneal tubercles. Palpable stiff cords or nodules within the fascia suggest plantar fascia spasm, Dupuytren's contractures tender under deep pressure, or plantar warts tender to pinching. A slight degree of swelling may be palpable. Tight plantar fascia raises the longitudinal arch. Callosities, like contractures, are tender to pressure but not to pinching. In acute cases, a slight degree of ecchymosis and severe tenderness may be exhibited at attachments, especially at the heel. Early roentgenographs are negative, but calcification may appear on later films.

Check carefully for possible cuboid or navicular subluxation. A temporary longitudinal arch support (or taping) and crutches are helpful during initial healing. Chronic low arches do not appear to be a precipitating factor.

Plantar Tension Test. The patient is placed supine and the involved foot and toes are dorsiflexed so that the plantar fascia is tensed. If pain occurs or if bead-like swellings and irregularities are found as the examiner deeply runs his thumb vertically along the plantar surface, plantar fascitis is suggested.

Trigger Points

The most common trigger points of the foot are of the short extensor and the abductor hallucis (Fig. 15.57).

Metatarsalgia[397–399]

Morton's syndrome (metatarsalgia) exhibits pain at a small spot near the proximal end of one of the three outer toes (Fig. 15.58). It is especially debilitating in occupations that require prolonged standing or walking and is almost always associated with compression of the foot by tight shoes resulting in pinching of the external plantar nerves between the metatarsal bones.

The syndrome triad consists of (1) a 1st

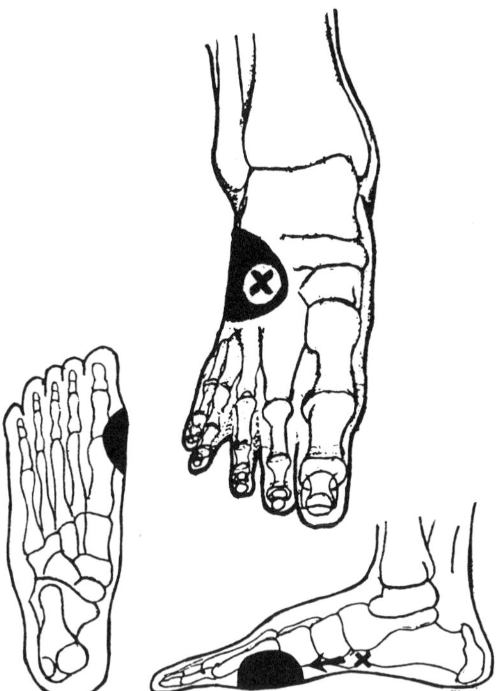

Figure 15.57. *Top*, short extensor trigger point; *X*, common site. *Blackened area* represents typical site of referred pain. *Bottom*, abductor hallucis trigger point; *left*, plantar aspect; *right*, medial aspect.

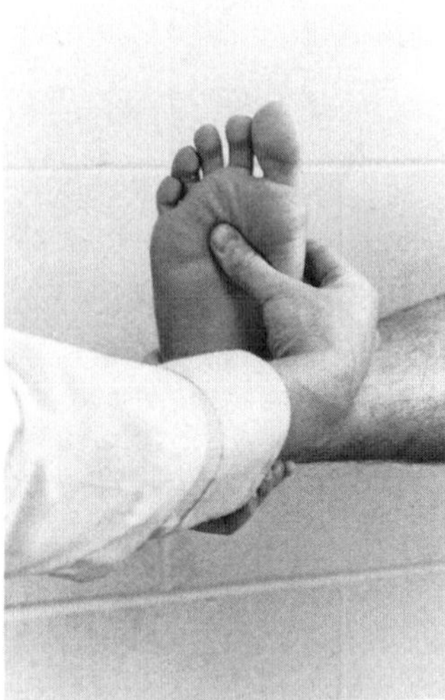

Figure 15.58. Palpation of the metatarsal heads. Each joint is palpated individually. Morton's neuroma is occasionally located, especially between the 3rd and 4th metatarsal heads.

metatarsal bone that is shorter than the 2nd, (2) hypermobility at the naviculocuneiform and medial- and inter-cuneiform articulations, and (3) posteriorly displaced sesamoids. Differentiation must be made from postural strains, neuroma, march fractures, subluxations, exostoses, and tendon avulsions.

The clinical picture includes toe pains, foot fatigue, and pronation complaints that are often associated with plantar callus patterns, bunion, corns, and intermetatarsal neuroma. The sesamoids are displaced posteriorly, there is hypertrophy of the 2nd metatarsal joint, the foot is pronated and the arch flattened. There is abnormal weight balance and distribution.

Strunsky's Test. This test is designed essentially for the recognition of lesions of the metatarsal arch. Under normal conditions when the toes are grasped and quickly flexed, the procedure is painless. Pain results if there is any inflammatory lesion of the metatarsal arch.

Morton's Test. In metatarsalgia, deep transverse pressure across the heads of the metatarsals causes a sharp pain, especially between the 2nd and 3rd metatarsal.

Supports. Physical care often includes joint mobilization, padding beneath the tongue of the shoe, and transverse arch support. A metatarsal crescent can be applied to the sole of the shoe or a felt pad placed just behind the plantar metatarsal heads involved. In either case, the object is to slightly lift the stressed joints during weight bearing. The patient should be advised to lace the front of the shoe loosely. Graduated tiptoe walking and walking on the lateral edge of the foot are most helpful to develop strength during rehabilitation.

Foot and Toe Sprains[400]

Rear Foot Sprains. These are usually chronic in nature and characterized by progressive pain and minimal swelling in the rear half of the foot during activity (Fig. 15.59). Talar subluxations and restrictions are often associated. In some cases, the cause will be traced to a low-grade tarsal synovitis from poor foot support on hard ground during strenuous activity.

Calcaneocuboid Sprain. This is usually the result of forceful internal rotation of the

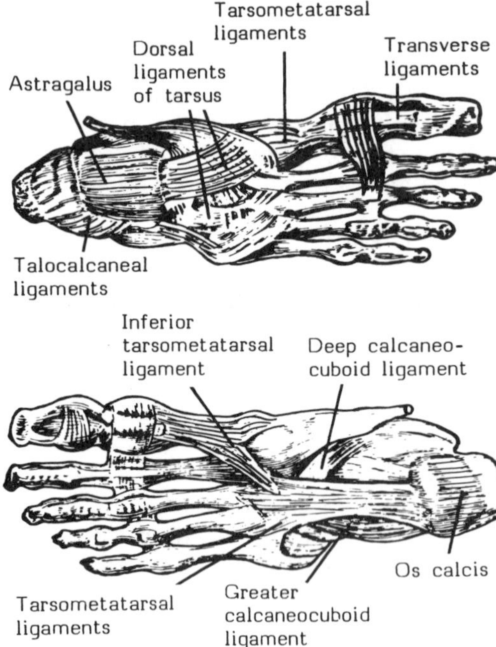

Figure 15.59. *Top*, major ligaments of the dorsal surface of the foot; *bottom*, major ligaments of the plantar surface of the foot.

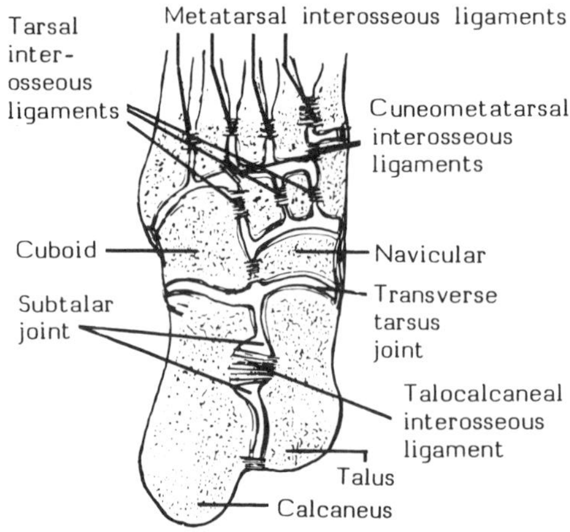

Figure 15.60. Oblique schematic section of the foot depicting the intertarsal joints and related structures.

foot on the talonavicular joint when the foot is inverted (Fig. 15.60). There is immediate severe pain, swelling over the calcaneocuboid area, and great disability.

Spring Ligament Sprain. Overstress of the plantar calcaneonavicular ligament is often associated with navicular subluxation. Symptoms of medial aching pain and tenderness deep within the plantar arch commonly arise after prolonged running when soft shoes are worn. Differentiation must be made from plantar fascitis which is more posterior and usually of a more acute nature.

Forefoot Sprains. Distal ache with tenderness under the 2nd and 3rd metatarsal heads is often the result of postural stress. As a consequence of severe eversion or inversion strain, avulsion of the insertion of the tibialis posterior may feature acute styloid tenderness.

Sprains of the Toes. The most common sprain of this area is that of the great toe, especially at the metatarsophalangeal joint as the result of forced plantar flexion or dorsiflexion. Sideward sprains are rarely witnessed. Swelling may be severe, but bony tenderness or crepitus is absent. Disability is severe because weight bearing is predominantly on the hallus.

Bruises of the Heel[401–403]

The area of the retrocalcaneal bursa located between the anterior surface of Achilles tendon and the top of the heel is palpated. The skin is lifted away from the tendon with one hand while the area anterior to the tendon is palpated. Then the calcaneal bursa situated between the insertion of Achilles tendon and the skin is checked. Both of these bursae are subject to inflammation from pressure or friction from poorly fitting shoes. Care must be taken not to confuse heel bursitis with avulsion of the Achilles insertion.

Hoffa's Sign. The patient is placed prone with the relaxed feet and ankles hanging over the edge of the table. A positive sign of an avulsion fracture of the calcaneus is found if the examiner by deep palpation finds that (1) the Achilles tendon is lax, (2) relaxed dorsiflexion is greater, and, possibly, (3) a bone fragment is felt behind either malleolus on the involved side.

Orthotics. One company has recently developed stabilizers that greatly reduce bone shock at heelstrike—a factor vitally important to the treatment of many athletic injuries of the lumbar spine, pelvis, and lower extremities. The stabilizers are constructed with Sorbothan II, a viscoelastic polymer that has the ability to accept pressure, shear, and torque forces synchronously without permanent distortion. Further information may be obtained from Foot Levelers, Inc, 1901 Rockdale Road, P.O. Box 272, Dubuque, Iowa 52004-9998.

Sesamoiditis[404]

Deep palpation within the flexor hallucis brevis tendon may locate the two sesamoids when signs of sesamoiditis exist. Sesamoid necrosis under the head of the 1st metatarsal within the tendon flexor hallucis longus tendon may show roentgenographic signs.

Common Subluxations of the Foot[405–410]

Lateral Cuboid Subluxation. This subluxation is usually associated with inversion sprain, lateral longitudinal arch pain and tenderness, and excessive pronation.

Inferior Cuboid Subluxation. The picture of an inferior cuboid subluxation is lateral longitudinal arch pains and excessive pronation or supination (Fig. 15.61).

Inferior-Medial Navicular Subluxation. This subluxation is associated with medial longitudinal arch pain, excessive pronation, and inversion or eversion ankle sprain.

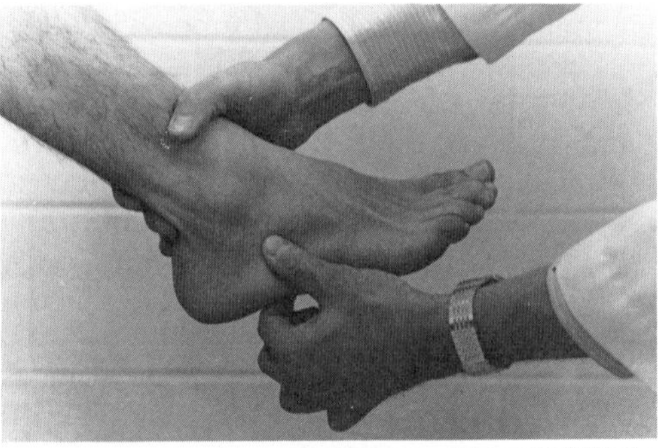

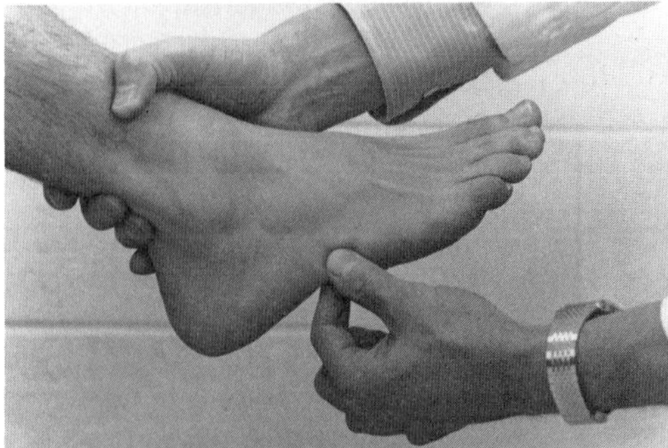

Figure 15.61. *Top*, palpation of the peroneus longus and brevis muscle tendons as they cross the peroneal tubercle; *bottom*, palpation of the styloid process of the 5th metatarsal.

Posterior Calcaneus Subluxation. This subluxation is usually associated with tarsal tunnel syndrome, excessive pronation, and pain sited inferiorly and slightly posterior to the medial malleolus.

Anterior Calcaneus Subluxation. The obvious signs of an anterior calcaneus subluxation include excessive supination and pes cavus.

Inferior Metatarsal Subluxation. The features of this subluxation are arch pain, ankle sprain, and excessive pronation or supination.

Superior Proximal-Metatarsal Subluxation. The characteristics of this type of subluxation are pain on the dorsum of the foot, inversion sprain resulting in a 1st metatarsal displaced superiorly, pronation syndrome with superior 1st and 5th metatarsals, and excessive supination.

Inferior Distal-Metatarsal Subluxation. This type of subluxation is commonly associated with excessive callus formation across the metatarsal heads, plantar forefoot pain, and excessive pronation.

Fatigue Fractures of the Foot[411,412]

These "march" fractures are characterized by point tenderness and sometimes a palpable bone callus. The onset of symptoms may be rapid or gradual. Diagnosis is made early by exclusion and late by roentgenographic findings. This rare condition is increasing in incidence among unconditioned joggers who run on hard surfaces. The second metatarsal is the site of the most common fatigue fractures seen in the foot. Various congenital or acquired factors such as Morton's toe, warts, and bunion may be the underlying factor in symptomatic runners.

Bowerman points out that chronic stress of the talus may produce marginal degenerative cysts similar to those seen in other weight-bearing joints (eg, knee, hip). Usually, but not always, the joint space near the cyst will be narrowed.[413]

Dancing Trauma

Dancing can take several forms. It can be conducted slowly with minimal movement and effort or involve considerable strength, endurance, control, coordination, and flexibility when intricate movements are required. Frequent, but usually minor, injuries can occur that are due to overuse, improper technique, poor training, poor conditions, and fatigue. Lindsay and Wheeler report that while the ankle and foot are commonly considered the most common sites of injury, the hip, knee, leg, or spine may be involved. In trained dancers, faulty technique appears to be the common cause of injury.[414]

Fixations

The bony complex of a foot (about 27 articulations) is a common site of single or multiple fixations that Gillet reports can frequently be linked to spinal fixations. In fact, Gillet looks to the feet as the functional base of the spine. He feels that the cause of many frequently recurring fixations in the spine or pelvis can be traced to a fixation in the feet. A high stiff arch that does not reduce somewhat during weight bearing is just as abnormal as a flattened arch.[389]

Fixation of the distal phalangeal joints is not common but fixation of those joints more proximal is. The metatarsophalangeal joint of the great toe is a common site, especially if plantar flexion is restricted. The intermetatarsal ligaments are frequently shortened. Partial or complete fixations are also found at the cuneiform-metatarsal, cuboid-metatarsal, cuneiform-navicular, intercuneiform, cuneiform-cuboid, navicular-cuboid, talus-navicular, and talus-cuboid articulations.

Gillet's studies showed a distinct relationship between phalangeal fixations and upper cervical fixations, metatarsal fixation and C3–C7 fixations, metatarsal-tarsal fixations and thoracic fixations, intermetatarsal fixations and costospinal subluxations, cuneiform-navicular or cuboid-calcaneus and lumbar fixations, and talus fixations and L5 fixations.[389] These findings are awaiting further confirmation, however.

Related Pathology and Deformities[415,416]

Plantar Neuroma[417,418]

A rare cause of metatarsalgia is Morton's neuroma: painful round "beads" found between the heads of the 1st through 4th metatarsals, especially between the 3rd and 4th. They are thought to be the effect of excessive foot rolling in which the plantar nerve is chronically impinged on taut fascia or bone and hypertrophy of the nerve sheath develops. There is an accompanying digital artery disorder. The shooting distal pain and sometimes numbness are severe but quickly relieved when the shoeless foot is rested. Roentgenographs are negative. Differentiation is necessary from postural strains and tendon avulsions that produce forefoot pain and plantar tenderness.

Neuroma Squeeze Test. If needle-like shooting pains occur when the forefoot is slowly squeezed, the probability of neuroma should be considered.

Heel Spurs[419,420]

A heel spur usually forms at the inferomedial aspect of the calcaneus from chronic traction of the plantar fascia upon calcaneal periosteum. Trauma is but one of the causes; biomechanical imbalance, focal infections, metabolic disturbances, and contracted plantar fascia may be involved.

The symptomatic picture presents a distinct limp, constant pain only during weight bearing, tenderness increased in dorsiflexion, and mild swelling along the medial aspect of the os calcis or plantar fascia attachments at the calcaneal tuberosity.

Exostoses

Bony overgrowth infrequently forms at the head of a metatarsal.[421] It is more common at the 1st metatarsal. Treatment is usually by exostectomy. However, what may at first appear to be an overgrowth during palpation (a knuckle-like prominence) may actually be a metatarsocuneiform subluxation. This can usually be demonstrated by roentgenography.

Anterior Compartment Syndrome

Tissues of the anterior compartment should normally feel soft and yielding; tautness suggests pathology such as in a compartment syndrome. The sinus tarsi area is often involved in ankle sprains wherein its normal concavity is swollen and tender (Fig. 15.62). Deep tenderness suggests arthritis, myositis, fracture, or spastic foot syndrome.

The pulse of the dorsal pedal artery can be felt between the extensor hallucis longus and extensor digitorum longus tendons of the dorsum of the foot. Being surrounded by bone, tendons, and fascia, it has diffi-

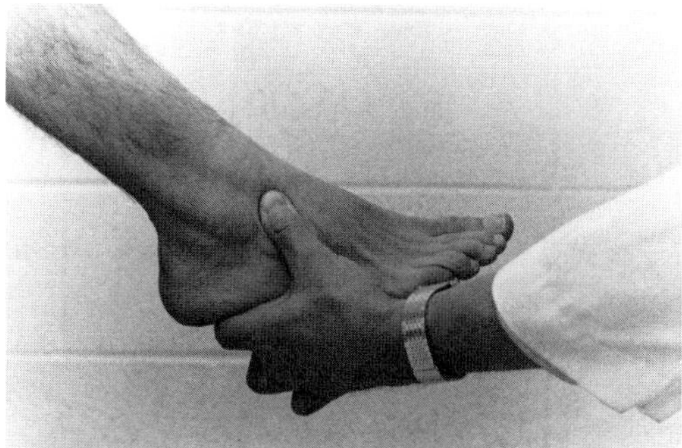

Figure 15.62. Palpation of the sinus tarsi.

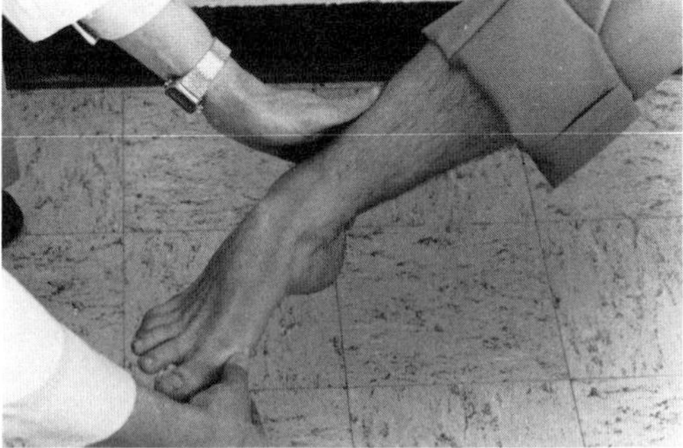

Figure 15.63. Checking for bursal formation over the head of the 1st metatarsal and the metatarsophalangeal joint.

culty in expanding during increased circulatory demands. This often produces swelling within the anterior compartment which leads to necrosis of vessels, muscles, and nerves, resulting in a foot-drop or an anterior compartment syndrome.

Toe Deformities[422–425]

Claw Toes. Claw toes, usually associated with pes cavus, feature flexed proximal and distal interphalangeal joints and hyperextended metatarsophalangeal joints. An early sign is callosities over the dorsal surface of the toes, on the tips of the toes, and on the plantar surface under the metatarsal heads.

Hammer Toe. A hammer toe presents flexion of the proximal interphalangeal joint and hyperextension of the metatarsophalangeal and distal interphalangeal joints. It is usually singular and associated with a callosity on top of the proximal interphalangeal joint. Predisposing factors include forceful plantar flexion of the metatarsal, pes cavus, short metatarsal, forefoot valgus, trauma, or pronation imbalance.

Mallet Toe. A mallet toe is a distal interphalangeal joint flexion contracture, which usually occurs in the smaller toes. It is less common than a hammer toe.

Hallux Valgus. This is a state of lateral deviation of the great toe, usually found in conjunction with a hypermobile pronated foot and the wearing of pointed-toe shoes, producing abuse to the medial aspect of the front foot. The 1st metatarsal becomes fixed in abduction and the hallux subluxates laterally. In time, the abductor hallucis becomes fixated in lateral displacement beneath the metatarsal head. The muscle becomes ineffective in maintaining abduction.

Bunion. A bunion is an effect of prolonged hallux valgus in which the great toe displaces laterally with rotation about the long axis so that the nail faces medially (Fig. 15.63). The sesamoid enlarges, and the soft tissues on the lateral aspect of the great toe enlarge. An adventitious bursa forms which often becomes tender and inflamed.

CONCLUSION

Through the study of clinical biomechanics, we can readily see that the axial skeleton from occiput to sacrum and the kinematic chains of the appendicular skeleton extending to the fingertips and to the toes comprise a marvelous design, an opus magnum carefully blending structure with function, notwithstanding certain areas of weakness that predispose to musculoskeletal and neurologic disorders, both directly and indirectly.

In the last decade or so, science, with the aid of advanced technology, has made rapid inroads in immunology. Forecasts predict that infectious processes and neoplasms may be eliminated as a major threat to humanity near the turn of the century. This is also true for the degenerative cardiovascular diseases. Through genetic manipulation, an answer to hereditary defects is approaching. However, musculoskeletal disorders will be with us as long as intrinsic forces must battle with the extrinsic forces of our environment. It is here that teamwork among engineer and physician will find its most humane contribution—and greatest challenge for the future.

REFERENCES

1. Hollingshead WH, Jenkins DB: *Functional Anatomy of the Limbs and Back.* Philadelphia, W.B. Saunders, 1981, pp 250–262, 270–284.
2. D'Ambrosia RD: The hip. In D'Ambrosia RD: *Musculoskeletal Disorders: Regional Examination and Differential Diagnosis.* Philadelphia, J.B. Lippincott, 1977, pp 298–403.
3. Morehouse LE, Cooper JM: *Kinesiology.* St. Louis, C.V. Mosby, 1950, pp 45–47, 76–81.
4. Kessler RM, Hertling D (eds): *Management of Common Musculoskeletal Disorders.* Philadelphia, Harper & Row, 1983, pp 368–377.
5. Esch D, Lepley M: *Musculoskeletal Function: An Anatomy and Kinesiology Laboratory Manual.* Minneapolis, University of Minnesota Press, 1974, pp 19–22.
6. Barham JN, Wooten EP: *Structural Kinesiology.* New York, Macmillan, 1973, pp 94–96.
7. Cailliet R: *Soft Tissue Pain and Disability.* Philadelphia, F.A. Davis, 1980, pp 196–197.
8. Hollingshead WH, Jenkins DB: *Functional Anatomy of the Limbs and Back.* Philadelphia, W.B. Saunders, 1981, pp 226, 236–240.
9. Kapandji IA: *Physiology of the Joints: Lower Limb,* ed 2. New York, Churchill Livingstone, 1981, vol 2, pp 10–23.
10. Hoppenfeld S: *Physical Examination of the Spine and Extremities.* New York, Appleton-Century-Crofts, 1976, pp 155–159.
11. Barham JN, Wooten EP: *Structural Kinesiology.* New York, Macmillan, 1973, pp 201–202, 224–229.
12. Cailliet R: *Soft Tissue Pain and Disability.* Philadelphia, F.A. Davis, 1980, pp 197–204.
13. D'Ambrosia RD: The hip. In D'Ambrosia RD: *Musculoskeletal Disorders: Regional Examination and Differential Diagnosis.* Philadelphia, J.B. Lippincott, 1977, pp 407–409.
14. Daniels L, Worthingham C: *Muscle Testing: Techniques of Manual Examination,* ed 4. Philadelphia, W.B. Saunders, 1980, pp 38–63.
15. Barham JN, Wooten EP: *Structural Kinesiology.* New York, Macmillan, 1973, pp 204–208, 219–223.
16. Hoppenfeld S: *Physical Examination of the Spine and Extremities.* New York, Appleton-Century-Crofts, 1976, pp 160–163.
17. Esch D, Lepley M: *Musculoskeletal Function: An Anatomy and Kinesiology Laboratory Manual.* Minneapolis, University of Minnesota Press, 1974, pp 54–64.
18. Goodheart GJ: *Applied Kinesiology.* City of publication not shown, published by the author, privately distributed, 1964, pp 21–22, 54–57, 63–65.
19. Goodheart GJ: The psoas muscle and the foot pronation problem. *Collected Published Articles and Reprints.* Montpellier, O, Williams County Publishing, 1969, pp 72–74.
20. Wheatley MD, Jahnke WD: Electromyographic study of the superficial thigh and hip muscles in normal individuals. *Archives of Physical Therapy* 31:508–522, 1951.
21. LaBan MM et al: Electromyographic study of function of iliopsoas muscles. *Archives of Physical Medicine and Rehabilitation* 46:676–679, 1965.
22. Schafer RC (ed): *Basic Chiropractic Procedural Manual,* ed 4. Arlington, Va, American Chiropractic Association, 1984, pp 291–294.
23. Esch D, Lepley M: *Evaluation of Joint Motion: Methods of Measurement and Recording.* Minneapolis, University of Minnesota Press, 1974, pp 33–37.
24. Gonzna ER, Harrington IJ (eds): *Biomechanics of Musculoskeletal Injury.* Baltimore, Williams & Wilkins, 1982, pp 39–40, 135–136, 144, 145–149.
25. LeVeau B: *Williams and Lissner: Biomechanics of Human Motion,* ed 2. Philadelphia, W.B. Saunders, 1977, pp 98–101.
26. D'Ambrosia RD: The hip. In D'Ambrosia RD: *Musculoskeletal Disorders: Regional Examination and Differential Diagnosis.* Philadelphia, J.B. Lippincott, 1977, pp 409–411.
27. Denham RA: Hip mechanics. *Journal of Bone and Joint Surgery (British)* 41:550–557, 1959.
28. Kessler RM, Hertling D (eds): *Management of Common Musculoskeletal Disorders.* Philadelphia, Harper & Row, 1983, pp 377–379.
29. Cailliet R: *Soft Tissue Pain and Disability.* Philadelphia, F.A. Davis, 1980, pp 204–215.
30. Scott WN, Nisonson B, Nicholas JA (eds): *Principles of Sports Medicine.* Baltimore, Williams & Wilkins, 1984, pp 245–263.
31. Hadler NM: *Medical Management of the Regional Musculoskeletal Diseases.* New York, Grune & Stratton, 1984, pp 229–247.
32. Wadsworth JB, Smidt GL, Johnston RC: Gait characteristics of subjects with hip disease. *Physical Therapy* 52:829–837, 1972.
33. Saunders JB, Inman VT, Eberhart HD: The major determinants of normal and pathological gait. *Journal of Bone and Joint Surgery* 35:543–558, 1953.
34. Grieve GP: *Common Vertebral Joint Problems.* New York, Churchill Livingstone, 1981, pp 334–335.
35. Mendler HM: Relationship to hip abductor muscles to posture. *Journal of American Physical Therapy Association* 44:98–102, 1964.
36. Barham JN, Wooten EP: *Structural Kinesiology.* New York, Macmillan, 1973, pp 224–230.
37. Daniels L, Worthingham C: *Therapeutic Exercise for Body Alignment and Function,* ed 2. Philadelphia, W.B. Saunders, 1977, pp 82–100.
38. Inman VT: Functional aspects of the abductor muscles of the hip. *Journal of Bone and Joint Surgery* 29:607–619, 1947.
39. Kaplan EB: The iliotibial tract. *Journal of Bone and Joint Surgery* 40A:817–832, 1958.
40. Black J, Dumbleton JH (eds): *Clinical Biomechanics: Case History Approach.* New York, Churchill Livingstone, 1981, pp 87–88.
41. LeVeau B: *Williams and Lissner: Biomechanics of Human Motion,* ed 2. Philadelphia, W.B. Saunders, 1977, pp 76–77, 101–102.
42. Blount WP: Don't throw away the cane. *Journal of Bone and Joint Surgery* 38:695, 1956.
43. Singleton MC, LeVeau BF: The hip joint: Struc-

ture, stability, and stress. *Physical Therapy* 55:957–973, 1975.
44. Barham JN, Wooten EP: *Structural Kinesiology.* New York, Macmillan, 1973, pp 232–233.
45. Hollingshead WH, Jenkins DB: *Functional Anatomy of the Limbs and Back.* Philadelphia, W.B. Saunders, 1981, p 289.
46. Hoppenfeld S: *Physical Examination of the Spine and Extremities.* New York, Appleton-Century-Crofts, 1976, p 262.
47. Cipriano JJ: *Photographic Manual of Regional Orthopaedic Tests.* Baltimore, Williams & Wilkins, 1985, p 103.
48. Mazion JM: *Illustrated Manual of Neurological Refexes/Signs/Tests, Orthopedic Signs/Tests/Maneuvers,* ed 2. Arizona City, published by the author, 1980, p 345.
49. Borrmann WR: Applied kinesiology of the hamstring muscles and related factors. *Wisconsin Chiropractic Association Journal* 28:15, April 1975.
50. Williams JGP, Sperryn PN (eds): *Sports Medicine,* ed 2. Baltimore, Williams & Wilkins, 1976, pp 438–439.
51. Hirata I Jr: *The Doctor and the Athlete,* ed 2. Philadelphia, J.B. Lippincott, 1974, pp 193–195, 199–211.
52. D'Ambrosia RD: The hip. In D'Ambrosia RD: *Musculoskeletal Disorders: Regional Examination and Differential Diagnosis.* Philadelphia, J.B. Lippincott, 1977, pp 429–430.
53. Nachemson AL: Electromyographical studies of the vertebral portion of the psoas muscle (with special reference to its stabilizing function of the lumbar spine). *Acta Orthopaedica Scandinavica* 37:177–190, 1966.
54. Ng YS: The significance of psoas myospasm in the lordotic compared to the kyphotic sacrolumbar spine. *ACA Journal of Chiropractic* October 1978.
55. Pace JB, Nagle D: Piriform syndrome. *Western Journal of Medicine* 124:435–439, 1976.
56. Van Dusen LG: *Chiropractic Relationship to Gravitational Force.* Sodus, NY, published by the author, 1968, pp 73–85, 89, 97–99.
57. Hoppenfeld S: *Physical Examination of the Spine and Extremities.* New York, Appleton-Century-Crofts, 1976, p 167.
58. Robertson WE, Robertson HF: *Diagnostic Signs, Reflexes, and Syndromes,* ed 3. Philadelphia, F.A. Davis, 1947, p 227.
59. Williams JGP, Sperryn PN (eds): *Sports Medicine,* ed 2. Baltimore, Williams & Wilkins, 1976, p 434.
60. D'Ambrosia RD: The hip. In D'Ambrosia RD: *Musculoskeletal Disorders: Regional Examination and Differential Diagnosis.* Philadelphia, J.B. Lippincott, 1977, pp 428–429.
61. Nash JM: Personal communication, Pasadena, Tex, 1985.
62. Klyop GW et al: Iliotibial band syndrome. *The Physician and Sports Medicine* 9(10):13, December 1981.
63. Hazel RH: Iliotibial band syndrome. *The Journal of the Council on Sports Injuries (ACA)* 1(4):12–14, September 1983.
64. Nobel CA: Iliotibial band friction syndrome in runners. *American Journal of Sports Medicine* 8:232–234, August 1980.
65. Gertler L: *Illustrated Manual of Extravertebral Technic,* ed 2. Bayside, NY, published by the author, 1978, pp 41–50.
66. Janse J, Houser RH, Wells BF: *Chiropractic Principles and Technic.* Chicago, National College of Chiropractic, 1947, pp 564–570.
67. Stierwalt DD: *Extremity Adjusting.* Davenport, Ia, published by the author, 1975, p 26.
68. Maitland GD: *Peripheral Manipulation.* London, Butterworths, 1976, pp 102–113.
69. Gonzna ER, Harrington IJ (eds): *Biomechanics of Musculoskeletal Injury.* Baltimore, Williams & Wilkins, 1982, pp 41–44, 153–158.
70. Williams JGP, Sperryn PN (eds): *Sports Medicine,* ed 2. Baltimore, Williams & Wilkins, 1976, pp 435–436.
71. Mazion JM: *Illustrated Manual of Neurological Reflexes/Signs/Tests, Orthopedic Signs/Tests/Maneuvers,* ed 2. Arizona City, published by the author, 1980.
72. Gozna ER: Biomechanics of pelvic and acetabular fractures. In Gonzna ER, Harrington IJ (eds): *Biomechanics of Musculoskeletal Injury.* Baltimore, Williams & Wilkins, 1982, pp 136–139.
73. D'Ambrosia RD: The hip. In D'Ambrosia RD: *Musculoskeletal Disorders: Regional Examination and Differential Diagnosis.* Philadelphia, J.B. Lippincott, 1977, pp 406–407, 434–438.
74. Holmes GW, Robbins LL: *Roentgen Interpretation,* ed 7. Philadelphia, Lea & Febiger, 1947, pp 51–53.
75. Iverson LD, Clawson DK: *Manual of Acute Orthopaedic Therapeutics.* Boston, Little, Brown, 1977, 187–199.
76. Holmes GW, Robbins LL: *Roentgen Interpretation,* ed 7. Philadelphia, Lea & Febiger, 1947, pp 58–60.
77. Gillet H, Liekens M: *Belgian Chiropractic Research Notes.* Huntington Beach, Cal, Motion Palpation Institute, 1981, pp 91–92.
78. Cyriax J: *Textbook of Orthopaedic Medicine. Vol. 1, Diagnosis of Soft Tissue Lesions,* ed 8. London, Bailliere Tindall, 1982, pp 297–298.
79. Helfet AJ, Gruebel Lee, DM: *Disorders of the Lumbar Spine.* Philadelphia, J.B. Lippincott, 1978, pp 24–25.
80. Hart FD (ed): *French's Index of Differential Diagnosis,* ed 12. Bristol, England, Wright, 1985, p 519.
81. Aiken P: Meralgia paresthetica. *Orthopedic Brief.* ACA Council on Orthopedics (undated).
82. James SL: The knee. In D'Ambrosia RD: *Musculoskeletal Disorders: Regional Examination and Differential Diagnosis.* Philadelphia, J.B. Lippincott, 1977, pp 440–446.
83. Hollingshead WH, Jenkins DB: *Functional Anatomy of the Limbs and Back.* Philadelphia, W.B. Saunders, 1981, pp 226, 241–248.
84. Morehouse LE, Cooper JM: *Kinesiology.* St. Louis, C.V. Mosby, 1950, pp 82–88.
85. Cailliet R: *Knee Pain and Disability.* Philadelphia, F.A. Davis, 1973, pp 1–31.
86. Kessler RM, Hertling D (eds): *Management of*

Common Musculoskeletal Disorders. Philadelphia, Harper & Row, 1983, pp 394–402.

87. Barham JN, Wooten EP: *Structural Kinesiology.* New York, Macmillan, 1973, p 193.
88. LeVeau B: *Williams and Lissner: Biomechanics of Human Motion,* ed 2. Philadelphia, W.B. Saunders, 1977, p 109.
89. Kapandji IA: *Physiology of the Joints: Lower Limb,* ed 2. New York, Churchill Livingstone, 1981, vol 2, pp 92, 96, 106, 114–119.
90. Cailliet R: *Soft Tissue Pain and Disability.* Philadelphia, F.A. Davis, 1980, pp 216–224.
91. Rosse C, Clawson DK (eds): *The Musculoskeletal System in Health and Disease.* Hagerstown, Md, Harper & Row, 1980, pp 277–282.
92. Barham JN, Wooten EP: *Structural Kinesiology.* New York, Macmillan, 1973, pp 199–200.
93. Esch D, Lepley M: *Musculoskeletal Function: An Anatomy and Kinesiology Laboratory Manual.* Minneapolis, University of Minnesota Press, 1974, pp 64–68.
94. Kapandji IA: *Physiology of the Joints: Lower Limb,* ed 2. New York, Churchill Livingstone, 1981, vol 2, pp 76–79, 88–90, 98–105, 128–134.
95. James SL: The knee. In D'Ambrosia RD: *Musculoskeletal Disorders: Regional Examination and Differential Diagnosis.* Philadelphia, J.B. Lippincott, 1977, pp 450–451, 452–455.
96. Cailliet R: *Knee Pain and Disability.* Philadelphia, F.A. Davis, 1973, pp 33–39.
97. Hoppenfeld S: *Physical Examination of the Spine and Extremities.* New York, Appleton-Century-Crofts, 1976, pp 187–189.
98. Rosse C, Clawson DK (eds): *The Musculoskeletal System in Health and Disease.* Hagerstown, Md, Harper & Row, 1980, pp 283–285.
99. Grice AS, Fligg DB: *Class Notes: Introductory Concepts to Clinical Analysis of Joint Movement and Muscle Testing.* Department of Biomechanics/Kinesiology, BK101. Toronto, Canadian Memorial Chiropractic College (undated) pp 57–69.
100. Hollingshead WH, Jenkins DB: *Functional Anatomy of the Limbs and Back.* Philadelphia, W.B. Saunders, 1981, pp 284–288.
101. Bierman W, Ralston MJ: Electromyographic study during passive and active flexion and extension of the knee of the normal human subject. *Archives of Physical Medicine and Rehabilitation* 46:71–75, January 1965.
102. Brewerton DA: The function of the vastus medialis muscle. *Annals of Physical Medicine* 2:164–168, 1955.
103. Barham JN, Wooten EP: *Structural Kinesiology.* New York, Macmillan, 1973, pp 199–200, 217–219.
104. Cailliet R: *Soft Tissue Pain and Disability.* Philadelphia, F.A. Davis, 1980, pp 228–233.
105. Hoppenfeld S: *Orthopaedic Neurology: A Diagnostic Guide to Neurologic Levels.* Philadelphia, J.B. Lippincott, 1977, p 194.
106. Barham JN, Wooten EP: *Structural Kinesiology.* New York, Macmillan, 1973, pp 204–206, 217–218.
107. Daniels L, Worthingham C: *Muscle Testing: Techniques of Manual Examination,* ed 4. Philadelphia, W.B. Saunders, 1980, pp 64–71.
108. Cailliet R: *Soft Tissue Pain and Disability.* Philadelphia, F.A. Davis, 1980, pp 224–227.
109. Hoppenfeld S: *Physical Examination of the Spine and Extremities.* New York, Appleton-Century-Crofts, 1976, pp 189–191.
110. Allington RO et al: Strengthening techniques of the quadriceps muscles: An electromyographic evaluation. *Physical Therapy* 46:1173–1176, November 1966.
111. Schafer RC (ed): *Basic Chiropractic Procedural Manual,* ed 4. Arlington, Va, American Chiropractic Association, 1984, p 294.
112. Esch D, Lepley M: *Evaluation of Joint Motion: Methods of Measurement and Recording.* Minneapolis, University of Minnesota Press, 1974, p 38.
113. Turek SL: *Orthopaedics: Principles and Their Application,* ed 3. Philadelphia, J.B. Lippincott, 1977, p 1192.
114. Williams M, Lissner HR: Biomechanical analysis of knee function. *Physical Therapy* 43:93–99, 1962.
115. Smidt GL: Biomechanical analysis of knee flexion and extension. *Journal of Biomechanics* 6:79–92, 1973.
116. Harrington IJ: Biomechanics of joint injuries. In Gonzna ER, Harrington IJ (eds): *Biomechanics of Musculoskeletal Injury.* Baltimore, Williams & Wilkins, 1982, pp 56–62.
117. LeVeau B: *Williams and Lissner: Biomechanics of Human Motion,* ed 2. Philadelphia, W.B. Saunders, 1977, pp 106–115.
118. Kapandji IA: *Physiology of the Joints: Lower Limb,* ed 2. New York, Churchill Livingstone, 1981, vol 2, pp 72–75.
119. Morrison JB: The mechanics of the knee joint in relation to normal walking. *Journal of Biomechanics* 3:51–61, 1970.
120. Kessler RM, Hertling D (eds): *Management of Common Musculoskeletal Disorders.* Philadelphia, Harper & Row, 1983, pp 402–410.
121. Hollingshead WH, Jenkins DB: *Functional Anatomy of the Limbs and Back.* Philadelphia, W.B. Saunders, 1981, pp 289–290.
122. Rosse C, Clawson DK (eds): *The Musculoskeletal System in Health and Disease.* Hagerstown, Md, Harper & Row, 1980, pp 285–286, 289–290.
123. Kapandji IA: *Physiology of the Joints: Lower Limb,* ed 2. New York, Churchill Livingstone, 1981, vol 2, pp 108–112, 120–126.
124. Kettlekamp DB: Clinical implications of knee biomechanics. *Archives of Surgery* 107:406–410, 1973.
125. Smith JW: Observations on the postural mechanism of the human knee joint. *Journal of Anatomy* 90:236–261, 1956.
126. Klein KK: The knee and the ligaments. *Journal of Bone and Joint Surgery* 44A:1191–1193, 1962.
127. James SL: The knee. In D'Ambrosia RD: *Musculoskeletal Disorders: Regional Examination and Differential Diagnosis.* Philadelphia, J.B. Lippincott, 1977, pp 456–462.
128. Hoppenfeld S: *Physical Examination of the Spine and Extremities.* New York, Appleton-Century-Crofts, 1976, pp 185–187, 191–194.
129. Grossman RB, Nicholas JA: Common disorders

of the knee. *Orthopaedic Clinics of North America* 8:619–640, 1977.

130. Eriksson E: Sports injuries of the knee ligaments: Their diagnosis, treatment, rehabilitation, and prevention. *Medical Science and Sports* 8:133–144, 1976.
131. Slocum D et al: Clinical test for anterolateral rotatory instability of the knee. *Clinical Orthopaedics* 118:63–69, 1976.
132. Marshall J et al: The anterior drawer sign: What is it? *American Journal of Sports Medicine* 3:152–158, 1975.
133. Kennedy JC, Fowler P: Medial and anterior instability of the knee. *Jouranl of Bone and Joint Surgery* 53A:1257–1270, 1971.
134. Dolan JP, Holladay LJ: *First-Aid Management*, ed 4, Danville, Ill, Interstate Printers & Publishers, 1974, pp 181–197.
135. Rosse C, Clawson DK (eds): *The Musculoskeletal System in Health and Disease.* Hagerstown, Md, Harper & Row, 1980, pp 286–289.
136. Cailliet R: *Soft Tissue Pain and Disability.* Philadelphia, F.A. Davis, 1980, pp 233–243.
137. Grice AS, Fligg DB: *Class Notes: Introductory Concepts to Clinical Analysis of Joint Movement and Muscle Testing.* Department of Biomechanics/Kinesiology, BK101. Toronto, Canadian Memorial Chiropractic College (undated), pp 72–78, 80–84.
138. Hadler NM: *Medical Management of the Regional Musculoskeletal Diseases.* New York, Grune & Stratton, 1984, pp 251–270.
139. Kessler RM, Hertling D (eds): *Management of Common Musculoskeletal Disorders.* Philadelphia, Harper & Row, 1983, pp 425–442.
140. Schneider RC, Kennedy JC, Plant ML (eds): *Sports Injuries: Mechanisms, Prevention, and Treatment.* Baltimore, Williams & Wilkins, 1985, pp 764–783.
141. Scott WN, Nisonson B, Nicholas JA (eds): *Principles of Sports Medicine.* Baltimore, Williams & Wilkins, 1984, pp 291–299, 303–336.
142. Kapandji IA: *Physiology of the Joints: Lower Limb*, ed 2. New York, Churhill Livingstone, 1981, vol 2, p 80.
143. James SL: The knee. In D'Ambrosia RD: *Musculoskeletal Disorders: Regional Examination and Differential Diagnosis.* Philadelphia, J.B. Lippincott, 1977, pp 476–481.
144. Barham JN, Wooten EP: *Structural Kinesiology.* New York, Macmillan, 1973, p 230
145. Cailliet R: *Knee Pain and Disability.* Philadelphia, F.A. Davis, 1973, pp 123–131.
146. Cailliet R: *Foot and Ankle Pain.* Philadelphia, F.A. Davis, 1979, pp 34–35.
147. Kendall HO, Kendall FP, Wadsworth GE: *Muscles: Testing and Function*, ed 2. Baltimore, Williams & Wilkins, 1971, pp 32–33.
148. Greenawalt, MH: *Spinal Pelvic Stabilization*, ed 2, Dubuque, Ia, Foot Levelers, 1978, pp 29–30.
149. Asher C: *Postural Variations in Childhood.* London, Butterworths, 1975, pp 54–72.
150. Asher C: *Postural Variations in Childhood.* London, Butterworths, 1975, pp 73–75.
151. Turek SL: *Orthopaedics: Principles and Their Application*, ed 3. Philadelphia, J.B. Lippincott, 1977, pp 1215–1216.
152. Asher C: *Postural Variations in Childhood.* London, Butterworths, 1975, pp 60–61.
153. Reider B, Marshall JL, Warren RF: Clinical characteristics of patellar disorders in young athletes. *American Journal of Sports Medicine* 9:270–274, 1981.
154. Insall JN: Patellar pain. *Journal of Bone and Joint Surgery* 64A:147–152, 1982.
155. Cailliet R: *Soft Tissue Pain and Disability.* Philadelphia, F.A. Davis, 1980, pp 244–245.
156. Cailliet R: *Knee Pain and Disability.* Philadelphia, F.A. Davis, 1973, pp 73–82.
157. Rosse C, Clawson DK (eds): *The Musculoskeletal System in Health and Disease.* Hagerstown, MD, Harper & Row, 1980, p 282.
158. Schafer RC: *Chiropractic Management of Sports and Recreational Injuries.* Baltimore, Williams & Wilkins, 1982, pp 474–475, 492–493.
159. Hoppenfeld S: *Physical Examination of the Spine and Extremities.* New York, Appleton-Century-Crofts, 1976, pp 194–196.
160. Hirata I Jr: *The Doctor and the Athelete*, ed 2. Philadelphia, J.B. Lippincott, 1974, pp 221–223.
161. Blits J: Ortho-differential diagnosis of popliteal swelling. *Ortho-Briefs* ACA Council on Orthopedics, 5(1):5, April 1983.
162. Gertler L: *Illustrated Manual of Extravertebral Technic*, ed 2. Bayside, NY, published by the author, 1978, p 21.
163. Maitland GD: *Peripheral Manipulation.* London, Butterworths, 1976, pp 122–124.
164. Stierwalt DD: *Extremity Adjusting.* Davenport, Ia, published by the author, 1975, p 27.
165. Schultz AL: *Athletic and Industrial Injuries of the Knee.* Mitchell SD, published by the author, 1951, pp 96–101.
166. Hirata I Jr: *The Doctor and the Athlete*, ed 2. Philadelphia, J.B. Lippincott, 1974, pp 227–228.
167. James SL: The knee. In D'Ambrosia RD: *Musculoskeletal Disorders: Regional Examination and Differential Diagnosis.* Philadelphia, J.B. Lippincott, 1977, pp 468–469.
168. Kettelkamp DB: Management of patellar malalignment. *Journal of Bone and Joint Surgery* 63A:1344–1347, 1981.
169. Houghston JC: Subluxation of the patella in athletes. *Symposium on Sports Medicine*, American Academy of Orthopaedic Surgeons, Oklahoma City, August 1967. St. Louis, C.V. Mosby, 1969, pp 162–177.
170. Goodrich TM: Analysis and treatment of common lesions of the knee. *ACA Journal of Chiropractic* January 1963.
171. Brantigan OC, Voshell AF: The mechanics of the ligaments and menisci of the knee joint. *Journal of Bone and Joint Surgery* 23(1):44–66, January 1941.
172. James SL: The knee. In D'Ambrosia RD: *Musculoskeletal Disorders: Regional Examination and Differential Diagnosis.* Philadelphia, J.B. Lippincott, 1977, pp 464–466.
173. Schultz AL: *Athletic and Industrial Injuries of the Knee.* Mitchell, SD, published by the author, 1951.

174. Barham JN, Wooten EP: *Structural Kinesiology.* New York, Macmillan, 1973, pp 231–232.
175. Cailliet R: *Soft Tissue Pain and Disability.* Philadelphia, F.A. Davis, 1980, pp 247
176. Cailliet R: *Knee Pain and Disability.* Philadelphia, F.A. Davis, 1973, pp 40–47, 62–71.
177. Bowerman JW: *Radiology and Injury in Sport.* New York, Appleton-Century-Crofts, 1977, pp 119–131.
178. Holmes GW, Robbins LL: *Roentgen Interpretation,* ed 7. Philadelphia, Lea & Febiger, 1947, pp 50–51.
179. Schafer RC: *Chiropractic Management of Sports and Recreational Injuries.* Baltimore, Williams & Wilkins, 1982, pp 478–479.
180. Williams JGP, Sperryn PN (eds): *Sports Medicine,* ed 2. Baltimore, Williams & Wilkins, 1976, pp 443–445.
181. Hirata I Jr: *The Doctor and the Athlete,* ed 2. Philadelphia, J.B. Lippincott, 1974, pp 215–216.
182. Teranel JA: *Chiropractic Orthopedics and Roentgenology.* Newark, NJ, Medusa Press, 1953, p 313.
183. Williams JGP, Sperryn PN (eds): *Sports Medicine,* ed 2. Baltimore, Williams & Wilkins, 1976, pp 440, 447, 449.
184. James SL: The knee. In D'Ambrosia RD: *Musculoskeletal Disorders: Regional Examination and Differential Diagnosis.* Philadelphia, J.B. Lippincott, 1977, pp 451–452.
185. Schafer RC: *Chiropractic Management of Sports and Recreational Injuries.* Baltimore, Williams & Wilkins, 1982, p 480.
186. Apley AG: The diagnosis of meniscal injuries. *Journal of Bone and Joint Surgery* 29:78–84, 1946.
187. James SL: The knee. In D'Ambrosia RD: *Musculoskeletal Disorders: Regional Examination and Differential Diagnosis.* Philadelphia, J.B. Lippincott, 1977, pp 467–468.
188. Cipriano JJ: *Photographic Manual of Regional Orthopaedic Tests.* Baltimore, Williams & Wilkins, 1985, pp 171, 173, 177.
189. Schafer RC: *Chiropractic Management of Sports and Recreational Injuries.* Baltimore, Williams & Wilkins, 1982, pp 480–482.
190. Williams JGP, Sperryn PN (eds): *Sports Medicine,* ed 2. Baltimore, Williams & Wilkins, 1976, pp 450–452.
191. Hirata I Jr: *The Doctor and the Athlete,* ed 2. Philadelphia, J.B. Lippincott, 1974, pp 217–218.
192. Bowerman JW: *Radiology and Injury in Sport.* New York, Appleton-Century-Crofts, 1977, pp 119–123.
193. Teranel JA: *Chiropractic Orthopedics and Roentgenology.* Newark, NJ, Medusa Press, 1953, pp 309–312.
194. Baker BE et al: Review of meniscal injury and associated sports. *American Journal of Sports Medicine* 13:1–4, 1985.
195. Schafer RC: *Chiropractic Management of Sports and Recreational Injuries.* Baltimore, Williams & Wilkins, 1982, p 482.
196. Teranel JA: *Chiropractic Orthopedics and Roentgenology.* Newark, NJ, Medusa Press, 1953, p 312.
197. Williams JGP, Sperryn PN (eds): *Sports Medicine,* ed 2. Baltimore, Williams & Wilkins, 1976, pp 449–450.
198. Torg J et al: Clinical diagnosis of anterior cruciate ligament instability in the athlete. *American Journal of Sports Medicine* 4:84–92, 1976.
199. Williams JGP, Sperryn PN (eds): *Sports Medicine,* ed 2. Baltimore, Williams & Wilkins, 1976, pp 452, 454.
200. Galway R et al: Pivot shift: A clinical sign of symptomatic anterior cruciate insufficiency. *Journal of Bone and Joint Surgery* 54B:763–764, 1974.
201. MacIntosch DL: The pivot shift and the anterior cruciate. Presented at the New York State Orthopaedic Society Meeting, New York, 1979.
202. Marshall J, Rubin R: Knee ligament injuries. *Orthopaedic Clinics of North America* 8:651–665, 1977.
203. Baltzell LG, Mackey RH (eds): *Firth's Technic Notes.* Publishing data not shown, 1967, pp 51–57. Available from National College of Chiropractic.
204. Janse J, Houser RH, Wells BF: *Chiropractic Principles and Technic.* Chicago, National College of Chiropractic, 1947, pp 570–582.
205. Gertler L: *Illustrated Manual of Extravertebral Technic,* ed 2. Bayside, NY, published by the author, 1978, pp 21–28.
206. Schultz AL: *Athletic and Industrial Injuries of the Knee.* Mitchell, SD, published by the author, 1951, pp 54–95, 104–109.
207. Maitland GD: *Peripheral Manipulation.* London, Butterworths, 1976, pp 114–129.
208. Stierwalt DD: *Extremity Adjusting.* Davenport, Ia, published by the author, 1975, pp 27–30.
209. Ogden JA: Subluxation and dislocation of the proximal tibiofibular joint. *Journal of Bone and Joint Surgery* 56A:145, 1974.
210. Williams JGP, Sperryn PN (eds): *Sports Medicine,* ed 2. Baltimore, Williams & Wilkins, 1976 pp 454–455.
211. Iverson LD, Clawson DK: *Manual of Acute Orthopaedic Therapeutics.* Boston, Little, Brown, 1977, p 235.
212. Vernon H: The Helfet test. *Journal of the CCA* December 1978, p 127.
213. Schafer RC: *Chiropractic Management of Sports and Recreational Injuries.* Baltimore, Williams & Wilkins, 1982, p 486.
214. Iverson LD, Clawson DK: *Manual of Acute Orthopaedic Therapeutics.* Boston, Little, Brown, 1977, pp 37–38.
215. Turek SL: *Orthopaedics: Principles and Their Application,* ed 3. Philadelphia, J.B. Lippincott, 1977, pp 617–618.
216. Bowerman JW: *Radiology and Injury in Sport.* New York, Appleton-Century-Crofts, 1977, pp 182, 219, 231, 273.
217. Zatzkin HR: *The Roentgen Diagnosis of Trauma.* Chicago, Year Book Medical Publishers, 1965.
218. James SL: The knee. In D'Ambrosia RD: *Musculoskeletal Disorders: Regional Examination and Differential Diagnosis.* Philadelphia, J.B. Lippincott, 1977, pp 481–485.
219. Zuidema GD, Rutherford RB, Ballinger WF (eds):

The Management of Trauma, ed 3. Philadelphia, W.B. Saunders, 1979, pp 645–650.

220. Gonzna ER, Harrington IJ (eds): *Biomechanics of Musculoskeletal Injury*. Baltimore, Williams & Wilkins, 1982, pp 60–62.
221. Cailliet R: *Knee Pain and Disability*. Philadelphia, F.A. Davis, 1973, pp 110–122.
222. Salter RB, Harris WR: Injuries involving the epiphyseal plate. *Journal of Bone and Joint Surgery* 45A:587, 1963.
223. Iverson LD, Clawson DK: *Manual of Acute Orthopaedic Therapeutics*. Boston, Little, Brown, 1977, pp 236–237.
224. Sisto J, Warren R: Complete knee dislocation. Presented at the American Orthopaedic Society for Sports Medicine, Anaheim, Cal, March 1983.
225. Gillet H, Liekens M: *Belgian Chiropractic Research Notes*. Huntington Beach, Cal, Motion Palpation Institute, 1981, p 91.
226. DePalma AI: *Diseases of the Knee*. Philadelphia, J.B. Lippincott, 1954.
227. Barham JN, Wooten EP: *Structural Kinesiology*. New York, Macmillan, 1973, pp 230–231.
228. Cailliet R: *Knee Pain and Disability*. Philadelphia, F.A. Davis, 1973, pp 77–82.
229. Wiles MR: Geriatric knee pain: Diagnosis and treatment. *Journal of Manipulative and Physiological Therapeutics* 2:93–98, 1979.
230. James SL: The knee. In D'Ambrosia RD: *Musculoskeletal Disorders: Regional Examination and Differential Diagnosis*. Philadelphia, J.B. Lippincott, 1977, pp 472–476.
231. Williams JGP, Sperryn PN (eds): *Sports Medicine*, ed 2. Baltimore, Williams & Wilkins, 1976, p 442.
232. Hirata I Jr: *The Doctor and the Athlete*, ed 2. Philadelphia, J.B. Lippincott, 1974, pp 229–230.
233. Cailliet R: *Soft Tissue Pain and Disability*. Philadelphia, F.A. Davis, 1980, p 248.
234. Williams JGP, Sperryn PN (eds): *Sports Medicine*, ed 2. Baltimore, Williams & Wilkins, 1976, pp 460–464.
235. James SL: The knee. In D'Ambrosia RD: *Musculoskeletal Disorders: Regional Examination and Differential Diagnosis*. Philadelphia, J.B. Lippincott, 1977, p 469.
236. Williams JGP, Sperryn PN (eds): *Sports Medicine*, ed 2. Baltimore, Williams & Wilkins, 1976, p 467.
237. Turek SL: *Orthopaedics: Principles and Their Application*, ed 3. Philadelphia, J.B. Lippincott, 1977, pp 1198–1199.
238. Schafer RC: *Chiropractic Management of Sports and Recreational Injuries*. Baltimore, Williams & Wilkins, 1982, pp 484–485.
239. Feldman F (ed): *Radiology, Pathology, and Immunology of Bones and Joints: A Review of Current Concepts*. New York, Appleton-Century-Crofts, 1978, pp 281–289.
240. Schafer RC: *Chiropractic Management of Sports and Recreational Injuries*. Baltimore, Williams & Wilkins, 1982, p 485.
241. Cailliet R: *Soft Tissue Pain and Disability*. Philadelphia, F.A. Davis, 1980, pp 248–250.
242. Hirata I Jr: *The Doctor and the Athlete*, ed 2. Philadelphia, J.B. Lippincott, 1974, pp 226–227, 230–231.
243. Maurer EL: Osteochondritis dissecans. *Success Express* 9(4):41–45. Published by Goals Unlimited International, Dubuque, Ia.
244. Giammarino MA: The adolescent knee. *Roentgenological Briefs* ACA Council on Roentgenology (undated).
245. Schafer RC: *Chiropractic Management of Sports and Recreational Injuries*. Baltimore, Williams & Wilkins, 1982, pp 494–495.
246. Rosse C, Clawson DK (eds): *The Musculoskeletal System in Health and Disease*. Hagerstown, Md, Harper & Row, 1980, p 291.
247. Asher C: *Postural Variations in Childhood*. London, Butterworths, 1975, pp 78–80.
248. Barham JN, Wooten EP: *Structural Kinesiology*. New York, Macmillan, 1973, pp 157–159, 162–166, 170–172.
249. Hollingshead WH, Jenkins DB: *Functional Anatomy of the Limbs and Back*. Philadelphia, W.B. Saunders, 1981, pp 226–227, 291–305, 319–321.
250. Esch D, Lepley M: *Musculoskeletal Function: An Anatomy and Kinesiology Laboratory Manual*. Minneapolis, University of Minnesota Press, 1974, pp 23–25.
251. Cailliet R: *Soft Tissue Pain and Disability*. Philadelphia, F.A. Davis, 1980, pp 252–261.
252. Grice AS, Fligg DB: *Class Notes: Introductory Concepts to Clinical Analysis of Joint Movement and Muscle Testing*. Department of Biomechanics/Kinesiology, BK101. Toronto, Canadian Memorial Chiropractic College (undated), pp 8–14, 25–31.
253. Morehouse LE, Cooper JM: *Kinesiology*. St. Louis, C.V. Mosby, 1950, pp 89–92.
254. Shoji H: The foot and ankle. In D'Ambrosia RD: *Musculoskeletal Disorders: Regional Examination and Differential Diagnosis*. Philadelphia, J.B. Lippincott, 1977, pp 487, 490–492.
255. Kessler RM, Hertling D (eds): *Management of Common Musculoskeletal Disorders*. Philadelphia, Harper & Row, 1983, pp 448–462.
256. Sutherland DH: An electromyographic study of the plantar flexors of the ankle in normal walking on the level. *Journal of Bone and Joint Surgery* 48A:66–71, January 1966.
257. Elfman H: Forces and energy changes in the leg during walking. *American Journal of Physiology* 125:339–356, 1959.
258. Esch D, Lepley M: *Musculoskeletal Function: An Anatomy and Kinesiology Laboratory Manual*. Minneapolis, University of Minnesota Press, 1974, pp 69–72.
259. Rosse C, Clawson DK (eds): *The Musculoskeletal System in Health and Disease*. Hagerstown, Md, Harper & Row, 1980, pp 295–297, 299–300.
260. Shephard E: Tarsal movements. *Journal of Bone and Joint Surgery* 33B:258–263, 1951.
261. Barham JN, Wooten EP: *Structural Kinesiology*. New York, Macmillan, 1973, pp 159–161, 177–178.
262. Shoji H: The foot and ankle. In D'Ambrosia RD: *Musculoskeletal Disorders: Regional Examination and Differential Diagnosis*. Philadelphia, J.B. Lippincott, 1977, p 500.

263. Kapandji IA: *Physiology of the Joints: Lower Limb*, ed 2. New York, Churchill Livingstone, 1981, vol 2, pp 136–142, 184–195.
264. Hoppenfeld S: *Physical Examination of the Spine and Extremities*. New York, Appleton-Century-Crofts, 1976, pp 223–225.
265. Morehouse LE, Cooper JM: *Kinesiology*. St. Louis, C.V. Mosby, 1950, pp 92–93.
266. Gowitzke BA, Milner M: *Understanding Scientific Basis of Human Movement*, ed 2. Baltimore, Williams & Wilkins, 1980, pp 23, 33.
267. Daniels L, Worthingham C: *Muscle Testing: Techniques of Manual Examination*, ed 4. Philadelphia, W.B. Saunders, 1980, pp 72–77.
268. Shoji H: The foot and ankle. In D'Ambrosia RD: *Musculoskeletal Disorders: Regional Examination and Differential Diagnosis*. Philadelphia, J.B. Lippincott, 1977, p 501.
269. Barham JN, Wooten EP: *Structural Kinesiology*. New York, Macmillan, 1973, pp 162–166, 176–177, 179.
270. Hoppenfeld S: *Physical Examination of the Spine and Extremities*. New York, Appleton-Century-Crofts, 1976, pp 227–229.
271. Dolan JP, Holladay LJ: *First-Aid Management*, ed 4. Danville, Ill, Interstate Printers & Publishers, 1974, pp 159–165.
272. Kirby JD: *Essentials of Physical Diagnosis*, North Hollywood, Cal, Chiropractic Business Services, 1978.
273. Schafer RC (ed): *Basic Chiropractic Procedural Manual*, ed 4. Arlington, Va, American Chiropractic Association, 1984, p 295.
274. Esch D, Lepley M: *Evaluation of Joint Motion: Methods of Measurement and Recording*. Minneapolis, University of Minnesota Press, 1974, pp 39–40.
275. Wiehe RJ: The importance of peripheral vascular diagnosis. *The Chiropractic Family Physician* 2(4):12–15, May 1980.
276. Jahn WF: Vascular disease and the chiropractic physician. *The Chiropractic Family Physician* 3(3):19–22, March 1981.
277. Cipriano JJ: *Photographic Manual of Regional Orthopedic Tests*. Baltimore, Williams & Wilkins, 1985.
278. Kessler RM, Hertling D (eds): *Management of Common Musculoskeletal Disorders*. Philadelphia, Harper & Row, 1983, pp 462–478.
279. Scott WN, Nisonson B, Nicholas JA (eds): *Principles of Sports Medicine*. Baltimore, Williams & Wilkins, 1984, pp 342–346, 348–358.
280. Barham JN, Wooten EP: *Structural Kinesiology*. New York, Macmillan, 1973, pp 178–183, 182–186.
281. Grice AS, Fligg DB: *Class Notes: Introductory Concepts to Clinical Analysis of Joint Movement and Muscle Testing*. Department of Biomechanics/Kinesiology, BK101. Toronto, Canadian Memorial Chiropractic College (undated) pp 37–42.
282. Harrington IJ: Biomechanics of joint injuries. In Gonzna ER, Harrington IJ (eds): *Biomechanics of Musculoskeletal Injury*. Baltimore, Williams & Wilkins, 1982, pp 62–66.
283. LeVeau B: *Williams and Lissner: Biomechanics of Human Motion*, ed 2. Philadelphia, W.B. Saunders, 1977, pp 113–114.
284. Kapandji IA: *Physiology of the Joints: Lower Limb*, ed 2. New York, Churchill Livingstone, 1981, vol 2, pp 146–152.
285. Dolan JP, Holladay LJ: *First-Aid Management*, ed 4. Danville, Ill, Interstate Printers & Publishers, 1974, pp 178–179.
286. Hirata I Jr: *The Doctor and the Athlete*, ed 2. Philadelphia, J.B. Lippincott, 1974, pp 234–236.
287. Herman R, Bragin SJ: Function of the gastrocnemius and soleus muscles. *Journal of the American Physical Therapy Association* 47:105–113, 1967.
288. Hirata I Jr: *The Doctor and the Athlete*, ed 2. Philadelphia, J.B. Lippincott, 1974, pp 236–237.
289. Michael RH, Holder LE: The soleus syndrome: A cause of medial tibial stress (shin splints). *The American Journal of Sports Medicine* 13(2):87, March/April 1985.
290. Bowerman JW: *Radiology and Injury in Sport*. New York, Appleton-Century-Crofts, 1977, pp 131–132.
291. Hirata I Jr: *The Doctor and the Athelete*, ed 2. Philadelphia, J.B. Lippincott, 1974, pp 238–240.
292. Craig TT (ed): *Comments in Sports Medicine*. Chicago, American Medical Association, 1973, p 33.
293. Williams JGP, Sperryn PN (eds): *Sports Medicine*, ed 2. Baltimore, Williams & Wilkins, 1976, pp 470–471.
294. Williams JGP, Sperryn PN (eds): *Sports Medicine*, ed 2. Baltimore, Williams & Wilkins, 1976, pp 471–472.
295. Hirata I Jr: *The Doctor and the Athlete*, ed 2. Philadelphia, J.B. Lippincott, 1974, p 241.
296. Iverson LD, Clawson DK: *Manual of Acute Orthopaedic Therapeutics*. Boston, Little, Brown, 1977, p 253.
297. Gollnick PD: Electrogoniometric study of walking on high heels. *Research Quarterly* American Association of Health and Physical Education, 35:370–378, 1964.
298. Williams JGP, Sperryn PN (eds): *Sports Medicine*, ed 2. Baltimore, Williams & Wilkins, 1976, pp 472–482.
299. Hirata I Jr: *The Doctor and the Athlete*, ed 2. Philadelphia, J.B. Lippincott, 1974, pp 240–241.
300. Dolan JP, Holladay LJ: *First-Aid Management*, ed 4. Danville, Ill, Interstate Printers & Publishers, 1974, pp 179, 132, 133–135.
301. Iverson LD, Clawson DK: *Manual of Acute Orthopaedic Therapeutics*. Boston, Little, Brown, 1977, pp 247–251.
302. Holmes GW, Robbins LL: *Roentgen Interpretation*, ed 7. Philadelphia, Lea & Febiger, 1947, pp 53–56.
303. Gonzna ER, Harrington IJ (eds): *Biomechanics of Musculoskeletal Injury*. Baltimore, Williams & Wilkins, 1982, pp 1–23.
304. Hirata I Jr: *The Doctor and the Athlete*, ed 2. Philadelphia, J.B. Lippincott, 1974, pp 232–234.
305. Cailliet R: *Foot and Ankle Pain*. Philadelphia, F.A. Davis, 1979, pp 117–124.
306. Cailliet R: *Soft Tissue Pain and Disability*. Philadelphia, F.A. Davis, 1980, pp 297–303.
307. Smith JW: The forces operating at the human

ankle joint during standing. *Journal of Anatomy* 91:545–564, 1957.
308. Williams JGP, Sperryn PN (eds): *Sports Medicine*, ed 2. Baltimore, Williams & Wilkins, 1976, pp 489–490.
309. Shoji H: The foot and ankle. In D'Ambrosia RD: *Musculoskeletal Disorders: Regional Examination and Differential Diagnosis*. Philadelphia, J.B. Lippincott, 1977, p 520.
310. Williams JGP, Sperryn PN (eds): *Sports Medicine*, ed 2. Baltimore, Williams & Wilkins, 1976, pp 482–485.
311. Iverson LD, Clawson DK: *Manual of Acute Orthopaedic Therapeutics*. Boston, Little, Brown, 1977, pp 251–253.
312. Hirata I Jr: *The Doctor and the Athlete*, ed 2. Philadelphia, J.B. Lippincott, 1974, pp 247–248, 250–251.
313. Schneider RC, Kennedy JC, Plant ML (eds): *Sports Injuries: Mechanisms, Prevention, and Treatment*. Baltimore, Williams & Wilkins, 1985, pp 788–790.
314. Dias LS: The lateral ankle sprain: An experimental study. *Journal of Trauma* 19:266–269, 1979.
315. Shoji H: The foot and ankle. In D'Ambrosia RD: *Musculoskeletal Disorders: Regional Examination and Differential Diagnosis*. Philadelphia, J.B. Lippincott, 1977, pp 500–501.
316. Hoppenfeld S: *Physical Examination of the Spine and Extremities*. New York, Appleton-Century-Crofts, 1976, pp 221–222.
317. Gonzna ER, Harrington IJ (eds): *Biomechanics of Musculoskeletal Injury*. Baltimore, Williams & Wilkins, 1982, pp 62–67.
318. Zuidema GD, Rutherford RB, Ballinger WF (eds): *The Management of Trauma*, ed 3. Philadelphia, W.B. Saunders, 1979, pp 652–658.
319. Janse J, Houser RH, Wells BF: *Chiropractic Principles and Technic*. Chicago, National College of Chiropractic, 1947, pp 583–587.
320. Stierwalt DD: *Extremity Adjusting*. Davenport, Ia, published by the author, 1975, pp 31–33.
321. Williams JGP, Sperryn PN (eds): *Sports Medicine*, ed 2. Baltimore, Williams & Wilkins, 1976, pp 485–486.
322. Shoji H: The foot and ankle. In D'Ambrosia RD: *Musculoskeletal Disorders: Regional Examination and Differential Diagnosis*. Philadelphia, J.B. Lippincott, 1977, pp 519–521.
323. Teranel JA: *Chiropractic Orthopedics and Roentgenology*. Newark, NJ, Medusa Press, 1953, pp 396–399.
324. Salter RB: Injuries of the ankle in children. *North American Clinical Orthopaedics* 5:147, 1974.
325. Schneider RC, Kennedy JC, Plant ML (eds): *Sports Injuries: Mechanisms, Prevention, and Treatment*. Baltimore, Williams & Wilkins, 1985, pp 793–794.
326. Dalinka MK: Ankle fractures. In Feldman F (ed): *Radiology, Pathology, and Immunology of Bones and Joints: A Review of Current Concepts*. New York, Appleton-Century-Crofts, 1978, pp 333–334.
327. Dalinka MK: Ankle fractures. In Feldman F (ed): *Radiology, Pathology, and Immunology of Bones and Joints: A Review of Current Concepts*. New York, Appleton-Century-Crofts, 1978, pp 329–334.
328. Bowerman JW: *Radiology and Injury in Sport*. New York, Appleton-Century-Crofts, 1977, pp 133–140.
329. Holmes GW, Robbins LL: *Roentgen Interpretation*, ed 7. Philadelphia, Lea & Febiger, 1947, pp 49–51.
330. Greenawalt MH: *Spinal Pelvic Stabilization*, ed 2. Dubuque, Ia, Foot Levelers, 1978, pp 38–44.
331. Shoji H: The foot and ankle. In D'Ambrosia RD: *Musculoskeletal Disorders: Regional Examination and Differential Diagnosis*. Philadelphia, J.B. Lippincott, 1977, p 502.
332. Greenawalt MH: *Spinal Pelvic Stabilization*, ed 2. Dubuque, Ia, Foot Levelers, 1978, p 31.
333. Turek SL: *Orthopaedics: Principles and Their Application*, ed 3. Philadelphia, J.B. Lippincott, 1977, pp 1272–1275.
334. Hadler NM: *Medical Management of the Regional Musculoskeletal Diseases*. New York, Grune & Stratton, 1984, pp 285–286.
335. Dolan JP, Holladay LJ: *First-Aid Management*, ed 4. Danville, Ill, Interstate Printers & Publishers, 1974, pp 130–131.
336. Asher C: *Postural Variations in Childhood*. London, Butterworths, 1975, pp 102–103.
337. Shoji H: The foot and ankle. In D'Ambrosia RD: *Musculoskeletal Disorders: Regional Examination and Differential Diagnosis*. Philadelphia, J.B. Lippincott, 1977, pp 488–490, 492–494.
338. Morehouse LE, Cooper JM: *Kinesiology*. St. Louis, C.V. Mosby, 1950, pp 94–98.
339. Cailliet R: *Soft Tissue Pain and Disability*. Philadelphia, F.A. Davis, 1980, pp 261–264.
340. Grice AS, Fligg DB: *Class Notes: Introductory Concepts to Clinical Analysis of Joint Movement and Muscle Testing*. Department of Biomechanics/Kinesiology, BK101. Toronto, Canadian Memorial Chiropractic College (undated), pp 15–22, 31–36.
341. Daniels L, Worthingham C: *Muscle Testing: Techniques of Manual Examination*, ed 4. Philadelphia, W.B. Saunders, 1980, pp 76–81.
342. Dempster WT: The range of motion of cadaver joints: The lower limb. *University of Michigan Medical Bulletin* 22:364–379, 1956.
343. Rosse C, Clawson DK (eds): *The Musculoskeletal System in Health and Disease*. Hagerstown, Md, Harper & Row, 1980, pp 293–294, 298, 300, 303–305.
344. Kapandji IA: *Physiology of the Joints: Lower Limb*, ed 2. New York, Churchill Livingstone, 1981, vol 2, pp 154–182.
345. Hollingshead WH, Jenkins DB: *Functional Anatomy of the Limbs and Back*. Philadelphia, W.B. Saunders, 1981, pp 307–311, 333–334.
346. Sheffield FJ, et al: Electromyographic study of the muscles of the foot in normal walking. *American Journal of Physical Medicine* 35:223–236, 1956.
347. Haxton HA: Absolute muscle force in the ankle flexors of man. *Journal of Physiology* 103:267–273, 1944.
348. Barham JN, Wooten EP: *Structural Kinesiology*. New York, Macmillan, 1973, pp 173, 177–178.

349. Lowman CL: Feet and body mechanics. *Journal of Health and Physical Education* 11:137, 1940.
350. Cailliet R: *Foot and Ankle Pain*. Philadelphia, F.A. Davis, 1979, pp 30–34.
351. Hoppenfeld S: *Physical Examination of the Spine and Extremities*. New York, Appleton-Century-Crofts, 1976, pp 225–227.
352. Daniels L, Worthingham C: *Muscle Testing: Techniques of Manual Examination*, ed 4. Philadelphia, W.B. Saunders, 1980, pp 82–87.
353. Barham JN, Wooten EP: *Structural Kinesiology*. New York, Macmillan, 1973, pp 173–179.
354. Cailliet R: *Soft Tissue Pain and Disability*. Philadelphia, F.A. Davis, 1980, pp 264–266.
355. Hoppenfeld S: *Physical Examination of the Spine and Extremities*. New York, Appleton-Century-Crofts, 1976, pp 227–230.
356. Karpovich PV, Wilklow LB: Goniometric study of the human foot in standing and walking. *Industrial Medicine and Surgery* 29:338–347, 1960.
357. Schafer RC (ed): *Basic Chiropractic Procedural Manual*, ed 4. Arlington, Va, American Chiropractic Association, 1984, pp 296–301.
358. O'Connell AL: Electromyographic study of certain leg muscles during movements of the free foot and during standing. *American Journal of Physical Medicine* 37:289–301, December 1958.
359. Smith JW: Muscular control of the arches of the foot in standing: An electromyographic assessment. *Journal of Anatomy* 88:152–162, 1954.
360. Hadler NM: *Medical Management of the Regional Musculoskeletal Diseases*. New York, Grune & Stratton, 1984, p 282.
361. Jones RJ: The human foot: An experimental study of its mechanics and the role of its muscles and ligaments in the support of the arch. *American Journal of Anatomy* 68:1–41, 1941.
362. Hollingshead WH, Jenkins DB: *Functional Anatomy of the Limbs and Back*. Philadelphia, W.B. Saunders, 1981, pp 334–335.
363. Daniels L, Worthingham C: *Therapeutic Exercise for Body Alignment and Function*, ed 2. Philadelphia, W.B. Saunders, 1977, pp 78, 100.
364. Cailliet R: *Foot and Ankle Pain*. Philadelphia, F.A. Davis, 1979, pp 45–56.
365. Teranel JA: *Chiropractic Orthopedics and Roentgenology*. Newark, NJ, Medusa Press, 1953, pp 285–286.
366. Greenawalt MH: *Spinal Pelvic Stabilization*, ed 2. Dubuque, Ia, Foot Levelers, 1978, pp 7–13.
367. Hollingshead WH, Jenkins DB: *Functional Anatomy of the Limbs and Back*. Philadelphia, W.B. Saunders, 1981, pp 227, 316–319, 321–333.
368. Kapandji IA: *Physiology of the Joints: Lower Limb*, ed 2. New York, Churchill Livingstone, 1981, vol 2, pp 196–204.
369. Asher C: *Postural Variations in Childhood*. London, Butterworths, 1975, pp 76–77.
370. Rosse C, Clawson DK (eds): *The Musculoskeletal System in Health and Disease*. Hagerstown, Md, Harper & Row, 1980, pp 306–307.
371. Daniels L, Worthingham C: *Therapeutic Exercise for Body Alignment and Function*, ed 2. Philadelphia, W.B. Saunders, 1977, pp 78–79.
372. Morehouse LE, Cooper JM: *Kinesiology*. St. Louis, C.V. Mosby, 1950, p 98.
373. Kapandji IA: *Physiology of the Joints: Lower Limb*, ed 2. New York, Churchill Livingstone, 1981, vol 2, pp 206–208.
374. Daniels L, Worthingham C: *Therapeutic Exercise for Body Alignment and Function*, ed 2. Philadelphia, W.B. Saunders, 1977, p 79.
375. Morehouse LE, Cooper JM: *Kinesiology*. St. Louis, C.V. Mosby, 1950, pp 98–100.
376. Cailliet R: *Soft Tissue Pain and Disability*. Philadelphia, F.A. Davis, 1980, pp 266–303.
377. Teranel JA: *Chiropractic Orthopedics and Roentgenology*. Newark, NJ, Medusa Press, 1953, pp 286–297.
378. Scott WN, Nisonson B, Nicholas JA (eds): *Principles of Sports Medicine*. Baltimore, Williams & Wilkins, 1984, pp 358–361.
379. Grice AS, Fligg DB: *Class Notes: Introductory Concepts to Clinical Analysis of Joint Movement and Muscle Testing*. Department of Biomechanics/Kinesiology, BK101. Toronto, Canadian Memorial Chiropractic College (undated), pp 42–44, 45–56.
380. Barham JN, Wooten EP: *Structural Kinesiology*. New York, Macmillan, 1973, pp 177, 182–181.
381. Kelly ED: A comparative study of structure and function of normal, pronated and painful feet among children. *Research Quarterly* American Association of Health and Physical Education, 18:291–312, 1947.
382. Daniels L, Worthingham C: *Therapeutic Exercise for Body Alignment and Function*, ed 2. Philadelphia, W.B. Saunders, 1977, pp 79–80, 90–99.
383. Gottlieb A: Flatfoot and its relation to the triceps surae muscle. *American Journal of Physical Therapy* 8:321–334, 1932.
384. Asher C: *Postural Variations in Childhood*. London, Butterworths, 1975, pp 80–82, 100.
385. Basmajian JV, Stecko G: The role of muscles in arch support of the foot. *Journal of Bone and Joint Surgery* 54A:1184–1190, 1963.
386. Cailliet R: *Foot and Ankle Pain*. Philadelphia, F.A. Davis, 1979, pp 42–44.
387. Rosse C, Clawson DK (eds): *The Musculoskeletal System in Health and Disease*. Hagerstown, Md, Harper & Row, 1980, p 308.
388. Kapandji IA: *Physiology of the Joints: Lower Limb*, ed 2. New York, Churchill Livingstone, 1981, vol 2, p 216.
389. Gillet H, Liekens M: *Belgian Chiropractic Research Notes*. Huntington Beach, Cal, Motion Palpation Institute, 1981, pp 85–88.
390. Asher C: *Postural Variations in Childhood*. London, Butterworths, 1975, pp 60, 70.
391. Shoji H: The foot and ankle. In D'Ambrosia RD: *Musculoskeletal Disorders: Regional Examination and Differential Diagnosis*. Philadelphia, J.B. Lippincott, 1977, p 521.
392. Barham JN, Wooten EP: *Structural Kinesiology*. New York, Macmillan, 1973, p 185.

393. Hollingshead WH, Jenkins DB: *Functional Anatomy of the Limbs and Back.* Philadelphia, W.B. Saunders, 1981, pp 335–337.
394. Williams JGP, Sperryn PN (eds): *Sports Medicine,* ed 2. Baltimore, Williams & Wilkins, 1976, pp 492–494.
395. Cailliet R: *Foot and Ankle Pain.* Philadelphia, F.A. Davis, 1979, pp 81–90.
396. Hadler NM: *Medical Management of the Regional Musculoskeletal Diseases.* New York, Grune & Stratton, 1984, pp 287–289.
397. Hirata I Jr: *The Doctor and the Athlete,* ed 2. Philadelphia, J.B. Lippincott, 1974, p 257.
398. Williams JGP, Sperryn PN (eds): *Sports Medicine,* ed 2. Baltimore, Williams & Wilkins, 1976, p 495.
399. Cailliet R: *Foot and Ankle Pain.* Philadelphia, F.A. Davis, 1979, pp 91–93.
400. Hirata I Jr: *The Doctor and the Athlete,* ed 2. Philadelphia, J.B. Lippincott, 1974, pp 259–260.
401. Greenawalt MH: Feet and the dynamic science of chiropractic. *ACA Journal of Chiropractic* May 1983.
402. Cailliet R: *Foot and Ankle Pain.* Philadelphia, F.A. Davis, 1979, pp 109–110, 112.
403. Hirata I Jr: *The Doctor and the Athlete,* ed 2. Philadelphia, J.B. Lippincott, 1974, pp 241–242.
404. Zange LL: Sesamoiditis: A sesamometatarsal lesion. *ACA Journal of Chiropractic* February 1982.
405. Baltzell LG, Mackey RH (eds): *Firth's Technic Notes.* Publishing data not shown, 1967, pp 63–71. Available from National College of Chiropractic.
406. Janse J, Houser RH, Wells BF: *Chiropractic Principles and Technic.* Chicago, National College of Chiropractic, 1947, pp 589–609.
407. Gertler L: *Illustrated Manual of Extravertebral Technic,* ed 2. Bayside, NY, published by the author, 1978, pp 8–20.
408. Stierwalt DD: *Extremity Adjusting.* Davenport, Ia, published by the author, 1975, pp 34–38.
409. Schultz AL: *Athletic and Industrial Injuries of the Knee.* Mitchell, SD, published by the author, 1951, pp 54–60.
410. Greenawalt MH: *Spinal Pelvic Stabilization,* ed 2. Dubuque, Ia, Foot Levelers, 1978, pp 63–72.
411. Williams JGP, Sperryn PN (eds): *Sports Medicine,* ed 2. Baltimore, Williams & Wilkins, 1976, pp 258, 494–495.
412. Hirata I Jr: *The Doctor and the Athlete,* ed 2. Philadelphia, J.B. Lippincott, 1974, pp 257–258.
413. Bowerman JW: *Radiology and Injury in Sport.* New York, Appleton-Century-Crofts, 1977, pp 139–140.
414. Wheeler LP: Common musculoskeletal dance injuries. In Coyle BA, Martinez DP: *Proceedings of the Second Conference on Current Topics in Chiropractic: Reviews of the Literature,* May 4–5, 1985. Sunnyvale, Cal, Palmer College of Chiropractic—West, 1985, section C3.
415. Barham JN, Wooten EP: *Structural Kinesiology.* New York, Macmillan, 1973, pp 183–184.
416. Shoji H: The foot and ankle. In D'Ambrosia RD: *Musculoskeletal Disorders: Regional Examination and Differential Diagnosis.* Philadelphia, J.B. Lippincott, 1977, pp 511–513.
417. Cailliet R: *Foot and Ankle Pain.* Philadelphia, F.A. Davis, 1979, p 129.
418. Hadler NM: *Medical Management of the Regional Musculoskeletal Diseases.* New York, Grune & Stratton, 1984, p 291.
419. Greenawalt MH: *Spinal Pelvic Stabilization,* ed 2. Dubuque, Ia, Foot Levelers, 1978, pp 34–35.
420. Cailliet R: *Foot and Ankle Pain.* Philadelphia, F.A. Davis, 1979, p 109.
421. Hadler NM: *Medical Management of the Regional Musculoskeletal Diseases.* New York, Grune & Stratton, 1984, pp 289–290.
422. Asher C: *Postural Variations in Childhood.* London, Butterworths, 1975, pp 105–107, 113.
423. Rosse C, Clawson DK (eds): *The Musculoskeletal System in Health and Disease.* Hagerstown, Md, Harper & Row, 1980, p 309.
424. Williams JGP, Sperryn PN (eds): *Sports Medicine,* ed 2. Baltimore, Williams & Wilkins, 1976, pp 496–497.
425. Cailliet R: *Foot and Ankle Pain.* Philadelphia, F.A. Davis, 1979, pp 99–106.

SUGGESTED READINGS

Black J, Dumbleton JH (eds): *Clinical Biomechanics: Case History Approach.* New York, Churchill Livingstone, 1981.

Close JR: *Motor Function in the Lower Extremity.* Springfield, Ill, Charles C Thomas, 1964.

Frankel VH, Burstein AH: *Orthopedic Biomechanics.* Philadelphia, Lea & Febiger, 1970.

Goss CM (ed): *Gray's Anatomy of the Human Body,* ed 29. Philadelphia, Lea & Febiger, 1973.

Granger CV: The clinical discernment of muscle weakness. *Archives of Physical Medicine* 44:430–438, 1963.

Hall MC: *The Locomotor System: Functional Anatomy.* Springfield, Ill, Charles C Thomas, Publishers, 1965.

Helfet AJ: *Disorders of the Knee,* ed 2. Philadelphia, J.B. Lippincott, 1982.

Inman VT: *The Joints of the Ankle.* Baltimore, Williams & Wilkins, 1976.

Jones FW: *Structure and Function as Seen in the Foot.* London, Bailliere, Tindall and Dox, 1944.

Karpovich PV, Sinning WE: *Physiology of Muscular Activity.* Philadelphia, W.B. Saunders, 1971.

Kelley DL: *Kinesiology: Fundamentals of Motion Descriptions.* Englewood Cliffs, NJ, Prentice-Hall, 1971.

Lewin P: *The Foot and Ankle,* ed 4. Philadelphia, Lea & Febiger, 1959.

Moore KL: *Clinically Oriented Anatomy.* Baltimore, Williams & Wilkins, 1980.

Morton DJ: *The Human Foot.* New York, Columbia University Press, 1935.

O'Donoghue DH: *Treatment of Injuries to Athletes,* ed 3. Philadelphia, W.B. Saunders, 1976.

Owen JD: Lower extremity problems relating to back problems. *ACA Journal of Chiropractic* February 1971.

Radin EL et al: *Practical Biomechanics for the Orthopaedic Surgeon.* New York, John Wiley & Sons, 1969.

Sante LR: *Principles of Roentgenological Interpretation.* Ann Arbor, Mich, Edwards Brothers, 1961.

Sills FD: Anthropometry in relation to physical performance. In Johnson WR (ed): *Science and Medicine or Exercise and Sports*. New York, Harper & Brothers, 1960.

Smillie IS: *Injuries of the Knee Joint*, ed 5. New York, Churchill Livingstone, 1978.

Strange FS: *The Hip*. Baltimore, Williams & Wilkins, 1965.

Straus RH: *Sports Medicine and Physiology*, Philadelphia, W.B. Saunders, 1979.

Travell J: Myofascial trigger points: Clinical view. In Bonica JJ, Albe-Fessard D (eds): *Advances in Pain Research and Therapy*. New York, Raven Press, 1976.

Wells KF: *Kinesiology: The Scientific Basis of Human Motion*, ed 5. Philadelphia, W.B. Saunders, 1971.

Index

A

Abbott-Saunders' test, 650–651
Abdomen
  posture, 94
  prevertebral function, 446–447
Acceleration
  angular, 65
  gait, 119
  law of, 44
  linear, 64–65
  measurement, 44
Action line(s), 47, 99–100, 483
Adams position, 460–463
Adductor reflex, 500
Adhesions, intrafascicular, 134
Adjustments, therapeutic, 281–283, 596
  cervical, upper, 283
  costotransverse, 423–425
  costovertebral, 423–425
  low-back pain, 491
  lumbar, 521–522, 526
  rib, 422, 424–425
  shoulder, 653–657
  temporomandibular joint, 399–400
Adolescence, 96
Adson's test, 373
Agility, 109
Alexander's technique, 101–102
Allis' knee sign, 708
Analyses
  free-body, 49–50
  kinematic, 66–67
  motion, 66–67
  plumb line, 98
Angle
  Cobb's, 591
  Q, 713–714
Anisotropism, 45
Ankle(s)
  Achilles tendon lesions, 738–740
  dislocations, 744–747
  dorsiflexion, 732–733
  eversion, 732–733
  flexion-extension during gait, 114
  fractures, 744–747
  gait disorders, 125
  innervation, 733
  instability, 743–744
  inversion, 732–733
  kinesiology, 732–733
  motion, 732–733
  pain during gait, 122
  plantar flexion, 732–733
  pronation, 620–622, 747
  pulse, 747
  rotation during gait, 115
  sprains, 742–744
  spurs, 747–748
  strains, 742
  subluxations, 744
  tourniquet test, 747
Ankylosis
  shoulder, 640
  thoracic, 435–436
Anterior drawer sign, 716
Anthropometry, 5, 30–36
Anulus, 212
Anvil test, 708
Ape hand, 377
Apley's test
  compression, 722
  distraction, 722–723
  scratch, 644
Arachnoiditis, adhesive, 557
Arch, foot, 750–751
Arm(s)
  circling exercise, 370
  drop test, 652
  swing, 114–115, 128
Artery, vertebral, 352, 373–374, 382
Arthritis
  psoriatic, 558
  rheumatoid, 389–390
  traumatic, 267, 647
Astrom's suspension test, 513
Asymmetry, 12–13
Atlas, 312–313, 322–323, 334–335
  aplasia, 392
  dislocation, 324–326
  fracture, 324–326
  palpation, 354–356
  visual subluxation patterns, 361–362
Atrophy, 163, 517
Autonomics, 225, 382
Avulsions, pelvic, 550–551
Axis (axes), 313–314
  body, 48–49
  fracture, 326–328
  neutral, 57
  odontoid anomalies, 392
  palpation, 354–355
  rotation, 63
  visual subluxation patterns, 361–362
Axon, 148, 149
Axonotmesis, 307

B

Balance, 104
  body, 110
  cervical righting mechanisms, 366
  effects of defects, 129–136
  heel alignment checks, 539
  lumbosacral, 457
  postural, 151
  recovery, 158
  spinal, 570–571
  sway, 101
Basal ganglia, 153
Base(s)
  segmental, 100
  support, 100–101
Basic technique, 583
Basilar
  anomaly, 210
  coarctation, 391–392
  impression, 392
Bearing, body, 86
Bechterew's test, 512

Beery's sign, 544, 706
Belt test, 544
Bending, biomechanical, 56–57
Bent-knee pull test, 519
Biceps
  stability test, 645
  syndrome, 649–650
  tendon dislocation, 650–651
Biodynamics, 5, 128
Biomechanics, concepts of, 4–6
Biometrics, 5
Bionergy, 4
Bionomy, 4
Biophysics, 4
Biostatistics, 5
Bipedism, 107, 130, 450, 522, 570
Body
  axes, 48–49
  balance, 98–99, 110
  bearings, 86
  bulk effects on posture, 109
  equilibrium, 98–99
  fat content, 32
  gravitational effects, 93–102
  gross movements, 24–25
  growth estimation, 34
  height, 31, 33, 103
  human potential, 54
  inspection, 93–95
  language, 360
  links, 67–68
  mass, 32–33
  maturity, 31–32
  mensuration, 33–34
  oscillation, 112–113
  oxygen intake variants, 32
  position changes, 98
  proportion, 33
  segmental centers of mass, 69
  size, 30–32
  speed, 161–162
  stability, 54, 98
  strength, 159–161
  types, 34–36, 130–132
  weight, 31–34, 56, 103
    bearing, 98
    development, 450
Bone(s)
  bruises, 266
  calcification disorders, 9–10
  cancellous, 7
  classifications, 6
  compact, 7–8
  cranial, involuntary motion, 398
  deformation in scoliosis, 588
  development, 8–9
  epiphyses, 9
  growth, 8–9
  infection, 268
  influences of stress, 8
  injuries, 266
  physical characteristics, 6–7
  prominences, 28
  structure, 7–8
  trauma, 10
Bonnet's sign, 520
Booth-Marvel's test, 645
Bounce home test, 712
Bracelet test, 679
Braces, 380, 595–598
Bragard's test, 518–519
Bryant's sign, 656
Buckling sign, 519
Buerger's test, 735
Buoyancy, 128–129
Bursae, 12
Bursitis
  heel, 754
  knee, 718
  olecranon, 668
  pelvic, 549
  subacromial, 646
  subdeltoid, 645–646
Buttock sign, 557–558

C

Calcification
  brachialis, 674
  supraspinatus, 646
  triceps brachii, 646–647
Calloway's sign, 656
Cane, use of, 702
Capsule, articular, 14–16
Capsulitis, 262, 647
Cartilage, 12
  aging effects, 87
  articular, 16, 84–88
  drug effects on, 88
  inflammation, 87
  nutrition, 87–88
  tension, 87
  trauma, 87
Carver, basic concepts of, 582–583
Casts, orthopedic, 595–596
Central nervous system, motor controls, 152–154
Cerebellum, 153–154
Cerebral cortex, 184–185
Cerebrospinal fluid, 243, 352
Chairs, 105–106
Chest
  expansion test, 435
  flail, 427
  referred symptoms, 276
Childress' duck waddle test, 723
Chondrification, spinal, 198
Circulation
  ankle pulse, 747
  cervical neurovascular deficit, 370–374
  leg, 735
  neural vs circulatory symptoms, 371
  postural, 134
  pulmonary, 438
  vertebrobasilar patency, 373–374
Clarke's sign, 730
Claudication test, 735
Clavicle, 633
  dislocations, 661
  fractures, 661
  injuries, 659–662
  subluxations, 660–661
Claw hand, 377
Clicks, joint, 19

Cobb's angle, 591
Coccyx (*see also* Pelvis)
  sprain, 550
  subluxation, 550
Codman's sign, 644–645
Collars, cervical, 379, 380
Colle's fracture, 677
Compression, 51
Concussion, spinal cord, 489
Connective tissue, 11–13
Contraction, muscle, 23–24, 73–74
Contractures
  forearm, 674
  hamstring, 704
  iliotibial band, 706
Contusions
  gluteal, 548
  peroneal nerve, 728
  pulmonary, 421
  rib, 422
  spinal cord, 489
Coordination, 108–109
Costoclavicular syndrome, 660
Coupling, 55–56
  cervical, lower, 332–333
  costotransverse, 415
  costovertebral, 415
  lumbosacral, 462
  scoliotic, 586
  shoulder, 652
  spinal, 201
  wrist and fingers, 671–672
Cozen's test, 667
Craniospinal mechanisms, 398
Craniospinal system, 228
Cranium, involuntary motion, 228, 398
Creep, biomechanical, 83, 596
  intervertebral disc, 217–218
Crohn's disease, 558
Curves, abnormal, types, 574–575
Cyst, Baker's, 719

D

Damping, 71–72
Dancing, trauma, 755–756
Dawbarn's test, 646
Deceleration, gait, 119
Deformation, biomechanical, 80, 85
Deformities
  knee, 717, 729
  rib, 592–593
  round back, 499–500
  spinal, classification, 580
  toe, 757
Dejerine's sign, 512–513
DeKleyn's test, 374
Demianoff's test, 519
Demifacets, thoracic, 412–413
Desks, 106
Development
  potential, 162–163
  progress, 95
  structural adaptations, 610
Deyelle-May test, 519
Disc(s)
  articular, 16–17
  intervertebral, 212–218
  knee menisci, 711, 722–725
  pressure, 104–105
  sternoclavicular, 660
Dislocations
  ankle, 744–747
  bicipital tendon, 650–651
  carpal, 677
  clavicle, 661
  elbow, 669
  finger, 686
  hip, 709–710
  knee, 729
  patella, 719
  shoulder, 655–657
  spine, lumbar, 488
  wrist, 675–677
Distortion
  pelvic, 611
  postural, 573–574
Double-leg-raise test, 500
Draw sign, 743–744
Dreyer's sign, 719–720
Ductility, 82
Dugas' test, 655–656
Dura mater, 222
Dynamometry, 683

E

Ectomorphism, 36, 131
Eden's test, 373
Effort, 72
  postural, 133
Elasticity, 81
Elbow(s)
  anatomy, 662
  dislocations, 669
  extension, 662, 663, 666
  flexion, 662, 663
  fractures, 669
  goniometry, 663
  growth centers, 665
  kinesiology, 663
  ligamentous stability test, 666–667
  medial epicondyle test, 668
  nerve compression, 669–670
  olecranon bursitis, 668
  pronation, 663
  radioulnar movements, 662–663
  roentgenography, 664–665, 667, 669
  sprains, 665–667
  strains, 665
  subluxations, 668–669
  supination, 663
  tennis, 667–668
Electromyography, 182–183, 581
Ely's test, 537
End-play, sacroiliac, 554
Endplates, 212, 514
Endomorphism, 36, 131–132
Endurance, 161
  biomechanical, 83–84
  postural, 133
Energy, 23, 43
Entrapment, nerve
  lumbar, 515

Entrapment, nerve—*continued*
  median, 677–679
  radial, 669–670
  ulnar, 670, 679
Epiphyses, 9, 199
Equilibrium
  cervical righting mechanisms, 366
  lumbosacral, 457
  postural, 159
  spinal, 576
  static, 49–50
  sway effects, 589
  swimming, 129
Erichsen's pelvic rock test, 542
Evaluation
  methodology, 36–37
  motor system, 180–185
Exercises
  cervical, posttraumatic, 367–369
  home, 287
  lumbar, 526–527
  temporomandibular joint, 401
  thoracic realignment, 438
Exostoses, foot, 756
Extensor digitorum communis test, 686
Eye dominance, 93

F

F-AB-ER-E, mnemonic for *f*lexed, *ab*ducted, *e*xternally *r*otated, and *e*xtended (*see also* Patrick's F-AB-ER-E test), 703
Facet(s)
  cervical, lower 331–332
  iliac, 465–466
  lumbar, 447–449, 524–525
  lumbosacral, 452–453, 498–499
  sacroiliac, 466–467, 553–556
  spinal, 207–208
  syndrome, 501–502
Fajersztajn's test, 519
Fascia, 12, 28
Fat pad(s), 18, 718
Fatigue
  biomechanical, 83–84
  intervertebral disc, 218
  muscle, 164–166
  postural, 133, 483–484
  sitting, 105
  strength, 160–161
  theory, 493
Feedback, electromyographic, 182–183
Feet (*see* Foot)
Femur
  dislocations, 709–710
  fixations, 710
  fractures, 709, 728–729
  subluxations, 707–708
Fibrocartilage, damage of, 17
Fibrositis, 261–262, 658–659
Fibula, subluxations, 727
Finger(s)
  abduction, 683
  adduction, 683
  anatomy, 681–682
  contractures, 686
  dislocations, 686
  extension, 682–683
  fixations, 684–685
  flexion, 682, 683
  fractures, 686
  goniometry, 684
  innervation, 683
  kinesiology, 682–683
  mallet, 685
  motions, 682–684
  trigger points, 684, 685–686
Finsterer's test, 677
Fixation(s)
  cervical, 353–360
  costovertebral, 434
  finger, 684–685
  foot, 756
  hip, 710
  intercostal, 433–434
  knee, 729
  ligament, 552–553
  lumbar, 495–496
  muscle, 552
  pelvic, 551–556
  pubic, 556
  sacral, 555–556
  sacroiliac, 557
  scapula, 659
  scoliosis, 587
  spinal, 277–280
  sternal, 433
Flail chest, 427
Flat hand, 377
Flatfoot, gait, 121
Flexibility, 81
Follow-through, 110–111
Foot
  anterior compartment syndrome, 756–757
  dancing trauma, 755–756
  exostoses, 756
  fascitis, 752
  fixations, 756
  flattened arch, 750–751
  flexion-extension during gait, 114
  fractures, 755
  gait clues, 751–752
  goniometry, 749
  kinesiology, 732–733, 748
  loading, 749–750
  metatarsalgia, 752–753
  motions, 748–749
  orthotics, 754–755
  plantar neuroma, 756
  posture, 95, 750
  pronation, 620–622
  rotation during gait, 115
  sesamoiditis, 755
  sprains, 753–754
  subluxations, 755
  supports, 753
  toe-in, 751
  trigger points, 752
  weight distribution, 750
Footflat, gait, 118
Footwork, 107
Force(s), 45
  cervical shear, 307
  characteristics, 47
  composition of, muscle, 76

concurrent, 51
coupling, 55–56
cervical, lower, 332–333
costotransverse, 415
costovertebral, 415
lumbosacral, 462
scoliotic, 586
shoulder, 652
spinal, 201
wrist and fingers, 671–672
direction of, 84–85
gravitational, 96–100
intervertebral disc, 213–218
linear, 50–51
muscle, 54, 73–74, 182
parallel, 52–58
pelvic, 471
reactive, 78
shear, 84
tensile, 84–85
types of, 45
Forearm
muscles, 664
roentgenography, 676–677
strains, 673–674
tenosynovitis, 675
Forestier's
bowstring sign, 435
test, 435
Fouchet's test, 730
Fracture(s)
ankle, 744–747
carpal, 677
clavicle, 661
Colle's, 676, 677
elbow, 669
fatigue, 84, 741–742, 755
femur, 709, 728–729
finger, 686
foot, 755
golfer's, 427
hip, 708
knee, 728–729
leg, 729, 740–742
meniscus, 724
patellar, 719
pelvic, 550–551
repair process, 10–11
rib, 426–427
sacral, 551
scapula, 659
shoulder, 657–658
spine, lumbar, 488
thoracic spine, 428–429
wrist, 675–677
Free bodies, joint, 20
Friction, 70–71
coefficient of, 70–71
intrinsic, 71
massage, 288–291
principles of, 71
Froment's test, 679

G

Gaenslen's test, 541
Gait(s), 102–109, 111–116
analysis, 465
antalgic, 121–122
anterior-posterior observation, 120–121
apraxia, 127
basal ganglia dysfunction, 123
base width, 121
cerebellar dysfunction, 123
cycle of, 111–112
effects of manipulation, 116
energy absorption, 118
examination of, 116–127
foot clues, 751–752
functionally inhibited, 127
iliotibial band syndrome, 707
lateral observation, 120
limp, 121
mensuration, 127
mowing, 123
muscle
analysis, 183–184
weakness, 124
neurologic, 122–123
paralytic, 123–124
proprioceptive impairment, 123
restricted motion, 126–127
sacroiliac motion, 475
senile, 126–127
steppage, 124–125
stress points, 113
waddling, 125
Ganglion, 675
subluxation irritation/compression, 241
Gauvain's sign, 708
Genes, 78, 163
Genu (*see* Knee)
George's test, 374
Giegel's (inguinal) reflex, 500
Gilcrest's sign, 645
Gills' test, 543
Goading, therapeutic, 436–437
Goldthwait's test, 543
Golfer's fracture, 427
Golgi tendon organs, 155–156
Goniometry
cervical, 302–303
elbow, 663
fingers, 684
foot, 749
hip, 700–701
joint, 20
knee, 713–714
shoulder, 639–640
thoracolumbar, 431
wrist, 672
Gout, sacroiliac, 558
Gower's maneuver, 501
Gravity, 3, 46, 77–78
center of, 97, 100, 104, 108
effect on diaphragm, 417
forces, 96–100
line, 97–98, 367
Groin, strains, 704–705
Growth, structural adaptations, 610

H

Hamilton's rules sign, 656
Hamstring reflex, 501

Hand
  grip strength, 683
  neuropathologic signs, 377
  trigger points, 681
Hangman's fracture, 327
Hautant's test, 374
Head
  motion, 107
  posture, 94
  weight, 100–101
Headaches, 275–276
  cervical originating, 352–353
  differentiation, 354
Healing, musculoskeletal, 257–258
Health, optimal, 37
Heat, muscle, 148
Heel
  bursitis, 754
  checks, 539
  lifts, 616–620
  spurs, 756
  walk test, 501
Heelstrike, gait, 117–118, 121
Height
  body, 31, 33, 103
  sitting, 105–106
  table, 105–106
Helfet's test, 727–728
Hemispheric dominance, 184–185
Hemivertebra, 210
Hennequin's sign, 708
Hernia, muscle, 173
Hibb's test, 542
High heels, posture and, 103
Hip(s)
  abduction, 697, 698, 699–700, 701
    stress test, 558
  adduction, 697, 698, 700, 701
    weakness, 702
  avulsions, 709
  conditioning, 702
  dislocations, 709–710
  epiphyseal slips, 709
  extension, 697, 698, 699, 701
  fixations, 710
  flexion, 697, 698–699, 700–701
  flexion-extension during gait, 114
  fractures, 708
  gait disorders, 125
  goniometry, 700–701
  impactions, 708–709
  joint, 696
  kinematic tests, 707
  kinesiology, 698–700
  loading, 701–702
  motion, 697–701
  pain during gait, 122
  roentgenography, 708–709
  rotation, 697–698, 701
  spasm, 537, 702–703
  sprain, 707
  trauma, 702–711
Hoffa's sign, 754
Homan's sign, 735
"Hot shot," 375
Hueter's sign, 645
Hughston's jerk sign, 715
Hyperextension tests, 501
Hyperkyphosis, 576–577
Hyperlordosis, lumbar, 500, 576–577
Hypertonicity, 277, 388–389, 493, 640–642
  lower cervical, 358–359
  thoracic, 426, 590
  upper cervical, 357–358
Hypolordosis, cervical, 333–335
Hysteresis, 83
  intervertebral disc, 218
Hysteria, 127

I

Iliac compression test, 542
Iliotibial band syndrome, 707
Immobilization, 9
Impact, 110
Impingement syndrome test, 651
Inertia, 57, 78
  area moment, 58
  law of, 44
  moment, 70
  polar moment, 58
Inspection, 93–95
  TMJ dysfunction, 396–397
Instability
  ankle, 743–744
  atlantoaxial, congenital, 392
  knee, 715–717
  lumbosacral, 497–499
  spinal, 259–261, 456–457
    cervical, 316, 330–331
    lumbar (*see* Spine, lumbar)
    thoracic, 421–422
Interaction, 44
Intervertebral disc(s), 212–218
  cervical, 380–386
  internal shifting, 513–515
  lumbar, 510–515
    syndromes, 511, 522–525
  nuclear shifting, 586–587
  nutrition of, 227–228
  occupational considerations, 273
  protruded, 271–273
  thoracic, 413–414
    disease, 439–440
    protrusion, 438–439
Intervertebral foramina, 208–210
  cervical, lower, 328
  encroachment, 273–274
  lumbar, 449–450
  spinal subluxation effects, 240–243
Ischemia, shoulder, 653
Ischial lifts, 616
Isotropism, 45

J

Jaw, temporomandibular joint disorders, 394–401
Jefferson fracture, 325–326
Joint(s)
  acromioclavicular, 633, 659–660
  apophyseal, 218–219
  architecture, 14
  articular
    capsule, 14–16

cartilage, 16
surfaces, 16
biaxial, 14
capsule tears, 15–16
circulation, 18
classification, 13–14
clicks, 19
costal, 414–415
costochondral, 415
degrees of freedom, 62–64
dysfunction, 20–21
fat pads, 18
fiber arrangement, 85
force, reactive, 78
free bodies, 20
goniometry, 20
hip, 696–698
history, 21
innervation, 15
interchondral, 415
intracapsular pinches, 16
knee, 711
locking, 727–728
intracapsular pinches, 718
lax shoulder, 649
ligaments, 18
loose bodies, 19–20
lubrication, 86–87
lumbar, hypomobile, 528
lumbosacral, 452–453
Luschka, 203, 329
mobility, 79
motion, 14, 15, 20, 62–64, 166
multiaxial, 14
nonaxial, 13
opposing forces on, 77–78
palsy, 18
receptors, 18, 156–157
restrictions, 19–20
sacrococcygeal, 470
sacroiliac, 465–476
shoulder, 633–634
spinal, 211–221
pathology, 266–268
sprains, 21–22
stability, 18–19, 79
sternoclavicular, 633, 660
sternocostal, 415
stiffness, 19
stress, 46
symphysis pubis, 470
synovial
fluid, 18
folds, 18
membrane, 17–18
zones, 17
temporomandibular (TMJ), 394–401
uniaxial, 13–14
Joint play, 280, 353
Jumping, 127–128

K

Kaplan's test, 668
Kemp's test, 512
Kernig's test
leg, 489
neck, 489
Kinematics, 64–68, 308
cervical, lower, 330–335
definition, 5
lumbar spine, 451–456
sacroiliac, 470–476
thoracic, 417–420
Kinesiology
ankle and foot, 732–733
applied, 583
definition, 5
elbow, 663
fingers, 682–683
foot, 748
hip, 698–700
knee, 713
shoulder, 636–639
spine
lumbar, 450–451
thoracic, 415–417
thumb, 679–680
wrist, 671
Kinetics, 5, 68–72
King concept, 583
Kleist's hooking sign, 686
Klippel-Feil syndrome, 393
Klippel-Weil's test, 686–687
Knee(s)
aneurysm, 719
Baker's cyst, 719
biomechanics, 714
bursitis, 718
collateral ligament stability tests, 721–722
deformities, 717, 729
dislocations, 729
distortions, functional, 717–718
effusion, 718, 729–730
extension, 712, 713
external rotation-recurvatum, 715
fixations, 729
flexion, 712, 713
flexion-extension during gait, 114
fractures, 728–729
genu
recurvatum, 717
valgum, 717
varum, 717
goniometry, 713–714
hemangioma, 719
hyperextension stress test, 715
hyperflexion stress test, 715
instability
anterolateral, 715–716
posterolateral, 717
joint, 711
locking, 727–728
kinesiology, 713
menisci, 722–725
menisci-coronary ligament relationship, 725–726
motion, 712–714
neoplasm, 719
osteochondritis dissecans, 731
osteochondromatosis, 730–731
pain during gait, 122

Knee(s)—*continued*
popliteal swelling, 719
roentgenography, 720, 731
rotation, 713
Sinding-Larsen-Johannson disease, 730
stability, 714–717
subluxations, 726–727
synovitis, 722
tests, general, 715
trauma, 720–725
Kyphosis, Scheuermann's, 440

L

Laguere's test, 707
Langoria's sign, 708
Lasègue
differential sign, 520
rebound test, 511
straight-leg-raising test, 511, 518, 519
standing test, 511–512
Law(s)
acceleration, 44
inertia, 44
Newton's, 43–49
reaction, 44–45
Wolff's, 8, 588
Lax capsule text, 649
Leg(s)
circulatory tests, 735
fractures, 729, 740–742
plantaris rupture, 738
posterior tibial compartment syndrome, 738
posture, 95
roentgenography, 741–742
rotation during gait, 114
short, 127, 609–610, 611
strains, 736–739
trigger points, 729
Lever(s), 52–54
arm length, 73
principle, 54
types of, 53–54
Leverage, 108
Lewin
knee sign, 706
punch test, 520
Lhermitte's sign, 382–383
Lifting, mechanics, 485–488
Lifts, shoe, 614, 616–620
Ligament(s), 12, 18
calcaneocuboid, 753–754
collateral, 711, 720–722
coronary, 711, 725
cruciate, 711, 725
dentate, 222–223
fixations, 552–553
iliofemoral, 457
iliolumbar, 552
lower cervical, 329–330
lumbosacral, static balance, 457
pain, 175
sacroiliac, 468, 552
sacrotuberous, 552–553
spinal, 219–221, 414, 433, 588
shortening
cervical, lower, 359
thoracic, 33
spring, 754
Limbic system, 154
Limp, gait, 121
Lindner's sign, 520
Line
action, 99–100, 483
Chamberlain's, 391–392
Ferguson's, 500
Fischgold-Metzger, 392
McGregor's, 391–392
Shenton's, 708–709
Links, body, 67–68
Lippman's test, 645
Loading
cartilage, 84–86
cyclic, 85–86
deformation, 85
external, 45–46
foot, 749–750
gait, 115–116
hip, 701–702
repetitive, 461
sacroiliac, 469
spinal, 46–47
disc, 214
lumbar, 502
vertebral body, 204–205
ultimate, 80
Locking position test, 651
Locomotion
early, 96
patterns, 154
Logan's rule, 611
Loose bodies, joint, 19–20
Lordosis, key, 582–583
Losee's test, 716
Lubrication, joint, 86–87
Lumbarization, 210
Lumbosacral instability, 497–499
Lumbosacropelvic rhythm, 461
Lungs
contusion, 421
pulmonary impairment, 438
Lust's sign, 728

M

Maigne's test, 374
Maisonneuve's sign, 677
Malformations, spine, upper, 391–394
Maneuver(s) (*see also* Test(s))
Gower's, 501
lumbar, painful, 526
Valsalva, 515
Manubrium, 410
fixation, 433
Mass, 43
body, 32–33
segments, 69
Massage, transverse friction, 288–291
McIntosh's test, 715
McKenzie's syndromes, 520–522
McMurray's test, 723
Mechanical advantage, 52–53, 73, 78
Mechanics, 4, 5
finger, 683–684

fluid, 128–129
lifting, 485–488
Newton's laws, 43–49
Medulla oblongata, 352
Meninges, 222
Mennel's test, 542
Meralgia paresthetica, 710–711
Mesomorphism, 35–36, 132
Metatarsalgia, 752–753
Midstance gait, 118, 121
Midswing gait, 119
Milgram's test, 489–490
Mills' test, 667–668
Minor's test, 519
Mobility, joint, 79
Modalities, 285–292, 310, 312, 436
Modulus, shear, 58
Moire topography, 581
Moment(s), 45
bending, 56–57
critical, 109
inertia, 56, 58, 70
polar, 58
Momentum, 68–70, 109
angular, 70
linear, 68
power and, 68–69
transference, 69–70
Morton's test, 753
Moskowicz's tourniquet test, 736
Motion(s)
ankle, 732–733
atlantoaxial, 319
barriers, 282
block, 460
elbow, 662–663
finger, 682–684
foot, 748–749
head, 107
joint, 62–64, 166
restricted, 19–20
kinematic analyses, 66–67
knee, 712–714
out of plane, 63
pelvic, 470–476
plane, 63
range of, 63–64, 73
respiratory movements, 416–417
sacroiliac, 553–556
shoulder, 634–640
spinal
cervical, 302–303, 359–360
cervicothoracic, 333
lumbar, 447
lumbosacral, 471
occipitoatlantal, 318
planes, 199
thoracic, 415–420
structural, 62–64
temporomandibular joint, 397–398
thumb, 679
trunk, 447
unit, vertebral, 203–204
wrist, 670–672
Motor
pathways, 153
system, evaluation, 180–185
Movement(s) (*see also* Motion)
ballistic, 25
gross, 24–25
postural, 24–25
tension, 25
voluntary control, 25
Muscle(s)
abdominal, 446–447
problems, 481–482
strains, 482
wall injury, 481–482
adaptation, 26–27
adductor strains, 549
analysis during gait, 183–184
angle of pull, 75
ankle, 732–733
antagonism, 26, 77
atrophy, 163
attachment site, 76–77
bands, 146
biceps, 649–651
biceps femoris, 705
blood supply, 144–145
brachialis, 653, 674
cervical
extensors, 367
flexors, 366–367
hypertonicity, 388–389
composition of forces, 76
conditioning (*see also* Exercises), 485
contraction, 23–24, 146–150
force, 73–74
speed, 75, 147–148
contractures, 173
control grading, 26
cramps, 170–172
deltoid, 588, 653
dysfunction, 28–30
elbow strains, 665
enlargement, 174, 492
erector spinae, 493
fatigue, 164–166
fiber length, 73–74
finger contractures, 686
fixations, pelvic, 552
force, 54, 73–75
forearm, 664
wasting, 674
function, 22–23
gastrocnemius, 737
gemelli, 535
gluteus, 532–533, 537–538, 548–549
gracilis, 706
hamstrings, 534–535, 552, 703–704
hernia, 173
hip
adductor weakness, 702
spasm, 537
hypertonicity, 493, 590
shoulder, 640–642
iliocostalis dorsi, 426
iliocostalis lumborum, 493
iliolumbar, 496
iliopsoas, 533–534, 536–537
imbalance, 606

Muscle(s)—*continued*
  injury, 28–30, 169
  innervation, 182
  interspinous, 359, 389, 432, 493, 495–496
  intertransverse, 358–359, 432, 496
  latissimus dorsi, 426, 493
  levator scapulae, 641
  longus capitis, 358
  longus colli, 357
  lumbar
    extensors, 552
    fixations, 495–496
  lymph dysfunction, 492–493
  macroanatomy, 27
  microstructure and function, 144–150
  motor units, 145–146
  multifidi, 359, 426, 493
  nerve supply, 145
  neuromuscular
    function, 143–144
    junction, 149–150
    mechanisms, 25–26
  neurotransmitters, 148–149
  obliques, abdominal, 446, 481
  obliquus capitis, 357, 388, 481
  obturator, 535
  pain, 492–494
    from lymph dysfunction, 174–175
  pectoralis, 433
  pelvic hypertonicity, 537–538
  piriformis, 533, 535–536
  plantar, 738, 752
  popliteus, 738
  postural, 108
  psoas, 493
  quadratus femoris, 535
  quadratus lumborum, 426, 446, 493, 496
  quadriceps, 705
  range of movement, 73–75
  reactive patterns, 639
  rectus abdominis, 446, 481, 482, 493
  rectus capitis, 357, 388–389
  rectus femoris, 705
  respiratory, 416–417
  rhomboids, 426, 433, 641–642
  rotator cuff, 651–653
  rotatores, 359, 432–433
  rupture, 172–173
  sacroiliac, 468–469
  sartorius, 706
  scalenus, 388
  semitendinosus, 706
  shortening in thigh, 705–706
  shoulder strains, 648–653
  skeletal classifications, 27
  soleus, 737
  soreness, 170
  spasm, 170–172, 492
    hip, 702–703
    lumbar, 528
    management, 642
    shoulder, 640–642
  spinal, 588–589
  splenius capitis, 388
  splinting, pelvic, 547
  stabilization, 24
  sternocleidomastoideus, 389
  stiffness, 170
  strains, 29
  strength evaluation, 181–182
  structural-functional relationships, 26
  structure, 144
  supraspinatus, 646
  synergism, 26, 77
  temporomandibular strength, 397–398
  tension, 262
  tensor fascia lata, 533, 538
  testing, 180–181
  thigh, 696–698
    hypertonicity, 705–706
  thoracic, 438
    hypertonicity, 426, 432–433
  thumb, 680
  tibialis anterior, 737–738
  tone, 24, 150–152, 163–164
  transversus abdominis, 446, 481
  trapezius, 389, 426, 641, 658
  trauma, 166–167
  triceps brachii, 646–647
  two-joint, 74–75
  upper extremity
    strengthening, 640, 642
    stretching, 640, 642
  vascularity, 28
  velocity, 75
  voluntary control, 25
  weakness, 166–169, 262, 599–600
  wrist, 671
Myalgia, 173–175, 261–262
Myelination, 145
Myotonicity, 163–164

N

Nachlas' test, 501
Naffziger's test, 512
Neck (*see also* Spine, cervical)
  cervical reflexes, 276
  exercises, posttraumatic, 367–369
  kinesiology, 299–303
  motion, 302–303
  musculoskeletal disorder classes, 348
  posterolateral injuries, 307–312
  posture, 94
  realignment exercises, 364–370
  sidebending, passive, 360
  torticollis, 386–389
  trigger points, 262–266
Neri's bowing sign, 706
Nerve(s)
  autonomic, 225, 382
  axonotmesis, 307
  axons, 149
  brachial plexus, 337, 374–378
  cervical, 306
    plexus, 320, 347–348
    receptors, 366
    root avulsion, 376
  femoral cutaneous, 556–557
  fiber degeneration, 178
  foraminal encroachment, 273–274
  lesions, 176–178

lumbar
distribution, 450
dorsal ramus, 518
impingement, 450, 528
radiculopathy, 516
receptors, 490
reflexes, 451
roots, 450, 515–520
lumbosacral plexus, 452
median entrapment at wrist, 677–679
neural vs circulatory symptoms, 371
neurapraxia, 307
neuromuscular junction, 149–150
neurotmesis, 307
obturator, 557
pedicular kinking, 274
peroneal injury, 728
pinch, 178, 375
plantar neuroma, 756
pressure, 241
radial compression at elbow, 669–670
regeneration changes, 178
root(s), 303
compression, 273
insults, cervical, 349–351
traction, 517
sacroiliac innervation, 469
sciatic compression, 556
sensory, 450, 517, 588
sensory-motor mechanisms, 150
solar plexus impaction, 481–482
stretch, 178, 375
synapses, 149
therapeutic stimulation, 437
ulnar compression
at elbow, 670
at wrist, 679
vagus, 352, 437
Neuralgia, postural, 133–134
Neurapraxia, 307
Neuroinhibition, 436–437
Neuromechanisms, 171
Neuron
motor, 151
structure, 148
Neurostimulation, 437
Neurotherapy, 436–437
Neurotmesis, 307
Neurotransmitters, 148–149
Newton's laws, 43–49
Newtons, 45
Node theory, 587
Nucleus pulposus, 212–213

O

Ober's test, 706
Obesity, 32–33
Occiput
basilar
coarctation, 391–392
impression, 392
condyles, 312
trauma, 324
occipitalization, 392
occipito-atlanto-axial complex, 323–324
palpation, 354–355
platybasia, 391–392
visual subluxation patterns, 361
Ochsner's clasping test, 678
O'Connell's test, 500–501
Ordinates, 48–49
Orthotics, foot, 754–755
Os odontoideum, 210
Ossification, 9
Achilles tendon, 740
spinal, 198–199
Oxygen intake variants, 32

P

Pain
ankle, during gait, 122
chemical, 491
control, 287
fatigue theory, 493
faulty body mechanics, 169
foot, 751–757
hip, during gait, 122
knee, during gait, 122
ligamentous, 175
lymph dysfunction, 492–493
mechanical, 490–491
muscle, 492–494
postexertion, 493
postural neuralgia, 133–134
referred, 274–277, 515, 517
segmental, locations, 278
shoulder, 640–647
spasm theory, 493–494
spinal, 245
during gait, 121–122
low-back, 487–488, 490–495
lumbar disc, 515, 522–525
lumbopelvic, nondisc, 483–484
lumbosacral syndromes, 500–501
scoliotic, 608
thoracic, 575
vertebrogenic, 285
tendon, 175
upper extremity, 640
Palmomental reflex, 687
Palpation
atlas, 354–356
axis, 355–356
cervical, 353–360
lower, 356–357
middle, 356–357
motion, 280
occiput, 354–355
sacroiliac, 553–556
temporomandibular joint, 396–397
thoracic, 434–435
Paralysis, 168–169
Patella, 711
altered position, 717–718
apprehension test, 720
bipartite, 731–732
chondromalacia, 730
dislocations, 719
fractures, 719
subluxations, 719–720
tendon, 718–719
trauma, 718–719

Patella—*continued*
  wobble sign, 719
Patrick's F-AB-ER-E test, 702–703
Patterns
  distortion, pelvic, 547
  lumbosacral distortion, kinetic tests, 456
  reactive muscles, 639
Payr's sign, 723
Pelvis
  angle, 457
  avulsions, 550–551
  bursitis, 549
  coccyx, 470
    sprain, 550
    subluxation, 550
  displacement during gait, 120–121
  distortion patterns, 547
  entrapment syndromes, 556–557
  fixations, 551–556
  fractures, 550–551
  heel alignment checks, 539
  height, 531–532
  hypertonicity, 537–538
  ilia, 465–466
    horizontal rotation, 554–555
  inflammations, 548–551
  irritation, 536–537
  ischia, 467
  kinematics, 470–476
  lateral
    flexion, 554
    inclination, 530–531
    sway during gait, 113–114
  lumbosacral angle syndromes, 496–503
  lumbosacral motion, 471
  muscle
    weakness, 532–535
    distortions, 538
  osteitis condensans ilii, 559
  osteomyelitis, 559
  posture, 94–95
    realignment, 529–539
  pubis
    fixation, 556
    sprain, 549–550
    subluxation
  reflexes, 538–539
  rotation
    gait, 113
    horizontal, 471–472
  sacroiliac joint(s)
    fixation, 557
    gout, 558
    infection, 557
    listings, 544–547
    palpation, 553–556
    pathology, 557–559
    psoriasis, 558
    spondylitis, 558
    sprain, 540–543
    subluxation, 543–548
  sacrum, 465–476
    extension, 554
    flexion, 554
    tumors of, 558–559
  strain, 547, 548–551
  structural asymmetry, 548
  three-joint complex, 471
  tilt, 103, 113, 471–472, 530, 608–610
  traumatic disorders, 539–551
  trigger points, 538
Periarthritis, 647
Periosteum, 8
Periostitis, 267
Peritendinitis, 262
  Achilles, 739–740
Perkin's patella grinding test, 730
Perry's technique, posture, 101–102
Perthe's tourniquet test, 735
Pettibon's approach, 584
Phalen's test, 678
Phelp's test, 706
Philosophy, 3–4, 5–6
Physical fitness, 159
Physique, 33
Piedallu's sign, 543–544
Pillows, cervical, 379–380
Pitres' (plumb line) chest sign, 421
Plantar
  lifts, 616
  tension test, 752
Plasticity, 81–82
Platybasia, 210, 391–392
Plumb line analyses, 98, 459
Poisson's ratio, 51
Pollicis longus tests, 686
Ponticulus, 210
Position
  Adams, 460–463
  prone, 463–464
  relief, 521–522
  standing, 458–463, 474
  supine, 464–465
Positioning, 108
Posterior drawer sign, 716
Posture, 491–492
  Alexander technique, 101–102
  analysis, 238–239
  balance, 151
  bulk effects, 109
  cervical realignment, 364–370
  changes during growth, 95–96
  circulation, 134
  developmental defects, 106–107
  distortion
    evaluation, 573–574
    phenomena, 167
  dynamic, 107–111
  effects on respiration, 417
  endurance, 133
  equilibrium, 159
  etiology of faults, 132
  evaluation of, 457–465
  faulty, visceral manifestations, 244
  feet realignment, 750
  good, definition, 574
  gross analyses, 93–95
  interspinal, 205–206
  leverage, 108
  low-back
    instability, 135–136
    pain syndrome, 520

lumbar realignment, 529–539
military, 103
occupational effects, 103
Perry's technique, 101–102
physiologic reactions, 132–133
plumb line analysis, 459
positioning, 108
pregnancy, 103
problems during youth, 484
proprioceptive mechanisms, 104
racial differences, 103
range of motion, 107–108
readiness, 104
reciprocal inhibition, 151–152
reclining, 106
respiratory considerations, 135
sitting, 102–107, 459–460, 476, 484
stabilization, 108, 588–589
stance and motion, 102–129
standing, 458–463, 474
standing surfaces, 103
static stance, 102–107
thoracic, 430–431
realignment, 438
tolerance, 133
tone, 151
upper extremity, 640
visceral implications, 134–135
Power, 68–69, 72
Pratt's tourniquet test, 735–736
Pressure, 50–51
disc, 104–105
monitoring, 183
therapeutic, 436–437
Process, paramastoid, 210
Pronation, effects, 620–622, 747
Proportionality, 44
Proprioception, 154–159, 365–366
Psychomotor responses, 167
Puberty, 96
Pubes, 467
fixation, 556
sprain, 549–550
subluxation, 549–550
Pulley systems, 55
Pushoff, gait, 119, 121

Q

Q angle, 713–714
Quadriceps hyperthyroidism test, 706

R

Radial/ulnar stress tests, 675
Radiculopathy, lumbar, 516
Rate, toppling, 99
Ratio, Poisson's, 51
Reaction, reciprocal, 44–45
Receptors
cervical, 158, 366
joint, 18, 156–157, 283–285
labyrinthine, 157–158
muscle and tendon, 155–156
nociceptive, lumbar, 490
skin, 157
Reflex(es)
adductor, 500
cervical, 276
craniosacral, 539
deep, 165
Giegel's (inguinal), 500
hamstring, 501
inverse myotatic, 170
irritations, 277
lumbar, 451, 517
muscle tone, 163–164
nocifensive, 152
palmomental, 687
pelvic, 538–539
perplexing, 178–180
referred, 274–277
righting, 589
sensory responses, 241
somatosomatic, 179
somatovisceral, 179
stretch, 155, 170, 171, 494
superficial, 165
tendon, 164
therapeutic technique, 285
viscerosomatic, 179–180, 538–539
viscerovisceral, 180
Reiter's syndrome, 558
Relaxation
biomechanical, 83, 596
intervertebral disc, 217–218
Repetitive heel raise test, 737
Respiration
craniosacral reflexes, 539
muscle action, 416–417
sacral motion, 476
Response(s)
psychomotor, 167
somatic and visceral, 167–168
Reticular activating system, 184–185
Retinacular test, 686
Rheumatism, psychogenic, 262
Rhythm, lumbosacropelvic, 461
Rib(s), 411–412
"bucket handle" complications, 425
bifid, 441
cervical, 210, 393–394
changes during spinal motion, 419–420
contusions, 422
dislocations, 427–428
distortion, measurement of, 458, 592–593
fixations, 433–434
fractures, 426–427
fused, 441
lumbar, 441
subluxations, 422–426
Rigidity, torsional, 58, 81
Rotator cuff, 651–653
Rule, Logan's, 611
Running, 127–128
Rupture, muscle, 172–173
plantaris, 738
popliteus, 738
supraspinatus, 653

S

Sacralization, 210
Sacroiliac stretch test, 543
Sacrum (*see also* Pelvis)

fixations, 555–556
fractures, 551
motion, involuntary, 228–229, 398
respiratory motion, involuntary, 476
Scapula(e), 458, 633
fixations, 659
fractures, 659
injuries, 658–659
prominent, 577–578
protraction, 634–635, 638–639
retraction, 634–635
Scapulocostal syndrome, 423
Schultz's test, 660
Sciatica, 503, 517–518
cervical subluxations and, 362
long-leg, 614
Sclerotome, 515, 517
Scoliometer, 614, 615
Scoliosis
acquired factors, 586
braces/casts, 595–596
cervical, 584–586
classifications, 578–580
Cobb's angle, 591
coupling factors, 586
course, 579, 581, 587
definitions, 572, 574–578
electrical stimulation, 596
electromyography, 581, 588
evaluative procedures, 581–589
fixation effects, 587
idiopathic, common causes, 461
incidence, 579, 581
key, 582
Lovett's principles, 605–608
lumbar, 605–608
mensuration of curve, 591–592
moire topography, 581
node theory, 587
orthopedic supports, 595–596
pain, scoliotic, 608
pelvis tilting, 608–610
prevalence, 579, 581
radius of curve, 589–590
range of curvature, 590–591
short-leg effect, 609–610
static vs dynamic, 611
subluxation patterns, 598–605, 611–614
terminology, 572, 574–578
thoracic, 586–605
hypertonicity, 590
tomography, 581–582
traction, 593, 595–596
Sesamoiditis, 755
Shear, 58, 79, 84
cervical, 307
intervertebral disc, 217
Shenton's line, 708–709
Shifting, 101
Shober's sign, 558
Shoe(s)
lifts, 118–119, 596, 614, 616–620
posture and, 103
Shoulder(s)
abduction, 634–637, 639
stress test, 644
adduction, 634, 637–639
ankylosis, 640
apprehension test, 655
depression, 372, 634–635, 638
dislocation, 655–657
elevation, 634–635, 638, 639
extension, 634, 636
flexion, 634, 636
fractures, 657–658
girdle, 633–634
goniometry, 639–640
injuries, 647–662
ischemia sites, 653
kinesiology, 636–639
lax joint, 649
motion, 634–640
pain, 640–647
posture, 94
referred symptoms, 276
roentgenography, 657, 658
rotation, 634–635, 638–640
rotator cuff, 651–653
shrugging exercise, 369–370
spasm, 640–642
sprains, 648–653
stability, 649
strains, 648–653
subluxations, 653–657
trigger points, 642–643
Sicard's sign, 520
Sign(s) (*see also* Test(s))
Allis' knee, 708
anterior drawer, 716
Beery's, 544, 706
Bonnet's, 520
Bryant's, 656
buckling, 519
buttock, 557–558
Calloway's, 656
Clarke's, 730
Codman's, 644–645
Dejerine's, 512–513
draw sign, 743–744
Dreyer's, 719–720
Forestier's, bowstring, 435
Gauvain's, 708
Gilcrest's, 645
Hamilton's ruler, 656
Hennequin's, 708
Hoffa's, 754
Homan's, 735
Hueter's, 645
Hughston's jerk, 715
Kleist's, hooking, 686
Langoria's, 708
Lasègue's differential, 520
Lewin's knee, 706
Lhermitte's, 382–383
Lindner's, 520
Lust's, 728
Maisonneuve's, 677
Neri's, bowing, 706
patella wobble, 719
Payr's, 723
Piedallu's, 543–544
Pitres' (plumb line), 421

posterior drawer, 716
Shober's, 558
Sicard's, 520
Steinmann's, 723
subacromial button, 646
Tinel's, 747
tripod, 706
Wartenburg's Oriental prayer, 678
Wilson's, 731
Simmond's test, 739
Sitting, 116
posture, 459–460
pressure points, 105
Skeleton, osteologic factors, 6–11
Skills, motor, 162
Slocum's test, 715–716
Smith-Peterson's test, 543
Soto-Hall's test, 428
Space, 48–49
Spasm, 19
hip, 537, 702–703
iliopsoas, 536–537
management, 171–172
piriformis, 535–536
shoulder, 640–642
temporomandibular, 400–401
Spasticity, 122–123, 171
Speed, body, 161–162
Spina bifida occulta, 211
Spinal cord, 223
cervical, 303–305
circulation, 227
concussion, 489
contusions, 489
lesions of, 176–178
maladaptation in scoliosis, 587
traction, pathologic, 489
Spindles, neuromuscular, 155
Spine
cervical, 206, 208–209
atlas, 312–313, 334–336
dislocation, 324–326
fracture, 324–326
visual subluxation patterns, 361–362
axis, 313–314, 354–355
fracture, 326–328
visual subluxation patterns, 362
brachial plexus, 337
canal, 303–305
cerebrospinal fluid circulation, 352
compression tests, 371–374
cord injury, 380
coupling, 332–333
curve reversal, 333–335
C5 vertebra, 389
deformities/anomalies, 391–394
disc and related disorders, 380–386
dislocations, 335–339
exercises, 364–370
posttraumatic, 367–369
extension, 300–302, 304, 306–310, 316–319, 332, 337–338, 367, 368
facet
action, 331–332
joints, 328–329
fixations, 353–360
flexion, 300, 302, 304, 306, 310, 316–319, 332, 337, 366–368
fractures, 335–339
goniometry, 302–303
hypertonicity, 357–359
inflammatory diseases, 389–391
instability, 316, 330–331
intervertebral foramina, 328
kinematics, 308, 330–335
kinesiology, 299–303
Klippel-Feil syndrome, 393
lateral flexion, 301–304, 307, 310, 317–319, 332, 338–339, 360, 368–369
ligaments, 329–330
lower
subluxations, 336
trauma, 335–339
medulla oblongata, 352
motion, 302, 332–333
measurements, 359–360
motion-unit dysfunction, 349
muscles (*see also* Muscle(s)), 301
nerves, 306
root insults, 349–351
vagus, 352
neural vs circulatory symptoms, 371
neurovascular deficit syndromes, 370–374
occipitoaxial locking, 358
occipitocervical ligaments, 314–315
occiput
condyles, 312
palpation, 354–355
subluxations, 320–322
visual subluxation patterns, 361
orthopedic supports, 379–380
plexus, 320
points of injury, 304
proprioception, 365–366
receptors, 158, 366
reflexes, 276
rib, 393–394
righting mechanisms, 366
roentgenography, 305–306
root avulsion, 376
rotation, 301–304, 307, 317, 319, 333, 339, 369
scoliosis, 584–586
secondary fixations, 358
spondylitis, 390–391
spondylosis, 383–386, 390
sprain, 307–310
sprain/strain management, 378–380
stenosis, congenital, 393
strain, 307–310
strength, 300–302
subluxation(s)
atlas, 322–323
neurovascular implications, 351–352
syndromes, 347–370
subluxation-induced reflexes, 351
thoracic outlet/inlet, 370–374
torticollis, 386–389
congenital, 393
traction, 362–364
trauma, 305–312
trigger points, 310
uncovertebral articulations, 329

Spine, cervical—*continued*
    upper, clinical biomechanics, 312–339
    upper
        kinematics, 315–319
        trauma, 319–320
    veins, 352
    vertebral artery, 352
    vertebral veins, 352
    vertebrobasilar patency, 373–374
    visual subluxation patterns, 360–362
    whiplash, 308–310, 378–380
  lumbar, 207, 209
    anatomy, 447–450
    balance, 457, 483–485
    cord injuries, 489–490
    dislocations, 488
    entrapment syndromes, 525–526
    equilibrium, 483–485
    extension, 447, 451, 454–455, 462–464, 496
    facets, 498–499
    fixations, 495–496
    flexion, 447, 451, 454, 461–462, 465, 496
    fractures, 488
    genetic defects, 450
    goniometry, 431
    hyperlordosis, 500, 576–577
    hypomobile, 528
    impingement, 503–529
    innervation, segmental, 451
    instability, 456–457, 497–499
    intervertebral discs, 446, 528
        syndromes, 510–515, 522–525
    intervertebral foramina, 449–450
    intradisc shifting, 513–515
    kinematics, 451–456
    kinesiology, 450–451
    lateral flexion, 447, 451, 453–454, 463, 496
    loading, 502
    lumbosacral stress, acute, 498–499
    management, 526–529
    muscle
        enlargement, 492
        weakness, 451
    nerve, 450, 451, 452
        lesion differentiation, 516
        roots, 450, 515–520
            traction, 517
    pain, 490–495
    palpation, 495–496
    posture, 491–492
        realignment, 482–485
    receptors, 490
    reflexes, 517
    roentgenography, 502, 508–509, 514–515, 525
    rotation, 447, 456, 462, 496
    scoliosis, 605–608
    segmental faults, 462
    slipped endplates, 514
    spasm, 492, 528
    spondylolisthesis, 503–506
    spondylolysis, 507–509
    spondylosis, 507–509
    sprain, 523
    stenosis, 509–510
    strain, 523
    subluxations, 488
    supports, 528–529
    traction, 527–528
    traumatic disorders, 485–490
    vertebra, 447–450
  thoracic, 206–207, 209
    anatomy, 410–420
    ankylosis, 435–436
    Calve's disease, 440
    collapse, 440
    deformities/anomalies, 440–441
    evaluation, gross, 429–431
    fixations, 431–436
    fracture, 440
    goniometry, 431
    hemivertebrae, 441
    hyperkyphosis, 576–577
    instability, 421–422
    intervertebral discs, 438–440
    kinematics, 417–420
    kinesiology, 415–417
    pain, 575
    palpation, 431–435, 438–440
    posttraumatic assessment, 420–421
    Scheuermann's kyphosis, 440
    scoliosis, 586–605
    spondylitis, 440
    sprains, 422–426
    stimulation, 437
    strains, 422–426
    subluxations, 423–426
    therapeutics, 436–438
    tuberculosis, 440
    unsegmented bar, 441
    wedged segments, 441
  thoracolumbar area
    extension, 415–418, 431, 435
    flexion, 415–418, 431, 435
    lateral flexion, 416, 418, 420, 431, 434–435
    rotation, 416, 418–420, 431, 435
Spinous processes, 202
  "kissing," 267–268
  thoracic, 413
Splinting, painful, 166
Spondylitis
  cervical, 390–391
  sacroiliac, 558
  thoracic spine, 440
Spondylolisthesis, 503–506
Spondylolysis, 211, 507–509
Spondyloschisis, 211
Spondylosis, 383–386, 390, 507–509
Spondylotherapy, 436–437
Sprain(s)
  acromioclavicular, 659–660
  ankle, 742–744
  calcaneocuboid, 753–754
  cervical, 378–380
  classification, 22
  coccyx, 550
  collateral ligaments, 720–722
  coronary ligament, 725
  costosternal, 422
  cruciate ligaments, 725
  elbow, 665–667
  foot, 753–754
  hip, 707

interphalangeal, 685
joint, 21–22
knee capsule, 722
low-back, 487–488
menisci, 722–726
metacarpophalangeal, 685
pubic, 549–550
sacroiliac, 540–543
shoulder, 649
spring liagment, 754
thoracic, 422–426
thumb, 681
toe, 753–754
wrist, 674–675
Sprengel's deformity, 211
Spurling's test, 372
Spurs
ankle, 747–748
heel, 756
Stability, 104
body, 54, 100–101
joint, 79
knee, 714–717
postural, 108
shoulder, 649
spinal, 231, 571–572
viscoelastic, 83
Stabilization, muscle testing, 181
Stance, 100, 112, 116–117, 121, 122
Standing posture, 458–459, 461–463
Statics, 49–50
Steinmann's sign, 723
Stenosis
cervical, congenital, 393
spinal, 509–510
Sternum, 410–411
fixations, 433
injury of, 426–427
Stiffness, 81
joint, 19
muscle, 170
spinal, posttraumatic, 250
Strain(s)
Achilles tendon, 738–740
adductor, 549
ankle, 742
biomechanical, 79–80
brachialis, 653
cervical, 378–380
classes, 29
deltoid, 653
elbow, 665
forearm, 673–674
gastrocnemius, 737
gluteal, 548–549
groin, 704–705
hamstring, 703–704
hip adductors, 704–705
leg, 736–739
low-back, 486–488
muscle and tendon, 29, 169–170
patella tendon, 718–719
plantar, 752
plantaris, 738
popliteus, 738
quadriceps, 705
rotator cuff, 651–653
soleus, 737
thoracic, 422–426
tibialis anterior, 737–738
trapezius, 658
Strength, 72, 159–161
cervical
extension, 367
flexion, 366–367
classifications, 159–160
development, 161
temporomandibular joint, 397–398
Stress
allowable, 82
biomechanical, 78–84
postural, 133
shear, 58
ultimate, 80
yield, 82
Strunsky's test, 753
Subacromial button sign, 646
Subluxation(s) (*see also* Fixation(s))
ankle, 744
atlantoaxial, rheumatoid, 390
clavicle, 660–661
elbow, 668–669
femur, 707
foot, 755
gross structural alterations, 237–239
induced reflexes, cervical, 351
knee, 726–727
neurovascular implications, 351–352
occipital, 320–322
visual patterns, 361
patella, 719–720
patterns, 598–605, 611–614
pubic, 549–550
rib
head, 424–425
pit, 422
sacroiliac, 543–548
shoulder, 653–657
spinal
atlas, 322–323
visual patterns, 361–362
axis, visual patterns, 361–362
biochemical reactions, 239
cerebrospinal fluid flow alterations, 243
cervical
lower, 336
patterns, 360–362
torticollis, 386–389
circulatory changes, 242–243
clinical classes, 233
costotransverse, 423–425
costovertebral, 423–425
distal neurologic manifestations, 243
effects of, 239–240
facets, 219
intervertebral foramina effects, 240–243
intraneural effects, 241
kinetic motion units, 236–237
lumbar, 488
meningeal irritations, 241–242
motion unit classes, 234–236
nerve root level, altered, 242

Subluxation(s), spinal—*continued*
paraforaminal adhesions, 242
precipitating factors, 239–244
somatic responses, 243
stress factors, 239
terminology, 233–234
thoracic, vertebral facet, 425–426
toxic effects, 243
visceromotor responses, 243–244
temporomandibular, 394–401
tibia, 727
Substitution, muscle, 181–182
Support, base of, 109–110
Supports
arch, 751
biomechanical, 287–288
cervical, orthopedic, 379–380
foot, 753
lumbar, 528–529
orthopedic, 595–598
pressure of, 50
Supraspinatus press test, 644
Sway, balance, 101
Swelling, popliteal, 719
Swing, gait, 112, 116–117, 121, 128, 183–184
Symmetry, 12–13
Synapses, 149
Syndrome(s)
anterior compartment, 756–757
Barré-Lieou, 373
bicipital, 649–650
carpal tunnel, 677–678
compartment, 29–30
costoclavicular, 660
derangement, 521–522
dysfunction, 520–521
entrapment, pelvic, 556–557
facet, 501–502
iliotibial band, 707
Klippel-Feil, 393
loose tendon, 650
lumbar
disc degeneration, 522–525
dorsal ramus, 518
entrapment, 525–526
intervertebral disc, 510–515
low-back pain, McKenzie's, 520–522
lumbosacral, 496–503
myofascial, shoulder, 642–643
nerve
pinch, 178, 375
stretch, 375
neurovascular deficit, 370–374
"9 to 5," 596–598
posterior tibial compartment, 738
postural, 520
referred spinal, 275
Reiter's, 558
scapulocostal, 423
short-leg, 127
shoulder pain, 643–647
stinger, 376
subluxation-induced reflexes, 351
tarsal tunnel, 747
thoracic
musculoskeletal, 421
outlet/inlet, 370
vertebral facet, 425–426
tibialis anterior, 737–738
trigger point, 263
Wallenberg's, 373
wrist, compression, 677–679
Synovia, 17–18

T

Talar slide test, 744
Tarsal tunnel syndrome, 747
Technique, Alexander's, 101–102
Tenderness, referred, 276–277
Tendinitis, 262
Achilles, 739
bicipital, 645
Tendon(s), 12, 28, 29
Achilles, 738–740
bicipital dislocation, 650
loose, 650
pain, 175
patella, 718–719
plantaris, 738
reflexes, 165
Tennis elbow, 667–668
Tenosynovitis
Achilles, 740
forearm, 675
TENS (*see* Transcutaneous electrical nerve stimulation)
Tension, 51
Test(s)
Abbott-Saunders', 650–651
Achilles tap, 739
active cervical rotary compression, 372
Adson's, 373
ankle tourniquet, 747
anvil, 708
Apley's
compression, 722
distraction, 722–723
scratch, 644
arm drop, 652
Astrom's suspension, 513
Bechterew's, 512
belt, 544
bent-knee pull, 519
biceps stability, 645
Booth-Marvel's, 645
bounce home, 712
bracelet, 679
Bragard's, 518–519
Buerger's, 735
cervical distraction, 372–373
Chapman's, 435
chest expansion, 435
Childress' duck waddle, 723
claudication, 735
Cozen's, 667
Dawbarn's, 646
DeKleyn's, 374
Demianoff's, 519
Deyelle-May, 519
double-leg-raise, 500

Dugas', 655–656
Eden's, 373
elbow
  ligamentous stability, 666–667
  medial epicondyle, 668
Ely's, 537
Erichsen's pelvic rock, 542
Fajersztajn's, 519
Finsterer's, 677
Forestier's, 435
Fouchet's, 730
Froment's, 679
Gaenslen's, 541
George's, 374
Gills', 543
Goldthwait's, 543
Hautant's, 374
heel walk, 501
Helfet's, 727–728
Hibb's, 542
hip
  abduction stress, 558
  kinematic, 707
hyperextension, 501
iliac compression, 542
impingement syndrome, 651
Kaplan's, 668
Kemp's, 512
Kernig's
  leg, 489
  neck, 489
kinetic, 456
knee
  collateral ligament stability, 721–722
  effusion, 718
  hyperextension stress, 715
Laguere's, 707
Lasègue's
  rebound, 511
  straight-leg-raising, 511, 518, 519
  standing, 511–512
lax capsule, 649
Lewin's
  punch, 520
  supine, 435–436
Lippman's, 645
locking position, 651
Losee's, 716
Maigne's, 374
McIntosh's, 715
McMurray's, 723
Mennel's, 542
Milgram's, 489–490
Mills', 667–668
Minor's, 519
Morton's, 753
Moskowicz's tourniquet, 736
Nachlas', 501
Naffziger's, 512
Ober's, 706
Ochsner's clasping, 678
O'Connell's, 500–501
passive cervical rotary compression, 372
patella apprehension, 720
Patrick's F-AB-ER-E, 702–703
pectoralis flexibility, 433
Perkin's patella grinding, 730
Perthe's tourniquet, 735
Phalen's, 678
Phelp's, 706
plantar tension, 752
Pratt's tourniquet, 735–736
quadriceps hyperthyroidism, 706
radial/ulnar stress, 675
repetitive heel raise, 737
retinacular, 686
sacroiliac stretch, 543
Schultz's, 660
shoulder
  abduction stress, 644
  apprehension, 655
  depression, 372
Simmond's, 739
Slocum's, 715–716
Smith-Peterson's, 543
Soto-Hall, 428
Spurling's, 372
Strunsky's, 753
supraspinatus press, 644
talar slide, 744
Thomas', 537
Thompson's, 739
Tinel's wrist, 678
toe walk, 501
Trendelenburg's hip, 709
Underburger's, 374
Wright's, 373
wrist
  flexion/extension stress, 674–675
  tourniquet, 678
Yeoman's, 542–543
Yergason's stability, 650
Therapy
  adjunctive, 37, 280–292, 310–312
  adjustive, 37, 281–282
  Oriental, 491
  spinal, 280–292
  temporomandibular joint, 399–401
  traction, cervical, 362–364
Thigh(s)
  meralgia paresthetica, 710–711
  muscles, 696–698
  rotation during gait, 114
  trigger points, 710
Thomas' test, 537
Thompson's test, 739
Thorax
  posture, 94
  spine (*see* Spine)
Thumb
  abduction, 679, 680
  adduction, 679–680
  extension, 679, 680
  flexion, 679, 680
  goniometry, 680–681
  innervation, 680
  motion, 679
  muscles, 680
  sprained, 681
Tibia
  rotation, 717–718
  subluxations, 727

Tibia—*continued*
  torsion, 717–718
Tinel's
  foot sign, 747
  wrist test, 678
TMJ (*see* Joint(s), temporomandibular)
Toe(s)
  bunion, 757
  claw, 757
  hallux valgus, 757
  hammer, 757
  mallet, 757
  sprains, 754
  walk test, 501
Tomography, 581–582
Tone, postural, 151
Toppling rate, 99
Torques, 99
  lumbopelvic, 483
Torsion, 57–58
  intervertebral disc, 217
Torticollis, 386–389
  congenital, 393
Tourniquet tests
  leg/ankle, 735–736, 747
  wrist, 678
Traction, 287
  brachial plexus, 374–378
  indications, 290
  lumbar cord, 489
  positional, 363
  therapeutic, 593–594
    cervical, 362–364
    lumbar, 527–528
Training, 159–163
Transcutaneous electrical nerve stimulation (TENS), 287
Transverse processes, thoracic, 413
Trendelenburg's hip test, 709
Triangle, lumbosacral, 498
Trigger points, 134, 175–176
  back, 262–266
  cervical, 310
  common, table, 263
  etiologic hypotheses, 264
  finger, 684
  foot, 752
  hand, 681
  leg, 729
  neck, 262–266
  pelvic, 538
  shoulder, 642–643
  temporomandibular, 400–401
  therapy for, 265–266
  thigh, 710
  thoracic, 575
  thoracolumbar, 494
Tripod sign, 706
Tropism, 211
Tuberculosis, spinal, 440
Tumors, sacral, 558–559

U

Ulnar tunnel triad, 679
Underburger's test, 374, 575

V

Vectors, 47–48
Veins
  cervical, 352
  vertebral, 352
Velocity, 65–66
  angular, 65–66
  instantaneous, 66
  linear, 65
  muscle, 75
Vertebra(e)
  fused, 211
  joints, 211
  occipital, 210
  plana, 440
  sagittal clefted, 210–211
  supernumerary segments, 211
  third condyle, 211
  thoracic, 412–414
Viscera, postural considerations, 134–135
Viscerosomatic reflexes, 538–539
Viscoelasticity, 82–83
Viscosity, 81, 87

W

Walking
  functions, 111–116
  patterns, 111
Wartenburg's Oriental prayer sign, 678
Weakness
  hip adductors, 702
  muscle, 166–169, 262, 599–600
  neuromuscular, 168
  pathologic, 168
  trunk, 451
Weight, 31–33, 43
  body, 32–34, 56, 103
    segments, 69
  effect on pelvis during development, 450
  foot distribution, 750
  head, 100–101
  lumbopelvic, 483
  lumbosacral, 485–488
  spinal distribution, 197
Wheel-and-axle mechanisms, 54
Whiplash, 173, 308–310, 378–380
Wilson's sign, 731
Wolff's law, 8, 588
Work, 72
  capacity, 72
  types of, 72
Wright's test, 373
Wrist(s)
  anatomy, 670
  biomechanics, 672–673
  carpal injury, 677
  compression syndromes, 677–679
  dislocations, 675–677
  drop, 377
  extension, 671
  flexion, 671
  flexion/extension stress tests, 674–675
  fractures, 675–677
  ganglion, 675

goniometry, 672
kinesiology, 671
lunate injury, 677
motion, 670–672
roentgenography, 676–677
sprain, 674–675
tourniquet test, 678
trauma, 673–674

Y

Yeoman's test, 542–543
Yergason's stability test, 650
Yield, biomechanical, 80–81, 82

Z

Zone, Head-McKenzie, 179